Clinical Pain Management

Chronic Pain

LEAD EDITOR

Andrew SC Rice MB BS MD FRCA
Reader in Pain Research, Department of Anaesthetics, Pain Medicine and Intensive Care
Imperial College London; and Honorary Consultant in Pain Medicine, Chelsea and
Westminster Hospital Foundation NHS Trust, London, UK

SERIES EDITORS

Douglas Justins MB BS FRCA
Fellow of the Faculty of Pain Medicine of the Royal College of Anaesthetists
Consultant in Pain Medicine and Anaesthesia
Pain Management Centre
St Thomas' Hospital
London, UK

Toby Newton-John BA(Hons) MPsych(Clin) PhD
Consultant Clinical Psychologist and Program Director
Innervate Pain Program and
Faculty of Medicine, University of Sydney
Australia

Richard F Howard BSc MB ChB FRCA
Fellow of the Faculty of Pain Medicine of the Royal College of Anaesthetists
Consultant in Paediatric Anaesthesia and Pain Management
Great Ormond Street Hospital for Children
London, UK

Christine A Miaskowski RN PhD FAAN
Professor and Associate Dean for Academic Affairs
Department of Physiological Nursing
UCSF School of Nursing
San Francisco, CA, USA

Acute Pain
Edited by Pamela E Macintyre, Suellen M Walker, and
David J Rowbotham

Chronic Pain
Edited by Peter R Wilson, Paul J Watson, Jennifer A Haythornthwaite, and
Troels S Jensen

Cancer Pain
Edited by Nigel Sykes, Michael I Bennett, and
Chun-Su Yuan

Practice and Procedures
Edited by Harald Breivik, William I Campbell, and
Michael K Nicholas

Clinical Pain Management

Chronic Pain

2nd edition

Edited by

Peter R Wilson
Professor of Pain Medicine
Mayo Clinic College of Medicine
Rochester, USA

Paul J Watson
Professor of Pain Management and Rehabilitation
Department of Health Sciences
University of Leicester
Leicester, UK

Jennifer A Haythornthwaite
Professor
Department of Psychiatry and Behavioral Sciences
Johns Hopkins Medical Institutions
Baltimore, USA

Troels S Jensen
Professor
Experimental and Clinical Pain Research
Department of Neurology and Danish Pain Research Center
Aarhus University
Denmark

HODDER ARNOLD
PART OF HACHETTE LIVRE UK

First published in Great Britain in 2003
This second edition published in 2008 by
Hodder Arnold, an imprint of Hodder Education,
part of Hachette Livre UK, 338 Euston Road, London NW1 3BH

http://www.hoddereducation.com

British Library Cataloguing in Publication Data
A catalogue record for this book is available from the British Library

Library of Congress Cataloging-in-Publication Data
A catalog record for this book is available from the Library of Congress

ISBN 978-0-340-94009-9 (Acute Pain)
ISBN 978-0-340-94008-2 (Chronic Pain)
ISBN 978-0-340-94007-5 (Cancer Pain)
ISBN 978-0-340-94006-8 (Practice and Procedures)
ISBN 978-0-340-93992-5 (4 vol set: Acute Pain/Chronic Pain/Cancer Pain/Practice and Procedures/Web edition)

1 2 3 4 5 6 7 8 9 10

Commissioning Editor: Joanna Koster
Project Editor: Zelah Pengilley
Production Controller: Joanna Walker
Cover Design: Helen Townson

Typeset in 10 pt Minion by Macmillan India
Printed and bound in the UK by MPG Books, Bodmin, Cornwall
Text printed on FSC accredited material

FSC
Mixed Sources
Product group from well-managed forests and other controlled sources
www.fsc.org Cert no. SA-COC-1565
© 1996 Forest Stewardship Council

Contents

Please note: The table of contents and a combined index for all four volumes in the series can be found on the Clinical Pain Management website at: www.clinicalpainmanagement.co.uk.

Contributors

Praveen Anand MA MD FRCP
Professor of Clinical Neurology
Division of Neuroscience and Mental Health, Imperial College London, Hammersmith Hospital, London, UK

Bradley E Aouizerat PhD MAS
Assistant Professor
School of Nursing and The Institute for Human Genetics
University of California, San Francisco, CA, USA

Charles E Argoff MD
Professor of Neurology
Albany Medical College
Director
Comprehensive Pain Program, Albany Medical College
New York, USA

Lene Baad-Hansen DDS PhD
Assistant Professor
Department of Clinical Oral Physiology, School of Dentistry
Faculty of Health Sciences, University of Aarhus
Aarhus, Denmark

Tanya Baqai MBChB MRCP
Specialist Registrar
Department of Rheumatology, Royal London Hospital
London, UK

Miles J Belgrade MD
Medical Director of Fairview Pain and Palliative Care Center
University of Minnesota Medical Center; and
Adjunct Professor
Department of Neurology, University of Minnesota Medical School, Minneapolis, USA

Nikolai Bogduk BSc(Med) MB BS PhD MD DSc Dip Anat MMed (Pain) FAFRM FFPM (ANZCA)
Conjoint Professor of Pain Medicine
University of Newcastle, Newcastle Bone and Joint Institute
Royal Newcastle Centre, Newcastle
New South Wales, Australia

Julie Bruce RGN BSc Msc PhD
MRC Senior Research Fellow
Department of Public Health, School of Medicine, College of Life Sciences and Medicine, University of Aberdeen
Aberdeen, UK

Serena F Carville PhD
Programme Manager
UK Age Research Forum, London, UK

Ernest H Choy MD FRCP
Reader in Rheumatology
Department of Academic Rheumatology, King's College London
London, UK

Sarah Cox MB BS BSc FRCP
Consultant in Palliative Medicine
Chelsea and Westminster Hospital NHS Foundation Trust; and Trinity Hospice, London, UK

Roy Croock BS
Research Assistant
Department of Epidemiology, The University of Texas MD Anderson Cancer Center, Houston, TX, USA

Chris Dodds MBBS MRCGP FRCA
Professor
Department of Anaesthesia, South Tees Hospitals NHS Trust
Middlesborough, UK

Christopher Eccleston PhD
Professor of Psychology and Director
Centre for Pain Research, The University of Bath, Bath, UK

Robert J Gatchel PhD ABPP
Chairman
Department of Psychology, College of Science at The University of Texas at Arlington; and
Director of Clinical Research
The Eugene McDermott Center for Pain Management
The University of Texas Southwestern Medical Center at Dallas
Arlington, TX, USA

Hanne Gottrup MD PhD
Department of Neurology and Danish Pain Research Center
Aarhus University Hospital, Århus, Denmark

C Roger Goucke MB ChB FANZCA FFPMANZCA
Head
Department of Pain Management, Sir Charles Gairdner Hospital
Nedlands, Western Australia

Kate Grady BSc FRCA
Consultant in Pain Medicine and Anaesthesia
University Hospital of South Manchester Foundation Trust
Wythenshawe, Manchester, UK

W Michael Hooten MD
Assistant Professor
Department of Anesthesiology, Department of Psychiatry and Psychology, Mayo Clinic College of Medicine
Rochester, MN, USA

John Hughes MBBS FRCA
Consultant in Anaesthetics and Pain Management
The James Cook University Hospital
Middlesbrough, UK

Marc A Huntoon MD
Associate Professor of Anesthesiology, Consultant in Pain Medicine
Mayo Clinic, Rochester, MN, USA

Ali Jawad MBChB FRCP
Honorary Senior Lecturer and Consultant
Department of Rheumatology, The Royal London Hospital
London, UK

Rigmor Jensen MD Dr Med Sci
Professor
Department of Neurology, University of Copenhagen
Glostrup, Denmark

Troels S Jensen MD PhD
Professor
Experimental and Clinical Pain Research, Department of Neurology and Danish Pain Research Center, Aarhus University
Denmark

Tim Johnson MB BS FRCA
Consultant in Pain Management
Manchester and Salford Pain Centre, Hope Hospital
Salford, UK

Robert W Johnson MD FRCA
Emeritus Consultant in Anaesthesia and Pain Medicine
United Bristol Hospitals and Senior Research Fellow
University of Bristol, Bristol, UK

K Riaz Khan MBBS MD FRCA
Clinical Fellow in Pain Medicine, St Thomas' Hospital
London, UK

Bruce Kidd DM FRCP FRACP
Professor of Clinical Rheumatology
Bone and Joint Research Unit, William Harvey Research Institute, Barts and The London, Queen Mary's School of Medicine and Dentistry, London, UK

Nancy D Kishino OTR CVE
West Coast Spine Restoration Center, Riverside, CA, USA

Signe Koch MD
Aarhus University Hospital, Aarhus, Denmark

Alyssa Lebel MD
Assistant Professor of Anesthesia
Children's Hospital Boston and Harvard Medical School
Boston, MA, USA

Allen H Lebovits PhD
Director
Psychological Services, Division of Neurology and Integrative Pain Medicine, ProHEALTH Care Associates, LLP; and
Adjunct Associate Professor
Department of Anesthesiology, NYU School of Medicine
New York, USA

Monica Lee MD
Fourth-year Resident in the Department of Obstetrics and Gynecology, David Geffen School of Medicine, UCLA, Center for Health Sciences, Los Angeles, CA, USA

William Macrae MB ChB FRCA
Consultant in Pain Medicine, Honorary Senior Lecturer
Ninewells Hospital and Medical School, Dundee, UK

Lance M McCracken PhD
Consultant Clinical Psychologist and Clinical Lead
Bath Centre for Pain Services, Royal National Hospital for Rheumatic Diseases NHS Foundation Trust; and
Senior Visiting Fellow
Department of Psychology, University of Bath
Bath, UK

Christine A Miaskowski PhD RN FAAN
Professor
School of Nursing, University of California
San Francisco, CA, USA

Stephen Morley PhD
Professor of Clinical Psychology
Leeds Institute of Health Sciences, University of Leeds
Leeds, UK

David B Morris PhD
University Professor (2002–2007) and Emeritus Professor of English
University of Virginia, Charlottesville, VA, USA

Paul R Nandi FRCP FRCA
Consultant Anaesthetist
University College London Hospitals Pain Management Centre
The National Hospital for Neurology and Neurosurgery
London, UK

Timothy J Ness MD PhD
Simon Gelman Endowed Professor of Anesthesiology
Department of Anesthesiology, University of Alabama at Birmingham, Birmingham, AL, USA

Lone Nikolajsen MD PhD
Consultant in Pain Medicine
Aarhus University Hospital, Aarhus, Denmark

Turo J Nurmikko
Professor of Pain Science
Pain Research Institute, University of Liverpool
Liverpool, UK

Ceri J Phillips BSc(Econ) MSc(Econ) PhD
Professor of Health Economics
Institute for Health Research, School of Health Science
Swansea University, Swansea, UK

Ivan N Ramos-Galvez FRCA
Consultant in Pain Medicine
Royal Berkshire NHS Foundation Trust, Reading, UK

Jon Raphael MB ChB MSc MD FRCA
Professor of Pain Medicine
Faculty of Health, Birmingham City University
Birmingham, UK

Andrea J Rapkin MD
Professor of Obstetrics and Gynecology
Department of Obstetrics and Gynecology, David Geffen School of Medicine, UCLA, Center for the Health Sciences
Los Angeles, CA, USA

Barry Rawicki MB BS FACRM FAFRM(RACP)
Associate Professor
Department of Medicine, Monash Medical Centre, Faculty of Medicine, Nursing and Health Sciences, Clayton, Victoria
Australia

Cielito Reyes-Gibby DrPh
Assistant Professor
Department of Epidemiology, The University of Texas MD Anderson Cancer Center, Houston, TX, USA

Andrew SC Rice MB BS MD FRCA
Reader in Pain Research
Department of Anaesthetics, Faculty of Medicine
Pain Medicine and Intensive Care, Imperial College; and
Honorary Consultant in Pain Medicine
Chelsea and Westminster Hospital Foundation NHS Trust
London, UK

Ben A Rich JD PhD
Professor of Internal Medicine and Anesthesiology and Pain Medicine, School of Medicine Alumni Association, Endowed Chair of Bioethics
University of California Davis School of Medicine
Sacramento, CA, USA

Katherine Roberts BSc
Division of Neuroscience and Mental Health, Imperial College London, Hammersmith Hospital, London, UK

Hans-Georg Schaible MD
Professor of Physiology
Department of Physiology, Friedrich-Schiller-University of Jena
Jena, Germany

Cassandra D Schamber MD
Staff Physician
Fairview Pain and Palliative Care Center, University of Minnesota Medical Center, Fairview, MN, USA

Lisa Scharff PhD
Assistant Professor of Psychology
Department of Psychiatry
Children's Hospital Boston and Harvard Medical School
Boston, MA, USA

Navil F Sethna MB ChB
Associate Professor of Anaesthesiology
Children's Hospital Boston and Harvard Medical School
Boston, USA

Randy A Shelerud MD
Assistant Professor
Department of Physical Medicine and Rehabilitation, Mayo Clinic College of Medicine; and
Director
Mayo Clinic Spine Center, Rochester, MN, USA

Ravikiran Shenoy MBBS MS DNB MRCS
Division of Neuroscience and Mental Health, Imperial College London, Hammersmith Hospital, London, UK

Philip J Siddall MBBS MM (Pain Mgt) PhD FFPMANZCA
Clinical Associate Professor
Pain Management Research Institute, University of Sydney
Royal North Shore Hospital, Sydney, Australia

Cathy Stannard MB ChB FRCA
Consultant in Pain Medicine
Pain Clinic, Macmillan Centre, Frenchay Hospital
Bristol, UK

Peter Svensson DDS PhD Dr Odont
Professor and Chairman
Department of Clinical Oral Physiology, School of Dentistry
Faculty of Health Sciences, University of Aarhus; and
Department of Oral and Maxillofacial Surgery
Aarhus University Hospital, Aarhus, Denmark

Peer Tfelt-Hansen MD Dr Med Sci
Consultant
Department of Neurology, University of Copenhagen
Glostrup Hospital, Glostrup, Denmark

Isabel Torres-Vigil DrPh
Instructor
Department of Health Disparities Research, The University of Texas MD Anderson Cancer Center, Houston, TX, USA

Glyn R Towlerton BSc MRCP FRCA FIPP
Consultant in Pain Medicine
Chelsea and Westminster Healthcare NHS Foundation Trust and
Royal Brompton Hospitals; and
Honorary Senior Lecturer
Imperial College, London, UK

Stephen P Tyrer MB BChir DPM MRCPsych LMCC MA FRCPsych
Professor
Department of Psychiatry, Royal Victoria Infirmary
University of Newcastle-upon-Tyne
Newcastle-upon-Tyne, UK

Eric J Visser MBBS FANZCA FFPMANZCA
Pain Medicine Specialist and Anaesthetist
Department of Anaesthesia and Pain Medicine
Royal Perth Hospital, Perth, Western Australia

Victoria CJ Wallace PhD
Post-Doctoral Research Fellow
Pain Medicine Research Associate, Department of Anaesthetics
Faculty of Medicine, Imperial College, Chelsea and Westminster
Hospital Campus, London, UK

James C Watson MD
Assistant Professor of Neurology, Consultant in Departments of
Neurology and Anesthesiology
Pain Division, Mayo Clinic College of Medicine
Rochester, MN, USA

Peter R Wilson MB BS PhD
Professor of Pain Medicine and Consultant in Anesthesiology
and Pain Medicine
Mayo Clinic College of Medicine, Rochester, MN, USA

Paul J Wrigley MBBS MM (Pain Mgt) PhD FANZCA FFPMANZCA
Clinical Senior Lecturer
Pain Management Research Institute, University of Sydney, Royal
North Shore Hospital, Sydney, Australia

Series preface

Since the successful first edition of *Clinical Pain Management* was published in 2002, the evidence base in many areas of pain medicine has changed substantially, thus creating the need for this second edition. We have retained the central ethos of the first volume in that we have continued to provide comprehensive coverage of pain medicine, with the text geared predominantly to the requirements of those training and practicing in pain medicine and related specialties. The emphasis continues to be on delivering this coverage in a format that is easily accessed and digested by the busy clinician in practice.

As before, *Clinical Pain Management* comprises four volumes. The first three cover the main disciplines of acute, chronic, and cancer pain management, and the fourth volume covers the practical aspects of clinical practice and research. The four volumes can be used independently, while together they give readers all they need to know to deliver a successful pain management service.

Of the 161 chapters in the four volumes, almost a third are brand new to this edition while the chapters that have been retained have been completely revised, in many cases under new authorship. This degree of change reflects ongoing progress in this broad field, where research and development provide a rapidly evolving evidence base. The international flavor of *Clinical Pain Management* remains an important feature, and perusal of the contributor pages will reveal that authors and editors are drawn from a total of 16 countries.

A particularly popular aspect of the first edition was the practice of including a system of simple evidence scoring in most of the chapters. This enables the reader to understand quickly the strength of evidence which supports a particular therapeutic statement or recommendation. This has been retained for the first three volumes, where appropriate. We have, however, improved the system used for scoring evidence from a three point scale used in the first edition and adopted the five point Bandolier system which is in widespread use and will be instantly familiar to many readers (www.jr2.ox.ac.uk/bandolier/band6/b6-5.html).

We have also retained the practice of asking authors to highlight the key references in each chapter. Following feedback from our readers we have added two new features for this edition: first, there are key learning points at the head of each chapter summarizing the most salient points within the chapter; and second, the series is accompanied by a companion website with downloadable figures.

This project would not have been possible without the hard work and commitment of the chapter authors and we are deeply indebted to all of them for their contributions. The volume editors have done a sterling job in diligently editing a large number of chapters, and to them we are also most grateful. Any project of this magnitude would be impossible without substantial support from the publishers – in particular we would like to acknowledge our debt to Jo Koster and Zelah Pengilley at Hodder. They have delivered the project on a tight deadline and ensured that a large number of authors and editors were kept gently, but firmly, "on track."

Andrew SC Rice, Douglas Justins, Toby Newton-John,
Richard F Howard, Christine A Miaskowski
London, Newcastle, and San Francisco

I would also like to add my personal thanks to the Series Editors who have given their time generously and made invaluable contributions through the whole editorial process from the very outset of discussions regarding a second edition in deciding upon the content of each volume and in selecting Volume Editors. More recently, they have provided an important second view in the consideration of all submitted chapters, not to mention stepping in and assisting with first edits where needed. The timely completion of the second edition would not have been possible without this invaluable input.

Andrew SC Rice
Lead Editor

Introduction to Clinical Pain Management: Chronic Pain

Chronic pain has traditionally had the negative connotation of psychogenic etiology and an arbitrary time domain. It has also been a pejorative term to the extent that chronic pain syndrome was deliberately omitted from the IASP *Taxonomy of Chronic Pain Syndromes*. This new volume gathers together the scientific and clinical evidence that confirms chronic pain as an identifiable syndrome, the final common path of many etiologies. Consistent with any clinical syndrome, there are common neurophysiological, neuroanatomical, and functional changes throughout the organism regardless of the precipitating factors. These changes are addressed in the early chapters of this volume. In addition, there is physical, psychological, and psychiatric deconditioning resulting from central and peripheral nervous system dysfunction. Socioeconomic impairment and reduction in quality of life almost invariably accompany these changes.

There has also been a recent paradigm shift from the curative medical model of pain in which symptoms are expected to resolve once the underlying pathologic process is treated medically or surgically to a model which emphasizes patient autonomy, symptom management, and functional restoration. This volume addresses this new model of chronic pain in those specific conditions where applicable. It also explores the conceptually distinct rehabilitation model, in which it is recognized that the underlying pathology may be incurable or untreatable. The goals now involve minimizing the adverse effects of the pain and maximizing function and quality of life.

Fundamental changes in practitioners' responsibilities to patients and society are occurring as a result of philosophical and legal advances related to chronic pain. Previously implied rights of patients now have been formalized in various intractable pain acts of several jurisdictions. The classical doctrine of *primum non nocere* (first do no harm) is being challenged ethically and legally under these circumstances. Experts in these fields explore these changing ethical and legal climates in early chapters.

This volume contains 46 chapters in three parts. The first part, General Considerations, comprises 14 chapters that cover subjects ranging from basic neurophysiology through clinical evaluation to the ethical, legal, and societal aspects of this disease as described above. Part II, entitled Management – therapies, contains 9 chapters that address pharmacological, psychological, behavioral, interventional (invasive) and alternative/complementary/placebo issues. Part III has 23 chapters that describe both specific and nonspecific pain syndromes and their management. The subjects discussed include general neuropathic pain syndromes, specific pain syndromes and regional pain (neck, back, joints, chest, abdomen, and pelvis), and issues related to pain at the extremes of age.

Chronic pain now covers a vast scientific and clinical arena, and has become a medical specialty in its own right. Scientific rationale and therapeutic options are much better described now than at any time in the past. This volume gathers the available evidence-based information on diagnosis and management in an accessible format without overwhelming detail. Where evidence-based data are not available, the authors provide thoughtful advice based on scientific experience and clinical wisdom. It is inevitable in a volume such as this that there will be omissions, for which we must accept responsibility. Nevertheless, we believe that this volume is an essential resource for all clinicians whose patients have chronic pain and scientists who challenge traditional assumptions.

Peter R Wilson, Paul J Watson, Jennifer A Haythornthwaite, and Troels S Jensen
Rochester, Leicester, Baltimore, and Aarhus

How to use this book

SPECIAL FEATURES

The four volumes of *Clinical Pain Management* incorporate the following special features to aid the readers' understanding and navigation of the text.

Key learning points

Each chapter opens with a set of key learning points which provide readers with an overview of the most salient points within the chapter.

Cross-references

Throughout the chapters in this volume you will find cross-references to chapters in other volumes in the *Clinical Pain Management* series. Each cross-reference will indicate the volume in which the chapter referred to is to be found.

Evidence scoring

In chapters where recommendations for surgical, medical, psychological, and complementary treatment and diagnostic tests are presented, the quality of evidence supporting authors' statements relating to clinical interventions, or the papers themselves, are graded following the Oxford Bandolier system by insertion of the following symbols into the text:

[I] Strong evidence from at least one published systematic review of multiple well-designed randomized controlled trials
[II] Strong evidence from at least one published properly designed randomized controlled trial of appropriate size and in an appropriate clinical setting
[III] Evidence from published well-designed trials without randomization, single group pre-post, cohort, time series, or matched case-controlled studies
[IV] Evidence from well-designed non-experimental studies from more than one center or research group
[V] Opinions of respected authorities, based on clinical evidence, descriptive studies or reports of expert consensus committees.

Oxford Bandolier system used by kind permission of Bandolier: www.jr2.ox.ac.uk/Bandolier

Where no grade is inserted, the quality of supporting evidence, if any exists, is of low grade only (e.g. case reports, clinical experience, etc).

Other textbooks devoted to the subject of pain include a tremendous amount of anecdotal and personal recommendations, and it is often difficult to distinguish these from those with an established evidence base. This text is thus unique in allowing the reader the opportunity to do this with confidence.

Reference annotation

The reference lists are annotated with asterisks, where appropriate, to guide readers to key primary papers, major review articles (which contain extensive reference lists), and clinical guidelines. We hope that this feature will render extensive lists of references more useful to the reader and will help to encourage self-directed learning among both trainees and practicing physicians.

A NOTE ON DRUG NAMES

The authors have used the international nonproprietary name (INN) for drugs where possible. If the INN name differs from the US or UK name, authors have used the INN name followed by the US and/or UK name in brackets on first use within a chapter.

Abbreviations

4-AP	4-aminopyridine
5-FU	5-fluorouracil
5-HT	5-hydroxytryptamine
ABC	American Botanical Council
ACC	anterior cingulate cortex
ACE	angiotensin-converting enzyme
Ach	acetylcholine
ACOG	American College of Obstetricians and Gynecologists
ACR	American College of Rheumatology
ACTH	adrenocortical trophic hormone
ACh	acetylcholine
ADL	activities of daily living
AED	antiepileptic drug
AFP	atypical facial pain
AHPA	American Herbal Products Association
AIDS	acquired immunodeficiency syndrome
ALJ	Administrative Law Judges
AMA	American Medical Association
AMPA	α-amino-3-hydroxyl-5-methyl-4-isoxazole
AO	atypical odontalgia
AOJ	atlanto-occipital joint
APC	adenoma prevention with celecoxib
APF	anti-proliferative factor
APPROVe	Adenomatous Polyp Prevention on Vioxx
ARF	acute renal failure
ASA	acetylsalicylic acid
ATN	antiretroviral toxic neuropathy
BDI	Beck Depression Inventory
BDNF	brain-derived neurotrophic factor
BDZ	benzodiazepine
BMS	burning mouth syndrome
BOI	burden of illness
BPI	Brief Pain Inventory
BSI	Brief Symptom Inventory
BTP	breakthrough pain
BZD	benzodiazepine
C	cytosine
CABG	coronary artery bypass graft
CAD	coronary atherosclerotic disease
CAM	complementary and alternative medicine
CARF	Commission on Accreditation of Rehabilitation Facilities
CART	Classification and Regression Tree
CBC	complete blood count
CBT	cognitive-behavioral therapy
CCI	chronic constriction injury
CCK	cholecystokinin
CCR2	chemotactic cytokine receptor 2
CD	Crohn's disease
cDNA	complementary DNA
CES	cauda equina syndrome
CES-D	Center for Epidemiological Studies-Depression
CFS	chronic fatigue syndrome
CGRP	calcitonin gene-related peptide
CHF	congestive heart failure
CI	confidence interval
CIN	cervical intraepithelial neoplasia
CLBP	chronic lower back pain
CMI	cell-mediated immunity
CMV	cytomegalovirus
CNCP	chronic noncancer pain
CNMP	chronic nonmalignant pain
CNS	central nervous system
COMM	current opioid misuse measure
COMT	catechol-O-methyltransferase
COOA	combined opioid–opioid analgesia
COPD	chronic obstructive pulmonary disease
COX	cyclooxygenase
CP/CPPS	chronic prostatitis/chronic pelvic pain syndrome
CPP	chronic pelvic pain
CPQ	Chronic Pain Questionnaire
CPSP	central poststroke pain; or chronic postsurgical pain
CRD	colorectal distension
CRP	chronic regional pain
CRPS	complex regional pain syndrome
CSA	Controlled Substances Act
CSF	cerebrospinal fluid
CSM	Committee on Safety of Medicines
CSQ	Coping Strategies Questionnaire
CT	computed tomography
CTN	classical trigeminal neuralgia

CTTH	chronic tension-type headache
CVA	cerebrovascular accident
CWP	chronic widespread pain
d4T	stavudine
DAP	depolarizing after potentials
DAS	Disease Assessment Score
DBS	Deep brain stimulation
ddC	zalcitabine
ddI	didanosine
DDwR	disk displacement with reduction
DDwoR	disk displacement without reduction
DEA	Drug Enforcement Administration
DHE	dihydroergotamine
DILS	diffuse infiltrative lymphocytosis
DLF	dorsolateral funiculus
DM	diabetes mellitus
DMARD	disease-modifying antirheumatic drugs
DMSO	dimethyl sulfoxide
DNA	deoxyribonucleic acid
DNIC	diffuse noxious inhibitory control
DPN	diabetic peripheral neuropathy
DREZ	dorsal root entry zone
DRG	dorsal root ganglion
DSM	Diagnostic and Statistical Manual of Mental Disorders
DSM-IV	Diagnostic and Statistical Manual of Mental Disorders IV
DSP	distal symmetrical polyneuropathy
EAA	excitatory amino acids
EDDP	ethylidine-dimethyl-diphenylpyrrolidine
EECP	enhanced external counter pulsation
EEG	electroencephalogram
ELBW	extremely low birth weight
EMDR	eye movement desensitization and reprocessing
EMG	electromyogram
EMLA	eutectic mixture of local anesthetics
EP	episodic pain
ERCP	endoscopic retrograde cholangiopancreatography
ERK	extracellular signal-regulated kinase
ES	effect size
ESBY	Electrical Stimulation versus Coronary Bypass Surgery
ESCOP	European Scientific Cooperative of Phytotherapy
ESR	erythrocyte sedimentation rate
ETTH	episodic tension-type headache
FABQ	Fear Avoidance Beliefs Questionnaire
FAP	functional abdominal pain
FBSS	failed back surgery syndrome
FCE	functional capacity evaluation
FDA	Food and Drug Administration
FDR	false discovery rate
FHM	familial hemiplegic migraine
fMRI	functional magnetic resonance imaging
FMS	fibromyalgia syndrome
FRA	flexor reflex afferents
FSH	follicle-stimulating hormone
G	guanine
GABA	gamma aminobutyric acid
GABA-A	gamma-aminobutyric acid A
GABA-b	gamma aminobutyric acid-b
GAD	generalized anxiety disorder; or glutamic acid decarboxylase
GBP	gabapentin
GBS	Guillain–Barré syndrome
GDNF	glial-derived neurotrophic factor
GH	growth hormone
GI	gastrointestinal
GnRH	gonadotropin-releasing hormone
gp120	glycoprotein 120
GP	general practitioner
GPRD	General Practice Research Database
GS	gastrocnemius-soleus
GTN	glyceryl trinitrate
HAART	highly active antiretroviral therapy
HADS	Hospital Anxiety and Depression Scale
HIV	human immunodeficiency virus
HIZ	high intensity zone
HLA	human leukocyte antigen
HMO	health maintenance organization
HPA	hypothalamic–pituitary–adrenal
HPV8	human papilloma virus 8
HRR	hazard rate ratio
HSAN	hereditary sensory and autonomic neuropathy
HTEA	high thoracic epidural anesthesia
HZ	herpes zoster
HZV	herpes zoster virus
IAP	intermittent acute porphyria
IASP	International Association for the Study of Pain
IBS	irritable bowel syndrome
IC	interstitial cystitis
ICD-10	International Classification of Diseases, 10th edition
ICER	incremental cost–effectiveness ratio
ICN	intercostobrachial neuralgia
ICU	intensive care unit
IDET	intradiscal electrothermotherapy
IGF	insulin-like growth factor
IHS	International Headache Society
IL-1β	interleukin-1β
IL-1Ra	interleukin-1 receptor antagonist
IL-6	interleukin-6
IMET	Individualized Medication Effectiveness Tests

INCB	International Narcotics Control Board
IP	incident pain
IRIS	immune reconstitution inflammatory syndrome
ISSVD	International Society for the Study of Vulvovaginal Disease
i.t.	intrathecal
ITB	intrathecal baclofen
ITDD	intrathecal drug delivery
IUD	intrauterine devices
IVOT	intravenous opioid (sensitivity) testing
IVR	intravenous regional
JCAHO	Joint Commission on the Accreditation of Healthcare Organizations
JFS	juvenile fibromyalgia syndrome
JNK	c-Jun-N-terminal kinase
LAAJ	lateral atlanto-axial joint
LANSS	Leeds Assessment of Neuropathic Symptoms and Signs
LBP	low back pain
LIF	leukemia inhibitory factor
LIMA	left internal mammary artery
Lng-IUS	levonorgestrol-releasing intrauterine system
LTP	long-term potentiation
LUNA	laparoscopic uterine nerve ablation
M6G	morphine-6-glucuronide
MBSR	mindfulness-based stress reduction
MCIC	minimum clinically important change
MCS	motor cortex stimulation
MCSF	macrophage colony-stimulating factor
MEDAL	Multinational Etoricoxib and Diclofenac Arthritis Long-term
MFP	myofascial pain
MMPI	Minnesota Multiphasic Personality Inventory
MOH	medication overuse headache
MPA	medroxyprogesterone acetate
MPI	Multidimensional Pain Inventory
MPQ	McGill Pain Questionnaire
MR	magnetic resonance
MRI	magnetic resonance imaging
mRNA	messenger RNA
MS	multiple sclerosis
MSP	musculoskeletal pain
MT	mindful therapies
MVAS	million visual analog scale
NAPQI	*N*-acetyl-*p*-benzoquinoneimine
NCPB	neurolytic celiac plexus block
NCS	nerve conduction studies
NE	noradrenaline; or norepinephrine
NGF	nerve growth factor
NHL	non-Hodgkin's lymphoma
NHS	National Health Service
NICE	National Institute for Clinical Excellence
NIH	National Institutes of Health
NMDA	*N*-methyl-D-aspartic acid
NNH	number needed to harm
NNT	number needed to treat
NO	nitric oxide
NOP	neuropathic orofacial pain
NPS	Neuropathic Pain Scale
NPV	negative predictive value
NRS	numeric rating scale
NRTI	nucleoside reverse transcriptase inhibitors
NSAID	nonsteroidal anti-inflammatory drug
NTG	nitroglycerin
NYHA	New York Heart Association
OA	osteoarthritis
OAM	Office of Alternative Medicine
OCP	oral contraceptive pill
ODER	opioid dose escalation rate
OECD	Organisation for Economic Cooperation and Development
OEI	opioid escalation index
OIH	opioid-induced hyperalgesia
OR	opioid rotation; or odds ratio
OT	opioid tolerance
PADT	Pain Assessment and Documentation Tool
PAG	periaqueductal gray
PAG/PVG	periaquaductal or periventricular gray
PAR	pain relief
PASS	Pain Anxiety Symptoms Scale
PCA	patient-controlled analgesia
PCPT	Posttraumatic Chronic Pain Test
PCR	polymerase chain reaction
PD	Parkinson's disease
PDN	painful diabetic neuropathy
PDPN	painful diabetic peripheral neuropathy
PDQ	Pain Disability Questionnaire
PENS	percutaneous electrical nerve stimulation
PET	positron emission tomography
PGIC	Patient Global Impression of Change
PHN	postherpetic neuralgia
PID	pelvic inflammatory disease
PKC	protein kinase C
PML	progressive multifocal leukoencephalopathy
PMP	Pain Management Program
PMR	percutaneous revascularization; or progressive muscle relaxation
PNL	partial sciatic nerve ligation
PNS	peripheral nervous system
POMS	Profile of Mood States
PPI	proton-pump inhibitors
PPV	positive predictive value
PT	physical therapy
PTSD	posttraumatic stress disorder
PVD	peripheral vascular disease

QALY	quality adjusted life year
QOL	quality of life
qPCR	quantitative polymerase chain reaction
QS	quality scale
QSART	quantitative sudomotor axon reflex test
QST	quantitative sensory testing
RA	rheumatoid arthritis
RAP	recurrent abdominal pain; or refractory angina pectoris
rCBF	regional cerebral blood flow
RCT	randomized controlled trial
RDC	research diagnostic criteria
RF	radiofrequency
rhNGF	recombinant human growth factor
RNA	ribonucleic acid
rRNA	ribosomal RNAs
RR	relative risk
RSD	reflex sympathetic dystrophy
RSO	resting sweat output
RVM	rostral ventromedial medulla
SCI	spinal cord injury
SCL-90R	Symptom Checklist 90-Revised
SCS	spinal cord stimulation
SDR	selective dorsal rhizotomy
SEP	somatosensory evoked potential
SF-36	Short-Form-36
SFS	Spinal Function Sort
SHBPS	Saskatchewan Health and Back Pain Survey
SIF	sacral insufficiency fracture
SIP	Sickness Impact Profile
SLE	systemic lupus erythematosus
SNF	skilled nursing facility
SNI	spared nerve injury
SNL	spinal nerve ligation
SNP	single nucleotide polymorphisms
SNRI	serotonin noradrenaline reuptake inhibitor
SNT	spinal nerve transection
SP	substance P
SPECT	single photon emission computed tomography
SPID	sum of the differences in pain intensity
SPS	Shingles Prevention Study
SR	sustained release
SSR	sympathetic skin response
SSRI	selective serotonin reuptake inhibitor
STAI	State-Trait Anxiety Inventory
STAR	Screening Tool for Addiction Risk
STN	symptomatic trigeminal neuralgia
SUPPORT	Study to Understand Prognosis, Preferences for Outcomes, and Risks of Treatment
T	thymine
TC	treatment control
TCA	trichloroacetic acid; or tricyclic antidepressant
tDCS	transcranial direct current stimulation
TDF	transdermal fentanyl
TENS	transcutaneous electrical nerve stimulation
TMD	temporomandibular disorder
TMJ	temporomandibular joint
TMR	transmyocardial revascularization
TN	trigeminal neuralgia
TNF	tumor necrosis factor
TNFα	tumor necrosis factor-α
TPBS	three-phase bone scan
TRP	transient receptor potential
TSK	Tampa Scale for Kinesiophobia
TST	thermoregulatory sweat test
TTH	tension-type headache
TTX	tetrodotoxin
TTX-r	tetrodotoxin-resistant
TTX-S	tetrodotoxin-sensitive channel
U	uracil
UC	ulcerative colitis
UMNS	upper motor neuron syndrome
VAS	visual analog scale
VC	ventrocaudalis
VDCC	voltage-dependent calcium channel
VMpo	ventral medial posterior
VPL	ventroposterolateral
VPM	ventroposteriomedial
VSCC	voltage-sensitive calcium channel
VZV	varicella zoster virus
WDR	wide dynamic range
WHO	World Health Organization
WHYMPI	West Haven-Yale Multidimensional Pain Inventory
WLC	waiting list control
WLQ	Work Limitations Questionnaire
WOMAC	Western Ontario and McMaster Universities Osteoarthritis Index
ZJ	zygapophysial joint

PART I

GENERAL CONSIDERATIONS

1

Applied physiology: neuropathic pain

VICTORIA CJ WALLACE AND ANDREW SC RICE

KEY LEARNING POINTS

- Much information about neuropathic pain models is gleaned from studies in animal models.
- Damage to peripheral nerves causes phenotypic and excitability changes.
- Inflammatory mediators can produce excitation of neurons in the peripheral nervous system (PNS) and central nervous system (CNS).
- Nerve injury can lead to cell death and anatomical reorganization.
- A loss of inhibitory mechanisms and increase in excitatory mechanisms are associated with increased activity in the spinal cord in neuropathic pain.
- Microglia are activated in neuropathic pain and release pronociceptive substances which can activate neurons in the spinal cord.
- Supraspinal sites have increased excitatory influences on spinal nociceptive processing following nerve injury.

INTRODUCTION

Neuropathic pain is a form of chronic pain defined as "Pain arising as a direct consequence of a lesion or disease affecting the somatosensory system."[1] The spectrum of neuropathic pain is associated with a variety of disease states (**Table 1.1**),[2, 3] but it is important to recognize that neuropathic pain is a relatively frequent, but unusual and by no means inevitable, consequence of those disorders.

Various patterns of neuropathic pain are recognized and it may be spontaneous in nature (continuous or paroxysmal) or evoked by sensory stimuli. These patterns may coexist in the same patient and are not necessarily unique to any disease entity. Neuropathic pain is also usually associated with various phenomena associated with disturbances in sensory function and it is possible to broadly classify neuropathic pain patients on the basis of their sensory phenotype, for example in postherpetic neuralgia.[4] Therefore, pain may exist in the context of sensory loss (anesthesia dolorosa) or more unusually in the presence of hypersensory phenomena (e.g. allodynia (**Figure 1.1**), hyperalgesia (**Figure 1.1**), and hyperpathia). Occasionally, a mixed picture of disordered sensory function may be evident depending on which areas are tested.

While the biological advantage to the organism of nociceptive pain is readily identifiable, it is less easy to do so for neuropathic pain and it is probable that, in broad terms, neuropathic pain is a result of a pathological process representing a disordered regenerative response to neuronal damage. For example, in patients with the hyper-sensory subtype of neuropathic pain, the mechanistic implication of allodynia is that elements of the sensory nervous system which normally signal innocuous

Table 1.1 A classification of the more frequent disorders associated with neuropathic pain, with examples.

Cause of neuropathy	Examples
Trauma	Phantom limb
	Spinal cord injury
	Surgical
	Peripheral nerve injury
Infection/inflammation	Postherpetic neuralgia
	HIV
Cancer	Invasion/compression of neural structures by tumor
Drugs	Vinca alkaloids
	Taxols
	Ethanol
	Antiretroviral drugs
Ischemic injury	Poststroke pain
	Metabolic neuropathies, i.e. diabetic neuropathy
Compression	Trigeminal neuralgia
	Sciatica
Demyelination	Multiple sclerosis
	Charcot–Marie–Tooth

sensation have begun to encode painful stimuli, while in hyperalgesia the structures which normally subserve nociception have become hyperexcitable.

Before exploring what is known about the pathophysiology of neuropathic pain, three major caveats as to the nature of the existing literature need to be stated. First, the overwhelming bulk of the literature related to neuropathic pain mechanisms has emerged from rodent studies in which the major outcome measure is hypersensitivity of spinal withdrawal reflexes evoked by sensory stimuli. Thus, in this chapter, it will actually only be possible to discuss the putative mechanisms of evoked hypersensitivity, a relatively minor component of the spectrum of clinical neuropathic pain. Second, since it is also not currently possible to directly measure pain in experimental animals, the putative pain mechanisms which are to be discussed can only be interpreted in the context of responses to nerve injury which are possibly, but not certainly, related to pain. Third, the vast majority of research into neuropathic pain mechanisms has concentrated on changes in the peripheral nerve or spinal cord following peripheral nerve injury. Although knowledge is accumulating regarding alterations in the brain following peripheral nerve injury, much less is known about the significance of these changes. Therefore, this chapter will focus mainly on peripheral and spinal mechanisms of neuropathic pain.

ANIMAL MODELS OF NEUROPATHIC PAIN

Unravelling the mechanisms involved in neuropathic pain requires the use of laboratory animal models that replicate as far as possible, with the above caveats, the different pathophysiological changes present in patients. For reasons of reproducibility and simplicity, most studies of neuropathic pain are based upon animal models of traumatic nerve injury, usually in the rat sciatic nerve (**Figure 1.2**).

Rodent models of neuropathy

The most commonly used nerve injury models are: the chronic constriction injury (CCI) of sciatic nerve,[7] the partial sciatic nerve ligation (PNL) model,[8] the spinal nerve ligation (SNL)/transection model (**Figure 1.2**),[9] and the spared nerve injury (SNI) model.[6] All models are associated with the development of hypersensitivity to thermal (heat and cold), and mechanical stimuli which are used experimentally as correlates of hyperalgesia and allodynia symptoms in neuropathic pain patients.[10] However, the relevance of these measures to the human condition is questionable.

The CCI model consists of the loose ligation of the sciatic nerve with chromic gut sutures. An inflammatory reaction develops and consequentially damage to most A-fibers and some C-fibers. It is likely that there is a significant inflammatory component in the development

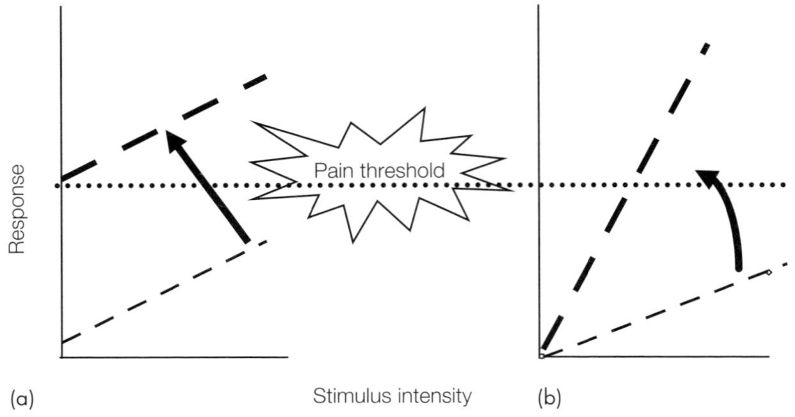

Figure 1.1 Graphical representation of (a) allodynia, a painful response to a normally innocuous stimuli and (b) hyperalgesia, an increased response to a normally painful stimulus. Stimulus intensity versus response relationship for noxious and innocuous stimuli. © The Board of Management and Trustees of the British Journal of Anaesthesia. Adapted from Bridges *et al.*, 2001[5] by permission of Oxford University Press/ British Journal of Anaesthesia.

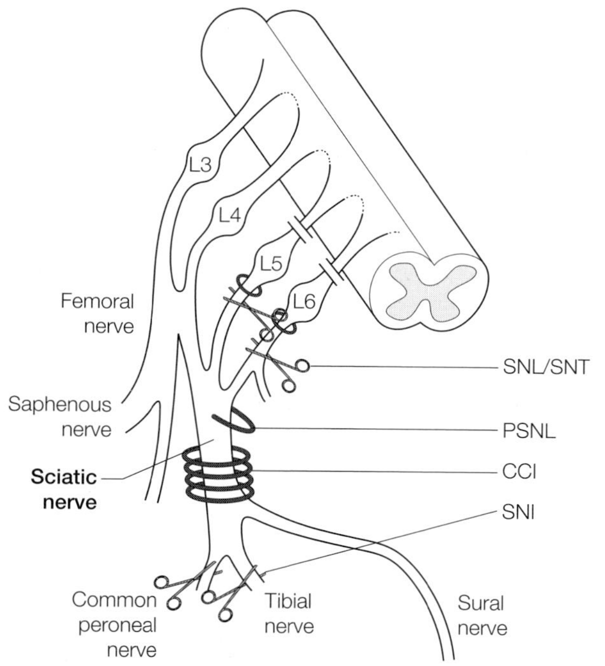

Figure 1.2 Rodent models of nerve injury. Many rodent models are based upon injury to the peripheral, usually sciatic, nerve. Schematic drawing of partial sciatic nerve injury (PSNL), chronic constriction injury (CCI), spared nerve injury (SNI), and spinal nerve ligation or transection (SNL/SNT) of the L5 and L6 spinal nerves. Adapted from Decosterd and Woolf, 2000[6] by permission of the International Association for the Study of Pain.

of the painful neuropathy.[11] In the PNL model, a tight ligation is created around 33–50 percent of the sciatic nerve, leaving the rest of the nerve "uninjured."[8] The SNL model traditionally consists of injury to the L5 and L6 spinal nerves, which contribute to the sciatic nerve.[9] However, a transection of the L5 spinal nerve alone results in comparative symptoms and hence some experimenters now use this as a modified SNL model.[5] This model is favorable to mixed injury models as it allows the examination of cellular responses of injured afferents (with cells in the L5/L6 dorsal root ganglia (DRG)) versus uninjured afferents (in the L4 DRG), and their relative importance in neuropathic pain.[12] The spared nerve injury model involves tight ligation and lesion of the tibial and common peroneal nerves.[6] This model allows testing of distinct regions of the hindpaw which are either innervated by injured or uninjured neurons, as well as separating degenerating neurons from uninjured neurons to a greater level.

Although commonly used and reproducible, there are shortcomings of these animal models which need to be considered. First, while neuropathic pain can be a devastating consequence of nerve injury in humans, the majority do not develop neuropathic pain following nerve injuries,[3] whereas most animals do develop reflex hypersensitivity in response to the above injuries. Therefore, the aforementioned animal models do not precisely mirror the "normal" human response to nerve injury. Second, for good ethical reasons, most animal models of neuropathic pain study the animals for a period of weeks, whereas the clinical course of neuropathic pain presenting to a pain relief clinic is often measured in years. Finally, as with all animal models, it is difficult to know what is actually perceived by the animal. To date, the behavioral manifestation of pain in rodent models of neuropathic pain has relied largely on measuring alterations in cutaneous sensory thresholds via measurement of reflex withdrawal thresholds to stimuli, such as punctuate mechanical (such as von Frey filaments),[13] which are not without their shortcomings, heat (such as the infrared heating device[14]) or cooling (such as the application of acetone) stimuli. Whilst these hypersensory phenomena do occur in a subset of humans with neuropathic pain, they are more usually observed in response to mechanical rather than thermal stimuli. (It must be noted that because the terms hyperalgesia and allodynia are defined in terms of pain, and we cannot yet measure pain in rodents, the use of these terms in the context of animal studies is inappropriate. We will therefore use the term "hypersensitivity" in the context of animal studies.)

Therefore, there is a need for the development of more clinically relevant animal models of neuropathic pain, as well as more complex behavioral tests designed to measure a spontaneous ongoing pain phenotype, and pain comorbidity.

Recent developments in rodent models of neuropathy

In recent years, scientists have worked to rectify the limitations of animal models, including development of models that more closely represent individual disease states. For example, as a model of peripheral diabetic neuropathy, a single injection of streptozotocin induces diabetes in the rat and is associated with the development of reflex hypersensitivity.[15] To model trigeminal neuralgia, chronic constriction injury of the infraorbital branch of the trigeminal nerve has been described.[16] In order to reproduce some features of postherpetic neuralgia, varicella zoster virus-infected fibroblasts are injected into the hindpaw and retrogradely transported to the cell bodies of sensory neurons in the DRG.[17,18,19] Similarly, the mechanisms by which the HIV virus could directly interact with the nervous system to produce peripheral neuropathic pain are being investigated by studying the effects of the HIV-envelope protein, glycoprotein 120 (gp120) *in vivo*.[20,21,22] Gp120 is thought to be key to the production of neurological disorders associated with HIV infection via the activation of the chemokine receptors CXCR4 and CCR5 expressed by neurons and glial cells.[23] Finally, drug-induced neuropathies are becoming more prevalent clinically with painful peripheral neuropathy presenting as an unfortunate side effect of treatment with chemotherapeutics, including taxols and vinca alkaloids, or with antiretroviral agents which form part of the highly active antiretroviral therapy (HAART) for the treatment of HIV disease. Rats treated systemically with such drugs develop signs of a neuropathic phenotype and are therefore important, clinically relevant models that are currently being investigated for the understanding of underlying mechanisms.[22, 24, 25, 26, 27] The aforementioned models are important as they model some aspects of the diseases most frequently associated with neuropathic pain.

The majority of neuropathic pain models were originally described in rats, but more recently have adapted to the mouse. The translation of these models from rat to mouse is important as novel transgenic tools, useful for the study of neuropathic pain, are further developed.

Behavioral tests of pain phenotype

In addition to new models, work is being conducted to improve the range of behavioral tests employed *in vivo* (**Figure 1.3**). For example, spontaneous exploratory activity assessed in the open field paradigm is classically used as a measure of anxiety-related behavior in rodents.[28] This test has been used as a measure of locomotor activity in pain models[29] and more recently, additional measures of thigmotactic behavior indicate the presence of altered exploratory behavior in rodent models of pain without the presence of locomotor deficits. This behavior is sensitive to clinically employed analgesics, such as gabapentin and morphine,[19, 27] suggesting the thigmotaxis to be correlated to a nonstimulus-evoked pain-like behavior in rodents be it spontaneous pain or pain comorbidities.

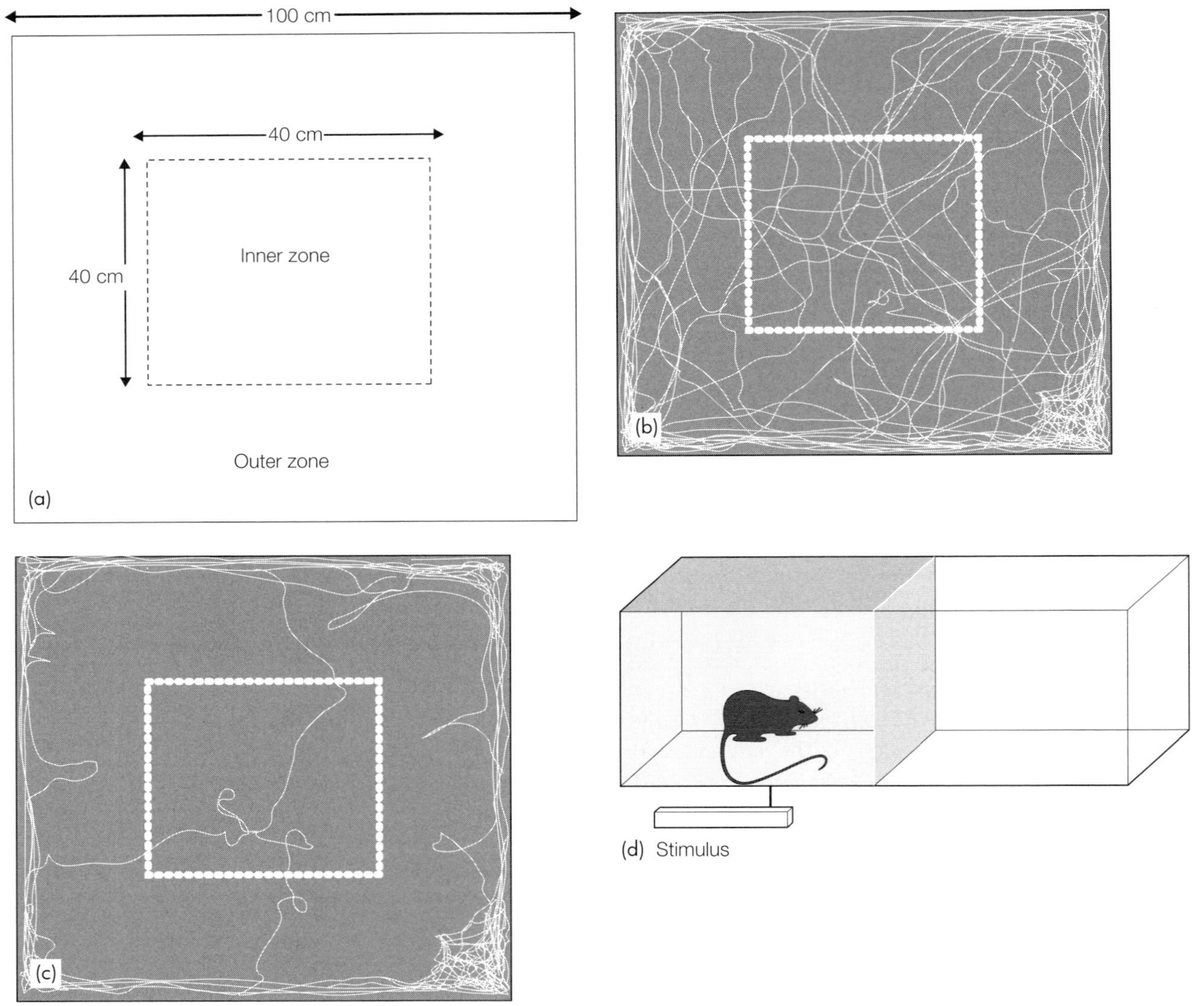

Figure 1.3 Examples of behavioral paradigms adapted for the assessment of pain conditions in rodents. (a–c) The open field paradigm in which neuropathic rats display thigmotactic (wall hugging) behavior: (a) open field arena; (b) naive rat; (c) rat with nerve injury. (d) The dark/light box: place preference paradigm in which rats chose between the aversive noxious stimulus or the aversive light compartment.

Further types of test involve active escape and avoidance of preferred environments (such as a dark versus light arena) in association with noxious stimuli.[30] These tests involve conflicting choices in which the animal must choose an adverse environment over the presence of a noxious stimulus and appear to respond well to analgesic drugs.[31] Alternatively, place preference paradigms associate a place with a preferable treatment such as delivery of an analgesic drug. However, the development of the latter paradigm in relation to neuropathic pain is ongoing and their utility remains to be proven. It is important to remember the effects of species variability[32] and therefore care must be taken to establish the suitability of tests in rodents.

MECHANISMS OF NEUROPATHIC HYPERSENSITIVITY

A variety of pain-related phenomena, both central and peripheral, have been associated with peripheral nerve injury (**Table 1.2**). These are generally not mutually exclusive and it is entirely possible that any one of these (or more likely a combination) contribute to symptomatology in individual patients suffering from neuropathic pain. It is therefore inappropriate to attempt to generate a unifying hypothesis of pathophysiology for all neuropathic pain states. The next challenge is to diagnose which of these phenomena may be operative in an individual patient and to interpret each symptom within the mechanistic framework arising from work with neuropathic pain models. In this regard, neuropathic pain is ideally suited to the mechanistic-based approach to treatment.[33, 34]

Peripheral mechanisms

PRIMARY AFFERENT EXCITABILITY

In normal primary afferent neurons, it is rare for firing threshold to be reached without the input of a stimulus.

Table 1.2 An overview of pathophysiological events which are likely to be related to the generation of neuropathic pain.

Peripheral nervous system	Central nervous system
Sensitization and spontaneous activity in sensory neurons	Central sensitization
Abnormal ion channel expression	Spinal reorganization
Altered neuronal biochemistry	Changes in inhibitory systems
Sensory neuron apoptosis	Glial cell activation
Immune–neuronal interactions	Alterations in descending modulation
Loss of trophic support for neurons	Cortical reorganization

However, following a nerve injury, many injured axons and associated cell bodies in the DRG undergo an increase in their intrinsic electrical excitability. As a result they begin to generate impulse discharge spontaneously or with only minimal stimulation linked to the injury site.[35] This has been termed ectopic discharge[36] and has also been demonstrated in humans, suffering from neuropathic pain.[37] Ectopic discharge originating in the peripheral nervous system (PNS) can result in excess spontaneous and stimulus-evoked electrical impulses feeding into the central nervous system (CNS) (**Figure 1.4**).[39] Ectopic afferent activity may also trigger and maintain central sensitization amplifying the afferent signal from the remaining afferents that innervate the partly denervated skin and deep tissues leading to tenderness to touch ("tactile allodynia").[38]

Furthermore, oscillations in resting membrane potential in primary sensory neurons are thought to contribute to their ectopic potential. A small number of A-fibers (10 percent) exhibit subthreshold membrane oscillations in their resting state or under depolarization conditions. An increase in these oscillations is observed in sensory neurons from axotomized rats.[40] Due to the sensitivity of such oscillations to tetrodotoxin (TTX), a role for changes in sodium channel function in the nerve in DRG has been proposed. Increases in oscillations lead to increased ectopic activity in these neurons that may underlie paresthesiae, dysesthesiae, as well as frank pain.

Abnormal discharges may also arise at the site of nerve injury, at other points along the nerves or in the cell body in the DRG.[41] Myelinated and unmyelinated primary afferent axons may become spontaneously active after nerve injury.[38, 42] Wallerian degeneration of an injured, spontaneously active myelinated fiber allows cross-excitation of neighboring unmyelinated fibers (termed "ephaptic transmission") inducing ectopic discharge even in an uninjured axon.[43, 44] Such ectopic discharge present in both low-threshold mechanoreceptors and in nociceptors may contribute to allodynia and hyperalgesic components of neuropathic pain.

Sodium channels

Sodium (Na^+) channels are critical to the physiology of excitable membranes. There are significant alterations in the expression of Na^+ channels in the cell bodies and the terminal neuroma of peripheral nerves following nerve injury. Such accumulation of Na^+ channels in the neuroma of cut sensory axons[45] are thought to generate ectopic discharge (**Figure 1.5**).[46]

There are many different and distinct voltage-gated Na^+ channels, of which at least six are expressed by primary afferent neurons within the DRG.[47] These can be defined by their sensitivity to TTX. In the DRG, TTX-sensitive channels (TTX-s) are expressed predominantly by A-fibers. In contrast, TTX-resistant (TTX-r) channels are expressed by a subset of primary afferent neurons specifically in the smaller C-fibers associated with

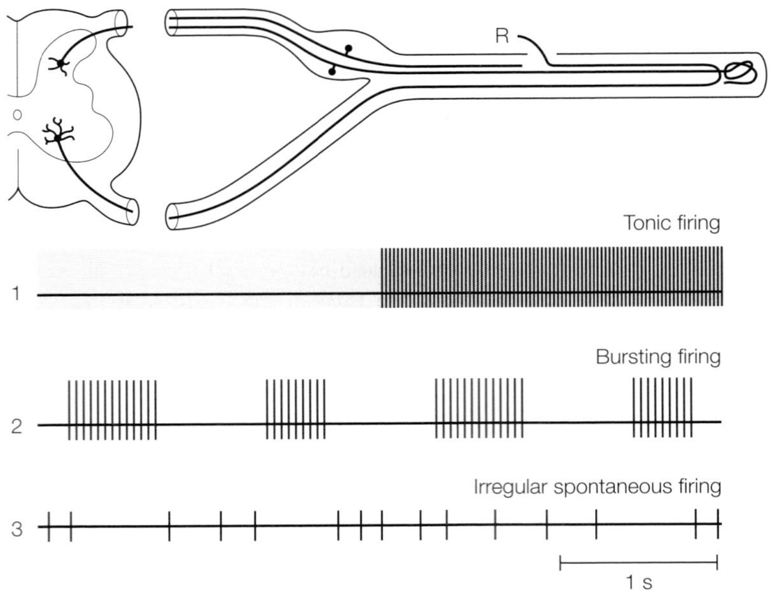

Figure 1.4 Patterns of spontaneous ectopic discharge recorded from sensory neurons ending in a neuroma. Fine axon bundles were microdissected from an injured nerve and placed on a recording electrode (R). Spontaneously active fibers fire tonically (1), in bursts (2), or irregularly (3). Intracellular recording from a dorsal root ganglion neuron with ectopic burst discharge (asterisks, spike height is truncated). One burst is shown in detail below. Bursts are triggered when ongoing membrane potential oscillations reach threshold and are maintained by postspike depolarizing after potentials (DAP). The burst initiates a hyperpolarizing shift which stops firing and resets the oscillations. Reprinted from Devor, *Melzack and Wall's Textbook of Pain*. 2005, 5th Edition © 2005 Elsevier Ltd,[38] adapted from Amir and Devor 1992.[39] Used with permission from The American Physiological Society and Elsevier.

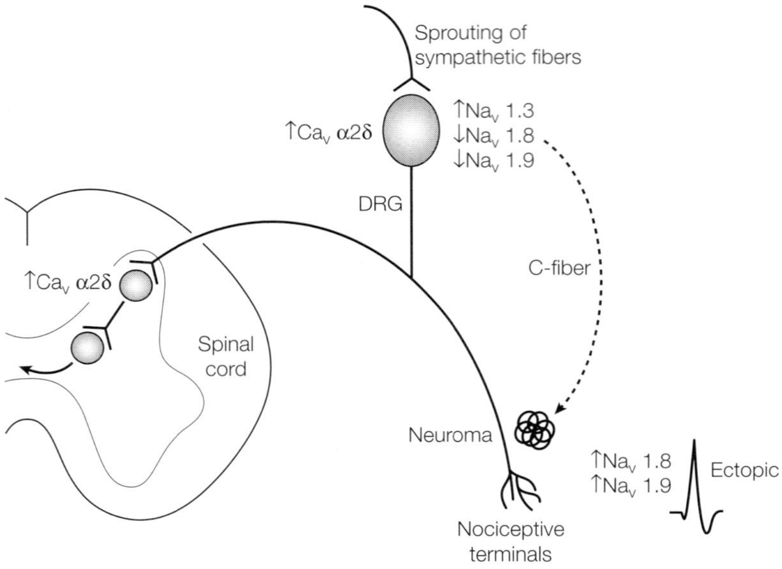

Figure 1.5 Alterations in Na^+ and Ca^{2+} channel subunits in the peripheral nervous system (PNS) following nerve injury. There is an increase in the expression of tetrodotoxin sensitive Nav1.3 channels and the calcium channel α2δ-1 (Cavα2δ-1) subunits in dorsal root ganglion (DRG) neuron cell bodies. The tetrodotoxin-resistant Na^+ channel subunits Nav1.8 and Nav1.9 decrease in the DRG and are also redistributed from the DRG neuron cell bodies to peripheral axons at the site of injury. Sprouting of sympathetic nerve fibers in the DRG also act to sensitize peripheral afferents. These changes are thought to result in spontaneous ectopic discharges and lower the threshold for mechanical activation that leads to hypersensitivity.

nociception.[48] Following peripheral nerve injury, there is a reorganization of ion channel expression in DRG neurons.[36] Some sodium channels subtypes are diminished, whilst others appear *de novo* and others are translocated to different parts of the neuron. For example, there is an up-regulation of the TTX-s channels $Na_v1.3$ (not normally expressed by DRG cells) and $Na_v1.7$, and a down-regulation of the TTX-r channels $Na_v1.8$ and $Na_v1.9$. As $Na_v1.8$ and $Na_v1.9$ produce slowly inactivating currents, their decreased expression may lead to a hyperpolarizing shift in resting potential, increasing the fraction of TTX-s channels available for activation.[47, 49] Electrophysiological studies demonstrate a reduced density of TTX-r currents and a shift in the voltage dependence of activation to a more negative potential in the following nerve injury.[49] In contrast, up-regulation of $Na_v1.3$ results in a switch in the properties of the TTX-s currents in DRG neurons, with the emergence of a rapidly repriming current, which could sustain frequent ectopic discharges and lead to hyperexcitability in the cell.[50] In support of this, TTX produces dose-dependent inhibition of ectopic activity[51] and reduced mechanical hypersensitivity in the spinal nerve transection (SNT) model.[52] In partial nerve injuries, the intact afferent neurons show little or no change in the expression of $Na_v1.8$, although there is a redistribution of these channels from their cell bodies in the DRG to their axons,[53] which may explain the neuroma hypersensitivity. These findings were corroborated in immunohistochemical studies of tissue taken from patients suffering from neuropathic pain following traumatic brachial plexus avulsion[54] and in human sensory nerves localized close to the injury site and within the neuroma.[55]

A Na^+ channel subunit that has received more attention in recent years is the $Na_v1.7$ channel. $Na_v1.7$ is expressed, almost exclusively, in DRG, particularly in small C-fiber nociceptors and to a lesser extent in medium-sized Aδ and large Aβ cells.[56] The $Na_v1.7$ channel underlies a fast TTX-s current with slow repriming kinetics and slow inactivation. Significantly, the $Na_v1.7$ channel has been localized to sensory endings, such that both its distribution and physiology may predispose it to a major role in transmitting painful stimuli. A mutation in the human gene encoding $Na_v1.7$ resulting in sensory neuron hyperexcitability is thought to be associated with the development of neuropathic pain in primary erythermalgia.[57, 58] However, experimentally the role for $Na_v1.7$ in neuropathic pain is unclear as mice lacking this channel develop signs of neuropathic pain as normal.[59]

The mechanism contributing to the changes in Na^+ channel expression in peripheral nerve injury is unclear, but the influence of growth factors appears to be a crucial factor. For example, in the absence of nerve growth factor (NGF), DRG neurons *in vitro* increase $Na_v1.3$ expression and decrease $Na_v1.8$ expression.[60] NGF is a member of the neurotrophin family of polypeptides, which are produced by peripheral target tissue during embryonic development, are required for peripheral sensory neurons for survival and can influence the morphology, excitability, and synaptic plasticity of sensory neurons in adulthood.[61] Additionally, glial-derived neurotrophic factor (GDNF), a member of a second family of growth factors, normalizes $Na_v1.3$ expression, reduces ectopic discharge in A-fibers, and reduces hypersensitivity[62] when delivered to the injured nerve. $Na_v1.9$ expression is similarly reliant on GDNF.

Therapeutic agents that exhibit use-dependent block of sodium channels show efficacy against painful peripheral neuropathy in the clinic. Systemic administration of lidocaine and other sodium-channel blockers relieves painful symptoms of postherpetic neuralgia, painful diabetic neuropathy, idiopathic trigeminal neuralgia, and other conditions.[63] Topical lidocaine also relieves pain in postherpetic neuralgia.[64] Sodium channel blockade is also a likely mechanism through which at least some drugs which also have efficacy in epilepsy (e.g. phenytoin and carbamazepine) might suppress neuropathic pain and the well-established efficacy of tricyclic antidepressants (TCA) may be due, at least in part, to their ability to block sodium channels.[65]

Potassium channels

There is a large variety of K^+ channels[66] and their significance in pain signaling is far from understood. Classic voltage-gated K^+ channels, often called delayed rectifiers, have six transmembrane domains and can be divided into nine gene subfamilies. The K_V1 subfamily is the most explored among subtypes of sensory neurons.[67] $K_V1.1$ and $K_V1.2$ are present in large-diameter sensory neurons, whereas $K_V1.4$ is present in most small sensory neurons that express $Na_V1.8$, making it the candidate nociceptive delayed rectifier. The activation of voltage-gated K^+ channels ultimately decreases the excitability of a cell. Thus, K^+ channels are prime molecular targets for suppressing hyperactive neurons, and might, therefore, prove useful in suppressing hypersensitivity.

Other K^+ channels that figure prominently in excitation of neurons, are the M channel (*KCNQ* gene), the H channel- (*HCN* gene) and calcium-activated K channels. All these channels are thought to be present on some populations of sensory neurons.[68, 69, 70] However, their relevance to pain is largely unknown.

Calcium channels

Activation of voltage-dependent calcium channels (VDCC) is critical for neurotransmitter release. Calcium ion channels have also been shown to influence the generation of hypersensitivity and in particular, a role for N-type Ca^{2+} channels has been shown. N-type, but not P- or Q-type, Ca^{2+} channel antagonists can attenuate hypersensitivity to mechanical and heat stimuli in models of neuropathic pain.[71, 72] Furthermore, cannabinoid receptor agonists, known to have analgesic effect in nerve injury models, attenuate Ca^{2+} flux at N-type channels.[73]

A calcium channel subunit that has received much attention of late is the $\alpha_2\delta$-1 subunit. This subunit is upregulated in rat DRG neurons, on central afferents terminals and on neurons within the spinal dorsal horn following nerve injury (**Figure 1.5**).[74, 75] This is correlated with pain behavior following peripheral nerve injury suggesting that $\alpha_2\delta$-1 may contribute to neuroplasticity in neuropathic pain. In support of this, transgenic mice that constitutively overexpress $\alpha_2\delta$-1 in neuronal tissues demonstrate pain behavior and exaggerated and prolonged dorsal horn neuronal responses to peripheral mechanical and thermal stimulation.[76] Furthermore, the $\alpha_2\delta$-1 subunit is thought to be the site of action of gabapentin[77, 78] and pregabalin,[79] which are effective in relieving signs of hypersensitivity in animal models[80] and neuropathic pain in man.[64, 81]

ALTERATIONS IN SENSITIVITY TO STIMULI

Transient receptor potential ion channels

Transient receptor potential (TRP) ion channels are sensory transducers, many of which are expressed in nociceptive primary sensory neurons where they are involved in generating chemical- and thermal-evoked pain sensations.[82] In particular, TRPV1 responds to noxious heat (temperatures $>43°C$) and the pungent ingredient in hot chilli peppers, capsaicin, producing the classic burning sensation. In contrast, TRPA1 responds to cold temperatures ($<18°C$) and to the irritant, mustard oil, also producing a burning sensation.

Following nerve injury, the phenotype of cells expressing TRP channels fundamentally changes so that TRPV1 and TRPA1 are also expressed by neurons of a non-nociceptive phenotype. Expression of TRPV1 has been shown to decrease in injured nociceptive neurons, while they increase in the neighboring uninjured neurons.[83] This includes novel expression in large diameter, low threshold A-fibers which may indicate a phenotypic switch contributing to symptoms of neuropathic pain. Similarly, TRPA1 expression is increased in a subset of small diameter primary sensory neurons following nerve injury likely inducing cold hypersensitivity.[84] Interfering with TRPA1 channel function using antisense knockdown technology abolishes hypersensitivity to a cold stimulus following spinal nerve ligation in the rat.[85] Therefore, targeting specific TRP channels may prove useful as analgesic strategies in the future.

THE ROLE OF PERIPHERAL INFLAMMATORY MEDIATORS

Nerve injury, trauma, and/or infection evoke a cascade of cellular events in the PNS, including a neuroinflammatory response with the release of chemical mediators, including many proinflammatory cytokines and chemokines.[86, 87] Cytokines and chemokines (small chemoattractant cytokines) are growth factor proteins secreted primarily from leukocytes as part of the immune and inflammatory response[88] and have been demonstrated to play a role in the pathogenesis of pain.[87] These factors can act on neurons to induce changes in gene expression, which in turn lead to the emergence of abnormal electrical activity, known to be essential for the manifestation of neuropathic pain behavior. Following nerve trauma, tumor necrosis factor-α (TNFα) is released from Schwann cells and infiltrating and resident macrophages, and in turn stimulates the sequential production and release of interleukin-1β (IL-1β) and interleukin-6 (IL-6) (**Figure 1.6**).[86] Accordingly, neutralizing antibodies to TNFα and IL-1β reduce behavioral signs of experimental neuropathic pain[90, 91] and IL-6 knockout mice fail to exhibit neuropathic pain after nerve injury.[92]

Intact and injured sensory neurons are known to express receptors which respond to TNFα, IL-1β, and IL-6. However, the direct mechanism of neuronal sensitization remains to be fully determined. Indirect evidence suggests an action of TNFα on neuronal sodium or calcium channels,[93] whereas IL-1β may be involved in a complex signaling cascade that leads to the production of pronociceptive compounds (such as nitric oxide, NGF, and prostaglandins) from immune cells or Schwann cells. Such substances lead to changes in gene expression and neuronal excitability in intact nociceptors.[94] The gp130 cytokines, IL-6 and leukemia inhibitory factor (LIF), have been shown to be crucial in the up-regulation of key modulators of sensory processing, such as brain-derived neurotrophic factor (BDNF), galanin, and substance P following nerve injury.[94] The chemokine CCL2 (MCP-1) is another injury-induced factor that accumulates within sensory neurons in models of neuropathic pain[22] and contributes to macrophage recruitment. CCL2 has been implicated in the maintenance of neuropathic pain and knockout mice for the receptor, CCR2, fail to develop signs of neuropathic pain.[95] Recent developments in the understanding of the importance of nonneuronal cells and inflammatory mediators in the response to damage of the peripheral nervous system has greatly aided the understanding of peripheral mechanisms of neuropathic pain.

CELL DEATH IN THE PNS

Many forms of nerve injury can also produce death of sensory neurons.[96] Apoptosis may be a result of mitochondrial dysfunction[97] and has been associated with a number of neuropathies.[96, 98, 99] Mitochondria-dependent apoptosis is activated by a number of factors including reactive oxygen species, ceramide, and nitric oxide,[100] which have been implicated in the pathophysiology of neuropathies. These factors cause the release of cytochrome C from mitochondria leading to the formation of the apoptosome complex and subsequent activation of effector caspases. Alternatively, apoptotic pathways can be activated via stimulation of death receptors, such as TNFR1[100] which can act via the JNK (c-Jun-N-terminal kinase) pathway to activate effector caspases. In support of this, TNFα is released in response to chemotherapeutic agents that produce painful peripheral neuropathy,[101] following direct nerve injury,[102] and in response to HIV-gp120 *in vitro*[103] and caspases have been shown to be important in neuropathic responses in various models of neuropathy.[20, 96, 104, 105] It is thought that the activation of these pathways may be involved in neuropathic pain even though there may be a prolonged latent phase of apoptosis, before cell death.

Spinal cord mechanisms

The sensory input from primary sensory neurons is transferred, via their central axons, to second-order neurons in the dorsal horn of the spinal cord. The synaptic contacts made between afferent central terminals and dorsal horn neurons are highly organized, both topographically and functionally to maintain accurate transfer of information regarding the peripheral noxious stimuli. Following peripheral nerve lesions, synaptic processing in the spinal cord can be subject to diverse forms of functional, chemical, and structural plasticity that are highly involved in the production of hypersensitivity to sensory input. Increased synaptic efficacy (the phenomenon of central sensitization), loss of inhibitory mechanisms, alterations in synaptic contacts, and the activation of nonneuronal cells all play major roles in producing increased pain sensitivity in neuropathic pain. This chapter will address each of these areas in turn.

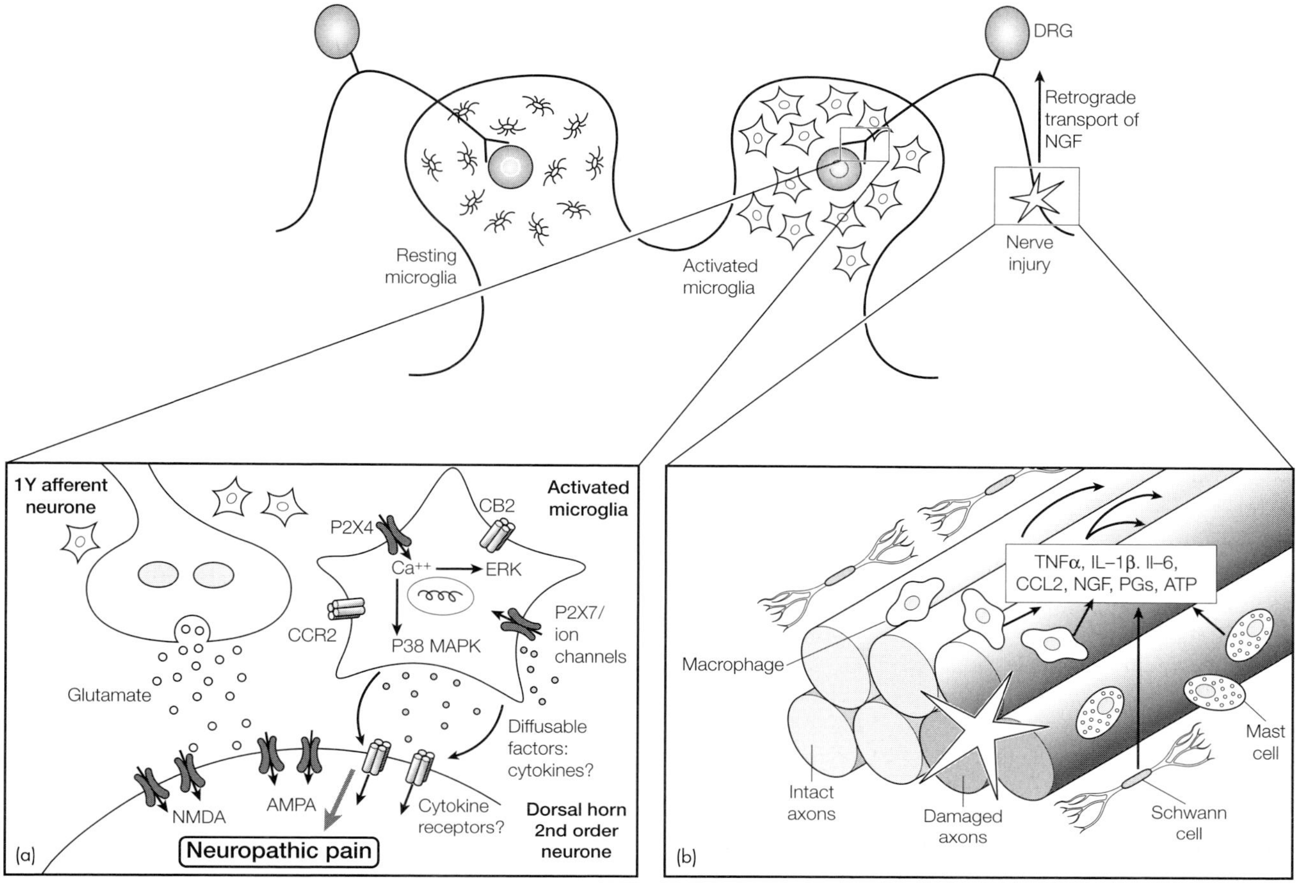

Figure 1.6 The immune system in neuropathic pain. Overview of the effect of the immune system on primary sensory neurons and the spinal cord after peripheral nerve injury. (a) Representation of a mixed nerve injury in which injured and uninjured axons are juxtaposed. The site of injury is typified by the recruitment and proliferation of nonneuronal elements (such as Schwann cells, mast cells, and macrophages), which release factors including the cytokines TNFα, IL-1δ, IL-6, the chemokine CCL2, prostaglandins (PGs) and growth factors, including nerve growth factor (NGF) that initiate and maintain sensory abnormalities after injury. These factors might either induce activity in the axons they act on or be transported retrogradely to cell bodies in the dorsal root ganglion (DRG), where they alter the gene expression of neurons. (b) The effect of the immune system in the spinal cord following peripheral nerve injury with a focus on microglial activation. A primary afferent neuron terminal is flanked by microglial cells that maintain and survey the environment in the spinal cord. In neuropathic pain states, the microglia are activated, probably by the release of transmitters or modulators from primary afferents. The activated microglia release several proinflammatory cytokines, chemokines, and other agents that modulate pain processing by affecting either presynaptic release of neurotransmitters and/or postsynaptic excitability. The release of inflammatory mediators (such as tumor necrosis factor-α (TNFα), interleukin-1β (IL-1β), interleukin-6 (IL-6), nitric oxide (NO), ATP, and prostaglandins (PGs) initiates a self-propagating mechanism of enhanced cytokine expression by microglial cells. This leads to an increase in intracellular calcium, and activation of the p38 and MAPK/ERK pathway. AMPA, α-amino-3-hydroxy-5-methyl-4-isoxazole propionic acid; CCR2, CCL2 receptor; CX3CR1, fractalkine receptor; EAA, excitatory amino acids; ERK, extracellular signal-regulated kinase; FPRL1, formyl peptide receptor-like 1; MHC, major histocompatibility complex; NGF, nerve growth factor; NK1R, neurokinin-1 receptor; NMDA, *N*-methyl-D-aspartic acid; P2 × 4, P2 × 7, ionotropic purinoceptors; p38MAPK, p38 mitogen-activated protein kinase. Adapted with permission from Macmillan Publishers Ltd: *Nature Reviews Neuroscience*[86] © 2005 and reprinted from *Trends in Neuroscience*, 28, Tsuda M, Inoue K, Salter MW, Neuropathic pain and spinal microglia: a big problem from molecules in "small" glia, 101–7, © 2005, with permission from Elsevier.[89]

EXCITATORY MECHANISMS

The afferent barrage associated with peripheral nerve injury is associated with the development of a sustained state of hyperexcitability of dorsal horn neurons, a process dubbed central sensitization.[106, 107] In addition to events such as lowering of activation thresholds of spinal neurons, central sensitization is characterized by the appearance of "wind-up."[108, 109, 110] Wind-up is characterized by an increasing response to repeated C-fiber volleys, and may contribute to hyperalgesia in humans. However, the exact relationship of the relatively short-lived phenomenon of wind-up and the persistent state of central sensitization remains to be fully elucidated.[111]

The excitatory amino acid glutamate is the major excitatory neurotransmitter released at the central terminals of primary afferent nociceptive neurons following noxious stimulation. Glutamate acts at a number of post-synaptic receptors, including metabotropic (mGluRs) and the ionotropic α-amino-3-hydroxyl-5-methyl-4-isoxazole (AMPA), kainate and *N*-methyl-D-aspartic acid (NMDA) receptors. A large body of evidence suggests that the NMDA receptor subtype is the most intimately involved in central sensitization associated with inflammation and nerve injury.[110] For glutamate to exert its effects, receptor phosphorylation and the removal of an Mg^{2+}-dependent ion channel block are critical events in activating the NMDA receptor. NK1 (substance P), AMPA (glutamate), and trkB (BDNF) receptors and the activation of intracellular serine/threonine and tyrosine kinase signalling cascades are all involved in this permissive process.[112, 113]

NMDA receptors are also involved in the maintenance of central sensitization. Nerve injury induces increased release of excitatory amino acids into the spinal dorsal horn which is associated, in an NMDA receptor-dependent manner, with increased intracellular calcium concentration ($[Ca^{2+}]_i$) in dorsal horn neurons.[114] Initial NMDA receptor activation contributes to further increased concentrations of glutamate and aspartate, representing a continual positive feedback loop which maintains sensitization. The increased $[Ca^{2+}]_i$ could also form a positive feedback loop, potentially through indirect activation of protein kinase C (PKC), a hypothesis supported by the antihypersensitivity effect of a PKC inhibitor in the SNL model of neuropathic pain,[115] as well as the evidence that deletion of genes for isoforms of adenylate cyclase, protein kinase A, and protein kinase C all impair the development of pain hypersensitivity in transgenic mice.[116, 117] Activity-dependent central sensitization is displayed by many cells in both the superficial and deep laminae of the dorsal horn. However, in the context of pain hypersensitivity, the effect of sensitization appears to be particularly important for lamina I spinothalamic or spinoparabrachial projection neurons, particularly those expressing the NK_1 receptor.[118, 119]

In addition to Ca^{2+} influx through the NMDA ion channel inducing heterosynaptic potentiation in dorsal horn neurons, activation of voltage-gated calcium channels can enhance excitatory transmission through NMDA receptor-independent mechanisms.[120] For example, neurotrophins such as BDNF, acting through their cognate Trk receptors, facilitate synaptic transmission,[121, 122] partly through a NMDA receptor independent mechanism. Synaptic transmission may also be enhanced by cytokines, such as TNFα, which may be released from glial cells in the dorsal horn.[123] Pharmacological studies support a role for NMDA receptors in neuropathic pain. Pre- and postinjury intraperitoneal administration of the NMDA receptor antagonist MK-801 prevented hypersensitivity in the CCI model[124] and electrophysiological data also demonstrates that MK-801 significantly reduces the hyperresponsiveness to noxious stimulation after peripheral nerve injury.[125]

The agonist action of glutamate at the NMDA receptor can be modulated by glycine.[126] Antagonizing the glycine modulatory site of the NMDA receptor prevents development of hypersensitivity following peripheral nerve injury and attenuates wind-up in isolated spinal cord neurons.[127] Coadministration of a glycine/NMDA receptor antagonist and morphine has also been demonstrated to attenuate pain behavior in an animal model of trigeminal neuralgia.[128]

SPINAL INHIBITORY SYSTEMS

γ-Aminobutyric acid and glycine

The γ-aminobutyric acid (GABA) pathway forms a major inhibitory neurotransmitter system in the CNS. Depression of such spinal inhibitory mechanisms are thought to be important for sustained enhancement of excitatory transmission and central sensitization.[129] In support of this, administration of GABA-mimetics reduces neuropathic hypersensitivity and antagonism of the GABA receptors is associated with hypersensitivity.[130] Moreover, peripheral nerve injury results in a substantial loss of GABA-mediated inhibitory currents,[131] decreased extracellular levels of GABA,[132] a decrease in dorsal horn levels of the GABA synthesizing enzyme glutamic acid decarboxylase (GAD) 65 kDa,[131] and decreased GABA receptor levels in the spinal cord, probably due to degeneration of the primary afferent neuron terminals on which the receptor is localized.[133] Apoptosis in the dorsal horn following nerve injuries may correlate to selective death of GABAergic inhibitory interneurons[131] due to excessive glutamate release or a result of cell death-inducing signals within the spinal cord.[134] All of the above factors likely promote a functional loss of GABAergic transmission in the superficial dorsal horn.

GABAergic and/or glycinergic inhibition are important factors in the maintenance of orderly information processing by preventing the generation of synchronized wave activity in the CNS. Synchronous neuronal activity leading to oscillatory Ca^{2+} waves can be evoked in the spinal dorsal horn network by the potassium channel blocker 4-aminopyridine (4-AP) after pretreatment with blockers of $GABA_A$, glycine, and AMPA/kainate receptors.[135] This may correlate to reduced inhibition and increased neuronal excitability observed in dorsal horns of animals with neuropathic pain.[136] Theoretically, such synchronous activation of larger parts of the dorsal horn network would lead to pain that violates the innervation patterns of peripheral nerves or dorsal roots characterized by violation of sensory modality borders (e.g. allodynia, where normally nonnoxious stimuli are perceived as painful) and somatotopic borders (radiating pain or mirror-image pain). Therefore, disinhibition as a result of altered GABA and glycine signaling may lead to waves of excitability and could underpin neuropathic pain. However, further studies will be required to evaluate under what physiological and pathophysiological conditions crossing of somatotopic and sensory modality borders occurs in spinal dorsal horn.[135]

Opioid system

The endogenous opioid system is also dysregulated following nerve injury. Evidence supports a loss of μ-opioid receptors in the DRG[137] and in the spinal cord following nerve injury.[40, 138, 139] Spinal opioid receptors are localized predominantly on the presynaptic terminals of primary afferents in the superficial dorsal horn[138] and therefore this may reflect degeneration of primary afferent neurons. Additionally, increased cholecystokinin (CCK) mRNA synthesis by DRG neurons[140] and increased expression of the CCK_B receptor in the superficial dorsal horn following peripheral axotomy may potentially decrease the antinociceptive effects of opioids due to opioid antagonistic properties of CCK.[141] These changes may all contribute to the reduced potency of peripherally or spinally delivered opioids in neuropathic pain (**Figure 1.7**).[142]

Cannabinoid system

The endogenous cannabinoid system has received much interest within the field of neuropathic pain due to the fact that unlike the opioid system, spinally expressed cannabinoid receptors are unaffected following nerve injury.[143] In such, manipulation of the cannabinoid system has been effective in alleviating signs of neuropathic pain in animal models of neuropathic pain[5, 22, 144, 145] representing a possible therapeutic advantage of cannabinoids over opioids in neuropathic pain.

ANATOMICAL REORGANIZATION

Tactile mechanical allodynia is thought to be mediated by Aβ-fiber afferents.[146] However, the mechanisms by which this occurs are yet to be fully understood. Several studies using bulk labeling and single afferent fiber-filling techniques have demonstrated that following a peripheral nerve lesion, the central axons of injured Aβ-fibers sprout from their normal termination sites in the deeper laminae of the dorsal horn (laminae II and IV) into lamina II of the dorsal horn, which is normally restricted to C-fiber and Aδ nociceptors.[147, 148] This synaptic rearrangement means that second-order dorsal horn neurons that normally receive predominantly high threshold sensory input, now receive inputs from low threshold mechanoreceptors. Such misinterpretation of information within the spinal cord may result in low threshold sensory information being interpreted as nociceptive, leading to the emergence of hypersensitivity after peripheral nerve injury. The outgrowth of central Aβ-fiber terminals is prevented by NGF and GDNF treatment, presumably by provision of trophic support for damaged C-fibers, suggesting an important role for neurotrophins in the regulation of this manifestation of structural plasticity.[149] However, some studies have raised concerns about the specificity of bulk-labeling techniques and the sampling of intracellular labeled intact and injured afferents,[150, 151] such that the labeling may actually be due to damaged C-fibers abnormally taking up the label. However, in favor of the sprouting theory, stimulation of Aβ-fibers in injured nerves can produce activation of neurons in lamina II measured electrophysiologically and by expression of c-Fos.[152, 153] Nevertheless, further work is required to resolve the basis for the differences in these anatomical studies, and to determine the extent to which sprouting of Aβ-fibers contributes to tactile hypersensitivity after peripheral nerve injury.

THE ROLE OF NONNEURONAL CELLS

Peripheral nerve injury produces molecular and cellular changes that result in multiple forms of neuronal plasticity and anatomical reorganization at various levels of the peripheral and central nervous systems. Oligodendrocytes, astrocytes, and microglia form a large group of CNS glial cells. Although often underappreciated, a substantial body of evidence has accumulated showing that peripheral nerve injury leads to activation of glia in the spinal cord implicating astrocytes and particularly microglia.[89, 123]

Microglia are immune-derived cells and represent 5–10 percent of glia in the CNS.[154] Microglia are said to be resting under normal conditions and do not actively influence nociceptive processing. However, microglia become activated by events such as CNS injury, microbial invasion, and in some pain states. Following peripheral nerve lesions, spinal microglia appear to migrate to the relevant spinal segments, thus increasing the local microglial population, and become activated involving a stereotypic series of changes including morphological alteration (they become hypertrophic and ameobiod), gene expression, and function. Moreover, activated microglia produce and release various chemical mediators, including proinflammatory cytokines, chemokines, and other potentially pain-producing substances, that can produce immunological actions and can also act on neurons to alter their function (**Figure 1.6**).[89, 155] The status of microglia in the spinal cord has been examined in a variety of nerve injury models and substantial evidence, both direct and indirect, indicates that microgliosis fundamentally contributes to the pathophysiology of neuropathic pain.[20, 22, 156, 157, 158] This is supported by several studies that have shown specific microglial inhibitors and/or modulators, such as fluorocitrate and minocycline block, and/or reverse neuropathic states.[21, 22, 159, 160]

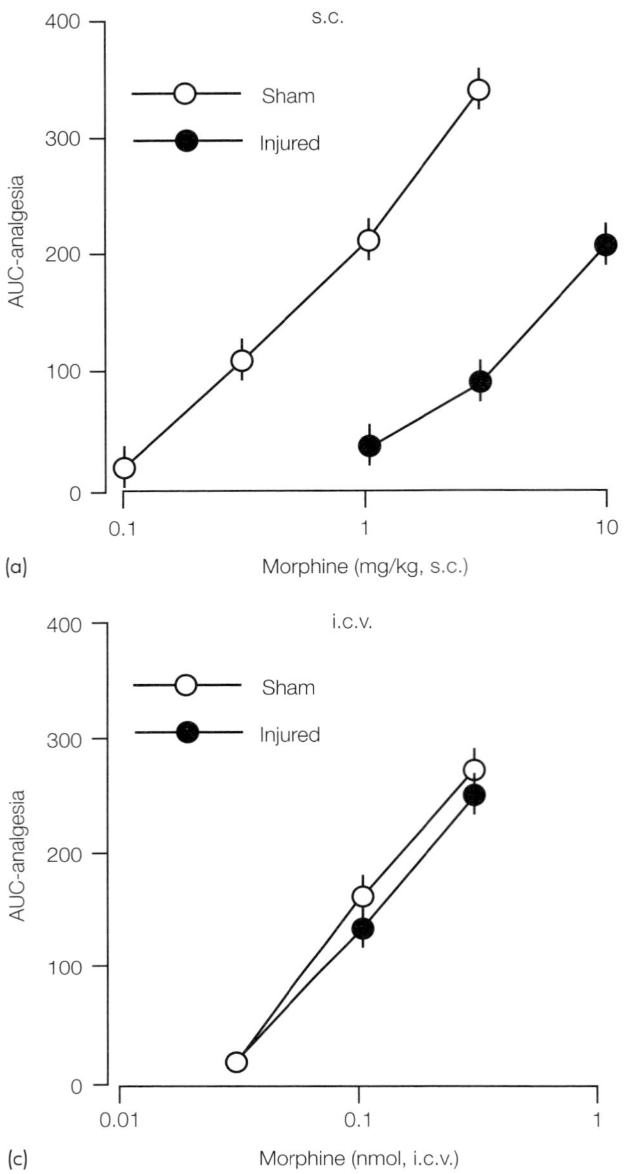

Figure 1.7 The effect of morphine in nerve-injured mice. Dose–response curves of morphine in sham-operated (sham) and nerve-injured (injured) mice after subcutaneous (s.c.), intrathecal (i.t.), and intracerebroventricular (i.c.v.) injection with the Hargreaves thermal paw withdrawal test. Graphs show dose–response curves of (a) s.c., (b) i.t., and (c) i.c.v. morphine in sham-operated and nerve-injured mice at seven days following nerve ligation. The data are presented as AUC analgesia. Each data point represents the mean s.e.m. from six mice. Redrawn from Rashid *et al.*, 2000[142] with permission from The American Society for Pharmacology and Experimental Therapeutics.

It is not clear what factors activate spinal microglia in peripheral neuropathic pain states. Several molecules have been implicated, including macrophage colony-stimulating factor (MCSF),[161] IL-6,[162] substance P, ATP, and the chemokines, fracktalkine,[163] and CCL2.[164] Activated microglia express various molecules allowing them to respond to such stimuli, including the ATP gated ligand-gated cation channels, P2 × 4,[165] and P2 × 7,[166] and the chemotactic cytokine receptor 2 (CCR2), a receptor for CCL2/MCP-1. Recent evidence suggests that ATP-stimulated microglia signal to lamina I neurons via their release of BDNF, causing a depolarizing shift in the neuronal anion reversal potential inverting the polarity of currents activated by GABA. This means that GABA now results in excitation of the cell as opposed to inhibition.[158] Evidence for a role of CCR2 in nerve injury-induced hypersensitivity[95] comes from mutant mice lacking the receptor. However, as CCR2 is also up-regulated in the peripheral nerve, at the site of the nerve injury and in the DRG, it is unclear whether spinal microglia expressed CCR2 is responsible. The cannabinoid receptor subtype CB_2 may also be expressed by spinal microglia after nerve injury and therefore cannabinoids may play a role as modulators of neuropathic pain via actions on microglia.[167] Accordingly, systemically administered CB_2 agonists can inhibit nerve injury-evoked pain behaviors.[95, 168] However, CB_2 agonists might act in the periphery and therefore the role of microglial CB_2 receptors is, at present, unclear.[169, 170]

The recruitment of microglia is commonly associated with the activation (phosphorylation) of p38 MAP (MAP) kinase and MAP kinase ERK (extracellular signal-regulated kinase) in the spinal cord. Phosphorylation of p38 is probably a key intracellular signal in the microglial response in neuropathic pain[157, 171] and the sequential activation of ERK in neurons, then microglia, and finally astrocytes in a neuropathic pain model[172] suggests that microglial activation might be the first step in a cascade of immune responses in the CNS.[86, 94] The aforementioned molecules expressed by activated microglia in neuropathic pain states, or associated intracellular signaling cascades may be potential analgesic targets.

Supraspinal mechanisms

DESCENDING MODULATION

In addition to the peripheral and spinal mechanisms discussed, supraspinal mechanisms are thought to play an important role in neuropathic pain.[173, 174] The periaqueductal gray (PAG) is the most characterized part of a CNS circuit that controls nociceptive transmission at the level of the spinal cord.[175] The PAG integrates inputs from areas such as the limbic forebrain, diencephalon, amygdala, and hippocampus with ascending nociceptive input from the dorsal horn[176] and is therefore associated with the affective and autonomic responses to pain.

The PAG is closely associated with the brainstem including the rostral ventromedial medulla (RVM), and is critical in the descending modulation of spinal activity through monoaminergic and other pathways.[177] Likely via anatomically distinct pathways, the PAG and RVM can exert both facilitatory and inhibitory influences on the spinal cord.[178] The balance of these two supraspinal pathways and primary afferent input, ultimately determines the excitability of spinal neurons.[174] Under pathological conditions, enhancement of descending facilitatory controls to the spinal cord are likely to allow excitatory influences to predominate to maintain spinal central sensitization (**Figure 1.8**).

Facilitatory cells within the RVM are classed as ON cells, whereas cells that have inhibitory influences on the spinal cord are termed OFF cells.[179] Following nerve injury, there is enhanced descending excitatory drive from the RVM[180] which may represent a central compensatory mechanism for the loss of normal sensory input following peripheral nerve damage.[174] The brainstem areas involved are also implicated in autonomic responses, emotions, and sleep. Therefore, these same pathways likely underpin the well-established links between these states and pain, and may provide a basis for an affective component of pain.[181]

Various transmitter pathways are implicated in descending control mechanisms. For example, CCK, an antianalgesic peptide, may contribute to RVM neuron excitability.[182] Intra-RVM CCK produces reversible thermal and tactile hypersensitivity in naive rats[141] and prevents both the activation of OFF cells and the antinociception produced by systemic morphine.[183] Additionally, although thought mainly to play an inhibitory role in supraspinal systems,[184] supraspinal serotonergic inputs to the spinal cord originating in the RVM may play a role in facilitatory influences following peripheral nerve injury.[185] The 5HT3 receptor, localized to a novel group of small diameter afferents, and a larger

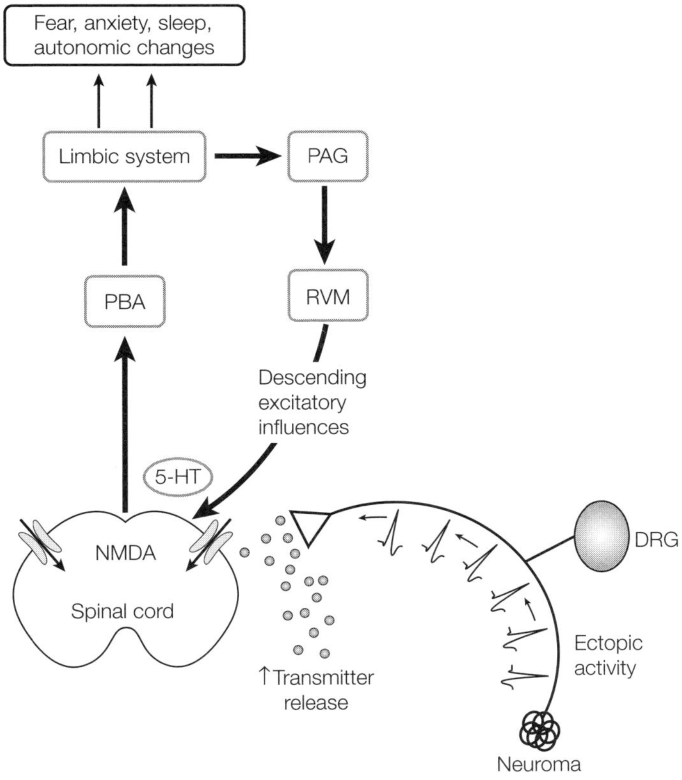

Figure 1.8 Overview of supraspinal involvement in neuropathic pain. Peripheral nerve injury induces spontaneous ectopic activity at the site of injury and the dorsal root ganglion (DRG) resulting in increased release of glutamate and neuropeptides (such as substance P) to the spinal cord, thereby promoting sensory transmission in the spinal cord. Centrally, there is increased function of the *N*-methyl-D-aspartic acid (NMDA) receptor and enhanced descending activity from the rostral ventromedial medulla (RVM) serotonergic excitatory pathways. All these mechanisms can contribute to the development of abnormal pain accompanying nerve injury. Plasticity is seen in the expression and function of ion channels (e.g. Na^+ channels) and neurotransmitters (e.g. substance P). Sprouting of sympathetic nerve fibers in the DRG act to sensitize peripheral afferents. Adapted from Suzuki and Dickenson, 2005,[174] by permission of S Karger AG, Basel.

number of presumed A-delta afferent fibers,[186] has been implicated as the target receptor of this system. Ondansetron, a $5HT_3$ antagonist exerts influences particularly on punctate mechanical responses after nerve injury.[187] Additionally, a preliminary clinical study suggests that block of $5HT_3$ receptors has clinical utility in the treatment of pain.[188]

Finally, evidence suggests that cannabinoids produce their antinociceptive effect at least in part by recruiting the PAG–RVM modulatory system.[189] CB_1 receptors are densely expressed in the PAG, and microinjection of CB_1 agonists into the PAG or RVM produces antinociception.[190] CB_1 receptors are also known to be expressed on rostrocaudally directed fibers in the dorsolateral funiculus, a major tract for descending control systems.[169, 170]

IMAGING OF THE BRAIN IN NEUROPATHIC PAIN

Recent advances in human brain imaging techniques offer an exciting opportunity to examine brain processes in experimental and clinical pain conditions. This has allowed insights into neural correlates of pain and led to a much greater understanding of the pain matrix,[191, 192] which includes brain structures, such as the anterior cingulate cortex (ACC), insula, frontal cortices, S1, second somatosensory cortex (S2), and amygdala.[193]

Neural correlates of allodynia have been examined in various conditions, including patients with neuropathic pain, central pain, or experimentally provoked allodynia. However, the existing data are controversial with some suggesting that allodynia is processed differently than nociceptive pain and others suggesting they share a common neural basis. Areas shown to be involved in allodynia include the parietal association cortex,[194] medial thalamus, putamen, and prefrontal cortex.[195] The ACC, which is almost always activated during acute pain in normal subjects and is involved in the affective (cognitive–evaluative) component of pain, has been differentially associated with processing of allodynia.[196, 197, 198, 199] This suggests that A-β-mediated pain may have a unique cortical representation in some situations which may aid further understanding of the phenomenon that is tactile allodynia. The amygdala, which plays an important role in fear-conditioning and affective disorders, such as anxiety and depression,[200] is activated by a diverse range of persistent nociceptive stimuli in the rat.[201, 202] Evidence suggests a role for the amygdala in the affective–emotional pain response in a rodent model of neuropathy involving GABAergic systems.[203] The amygdala has also been linked to spontaneous pain in humans suffering from postherpetic neuralgia.[204] Such studies highlight the involvement of a number of brain areas in pain responses in neuropathic pain conditions. However, further work using brain imaging techniques is required before our understanding of such systems is complete.

CONCLUSIONS

This brief overview of mechanisms of neuropathic pain outlines the complex nature of the response of the nervous system to a peripheral nerve injury. There is little doubt that a combination of mechanisms, involving peripheral, spinal, and supraspinal mediated events, contribute to the manifestation of neuropathic pain in any one individual. Eventually, it may be possible to improve the ethos of clinical management protocols so that they will move away from disease-based treatment towards symptom or, ultimately, mechanism-based therapies.[34] However, this will require a better understanding of mechanisms involved in neuropathic pain and reliable convenient tools for their assessment in the clinic.[33] It must be emphasized that the majority of preclinical studies employ animal models of nerve injury and measure associated hypersensitivity, which is only evident in a subset of patients with neuropathic pain. Therefore, improvement of animal models and behavioral tests will possibly unravel more therapeutically relevant mechanisms. Advances in technology have led to new approaches for the identification of novel targets involved in neuropathic pain. For example, microarray technology generates data regarding a large number of genes which can lead to the investigation of promising novel targets in neuropathic pain.[205] Additionally, our understanding of genetics may uncover genetic variation in the susceptibility of individuals to develop neuropathic pain,[206] which can also aid our understanding of specific mechanistic alterations and "genetically tailor" analgesics based on an individual's pharmacogenetic profile.

REFERENCES

* 1. Treede RD, Jensen TS, Campbell JN *et al.* Neuropathic pain. Redefinition and a grading system for clinical and research purposes. *Neurology.* 2008; **70**: 1630–5.
* 2. Dworkin RH, Backonja M, Rowbotham MC *et al.* Advances in neuropathic pain: diagnosis, mechanisms, and treatment recommendations. *Archives of Neurology.* 2003; **60**: 1524–34.

3. Hansson P. Neuropathic pain: clinical characteristics and diagnostic workup. *European Journal of Pain.* 2002; **6** (Suppl. A): 47–50.
4. Fields HL, Rowbotham M, Baron R. Postherpetic neuralgia: irritable nociceptors and deafferentation. *Neurobiology of Disease.* 1998; **5**: 209–27.
5. Bridges D, Ahmad K, Rice AS. The synthetic cannabinoid WIN55,212-2 attenuates hyperalgesia and allodynia in a rat model of neuropathic pain. *British Journal of Pharmacology.* 2001; **133**: 586–94.
6. Decosterd I, Woolf CJ. Spared nerve injury: an animal model of persistent peripheral neuropathic pain. *Pain.* 2000; **87**: 149–58.

7. Bennett GJ, Xie YK. A peripheral mononeuropathy in rat that produces disorders of pain sensation like those seen in man. *Pain.* 1988; **33**: 87–107.
8. Seltzer Z, Dubner R, Shir Y. A novel behavioral model of neuropathic pain disorders produced in rats by partial sciatic nerve injury. *Pain.* 1990; **43**: 205–18.
9. Kim SH, Chung JM. An experimental model for peripheral neuropathy produced by segmental spinal nerve ligation in the rat. *Pain.* 1992; **50**: 355–63.
* 10. Mogil JS, Crager SE. What should we be measuring in behavioral studies of chronic pain in animals? *Pain.* 2004; **112**: 12–15.
11. Wagner R, Janjigian M, Myers RR. Anti-inflammatory interleukin-10 therapy in CCI neuropathy decreases thermal hyperalgesia, macrophage recruitment, and endoneurial TNF-alpha expression. *Pain.* 1998; **74**: 35–42.
12. Li Y, Dorsi MJ, Meyer RA, Belzberg AJ. Mechanical hyperalgesia after an L5 spinal nerve lesion in the rat is not dependent on input from injured nerve fibers. *Pain.* 2000; **85**: 493–502.
13. Bove G. Mechanical sensory threshold testing using nylon monofilaments: the pain field's "tin standard". *Pain.* 2006; **124**: 13–17.
14. Hargreaves K, Dubner R, Brown F *et al.* A new and sensitive method for measuring thermal nociception in cutaneous hyperalgesia. *Pain.* 1988; **32**: 77–88.
15. Malcangio M, Tomlinson DR. A pharmacologic analysis of mechanical hyperalgesia in streptozotocin/diabetic rats. *Pain.* 1998; **76**: 151–7.
16. Idanpaan-Heikkila JJ, Guilbaud G. Pharmacological studies on a rat model of trigeminal neuropathic pain: baclofen, but not carbamazepine, morphine or tricyclic antidepressants, attenuates the allodynia-like behaviour. *Pain.* 1999; **79**: 281–90.
17. Fleetwood-Walker SM, Quinn JP, Wallace C *et al.* Behavioural changes in the rat following infection with varicella-zoster virus. *Journal of General Virology.* 1999; **80**: 2433–6.
18. Garry EM, Delaney A, Anderson HA *et al.* Varicella zoster virus induces neuropathic changes in rat dorsal root ganglia and behavioral reflex sensitisation that is attenuated by gabapentin or sodium channel blocking drugs. *Pain.* 2005; **118**: 97–111.
19. Hasnie FS, Breuer J, Parker S *et al.* Further characterization of a rat model of varicella zoster virus-associated pain: Relationship between mechanical hypersensitivity and anxiety-related behavior, and the influence of analgesic drugs. *Neuroscience.* 2006; **144**: 1495–508.
20. Wallace VC, Blackbeard J, Pheby T *et al.* Pharmacological, behavioural and mechanistic analysis of HIV-1 gp120 induced painful neuropathy. *Pain.* 2007; **133**: 47–63.
21. Milligan ED, Mehmert KK, Hinde JL *et al.* Thermal hyperalgesia and mechanical allodynia produced by intrathecal administration of the human immunodeficiency virus-1 (HIV-1) envelope glycoprotein, gp120. *Brain Research.* 2000; **861**: 105–16.
22. Wallace VC, Blackbeard J, Segerdahl AR *et al.* Characterization of rodent models of HIV-gp120 and anti-retroviral-associated neuropathic pain. *Brain.* 2007; **130**: 2688–702.
23. Gonzalez-Scarano F, Martin-Garcia J. The neuropathogenesis of AIDS. *Nature Reviews. Immunology.* 2005; **5**: 69–81.
24. Authier N, Gillet JP, Fialip J *et al.* An animal model of nociceptive peripheral neuropathy following repeated cisplatin injections. *Experimental Neurology.* 2003; **182**: 12–20.
25. Polomano RC, Mannes AJ, Clark US, Bennett GJ. A painful peripheral neuropathy in the rat produced by the chemotherapeutic drug, paclitaxel. *Pain.* 2001; **94**: 293–304.
26. Joseph EK, Chen X, Khasar SG, Levine JD. Novel mechanism of enhanced nociception in a model of AIDS therapy-induced painful peripheral neuropathy in the rat. *Pain.* 2004; **107**: 147–58.
27. Wallace VC, McMahon SB, Rice AS. The characterisation of a rodent model of antiretroviral-associated painful peripheral neuropathy. Presented as a poster at Society for Neuroscience, Atlanta, GA, 2006.
* 28. Cryan JF, Holmes A. The ascent of mouse: advances in modelling human depression and anxiety. *Nature Reviews. Drug Discovery.* 2005; **4**: 775–90.
29. Morgan MM, Whitney PK. Immobility accompanies the antinociception mediated by the rostral ventromedial medulla of the rat. *Brain Research.* 2000; **872**: 276–81.
30. LaBuda CJ, Fuchs PN. A behavioral test paradigm to measure the aversive quality of inflammatory and neuropathic pain in rats. *Experimental Neurology.* 2000; **163**: 490–4.
31. Pedersen LH, Blackburn-Munro G. Pharmacological characterisation of place escape/avoidance behaviour in the rat chronic constriction injury model of neuropathic pain. *Psychopharmacology (Berlin).* 2006; **185**: 208–17.
32. Hasnie FS, Wallace VC, Hefner K *et al.* Mechanical and cold hypersensitivity in nerve-injured C57BL/6J mice is not associated with fear-avoidance- and depression-related behaviour. *British Journal of Anaesthesia.* 2007; **98**: 816–22.
* 33. Finnerup NB, Jensen TS. Mechanisms of disease: mechanism-based classification of neuropathic pain – a critical analysis. *Nature Clinical Practice. Neurology.* 2006; **2**: 107–15.
* 34. Woolf CJ, Mannion RJ. Neuropathic pain: aetiology, symptoms, mechanisms, and management. *Lancet.* 1999; **353**: 1959–64.
* 35. Wall PD, Gutnick M. Ongoing activity in peripheral nerves: the physiology and pharmacology of impulses originating from a neuroma. *Experimental Neurology.* 1974; **43**: 580–93.
* 36. Devor M. Sodium channels and mechanisms of neuropathic pain. *Journal of Pain.* 2006; **7**: S3–12.
37. Nordin M, Nystrom B, Wallin U, Hagbarth KE. Ectopic sensory discharges and paresthesiae in patients with

disorders of peripheral nerves, dorsal roots and dorsal columns. *Pain.* 1984; **20**: 231–45.

38. Devor M. Response of nerves to injury in relation to neuropathic pain. In: McMahon SB, Koltzenburg M (eds). *Melzack and Wall's textbook of pain*, 5th edn. London: Churchill-Livingstone, 2005: 905–28.

* 39. Amir R, Devor M. Axonal cross-excitation in nerve-end neuromas: comparison of A- and C-fibers. *Journal of Neurophysiology.* 1992; **68**: 1160–6.

40. Amir R, Michaelis M, Devor M. Membrane potential oscillations in dorsal root ganglion neurons: role in normal electrogenesis and neuropathic pain. *Journal of Neuroscience.* 1999; **19**: 8589–96.

41. Wall PD, Devor M. Sensory afferent impulses originate from dorsal root ganglia as well as from the periphery in normal and nerve injured rats. *Pain.* 1983; **17**: 321–39.

42. Michaelis M, Liu X, Janig W. Axotomized and intact muscle afferents but no skin afferents develop ongoing discharges of dorsal root ganglion origin after peripheral nerve lesion. *Journal of Neuroscience.* 2000; **20**: 2742–8.

* 43. Wu G, Ringkamp M, Hartke TV *et al.* Early onset of spontaneous activity in uninjured C-fiber nociceptors after injury to neighboring nerve fibers. *Journal of Neuroscience.* 2001; **21**: RC140.

* 44. Wu G, Ringkamp M, Murinson BB *et al.* Degeneration of myelinated efferent fibers induces spontaneous activity in uninjured C-fiber afferents. *Journal of Neuroscience.* 2002; **22**: 7746–53.

45. Devor M, Keller CH, Deerinck TJ *et al.* Na+ channel accumulation on axolemma of afferent endings in nerve end neuromas in Apteronotus. *Neuroscience Letters.* 1989; **102**: 149–54.

46. Matzner O, Devor M. Hyperexcitability at sites of nerve injury depends on voltage-sensitive Na+ channels. *Journal of Neurophysiology.* 1994; **72**: 349–59.

47. Waxman SG, Cummins TR, Dib-Hajj SD, Black JA. Voltage-gated sodium channels and the molecular pathogenesis of pain: a review. *Journal of Rehabilitation Research and Development.* 2000; **37**: 517–28.

* 48. Akopian AN, Sivilotti L, Wood JN. A tetrodotoxin-resistant voltage-gated sodium channel expressed by sensory neurons. *Nature.* 1996; **379**: 257–62.

49. Dib-Hajj SD, Fjell J, Cummins TR *et al.* Plasticity of sodium channel expression in DRG neurons in the chronic constriction injury model of neuropathic pain. *Pain.* 1999; **83**: 591–600.

* 50. Waxman SG, Dib-Hajj S, Cummins TR, Black JA. Sodium channels and pain. *Proceedings of the National Academy of Sciences of the United States of America.* 1999; **96**: 7635–9.

51. Omana-Zapata I, Khabbaz MA, Hunter JC *et al.* Tetrodotoxin inhibits neuropathic ectopic activity in neuromas, dorsal root ganglia and dorsal horn neurons. *Pain.* 1997; **72**: 41–9.

52. Lyu YS, Park SK, Chung K, Chung JM. Low dose of tetrodotoxin reduces neuropathic pain behaviors in an animal model. *Brain Research.* 2000; **871**: 98–103.

53. Novakovic SD, Tzoumaka E, McGivern JG *et al.* Distribution of the tetrodotoxin-resistant sodium channel PN3 in rat sensory neurons in normal and neuropathic conditions. *Journal of Neuroscience.* 1998; **18**: 2174–87.

54. Coward K, Plumpton C, Facer P *et al.* Immunolocalization of SNS/PN3 and NaN/SNS2 sodium channels in human pain states. *Pain.* 2000; **85**: 41–50.

55. Yiangou Y, Birch R, Sangameswaran L *et al.* SNS/PN3 and SNS2/NaN sodium channel-like immunoreactivity in human adult and neonate injured sensory nerves. *FEBS Letters.* 2000; **467**: 249–52.

56. Rogers M, Tang L, Madge DJ, Stevens EB. The role of sodium channels in neuropathic pain. *Seminars in Cell and Developmental Biology.* 2006; **17**: 571–81.

57. Rush AM, Dib-Hajj SD, Liu S *et al.* A single sodium channel mutation produces hyper- or hypoexcitability in different types of neurons. *Proceedings of the National Academy of Sciences of the United States of America.* 2006; **103**: 8245–50.

58. Harty TP, Dib-Hajj SD, Tyrrell L *et al.* Nav1.7 mutant A863P in erythromelalgia: effects of altered activation and steady-state inactivation on excitability of nociceptive dorsal root ganglion neurons. *Journal of Neuroscience.* 2006; **26**: 12566–75.

* 59. Nassar MA, Levato A, Stirling LC, Wood JN. Neuropathic pain develops normally in mice lacking both Nav1.7 and Nav1.8. *Molecular Pain.* 2005; **1**: 24.

60. Black JA, Langworthy K, Hinson AW *et al.* NGF has opposing effects on Na+ channel III and SNS gene expression in spinal sensory neurons. *Neuroreport.* 1997; **8**: 2331–5.

* 61. Pezet S, McMahon SB. Neurotrophins: mediators and modulators of pain. *Annual Review of Neuroscience.* 2006; **29**: 507–38.

* 62. Boucher TJ, Okuse K, Bennett DL *et al.* Potent analgesic effects of GDNF in neuropathic pain states. *Science.* 2000; **290**: 124–7.

63. Amir R, Argoff CE, Bennett GJ *et al.* The role of sodium channels in chronic inflammatory and neuropathic pain. *Journal of Pain.* 2006; **7**: S1–29.

* 64. Hempenstall K, Nurmikko TJ, Johnson RW *et al.* Analgesic therapy in postherpetic neuralgia: a quantitative systematic review. *PLoS Medicine.* 2005; **2**: e164.

65. Gerner P, Mujtaba M, Sinnott CJ, Wang GK. Amitriptyline versus bupivacaine in rat sciatic nerve blockade. *Anesthesiology.* 2001; **94**: 661–7.

66. Gutman GA, Chandy KG, Adelman JP *et al.* International Union of Pharmacology. XLI. Compendium of voltage-gated ion channels: potassium channels. *Pharmacological Reviews.* 2003; **55**: 583–6.

* 67. Rasband MN, Park EW, Vanderah TW *et al.* Distinct potassium channels on pain-sensing neurons. *Proceedings of the National Academy of Sciences of the United States of America.* 2001; **98**: 13373–8.

68. Doan TN, Stephans K, Ramirez AN *et al.* Differential distribution and function of hyperpolarization-activated

channels in sensory neurons and mechanosensitive fibers. *Journal of Neuroscience.* 2004; **24**: 3335–43.

69. Passmore GM, Selyanko AA, Mistry M *et al.* KCNQ/M currents in sensory neurons: significance for pain therapy. *Journal of Neuroscience.* 2003; **23**: 7227–36.
70. Boettger MK, Till S, Chen MX *et al.* Calcium-activated potassium channel SK1- and IK1-like immunoreactivity in injured human sensory neurones and its regulation by neurotrophic factors. *Brain.* 2002; **125**: 252–63.
71. Xiao WH, Bennett GJ. Synthetic omega-conopeptides applied to the site of nerve injury suppress neuropathic pains in rats. *Journal of Pharmacology and Experimental Therapeutics.* 1995; **274**: 666–72.
72. White DM, Cousins MJ. Effect of subcutaneous administration of calcium channel blockers on nerve injury-induced hyperalgesia. *Brain Research.* 1998; **801**: 50–8.

✻ 73. Pertwee RG. Pharmacology of cannabinoid CB1 and CB2 receptors. *Pharmacology and Therapeutics.* 1997; **74**: 129–80.

✻ 74. Luo ZD, Chaplan SR, Higuera ES *et al.* Upregulation of dorsal root ganglion (alpha)2(delta) calcium channel subunit and its correlation with allodynia in spinal nerve-injured rats. *Journal of Neuroscience.* 2001; **21**: 1868–75.

✻ 75. Li CY, Song YH, Higuera ES, Luo ZD. Spinal dorsal horn calcium channel alpha2delta-1 subunit upregulation contributes to peripheral nerve injury-induced tactile allodynia. *Journal of Neuroscience.* 2004; **24**: 8494–9.

76. Li CY, Zhang XL, Matthews EA *et al.* Calcium channel alpha(2)delta(1) subunit mediates spinal hyperexcitability in pain modulation. *Pain.* 2006; **125**: 20–34.
77. Gee NS, Brown JP, Dissanayake VU *et al.* The novel anticonvulsant drug, gabapentin (Neurontin), binds to the alpha2delta subunit of a calcium channel. *Journal of Biological Chemistry.* 1996; **271**: 5768–76.
78. Marais E, Klugbauer N, Hofmann F. Calcium channel alpha(2)delta subunits-structure and Gabapentin binding. *Molecular Pharmacology.* 2001; **59**: 1243–8.
79. Field MJ, Cox PJ, Stott E *et al.* Identification of the {alpha}2-{delta}-1 subunit of voltage-dependent calcium channels as a molecular target for pain mediating the analgesic actions of pregabalin. *Proceedings of the National Academy of Sciences of the United States of America.* 2006; **103**: 17537–42.
80. Gilron I, Flatters SJ. Gabapentin and pregabalin for the treatment of neuropathic pain: A review of laboratory and clinical evidence. *Pain Research and Management.* 2006; **11** (Suppl A): 16A–29A.

✻ 81. Finnerup NB, Otto M, McQuay HJ *et al.* Algorithm for neuropathic pain treatment: an evidence based proposal. *Pain.* 2005; **118**: 289–305.

✻ 82. Wang H, Woolf CJ. Pain TRPs. *Neuron.* 2005; **46**: 9–12.

83. Hudson LJ, Bevan S, Wotherspoon G *et al.* VR1 protein expression increases in undamaged DRG neurons after partial nerve injury. *European Journal of Neuroscience.* 2001; **13**: 2105–14.

✻ 84. Obata K, Yamanaka H, Fukuoka T *et al.* Contribution of injured and uninjured dorsal root ganglion neurons to pain behavior and the changes in gene expression following chronic constriction injury of the sciatic nerve in rats. *Pain.* 2003; **101**: 65–77.

85. Katsura H, Obata K, Mizushima T *et al.* Antisense knock down of TRPA1, but not TRPM8, alleviates cold hyperalgesia after spinal nerve ligation in rats. *Experimental Neurology.* 2006; **200**: 112–23.

✻ 86. Marchand F, Perretti M, McMahon SB. Role of the immune system in chronic pain. *Nature Reviews. Neuroscience.* 2005; **6**: 521–32.

✻ 87. White FA, Bhangoo SK, Miller RJ. Chemokines: integrators of pain and inflammation. *Nature Reviews. Drug Discovery.* 2005; **4**: 834–44.

88. Vilcek J. The cytokines: an overview. In: Thomson A (ed.). *The cytokine handbook*, 3rd edn. San Diego: Academic Press, 1998: 1–20.

✻ 89. Tsuda M, Inoue K, Salter MW. Neuropathic pain and spinal microglia: a big problem from molecules in "small" glia. *Trends in Neuroscience.* 2005; **28**: 101–7.

90. Sommer C, Petrausch S, Lindenlaub T, Toyka KV. Neutralizing antibodies to interleukin 1-receptor reduce pain associated behavior in mice with experimental neuropathy. *Neuroscience Letters.* 1999; **270**: 25–8.
91. Schafers M, Brinkhoff J, Neukirchen S *et al.* Combined epineurial therapy with neutralizing antibodies to tumor necrosis factor-alpha and interleukin-1 receptor has an additive effect in reducing neuropathic pain in mice. *Neuroscience Letters.* 2001; **310**: 113–16.
92. Ramer MS, Murphy PG, Richardson PM, Bisby MA. Spinal nerve lesion-induced mechanoallodynia and adrenergic sprouting in sensory ganglia are attenuated in interleukin-6 knockout mice. *Pain.* 1998; **78**: 115–21.
93. Wilkinson MF, Earle ML, Triggle CR, Barnes S. Interleukin-1beta, tumor necrosis factor-alpha, and LPS enhance calcium channel current in isolated vascular smooth muscle cells of rat tail artery. *FASEB Journal.* 1996; **10**: 785–91.

✻ 94. McMahon SB, Cafferty WB, Marchand F. Immune and glial cell factors as pain mediators and modulators. *Experimental Neurology.* 2005; **192**: 444–62.

95. Abbadie C, Lindia JA, Cumiskey AM *et al.* Impaired neuropathic pain responses in mice lacking the chemokine receptor CCR2. *Proceedings of the National Academy of Sciences of the United States of America.* 2003; **100**: 7947–52.
96. Joseph EK, Levine JD. Caspase signalling in neuropathic and inflammatory pain in the rat. *European Journal of Neuroscience.* 2004; **20**: 2896–902.
97. Lorenzo HK, Susin SA. Mitochondrial effectors in caspase-independent cell death. *FEBS Letters.* 2004; **557**: 14–20.
98. Inoue S, Salah-Eldin AE, Omoteyama K. Apoptosis and anticancer drug resistance. *Human Cell.* 2001; **14**: 211–21.
99. Cossarizza A, Moyle G. Antiretroviral nucleoside and nucleotide analogues and mitochondria. *AIDS.* 2004; **18**: 137–51.

*100. Benn SC, Woolf CJ. Adult neuron survival strategies – slamming on the brakes. *Nature Reviews. Neuroscience.* 2004; **5**: 686–700.

101. Tonini G, Santini D, Vincenzi B *et al.* Oxaliplatin may induce cytokine-release syndrome in colorectal cancer patients. *Journal of Biological Regulators and Homeostatic Agents.* 2002; **16**: 105–9.

102. George A, Schmidt C, Weishaupt A *et al.* Serial determination of tumor necrosis factor-alpha content in rat sciatic nerve after chronic constriction injury. *Experimental Neurology.* 1999; **160**: 124–32.

103. Keswani SC, Polley M, Pardo CA *et al.* Schwann cell chemokine receptors mediate HIV-1 gp120 toxicity to sensory neurons. *Annals of Neurology.* 2003; **54**: 287–96.

104. Jiang Y, Zhang JS, Jakobsen J. Differential effect of p75 neurotrophin receptor on expression of pro-apoptotic proteins c-jun, p38 and caspase-3 in dorsal root ganglion cells after axotomy in experimental diabetes. *Neuroscience.* 2005; **132**: 1083–92.

105. Jin HW, Ichikawa H, Fujita M *et al.* Involvement of caspase cascade in capsaicin-induced apoptosis of dorsal root ganglion neurons. *Brain Research.* 2005; **1056**: 139–44.

*106. Coderre TJ, Katz J, Vaccarino AL, Melzack R. Contribution of central neuroplasticity to pathological pain: review of clinical and experimental evidence. *Pain.* 1993; **52**: 259–85.

*107. Wall PD. Neuropathic pain and injured nerve: central mechanisms. *British Medical Bulletin.* 1991; **47**: 631–43.

108. Mendell LM. Physiological properties of unmyelinated fiber projection to the spinal cord. *Experimental Neurology.* 1966; **16**: 316–32.

109. Wall PD, Woolf CJ. The brief and the prolonged facilitatory effects of unmyelinated afferent input on the rat spinal cord are independently influenced by peripheral nerve section. *Neuroscience.* 1986; **17**: 1199–205.

110. Doubell TP, Mannion RJ, Woolf CJ. The dorsal horn: state-dependent sensory processing, plasticity and the generation of pain. In: Wall PD, Melzack R (eds). *Textbook of pain*, 4th edn. London: Churchill Livingstone, 1999: 165–82.

*111. Woolf CJ. Windup and central sensitization are not equivalent. *Pain.* 1996; **66**: 105–08.

112. Thompson SW, Bennett DL, Kerr BJ *et al.* Brain-derived neurotrophic factor is an endogenous modulator of nociceptive responses in the spinal cord. *Proceedings of the National Academy of Sciences of the United States of America.* 1999; **96**: 7714–18.

*113. Woolf CJ, Salter MW. Neuronal plasticity: increasing the gain in pain. *Science.* 2000; **288**: 1765–9.

114. Kawamata M, Omote K. Involvement of increased excitatory amino acids and intracellular Ca^{2+} concentration in the spinal dorsal horn in an animal model of neuropathic pain. *Pain.* 1996; **68**: 85–96.

115. Hua XY, Chen P, Yaksh TL. Inhibition of spinal protein kinase C reduces nerve injury-induced tactile allodynia in neuropathic rats. *Neuroscience Letters.* 1999; **276**: 99–102.

116. Malmberg AB, Brandon EP, Idzerda RL *et al.* Diminished inflammation and nociceptive pain with preservation of neuropathic pain in mice with a targeted mutation of the type I regulatory subunit of cAMP-dependent protein kinase. *Journal of Neuroscience.* 1997; **17**: 7462–70.

117. Wei F, Qiu CS, Kim SJ *et al.* Genetic elimination of behavioral sensitization in mice lacking calmodulin-stimulated adenylyl cyclases. *Neuron.* 2002; **36**: 713–26.

118. Honor P, Menning PM, Rogers SD *et al.* Spinal substance P receptor expression and internalization in acute, short-term, and long-term inflammatory pain states. *Journal of Neuroscience.* 1999; **19**: 7670–8.

119. Mantyh PW, Rogers SD, Honore P *et al.* Inhibition of hyperalgesia by ablation of lamina I spinal neurons expressing the substance P receptor. *Science.* 1997; **278**: 275–9.

120. Koltzenburg M, Lundberg LE, Torebjork HE. Dynamic and static components of mechanical hyperalgesia in human hairy skin. *Pain.* 1992; **51**: 207–19.

121. Kerr BJ, Bradbury EJ, Bennett DL *et al.* Brain-derived neurotrophic factor modulates nociceptive sensory inputs and NMDA-evoked responses in the rat spinal cord. *Journal of Neuroscience.* 1999; **19**: 5138–48.

122. Mannion RJ, Costigan M, Decosterd I *et al.* Neurotrophins: peripherally and centrally acting modulators of tactile stimulus-induced inflammatory pain hypersensitivity. *Proceedings of the National Academy of Sciences of the United States of America.* 1999; **96**: 9385–90.

*123. Watkins LR, Milligan ED, Maier SF. Glial activation: a driving force for pathological pain. *Trends in Neuroscience.* 2001; **24**: 450–5.

124. Davar G, Hama A, Deykin A *et al.* MK-801 blocks the development of thermal hyperalgesia in a rat model of experimental painful neuropathy. *Brain Research.* 1991; **553**: 327–30.

125. Sotgiu ML, Biella G. Differential effects of MK-801, a *N*-methyl-D-aspartate non-competitive antagonist, on the dorsal horn neuron hyperactivity and hyperexcitability in neuropathic rats. *Neuroscience Letters.* 2000; **283**: 153–6.

126. Corsi M, Fina P, Trist DG. Co-agonism in drug-receptor interaction: illustrated by the NMDA receptors. *Trends in Pharmacological Sciences.* 1996; **17**: 220–2.

127. Quartaroli M, Carignani C, Dal Forno G *et al.* Potent antihyperalgesic activity without tolerance produced by glycine site antagonist of *N*-methyl-D-aspartate receptor GV196771A. *Journal of Pharmacology and Experimental Therapeutics.* 1999; **290**: 158–69.

128. Christensen D, Kayser V. The development of pain-related behaviour and opioid tolerance after neuropathy-inducing surgery and sham surgery. *Pain.* 2000; **88**: 231–8.

129. Sivilotti L, Woolf CJ. The contribution of GABAA and glycine receptors to central sensitization: disinhibition and touch-evoked allodynia in the spinal cord. *Journal of Neurophysiology.* 1994; **72**: 169–79.

130. Malan TP, Mata HP, Porreca F. Spinal GABA(A) and GABA(B) receptor pharmacology in a rat model of neuropathic pain. *Anesthesiology.* 2002; **96**: 1161–7.

*131. Moore KA, Kohno T, Karchewski LA *et al.* Partial peripheral nerve injury promotes a selective loss of GABAergic inhibition in the superficial dorsal horn of the spinal cord. *Journal of Neuroscience*. 2002; **22**: 6724–31.

132. Stiller CO, Cui JG, O'Connor WT *et al.* Release of gamma-aminobutyric acid in the dorsal horn and suppression of tactile allodynia by spinal cord stimulation in mononeuropathic rats. *Neurosurgery*. 1996; **39**: 367–74.

133. Castro-Lopes JM, Malcangio M, Pan BH, Bowery NG. Complex changes of GABAA and GABAB receptor binding in the spinal cord dorsal horn following peripheral inflammation or neurectomy. *Brain Research*. 1995; **679**: 289–97.

134. Scholz J, Broom DC, Youn DH *et al.* Blocking caspase activity prevents transsynaptic neuronal apoptosis and the loss of inhibition in lamina II of the dorsal horn after peripheral nerve injury. *Journal of Neuroscience*. 2005; **25**: 7317–23.

*135. Ruscheweyh R, Sandkuhler J. Long-range oscillatory Ca^{2+} waves in rat spinal dorsal horn. *European Journal of Neuroscience*. 2005; **22**: 1967–76.

136. Woolf CJ. Dissecting out mechanisms responsible for peripheral neuropathic pain: implications for diagnosis and therapy. *Life Science*. 2004; **74**: 2605–10.

137. Zhang X, Bao L, Shi TJ *et al.* Down-regulation of mu-opioid receptors in rat and monkey dorsal root ganglion neurons and spinal cord after peripheral axotomy. *Neuroscience*. 1998; **82**: 223–40.

138. Besse D, Lombard MC, Besson JM. Autoradiographic distribution of mu, delta and kappa opioid binding sites in the superficial dorsal horn, over the rostrocaudal axis of the rat spinal cord. *Brain Research*. 1991; **548**: 287–91.

139. Besse D, Lombard MC, Perrot S, Besson JM. Regulation of opioid binding sites in the superficial dorsal horn of the rat spinal cord following loose ligation of the sciatic nerve: comparison with sciatic nerve section and lumbar dorsal rhizotomy. *Neuroscience*. 1992; **50**: 921–33.

140. Xu XJ, Puke MJ, Verge VM *et al.* Up-regulation of cholecystokinin in primary sensory neurons is associated with morphine insensitivity in experimental neuropathic pain in the rat. *Neuroscience Letters*. 1993; **152**: 129–32.

141. Kovelowski CJ, Ossipov MH, Sun H *et al.* Supraspinal cholecystokinin may drive tonic descending facilitation mechanisms to maintain neuropathic pain in the rat. *Pain*. 2000; **87**: 265–73.

*142. Rashid MH, Inoue M, Toda K, Ueda H. Loss of peripheral morphine analgesia contributes to the reduced effectiveness of systemic morphine in neuropathic pain. *Journal of Pharmacology and Experimental Therapeutics*. 2004; **309**: 380–7.

143. Farquhar-Smith WP, Egertova M, Bradbury EJ *et al.* Cannabinoid CB(1) receptor expression in rat spinal cord. *Molecular and Cellular Neurosciences*. 2000; **15**: 510–21.

144. Herzberg U, Eliav E, Bennett GJ, Kopin IJ. The analgesic effects of R(+)-WIN 55,212-2 mesylate, a high affinity cannabinoid agonist, in a rat model of neuropathic pain. *Neuroscience Letters*. 1997; **221**: 157–60.

145. Wallace VC, Cottrell DF, Brophy PJ, Fleetwood-Walker SM. Focal lysolecithin-induced demyelination of peripheral afferents results in neuropathic pain behavior that is attenuated by cannabinoids. *Journal of Neuroscience*. 2003; **23**: 3221–33.

146. Campbell JN, Raja SN, Meyer RA, Mackinnon SE. Myelinated afferents signal the hyperalgesia associated with nerve injury. *Pain*. 1988; **32**: 89–94.

147. Koerber HR, Mirnics K, Brown PB, Mendell LM. Central sprouting and functional plasticity of regenerated primary afferents. *Journal of Neuroscience*. 1994; **14**: 3655–71.

*148. Woolf CJ, Shortland P, Coggeshall RE. Peripheral nerve injury triggers central sprouting of myelinated afferents. *Nature*. 1992; **355**: 75–8.

149. Bennett DL, French J, Priestley JV, McMahon SB. NGF but not NT-3 or BDNF prevents the A fiber sprouting into lamina II of the spinal cord that occurs following axotomy. *Molecular and Cellular Neurosciences*. 1996; **8**: 211–20.

150. Hughes DI, Scott DT, Todd AJ, Riddell JS. Lack of evidence for sprouting of Abeta afferents into the superficial laminas of the spinal cord dorsal horn after nerve section. *Journal of Neuroscience*. 2003; **23**: 9491–9.

*151. Tong YG, Wang HF, Ju G *et al.* Increased uptake and transport of cholera toxin B-subunit in dorsal root ganglion neurons after peripheral axotomy: possible implications for sensory sprouting. *Journal of Comparative Neurology*. 1999; **404**: 143–58.

152. Okamoto M, Baba H, Goldstein PA *et al.* Functional reorganization of sensory pathways in the rat spinal dorsal horn following peripheral nerve injury. *Journal of Physiology*. 2001; **532**: 241–50.

153. Bester H, Beggs S, Woolf CJ. Changes in tactile stimuli-induced behavior and c-Fos expression in the superficial dorsal horn and in parabrachial nuclei after sciatic nerve crush. *Journal of Comparative Neurology*. 2000; **428**: 45–61.

154. Gehrmann J, Matsumoto Y, Kreutzberg GW. Microglia: intrinsic immuneffector cell of the brain. *Brain Research. Brain Research Reviews*. 1995; **20**: 269–87.

155. Stoll G, Jander S. The role of microglia and macrophages in the pathophysiology of the CNS. *Progress in Neurobiology*. 1999; **58**: 233–47.

156. Raghavendra V, Tanga FY, DeLeo JA. Complete Freunds adjuvant-induced peripheral inflammation evokes glial activation and proinflammatory cytokine expression in the CNS. *European Journal of Neuroscience*. 2004; **20**: 467–73.

157. Tsuda M, Mizokoshi A, Shigemoto-Mogami Y *et al.* Activation of p38 mitogen-activated protein kinase in spinal hyperactive microglia contributes to pain hypersensitivity following peripheral nerve injury. *Glia*. 2004; **45**: 89–95.

*158. Coull JA, Beggs S, Boudreau D *et al.* BDNF from microglia causes the shift in neuronal anion gradient underlying neuropathic pain. *Nature*. 2005; **438**: 1017–21.

159. Ledeboer A, Sloane EM, Milligan ED *et al.* Minocycline attenuates mechanical allodynia and proinflammatory

cytokine expression in rat models of pain facilitation. *Pain.* 2005; **115**: 71–83.

160. Raghavendra V, Tanga F, DeLeo JA. Inhibition of microglial activation attenuates the development but not existing hypersensitivity in a rat model of neuropathy. *Journal of Pharmacology and Experimental Therapeutics.* 2003; **306**: 624–30.

161. Kalla R, Liu Z, Xu S *et al.* Microglia and the early phase of immune surveillance in the axotomized facial motor nucleus: impaired microglial activation and lymphocyte recruitment but no effect on neuronal survival or axonal regeneration in macrophage-colony stimulating factor-deficient mice. *Journal of Comparative Neurology.* 2001; **436**: 182–201.

162. Klein MA, Moller JC, Jones LL *et al.* Impaired neuroglial activation in interleukin-6 deficient mice. *Glia.* 1997; **19**: 227–33.

163. Milligan ED, Zapata V, Chacur M *et al.* Evidence that exogenous and endogenous fractalkine can induce spinal nociceptive facilitation in rats. *European Journal of Neuroscience.* 2004; **20**: 2294–302.

164. Zhang J, Koninck Y. Spatial and temporal relationship between monocyte chemoattractant protein-1 expression and spinal glial activation following peripheral nerve injury. *Journal of Neurochemistry.* 2006; **97**: 772–83.

165. Tsuda M, Shigemoto-Mogami Y, Koizumi S *et al.* P2 × 4 receptors induced in spinal microglia gate tactile allodynia after nerve injury. *Nature.* 2003; **424**: 778–83.

166. Le Feuvre RA, Brough D, Iwakura Y *et al.* Priming of macrophages with lipopolysaccharide potentiates P2 × 7-mediated cell death via a caspase-1-dependent mechanism, independently of cytokine production. *Journal of Biological Chemistry.* 2002; **277**: 3210–8.

167. Walter L, Franklin A, Witting A *et al.* Nonpsychotropic cannabinoid receptors regulate microglial cell migration. *Journal of Neuroscience.* 2003; **23**: 1398–405.

168. Cravatt BF, Lichtman AH. The endogenous cannabinoid system and its role in nociceptive behavior. *Journal of Neurobiology.* 2004; **61**: 149–60.

169. Malan Jr TP, Ibrahim MM, Lai J *et al.* CB2 cannabinoid receptor agonists: pain relief without psychoactive effects? *Current Opinion in Pharmacology.* 2003; **3**: 62–7.

170. Ibrahim MM, Deng H, Zvonok A *et al.* Activation of CB2 cannabinoid receptors by AM1241 inhibits experimental neuropathic pain: pain inhibition by receptors not present in the CNS. *Proceedings of the National Academy of Sciences of the United States of America.* 2003; **100**: 10529–33.

171. Jin SX, Zhuang ZY, Woolf CJ, Ji RR. p38 mitogen-activated protein kinase is activated after a spinal nerve ligation in spinal cord microglia and dorsal root ganglion neurons and contributes to the generation of neuropathic pain. *Journal of Neuroscience.* 2003; **23**: 4017–22.

*172. Zhuang ZY, Gerner P, Woolf CJ, Ji RR. ERK is sequentially activated in neurons, microglia, and astrocytes by spinal nerve ligation and contributes to mechanical allodynia in this neuropathic pain model. *Pain.* 2005; **114**: 149–59.

*173. Ossipov MH, Lai J, Malan Jr TP, Porreca F. Spinal and supraspinal mechanisms of neuropathic pain. *Annals of the New York Academy of Sciences.* 2000; **909**: 12–24.

*174. Suzuki R, Dickenson A. Spinal and supraspinal contributions to central sensitization in peripheral neuropathy. *Neurosignals.* 2005; **14**: 175–81.

175. Fields HL, Heinricher MM, Mason P. Neurotransmitters in nociceptive modulatory circuits. *Annual Review of Neuroscience.* 1991; **14**: 219–45.

176. Bandler R, Keay KA. Columnar organization in the midbrain periaqueductal gray and the integration of emotional expression. *Progress in Brain Research.* 1996; **107**: 285–300.

177. Millan MJ. Descending control of pain. *Progress in Neurobiology.* 2002; **66**: 355–474.

178. Zhuo M, Gebhart GF. Biphasic modulation of spinal nociceptive transmission from the medullary raphe nuclei in the rat. *Journal of Neurophysiology.* 1997; **78**: 746–58.

*179. Fields HL, Malick A, Burstein R. Dorsal horn projection targets of ON and OFF cells in the rostral ventromedial medulla. *Journal of Neurophysiology.* 1995; **74**: 1742–59.

180. Burgess SE, Gardell LR, Ossipov MH *et al.* Time-dependent descending facilitation from the rostral ventromedial medulla maintains, but does not initiate, neuropathic pain. *Journal of Neuroscience.* 2002; **22**: 5129–36.

181. Monassi CR, Bandler R, Keay KA. A subpopulation of rats show social and sleep-waking changes typical of chronic neuropathic pain following peripheral nerve injury. *European Journal of Neuroscience.* 2003; **17**: 1907–20.

*182. Porreca F, Ossipov MH, Gebhart GF. Chronic pain and medullary descending facilitation. *Trends in Neuroscience.* 2002; **25**: 319–25.

183. Heinricher MM, McGaraughty S, Tortorici V. Circuitry underlying antiopioid actions of cholecystokinin within the rostral ventromedial medulla. *Journal of Neurophysiology.* 2001; **85**: 280–6.

184. Le Bars D. Neuronal serotonin. In: Osborne NMHM (ed.). *Serotonin and pain.* New York: John Wiley, 1988: 171–226.

185. Rahman W, Suzuki R, Webber M *et al.* Depletion of endogenous spinal 5-HT attenuates the behavioural hypersensitivity to mechanical and cooling stimuli induced by spinal nerve ligation. *Pain.* 2006; **123**: 264–74.

186. Zeitz KP, Guy N, Malmberg AB *et al.* The 5-HT3 subtype of serotonin receptor contributes to nociceptive processing via a novel subset of myelinated and unmyelinated nociceptors. *Journal of Neuroscience.* 2002; **22**: 1010–19.

187. Suzuki R, Rahman W, Hunt SP, Dickenson AH. Descending facilitatory control of mechanically evoked responses is enhanced in deep dorsal horn neurones following peripheral nerve injury. *Brain Research.* 2004; **1019**: 68–76.

188. McCleane GJ, Suzuki R, Dickenson AH. Does a single intravenous injection of the 5HT3 receptor antagonist ondansetron have an analgesic effect in neuropathic pain? A double-blinded, placebo-controlled cross-over study. *Anesthesia and Analgesia.* 2003; **97**: 1474–8.

189. Fields HL, Basbaum AI, Heinricher MM. Central nervous system mechanisms of pain modulation. In: Koltzenburg M, McMahon SB (eds). *Melzack and Wall's textbook of pain.* London: Elsevier, 2005: 125–42.
190. Meng ID, Manning BH, Martin WJ, Fields HL. An analgesia circuit activated by cannabinoids. *Nature.* 1998; **395**: 381–3.
191. Ingvar M. Pain and functional imaging. *Philosophical Transactions of the Royal Society of London. Series B, Biological Sciences.* 1999; **354**: 1347–58.
*192. Brooks J, Tracey I. From nociception to pain perception: imaging the spinal and supraspinal pathways. *Journal of Anatomy.* 2005; **207**: 19–33.
193. Peyron R, Garcia-Larrea L, Gregoire MC *et al.* Parietal and cingulate processes in central pain. A combined positron emission tomography (PET) and functional magnetic resonance imaging (fMRI) study of an unusual case. *Pain.* 2000; **84**: 77–87.
194. Witting N, Kupers RC, Svensson P *et al.* Experimental brush-evoked allodynia activates posterior parietal cortex. *Neurology.* 2001; **57**: 1817–24.
195. Lorenz J, Cross D, Minoshima S *et al.* A unique representation of heat allodynia in the human brain. *Neuron.* 2002; **35**: 383–93.
196. Iadarola MJ, Berman KF, Zeffiro TA *et al.* Neural activation during acute capsaicin-evoked pain and allodynia assessed with PET. *Brain.* 1998; **121**: 931–47.
197. Peyron R, Schneider F, Faillenot I *et al.* An fMRI study of cortical representation of mechanical allodynia in patients with neuropathic pain. *Neurology.* 2004; **63**: 1838–46.
198. Petrovic P, Ingvar M, Stone-Elander S *et al.* A PET activation study of dynamic mechanical allodynia in patients with mononeuropathy. *Pain.* 1999; **83**: 459–70.
199. Baron R, Baron Y, Disbrow E, Roberts TP. Activation of the somatosensory cortex during Abeta-fiber mediated hyperalgesia. A MSI study. *Brain Research.* 2000; **871**: 75–82.
200. LeDoux JE. Emotion circuits in the brain. *Annual Review of Neuroscience.* 2000; **23**: 155–84.
201. Stam R, Ekkelenkamp K, Frankhuijzen AC *et al.* Long-lasting changes in central nervous system responsivity to colonic distention after stress in rats. *Gastroenterology.* 2002; **123**: 1216–25.
202. Tanimoto S, Nakagawa T, Yamauchi Y *et al.* Differential contributions of the basolateral and central nuclei of the amygdala in the negative affective component of chemical somatic and visceral pains in rats. *European Journal of Neuroscience.* 2003; **18**: 2343–50.
203. Pedersen LH, Scheel-Kruger J, Blackburn-Munro G. Amygdala GABA-A receptor involvement in mediating sensory-discriminative and affective-motivational pain responses in a rat model of peripheral nerve injury. *Pain.* 2006; **127**: 17–26.
204. Geha PY, Baliki MN, Chialvo DR *et al.* Brain activity for spontaneous pain of postherpetic neuralgia and its modulation by lidocaine patch therapy. *Pain.* 2006; **128**: 88–100.
*205. Tegeder I, Costigan M, Griffin RS *et al.* GTP cyclohydrolase and tetrahydrobiopterin regulate pain sensitivity and persistence. *Nature Medicine.* 2006; **12**: 1269–77.
*206. Mogil JS, Grisel JE. Transgenic studies of pain. *Pain.* 1998; **77**: 107–28.

2

Applied physiology: persistent musculoskeletal pain

HANS-GEORG SCHAIBLE

KEY LEARNING POINTS

- In normal joint and muscle, pain is only elicited by intense tissue-threatening (noxious) stimuli. Inflammation and other deep tissue pathologies cause a state of hyperalgesia and pain that often becomes chronic. Under these conditions, pain is elicited by physiological stimuli.
- Muscle and joint nerves possess nociceptors which are exclusively or preferentially excited by noxious stimuli, and silent nociceptors which do not respond to stimuli under normal conditions.
- During pathological processes, such as inflammation muscle and joint nociceptors, are sensitized to mechanical stimuli. This peripheral sensitization is an important mechanism of primary hyperalgesia.
- Peripheral sensitization is induced and maintained by inflammatory mediators acting on the nociceptive terminals, and by changes of the intrinsic response properties of the neurons.
- In the central nervous system, nociceptive stimulation of deep tissue is encoded in neurons exclusively driven by deep input, and by neurons that show convergent inputs from deep tissue and skin.
- Peripheral sensitization induces a state of hyperexcitability in the central nociceptive system (central sensitization) that increases the gain of central nociceptive processing at spinal, thalamic, and cortical levels. Spinal hyperexcitability contributes to primary and accounts for secondary hyperalgesia.
- Descending systems control the nociceptive processing at the spinal level. During peripheral inflammation descending inhibition increases and reduces central sensitization. Descending facilitation may support secondary hyperalgesia.
- Pain treatment should target peripheral, as well as central, sensitization.

PAIN IN THE MUSCULOSKELETAL SYSTEM

Pain in the musculoskeletal system is of major clinical importance because it is frequent and often chronic. In general, the deep somatic tissue is a major site of injury (e.g. sport injuries), acute and chronic inflammatory processes (e.g. rheumatoid arthritis), and degenerative disease (e.g. osteoarthritis, osteoporosis). Because many of the pathological changes in the musculoskeletal system are not reversible, symptomatic pain treatment is one of the most important tasks in clinical medicine. It should limit suffering and maintain the ability to use the motor system properly.

Pain sensation in muscle and joint

The major sensation from deep tissue, such as joint and muscle, is pain. In the absence of disease, we are not aware of sensory processes in the deep tissue. However, sensory information from muscle and joint continuously controls the activity of the motor system and is involved in the sense of movement and position.[1] Pain significantly influences the motor control system and usually forces the patient to restrict movements.

Deep tissue pain is often dull and aching, and poorly localized, and is thus different from cutaneous pain which may be sharp and precisely localized.[2] In particular, muscle pain is often aching and cramping and often referred to other deep tissue, such as other muscles, tendon, fascia, joint, and ligaments.[3] In the normal deep tissue, acute and short-lasting pain sensations can be elicited by tissue-threatening mechanical stimuli, showing the excitation of nociceptors in deep tissue structures (see below under Nociceptors of deep tissue and peripheral sensitization). Clinically relevant pain in deep tissue is different. It usually appears as hyperalgesia or persistent pain at rest.[2, 4, 5, 6] In the state of hyperalgesia, noxious stimuli cause stronger pain than normal, and pain is even evoked by mechanical stimuli whose intensity does not normally elicit pain, i.e. movements in the working range and gentle pressure, e.g. during palpation. Clinically relevant muscle pain often appears as a combination of ongoing muscle pain, tenderness, soreness (tenderness and stiffness), weakness, and paresthesias (sensation of pressure and tension) in the muscle.[7, 8]

Some decades ago and again more recently, in order to gain more insight into the nature and origin of deep tissue pain, experimental invasive sensory testing was carried out in conscious humans. For example, pain in the normal joint can be elicited when noxious mechanical and chemical stimuli are directly applied to the fibrous structures, such as ligaments and fibrous capsule. No pain is elicited by stimulation of cartilage and stimulation of normal synovial tissue rarely evokes pain.[5] Stimulation of fibrous structures with innocuous mechanical stimulation can evoke pressure sensations.[5] In the muscle, pain can be elicited by noxious mechanical stimulation and also by high intensity thermal stimulation (48°C).[9] Collectively these data show good correlation between the impact of noxious stimuli and the evoked pain sensations at least in the normal deep tissue. Accordingly, recordings from deep tissue afferents have revealed that deep tissue nociceptors reliably encode noxious stimuli.

Differences between cutaneous and deep tissue pain sensations have been pointed out. In addition to differences in pain sensation, autonomic responses to noxious stimuli can be different. In contrast to cutaneous pain, muscle pain typically elicits a drop in blood pressure, as well as sweating and nausea.[10]

Causes of clinically relevant pain in deep tissue

Considerations on clinically relevant pain in the deep tissues include several questions: (1) Which pathological processes cause pain? (2) From which structures is pain evoked? This is being particularly discussed for osteoarthritic pain. (3) Does pain reflect nociception and how much is it associated with psychological and social factors? This seems to be extremely relevant for the large number of patients with low back pain.

In general, inflammatory conditions cause similar pain symptoms in all somatic deep tissues, namely hyperalgesia with increased responses to noxious stimuli and occurrence of pain upon innocuous mechanical stimulation. Inflammatory conditions are frequent in joints and often chronic, such as during rheumatoid arthritis. Initially, the synovial tissue and the articular and periarticular soft tissues are the most important sites of inflammation, but with time the joint undergoes structural changes, such as cartilage degradation, pannus formation, and bone deformation. Presumably all of these changes may contribute to pain generation, and mechanical as well as inflammatory factors may contribute to the activation of the nociceptive system.

Pain during degenerative osteoarthritis (OA) shows similarities and differences to inflammatory arthritic pain. Osteoarthritic pain is usually localized to the joint with OA, but it can be referred (e.g. hip OA may cause knee pain). It varies in intensity and is usually worsened by exercise (weight-bearing, movement) and relieved at rest. It is usually episodic, but may be constantly present in advanced OA. A particular quality of OA pain is pain at night.[11] The site of OA pain and the nature of OA pain are under discussion because the cartilage is not innervated[12] and because there is a poor correlation between radiological signs (narrow joint space and osteophytes) and the occurrence of joint pain.[11] Some recent studies used magnetic resonance (MR) imaging and found that painful OA knee joints exhibit more MR abnormalities than nonpainful OA joints. These are synovial hypertrophy and synovial effusions, as well as subchondral bone marrow edema lesions (which may increase intraosseal pressure).[13] These data and the observation of inflammatory cells in the sublining tissue[11] suggest that pain may be evoked by inflammatory mechanisms that appear from time to time (possibly corresponding to painful episodes in chronic OA). At later stages, capsular fibrosis and muscle contracture around the joint may contribute to OA pain. Quite clearly, however, factors such as obesity, perceived helplessness, and other psychological factors influence OA pain as well.[11]

Specific causes of muscle pain are acute trauma (tear and blow), overload (e.g. exercise, particularly eccentric contraction), and myositis. Muscle pain is also elicited by ischemic contractions and by muscle spasm. A particular muscle pain syndrome is the referred pain elicited from painful trigger points in the muscle. Pain syndromes involving muscular pain are fibromyalgia and the myofascial pain syndrome, but in these cases no clear muscle pathophysiology has been established. On the other hand, significant muscular diseases, such as slow cell death in muscle during muscle dystrophy do not cause pain.[10, 11]

Another site of clinically relevant pain in deep tissue is the bone. Frequent causes of bone pain are trauma, fracture, and also degenerative disorders, such as osteoporosis and bone metastases.[14, 15] Research into neuronal mechanisms of bone pain has been very sporadic. However, recent studies on cancer pain have focused on mechanisms of bone pain,[14] and the bone near the joint may be one site at which osteoarthritic pain is generated, as mentioned above.[11, 13]

INNERVATION OF JOINT, MUSCLE, AND BONE

Joints are supplied by branches descending from main nerve trunks or their muscular, cutaneous, and periosteal branches. A typical joint nerve contains thick myelinated Aβ- (group II), thinly myelinated Aδ- (group III), and a high proportion (~80 percent) of unmyelinated C- (group IV) fibers. The latter are either sensory afferents or sympathetic efferents (each ~50 percent).[12] Aβ fibers terminate as corpuscular endings of the Ruffini-, Golgi-, and Pacini-type in fibrous capsule, articular ligaments, menisci, and adjacent periosteum.[1] Articular Aδ- and C-fibers terminate as noncorpuscular or free nerve endings in the fibrous capsule, adipose tissue, ligaments, menisci, and the periosteum.[16] Using staining for nerve fibers and neuropeptides, endings were also identified in the synovial layer. The cartilage is not innervated.[12]

Muscle nerves contain axons from motoneurons, sensory neurons, and postganglionic sympathetic neurons. For example, in the nerve of cat gastrocnemius-soleus (GS) muscle, about one-third of the axons are myelinated (~60 percent of these are from motoneurons and ~40 percent are sensory) and two-thirds of the fibers are unmyelinated. In the latter group, ~50 percent of the units are sensory and ~50 percent are sympathetic efferent. Thick myelinated afferents terminate as organized endings (muscle spindles, tendon organs), whereas Aδ- and C-fibers terminate as free nerve endings. Most of these endings are located in the wall of arterioles in the muscle belly and in the surrounding connective tissue.[7]

A large proportion of articular and muscular sensory neurons are peptidergic. The major neuropeptides in joint and muscle nerves are substance P, calcitonin gene-related peptide (CGRP), and somatostatin. Neurokinin A, galanin, enkephalins, and neuropeptide Y have also been localized in joint afferents. Neuropeptides influence the inflammatory process in the periphery and modify spinal processing of joint and muscle input. They may also act on the primary afferent neurons themselves (see below under Molecular mechanisms of peripheral sensitization). However, these neuropeptides are not specific for deep afferents.[7, 12]

ACTIVATION OF THE NOCICEPTIVE SYSTEM BY NOXIOUS DEEP TISSUE STIMULATION UNDER NORMAL AND INFLAMMATORY CONDITONS

Nociceptors of the deep somatic tissue encode noxious stimuli applied to the normal tissue. This is important for the protection of the tissue against damage. Noxious stimuli, such as twisting of a joint, cause immediate motor responses and a conscious pain experience both of which are parts of a strategy to avoid further damage. It is thought that loss of sensory mechanisms causes damage of the joint such as in Charcot's joint. Essentially, treatment of joint pain should not impair the normal nociceptive function.

Importantly, significant changes of the nociceptive processing are induced by inflammation and tissue injury which are called peripheral sensitization (sensitization of primary afferents) and central sensitization (development of hyperexcitability of nociceptive neurons in the central nervous system). **Figure 2.1** summarizes the structures of the nociceptive system and the sequence of inflammation-evoked events in the nociceptive system. Inflammation leads to peripheral sensitization which in turn causes the development of hyperexcitability in the spinal cord.[7, 12] Ascending axons in the spinothalamic tract activate the lateral and medial thalamocortical system which evoke the conscious pain sensation with its sensory discriminative and the affective components.[17] In parallel, ascending projections to the brainstem are activated. The activation of the brainstem contributes to the activation of the brain by noxious stimuli, but it also acts back on the spinal cord through descending systems.[18, 19, 20]

NOCICEPTORS OF DEEP TISSUE AND PERIPHERAL SENSITIZATION

Mechanosensitivity of peripheral nociceptors in the normal joint and muscle

In single-fiber recordings, primary afferent neurons have been classified according to their mechanosensitivity. These recordings showed types of primary afferent neurons that encode noxious stimuli applied to joint and muscle and are thus suitable for signaling noxious

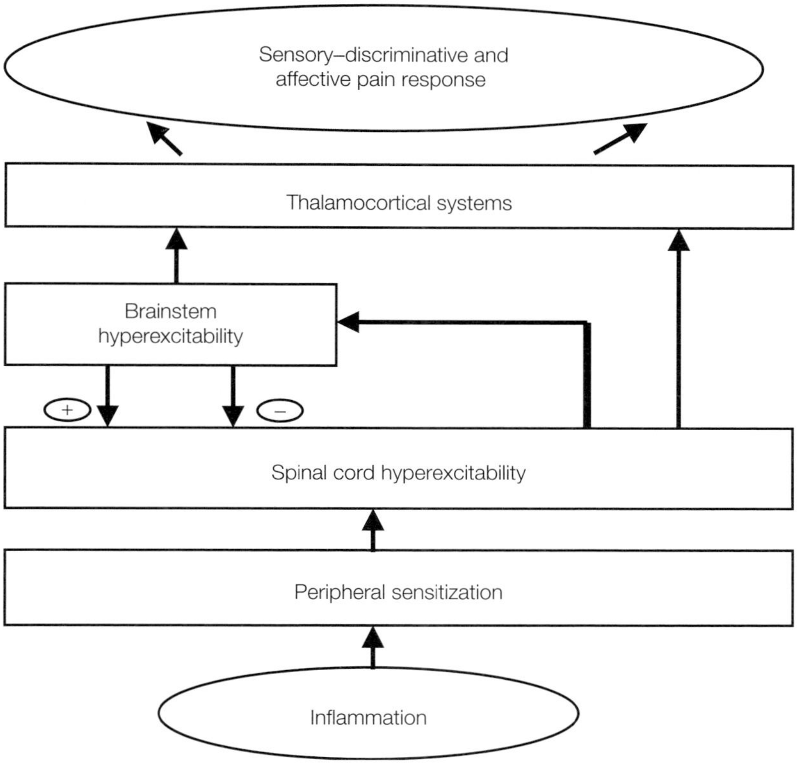

Figure 2.1 Sequence of neuronal events induced by inflammation in deep tissue.

mechanical events which cause pain sensations in awake individuals.

In the joint nerve, more than 50 percent of the Aδ-fibers and most C-fibers with a detectable receptive field are able to encode noxious mechanical stimuli applied to the joint. These fibers are either weakly activated by innocuous stimuli and strongly activated by noxious stimuli, or they are exclusively activated by noxious stimuli.[21, 22] Innocuous stimuli are light to moderate pressure and movements within the normal working range of the joint. Noxious stimuli are high-intensity pressure (that causes pain when applied to humans) and movements against the resistance of the tissue beyond the limit of the normal working range. Fibers activated by these noxious mechanical stimuli are thought to be the nociceptors which cause pain upon twisting the normal joint against the resistance of the tissue. Some Aδ-fibers and a significant proportion of C-fibers do not respond to any mechanical stimulus applied to the normal joint. These fibers are "initially mechanoinsensitive" or "silent nociceptors" that are only activated during inflammation (see below under Changes of mechanosensitivity during inflammation (peripheral sensitization)).[23, 24, 25] In contrast, most Aβ-fibers and about half of the Aδ-fibers are low threshold units that are strongly activated by innocuous pressure, such as light pressure and movements in the working range.[26, 27] Their responses to innocuous stimuli might be used to control movements and to prevent unphysiological movements. Although these units may show their highest discharge rate upon noxious stimuli, they do not discriminate between innocuous and noxious stimuli. In fact, the most adequate innocuous mechanical stimulus can evoke a stronger response than a noxious mechanical stimulus, e.g. a noxious movement into another direction.[26, 27]

In the muscle nerve, numerous sensory Aδ- and C-fibers are only activated by noxious mechanical stimuli. These muscle nociceptors do not respond to everyday stimuli, such as weak local pressure, contractions, and muscle stretch within the physiological range. They require potentially noxious stimuli to be readily activated, and the best stimulus is noxious squeezing of the muscle belly or tendon at intensities that elicit pain in humans. Nociceptors may also respond to unphysiological stretch and maximal contraction. The threshold of a nociceptor may lay below frankly tissue-damaging intensities (small response to moderate pressure). Similar units have been found in the cat, dog, rat, and humans.[28, 29, 30, 31, 32, 33] Electrical stimulation of such nerve fibers in human muscle nerves evokes cramp-like sensations. Electrical stimulation frequencies of 5–6 Hz are required to elicit pain sensations.[34] Why such high frequencies are needed is unknown. It may be speculated that a small number of muscle afferents drive spinal cord neurons only during temporal facilitation, either because they form fewer synapses on neurons than cutaneous afferents or because descending inhibition of nociceptive spinal cord neurons is stronger for deep input than for cutaneous input (see below under Descending influences on spinal neurons with deep input).

Only a proportion of the sensory units with free nerve endings in muscle nerves are nociceptors. Other slowly conducting units are more sensitive and respond strongly to physiological stimuli, such as stretch and contraction. These low threshold units are considered to be ergoreceptors. Presumably they are important for respiratory and circulatory adjustments during physical exercise.[7] In addition, as in the joint nerve, some units are mechanoinsensitive and may thus be silent nociceptors, because they respond to intra-arterial injection of bradykinin into the muscle.

Changes of mechanosensitivity during inflammation (peripheral sensitization)

An inflamed joint hurts during movements in the working range and during palpation, and pain may occur under resting conditions. An inflamed muscle exhibits tenderness. An important mechanism for the heightened pain sensitivity is an increase of mechanosensitivity in afferent fibers supplying inflamed tissue. During development of inflammation in the joint, some low threshold Aβ-fibers show transiently increased responses to joint movements in the initial hours of inflammation. They do not develop resting discharges. Importantly, the majority of Aδ- and C-fibers show increased mechanosensitivity. Many low threshold Aδ- and C-fibers show increased responses to movements in the working range and to noxious movements. Most strikingly, a large proportion of high threshold afferents are sensitized such that they begin to respond to movements in the working range of the joint. The units may develop ongoing discharges in the resting position.[23, 24, 25] Increased mechanosensitivity has also been found during chronic forms of arthritis, suggesting that mechanical sensitization is an important neuronal basis for chronic persistent hyperalgesia of the inflamed joint.[35]

Furthermore, initially mechanoinsensitive afferents (silent nociceptors) are sensitized and become mechanosensitive.[23, 24, 25] While these fibers are not activated even by noxious mechanical stimulation of the normal joint, they can develop mechanosensitivity within one to four hours after onset of inflammation. Then they show responses to movements of the joint, even to innocuous ones, and one can identify a receptive field upon mechanical stimulation of the inflamed tissue. Thus, during inflammation, there is a recruitment of further nociceptive sensory neurons for signaling of noxious events. Silent nociceptors have also been identified in cutaneous nerves in humans and in visceral nerves.[36, 37, 38] In particular, studies in skin nerves of humans have shown that silent nociceptors are particularly important for neurogenic inflammation and for the induction of central sensitization.[39, 40]

In muscle nerve, inflammation enhances the proportion of Aδ-fibers showing resting discharges, as well as the discharge rate in spontaneously active fibers. It is likely that these changes produce spontaneous pain and dysesthesias of the inflamed muscle. In addition, mechanical threshold significantly drops in numerous sensory C-fibers.[41] Thus, similar processes are seen as in afferent fibers of the joint. In addition, in the muscle, ischemic conditions may play an important role in pain generation. Interruption of blood supply to a resting muscle is not painful unless it lasts for long periods of time. Indeed, ligation of arteries to the muscle does not activate Aδ- and C-fibers within the first five minutes.[42] Long-lasting complete interruption of blood supply may cause resting discharges in muscle afferents within 15–60 minutes followed by a block of action potential generation or conduction.[7] However, if the muscle is forced to contract under ischemic conditions, severe pain develops rapidly. During ischemia, a small percentage of sensory C-fibers respond to contraction, although these units do not or only minimally respond to contraction when the blood supply is intact.[42, 43]

Molecular mechanisms of peripheral sensitization

Primary afferent neurons are equipped with numerous ion channels and receptors for mediators. Stimuli applied to the sensory endings open ion channels, and the resulting ion currents depolarize the endings. The generation of this receptor potential is called transduction. When the depolarization reaches a certain threshold, voltage-gated ion channels are opened that generate action potentials which are conducted along the axon to the spinal cord. The generation of the action potential is called transformation. Thus, the responsiveness of neurons depends on transduction mechanisms and on the triggering of action potentials.[44, 45]

The elicitation of an action potential by a stimulus is called activation. The previous sections have described changes of mechanosensitivity upon inflammation which are called sensitization (see above under Nociceptors of deep tissue and peripheral sensitization). After sensitization, action potentials are elicited at lower stimulus energies, and thus a nociceptive neuron may respond to normally innocuous stimuli, in addition to showing an augmented response to noxious stimuli.

Sensitization involves a number of different molecular mechanisms. It results from the effect of numerous inflammatory mediators that bind to receptors in the membrane of the sensory endings, but changes of the intrinsic properties of the neurons also contribute to sensitization. The latter conclusion is derived from findings that dorsal root ganglion or trigeminal neurons from inflamed tissue maintain enhanced excitability even when the neurons are removed from the ganglion and acutely dissociated several days after inflammation of joint[46] or muscle.[47] In whole cell patch clamp recordings from these neurons, enhanced excitability could be identified by a decrease of the rheobase, an increase in the slope of the stimulus response function assessed with depolarizing current injection, and a decrease in the duration of the action potential after hyperpolarization. Most likely, changes in the activation of voltage-gated K^+ currents play an important role.[46, 47]

As mentioned, nociceptors are equipped with numerous receptors for inflammatory mediators. Binding of mediators to membrane receptors (many of which are coupled to G proteins) activates intracellular second messenger systems. These in turn activate intracellular processes that increase the sensitivity of the ion channels that are involved in stimulus transduction and/or transformation. Mediators are thus able to excite and/or sensitize primary afferent neurons for mechanical and chemical stimuli. These mediators also produce vascular and other changes in the tissue and thus contribute to the inflammatory process itself.

Effects of mediators on joint afferents have been previously summarized in detail elswhere.[48] As far as it has been tested, the effects on muscular afferents are comparable. Mediators that have effects on joint afferents include classical inflammatory mediators such as bradykinin, prostaglandins E_2 and I_2, and serotonin, purinergic compounds, neuropeptides, cytokines, and others. Common observations are that these mediators (1) affect Aδ- and/or C-fibers, not Aβ-fibers, (2) have an effect only in subpopulations of the units, (3) may or may not affect high threshold, as well as low threshold Aδ- and C-fibers, and (4) cause some initially mechanoinsensitive afferent fibers to be sensitized and become mechanosensitive.

Bolus injection of bradykinin, an algesic mediator, into joint and muscle arteries may cause an immediate short-lasting activation (less than one minute) of joint and muscle afferents, but thereafter there is a sensitization for mechanical stimuli of joint and muscle afferents that lasts minutes even when bradykinin did not excite the neuron.[49, 50] Both PGE_2 and PGI_2 cause ongoing discharges and/or sensitization to mechanical stimulation of the joint. The effect of PGE_2 has a slow onset and a duration of minutes, the action of PGI_2 begins quickly and has a short duration.[51, 52, 53, 54] In addition, these PGs sensitize joint and muscle afferents to the effects of bradykinin whether or not they have an excitatory effect by themselves.[42, 55] PGE_2 and bradykinin together can cause a stronger sensitization to mechanical stimulation than bradykinin or PGE_2 alone.[49] Conversely, nonsteroidal anti-inflammatory drugs (NSAID), such as aspirin and indometacin, which block PG synthesis, reduce spontaneous discharges from acutely and chronically inflamed joints, and attenuate the responses to mechanical stimulation.[56, 57] Serotonin also sensitizes joint afferents to mechanical stimuli,[58, 59] and Aδ- and C-fibers muscle afferents to the action of bradykinin and to excitation by mechanical stimuli.[55] Combined i.m. application of bradykinin and serotonin causes muscle pain in humans.[60]

ATP,[61, 62] adenosine,[62] capsaicin, and anandamide[63, 64] excite a proportion of joint afferents (the latter indicate the presence of the TRPV1 receptor). Capsaicin also causes muscle pain in humans.[65] Effects have also been observed for neuropeptides. Indeed, substance P[66] and VIP[67, 68] increased, whereas somatostatin[69] and endomorphin[70] reduced mechanosensitivity in numerous afferents; the peptides galanin,[71] neuropeptide Y,[72] and nociceptin[73] sensitized some neurons and reduced responses in other neurons. Whether the different patterns of peptide effects (excitation or inhibition) are dependent on the functional state of the neuron is not known at the moment. It was proposed that the simultaneous presence of different neuropeptides regulates excitability of the afferent fibers.

Of particular importance for the progress of arthritis are cytokines such as TNFα, interleukin-1β, and interleukin-6. Cytokines play an important role in neuropathic pain,[74] but, for example, IL-6 is also able to induce a long-lasting sensitization of C-fibers of the joints to mechanical stimulation.[75] Finally, mechanosensitivity can also be influenced by quite different compounds. For example, it was shown that responses of nociceptive articular afferents are reduced by gabapentin,[76] a compound used for the treatment of neuropathic pain, and by intra-articular injection of elastoviscous hyaluronan solutions.[77]

Recordings from afferent fibers from inflamed joints revealed that the proportion of neurons that show an effect of a given mediator can be different from the proportion of responsive afferents from normal joints. This may result from changes of receptor expression. Some data indicate that receptor expression in dorsal root ganglion (DRG) neurons can change in the course of arthritis (e.g. down-regulation of mu-opioid receptors[70] or biphasic regulation of somatostatin receptors[78]). However, changes of the neurons may also result from changes of the milieu in the tissue innervated. Disease processes are dynamic and, therefore, it is likely that different cells and molecules are important at different times in a chronic inflammatory or degenerative process[11] or during growth of bone cancer.[14] Hence the molecular mechanism of nociception may change over time. This aspect needs much more attention.

SPINAL PROCESSING OF INPUT FROM DEEP TISSUE AND CENTRAL SENSITIZATION

Nociceptive spinal cord neurons with joint and muscle input

Neurons with input from joint and muscle are located in the superficial and deep dorsal horn. This distribution matches the spinal termination of joint and muscle afferents which project to the superficial dorsal horn and, in particular Aβ- and Aδ-fibers, to the deep dorsal horn.[7, 12] Neurons with nociceptive information from joint[12, 79, 80] and muscle[81, 82, 83, 84] are either exclusively driven by input from deep tissue, or they exhibit convergent inputs from skin and deep structures. Neurons exclusively driven from deep tissue are excited by pressure applied to the deep tissue, but not by mechanical stimulation of the overlying skin. Their receptive fields are not restricted to a specific structure such as only a joint or a muscle belly. Rather they include a joint and adjacent muscles. Many of these neurons are high-threshold and require noxious pressure onto joint and/or muscle to be activated. Neurons with joint input may be activated by noxious movements, such as twisting of the joint against resistance of the tissue, like the articular nociceptors. The remaining neurons are wide dynamic range neurons which respond with increasing frequency when stimulus intensity is increased from the innocuous to the noxious range. Neurons with convergent inputs from deep tissue and skin are excited by mechanical stimuli applied to deep tissue (muscle, tendons, joint structures) and by mechanical stimulation of the skin. Often receptive fields in the deep tissue are located more rostral than cutaneous receptive fields thus allowing determination of both receptive fields. Most of these neurons are wide dynamic range neurons which respond to innocuous and noxious pressure onto deep tissue in a graded fashion. They may be activated by movements in the working range, but show much stronger responses to painful movements.

Neurons with input from joint and muscle project to different supraspinal sites (cerebellum, spinocervical nucleus, thalamus, reticular formation) subserving the generation of the conscious pain response and adaptations to pain (see **Figure 2.1**), or they project to intraspinal (segmental) interneurons and motoneurons.[7, 12] Spinal and supraspinal motor reflexes regulate movements and exert protective functions including flexor reflexes upon nociceptive stimulation.[1] Noxious stimulation of joint afferents[12, 85] and muscle afferents[7, 8] can evoke nociceptive withdrawal reflexes. During acute chemical stimulation of the knee and electrical stimulation of muscle nerves[86] and during inflammation in the joint,[85, 87] spinal motor reflexes are enhanced. In line with this, it has been thought that noxious stimulation of the muscle causes reflex muscle spasms and that muscle spasms will enhance the pain in the muscle – thus establishing a vicious circle. However, during myositis, a decrease rather than an increase of the reflex activation of motoneurons was observed,[8] and during experimental joint inflammation some γ-motoneurons developed progressive inhibition rather than facilitation.[87] Thus, the reflex pattern is modified during inflammation. Patients with painful muscles exhibit low rather than enhanced EMG activity[8] indicating that prolonged nociceptive stimulation actually induces a reduction of motor reflexes, followed by atrophy and loss of force.[8, 12] However, muscle spasms may be elicited from painful trigger points in adjacent muscles, and by articular dysfunction and ligamentous strain.[8]

Development of spinal hyperexcitability during peripheral inflammation

In the course of joint or muscle inflammation, spinal cord neurons with deep input develop a state of hyperexcitability, which is also called central sensitization (see **Figure 2.1**). Central sensitization is characterized by typical neuronal changes: (1) Spinal cord neurons with high threshold show a decrease of their excitation threshold, such that they are activated by innocuous stimuli applied to the inflamed tissue. (2) Both high threshold and wide dynamic range neurons show a marked increase of their responses to noxious stimulation of the inflamed tissue. This increased responsiveness to stimuli applied to inflamed tissue contributes to primary hyperalgesia at the site of inflammation. (3) With a similar time course, the neurons also show enhanced responses to mechanical stimuli applied to adjacent and even remote healthy tissue, and the total receptive field may expand.[80, 88, 89] These changes indicate that the sensitivity of the spinal cord neuron is increased so that previous subthreshold inputs are now sufficient to excite the neuron. The sensitization of neurons with expansion of receptive fields has the consequence that a stimulus activates more neurons in a segment.[90] Central sensitization can persist during chronic inflammation. In rats with unilateral arthritis,[79] as well as in rats suffering from chronic polyarthritis,[91] spinal cord neurons appear on average more sensitive and have expanded receptive fields in deep tissue and skin.

Pronounced spinal changes evoked by persistent inflammation were also observed when c-Fos was used to label activated neurons. During polyarthritis induced by injection of Freund's complete adjuvcant, numerous neurons in the dorsal and also in the ventral horn of several segments expressed c-Fos.[92] Increased c-Fos staining was also elicited by palpation of bones that were infiltrated with cancer cells, thus strongly suggesting that central sensitization is involved in bone pain.[14]

The changes described in the spinal cord are likely to account for deep referred pain and secondary hyperalgesia that are induced in humans by noxious stimulation of deep tissue.[93] Numerous pathological conditions, such as inflammation and osteoarthritis, seem to be associated with central sensitization. When a noxious stimulus, e.g. intramuscular injection of 6 percent NaCl, is applied to a muscle, the area in which pain is felt is larger during pathological conditions, such as osteoarthritis.[94] This suggests that the spinal cord is indeed in a state of hyperexcitability.

Sensitized nociceptive afferents from inflamed tissue play a key role in initial sensitization. Obviously these afferents not only evoke enhanced synaptic activation of spinal cord neurons to stimulation of inflamed tissue, but they also trigger the processes that increase sensitivity of spinal cord neurons. Interestingly, the stimulation of primary afferents from deep tissue (muscle and joint) evokes more prolonged facilitation of a nociceptive flexor reflex than stimulation of cutaneous afferents,[86] and capsaicin injection into deep tissue elicits more prolonged hyperalgesia than injection of capsaicin into the skin,[95] suggesting that deep input is particularly able to induce long-term changes in the nociceptive system. In addition to afferent and spinal mechanisms, descending pathways influence central sensitization.

Molecular mechanisms of spinal sensitization

In experiments, central sensitization has been observed during peripheral inflammation and also in models of neuropathic pain. Research in humans suggests that central sensitization may indeed be present in a number of different pain states, such as inflammation, osteoarthritis, fibromyalgia, migraine attacks, and others. Concerning molecular mechanisms of central sensitization, several points must be made. First, an important basis for central sensitization is the potential of nociceptive spinal cord neurons to undergo neuroplastic changes. The latter can, for example, be shown with defined protocols of electrical nerve stimulation. Electrical stimulation of C-fibers can induce wind-up of the responses to electrical nerve stimulation[96] (a short-lived increase of responsiveness, however, not outlasting the stimulation protocol) or a long-term potentiation[97] (a persistent increase of synaptic responses to electrical stimulation outlasting the conditioning stimulus). Second, while for central sensitization under inflammatory conditions mainly an increase of excitatory mechanism is being discussed, in the case of neuropathic pain loss of inhibition (e.g. by apoptosis of inhibitory interneurons) has been proposed as an important mechanism.[98] Third, again in studies on neuropathic pain, an involvement of both neurons and glial cells has been shown.[99] These data suggest that different mechanisms may contribute to central sensitization in different pain states. Ongoing research has to dissect out which mechanisms are particularly important for different pain states.

In the case of inflammation in joint and muscle, the contribution of transmitters and receptors to central sensitization has mainly been studied. Once inflammation develops in the joint, the intraspinal release of glutamate[100] (the main transmitter of nociceptive afferents) and neuropeptides (cotransmitters in primary afferents and interneurons) is enhanced. While only noxious compression of the normal joint enhances the intraspinal release of substance P, neurokinin A, and CGRP above baseline, these excitatory peptides are intraspinally released even by innocuous compression when the joint is inflamed.[101, 102, 103] Intraspinal release of substance P is also evoked by palpation of bone with cancer.[14] In addition, the intraspinal milieu is altered by (enhanced) release of further mediators. For example, prostaglandin E_2 is tonically released above baseline within the dorsal and ventral horn.[104] This is likely to result from an up-regulation of spinal COX-2, that is already present at three hours after induction of knee joint inflammation.[104] Thus, as a presynaptic mechanism, a cocktail of transmitters and/or modulators is released in the spinal cord under inflammatory conditions that is likely to influence the synaptic processing.

Glutamate activates AMPA/kainate (non-*N*-methyl-D-aspartic acid (NMDA)) receptors and NMDA receptors. Both glutamate receptor types have been implicated in the generation and maintenance of inflammation-induced spinal hyperexcitability. Application of antagonists at AMPA/kainate and NMDA receptors prevents the development of hyperexcitability in the course of joint inflammation[80] and muscle inflammation.[8] Importantly, antagonists at both receptor types can also reduce responses of the neurons to mechanical stimulation of the joint after inflammation is established,[80] even in a chronic model of inflammation.[12] The excitatory neuropeptides facilitate the responses of spinal cord neurons to mechanical stimulation of joint and muscle, further the development of inflammation-evoked hyperexcitability, and "open" synaptic pathways such that more neurons respond to stimulation.[8] However, antagonists at neuropeptide receptors are less antinociceptive than antagonists at glutamate receptors.[105, 106, 107] Topical application of PGE_2 to the spinal cord surface facilitates the responses of spinal cord neurons to mechanical stimulation of the joint similar to knee joint inflammation.[108] Topical application of the COX inhibitor indometacin to the spinal cord before inflammation attenuated the development of hyperexcitability.[108] Thus spinal PGs are involved in inflammation-evoked spinal hyperexcitability.

DESCENDING INFLUENCES ON SPINAL NEURONS WITH DEEP INPUT

From brainstem nuclei, impulses "descend" onto the spinal cord and influence the transmission of pain signals at the dorsal horn.[18, 19, 20] The periaqueductal gray (PAG) matter is a key region for descending inhibition. It receives inputs from the hypothalamus, cortical regions, and the limbic system and projects to the rostral ventromedial medulla (RVM), which includes several subnuclei. Neurons in RVM then project along the dorsolateral funiculus (DLF) to the dorsal horn. OFF cells of RVM exert descending inhibition of nociception, but ON cells facilitate nociceptive mechanisms at the spinal dorsal horn. Spinobulbospinal loops are significant in setting the gain of spinal processing.[19]

A particular form of descending inhibition of wide dynamic range neurons is the diffuse noxious inhibitory controls (DNIC). When a strong noxious stimulus is applied to a given body region, nociceptive neurons with input from that body region send impulses to structures located in the caudal medulla (caudal to RVM) and this triggers a centrifugal inhibition (DNIC) of nociceptive wide dynamic range neurons located throughout the neuraxis.[109]

Most spinal cord neurons with joint and muscle input are tonically inhibited by descending inhibitory systems that modulate spinal cord activity.[81, 110] These neurons are also inhibited by DNIC.[109] Tonic descending inhibition,[110] as well as DNIC,[109, 111] are increased during acute inflammation, but may be normalized in the chronic stage of inflammation.[111, 112] Interestingly, inhibition is mainly observed on neurons with input from the inflamed region (thus attenuating primary hyperalgesia), but processing in neurons with input from neighboring tissues may rather be enhanced, thus facilitating secondary hyperalgesia.[19]

SUPRASPINAL NEURONS WITH INPUT FROM JOINT AND MUSCLE

The thalamus and cortex contain nociceptive neurons that are activated by nociceptive deep input from muscles and joints. Most of these neurons have convergent inputs from skin and deep tissue, but small proportions of neurons respond only to noxious stimulation of muscle and tendon.[113, 114, 115] In the thalamus, such neurons are located in the ventrobasal complex, in the posterior complex[114] and in the medial nucleus.[116] Similarly, the somatosensory cortex contains a large proportion of neurons that respond to noxious stimulation, and a small proportion of these neurons is driven by deep input.[7, 117]

In polyarthritic rats, a large proportion of neurons in the ventrobasal complex respond to movements and gentle pressure on to inflamed joints and often long-lasting discharges were noted, whereas only few neurons respond to these stimuli in normal rats. Some neurons also displayed paroxysmal discharges. Furthermore, neurons in the nucleus centralis lateralis acquire input from the inflamed joint which is not present in normal animals.[118] Similarly, neurons in superficial cortical layers that do not respond to joint stimulation in normal rats start to respond to joint stimulation in polyarthritic rats.[119, 120] These findings indicate substantial neuroplasticity at the thalamocortical level that may contribute to inflammatory deep tissue pain. It is unknown whether these alterations mirror the altered spinal processing or whether additional elements of neuroplasticity are generated in the thalamus and cortex themselves.

CONCLUSIONS

There is considerable experimental evidence for substantial changes in the nociceptive processing during disease processes in the deep tissue such as joint, muscle, and bone. Available data from patients show considerable convergence of experimental and clinical data, and they indicate that different levels of the neuraxis are rational targets for analgesic treatment. Still much more research is required in order to better understand and treat chronic pain because current treatments are often not sufficient. There may be several reasons for that. Long-term molecular changes in the nociceptive systems are still poorly understood. Furthermore, chronic pain often seems to be a state in which nociceptive and neuropsychological components interact. This interaction should be better explored and form the basis of an "integrative" treatment strategy.

REFERENCES

1. Johannson H, Sjölander P, Sojka P. Receptors in the knee joint ligaments and their role in biomechanics of the joint. *Critical Reviews in Biomedical Engineering.* 1991; **18**: 341–68.
2. Lewis T. Suggestions relating to the study of somatic pain. *British Medical Journal.* 1938; **1**: 321–5.
3. Kellgren JH. Observations on referred pain arising from muscle. *Clinical Science.* 1938; **3**: 175–90.
4. Lewis T. *Pain.* London: Macmillan, 1942.
5. Kellgren JH, Samuel EP. The sensitivity and innervation of the articular capsule. *Journal of Bone and Joint Surgery.* 1950; **32B**: 84–91.
6. Kellgren JH. Some painful joint conditions and their relation to osteoarthritis. *Clinical Science.* 1939; **4**: 193–205.
7. * Mense S. Nociception from skeletal muscle in relation to clinical muscle pain. *Pain.* 1993; **54**: 241–89.
8. * Mense S. Pathophysiologic basis of muscle pain syndromes. In: Fischer AA (ed.). *Myofascial pain: update in diagnosis and treatment.* Philadelphia: WB Saunders, 1997: 23–53.
9. Graven-Nielsen T, Arendt-Nielsen L, Mense S. Thermosensitivity of muscle: high intensity thermal stimulation of muscle induces muscle pain in humans. *Journal of Physiology.* 2002; **540**: 647–56.
10. Feinstein B, Langton JNK, Jameson RM *et al.* Experiments on pain referred from deep somatic tissues. *Journal of Bone and Joint Surgery.* 1954; **36**: 981–97.
11. * Scott DL. Osteoarthritis and rheumatoid arthritis. In: McMahon SB, Koltzenburg M (eds). *Wall and Melzack's textbook of pain*, 5th edn. Elsevier, 2006: 653–67.
12. * Schaible H-G, Grubb BD. Afferent and spinal mechanisms of joint pain. *Pain.* 1993; **55**: 5–54.
13. * Felson DT. The sources of pain in knee osteoarthritis. *Current Opinion in Rheumatology.* 2005; **17**: 624–8.
14. * Mantyh PW. Cancer pain: causes, consequences and therapeutic opportunities. In: McMahon SB, Koltzenburg M (eds). *Wall and Melzack's textbook of pain*, 5th edn. Elsevier, 2006: 1087–97.
15. Cherny NI. The assessment of cancer pain. In: McMahon SB, Koltzenburg M (eds). *Wall and Melzack's textbook of pain*, 5th edn. Elsevier, 2006: 1099–125.

16. Heppelmann B, Messlinger K, Neiss W *et al.* Ultrastructural three-dimensional reconstruction of group III and group IV sensory nerve endings (free nerve endings) in the knee joint capsule of the rat: evidence for multiple receptive sites. *Journal of Comparative Neurology.* 1990; **292**: 103–16.

* 17. Vogt BA. Pain and emotion. Interactions in subregions of the cingulate gyrus. *Nature Reviews. Neuroscience.* 2005; **6**: 533–44.

* 18. Porreca F, Ossipov MH, Gebhart GF. Chronic pain and medullary descending facilitation. *Trends in Neuroscience.* 2002; **25**: 319–25.

* 19. Vanegas H, Schaible H-G. Descending control of persistent pain: inhibitory or facilitatory? *Brain Research Reviews.* 2004; **46**: 295–309.

20. Ossipov MH, Porreca F. Descending modulation of pain. In: Merskey H, Loeser JD, Dubner R (eds). *The paths of pain 1975–2005.* Seattle: IASP Press, 2005: 117–30.

21. Schaible H-G, Schmidt RF. Activation of groups III and IV sensory units in medial articular nerve by local mechanical stimulation of knee joint. *Journal of Neurophysiology.* 1983; **49**: 35–44.

22. Schaible H-G, Schmidt RF. Responses of fine medial articular nerve afferents to passive movements of knee joint. *Journal of Neurophysiology.* 1983; **49**: 1118–26.

23. Schaible H-G, Schmidt RF. Effects of an experimental arthritis on the sensory properties of fine articular afferent units. *Journal of Neurophysiology.* 1985; **54**: 1109–22.

24. Schaible H-G, Schmidt RF. Time course of mechanosensitivity changes in articular afferents during a developing experimental arthritis. *Journal of Neurophysiology.* 1988; **60**: 2180–95.

25. Grigg P, Schaible H-G, Schmidt RF. Mechanical sensitivity of group III and IV afferents from posterior articular nerve in normal and inflamed cat knee. *Journal of Neurophysiology.* 1986; **55**: 635–43.

26. Dorn T, Schaible H-G, Schmidt RF. Response properties of thick myelinated group II afferents in the medial articular nerve of normal and inflamed knee joints of the cat. *Somatosensory and Motor Research.* 1991; **8**: 127–36.

27. Krauspe R, Schmidt M, Schaible H-G. Sensory innervation of the anterior cruciate ligament: An electrophysiological study of the response properties of single identified mechanoreceptors in the cat. *Journal of Joint and Bone Surgery.* 1992; **7**: 390–7.

28. Bessou P, Laporte Y. Activation des fibres afferentes myelinisees de petit calibre d'órigine musculaire (fibres du group III). *Journal of Physiology (Paris).* 1960; **52**: 19–20.

29. Paintal AS. Funtional analysis of group III afferent fibres of mammalian muscles. *Journal of Physiology.* 1960; **152**: 250–70.

30. Iggo A. Non-myelinated afferent fibres from mammalian skeletal muscle. *Journal of Physiology.* 1961; **155**: 52–3.

31. Kumazawa T, Mizumura K. Thin-fibre receptors responding to mechanical, chemical and thermal stimulation in the skeletal muscle of the dog. *Journal of Physiology.* 1977; **273**: 179–94.

32. Kaufman MP, Iwamoto GA, Longhurst JC *et al.* Effects of capsaicin and bradykinin on afferent fibres with endings in skeletal muscle. *Circulation Research.* 1982; **50**: 133–9.

33. Mense S, Meyer H. Different types of slowly conducting afferent units in cat skeletal muscle and tendon. *Journal of Physiology.* 1985; **363**: 403–17.

34. Simone DA, Marchettini P, Caputi G *et al.* Identification of muscle afferents subserving sensation of deep pain in humans. *Journal of Neurophysiology.* 1994; **72**: 883–9.

35. Guilbaud G, Iggo A, Tegner R. Sensory receptors in ankle joint capsules of normal and arthritic rats. *Experimental Brain Research.* 1985; **58**: 29–40.

36. Weidner C, Schmelz M, Schmidt R *et al.* Functional attributes discriminating mechano-insensitive and mechano-responsive C nociceptors in human skin. *Journal of Neuroscience.* 1999; **19**: 10184–90.

37. Campbell JN, Meyer RA. Neuropathic pain: from the nociceptor to the patient. In: Merskey H, Loeser JD, Dubner R (eds). *The paths of pain 1975–2005.* Seattle: IASP Press, 2005: 229–42.

38. Häbler H-J, Jänig W, Koltzenburg M. A novel type of unmyelinated chemosensitive nociceptor in the acutely inflamed urinary bladder. *Agents and Actions.* 1988; **25**: 219–21.

39. Schmelz M, Michael K, Weidner C *et al.* Which nerve fibers mediate the axon reflex flare in human skin? *Neuroreport.* 2000; **11**: 645–8.

40. Klede M, Handwerker HO, Schmelz M. Central origin of secondary mechanical hyperalgesia. *Journal of Neurophysiology.* 2003; **90**: 353–9.

41. Berberich P, Hoheisel U, Mense S. Effects of a carrageenan-induced myositis on the discharge properties of group III and IV muscle receptors in the cat. *Journal of Neurophysiology.* 1988; **59**: 1395–409.

42. Mense S, Stahnke M. Responses in muscle afferent fibres of slow conduction velocity to contractions and ischemia in the cat. *Journal of Physiology.* 1983; **342**: 383–97.

43. Bessou P, Laporte Y. Activation des fibres afferentes amyeliniques d'órigine musculaire. *Comptes Rendus des Séances de la Société de Biologie et de ses Filiales.* 1958; **152**: 1587–90.

* 44. McCleskey EW, Gold MS. Ion channels of nociception. *Annual Review of Physiology.* 1999; **61**: 835–56.

* 45. Gold MS. Molecular basis of receptors. In: Merskey H, Loeser JD, Dubner R (eds). *The paths of pain 1975–2005.* Seattle: IASP Press, 2005: 49–67.

46. Flake NM, Gold MS. Inflammation alters sodium currents and excitability of temporomandibular joint afferents. *Neuroscience Letters.* 2005; **384**: 294–9.

47. Harriott AM, Dessem D, Gold MS. Inflammation increases the excitability of masseter muscle afferents. *Neuroscience.* 2006; **141**: 433–42.

* 48. Schaible H-G. Basic mechanisms of deep somatic pain. In: McMahon SB, Koltzenburg M (eds). *Wall and Melzack's textbook of pain*, 5th edn. Elsevier, 2006: 621–33.

49. Neugebauer V, Schaible H-G, Schmidt RF. Sensitization of articular afferents for mechanical stimuli by bradykinin. *Pflügers Archiv.* 1989; **415**: 330–5.
50. Mense S, Meyer H. Bradykinin-induced modulation of the response behaviour of different types of feline group III and IV muscle receptors. *Journal of Physiology.* 1988; **398**: 49–63.
51. Grubb BD, Birrell J, McQueen DS *et al.* The role of PGE_2 in the sensitization of mechanoreceptors in normal and inflamed ankle joints of the rat. *Experimental Brain Research.* 1991; **84**: 383–92.
52. Schaible H-G, Schmidt RF. Excitation and sensitization of fine articular afferents from cat's knee joint by prostaglandin E_2. *Journal of Physiology.* 1988; **403**: 91–104.
53. Schepelmann K, Messlinger K, Schaible H-G *et al.* Inflammatory mediators and nociception in the joint: Excitation and sensitization of slowly conducting afferent fibers of cat's knee by prostaglandin I_2. *Neuroscience.* 1992; **50**: 237–47.
54. Birrell GJ, McQueen DS, Iggo A *et al.* PGI_2-induced activation and sensitization of articular mechanoreceptors. *Neuroscience Letters.* 1991; **124**: 5–8.
55. Mense S. Sensitization of group IV muscle receptors to bradykinin by 5-hydroxytryptamine and prostaglandin E_2. *Brain Research.* 1981; **225**: 95–105.
56. Guilbaud G, Iggo A. The effect of acetylsalicylate on joint mechanoreceptors in rats with polyarthritis. *Experimental Brain Research.* 1985; **61**: 164–8.
57. Heppelmann B, Pfeffer A, Schaible HG *et al.* Effects of acetylsalicylic acid (ASA) and indomethacin on single groups III and IV units from acutely inflamed joints. *Pain.* 1986; **26**: 337–51.
58. Birrell GJ, McQueen DS, Iggo A *et al.* The effect of 5-HT on articular sensory receptors in normal and arthritic rats. *British Journal of Pharmacology.* 1990; **101**: 715–21.
59. Herbert MK, Schmidt RF. Activation of normal and inflamed fine articular afferent units by serotonin. *Pain.* 1992; **50**: 79–88.
60. Babenko V, Graven-Nielsen T, Svensson P *et al.* Experimental human muscle pain and muscular hyperalgesia induced by combinations of serotonin and bradykinin. *Pain.* 1999; **82**: 1–8.
61. Dowd E, McQueen DS, Chessell IP *et al.* P2X receptor-mediated excitation of nociceptive afferents in the normal and arthritic rat knee joint. *British Journal of Pharmacology.* 1998; **125**: 341–6.
62. Dowd E, McQueen DS, Chessell IP *et al.* Adenosine A1 receptor-mediated excitation of nociceptive afferents innervating the normal and arthritic rat knee joint. *British Journal of Pharmacology.* 1998; **125**: 1267–71.
63. He X, Schepelmann K, Schaible H-G *et al.* Capsaicin inhibits responses of fine afferents from the knee joint of the cat to mechanical and chemical stimuli. *Brain Research.* 1990; **530**: 147–50.
64. Gauldie SD, McQueen DS, Pertwee R *et al.* Anandamide activates peripheral nociceptors in normal and arthritic rat knee joints. *British Journal of Pharmacology.* 2001; **132**: 617–21.
65. Witting N, Svensson P, Gottrup H *et al.* Intramuscular and intradermal injection of capsaicin: a comparison of local and referred pain. *Pain.* 2000; **84**: 407–12.
66. Heppelmann B, Pawlak M. Sensitisation of articular afferents in normal and inflamed knee joints by substance P in the rat. *Neuroscience Letters.* 1997; **223**: 97–100.
67. McDougall JJ, Watkins L, Li Z. Vasoactive intestinal peptide (VIP) is a modulator of joint pain in a rat model of osteoarthritis. *Pain.* 2006; **123**: 98–105.
68. Schuelert N, McDougall JJ. Electrophysiological evidence that the vasoactive intestinal peptide receptor antagonist VIP(6-28) reduces nociception in an animal model of osteoarthritis. *Osteoarthritis Cartilage.* 2006; **14**: 1155–62.
69. Heppelmann B, Pawlak M. Inhibitory effect of somatostatin on the mechanosensitivity of articular afferents in normal and inflamed knee joints of the rat. *Pain.* 1997; **73**: 377–82.
70. Li Z, Proud D, Zhang C *et al.* Chronic arthritis down-regulates peripheral mu-opioid receptor expression with concomitant loss of endomorphin 1 antinociception. *Arthritis and Rheumatism.* 2005; **52**: 2955–9.
71. Heppelmann B, Just S, Pawlak M. Galanin influences the mechanosensitivity of sensory endings in the rat knee joint. *European Journal of Neuroscience.* 2000; **12**: 1567–72.
72. Just S, Heppelmann B. Neuropeptide Y changes the excitability of fine afferent units in the rat knee joint. *British Journal of Pharmacology.* 2001; **132**: 703–8.
73. McDougall JJ, Pawlak M, Hanesch U *et al.* Peripheral modulation of rat knee joint afferent mechanosensitivity by nociceptin/orphanin FQ. *Neuroscience Letters.* 2000; **288**: 123–6.
74. Marchand F, Perretti M, McMahon SB. Role of the immune system in chronic pain. *Nature Reviews. Neuroscience.* 2005; **6**: 521–32.
75. Brenn D, Richter F, Schaible H-G. Sensitization of unmyelinated sensory fibres of the joint nerve for mechanical stimuli by interleukin-6. *Arthritis and Rheumatism.* 2007; **56**: 351–9.
76. Hanesch U, Pawlak M, McDougall JJ. Gabapentin reduces the mechanosensitivity of fine afferent nerve fibres in normal and inflamed rat knee joint. *Pain.* 2003; **104**: 363–6.
77. Gomis A, Pawlak M, Balazs EA *et al.* Effects of different molecular weight elastoviscous hyaluronan solutions on articular nociceptive afferents. *Arthritis and Rheumatism.* 2004; **50**: 314–26.
78. Bär K-J, Schurigt U, Scholze A *et al.* The expression and localisation of somatostatin receptors in dorsal root ganglion neurons of normal and monoarthritic rats. *Neuroscience.* 2004; **127**: 197–206.
79. Grubb BD, Stiller RU, Schaible H-G. Dynamic changes in the receptive field properties of spinal cord neurons with ankle input in rats with unilateral adjuvant-induced

inflammation in the ankle region. *Experimental Brain Research*. 1993; **92**: 441–52.
80. Neugebauer V, Lücke T, Schaible H-G. *N*-methyl-D-aspartate (NMDA) and non-NMDA receptor antagonists block the hyperexcitability of dorsal horn neurons during development of acute arthritis in rat's knee joint. *Journal of Neurophysiology*. 1993; **70**: 1365–77.
81. Pomeranz B, Wall PD, Weber WV. Cord cells responding to fine myelinated afferents from viscera, muscle and skin. *Journal of Physiology*. 1968; **199**: 511–32.
82. Craig AD, Kniffki K-D. Spinothalamic lumbosacral lamina I cells responsive to skin and muscle stimulation in the cat. *Journal of Physiology*. 1985; **365**: 197–221.
83. Hoheisel U, Mense S. Response behavior of cat dorsal horn neurones receiving input from skeletal muscle and other deep somatic tissues. *Journal of Physiology*. 1990; **426**: 265–80.
84. Yu X-M, Mense S. Response properties and descending control of rat dorsal horn neurons with deep receptive fields. *Neuroscience*. 1990; **39**: 823–31.
85. Ferrell WR, Wood L, Baxendale RH. The effect of acute joint inflammation on flexion reflex excitability in the decerebrate, low spinal cat. *Quarterly Journal of Experimental Psychology*. 1988; **373**: 353–65.
86. Woolf CJ, Wall PD. Relative effectiveness of C primary afferent fibres of different origins in evoking a prolonged facilitation of the flexor reflex in the rat. *Journal of Neuroscience*. 1986; **6**: 1433–42.
87. He X, Proske U, Schaible H-G *et al*. Acute inflammation of the knee joint in the cat alters responses of flexor motoneurones to leg movements. *Journal of Neurophysiology*. 1988; **59**: 326–40.
88. Schaible H-G, Schmidt RF, Willis WD. Enhancement of the responses of ascending tract cells in the cat spinal cord by acute inflammation of the knee joint. *Experimental Brain Research*. 1987; **66**: 489–99.
89. Neugebauer V, Schaible H-G. Evidence for a central component in the sensitization of spinal neurons with joint input during development of acute arthritis in cat's knee. *Journal of Neurophysiology*. 1990; **64**: 299–311.
90. Hoheisel U, Koch K, Mense S. Functional reorganization in the rat dorsal horn during an experimental myositis. *Pain*. 1994; **59**: 111–8.
91. Menetréy D, Besson J-M. Electrophysiological characteristics of dorsal horn cells in rats with cutaneous inflammation. *Pain*. 1982; **13**: 343–64.
92. Abbadie C, Besson J-M. C-fos expression in rat lumbar spinal cord during the development of adjuvant-induced arthritis. *Neuroscience*. 1992; **48**: 985–93.
93. Arendt-Nielsen L, Laursen RJ, Drewes AM. Referred pain as an indicator for neural plasticity. *Progress in Brain Research*. 2000; **129**: 343–56.
94. Bajaj P, Bajaj P, Graven-Nielsen T, Arendt-Nielsen L. Osteoarthritis and its association with muscle hyperalgesia: an experimental controlled study. *Pain*. 2001; **93**: 107–14.
95. Sluka KA. Stimulation of deep somatic tissue with capsaicin produces long-lasting mechanical allodynia and heat hypoalgesia that depends on early activation of the cAMP pathway. *Journal of Neuroscience*. 2002; **22**: 5687–93.
96. Mendell LM, Wall PD. Responses of single dorsal cord cells to peripheral cutaneous unmyelinated fibers. *Nature*. 1965; **206**: 97–9.
97. Sandkühler J. Learning and memory in pain pathways. *Pain*. 2000; **88**: 113–8.
98. Schaible HG. Peripheral and central mechanisms of pain generation. In: Stein C (ed.). *Handbook of experimental pharmacology*, vol 177. Berlin: Springer-Verlag, 2006: 4–28.
99. Watkins LR, Maier SF. Glia and pain: past, present, and future. In: Merskey H, Loeser JD, Dubner R (eds). *The paths of pain 1975–2005*. Seattle: IASP Press, 2005: 165–75.
100. Sorkin LS, Westlund KN, Sluka KA *et al*. Neural changes in acute arthritis in monkeys. IV: Time course of amino acid release into the lumbar dorsal horn. *Brain Research Reviews*. 1992; **17**: 39–50.
101. Hope PJ, Jarrott B, Schaible H-G *et al*. Release and spread of immunoreactive neurokinin A in the cat spinal cord in a model of acute arthritis. *Brain Research*. 1990; **533**: 292–9.
102. Schaible H-G, Jarrott B, Hope PJ *et al*. Release of immunoreactive substance P in the cat spinal cord during development of acute arthritis in cat's knee: A study with antibody bearing microprobes. *Brain Research*. 1990; **529**: 214–23.
103. Schaible H-G, Freudenberger U, Neugebauer V *et al*. Intraspinal release of immunoreactive calcitonin gene-related peptide during development of inflammation in the joint *in vivo* – a study with antibody microprobes in cat and rat. *Neuroscience*. 1994; **62**: 1293–305.
104. Ebersberger A, Grubb BD, Willingale HL *et al*. The intraspinal release of prostaglandin E_2 in a model of acute arthritis is accompanied by an upregulation of cyclooxygenase-2 in the rat spinal cord. *Neuroscience*. 1999; **93**: 775–81.
105. Neugebauer V, Weiretter F, Schaible H-G. The involvement of substance P and neurokinin-1 receptors in the hyperexcitability of dorsal horn neurons during development of acute arthritis in rat's knee joint. *Journal of Neurophysiology*. 1995; **73**: 1574–83.
106. Neugebauer V, Rümenapp P, Schaible H-G. The role of spinal neurokinin-2 receptors in the processing of nociceptive information from the joint and in the generation and maintenance of inflammation-evoked hyperexcitability of dorsal horn neurons in the rat. *European Journal of Neuroscience*. 1996; **8**: 249–60.
107. Neugebauer V, Rümenapp P, Schaible H-G. Calcitonin gene-related peptide is involved in the generation and maintenance of hyperexcitability of dorsal horn neurons observed during development of acute inflammation in rat's knee joint. *Neuroscience*. 1996; **71**: 1095–109.

108. Vasquez E, Bär K-J, Ebersberger A *et al.* Spinal prostaglandins are involved in the development but not the maintenance of inflammation-induced spinal hyperexcitability. *Journal of Neuroscience.* 2001; **21**: 9001–8.
109. Calvino B, Villanueva L, LeBars D. Dorsal horn (convergent) neurones in the intact anaesthetized arthritic rat. II. Heterotopic inhibitory influences. *Pain.* 1987; **31**: 359–79.
110. Schaible H-G, Neugebauer V, Cervero F *et al.* Changes in tonic descending inhibition of spinal neurons with articular input during the development of acute arthritis in the cat. *Journal of Neurophysiology.* 1991; **66**: 1021–32.
111. Danziger N, Weil-Fugazza J, LeBars D *et al.* Alteration of descending modulation of nociception during the course of monoarthritis in the rat. *Journal of Neuroscience.* 1999; **19**: 2394–400.
112. Danziger N, Weil-Fugazza J, LeBars D *et al.* Stage-dependent changes in the modulation of nociceptive neuronal activity during the course of inflammation. *European Journal of Neuroscience.* 2001; **13**: 230–40.
113. Kniffki K-D, Mizumura K. Responses of neurons in VPL and VPL-VL region of the cat to algesic stimulation of muscle and tendon. *Journal of Neurophysiology.* 1983; **49**: 649–61.
114. Hutchison WD, Lühn MA, Schmidt RF. Knee joint input into the peripheral region of the ventral posterior lateral nucleus of cat thalamus. *Journal of Neurophysiology.* 1992; **67**: 1092–104.
115. Guilbaud G, Peschanski M, Gautron M *et al.* Neurones responding to noxious stimulation in VB complex and caudal adjacent regions in the thalamus of the rat. *Pain.* 1980; **8**: 303–18.
116. Dong WK, Ryu H, Wagman IH. Nociceptive responses of neurons in medial thalamus and their relationship to spinothalamic pathways. *Journal of Neurophysiology.* 1978; **41**: 1592–613.
117. Heppelmann B, Pawlak M, Just S, Schmidt RF. Cortical projection of the rat knee joint innervation and its processing in the somatosensory areas SI and SII. *Experimental Brain Research.* 2001; **141**: 501–6.
118. Gautron M, Guilbaud G. Somatic responses of ventrobasal thalamic neurones in polyarthritic rats. *Brain Research.* 1982; **237**: 459–71.
119. Lamour Y, Willer JC, Guilbaud G. Rat somatosensory (Sm I) cortex. II. Laminar and columnar organization of noxious and non-noxious inputs. *Experimental Brain Research.* 1983; **49**: 46–54.
120. Lamour Y, Willer JC, Guilbaud G. Altered properties and laminar distribution of neuronal responses to peripheral stimulation in the Sm I cortex of the arthritic rat. *Brain Research.* 1983; **273**: 183–7.

3

Applied physiology: persistent visceral pain

TIMOTHY J NESS

KEY LEARNING POINTS

- Persistent visceral pain is common and represents a state of hypersensitivity.
- The substrates of visceral sensation differ from cutaneous sensation.
- Inflammation, stress, and altered neurological substrates due to neuropathic or developmental processes can all lead to visceral hypersensitivity.

INTRODUCTION

Persistent visceral pain is a common clinical experience, but only recently have scientific studies defined its mechanisms. It is poorly understood and much of our knowledge of it is an extrapolation from acute pain studies. Pain arising from the internal organs of the body is uniquely different from pain that arises from the surface of the body in relation to the neuroanatomical substrates involved, in relation to the responses evoked by visceral stimuli, and in relation to the modifying effects of both internal and external factors. Most painful disorders associated with the viscera represent conditions of hypersensitivity made manifest by these same internal and external factors. There are underlying similarities that have been observed between multiple visceral sensory systems such that an understanding of one particular system may improve understanding of other systems. This chapter attempts to summarize what is known about persistent visceral pain by placing an emphasis on the mechanisms of visceral hypersensitivity. These mechanisms will be contrasted and compared with what is known about the more extensively studied superficial pains. This summary builds on previous reviews by this author of similar topics and general statements are referred to those reviews.[1, 2, 3, 4]

THE EXPERIENCE OF VISCERAL PAIN

When visceral pains are experienced, they are often associated with poor and unreliable localization. They are generally deep and diffuse and often the only localization of pathology comes with a physical examination in which manipulations directly stimulate the painful organ. Whereas superficial sensations from a specific site are always reliably localized to the same site and do not migrate to other body areas in the absence of nerve injury, the same cannot be said for visceral pain. Visceral pain can be felt in several different areas at the same time or can migrate throughout a region even though pathology is localized within a single organ. Visceral pain is classically described as being referred to other sites and this referral has two separate components: (1) the sensation is transferred to another site (e.g. angina can be felt in the neck and arm) and (2) other sites become more sensitive to inputs applied directly to those other sites (e.g. flank muscle becomes sensitive to palpation when passing a kidney stone). This latter phenomenon is a form of secondary hyperalgesia which can involve both somatic and other visceral structures.

Based on clinical experience, stimuli which can lead to the production of pathological visceral pain can be categorized into four groups:

1. acute mechanical stretch/distension of visceral structures;
2. ischemia of visceral structures;
3. chemical stimuli from a local pathological process (e.g. an infiltrating tumor);
4. functional alterations leading to atypical patterns of afferent activity.

Visceral pains may also occur secondary to iatrogenic damage of the viscera and their associated nerves produced by interventional therapies, surgery, chemotherapy, and/or radiation. There is a poor correlation between the amount of visceral pathology and the intensity of associated pain. For example, very extensive processes with ongoing tissue damage (e.g. ulcerative colitis or gastric perforation) may produce little or no pain in some individuals, while minimally discernable pathology may produce out-of-control pain in others.

VISCERAL HYPERSENSITIVITY DISORDERS

The observation that pathology and symptomatology may not correlate is readily apparent in numerous visceral pain disorders. Some disorders, such as chronic pancreatitis, have definable pathology, but alterations in pain appear out of proportion to objective radiographic or laboratory findings. Other disorders, such as irritable bowel syndrome, noncardiac chest pain, and postcholecystectomy syndrome, appear to have no grossly apparent histopathological basis for the discomfort and pain. Instead, visceral discomfort and pain in such conditions are termed functional and are associated with altered patterns/pressures associated with motility, production of gas, and ingestion of food or beverage. Hence, natural visceral stimuli in the physiologic range can be associated with discomfort and pain in the absence of obvious visceral pathology.

Hypersensitivity to somatically applied stimuli is typically associated with histological evidence of ongoing tissue damage/inflammation. Exception to this statement are neuropathic pain disorders in which there may be a history of nerve injury, but no apparent local histopathological changes. In this case, routine tissue examination would suggest that neuropathic pain disorders are functional.

With an increased sophistication of testing related to visceral disorders, there may prove to be identifiable markers or imaging studies that allow for a reduced reliance on subjective reports of sensation. An example of this comes from the painful bladder disorder, interstitial cystitis (IC). In general, the urothelium of patients with the nonulcerative form of IC appears normal on routine cystoscopic and microscopic examination. It takes a highly sophisticated analysis to discern any quantitative differences between the tissues of IC patients and normal healthy controls such that most measures have been deemed to be of little use in diagnosis. However, when the urothelium of IC patients is examined using a scanning electron microscope, defects in the urothelial surface and tight junctions are common[5] and a laboratory marker for a factor that suppresses urothelial cell proliferation may prove diagnostic for the disorder.[6] Until similar subtleties of evaluation become routine, the current state-of-the-art for diagnosis of painful visceral disorders requires full consideration of the entire constellation of signs, symptoms, and tests.

Psychophysical studies have demonstrated evidence for hypersensitivity in virtually all clinically relevant visceral pain disorders. This includes hypersensitivity to gastric distension in patients with functional dyspepsia,[7] intestinal and rectal distension in patients with irritable bowel syndrome,[8, 9] biliary and/or pancreatic duct distension in patients with postcholecystectomy syndrome or chronic pancreatitis,[10] and bladder distension in patients with interstitial cystitis.[11] In these studies, pain could be evoked at intensities of stimulation lower than those required to produce the same quality and intensity of sensation in a healthy population. A more sophisticated testing of visceral sensitivity using random order, graded distension of the rectum in irritable bowel patients suggest that the population of subjects is heterogenous,[12] with subgroups demonstrating hypersensitivity and others hypervigilance.

Dissociating potential psychological modifiers of sensory reports from other more physiological pathologies has proven to be difficult. It represents a sometimes insurmountable methodological problem and, perhaps more importantly, due to observations related to the phenomenon of stress-induced hyperalgesia (where psychological factors alter physiological responses) it may not be appropriate to perform such a dissociation. Psychophysical studies related to visceral sensation in normal healthy subjects have suggested a basis for some of the emotional factors that may affect pain reports. Strigo *et al.*[13] compared sensations evoked by balloon distension of the esophagus with thermal stimulation of the skin overlying the sternum and found that greater anxiety was evoked by esophageal distension. Furthermore, they found unpleasantness ratings were higher when the esophageal stimulus was administered and a stronger affective component to the visceral sensation was measured using the McGill Pain Questionnaire.

Other psychophysical studies of experimental visceral pain sensation in humans have identified that a sensitization process occurs with repeated stimulation of the gut[14, 15] and of the urinary bladder[16] consistent with observations in nonhuman animals, where repeated presentation of the same visceral stimuli produces increasing vigor of neuronal, cardiovascular, and visceromotor reflex responses.[17, 18]

Clinically, there are three entities that are accepted as potential sources of painful hypersensitivity: (1) inflammation; (2) stress (anxiety); and (3) altered neural function that may be due to injury during critical periods of development (e.g. the neonatal period) or more direct neuropathic processes. These will be discussed below after a description of the anatomy of visceral pain.

SUBSTRATES OF SENSATION

Peripheral pathways

The peripheral nervous system pathways of abdominal visceral sensation have been defined in humans and are summarized in **Figure 3.1**. Most viscera have a dual, or in some cases triple, source of afferents travelling via the vagus nerve, the pelvic nerve, and/or via the splanchnics (nerves travelling in association with sympathetic efferent fibers). Spinal visceral afferent fibers have their cell bodies in dorsal root ganglia and central terminals in the superficial dorsal horn of the spinal cord (lamina I and II), deeper laminae (IV, V), the intermediolateral cell column and sacral parasympathetic nucleus (pelvic nerve), and in the area around and dorsal to the central canal (lamina X). It is notable that visceral primary afferents differ significantly from cutaneous primary afferents in both number and pattern of distribution. Grossly, peripheral axons of visceroceptive primary afferents are diffusely organized into web-like plexuses rather than forming distinct peripheral nerve entities. Afferents with endings in a specific visceral site may have cell bodies in the dorsal root ganglia of ten or more spinal levels in a bilaterally distributed fashion. In contrast, afferents arising in cutaneous structures travel to a limited number (three to five levels) of unilaterally located dorsal root ganglia. Individual visceroceptive afferent C-fibers have been demonstrated to branch within the spinal cord and to spread over ten or more spinal segments and to branch into superficial, deep, and even contralateral spinal dorsal horn laminae.[19] Individual cutaneous afferent C-fibers, on the other hand, have been demonstrated to form tight unilateral baskets of input to localized spinal cord segments and terminate predominantly in superficial laminae.[19]

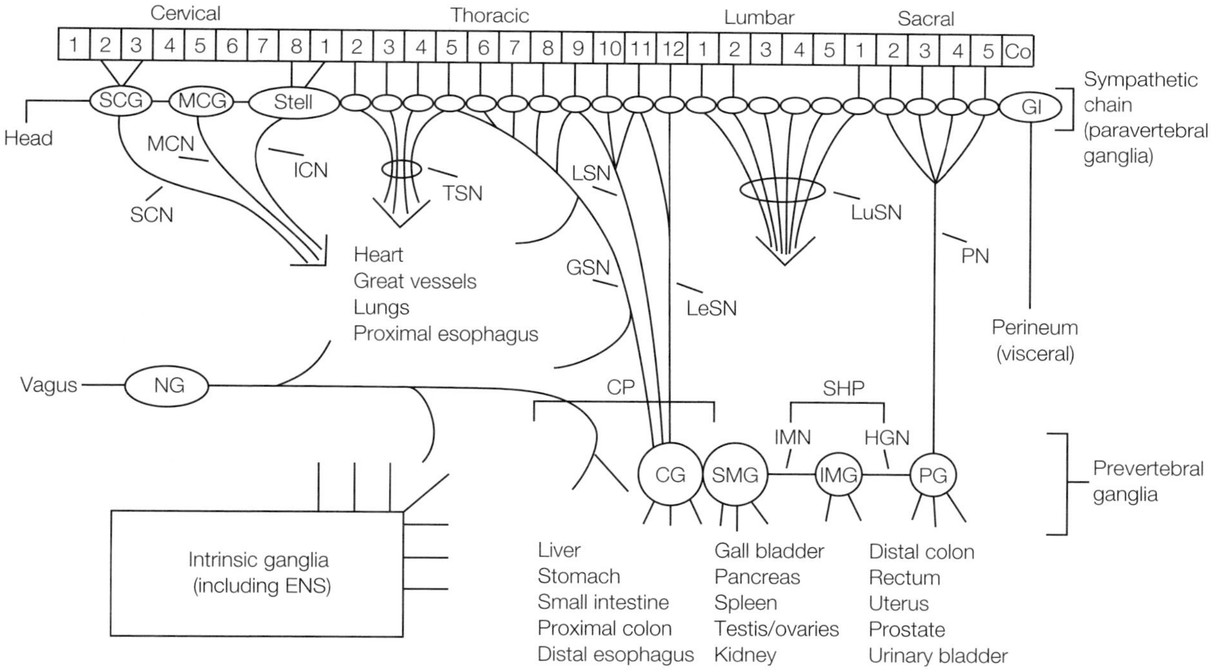

Figure 3.1 The nervous supply of the viscera in humans. Abbreviations are as follows: SCN, MCN, ICN, superior middle and inferior cardiac nerves; TSN, GSN, LSN, LeSN, LuSN, thoracic, greater, lesser, least, lumbar splanchnic nerves; PN, pelvic nerve; IMN, intermesenteric nerve; HGN, hypogastric nerve; SCG, MCG, superior and middle cervical ganglia; Stell: stellate ganglion; CG, celiac ganglion; SMG, IMG, superior and inferior mesenteric ganglia; PG, pelvic ganglion; GI, ganglion impar; CP, SHP, celiac and superior hypogastric plexuses; NG, nodose ganglion; ENS, enteric nervous system. Adapted from Ness and Gebhart, 1990.[1]

Spinal dorsal horn neurons

When quantitatively examined, spinal dorsal horn neurons with visceral inputs are located in the dorsal horn of the spinal cord (lamina I, II, V), the intermediolateral cell column and sacral parasympathetic nucleus (pelvic nerve), and in lamina X. These neurons have multiple, convergent inputs from other viscera, from joints, from muscle, and from cutaneous structures. Convergent receptive fields for these neurons are therefore large with diffuse inputs. This is considered the basis of referral of visceral sensation to somatic sites (e.g. myocardial ischemia typically radiates to the left shoulder and upper arm; the pain is not felt at the source – the heart). In contrast, neurons with exclusively cutaneous input are commonly identified in the spinal dorsal horn, in particular from glabrous skin. Taken together, these results suggest an imprecise organization of visceral primary inputs that would be consistent with an imprecise localization by the central nervous system. Viscero–visceral convergence and secondary hyperalgesia are common enough phenomena that, when coupled with the baseline diffuse character of visceral sensations, there prove to be diagnostic difficulties for both patients and physicians when the possibility of more than one pathology exists.

Unique spinal pathway

The traditional pain pathway for the transmission of information from the dorsal horn of the spinal cord to the brain is via the anterolateral quadrant white matter of the spinal cord. Based on lesion and tracing studies, tracts located within these sites include the spinothalamic, spinoreticular, spinomesencephalic, and spinohypothalamic tracts. This area is clearly important for cutaneous pain sensation because lesions of the anterolateral spinal white matter lead to pinprick analgesia in contralateral dermatomes below the level of the lesion. However, recently researchers have demonstrated that surgical lesions of the dorsal midline of the spinal cord have profound effects on visceral pain-related responses in humans, primates, and rodents. Specifically, a punctate thoracic midline myelotomy in humans has been demonstrated to relieve cancer-related pelvic and abdominal pain.[20, 21, 22, 23, 24, 25] Similar lesions in nonhuman primates reduce the activity of thalamic neurons evoked by colorectal distension[26] and in rats, similar lesions reduce or abolish thalamic neuronal responses and/or behavioral responses to colorectal distension,[27, 28] duodenal distension,[29] pancreatic stimulation,[30] and hypersensitivity following lower extremity osteotomy.[31] Not all ascending information related to the viscera travels by this midline route: dorsal midline lesions abolished visceral inputs to the nucleus gracilis of the medulla,[32] but did not affect inputs to the ventrolateral medulla.[28] Spinal neurons with viscerosomatic convergence and axonal extensions into the dorsal columns have been demonstrated for primates[33] and rats.[20, 32] In rats, acute inflammation of the colon, produced by the topical application of mustard oil, resulted in increased responses of these postsynaptic dorsal column neurons to colorectal distension.[34] Using that model, Palacek and Willis[35] demonstrated that the dorsal midline pathway may be necessary for the augmentation of reflex responses that occur secondary to visceral inflammation, but not for the basal reflex responses.

Supraspinal terminations of visceral input

Standard anatomical and electrophysiological tracing methods have established widespread distribution of visceral input to the brain. The axons of second-order spinal neurons that receive visceral input have been shown to ascend the spinal cord to the brain with sites of termination in the medulla, pons, mesencephalon, hypothalamus, and thalamus. Neurons excited by visceral stimuli have likewise been identified at these same sites with extensive characterizations of neurons located within the ventral posterolateral, dorsomedial, and submedius nuclei of the thalamus, the locus coeruleus, parabrachial nucleus, ventrolateral medulla, and numerous brain stem and limbic sites.[36, 37, 38, 39, 40, 41, 42] Higher-order neurons excited by visceral stimuli have also been demonstrated to be present in the somatosensory and ventrolateral orbital cerebral cortices.[43, 44, 45] A lack of visceral sensation has been noted in neurosurgical patients who have sustained damage to their frontal lobes.[46, 47, 48]

Functional imaging of humans during visceral stimulation has revealed some consistencies, but the most common finding is that there is a multitude of sites which demonstrate increased regional blood flow in response to visceral stimulation. Rectal distension and urinary bladder distension both produce increased bloodflow in select areas of the thalamus, hypothalamus, mesencephalon, pons, and medulla (for example, Ref. 49). Cortical sites of processing include the anterior and midcingulate cortex, the frontal and parietal cortices and in the cerebellum.[50] The most illustrative imaging study to date comparing visceral pain sensation with cutaneous pain sensation is that of Strigo *et al.*[51] These investigators matched the intensity of pain sensation produced by esophageal distension with that produced by heating of the skin overlying the sternum. Whereas both cutaneous and esophageal pain sensations were associated with activation of the secondary somatosensory cortex, the parietal cortex, the thalamus, basal ganglia, and cerebellum, there was a higher activation of the anterior insular cortex bilaterally when cutaneous stimuli were used and the esophageal stimulus selectively activated the ventrolateral prefrontal cortex. Esophageal pain produced a broader bilateral cortical activation and produced activation of a more anterior locus of the anterior cingulate cortex than cutaneous pain. This all suggests some shared components of sensation from the same segmental structures, but also a selective activation of some structures by different types of pain.

MODELS OF VISCERAL PAIN

Human models

Stimuli which have been employed in experimental studies of visceral nociception in human subjects include electrical stimuli, chemical stimuli, thermal stimuli, ischemia, and mechanical stimuli. Electrical stimulation produces reports of pain in humans and has been used to evoke cerebral potentials, in order to assess visceral sensory pathways. Chemical stimuli have been applied topically, intravascularly, or via physiological pathways (e.g. excreted agents) in order to define the endogenous substances responsible for an altered sensitivity to mechanical or environmental stimuli (e.g. acidity of urine) which may occur spontaneously or secondary to inflammation. Thermal stimuli (hot or cold) have been administered using hot or cold solutions instilled into visceral lumens and utilized to test for normal sensation and function, but rarely have been sources of clinical pain.[52] Ischemia of visceral structures has been produced by the occlusion of visceral vasculature. Experimentally and clinically, the effects of such occlusion are dependent upon collateral bloodflow and metabolic activity of the selected organ. Venous congestion has mixed ischemic and mechanical components and so could also be a source of pain. The most commonly utilized experimental visceral stimuli are mechanical stimuli, such as the probing and stretch of visceral structures or the distension of hollow organs using fluids or foreign bodies. Mechanical stimuli may mimic what is observed in certain pathological pain states (e.g. bowel obstruction) and the pattern of mechanical stimulation may be important as it has been proposed to be the source of pain in functional bowel disorders.

Due to the fact that the hollow organs of the gastrointestinal tract are readily accessible through natural orifices, the earliest clinical studies of visceral sensation used balloon distension of esophagus, stomach, small bowel, large bowel, and rectum as their visceral stimuli. The advantages of balloon distension of hollow organs are many, foremost being that balloon distension reproduces pathologically experienced pain in humans in terms of intensity, quality, and area to which the sensation is referred. Hollow organ distension at constant pressure produces sensations and responses that are reliably reproducible and easily controlled by the experimenter.

Nonhuman animal models

There are over 50 different models of visceral pain that have been described, but only a few have been utilized in more than one laboratory.[2] The recent past has seen a development of models that approximate physiological and behavioral responses similar to that of human visceral pain. One of the earliest models, the chemically induced writhing model in rodents, is produced by injecting irritant chemicals into the peritoneal cavity. This model has found less utility with the development of other models since the intraperitoneal injections did not selectively activate specific viscera, frequently yielded false positives when used to screen potential analgesic drugs, and are ethically questionable as they are associated with a persistent stimulus from which the animal cannot escape. Current models of visceral pain are more likely to utilize mechanical (e.g. distending) stimuli of controllable duration or chemical stimuli applied directly to relevant targets, thus permitting selectivity with respect to site of stimulation.

Balloon distension of hollow organs, principally along the gastrointestinal tract, is the most widely used experimental stimulus of the viscera. As noted above, experimental balloon distension of the gastrointestinal tract in humans has been established to reproduce pathologically experienced pain in terms of intensity, quality, and the area to which the sensation is referred. Whereas distending stimuli have been established as adequate for hollow organs, occlusive, ischemic, and irritant stimuli have been tested as adequate stimuli in other organs. Because inflammation of the urinary bladder is commonly associated with reports of pain and urgency in humans, experimental models of bladder irritation, including a model of cystitis, have been developed in rodents.[53] Kidney stones are undeniably painful in humans and a model of artificial ureteral calculosis has been developed in rats.[54] Occlusion of blood supply to most viscera is associated with pain and ischemia/anoxia is thus considered an adequate stimulus in the viscera. Accordingly, models of coronary artery occlusion and ischemia of abdominal visceral organs have been reported.[55]

Visceral pain is not a unitary entity and so there is a need for more than one visceral pain model. It is difficult to equate pain due to infection of the normally sterile urinary bladder with painless colons containing a sewer of the same infective organisms. Some differences between organ systems are clearly developmental in that organs which derive from midline structures (i.e. the gut) are associated with bilateral sensations, highly generalized responses and processing bilaterally within the spinal dorsal horn. In contrast, those organs which derive from unilateral structures (i.e. kidneys, ureters) generally have lateralized sensations, more regionalized responses, and lateralized spinal processing. The use of multiple models and multiple types of noxious stimuli applied to different organ systems allow us to distinguish the generalities of visceral pain from its mechanistic specifics.

MECHANISMS OF VISCERAL HYPERSENSITIVITY

Inflammation as a mechanism

A potent modifier of behavioral, neuronal, autonomic, and motor responses to visceral stimulation in experimental models inflammation has been commonly used to produce visceral hypersensitivity. The presence of inflammation in visceral structures frequently, but not universally, leads to reports of pain and sensitivity to mechanical and chemical stimuli. Cystitis, esophagitis, gastritis, duodenitis, ileitis, colitis, and proctitis all have evidence of mucosal inflammatory changes, as a hallmark finding. However, profound inflammatory changes of the mucosal lining, such as occurs with ulcerative colitis, may present with nonpainful, bloody stools.

Inflammation produces profound changes in the responsiveness of subsets of previously unresponsive visceral primary afferents and the term "silent" afferents has been coined.[56] These afferents are normally nonreactive to most stimuli, but in the presence of products of inflammation become spontaneously active and highly reactive to mechanical stimuli, such as distension. Silent afferents have been frequently noted in visceral structures forming up to 50 percent of the neuronal sample,[57] but are only infrequently noted in cutaneous structures. The lack of sensitivity of the viscera at baseline may relate to the sparcity of active visceral afferents which are quantitatively fewer per unit area than similar measures of cutaneous afferents. Because they are few, increased activity may be necessary in order to cross a threshold for perception.

Spinal neurons responsive to visceral stimuli also change their responsiveness to visceral stimuli in the presence of inflammation and when other sensitizing manipulations have been performed (see, for example, Refs 58, 59). Whether this is due to increased afferent activity, altered intrinsic properties of dorsal horn neurons, or altered modulatory influences within the central nervous system is unknown. It is likely that all of these separate mechanisms contribute in some way to the final sensitized state.

Whereas acute inflammation is often obvious with the hallmark features of redness, swelling, pain, and warmth, the more subtle changes related to chronic inflammation are often difficult to identify. Progressive fibrosis, mast cell infiltration, and altered oxidative stress markers all suggest that an ongoing indolent inflammatory process may be present that has sensory consequences equal to that of acute inflammation. Mast cell infiltration has been implicated in the hypersensitivity states of irritable bowel syndrome[60] and interstitial cysititis,[61] which has, in turn, prompted treatment with antihistamines and cromolyn-related compounds with mixed benefits. Mast cells have been observed to cluster around nerve bundles[62] and have been noted to express estrogen receptors[63] which, in turn, suggests a mechanism for menstrual cycle-associated exacerbations of some visceral pains.

More subtle than the histologically identifiable alterations in cell distribution are the biochemical changes that indicate a low level of chronic inflammation. Alterations in measures of oxidative stress have been observed in several hypersensitivity disorders, such as fibromylagia[64] and chronic fatigue syndrome,[65] and form a basis for sensory changes in the absence of histological changes. Use of antioxidant/micronutrient therapies (e.g. vitamins C and E, selenium) has had reported utility in the treatment of painful visceral disorders, such as chronic pancreatitis.[66]

Stress as a mechanism

Cutaneous and visceral sensation appears to differ in relation to the effect of stress on the magnitude of responses to stimulation. Although stress-induced analgesia (or hypoalgesia) has been a long-recognized phenomenon associated with cutaneous sensation, it would appear that stress-induced hyperalgesia is the correlate phenomenon associated with visceral sensation. Clinically, stressful life events have been viewed as classic triggers for the evocation of diffuse abdominal complaints of presumed visceral origin.[9] It is the rule, rather than the exception, that stressful life events, unless coupled with other major physiological events such as pregnancy, lead to an exacerbation of underlying pain disorders. A prominent role for stress in the pathophysiology and presentation of multiple clinical pain states, including irritable bowel syndrome, Crohn's disease, interstitial cystitis, rheumatoid arthritis, and psoriasis, has been well documented.[67, 68, 69, 70, 71] Using IC as a specific example, more than 60 percent of IC patients report symptom exacerbation by both acute and chronic stress, and clinical studies have shown that acute stress increases bladder pain and urgency in these individuals.[72, 73, 74, 75, 76] Not only is there a significant positive relationship between stress and the IC symptoms of pain and urgency, but as severity of the disease increases, the relationship between stress and symptom manifestation becomes even more evident.[76]

In nonhuman animal models, acute exposure to numerous stressors (footshock, water avoidance, forced swimming, cold water swim) can produce stress-induced analgesia.[77] However, in these same model systems when the stress is perceived as uncontrollable, chronic, or unpredictable, it may induce long-term pathophysiological changes presumed to be the mechanisms of stress-induced hyperalgesia. It is notable that stress-induced analgesia and stress-induced hyperalgesia can be apparently coexistent. Classic behavioral stressors, such as restraint or cold-water swim, produce an elevation in thresholds for the evocation of responses to thermal stimuli (stress-induced analgesia), but the same animals have an increased vigor of visceromotor responses to colorectal distension (visceral hyperalgesia[78, 79]). This phenomenon appears to be associated with early-in-life events,[78] genetics,[80] and can be modified by gonadal hormones, neurokinins, corticotrophin-releasing factor, and mast cell function. Robbins *et al.*[81] has demonstrated similar phenomena in association with urinary bladder sensation and function.

A neurophysiological correlate of the phenomenon of stress-induced hyperalgesia was demonstrated by Qin *et al.*[82, 83, 84] In their studies, they injected glucocorticoids or aldosterone into the amygdala, manipulations which are known to produce increased measures of anxiety in animal subjects. These manipulations also produced a hypersensitivity to visceral stimulation as measured by an increased vigor of both visceromotor responses and responses of spinal dorsal horn neurons to colon or urinary bladder distension. This suggests the potential for a chicken–egg relation, where visceral pain (which produces anxiety) may activate the mechanisms of stress-induced hyperalgesia, thereby leading to visceral hypersensitivity which produces more anxiety, and on and on. Logically, a cotreatment of both pain and anxiety would seem to have the greatest utility.

Developmental changes as a mechanism

The neonatal period is a critical period of development related to visceral sensation and function. Multiple lines of convergent evidence suggest that neural monitoring and control systems are rapidly developing at both peripheral and central sites during the mid- to late-neonatal period. For example, in rats, the spinobulbospinal reflexes associated with micturition develop at two to three weeks postpartum and are associated with alterations in transient glutamatergic receptor expression.[85] Neurotrophins, which in rats are at minimal levels at birth in visceral tissues such as the urinary bladder, increase during development and have maximal levels present two weeks after birth with subsequent reductions with additional development.[86] Taken together, these findings indicate that the viscera and the neural structures associated with sensation and motor function are rapidly changing in the neonatal period and infancy periods and, as such, are susceptible to modifications by factors, such as inflammation. Control systems related to nociceptive processing are also developing at the same time[87] and are associated with progressive increases in glycinergic and GABAergic spinal inhibitory influences from birth through infancy.[88] A postnatal switch in GABAergic control of nociceptive reflexes has been observed to occur[89] and altered expression of μ-opioid receptors occurs in the same time period.[90] In rats, inflammation of the hindpaw has been demonstrated to produce primary afferent terminal expansion within lamina II,[91] III, and IV[92] of the spinal dorsal horn when performed in the neonatal, but not adult periods, and so a similar expansion of primary afferent terminals due to visceral inflammation would seem likely. A series of studies by Al-Chaer *et al.*,[93, 94] demonstrated that similar long-lasting effects resulting from neonatal exposure to nociceptive stimuli also occur in visceral pain systems: neonatal exposure to either repetitive colorectal distension (CRD) or repetitive application of mustard oil to the colorectal region resulted in increased abdominal withdrawal reflexes to CRD, increased responses of primary afferents to CRD, and increased spinal neuronal responses to CRD in rats tested as adults. Importantly, these effects did not require an identifiable change in colonic histopathology in the adult animals. Randich *et al.*[95] noted similar persistent developmental and experiential influences following neonatal inflammation of the bladder.

At the present time, there has been only a limited amount of work performed in humans, but seminal studies by Fitzgerald,[96, 97] and expanded on by others (for review, see Ref. 98), have provided evidence that early-in-life exposure to painful cutaneous stimuli can lead to later-in-life increases in sensitivity to the same stimuli. For example, extremely low birth weight (ELBW) infants who received multiple painful procedures as part of their neonatal care demonstrated some characteristics of autonomic hyperresponsiveness to needle sticks or other painful stimuli,[99] were more prone to clinical somatization,[100] and reported more pain as a component of their overall health status during adolescence.[101] These findings coupled with the nonhuman animal data are consistent with the view that neonatal events could prime an organism to respond with enhanced sensory reactions to inflammation and related painful stimuli as adults.

Neuropathic changes as a mechanism

A possible source of visceral hypersensitivity could be previous injury of the nerve pathways associated with visceral sensation. Interventional neurolytic procedures and intra-abdominal surgical interventions undoubtedly injure these nerve pathways, but there has been a long-unstated assumption that this form of nerve injury is without perceived consequence. The validity of such an assumption is certainly not established and there is evidence of visceral sensory consequences in models of neuropathic pain.[102] It will take future epidemiologic studies to properly assess such possibilities.

CONCLUSIONS

Visceral pain differs from other pains in many ways. This is not to say that there are no similarities. Primary afferent cell bodies associated with visceral nociception reside within dorsal root ganglia and the initial processing of sensory information occurs at the level of the dorsal horn of the spinal cord or in the brain stem (e.g. vagal and trigeminal inputs). Many sites of higher processing in the brain are activated by both noxious visceral and noxious somatic stimuli. Where visceral pains differ from somatic pain is in the encoding properties of visceral primary afferent transducers and in their distribution to and within the central nervous system. The final consequence of these dissimilarities is a difference in localization and a difference in the magnitude of emotional and autonomic responses to visceral stimuli. Persistent visceral pain is also different from other pains in that it represents a hypersensitivity state that may be induced/exacerbated by inflammation, stress, developmental changes, and/or nerve injury. Due to its differences from other types of pain, the treatment of visceral pain may need to differ and may need to address the mechanisms of hypersensitivity rather than simple organ pathology. At present, clinical practice is the use of the same therapeutics for pain of any type. With additional information, it may become possible to determine treatments that are selective for persistent visceral pains.

REFERENCES

1. Ness TJ, Gebhart GF. Visceral pain: a review of experimental studies. *Pain*. 1990; **41**: 167–234.
2. Ness TJ. Models of visceral nociception. *ILAR Journal*. 1999; **40**: 119–28.
3. Ness TJ, Gebhart GF. Mechanisms of visceral pain. In: Pappagallo M (ed.). *The neurological basis of pain*. New York: McGraw-Hill, 2004: 95–103.
4. Ness TJ. Visceral pain. In: de Leon-Casasola OA (ed.). *Cancer pain: pharmacologic, interventional, and palliative approaches*. New York: Saunders, 2006: 85–94.
5. Elbadawi AE, Light JK. Distinctive ultrastructural pathology of nonulcerative interstitial cystitis: new observations and their potential significance to pathogenesis. *Urologia Internationalis*. 1996; **56**: 137–62.
6. Keay SK, Szekely Z, Conrads TP *et al.* An antiproliferative factor from interstitial cystitis patients is a frizzled 8 protein-related sialoglycopeptide. *Proceedings of the National Academy of Sciences of the United States of America*. 2004; **101**: 11803–08.
7. Salet GA, Samsom M, Roelofs JM *et al.* Responses to gastric distension in functional dyspepsia. *Gut*. 1998; **42**: 823–9.

* 8. Ritchie J. Pain from distension of the pelvic colon by inflating a balloon in the irritable colon syndrome. *Gut*. 1973; **14**: 125–32.

9. Mertz H. Visceral hypersensitivity. *Alimentary Pharmacology and Therapeutics*. 2003; **17**: 623–33.

* 10. Corazziari E, Shaffer EA, Hogan WJ *et al.* Functional disorders of the biliary tract and pancreas. *Gut*. 1999; **45** (Suppl. 2): II48–54.

* 11. Ness TJ, Powell-Boone T, Cannon R *et al.* Psychophysical evidence of hypersensitivity in subjects with interstitial cystitis. *Journal of Urology*. 2005; **73**: 1983–7.

12. Naliboff BD, Munakata J, Fullerton S *et al.* Evidence for two distinct perceptual alterations in irritable bowel syndrome. *Gut*. 1997; **41**: 505–12.
13. Strigo IA, Bushnell MC, Boivin M *et al.* Psychophysical analysis of visceral and cutaneous pain in human subjects. *Pain*. 2002; **97**: 235–46.
14. Ness TJ, Metcalf AM, Gebhart GF. A psychophysiological study in humans using phasic colonic distension as a noxious visceral stimulus. *Pain*. 1990; **43**: 377–86.
15. Munakata J, Naliboff B, Harraf F *et al.* Repetitive sigmoid stimulation induces rectal hyperalgesia in patients with irritable bowel syndrome. *Gastroenterology*. 1997; **112**: 55–63.
16. Ness TJ, Richter HE, Varner RE *et al.* A psychophysical study of discomfort produced by repeated filling of the urinary bladder. *Pain*. 1998; **76**: 61–9.
17. Ness TJ, Gebhart GF. Colorectal distension as a noxious visceral stimulus: physiologic and pharmacologic characterization of pseudaffective reflexes in the rat. *Brain Research*. 1988; **450**: 153–69.
18. Ness TJ, Lewis-Sides A, Castroman P. Characterization of pressor and visceromotor reflex responses to bladder distension in rats: sources of variability and effect of analgesics. *Journal of Urology*. 2001; **165**: 968–74.
19. Sugiura Y, Terui N, Hosoya Y *et al.* Quantitative analysis of central terminal projections of visceral and somatic unmyelinated (C) primary afferent fibers in the guinea pig. *Journal of Comparative Neurology*. 1993; **332**: 315–25.

* 20. Hirshberg RM, Al-Chaer ED, Lawand NB *et al.* Is there a pathway in the posterior funiculus that signals visceral pain? *Pain*. 1996; **67**: 291–305.

21. Nauta HJW, Hewitt E, Westlund KN *et al.* Surgical interruption of a midline dorsal column visceral pain pathway. *Journal of Neurosurgery*. 1997; **86**: 538–42.
22. Nauta HJ, Soukup VM, Fabian RH *et al.* Punctate midline myelotomy for the relief of visceral cancer pain. *Journal of Neurosurgery*. 2000; **92**: 125–30.
23. Kim YS, Kwon SJ. High thoracic midline dorsal colum myelotomy for severe visceral pain due to advanced stomach cancer. *Neurosurgery*. 2000; **46**: 85–92.
24. Becker R, Gatscher S, Sure U, Bertalanffy H. The punctuate midline myelotomy concept for visceral cancer pain control – case report and review of the literature. *Acta Neurochirurgica. Supplement*. 2002; **79**: 77–8.
25. Hong D, Andren-Sandberg A. Punctate midline myelotomy: a minimally invasive procedure for the treatment of pain in inextirpable abdominal and pelvic cancer. *Journal of Pain and Symptom Management*. 2007; **33**: 99–109.
26. Al-Chaer ED, Feng Y, Willis WD. A role for the dorsal column in nociceptive visceral input into the thalamus of primates. *Journal of Neurophysiology*. 1998; **79**: 3143–50.
27. Al-Chaer ED, Westlund KN, Willis WD. Nucleus gracilis: an integrator for visceral and somatic information. *Journal of Neurophysiology*. 1997; **78**: 521–7.

28. Ness TJ. Evidence for ascending visceral nociceptive information in the dorsal midline and lateral spinal cord. *Pain.* 2000; **87**: 83–8.
29. Feng Y, Cui M, Al-Chaer ED *et al.* Epigastric antinociception by cervical dorsal column lesions in rats. *Anesthesiology.* 1998; **89**: 411–20.
30. Houghton AK, Wang CC, Westlund KN. Do nociceptive signals from the pancreas travel in the dorsal column? *Pain.* 2001; **89**: 207–20.
31. Houghton AK, Hewitt E, Westlund KN. Dorsal column lesions prevent mechanical hyperalgesia and allodynia in osteotomy model. *Pain.* 1999; **82**: 73–80.
32. Al-Chaer ED, Lawand NB, Westlund KN *et al.* Pelvic visceral input into the nucleus gracilis is largely mediated by the postsynaptic dorsal column pathway. *Journal of Neurophysiology.* 1996; **76**: 2675–90.
33. Al-Chaer ED, Feng Y, Willis WD. Comparative study of viscerosomatic input onto postsynaptic dorsal column and spinothalamic tract neurons in the primate. *Journal of Neurophysiology.* 1999; **82**: 1876–82.
34. Al-Chaer ED, Westlund KN, Willis WD. Potentiation of thalamic responses to colorectal distension by visceral inflammation. *Neuroreport.* 1996; **7**: 1635–9.
35. Palacek J, Willis WD. The dorsal column pathway facilitates visceromotor responses to colorectal distension after colon inflammation in rats. *Pain.* 2003; **104**: 501–07.
36. Bruggemann J, Shi T, Apkarian AV. Viscerosomatic interactions in the thalamic ventral posterolateral nucleus (VPL) of the squirrel monkey. *Brain Research.* 1998; **787**: 269–76.
37. Elam M, Thoren P, Svensson TH. Locus coeruleus neurons and sympathetic nerves: activation by visceral afferents. *Brain Research.* 1986; **375**: 117–25.
38. Traub RJ, Silva E, Gebhart GF *et al.* Noxious colorectal distension induced c-fors protein in limbic brain structures in the rat. *Neuroscience Letters.* 1996; **215**: 165–8.
39. Almeida A, Lima D. Activation by cutaneous or visceral noxious stimulation of spinal neurons projecting in the medullary dorsal reticular nucleus in the rat: a c-fos study. *European Journal of Neuroscience.* 1997; **9**: 686–95.
40. Ness TJ, Follett KA, Piper JG *et al.* Characterization of neurons in the area of the medullary lateral reticular nucleus responsive to noxious visceral and cutaneous stimuli. *Brain Research.* 1998; **802**: 163–74.
41. Lanteri-Minet M, Bon K, de Pommery J *et al.* Cyclophosphamide cystitis as a model of visceral pain in rats: model elaboation and spinal structures involved as revealed by the expression of c-fos and Krox-24 proteins. *Experimental Brain Research.* 1995; **105**: 220–32.
42. Bon K, Lanteri-Minet M, Michiels JF *et al.* Cyclophosphamide cystitis as a model of visceral pain in rats: a c-fos and Krox-24 study at telencephalic levels, with a note on pituitary adenylate cyclase activating polypeptide (PACAP). *Experimental Brain Research.* 1998; **122**: 165–74.
43. Follett KA, Dirks B. Characterization of responses of primary somatosensory cerebral cortex neurons to noxious visceral stimulation in the rat. *Brain Research.* 1994; **656**: 27–32.
44. Follett KA, Dirks B. Responses of neurons in ventrolateral orbital cortex to noxious visceral stimulation in the rat. *Brain Research.* 1995; **669**: 157–62.
45. Snow PJ, Lumb BM, Cervero F. The representation of prolonged and intense, noxious somatic and visceral stimuli in the ventrolateral orbital cortex of the cat. *Pain.* 1992; **48**: 89–99.
46. Andrew J, Nathan PW. Lesions of the anterior frontal lobes and disturbances of micturition and defaecation. *Brain.* 1964; **87**: 233–62.
47. Andrew J, Nathan PW, Spanos NC. Disturbances of micturition and defaecation due to aneurysms of anterior communicating or anterior cerebral arteries. *Journal of Neurosurgery.* 1966; **24**: 1–10.
48. Nathan P. Lesions of the anterior frontal lobes and disturbances of micturition and defaecation. *Neurologia.* 1963; **5**: 9–17.
49. Blok BFM. Central pathways controlling micturition and urinary continence. *Urology.* 2002; **59** (Suppl 5A): 13–17.
50. Athwal BS, Berkley KJ, Hussain I *et al.* Brain responses to changes in bladder volume and urge to void in healthy men. *Brain.* 2001; **124**: 369–77.
51. * Strigo IA, Duncan GH, Boivin M, Bushnell MC. Differentiation of visceral and cutaneous pain in the human brain. *Journal of Neurophysiology.* 2003; **89**: 3294–303.
52. Mukerji G, Waters J, Chessell IP *et al.* Pain during ice water test distinguishes clinical bladder hypersensitivity from overactivity disorders. *BMC Urology.* 2006; **6**: 31.
53. * McMahon SB, Abel C. A model for the study of visceral pain states: chronic inflammation of the chronic decerebrate rat urinary bladder by irritant chemicals. *Pain.* 1987; **28**: 109–32.
54. Giamberardino MA, Valente R, de Bigontina P, Vecchiet L. Artificial ureteral calculosis in rats: behavioural characterization of visceral pain episodes and their relationship with referred lumbar muscle hyperalgesia. *Pain.* 1995; **61**: 459–69.
55. Foreman RD, Ohata CA. Effects of coronary artery occlusion on thoracic spinal neurons receiving viscerosomatic inputs. *American Journal of Physiology.* 1980; **238**: H667–778.
56. Michaelis M, Habler HJ, Jänig W. Silent afferents: a separate class of primary afferents? *Clinical and Experimental Pharmacology and Physiology.* 1996; **23**: 99–105.
57. Habler HJ, Jänig W, Koltzenberg M. Activation of unmyelinated afferent fibres by mechanical stimuli and inflammation of the urinary bladder in the cat. *Journal of Physiology.* 1990; **425**: 545–60.
58. Olivar T, Cervero F, Laird JM. Responses of rat spinal neurons to natural and electrical stimulation of colonic afferents: effects of inflammation. *Brain Research.* 2000; **866**: 168–77.

59. Ness TJ, Gebhart GF. Inflammation enhances reflex and spinal neuron responses to noxious visceral stimulation in rats. *American Journal of Physiology.* 2001; **280**: G649–57.
60. Barbara G, Wang B, Stanghellini V *et al.* Mast cell dependent excitation of visceral-nociceptive sensory neurons in irritable bowel syndrome. *Gastroenterology.* 2007; **132**: 26–37.
61. Sant GR, Kempuraj D, Marchand JE, Theoharides TC. The mast cell in interstitial cystitis: role in pathophysiology and pathogenesis. *Urology.* 2007; **69** (Suppl. 4): 34–40.
62. Letourneau R, Pang X, Sant GR, Theoharides TC. Intragranular activation of bladder mast cells and their association with nerve processes in interstitial cystitis. *British Journal of Urology.* 1996; **77**: 41–54.
63. Pang X, Cotreau-Bibbo MM, Sant GR, Theoharides TC. Bladder mast cell expression of high affinity oestrogen receptors in patients with interstitial cystitis. *British Journal of Urology.* 1995; **75**: 154–61.
64. Ozgocmen S, Ozyurt H, Sogut S, Akyol O. Current concepts in the pathophysiology of fibromyalgia: the potential role of oxidative stress and nitric oxide. *Rheumatology International.* 2006; **26**: 585–97.
65. Kennedy G, Spence VA, McLaren M *et al.* Oxidative stress levels are raised in chronic fatigue syndrome and are associated with clinical symptoms. *Free Radical Biology and Medicine.* 2005; **39**: 584–9.
66. Kirk GR, White JS, McKie L *et al.* Combined antioxidant therapy reduces pain and improves quality of life in chronic pancreatitis. *Journal of Gastrointestinal Surgery.* 2006; **10**: 499–503.
67. Farber EM, Nickoloff BJ, Recht B, Fraki JE. Stress, symmetry and psoriasis: possible role of neuropeptides. *Journal of the American Academy of Dermatology.* 1986; **2**: 305–12.
68. Thomason BT, Brantley PJ, Jones GN *et al.* The relation between stress and disease activity in rheumatoid arthritis. *Journal of Behavioral Medicine.* 1992; **15**: 215–20.
69. Zautra AJ, Hoffman J, Potter P *et al.* Examination of changes in interpersonal stress as a factor in disease exacerbations among women with rheumatoid arthritis. *Annals of Behavioral Medicine.* 1997; **19**: 279–86.
70. Dancey CP, Taqhavi M, Fox RJ. The relationship between daily stress and symptoms of irritable bowel. *Journal of Psychosomatic Research.* 1998; **44**: 537–45.
71. Garrett VD, Brantley PJ, Jones GN, McKnight GT. The relation between daily stress and Crohn's disease. *Journal of Behavioral Medicine.* 1991; **14**: 87–96.
72. Macaulay AJ, Stern RS, Holmes DM, Santon SL. Micturition and the mind: psychological factors in the aetiology and treatment of urinary symptoms in women. *British Medical Journal.* 1987; **294**: 540–3.
73. Baldoni F, Ercolani M, Baldaro B, Trombini G. Stressful events and psychological symptoms in patients with functional urinary disorders. *Perceptual and Motor Skills.* 1995; **80**: 605–06.
74. Koziol JA, Clark DC, Gittes RF, Tan EM. The natural history of interstitial cystitis: a survey of 374 patients. *Journal of Urology.* 1993; **149**: 465–9.
* 75. Lutgendorf SK, Kreder KJ, Rothrock NE *et al.* Stress and symptomatology in patients with interstitial cystitis: a laboratory stress model. *Journal of Urology.* 2000; **164**: 1265–9.
76. Rothrock NE, Lutgendorf SK, Kreder KJ *et al.* Daily stress and symptom exacerbation in interstitial cystitis patients. *Urology.* 2001; **57**: 422–7.
77. Amit Z, Galina ZH. Stress-induced analgesia: adaptive pain suppression. *Physiological Reviews.* 1986; **66**: 1091–120.
* 78. Coutinho SV, Plotsky PM, Sablad M *et al.* Neonatal maternal separation alters stress-induced responses to viscerosomatic nociceptive stimuli in rats. *American Journal of Physiology.* 2002; **282**: G307–16.
79. Bradesi S, Eutamene H, Fioramonti J, Bueno L. Acute restraint stress activates functional NK1 receptor in the colon of female rats: involvement of steroids. *Gut.* 2002; **50**: 349–54.
80. Gunter WD, Shepard JD, Foreman RD *et al.* Evidence for visceral hypersensitivity in high-anxiety rats. *Physiology and Behavior.* 2000; **69**: 379–82.
81. Robbins MT, DeBerry J, Ness TJ. Chronic psychological stress enhances nociceptive processing in the urinary bladder in high-anxiety rats. *Physiology and Behavior.* 2007; **91**: 544–50.
82. Qin C, Greenwood-Meerveld B, Foreman RD. Spinal neuronal responses to urinary bladder stimulation in rats with corticosterone or aldosterone onto the amygdala. *Journal of Neurophysiology.* 2003; **90**: 2180–9.
83. Qin C, Greenwood-Meerveld B, Foreman RD. Visceromotor and spinal neuronal responses to colorectal distension in rats with aldosterone onto the amygdala. *Journal of Neurophysiology.* 2003; **90**: 2–11.
84. Greenwood-Van Meerveld B, Gibson M, Gunter W *et al.* Stereotaxic delivery of corticosterone to the amygdale modulates colonic sensitivity in rats. *Brain Research.* 2001; **893**: 135–42.
85. de Groat WC, Araki I, Vizzard MA *et al.* Developmental and injury induced plasticity in the micturition reflex pathway. *Behavioral Brain Research.* 1998; **92**: 127–40.
86. Vizzard MA, Wu KH, Jewett IT. Developmental expression of urinary bladder neurotrophic factor mRNA and protein in the neonatal rat. Brain Research. *Developmental Brain Research.* 2000; **119**: 217–24.
87. Boucher T, Jennings E, Fitzgerald M. The onset of diffuse noxious inhibitory controls in postnatal rat pups: a C-Fos study. *Neuroscience Letters.* 1998; **257**: 9–12.
88. Baccei ML, Fitzgerald M. Development of GABAergic and glycinergic transmission in the neonatal rat dorsal horn. *Journal of Neuroscience.* 2004; **24**: 4749–57.
89. Hathway G, Harrop E, Baccei M *et al.* A postnatal switch in GABAergic control of spinal cutaneous reflexes. *European Journal of Neuroscience.* 2006; **23**: 112–18.
90. Nandi R, Fizgerald M. Opioid analgesia in the newborn. *European Journal of Pain.* 2005; **9**: 105–08.

91. Walker SM, Meredith-Middleton J, Cooke-Yarborough C, Fitzgerald M. Neonatal inflammation and primary afferent terminal plasticity in the rat dorsal horn. *Pain*. 2003; **105**: 185–95.
92. Ling QD, Chien CC, Wen YR *et al*. The pattern and distribution of calcitonin gene-related peptide (CGRP) terminals in the rat dorsal horn following neonatal peripheral inflammation. *Neuroreport*. 2003; **14**: 1919–21.
* 93. Al-Chaer ED, Kawasaki M, Pasricha PJ. A new model of chronic visceral hypersensitivity in adult rats induced by colon irritation during postnatal development. *Gastroenterology*. 2000; **119**: 1276–85.
94. Lin C, Al-Chaer ED. Long-term sensitization of primary afferents in adult rats exposed to neonatal colon pain. *Brain Research*. 2003; **971**: 73–82.
* 95. Randich A, Uzzel T, DeBerry JJ, Ness TJ. Neonatal urinary bladder inflammation produces adult bladder hypersensitivity. *Journal of Pain*. 2006; **7**: 469–79.
96. Grunau RE, Oberlander TF, Whitfield MF *et al*. Demographic and therapeutic determinants of pain reactivity in very low birth weight neonates at 32 weeks' postconceptional age. *Pediatrics*. 2001; **107**: 105–12.
97. Pattinson D, Fitzgerald M. The neurobiology of infant pain: development of excitatory and inhibitory neurotransmission in the spinal dorsal horn. *Regional Anesthesia and Pain Medicine*. 2004; **29**: 36–44.
98. Lidow MS. Long-term effects of neonatal pain on nociceptive systems. *Pain*. 2002; **99**: 377–83.
99. Oberlander TF, Grunau RE, Whitfield MF *et al*. Biobehavioral pain responses in former extremely low birth weight infants at four months' corrected age. *Pediatrics*. 2000; **105**: e6.
100. Grunau RE, Whitfield MF, Petrie JH, Fryer EL. Early pain experience, child and family factors, as precursors of somatization: a prospective study of extremely premature and fullterm children. *Pain*. 1994; **56**: 353–9.
101. Saigal S, Feeny D, Rosenbaum P *et al*. Self-perceived health status and health-related quality of life of extremely low-birth-weight infants at adolescence. *Journal of the American Medical Association*. 1996; **276**: 453–9.
102. Shin SW, Eisenach JC. Peripheral nerve injury sensitizes the responses to visceral distension but not its inhibition by the antidepressant milnacipran. *Anesthesiology*. 2004; **100**: 671–3.

4

Genetics of chronic pain: crucial concepts in genetics and research tools to understand the molecular biology of pain and analgesia

BRADLEY E AOUIZERAT AND CHRISTINE A MIASKOWSKI

KEY LEARNING POINTS

- The genetics of pain is a complex trait, due to a combination of genetic and environmental factors.
- Methodological and technological developments in genetics make the study of the genetics of pain tenable.
- Measurement in pain genetics research is a unique and critical consideration.
- Common genetic influences on analgesic drugs are a critical field of pain research.

NOTE

This chapter is organized into two sections: the first section provides an introduction to concepts of and tools for the study of genetics and genomics; the second section delves into research-related issues unique to the study of pain.

CONCEPTS AND TOOLS IN GENETICS AND GENOMICS

INTRODUCTION

With few exceptions, all of the cells in the human body contain the same genetic material in the form of deoxyribonucleic acid (DNA). DNA is composed of a collection of functional units termed *genes* (collectively referred to as a *genome*) that provide the instructions for the synthesis of all ribonucleic acid (RNA)-based transcripts (an intermediary of most gene expression). In turn, these RNA transcripts provide the basis for the translation of all human proteins. However, different cell types each synthesize (or "express") a unique subset of the total possible RNA species and proteins encoded for by DNA. These differences in expression are the primary basis for the different cell types (as defined both in terms of their structure and function), as well as the cooperative assembly of various cell types into tissues and organs. The occurrence of changes in the nucleotide composition of a DNA molecule (a nucleotide is the "quantum unit" of

DNA), either through variations or mutations, can modify gene expression and resultant protein synthesis, thus altering cell structure and function. These genotypic changes lead to phenotypic changes that are observed as neuronal abnormalities, altered pain sensations, and/or a variety of medical conditions.

The Human Genome Project has increased our understanding of the contribution of genetics to health and human disease. While its initial goal was the mapping of the human genome, the project has expanded to map the genomes of many organisms. In addition, the Human Genome Project will determine the common population variations in given genomes, as well as their expression at both the RNA (transcriptome) and protein (proteome) levels. An in-depth description of the Human Genome Project can be found at www.genome.gov.

GENES AND CHROMOSOMES

Genes determine hereditary traits through the provision of precise instructions for cellular activity. Genes are both the functional and physical unit of heredity passed from parent to offspring. A gene is composed of a linear segment of DNA that encodes instructions for the synthesis of RNA molecules, which in turn provide the instructions for the synthesis of proteins. Each DNA molecule contains from tens to thousands of genes.

The nucleic acid sequence of a DNA molecule is encoded by four repeating nucleotide bases: adenine (A), cytosine (C), guanine (G), and thymine (T) (**Figure 4.1**). A DNA molecule is composed of two strands of nucleotides with the nucleic acids facing inward in an antiparallel fashion and the sugar-phosphate backbone forming a ladder-like structure which twists for stability. Nucleotide bases on each side of the ladder are linked by hydrogen bonds to form a base pair, with adenine coupled with thymine and guanine coupled with cytosine.

DNA molecules are wound around histone protein complexes that provide structural support and regulatory functions. This structure permits a remarkable amount of compaction, which results in condensed superstructures called chromosomes. Nucleated cells of humans have 23 pairs of morphologically distinct chromosomes, with one chromosome of a pair inherited from each parent. There are 22 autosomes and a pair of sex chromosomes. The chromosomes that form each pair are termed *homologs*, and with the exception of a set of genes harbored in the sex chromosomes, each chromosome pair provides two copies of each gene. The two copies of the gene are called *alleles*. The two alleles are referred to as *homozygous* if their sequence is the same and *heterozygous* if each allele's sequence is different. Chromosomes can be isolated from cells, stained and visualized by microscopy with the total chromosomal set of a cell termed a *karyotype* (**Figure 4.2**). Publication of the human genome sequence in 2000 provided more precise estimates of the position of genes and has largely superseded the use of karyotype analysis (i.e. chromosome banding). However, gross chromosomal abnormalities such as extra, missing, or broken chromosomes are still commonly identified by examining the karyotype.

In addition to the nuclear genome, DNA is contained in mitochondria. The mitochondrial genome is a compact circular DNA molecule and exists in multiple copies within each mitochondrion. The number of mitochondria found in each cell type is dependent on the energy requirements of that cell. Neurons are among the most mitochondrion-rich cell types. The human mitochondrial genome is composed of 37 genes, including 24 genes that encode RNA end-products (2 ribosomal RNAs (rRNA) and 22 transfer RNAs (tRNA)). Mitochondrial genomes are transmitted matrilineally to offspring as the only gamete that contains both cytoplasm and organelles is the human egg.

GENE EXPRESSION AND PROTEIN SYNTHESIS – REGULATION OF GENE EXPRESSION

Genes are transcribed into complementary single-stranded molecules of genetic material composed of RNA (**Figure 4.1**). The primary differences between DNA and RNA are the presence of a hydroxyl group at the 2′-position of the ribose sugar and the use of uracil (U) to replace thymine as the base complementary to adenine. Messenger RNA is then translated into the amino acid sequence of a protein at a cellular structure called the ribosome.

Subsets of RNA molecules serve as the end-product of gene expression. One subset, the rRNA genes, expresses only RNA which combines with proteins to form ribosomes that participate in protein translation of messenger RNA (mRNA). The other subset is tRNA genes whose products participate in protein synthesis by donating amino acids to a growing protein polypeptide chain. Only a small fraction of each RNA transcript is translated.

Most genes are organized into two main regions, the promoter and the coding regions. The promoter region lies immediately upstream of the coding region. A specific sequence of nucleotides in the promoter region interacts with protein complexes termed transcription factors in a dynamic manner to determine each gene's unique expression pattern (i.e. timing, quantity). In addition, transcription factors provide genes with the ability to interact with and respond to changes in the cellular environment.

The coding region is composed of exons (i.e. the portions of genes that are included in the mature mRNA) and introns (i.e. the portions of genes that are initially transcribed but are later processed, or spliced, out of the mature mRNA). The outer ends of genes are often untranslated and are termed the 5′- (the upstream or beginning) and 3′- (the downstream or end) regions

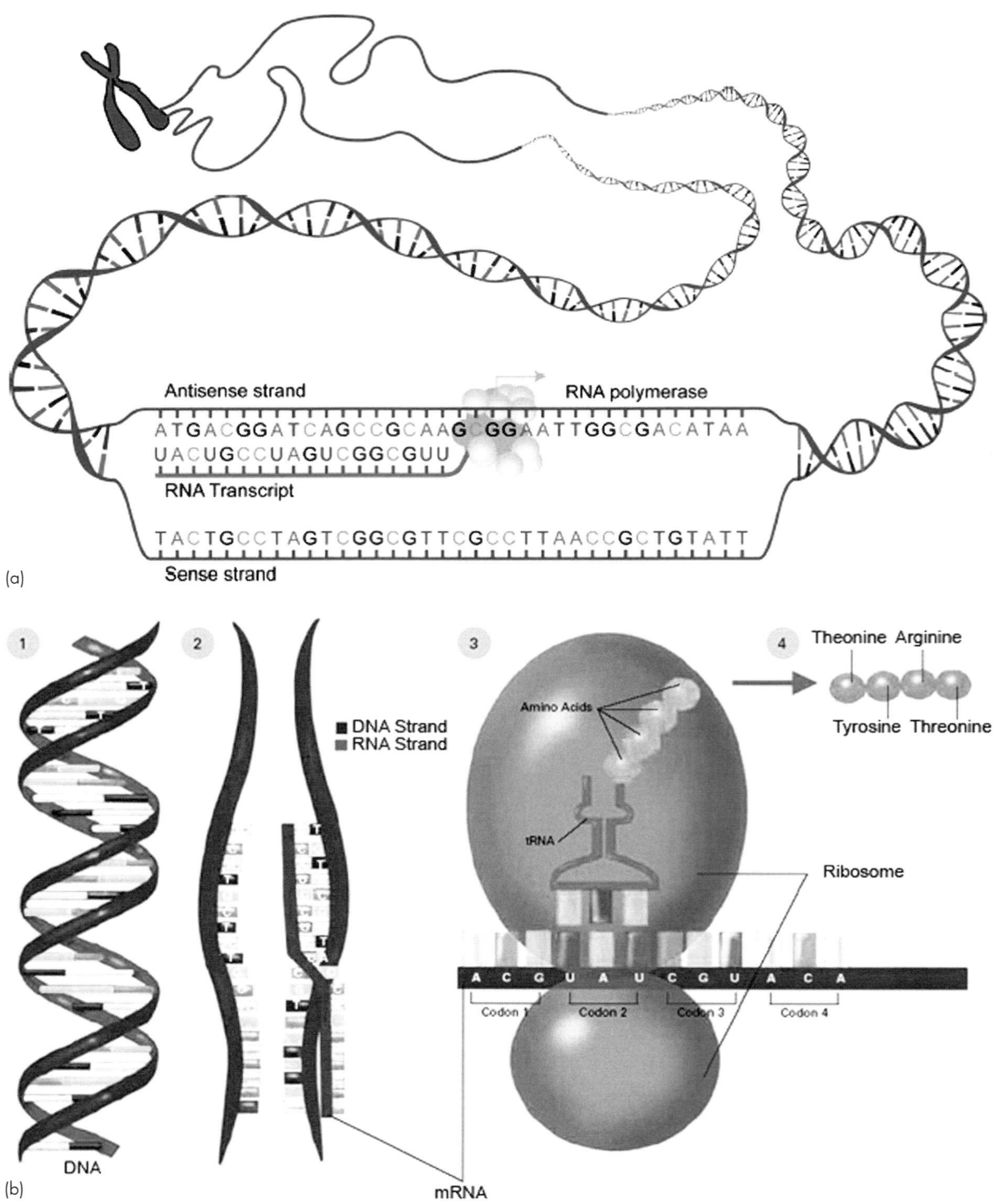

Figure 4.1 The structure of DNA contains information that is *transcribed* into RNA and subsequently *translated* into proteins. (a) The DNA molecule consists of two long strands of nucleotides that are complementary and which coil into a double helix for stability. The two strands (i.e. sense, antisense) are held together by hydrogen bonds between complementary nucleic acid bases: A with T, G with C. The double helix opens and one side is transcribed into a single complementary strand of mRNA. (b) The resulting mRNA is then translated into amino acids (read in units of three adjacent nucleotides, or *codons*) and a peptide chain is formed at a cell structure called the ribosome. The amino acid chain may be further processed to form a mature protein. (a) Reprinted from National Human Genome Research Institute. *Online Education Kit: Bioinformatics: Finding Genes.* Bethesda, MD, USA: National Human Genome Research Institute, last updated: April 27, 2007. Available from: www.genome.gov/25020001. (b) Reprinted from National Institute of General Medical Sciences. The New Genetics. Bethesda, MD, USA: National Institute of General Medical Sciences, 2006: 13. Available from: http://publications.nigms.nih.gov/thenewgenetics/index.html.

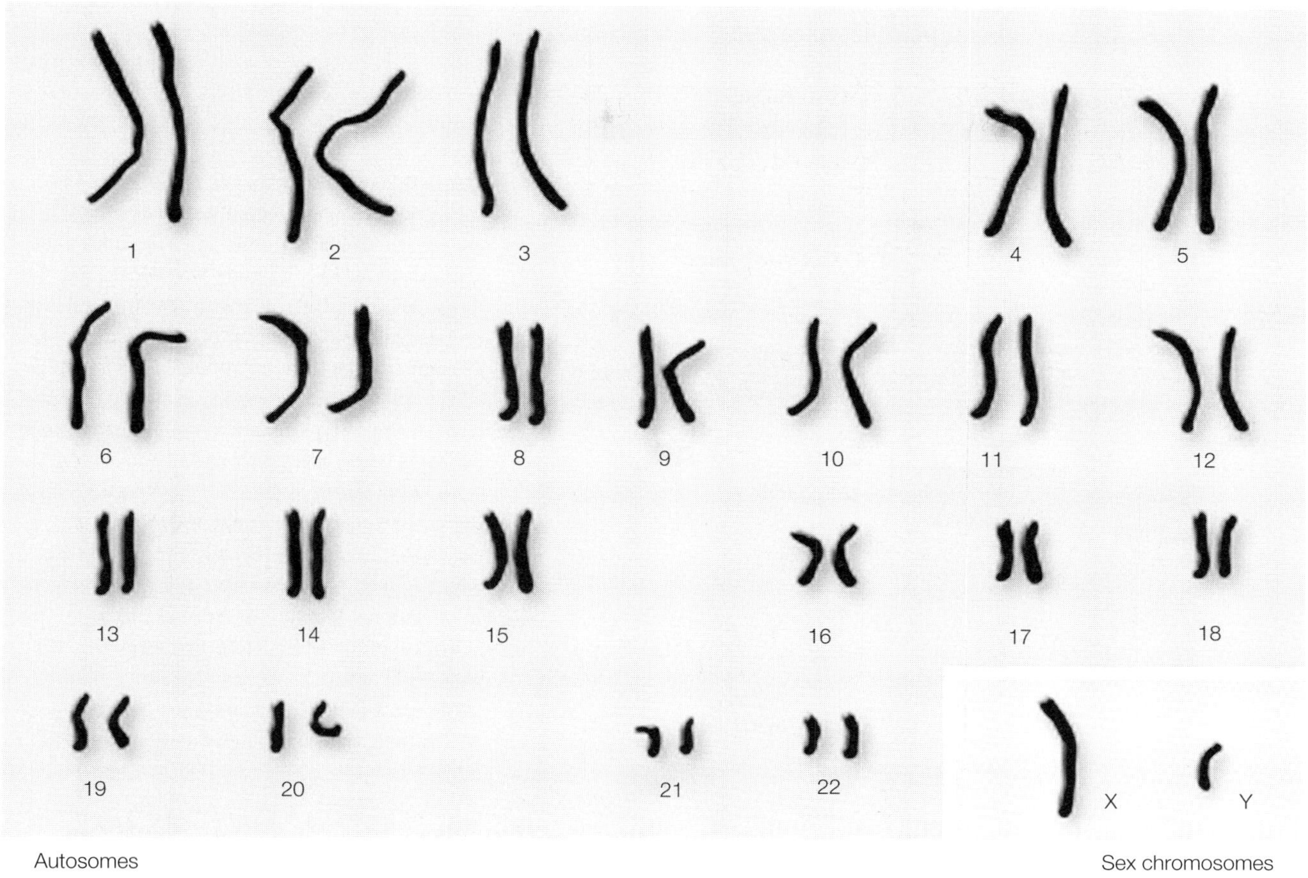

Figure 4.2 The human karyotype. There are 22 autosomal chromosomes or *autosomes*. The autosomal chromosomes are numbered from 1 to 22. Each of the chromosomes can be recognized by its size, shape, staining pattern, and the position of the centromere (the constriction at which sister chromatids are anchored prior to cell division). The largest autosome is number 1, and the smallest is number 21. Historically, the second smallest chromosome has been designated number 22. Y chromosome is about the same size as chromosome 22 and the X chromosome is larger than the Y chromosome. Reprinted from US National Library of Medicine. *Handbook: Help Me Understand Genetics*. Bethesda, MD, USA: US National Library of Medicine. Available from: http://ghr.nlm.nih.gov/handbook/basics/howmanychromosomes.

(**Figure 4.3**). In addition, an entire complement of exons encoded in a given gene need not be expressed, resulting in different species of RNA. These RNA species, generated by a process termed alternative splicing, can lead to different forms of proteins with associated functions.

Transcripts are threaded into ribosomes and are read in groups of three nucleotides termed codons. These codons interact with a tRNA that bears a complementary anti-codon to which is tethered an amino acid. Each codon is read in turn and the corresponding amino acid is added to the growing polypeptide chain (**Figure 4.1**). Though there are 64 possible codons (4^3 – four nucleotides read in groups of three), only 20 amino acids serve as the building blocks of proteins (**Figure 4.4**).

Gene expression is a dynamic and exquisitely regulated process. In each cell, a subset of genes is expressed at a basal level or is modulated while others are not expressed. Extracellular signals such as hormones, neurotransmitters, nutrients, and proteins can modulate gene expression. Differentiation of cell structure and function results from, and is influenced by, regulation of gene expression at the transcriptional, translational, and post-translational levels. Both innate and acquired changes (e.g. gene mutations, variations) in transcription factors, cofactors, signaling molecules, promoters, or coding regions of a gene can result in susceptibility to disease.

DNA AND HUMAN DIVERSITY

Though individuals can differ greatly in appearance and risk for disease, they are surprisingly alike at the genetic level, sharing approximately 99.9 percent of their genomes in common. This statistic is somewhat misleading in that the approximate 0.1 percent difference is comprised of as many as four million mutations and variations spanning approximately 12 million base pairs.[1] As opposed to mutations which occur in individuals or even

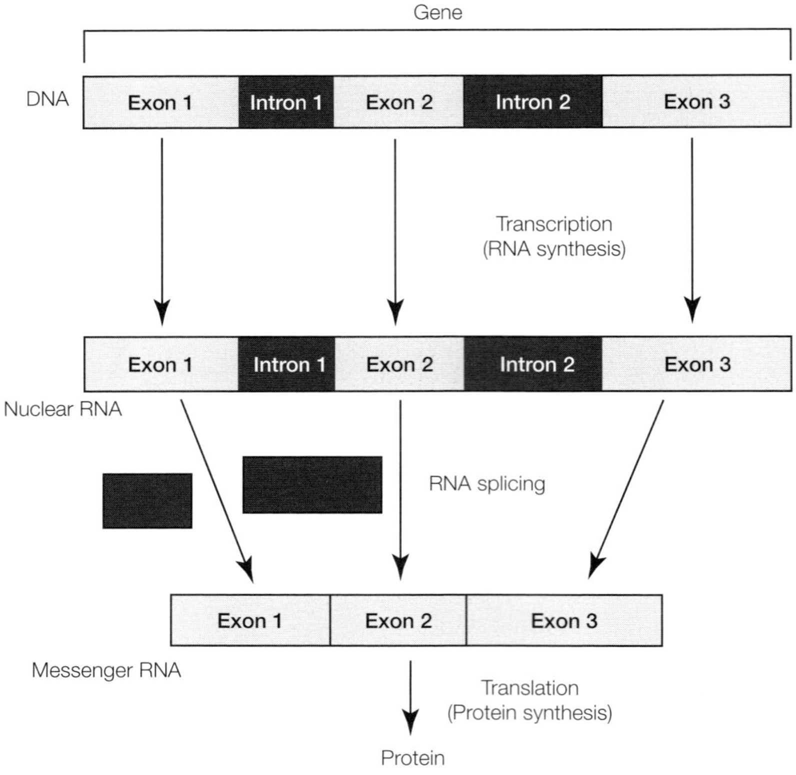

Figure 4.3 Transcription unit of a gene. The transcription unit of a gene has nucleotides providing information other than the nucleotide triplicates (codon) that code for amino acids. The promoter area is involved with regulation of the rate and tissue distribution of transcription. The initiator site and the initiation codon indicate where transcription and translation begins, respectively. The termination site and stop codon indicates where transcription and translation stops, respectively. Genes often have areas that are not included in the final mRNA (introns); exons are spliced together to form the mRNA, which is then translated into a protein. Reprinted from National Institute of General Medical Sciences. The New Genetics. Bethesda, MD, USA: National Institute of General Medical Sciences, 2006: 15. Available from: http://publications.nigms.nih.gov/thenewgenetics/index.html.

First (5') letter	Second letter: U		C		A		G		Third (3') letter
U	UUU	Phe	UCU	Ser	UAU	Tyr	UGU	Cys	U
	UUC		UCC		UAC		UGC		C
	UUA	Leu	UCA		UAA	Ochre#	UGA	Opal #	A
	UUG		UCG		UAG	Amber#	UGG	Trp	G
C	CUU	Leu	CCU	Pro	CAU	His	CGU	Arg	U
	CUC		CCC		CAC		CGC		C
	CUA		CCA		CAA	Gln	CGA		A
	CUG		CCG		CAG		CGG		G
A	AUU	Ileu	ACU	Thr	AAU	Asn	AGU	Ser	U
	AUC		ACC		AAC		AGC		C
	AUA		ACA		AAA	Lys	AGA	Arg	A
	AUG	Met*	ACG		AAG		AGG		G
G	GUU	Val	GCU	Ala	GAU	Asp	GGU	Gly	U
	GUC		GCC		GAC		GGC		C
	GUA		GCA		GAA	Glu	GGA		A
	GUG		GCG		GAG		GGG		G

Figure 4.4 Each codon in messenger RNA specifies the initiation signal, amino acid or termination signal called for in a given polypetide chain, or *protein*. * Initiation codon, # termination codons. Amino acid three-letter and single-letter abbreviations: alanine, Ala(A); arginine, Arg(R); aspartic acid, Asn(N); asparagine, Asx(B); cysteine, Cys(C); glutamine, Gln(Q); glutamic acid, Glu(E); glutamine, Glx(Z); glycine, Gly(G); histidine, His(H); isoluecine, Iso(I); leucine, Leu(L); lysine, Lys(K); methionine, Met(M); phenylalanine, Phe(F); proline, Pro(P); serine, Ser(S); threonine, Thr(T); tryptophan, Trp(W); tyrosine, Tyr(Y); valine, Val(V).

a family, sequence variations occur at frequencies ranging from 1 to 50 percent in the general population. These variations have the potential to influence many aspects of biology, health, and disease. The majority of these variations do not occur within the coding regions of the estimated 20,000 to 25,000 genes in the human genome. However, the remaining subset of variations that do occur in gene regions result in different alleles that provides a rich tool for human genetic investigation.

Genetic variations, also referred to as polymorphisms, occur in many forms and include: single nucleotide polymorphisms (SNPs), small-scale insertions/deletions, and repetitive elements (e.g. satellite DNA). Satellite DNA is common throughout the genome. These groups of variations are segments of DNA which are repeated in tandem and result in many alleles in the population. Historically, these satellite DNA have proven quite useful in the mapping of disease-causing genes in the human genome[2, 3] and to differentiate individuals (e.g. paternity testing[4]). By far the most common variations are SNPs. Polymorphisms (e.g. SNPs) can change a gene's transcript or protein product, alter a gene's temporal or spatial expression, or silence its expression altogether.

The impact of a mutation or a polymorphism on the phenotype of an individual depends on many factors. Phenotype refers to a characteristic or trait of an individual that is observable or measurable. One's genetic constitution, or genotype, is a major determinant of phenotype. For example, an individual heterozygous for a deleterious allele is likely to display an intermediate phenotype in comparison to an individual homozygous for this deleterious allele. Another factor that impacts a phenotype is whether an allele exerts a dominant, a recessive, or an additive influence. In the case of autosomal dominant inheritance, it takes only one mutated allele to express a trait. In the case of autosomal recessive inheritance, only an individual homozygous for the recessive allele will express the trait. Whether a trait is dominant or recessive in its inheritance depends in part on whether the functional effect of the mutation or variation can be compensated for by other factors. In the case of additive inheritance, each additional allele contributes incrementally to a trait.

A pedigree diagram is often used to visually represent the genetic history of a family for a given disease or trait (**Figure 4.5**). Pedigree charts are used to determine patterns of inheritance, as well as the risk that a specific individual will develop a trait or disease. Dominant and recessive patterns of inheritance can occur with the sex chromosomes and are termed X-linked or Y-linked dominant or recessive. Examples of autosomal dominant, autosomal recessive, and X-linked recessive inheritance are illustrated in **Figure 4.5a, 4.5b,** and **4.5c**, respectively. A less common pattern of inheritance is mitochondrial inheritance. Transmission is maternal and thus affected men do not pass on the trait.

A subset of individuals that carry a specific disease-causing genotype do not display the trait or disease because the disease or even the specific allele displays incomplete penetrance. Of note, a certain degree of penetrance is explained in part by the sensitivity of the measure of a phenotype. Variations in penetrance and phenotypic expression of a gene may be related to gene–gene interactions (i.e. one gene modulates the expression of another) or environment–gene interactions (i.e. environmental factors modulate the expression of a gene).

COMPLEX, MULTIFACTORIAL DISORDERS

Single gene (i.e. "Mendelian") disorders follow the patterns of inheritance discussed above under DNA and human diversity. However, many diseases are due to the combination of the inheritance of alleles with suboptimal function with environmental risk factors. These diseases or conditions are termed multifactorial. Each component allelic mutation or polymorphism displays varying degrees of penetrance. Therefore, the contribution of each polymorphism may be subtle and the severity of a trait will depend on the number of genes and alleles involved. Gene polymorphisms associated with altered risk for a disease are termed "susceptibility genes." The discovery and characterization of susceptibility genes and alleles for a number of medical conditions has accelerated since the Human Genome Project yielded both a draft sequence of the human genome and a growing compendium of SNPs. These SNPs can be used to screen for potential involvement of a polymorphism in a trait of interest.

Complex traits cluster in families and rarely appear to follow Mendelian patterns of inheritance. However, each component allele does follow a Mendelian pattern of inheritance but the component patterns are difficult to discern when classical genetics approaches (e.g. pedigree analysis) are used to analyze a genetic disorder.[5] Multifactorial traits emerge when genetic and environmental risk factors interact and surpass a critical threshold, resulting in a disease or medical condition defined by specific phenotypic characteristics (e.g. clinical criteria).

The impact of environmental and lifestyle factors on the disease phenotype is complicated and difficult to predict. This complexity arises from the fact that environmental factors interact with individual susceptibility genes in different ways, which influences the contribution of each susceptibility gene to the risk for a trait or disease. In addition, the amount of exposure to environmental factors varies among individuals and is often difficult to quantify accurately, further complicating estimates of risk. Environmental factors may include pathogens, lifestyle factors (e.g. diet, exercise, stress), injury (e.g. surgery, infection), and toxins. Environmental factors can act at the genetic (i.e. DNA-damaging agents), expression (i.e. influencing RNA stability or turnover), and protein levels. Because RNA and proteins act as the molecular machinery of the cell, they mediate cellular phenotype and the balance between health and disease.

Environmental factors can influence biologic processes in a number of ways, including:

- acting as a signal that is transduced through cellular machinery (i.e. receptor-mediated signal transduction);
- by modifying or interacting with a protein that influences the protein's action;
- by modifying the effect of other signals.

APPROACHES USED TO CONDUCT GENETIC STUDIES

Depending on clinical characteristics, population frequency, and methods of measurement for specific trait(s), research designs may be either observational or

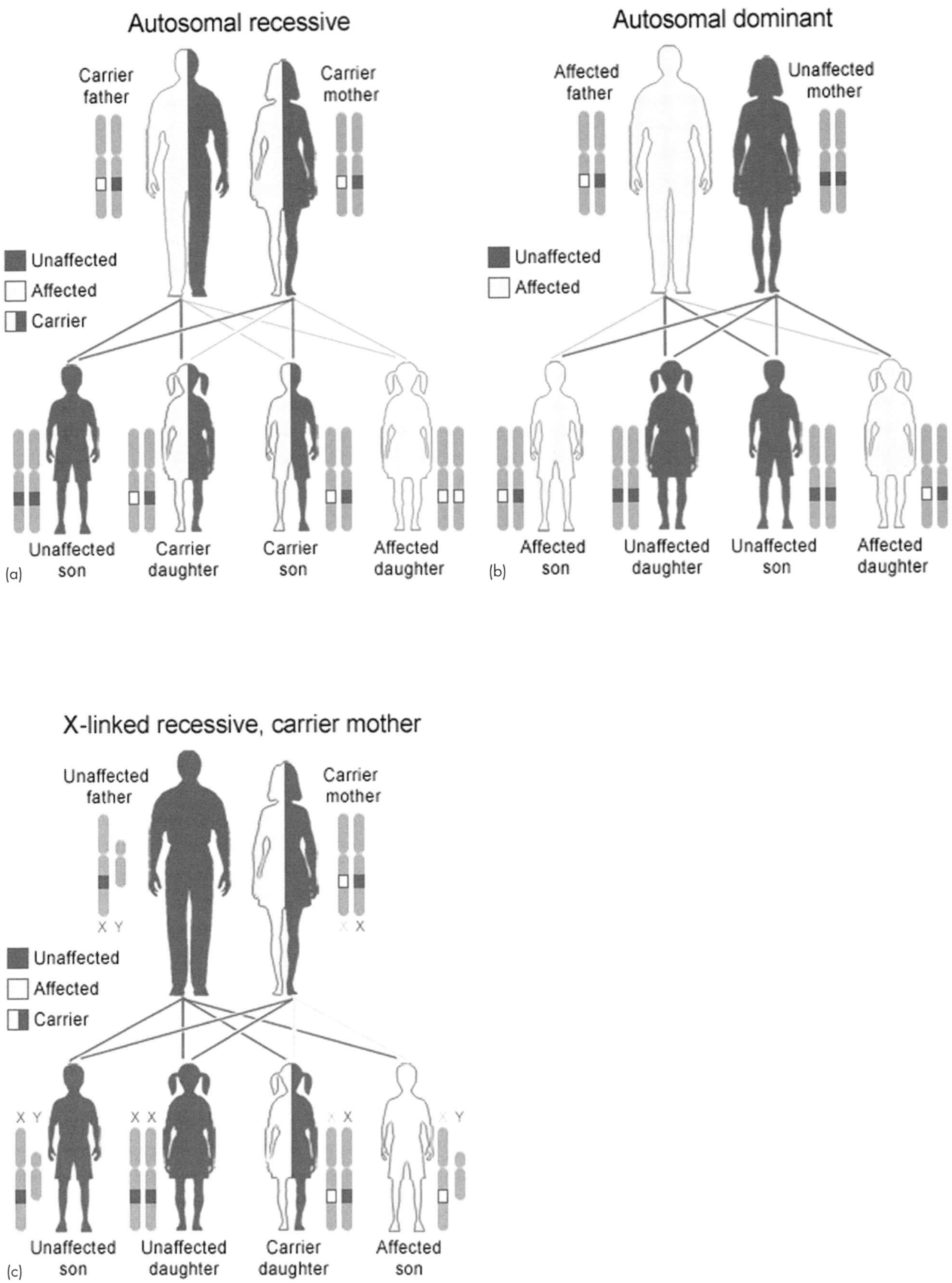
Autosomal recessive
Carrier father
Carrier mother
Unaffected
Affected
Carrier
Unaffected son
Carrier daughter
Carrier son
Affected daughter
(a)
Autosomal dominant
Affected father
Unaffected mother
Unaffected
Affected
Affected son
Unaffected daughter
Unaffected son
Affected daughter
(b)
X-linked recessive, carrier mother
Unaffected father
X Y
Carrier mother
X X
Unaffected
Affected
Carrier
X Y
X X
X X
X Y
Unaffected son
Unaffected daughter
Carrier daughter
Affected son
(c)

experimental (**Table 4.1**). Experimental methods can be employed to study groups of individuals (e.g. clinical trial, cohort),[18] animal models (e.g. knock-out, knock-in, knock-down, knock-up, transgenic animal models),[19] cells (e.g. cell culture),[20] or specific proteins (e.g. biochemical assay). Observational methods usually involve groups of individuals (e.g. case–control, cohort, family-based).[5, 18] Given the uncertainty surrounding the accuracy of characterizing a trait in terms of measurement of the phenotype (e.g. self-report of pain intensity), a combination of approaches is often pursued. For example, animal models are used to study the pathophysiology of a pain condition and to identify potential genes and pathways. These findings are then used to guide the design and execution of studies in humans.

Genetic epidemiology

Epidemiology is the study of factors that contribute to health and disease in the population with the goal of disease prevention.[18] Genetic epidemiology focuses on the identification of genetic and environmental risk factors that predispose individuals in families and populations to disease.[5] Genetic epidemiology generally follows three steps:

1. providing evidence that a genetic component exists for the trait of interest;
2. estimating the relative size of said genetic component in relation to other factors that influence the trait (e.g. environmental factors, other genetic factors);
3. identifying the gene(s) that underlie the genetic component of the disease.

These three steps can be pursued by either population studies (termed association studies) or family studies which can involve genetic risk, segregation, linkage, or association analyses.

Genetic studies, step 1: evidence of heritability

Genetic risk studies evaluate the contribution of genetics to a trait as compared to the environment and are pursued by family-based, twin, or adoption studies.[21] Twin studies compare the degree to which monozygotic twins (who share 100 percent of their genes) are concordant for a specific trait as compared to dizygotic twins (who share 50 percent of their genes in common). The greater the similarity between monozygotic twins compared to dizygotic twins, the greater the evidence of a heritable component to a medical condition.

Genetic studies, step 2: estimating the pattern of inheritance

Segregation analysis employs multigenerational families to fit a model for the genetic component of interest (e.g. autosomal recessive, X-linked, or environmental (no evidence of genetic component)).[21] It is most useful in Mendelian disorders. It is a less powerful technique in the analysis of complex traits when multiple genes each with multiple alleles are involved. Segregation analysis is a prerequisite for parametric linkage analyses.

Genetic studies, step 3: identifying genes that cosegregate with a phenotype

Initially, linkage studies can be used in a hypothesis-based evaluation of the cosegregation of gene variations in "candidate genes" with a trait.[22] A candidate gene is defined as a gene that may contribute to a trait based on

Figure 4.5 A pedigree is a diagram of a family's members and their relationship to the member who was identified as having a genetic trait of interest (the proband). Typically, three generations or more are collected by a medical geneticist, advanced practice nurse, genetic counselor, or geneticist. (a) A pedigree of autosomal recessive inheritance. In this example, two unaffected parents each carry one copy of a gene mutation (they are each heterozygous) for an autosomal recessive disorder. They have one affected child (homozygous) and three unaffected children, two of which carry one copy of the gene mutation (again, they are heterozygous). Each offspring's risk of receiving a recessive allele is one half from each parent. Therefore, each offspring of two carriers has a 25 percent chance of being affected, a 50 percent of chance of being a carrier, and a 25 percent chance of inheriting neither mutant allele. Both genders are equally likely to be affected. (b) A pedigree of autosomal dominant inheritance. In this example, a man with an autosomal dominant disorder has two affected children and two unaffected children. In a typical autosomal dominant inheritance, every affected individual in a pedigree has an affected parent, who also has an affected parent. It also affects several generations. Both sexes are equally likely to be affected and a male-to-male transmission exists. Each offspring of an affected parent has a 50 percent chance of being affected. (c) A pedigree of X-linked recessive inheritance. In this example, an unaffected woman carries one copy of a gene mutation for an X-linked recessive disorder. She has an affected son, an unaffected daughter who carries one copy of the mutation, and two unaffected children who do not have the mutation. There is no male-to-male transmission. All daughters of an affected male are carriers. Sons of a carrier mother have a 50 percent chance of being affected. Daughters of a carrier mother have a 50 percent chance of being carriers. Reprinted from US National Library of Medicine. Handbook: Help Me Understand Genetics. Bethesda, MD, USA: US National Library of Medicine. Available from: http://ghr.nlm.nih.gov/handbook/inheritance.

Table 4.1 Examples of pain research that used different study designs.

Category	Type	Author	Purpose
Experimental studies	Clinical trial	Hudcova *et al.*[6]	To conduct a meta-analysis to evaluate the efficacy of patient-controlled analgesia (PCA) versus conventional analgesia (e.g. a nurse administering an analgesic upon a patient's request) for postoperative pain control
		Huas *et al.*[7]	To evaluate the impact of using pain assessment scales on the management of musculoskeletal chronic pain employing a cluster-randomized controlled multicenter trial with practices randomized by region before patient recruitment
		Linde *et al.*[8]	To compare patient characteristics and outcomes between a randomized controlled trial and an observational study of acupuncture treatment in patients with migraine
	Cohort	Ives *et al.*[9]	To estimate the incidence and risk factors for opioid misuse in patients with chronic pain in a prospective cohort study of patients enrolled in a chronic pain disease management program within an academic internal medicine practice
	Animal model	Lichtman *et al.*[10]	To test whether anandamide and other non-cannabinoid fatty amides modulate nociception in a fatty acid amide hydrolase FAAH deficient mouse model as compared to FAAH positive mice employing a series of tests (i.e. tail immersion, hot plate, formalin tests, thermal hyperalgesia in the carrageenan, chronic constriction injury)
		Al-Khrasani, *et al.*[11]	To examine the antinociceptive effects of peripheral micro-opioid receptor agonists (e.g. 14-O-methyloxymorphone, DAMGO and morphine) were evaluated in a mouse model of visceral pain
	In vitro	Huang *et al.*[12]	To understand whether the proton-sensing G-protein-coupled receptors (PS-GPCR) are expressed in nociceptors, four PS-GPCR (i.e. OGR1, GPR4, G2A, TDAG8) were cloned, their tissue distribution examined, and their localization in pain-relevant loci (i.e. the dorsal root ganglion) determined
Observational studies	Case–control	Kang *et al.*[13]	To investigate the association between an estrogen receptor alpha polymorphism and pain susceptibility in a case-control study of female symptomatic temporomandibular joint osteoarthritis
	Cohort	Diatchenko *et al.*[14]	In order to identify genes that contribute to interindividual variability on pain sensitivity a cohort of healthy pain-free females were assessed for pain perception thresholds and genotyped for candidate genes
		Gansky *et al.*[15]	To assess the distribution of widespread pain, tender points, and fibromyalgia in young African American and Caucasian women in a community population of young women
	Family-based	Indo *et al.*[16]	To identify mutations in the nerve growth factor receptor tyrosine kinase (NTRK1) that underlie congenital insensitivity to pain in nine families
	Animal model	Chesler *et al.*[17]	To examine the heritability of sensitivity to analgesia from gabapentin and pregabalin as a precursor to linkage mapping efforts, 11 inbred mouse strains were tested for inhibition of nociception by gabapentin or pregabalin in two different preclinical assays of inflammatory pain (i.e. formalin test, zymosan thermal hyperalgesia on the paw-withdrawal test)

the biochemical properties of its gene product. Alternatively, one can identify genes in a hypothesis-free manner by screening a set of genetic markers that span the entire genome or discrete chromosomal segments. Linkage studies attempt to locate gene(s) that underlie the trait(s) of interest.[5] Linkage approaches can be used in any organism for which pedigrees can be collected and in which a genetic marker set of sufficient density is available (e.g. human, mouse,[23] dog,[24] fruit fly,[25, 26] zebrafish[27, 28]) to interrogate the genome.

Linkage analysis examines the cosegregation of genetic markers (e.g. SNPs) within families whereas association is meant to provide information on the involvement of specific alleles in a trait of interest in a group of unrelated individuals.[21] One potential weakness of association studies is the fact that cryptic relatedness or population substructure (e.g. self-reported ethnicity may not adequately capture different subpopulations that may self-identify as the same ethnicity and could result in chance differences in the proportions of such subpopulations between cases and controls) thereby confounding the results. Although association studies are susceptible to confounding due to differences in population substructure, they have several advantages over linkage analysis, including:

- the need to recruit multigenerational families where the contribution of family members to the analysis is difficult to ascertain a priori is obviated;
- the power to detect alleles with weak effects, and the ability to provide estimates of the relative magnitude of the effects of multiple alleles.

Several variations and mixtures of the above-mentioned study designs and statistical genetic analyses exist, but are beyond the scope of this chapter. For an in-depth review of these methods and analyses, the reader is directed to *Analysis of human genetic linkage*.[29] An in-depth exploration of the use of murine models is provided by Lee Silver.[30] An excellent description of the use of mammalian models in the study of the genetics of pain is available.[23]

EXPRESSION ANALYSES: RNA-BASED STUDIES

Gene expression is a complex and exquisitely regulated process that enables cells, tissues, systems, and even the entire organism to respond dynamically to both internal and external stimuli. While all nucleated cells each contain a copy of the entire genome, only a subset of its genes is expressed. Such cell- or even tissue-specific gene expression results in the production of a different set of proteins. This genetic expression renders the identity of these cells, as well as how they interact with their environment. In as much as one can isolate the cell- or tissue-type(s) of interest, the study of gene expression can provide unique and vital insights into biologic function and even the pathophysiology of disease. Expression analyses involve not only the presence or absence of gene expression, but the quantification of the level of expression. This approach provides more information than genetic analyses alone.

While the study of a single or a small set of genes expression has been possible for over three decades, recent technological advances have permitted the study of vast if not global patterns of gene expression (i.e. the sum total of a cell's gene expression termed the "transcriptome"). In addition, new technologies provide a level of both sensitivity and specificity hitherto unavailable using classical electrophoresis gel-based methods.

Perhaps the two most influential technological developments in molecular biology are the availability of quantitative real-time PCR (see **Box 4.1**) and the development of high-density arrays of oligonucleotides that are complementary to a large fraction of the RNA species

Box 4.1 Quantitative polymerase chain reaction

The most common method of DNA analysis is based on the amplification of segments of DNA from a small amount of DNA. The technology, polymerase chain reaction (PCR), is an enzymatic process that results in site-specific DNA replication by the inclusion of a specific set of small nucleotide sequences (termed primers) that flank a sequence of interest, an excess of nucleotide building blocks [A, T, G, C], and a heat-resistant form of DNA polymerase that can be manipulated thermally to rapidly replicate a sequence of interest. Because DNA replication results in a doubling of the target region with every cycle of the reaction, PCR results in the exponential amplification of a region of interest. This approach results in hundreds of millions of replicated copies within 35–40 cycles of PCR carried out over the period of a few hours. Resulting PCR products (termed amplicons) can be visualized using a host of solid-state (e.g. gel electrophoresis, oligonucleotide hybridization) or fluidic (e.g. florescence-resonance energy transfer) processes. Both DNA and RNA can be readily analyzed by this method.

Quantitative polymerase chain reaction (qPCR) is a modification of PCR that allows for the florescent quantitation of PCR amplicons at each cycle of the reaction. Where PCR is only semi-quantitative in nature (since PCR-amplification is approximately exponential, the number of amplification cycles and the amount of amplicons measured after the last cycle can be used to derive the approximate initial concentration of starting material), qPCR measures the concentration of amplicons at each cycle and can more accurately estimate the starting concentrations of targets of interest (termed real-time PCR). RNA can be similarly estimated by first adding reverse transcriptase, which results in a complementary DNA molecule that can then be measured as described above (termed real-time (RT-PCR)).

transcribed in a cell. These arrays, termed microarrays, allow for the rapid, efficient, and simultaneous analysis of almost the entire transcriptome of an organism of interest. RNA analysis has always relied on the property of genetic material to recognize, or hybridize, its reverse complement (e.g. AGTTAC will recognize and hybridize to TCAATG). Microarray technology exploits this property on a solid support (e.g. a membrane or even a small glass microscope slide) and at an impressively high density to allow for the simultaneous analysis of hundreds to tens of thousands of RNA species in a single experiment.

Typically, experiments involving gene expression microarrays adopted one of two designs. In the first experimental design, the RNA from two different cell types (e.g. cells exposed to two different stimuli, cells from an individual with and an individual without a trait or disease, or even cells followed over time) serve as the template for the synthesis of complementary DNA (cDNA) labeled with differentiating chromogenic reagents. The two cDNA pools are mixed and allowed to compete for the same target sequences on the array. The excess cDNA (i.e. the RNA surrogate) from one or the other comparison group results in an increase in the amount of that chromogen bound to the target sequence (**Figure 4.6**). In the second design, the cDNA from each tissue being compared is hybridized to different chips and the absolute levels of each RNA species bound to the target sequence are compared. Common uses of expression analyses include susceptibility gene discovery, drug development, drug response, and therapy development.

DNA microarrays refer to the class of high-throughput technologies that permit the screening of hundreds to hundreds of thousands of variant sequences (e.g. SNPs, copy number variations). DNA from an individual or organism under study is applied to the microarray. Complementary sequences hybridize to their target, which

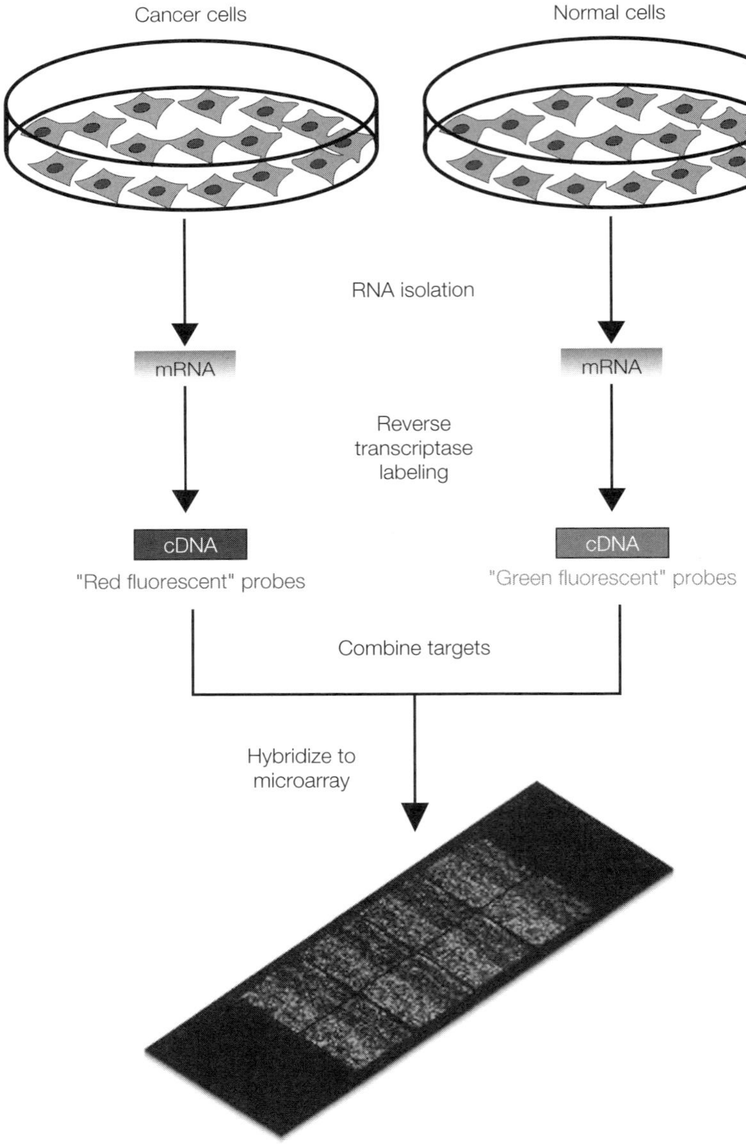

Figure 4.6 Two different tissues are isolated and rendered for their RNA. The RNA is reverse-transcribed into cDNA and each pool of RNA is labeled with a different chromogenic agent (i.e. red, green). The labeled specimens are mixed and allowed to compete for the same target sequences imbedded on the microarray. When a specific cDNA from a given pool is present at a greater concentration than the comparison group (e.g. green-labeled cDNA), more labeled cDNA species will hybridize to the target sequence and that "spot" on the microarray will fluoresce green not red. Thus, green spots indicate higher levels of a given cDNA from the green pool. Red spots indicate higher levels of a given cDNA from the pool labeled with the red chromogenic agent. Yellow spots indicate equal levels of each cDNA species. And black spots mean no cDNA from either pool was present in sufficient levels to bind a target sequence. Reprinted from http://en.wikipedia.org/wiki/Image:Microarray-schema.jpg.

permits simultaneous assay of all of the sequences (i.e. polymorphisms) featured on the microarray. Common uses of DNA microarrays include susceptibility gene discovery and drug development. Recent success in the application of DNA microarray-based gene discovery for migraine suggest that population genetic studies of pain phenotypes are now tenable.[31] In addition, the recent release of commercial DNA microarray-based pain candidate gene panels (http://www.congenics.com) represents an intriguing research tool to explore inter-individual variation in pain, analgesia, and allodynia in human populations.

Both DNA and RNA expression arrays are visualized in a similar manner following hybridization. DNA microarrays are biotin-labeled and are recorded in black and white, with lack of hybridization recorded as black. With RNA expression arrays, the chromogenic agents are usually red and green. A red fluorescent signal indicates that there is excess of the RNA species labeled with the red chromogenic agent. A green fluorescent signal indicates that there is excess of the RNA species labeled with the green chromogenic agent. A yellow fluorescent signal indicates equal levels of each cell's RNA species binding to a given spot and black indicates lack of hybridization to a spot.

Microarrays are placed into a reader or scanner where a laser excites the chromomeric label and a microscope fitted with a high-resolution digital camera records the digital image of the array. The hybridization data are analyzed by computer software which processes the hybridization signals, as well as various quality control indicators imbedded on the array, to provide semi-quantitative (e.g. DNA genotypes) or quantitative (e.g. RNA transcript level) information for each spot on the microarray. The algorithms used by microarray analysis software are evolving. Gene expression profiles are generated that can be used to examine differences in the level of single transcripts, differences in gene expression of an entire pathway, or even a series of pathways.

While microarrays allow for comprehensive surveys of gene expression, many challenges remain in how to interpret microarray data. The optimal method of statistical analysis is a subject of ongoing research and debate. Moreover, the expression profiles of a pathophysiologic process can only be studied if the tissue in question can be assessed directly. This requirement is a near impossible proposition for many human diseases and for many painful conditions where central nervous system tissue is involved in the pathophysiological process. Lastly, the function and catalog of genes and their expressed products is incomplete, which leaves many expression profiles difficult to interpret. Ultimately, as more information accumulates, microarray technology will allow for the pursuit of increasingly more complex questions. An active area of development is the combination of both DNA microarrays and gene expression microarrays in order to integrate the role of common gene variations with associated differences in gene expression.[32]

One could imagine that the identification of genes associated with a pain phenotype in a study population could be coupled with RNA expression profiles generated from tissue isolated from the same population. These data would be used to identify entire pathways of genes whose expression changes in individuals that carry specific gene variations associated with pain sensitivity. These observations could be used to identify specific genes whose expression may be rate-limiting for pain. Alternatively, some genes suggested by this approach may provide better targets for pharmacotherapy based on the population prevalence of a gene variation and its associated influence on gene expression. This combined comprehensive analysis is termed "systems biology."

PROTEOME ANALYSES: PROTEIN-BASED STUDIES

The term proteome is a blend of the words "proteins" and "genome." Initially, it was meant to describe the entire complement of proteins expressed by a genome, cell, tissue, or organism. However, the term is now used to refer to all of the expressed proteins at a given time point under defined conditions by a genome, cell, tissue, or organism. For example, a cellular proteome refers to the collection of proteins in a specific cell type under particular environmental conditions. Due to the fact that many of the genes in a genome can form different proteins due to alternative splicing; that proteins can be modified after their synthesis (termed, post-translational modifications); and that combinations of proteins can form larger multimeric complexes, the proteome is generally considered to be larger than the genome.

Historically, the study of the proteome, termed proteomics, was pursued through the electrophoretic separation of proteins using a gel matrix. Initially, these gels were carried out in one dimension (e.g. based on protein size, shape, or charge). Currently, two-dimensional gel electrophoresis is the standard approach. Proteins are separated based on charge in the first dimension through a slab of gel that is then turned 90° and loaded onto a second gel that separates proteins based on their molecular weight. The gel is then treated with a dye or stain used to visualize all of the proteins in the gel. These two-dimensional profiles are photographed and compared. Specific spots can be excised for further analysis (e.g. a spot that is present, absent, or occurs at a different concentration than another sample's two-dimensional profile). This excised material can be submitted to a subsequent round of two-dimensional analysis to further separate the proteins. Alternatively, the material can be sequenced in order to identify the specific protein(s).

More recently, mass spectroscopy promises to advance the field of proteomics. Two different methods of mass spectroscopy are being applied: peptide mass fingerprinting and tandem mass spectroscopy. Peptide mass fingerprinting identifies a protein by cleaving it into short peptides and uses a peptide sequence database to align the short peptides and then deduce the protein's identity by matching it against proteins in the database. By comparison, tandem mass spectrometry derives sequence information from individual peptides that are isolated and then collided with a nonreactive gas. Data on the array of fragment ions produced is recorded and analyzed. Unlike genome- and transcriptome-based methods, proteomic analyses struggle to attain the same level of throughput. The major limitation is that proteins cannot be amplified in a manner similar to nucleic acid amplification and the cost of mass spectroscopy is prohibitive.

THE NEW FRONTIER: SYSTEMS BIOLOGY

Systems biology focuses on the study of emergent properties, defined as important features of biologic systems that are often discerned only by examination of the system as a whole. Until recently, the study of the genetic component in the etiology of disease was limited to the study of single genes, their message, and/or its protein. The advent of high throughput methods made possible by both advances in data analysis and technology allows for the interrogation of entire genomes and their expression (i.e. the transcriptome, the proteome). Such systems-level approaches are being applied in ever-evolving and innovative ways, to the study of organisms, tissues, cells, and even organelles. Of particular interest is the growing focus on systems biology, where the findings from several lines of inquiry (e.g. a genome search and a gene expression analysis) are integrated to gain further insight into a biologic process, be it physiologic or pathophysiologic. A goal of this approach is to construct networks of genes, proteins, even metabolites, that act in concert to create a biological process. For an in-depth review, see Ref. 32.

RESEARCH-RELATED ISSUES UNIQUE TO THE STUDY OF PAIN ALLELES

GENETICS AND PAIN SENSITIVITY

Despite the challenges in the measurement of pain, the discovery of genes and gene variations involved in pain sensitivity is advancing. Clinical characteristics, population frequency, and methods of measurement for specific trait(s) continue to play important roles in the research design of studies of pain (**Table 4.1**). For example, an estimate of the heritability of pain sensitivity in humans was recently explored by studying a group of 51 monozygotic and 47 dizygotic female twins.[33] Evidence for a genetic component for a range of painful stimuli (e.g. heat pain threshold, the pain rating during induction of a thermal burn) was observed with estimates ranging between 22 and 55 percent. Of note, not all phenotypic measurements of pain provided evidence of a genetic component. The area of skin flare following thermal burn induction did not have a significant genetic component. This finding indicates that careful assessment of the painful phenotype is critical for any genetic study.

A striking demonstration of the role of genetics in the control of human pain was demonstrated by Cox and colleagues.[34] Three distinct mutations in the sodium channel N9A (SCN9A) gene that encodes the alpha subunit of the voltage-gates sodium channel (Nav1.7) result in a rare and complete inability to sense pain and exhibit an autosomal recessive pattern of inheritance.[34] Nav1.7 is highly expressed in nociceptive neurons.

Of note, genetic modulation of pain is not limited to the nuclear genome. Several human diseases (e.g. cardiomyopathy, neuropathy, deafness) are caused by mitochondrial gene mutations. In addition, acquired deficiencies in mitochondrial function are thought to lead to some forms of neuropathy.

The elegant control of a gene's expression is also fertile ground for the characterization of the mechanisms that control pain. For example, the mu opioid receptor, the endogenous receptor for opioid drugs, has several functional splice variants in mammals.[35,36] Of note, each splice variant displays a different affinity for exogenous opioid ligands (e.g. mu, kappa, delta opioids).

THE COMPLEXITIES OF DETERMINING GENETIC RISK FACTORS FOR CHRONIC PAIN

The concept of complex traits is particularly relevant to the study of pain. Indeed, researchers and clinicians have long appreciated that sensitivity to pain and pain-related traits (e.g. response to analgesics) are highly variable. Both classic and novel genetic techniques are essential tools to study the genetics of pain in both animals and humans. These approaches will be enhanced through the use of precise measures to characterize a particular painful condition (i.e. the "pain" phenotype) or pain management intervention (**Table 4.2**). While the investigation of specific traits such as sensitivity to pain or opioids has met with some success (for a review see Mogil *et al.*[37]), systematic investigations of the role of genetics in pain perception, painful conditions, and responses to pain management interventions are still in their infancy.

An additional caveat to assessment of familial aggregation is that environmental or cultural factors can lead to familial clustering and risk in the absence of a genetic component. Both acute and chronic pain states are known to be influenced by a variety of environmental, social, and cultural factors. Therefore, these factors will need to be considered and measured as part of studies that evaluate the genetics of pain and pain treatments. Currently, there are no published reports of multigenerational family studies of pain. This approach might

Table 4.2 Examples of measurements used in pain research.

Class	Organism	Methods	Pros	Cons
In vivo	Human	Physiological measurement Self-report instruments	Understanding interindividual differences in response to pain in humans is the goal of the field	Physiological measures of pain still require a verbal response, introducing an unknown level of imprecision Self-report measures are subjective in nature, introducing an unknown level of imprecision
	Animal model	Physiological measurement	Use of inbred strains of animals for genetic studies is a proven tool in the dissection of genetic traits	The study of the genetics of pain in animal models may be difficult to translate to human pain biology
	Other models	*Drosophila melanogaster* (fruitfly) genetic studies	Use of *D. melanogaster* for genetic studies is a proven tool in the dissection of genetic traits	The study of the genetics of pain in *D. melanogaster* may be difficult to translate to human pain biology
In vitro	Various (e.g. human, animal, other)	Cell culture	Permits exquisite control of the cellular environment and manipulation of exposures to test hypotheses	May provide limited insight into the dynamic physiologic environment *in vivo* Some tissue models cannot be emulated *in vitro* (e.g. complex interactions between cell types)
In silico	–	Data mining	Relatively inexpensive to mine databases for DNA, RNA, protein, and interaction data	Requires an understanding of bioinformatics

be useful to investigate the genetic basis for chronic pain problems that appear to occur in family members (e.g. chronic low back pain,[38, 39] fibromyalgia[40]).

PHARMACOGENETICS AND ANALGESIC DRUGS

Drug response is a complex trait that is governed by many processes and is multifactorial. The study of the genes that influence drug response is termed pharmacogenetics. The study of the entire complement of genes that influence drug response in an individual is termed pharmacogenomics. Though drug discovery progressively incorporates knowledge of the genetic factors that influence their metabolism, genetic tests that can predict an individual's response to a specific drug remain limited. Improvements in both the assessment of gene variations (e.g. microarray methods) and in an understanding of the genes and metabolic pathways that dictate the pharmacokinetics and the pharmacodynamics of drugs are contributing greatly to the development of genetic tests that may predict an individual's response to a drug (e.g. positive, negative). Examples of the pharmacogenetic discoveries in pain and analgesia are listed in **Table 4.3**.

The potential benefits of pharmacogenomics are manifold. In addition, to being able to identify individuals who will or will not respond adversely to a particular drug, the identification of individuals who may need a different dose will minimize the amount of titration required to obtain the optimal effect and perhaps reduce the number and severity of adverse effects. An additional benefit would be in the area of drug development, where specific pharmacogenetic entry criteria for clinical trials would limit the sample to persons more likely to respond to the test drug. This approach would increase the chance that a given drug would make it to market. In addition, clinical trials would require fewer participants thus reducing cost, decreasing the time to conduct a trial, and reducing the risk to participants. Presumably, this approach would culminate in a reduction in drug costs and allow physicians to prescribe the drug to the patients who would most likely benefit from it.

Table 4.3 Pharmacogenetic candidate genes.

Gene	Name	Trait	Reference
OPRM1	Mu-opioid receptor	Presence of the G allele for rs17181017 is associated with a difference in the standard dose in order to obtain similar effects as those individuals that carry the common allele. Affected analgesics include: afentanil, morphine, M6G, and levomethadone	41, 42, 43
COMT	Catechol-*O*-methyl transferase	Presence of the A allele for rs4680 is associated with a difference in the standard dose of morphine in order to obtain similar effects as those individuals that carry the common allele	44
MC1R	Melanocortin-1-receptor	Three polymorphisms associated with a difference in the standard dose of an analgesic in order to obtain similar effects as those individuals that carry the common allele. Affected analgesics include: morphine (polymorphism: 29insA), M6G (polymorphism: rs1805007), and pentazocine (polymorphism: rs1805008; women only)	45
CYP2D6	Cytochrome P450 2D6	Various polymorphisms and genetic lesions have been associated with altered drug metabolism. Affected analgesics include: tramadol and codeine	46

Adapted from Lotsch *et al.*[47]

Table 4.4 Tools available for the study of the genetics of pain.

Level of inquiry	Approach (methods)	Advantages	Disadvantages
DNA	DNA re-sequencing	DNA is relatively stable and easy to obtain sufficient quantities for analysis	Many DNA variations are of unknown function and may act as surrogates for the causal DNA variation
	DNA polymorphism (Southern blot)		Multiplex analyses can be cost-prohibitive
	Microarray (multiplex) analysis		Multiplex approaches require expensive equipment and specialized training (best pursued via core facilities)
RNA	RNA levels (northern blot)	Differences in RNA level may be more closely linked to pathophysiology	RNA is more labile than DNA
	cDNA re-sequencing	Multiplex (e.g. microarray) approaches may provide information on pathways of gene expression that are altered in trait of interest, providing greater insight into (patho)physiology	Expression analyses require tissue affected by the trait in question
	Microarray (multiplex) analysis		Heterogeneous composition of target tissue makes isolation of relevant RNA pool difficult and susceptible to artifact
			Multiplex analyses can be cost-prohibitive
			Multiplex approaches require expensive equipment and specialized training (best pursued via core facilities)
Protein	Protein levels (western blot)	Differences in RNA level may be more closely linked to pathophysiology	Protein can be more labile than DNA
	Peptide sequencing	Multiplex (e.g. microarray) approaches may provide information on pathways of gene or protein expression that are altered in trait of interest, providing greater insight into (patho)physiology	Expression analyses require tissue affected by the trait in question
	Multiplex protein analysis		Heterogeneous composition of target tissue makes isolation of relevant protein(s) difficult and susceptible to artifact
			Multiplex analyses are cost-prohibitive
			Multiplex approaches require expensive equipment and specialized training (best pursued via core facilities)

Notes: Other levels of inquiry include the metabolome, posttranslational modifications, alternative splicing.

MOLECULAR BIOLOGIC TOOLS IN THE ELUCIDATION OF PAIN MECHANISMS AND DRUG DISCOVERY

Though rooted in the basic principles of molecular biology, advances in both technology and biostatistical methods continue to yield an ever-evolving array of tools for the examination of DNA, RNA, and protein (**Table 4.4**). Though population studies are of interest to the pain research community as a means of identifying common genetic risk factors for pain sensitivity, a useful tool for the discovery and characterization of genetic risk factors continues to involve studies of gene and protein expression (**Table 4.2**). Common uses of expression analyses include causal and susceptibility gene discovery, drug development, drug response, and therapy development. The study of gene expression requires obtaining RNA from specific tissues (e.g. neurons, sensory ganglia, central nervous system, brain). To date, because of this need for target tissue, the majority of expression microarray pain research is limited to animal models. However, novel minimally invasive methods (e.g. laser capture microdissection) may increase the opportunity to study gene expression in human tissues that are readily accessible.[48]

Though lagging behind the study of the human genome (i.e. DNA) and transcriptome (i.e. RNA), the proteome (i.e. protein) is a frontier of great interest. Whereas individual proteins can be readily studied given sufficient quantities and purity, more high-throughput approaches (i.e. analogous to gene expression arrays) is still cost-prohibitive. This approach suffers from the same limitations as RNA-based methods (i.e. access to tissue); however, recent proteomic analysis of spinal protein expression in rats exposed to morphine suggests that this approach will provide a novel tool in pain research.[49]

REFERENCES

* 1. Levy S, Sutton P, Ng PC *et al.* The diploid genome sequence of an individual human. *PLoS Biology.* 2007; **5**: e254.
* 2. Dearlove AM. High throughput genotyping technologies. *Briefings in Functional Genomics and Proteomics.* 2002; **1**: 139–50.
3. Fan H, Chu JY. A brief review of short tandem repeat mutation. *Genomics, Proteomics and Bioinformatics.* 2007; **5**: 7–14.
4. Pena SD, Chakraborty R. Paternity testing in the DNA era. *Trends in Genetics.* 1994; **10**: 204–09.
5. Khoury MJ, Beaty TH, Cohen BH. *Fundamentals of genetic epidemiology. Monographs in epidemiology and biostatistics*, Vol 19. New York: Oxford University Press, 1993.
6. Hudcova J, McNicol E, Quah C *et al.* Patient controlled opioid analgesia versus conventional opioid analgesia for postoperative pain. *Cochrane Database of Systematic Reviews.* 2006; **CD003348**.
7. Huas D, Pouchain D, Gay B *et al.* Assessing chronic pain in general practice: are guidelines relevant? A cluster randomized controlled trial. *European Journal of General Practice.* 2006; **12**: 52–7.
8. Linde K, Streng A, Hoppe A *et al.* Randomized trial vs. observational study of acupuncture for migraine found that patient characteristics differed but outcomes were similar. *Journal of Clinical Epidemiology.* 2007; **60**: 280–7.
9. Ives TJ, Chelminski PR, Hammett-Stabler CA *et al.* Predictors of opioid misuse in patients with chronic pain: a prospective cohort study. *BMC Health Services Research.* 2006; **6**: 46.
10. Lichtman AH, Shelton CC, Advani T, Cravatt BF. Mice lacking fatty acid amide hydrolase exhibit a cannabinoid receptor-mediated phenotypic hypoalgesia. *Pain.* 2004; **109**: 319–27.
11. Al-Khrasani M, Spetea M, Friedmann T *et al.* Furst, DAMGO and 6beta-glycine substituted 14-O-methyloxymorphone but not morphine show peripheral, preemptive antinociception after systemic administration in a mouse visceral pain model and high intrinsic efficacy in the isolated rat vas deferens. *Brain Research Bulletin.* 2007; **74**: 369–75.
12. Huang CW, Tzeng JN, Chen YJ *et al.* Nociceptors of dorsal root ganglion express proton-sensing G-protein-coupled receptors. *Molecular and Cellular Neurosciences.* 2007; **36**: 195–210.
13. Kang SC, Lee DG, Choi JH *et al.* Association between estrogen receptor polymorphism and pain susceptibility in female temporomandibular joint osteoarthritis patients. *International Journal of Oral and Maxillofacial Surgery.* 2007; **36**: 391–4.
* 14. Diatchenko L, Slade GD, Nackley AG *et al.* Genetic basis for individual variations in pain perception and the development of a chronic pain condition. *Human Molecular Genetics.* 2005; **14**: 135–43.
15. Gansky SA, Plesh O. Widespread pain and fibromyalgia in a biracial cohort of young women. *Journal of Rheumatology.* 2007; **34**: 810–17.
16. Indo Y. Molecular basis of congenital insensitivity to pain with anhidrosis (CIPA): mutations and polymorphisms in TRKA (NTRK1) gene encoding the receptor tyrosine kinase for nerve growth factor. *Human Mutation.* 2001; **18**: 462–71.
17. Chesler EJ, Ritchie J, Kokayeff A *et al.* Genotype-dependence of gabapentin and pregabalin sensitivity: the pharmacogenetic mediation of analgesia is specific to the type of pain being inhibited. *Pain.* 2003; **106**: 325–35.
* 18. Hulley SB, Cummings SR. *Designing clinical research: an epidemiologic approach.* Baltimore: Williams and Wilkins, 1988.
19. Capecchi MR. Cold Spring Harbor Laboratory. *Molecular genetics of early Drosophila and mouse development. Current communications in molecular biology.* Cold Spring Harbor, NY: Cold Spring Harbor Laboratory Press, 1989.

20. He Y, Baas PW. Growing and working with peripheral neurons. *Methods in Cell Biology.* 2003; **71**: 17–35.

* 21. Haines JL, Pericak-Vance MA. *Genetic analysis of complex diseases*, 2nd edn. Hoboken, NJ: Wiley-Liss, 2006.

22. Daly AK. Candidate gene case-control studies. *Pharmacogenomics.* 2003; **4**: 127–39.

* 23. Mogil JS. International Association for the Study of Pain. *The genetics of pain. Progress in pain research and management.* Seattle: IASP Press, 2004.

24. Parker HG, Ostrander EA. Canine genomics and genetics: running with the pack. *PLoS Genetics.* 2005; **1**: e58.

25. Aquadro CF, Bauer DuMont V, Reed FA. Genome-wide variation in the human and fruitfly: a comparison. *Current Opinion in Genetics and Development.* 2001; **11**: 627–34.

26. Zhai RG, Hiesinger PR, Koh TW *et al.* Mapping Drosophila mutations with molecularly defined P element insertions. *Proceedings of the National Academy of Sciences of the United States of America.* 2003; **100**: 10860–5.

27. Avanesov A, Malicki J. Approaches to study neurogenesis in the zebrafish retina. *Methods in Cell Biology.* 2004; **76**: 333–84.

28. Dooley K, Zon LI. Zebrafish: a model system for the study of human disease. *Current Opinion in Genetics and Development.* 2000; **10**: 252–6.

29. Ott J. *Analysis of human genetic linkage*, 3rd edn. Baltimore: Johns Hopkins University Press, 1999.

* 30. Silver LM. *Mouse genetics: concepts and applications.* New York: Oxford University Press, 1995.

31. Estevez M, Gardner KL. Update on the genetics of migraine. *Human Genetics.* 2004; **114**: 225–35.

* 32. Lusis AJ. A thematic review series: systems biology approaches to metabolic and cardiovascular disorders. *Journal of Lipid Research.* 2006; **47**: 1887–90.

33. Norbury TA, MacGregor AJ, Urwin J *et al.* Heritability of responses to painful stimuli in women: a classical twin study. *Brain.* 2007; **130**: 3041–9.

* 34. Cox JJ, Reimann F, Nicholas AK *et al.* An SCN9A channelopathy causes congenital inability to experience pain. *Nature.* 2006; **444**: 894–8.

35. Doyle GA, Sheng XR, Lin SS *et al.* Identification of five mouse mu-opioid receptor (MOR) gene (Oprm1) splice variants containing a newly identified alternatively spliced exon. *Gene.* 2007; **395**: 98–107.

36. Pan YX, Xu J, Bolan E *et al.* Identification and characterization of three new alternatively spliced mu-opioid receptor isoforms. *Molecular Pharmacology.* 1999; **56**: 396–403.

* 37. Mogil JS, Wilson SG, Chesler EJ *et al.* The melanocortin-1 receptor gene mediates female-specific mechanisms of analgesia in mice and humans. *Proceedings of the National Academy of Sciences of the United States of America.* 2003; **100**: 4867–2.

38. Katon W, Egan K, Miller D. Chronic pain: lifetime psychiatric diagnoses and family history. *American Journal of Psychiatry.* 1985; **142**: 1156–60.

39. Reis S, Hermoni D, Borkan JM *et al.* A new look at low back complaints in primary care: a RAMBAM Israeli Family Practice Research Network study. *Journal of Family Practice.* 1999; **48**: 299–303.

40. Pellegrino MJ, Waylonis GW, Sommer A. Familial occurrence of primary fibromyalgia. *Archives of Physical Medicine and Rehabilitation.* 1989; **70**: 61–3.

41. Lotsch J, Zimmermann M, Darimont J *et al.* Does the A118G polymorphism at the mu-opioid receptor gene protect against morphine-6-glucuronide toxicity? *Anesthesiology.* 2002; **97**: 814–19.

42. Romberg R, Olofsen E, Sarton E *et al.* Pharmacokinetic-pharmacodynamic modeling of morphine-6-glucuronide-induced analgesia in healthy volunteers: absence of sex differences. *Anesthesiology.* 2004; **100**: 120–33.

43. Skarke C, Darimont J, Schmidt H *et al.* Analgesic effects of morphine and morphine-6-glucuronide in a transcutaneous electrical pain model in healthy volunteers. *Clinical Pharmacology and Therapeutics.* 2003; **73**: 107–21.

44. Rakvag TT, Klepstad P, Baar C *et al.* The Val158Met polymorphism of the human catechol-O-methyltransferase (COMT) gene may influence morphine requirements in cancer pain patients. *Pain.* 2005; **116**: 73–8.

45. Mogil JS, Ritchie J, Smith SB *et al.* Melanocortin-1 receptor gene variants affect pain and mu-opioid analgesia in mice and humans. *Journal of Medical Genetics.* 2005; **42**: 583–7.

46. Stamer UM, Lehnen K, Hothker F *et al.* Impact of CYP2D6 genotype on postoperative tramadol analgesia. *Pain.* 2003; **105**: 231–8.

* 47. Lotsch J, Geisslinger G. Current evidence for a genetic modulation of the response to analgesics. *Pain.* 2006; **121**: 1–5.

48. Reilly SC, Cossins AR, Quinn JP, Sneddon LU. Discovering genes: the use of microarrays and laser capture microdissection in pain research. *Brain Research. Brain Research Reviews.* 2004; **46**: 225–33.

49. Shui HA, Ho ST, Wang JJ *et al.* Proteomic analysis of spinal protein expression in rats exposed to repeated intrathecal morphine injection. *Proteomics.* 2007; **7**: 796–803.

5

Epidemiology of chronic pain: classical to molecular approaches to understanding the epidemiology of pain

CIELITO REYES-GIBBY, ISABEL TORRES-VIGIL, AND ROY CROOCK

KEY LEARNING POINTS

- Epidemiology provides a framework for determining the prevalence, incidence, and risk of pain in populations.
- Measures of risk typically include the absolute risk, relative risk, and odds ratio.
- The three principal observational designs used by epidemiologists are cross-sectional, case-control (or group comparison), and cohort studies.
- Classical epidemiology approaches have resulted in the identification of subgroups that are at higher risk for pain (by sex, age, and ethnicity).
- The new molecular epidemiology paradigm integrates the use of biological markers that indicate events at the physiological, cellular, and molecular levels.
- The principal molecular epidemiology approaches are candidate gene, pathway-based, and genome-wide scanning approaches.
- The statistical analyses performed in genetic association studies of pain follow traditional parametric and nonparametric statistical procedures. However, approaches such as pathway-based analyses and classification and regression tree analyses have gained considerable attention as well.
- Special considerations in the conduct of genetic association studies of pain include issues of multiple comparisons and population stratification.

INTRODUCTION

Epidemiology provides a framework for determining the prevalence, incidence, and risk of pain in populations. Epidemiological studies use the paradigm of exposure–disease assessment. Classical epidemiological research focuses on the distribution of diseases and their determinants within populations and relies on field-tested measures of exposure (usually self-reported) in defining disease–exposure associations. More recently, advances in molecular technology have made possible the measurement of genetic markers of disease, prognosis, and therapeutic response. This newer molecular epidemiology paradigm represents the confluence of sophisticated advances in molecular biology and field-tested epidemiological methodologies. Currently, interest in the use of biological markers in epidemiology to enhance assessment of exposures to disease, provide insight into disease mechanisms, understanding susceptibility to diseases, and refining assessment of risk of disease is increasing. In this chapter we present the results of studies of the epidemiology of pain using classical epidemiological methods; describe the basic principles of epidemiology; and introduce the concepts and approaches for exploring the molecular epidemiology of pain.

PREVALENCE OF PAIN

As many as 11 to 60 percent of general adult populations suffer from chronic pain[1, 2, 3, 4, 5, 6, 7, 8, 9, 10, 11, 12, 13, 14, 15, 16, 17, 18, 19] (**Table 5.1**). It should be noted that estimates of the prevalence of pain have varied widely, mainly because of a lack of uniformity or standardization in the definitions of and assessment measures used for pain (i.e. no gold standard exists) and the heterogeneity of pain conditions (nociceptive versus neuropathic). Other factors contributing to the wide variation in results include, but are not limited to, the heterogeneity of disease conditions and the types of treatment settings (outpatient versus inpatient versus community) in which the studies were conducted.

Adverse impact of pain

Left untreated, pain adversely affects function and daily activity. One study showed that individuals with persistent pain were more likely to experience severe activity limitations than those without persistent pain (odds ratio, 1.63; 95 percent confidence interval, 1.41–1.89).[20] Another study found that among individuals with abdominal pain, more than 65 percent reported some activity limitations.[21] Up to 20 percent of older adults in the general population in the United States have reported significant pain resulting in activity limitations.[22]

The adverse impact of pain is not limited to function. For example, individuals with chronic pain have up to a four-fold increase in the incidence of psychological disorders when compared with those without chronic pain.[20, 23, 24] Pain is predictive of the development of depression.[25] Several studies have addressed the relationship between depression and pain and found that depression has either a causal or mediating effect on pain. One study in particular found a strong correlation between pain severity and depression in older patients but a weak and insignificant correlation between the two in younger patients.[26] Although the causal relationship between depression and pain remains debatable, at least in primary care settings, studies have shown that symptoms such as pain are in fact associated with depressive disorders or psychological distress and anxiety.[27, 28, 29]

Pain has a significant economic impact. In the United States alone, lost productive time resulting from common pain conditions among active workers costs an estimated $61.2 billion annually.[30] An estimated 2.9 million Americans (1.1 percent of the population) receive treatment annually from chronic pain specialists. In the United Kingdom, the mean cost per adolescent experiencing chronic pain was approximately £8000 per year, including direct and indirect costs.[31]

Variance in pain by age, sex, and ethnicity/culture/race

Although the pattern of pain prevalence in older individuals is unclear, several community-based studies of pain suggest that pain prevalence increases from the early adult years up to approximately 60 years of age[32, 33] and thereafter reaches a plateau and may even decline in extreme old age. It is generally accepted that increased pathological load is an overriding factor contributing to increased pain complaints with advancing age,[33] as older adults are at greater risk for diseases that cause pain, such as arthritis and cancer. Patients older than 60 years of age have a two-fold increase in the incidence of painful conditions relative to younger patients[34] and older patients are less likely to receive adequate analgesic treatment.[35] Furthermore, although they are more likely to experience pain than younger individuals, older adults tend to be less likely to complain of pain.[36] Factors such as other medical problems, cognitive and sensory impairment, and depression are possible contributors to the underreporting of pain among older adults.

Women have a greater risk of pain and report more severe pain, more frequent pain, and longer pain durations than men do.[37] These differences are partially attributed to the action of sex hormones, which may influence central and peripheral mechanisms of nociceptive pain transmission, pain sensitivity, and pain perception.[38] Studies have also shown sex differences in responses to treatment with analgesics, especially opioids.[39]

The epidemiology of pain in ethnic minority communities has been a matter of intense investigation in racially and culturally diverse countries such as the United States. Studies of chronic pain conditions showed that African Americans consistently reported greater pain severity and disability than did those in other racial and ethnic groups.[40, 41] A recent study of a nationally representative sample of adults in the United States showed that Latino (Hispanic people) and Anglos (non-Hispanic white people) reported lower rates of activity impairment resulting from pain than did African Americans (non-Hispanic black people).[42] Also, more African Americans than Anglos and Latinos reported functional impairment

Table 5.1 Population-based studies of chronic pain.

Author	Country	Study design	Setting	Age range (years)	Number of subjects	Data collection methods: pain assessment tools	Pain prevalence (type)
Andersson[1]	Sweden	Cross-sectional	Two primary health care districts, rural areas	25–74	1625	Mailed questionnaire	55.0% and 49.0% (chronic)
Bergman *et al.*[2]	Sweden	Cross-sectional	West coast of Sweden, community-based	20–74	2425	Mailed questionnaire	23.9% (CRP); 11.4% (CWP)
Blyth *et al.*[3]	Australia	Cross-sectional	Nationwide, community-based	≥16	17,543	Computer-assisted telephone interview	17.1% male, 20.0% female
Blyth *et al.*[4]	Australia	Cross-sectional	Northern Sydney, community-based	≥18	2092	Telephone survey	22.1% (chronic)
Breivik *et al.*[5]	Fifteen European countries[a] and Israel	Cross-sectional	Community-based	≥18	46,394	Screening questionnaire	19.0% (chronic); half reported having received inadequate treatment
Cassidy *et al.*[6]	Canada	Cross-sectional	Nationwide, community-based	20–69	1131	SHBPS	22.2% (depressive symptomatology)
Catala *et al.*[7]	Spain	Cross-sectional	Nationwide, general population	18–95	5000	Telephone survey	54.0% (chronic); 23.4 % of population
Chrubasik *et al.*[8]	Germany	Cross-sectional	Regierungsbezirk Karlsruhe County, general population	18–80	1304	Mailed survey	47.0% (unduly prolonged pain)
Croft et al.[9]	England	Cross-sectional	Northern England, general population	≥18	2034	Mailed survey	11.2% (chronic)
Elliot *et al.*[10]	United Kingdom	Cross-sectional	Grampian region, sample of patients from 29 general practice/ primary care facilities	≥25	3605	Chronic Pain Grade questionnaire	50.4% (chronic), 16.0% (back), and 15.8% (arthritis)
Eriksen *et al.*[11]	Denmark	Cross-sectional	Nationwide, random sample, patients without cancer	≥16	10,066	SF-36	16.0% male, 21.0% female (chronic)
Hassan *et al.*[12]	Saudi Arabia	Cross-sectional	Ten regional health care centers		100		41.0% (neuropathic), 59.0% (nociceptive)

(*Continued over*)

Table 5.1 Population-based studies of chronic pain (continued).

Author	Country	Study design	Setting	Age range (years)	Number of subjects	Data collection methods: pain assessment tools	Pain prevalence (type)
Moulin *et al.*[13]	Canada	Cross-sectional	Nationwide, random samples and patients prescribed pain medication	≥ 18	2012	Telephone survey	29.0% (chronic, not cancer-related)
Ng *et al.*[14]	China	Cross-sectional	Hong Kong, random sample	≥ 18	1051	Telephone interview	10.8% (chronic)
Rustoen *et al.*[15]	Norway	Cross-sectional	Nationwide, general population	18–91	1912	Mailed questionnaire	24.4% (chronic)
Saastamoinen *et al.*[16]	Finland	Cross-sectional	Helsinki, city employees	40, 45, 50, 55, and 60	6010	Chronic Pain Grade questionnaire	24.0% male, 29.0% female (chronic)
Taylor[17]	New Zealand	Cross-sectional	North Island, general population	≥ 18	329	Mailed questionnaire	40.0–60% musculoskeletal
Torrance *et al.*[18]	United Kingdom	Cross-sectional	Aberdeen, Leeds, and London; random samples generated by six family practices	≥ 18	3120	S-LANSS	48.0% (chronic)
Yu *et al.*[19]	Taiwan	Cross-sectional	Taipei City, multiple-stage random sampling technique	≥ 65	219	Interview	42.0% (chronic)

[a]The 15 European countries were Finland, Norway, Sweden, France, Belgium, Spain, Italy, Poland, Ireland, Denmark, The Netherlands, United Kingdom, Switzerland, Austria, and Germany.
CRP, chronic regional pain; CWP, chronic widespread pain; SF-36, Short-Form-36; SHBPS, Saskatchewan Health and Back Pain Survey; S-LANSS, Leeds Assessment of Neuropathic Symptoms and Signs score.

as a result of pain, a result that approached statistical significance at mild levels of pain severity.

Many have argued that the association between race/ethnicity and poor health is largely a result of poor socioeconomic conditions among racial and ethnic minorities.[43, 44, 45] A report from the Institute of Medicine[45] in the United States suggested that factors such as stereotyping and bias on the part of healthcare providers, the clinical appropriateness of care, and persistent racial and ethnic discrimination are among the reasons for racial and ethnic disparities in health care.

UNDERSTANDING THE BASIC PRINCIPLES OF EPIDEMIOLOGY

Epidemiological studies identify associations between risk factors and disease outcomes. Identifying these associations can be useful for classifying individuals into risk sets whether or not a causal relationship between the disease and its correlate can be established. Measures of risk typically include the absolute risk, relative risk, and odds ratio. These three risk measures are described briefly below, but much more detail on them can be found in standard epidemiological reference texts such as those by Rothman[46] and Selvin.[47]

Absolute risk is the most easily interpreted risk measure. It is usually specified in terms of risk per time unit per individual. Using the cells in **Table 5.2**, the absolute risk in individuals exposed to a risk factor per time unit is $(a)/(a+c)$. An example for this type of analysis was conducted using the population-based ($n=1387$) Longitudinal Study of Aging Danish Twins. The authors assessed the influence of physical activity as a risk factor for incident low back pain among seniors aged 70–100 years. They found that active lifestyle protects against incident low back pain. Absolute risk estimates for incident low back pain among participants with below average strength score engaged in strenuous physical activity and those with below average strength score not engaged in strenuous physical activity were 10 and 21 percent, respectively.[48]

The relative risk is the risk of disease in individuals who have been exposed to a risk factor divided by the risk of disease in individuals who have not been exposed to that risk factor. Again using the cells in **Table 5.2**, the relative risk in individuals exposed to a risk factor is $((a)/(a+c))/((b)/(b+d))$. The relative risk for developing chronic pain from work-related stress was assessed using longitudinal data from the National Population Health Survey in Canada ($n=6571$). The investigators found that relative risk for developing chronic pain was 1.39 (95 percent CI = 1.01–1.91) for medium stress and 1.80 (95 percent CI = 1.28–2.52) for high stress.[49]

Table 5.2 Parameters for calculating risk in epidemiological studies.

	Exposed	Not exposed	
Diseased	a	b	a+b
Not diseased	c	d	c+d
	a+c	b+d	–

Finally, the odds ratio is the ratio of the probability of exposure to a risk factor in diseased patients to the probability of exposure to a risk factor in nondiseased patients divided by the probability of nonexposure to a risk factor in diseased patients divided by the probability of nonexposure to a risk factor in nondiseased patients. Using the cells in **Table 5.2**, this ratio is $((a)/(c))/((b)/(d))$.

When the prevalence of cases of pain in a population is low, the odds ratio approximates the relative risk (i.e. $a+c \cong d$ and $b+d \cong d$). For relative risks greater than 1, the odds ratio overestimates the relative risk; however, the odds ratio is nearly unbiased when studying uncommon events such as the risk of neuropathic pain. The odds ratio is a measure used to estimate the relative risk for several reasons. For example, in case–control studies, if a disease is uncommon, the odds ratio gives a nearly unbiased estimate of its relative risk. Also, commonly used data analysis tools, such as logistic regression, readily provide estimates of odds ratios.

BASIC DESIGNS OF EPIDEMIOLOGICAL STUDIES

Epidemiologists typically identify two major types of study designs: experimental and observational. The principal distinction is whether the treatment or intervention is under the control of the investigator. In experimental studies, the investigator introduces a factor or intervenes in the environment of the study subjects and observes the impact of the intervention on the study subjects. In observational studies, the investigators describe the events that naturally occur without their direct intervention. The three principal observational designs used by epidemiologists, cross-sectional, case–control (or group comparison), and cohort studies, are described below.

Cross-sectional studies

Studies of chronic pain are predominantly cross-sectional studies. In these studies, participants are sampled, and information related to pain and its risk factors is measured at a single point in time. Prevalence is estimated as the proportion of subjects with pain in the whole study sample. Because information relating to the disease state and risk factors is assessed at the same point in time, causality cannot be inferred, and biases regarding exposure exist. There are several data collection methods used in cross-sectional studies including in-person/household surveys and telephone and postal surveys (**Table 5.1**).

Case–control studies

Epidemiologists often perform case–control studies because they are relatively easy to conduct. In these studies, cases are sampled according to a predetermined protocol, and the controls selected must be comparable with the cases.[50, 51, 52] However, identifying a suitable control population is often difficult for two reasons: (1) identifying the characteristics that ensure comparability with the cases is often difficult, and (2) to avoid selection biases, one must sample the participants from the control population according to a well-controlled scheme. To ensure random sampling, researchers must select controls at random. Often, investigators match controls with the cases according to criteria that are known to be associated with disease risk. Matching cases and controls minimizes the variability among the subjects according to known risk factors that may not be of interest. For instance, controls may be grouped with cases according to demographic characteristics such as age, ethnicity, and sex. In such instances, researchers usually perform a conditional analysis, in which each case is matched with a control or set of controls.

The control population should be comparable with the case population in terms of socioeconomic status and other unmeasured factors. Several methods of accruing controls can be used. One is random-digit telephone dialing. However, one should note that one fourth of all residential telephone subscribers use caller identification devices and thus are able to screen out unfamiliar callers. As a result, using this method would increase the potential for sample bias. Another popular method for selecting controls in the United States has been the use of data tapes obtained from motor vehicle bureaus, but because older adults may no longer have driver's licenses, this method may exclude potential controls. Furthermore, several states have passed legislation banning distribution of lists of registered drivers containing their names and addresses.

One may have to make a tradeoff when performing case–control epidemiological studies. Although population-based studies are inarguably the gold standard for modern epidemiological case–control research, one may be unable to conduct population-based studies for practical reasons. For example, population-based research may not be feasible when studying very rare pain conditions (e.g. neuropathic pain) for which the catchment population is prohibitively large or when studying pain conditions associated with very lethal diseases (e.g. cancer-related pain) because the population-based ascertainment may fail to provide a representative sample of cases as a result of patient deaths prior to enrollment.

Cohort studies

Prospective cohort studies identify groups of subjects and collect samples and/or data from the subjects at baseline and thereafter until a specific point in time. The advantages of this design are that one can establish temporal relationships between events and exposure and that biases relating to incomplete recall of exposures are minimized. In addition, both absolute and relative risk measures of disease can be estimated. The disadvantages of this design include difficulty in maintaining follow-up for the study subjects and potential inefficiency if the disease outcome of interest is rare or infrequent in the study population (e.g. neuropathic pain).

An approach to limiting the cost of prospective cohort studies is to set up the cohort and then only conduct laboratory analyses for study subjects who become affected with the disease of interest along with a matched set of study subjects who do not become affected. This is called a nested case–control design because it is a case–control study nested within a cohort.

MOLECULAR EPIDEMIOLOGY

Geneticists have historically used genetic mapping of trait causing genes to chromosomal locations in experimental organisms (nematodes worms, fruit flies, etc.). However, genetic mapping was not used for the study of humans due to the lack of an abundant supply of genetic markers with which to study inheritance and the inability to arrange human crosses to suit experimental crosses. A key breakthrough in genetic studies of human diseases was the recognition that naturally occurring DNA sequence variation provide an unlimited supply of genetic markers. The completion of the human genome sequence was a further impetus to the exploration of genes as predictors of disease states and clinical response to treatment. There is now much scientific interest in examining the role of genes and their products in the expression of pain. Identifying markers of genetic susceptibility to pain will facilitate the early detection of patients at high risk for pain, prompt treatment, and the development of targeted pain therapies.

Whereas classical epidemiology approaches have resulted in the identification of subgroups that are at higher risk for pain (by gender, age-groups, and racial/ethnic groups), molecular epidemiology integrates the use of biological markers that indicate events at the physiological, cellular, and molecular levels. Thus, although studies have generally established that individual and group risk assessments are possible using classical epidemiology methods, integrating the use of molecular epidemiology methods enhances individual and group risk assessments by providing more person-specific information (genetic profile). Furthermore, the use of molecular epidemiological methods can also reduce misclassification of exposure (avoiding recall bias in exposure identification) and, importantly, provide information about when interventions can be most effective (pharmacogenetics).

The classic central dogma regarding the genome is that DNA in the nucleus directs the production of proteins. Proteins carry out several life functions through the RNA. By analyzing the DNA, we are able to understand the variability in the genome and the extent to which this variability contributes to physiological traits, including disease susceptibility. Several types of variations exist in the human genome. Of these variations, single nucleotide polymorphisms (SNPs) are the most common and easiest to measure, and are used more frequently in pain research. Several approaches to exploring the molecular epidemiology of pain are currently in use. Advances in molecular technology are expected to lead to improvements in the different approaches currently used in pain research. Three of these approaches are described below.

Candidate gene approach

Many studies have reported associations between genetic polymorphisms and susceptibility to common complex diseases and conditions such as pain, most of which have used the candidate gene approach. In this hypothesis-driven approach, one or a few selected polymorphisms are investigated at a time. Although researchers use a priori knowledge of polymorphisms and gene functions in the candidate gene approach, these studies have yielded informative but conflicting results. For example, an initial report suggested that an SNP of catechol-*O*-methyltransferase gene inducing amino acid change at codon 158 from valine to methionine significantly increased pain response to an experimental stimulus.[53] However, this association was not replicated by other investigators using larger sample sizes.[54, 55] The opposite influence has also been reported for this SNP as patients with the methionine allele require a lower amount of morphine compared to those with the valine allele to treat pain due to cancer.[56, 57] Among the reasons for the lack of consistency in the results are the use of small sample sizes, use of inadequate statistical methods, and failure to evaluate the effect of multiple pathophysiologically related genes. Importantly, one should recognize that because pain is a complex human trait, the interaction of multiple genes, each with small individual effects, rather than a few genes alone likely influences the experience of pain.

Pathway-based approach

Because of the limitations of the candidate gene approach, researchers have introduced other approaches to understand the epidemiology of complex diseases. For example, investigators have used a pathway-based multigenic genotyping approach to assess the combined effects of a panel of polymorphisms that act in the same pathway, thus enhancing the effects of the individual polymorphisms. Although application of the pathway-based approach in pain research has been limited, several studies of complex diseases such as cancer have shown the usefulness and encouraging results of this approach. For example, Wu and colleagues[58] assessed a comprehensive panel of 44 selected polymorphisms in two pathways, DNA repair and cell-cycle control for bladder cancer risk and found that individuals with a higher number of genetic variations in DNA-repair and cell-cycle control genes are at an increased risk for bladder cancer. However, although comprehensive, the pathway-based approach still relies on a priori knowledge of SNPs and gene functions and on biological plausibility.

High-density genome-wide scanning approach

Rapid advances in molecular and genetic technology coupled with cost reductions and the progress of the International HapMap Project have led to the application of genome-wide scanning approaches to understanding the molecular epidemiology of complex diseases. Whereas candidate gene and pathway-based approaches use information about several SNPs, whole genome (genome-wide) scanning approaches allow for the examination of thousands of SNPs at a time. With the inclusion of up to several thousand SNPs in a single DNA chip, more genetic markers throughout the genome are analyzed efficiently.

Affymetrix (Santa Clara, CA) produced one of the first generation DNA array chips. They use a restriction enzyme-based adaptor ligation polymerase chain reaction procedure in which the genomic complexity is first reduced by restriction enzymes followed by the addition of universal primers and polymerase chain reaction amplification of digested genomic portions. More recently, Illumina (San Diego, CA) launched a series of whole-genome SNP array chips. In contrast with the Affymetrix approach, in which the ability to choose SNPs is limited because it requires SNPs to be present in the amplified representation, Illumina's Infinium assay allows for accurate and robust genotyping in the context of full genomic complexity and enables selection of SNPs anywhere in the genome. Studies using whole-genome (genome-wide) scanning approaches in uncovering genes for pain are under way.

Statistical approaches

The statistical analyses performed in genetic association studies of pain follow traditional parametric and non-parametric statistical procedures. However, approaches such as pathway-based analyses and classification and regression tree analyses have gained considerable attention as well.

Pathway-based association test: This test has been used to test the overall association of sets of SNPs. With this data-driven approach, a model with complex combination of SNPs will be derived based on all SNPs in the set. A recently developed method to jointly incorporate several polymorphisms or pathways[59, 60] uses Tukey's 1-degree-of-freedom model of interaction.[61] The model specifically tests if SNPs within genes are associated with disease through a common biological pathway. This model is computationally a simple generalized test of association that can simultaneously capture both the main effects of the variants within a genomic region and their interactions with the variants in another region or with other covariates. The first level models the associations between the markers and the underlying biological variables with a linear model. The second level models the risk of outcome (severe pain versus nonsevere, for example) with a logistic model that depends on the biological variables from the first level. The method is flexible since it also allows the causal SNPs in the logistic model.

CART analysis: Classification and regression tree (CART) modeling are also performed for genetic association studies of symptoms. Tree-based modeling is an exploratory technique for uncovering structure in data. Tree-based models use both categorical variables (i.e. marker genotypes) and continuous variables (i.e. age). The classification tree divides the study sample into a number of homogenous subgroups (nodes) based on risk factors. At each node, all possible splits for all of the included covariates are evaluated and compared and the covariate that has the best split point of the response is chosen. The recursive procedure is continued to produce subsequent nodes that are more homogenous (with respect to the response variable) than the original node. The final model is a tree-structure with numerous binary splits.

Special considerations

Multiple comparisons and controlling for false discovery rate: False positive findings become a problem when the associations between multiple genetic loci are tested against multiple clinical endpoints. However, corrective methods for multiple testing, such as Bonferroni's corrections, increase the risk of false negative errors. Benjamini and Hochberg[62] proposed a novel approach, the false discovery rate (FDR), to account for multiple comparisons. The FDR controls the expected proportion of incorrectly rejected null hypotheses in a list of rejected hypotheses. The Bonferroni correction is very conservative and permutation-based methods such as the re-sampling method of Westfall and Young,[63] are computationally very intensive. The FDR method has been refined to increase its accuracy, applicability, and power.[64, 65] Thus, calculating the FDR-adjusted *p*-values will help determine whether the observed *p*-values are still significant after taking into account multiple comparisons.

Population stratification: Population stratification (different racial/ethnic distribution) can be a confounding factor in genetic studies. As an example, haplotype blocks in African populations are shorter than those in Caucasians. Further, the linkage disequilibrium between investigated SNPs are usually different between ethnic populations (http://www.hapmap.org/). Therefore, a mixed population cannot be analyzed together for the association with pain phenotypes. It is generally recommended to genotype a number (preferably >100) of widely spaced null SNPs (preferably ancestry informative markers) in addition to the candidate SNPs.

FUTURE DIRECTIONS

Studies of the incidence, prevalence, severity, and treatment of pain have a number of shortcomings. Often, pain is evaluated and reported without stratifying for heterogeneity with respect to pain type, disease type, disease treatment, and response to treatment. Durations of pain may be days, months, or years, but assessments often are performed cross-sectionally rather than longitudinally, thus failing to assess patterns and trajectories. Cohort studies that will provide clinicians with information regarding the incidence, severity, and duration of pain will be useful in determining the epidemiology of pain.

Furthermore, there is a need to recognize and apply the rapidly emerging wealth of genetic information for improving pain management and control. Pain research and genetic research are both in an early stage of investigation and a particular challenge for epidemiologists is to incorporate molecular epidemiology methods to pain research. Epidemiologists will increasingly be called upon to identify genetically high-risk (susceptible) subgroups that disproportionately suffer from pain, and could greatly benefit from early pain interventions. Nevertheless, further integration of molecular epidemiology methods to pain research, coupled with incorporating knowledge about pain from other disciplines can lead to a better understanding of chronic pain in populations and potentially for individualizing pain therapy.

REFERENCES

1. Andersson HI. The epidemiology of chronic pain in a Swedish rural area. *Quality of Life Research*. 1994; **3**: S19–26.
2. Bergman S, Herrstrom P, Hogstrom K *et al.* Chronic musculoskeletal pain, prevalence rates, and sociodemographic associations in a Swedish population study. *Journal of Rheumatology*. 2001; **28**: 1369–77.

3. Blyth FM, March LM, Brnabic AJM *et al.* Chronic pain in Australia: a prevalence study. *Pain.* 2001; **89**: 127–34.
4. Blyth FM, March LM, Cousins MJ. Chronic pain-related disability and use of analgesia and health services in a Sydney community. *Medical Journal of Australia.* 2003; **179**: 84–7.
5. Breivik H, Collett B, Ventafridda V *et al.* Survey of chronic pain in Europe: Prevalence, impact on daily life, and treatment. *European Journal of Pain.* 2006; **10**: 287–333.
6. Cassidy JD, Carroll LJ, Cote P. The Saskatchewan health and back pain survey – The prevalence of low back pain and related disability in Saskatchewan adults. *Spine.* 1998; **23**: 1860–6.
7. Catala E, Reig E, Artes M *et al.* Prevalence of pain in the Spanish population: telephone survey in 5000 homes. *European Journal of Pain – London.* 2002; **6**: 133–40.
8. Chrubasik S, Junck H, Zappe HA, Stutzke O. A survey on pain complaints and health care utilization in a German population sample. *European Journal of Anaesthesiology.* 1998; **15**: 397–408.
9. Croft P, Rigby AS, Boswell R *et al.* The prevalence of chronic widespread pain in the general-population. *Journal of Rheumatology.* 1993; **20**: 710–13.
10. Elliott AM, Smith BH, Penny KI *et al.* The epidemiology of chronic pain in the community. *Lancet.* 1999; **354**: 1248–52.
11. Eriksen J, Jensen MK, Sjogren P *et al.* Epidemiology of chronic non-malignant pain in Denmark. *Pain.* 2003; **106**: 221–8.
12. Hassan AE, Saleh HA, Baroudy YM *et al.* Prevalence of neuropathic pain among patients suffering from chronic low back pain in Saudi Arabia. *Saudi Medical Journal.* 2004; **25**: 1986–90.
13. Moulin DE, Clark AJ, Speechley M, Morley-Forster PK. Chronic pain in Canada – prevalence, treatment, impact and the role of opioid analgesia. *Pain Research and Management.* 2002; **7**: 179–84.
14. Ng KF, Tsui SL, Chan WS. Prevalence of common chronic pain in Hong Kong adults. *Clinical Journal of Pain.* 2002; **18**: 275–81.
15. Rustoen T, Wahl AK, Hanestad BR *et al.* Prevalence and characteristics of chronic pain in the general Norwegian population. *European Journal of Pain.* 2004; **8**: 555–65.
16. Saastamoinen P, Leino-Arjas P, Laaksonen M, Lahelma E. Socio-economic differences in the prevalence of acute, chronic and disabling chronic pain among ageing employees. *Pain.* 2005; **114**: 364–71.
17. Taylor WJ. The frequency and impact of musculoskeletal pain in the adult New Zealand general population. *Annals of the Rheumatic Diseases.* 2005; **64**: 548.
18. Torrance N, Smith BH, Bennett MI, Lee AJ. The epidemiology of chronic pain of predominantly neuropathic origin. Results from a general population survey. *Journal of Pain.* 2006; **7**: 281–9.
19. Yu HY, Tang FI, Kuo BIT, Yu S. Prevalence, interference, and risk factors for chronic pain among Taiwanese community older people. *Pain Management Nursing.* 2006; **7**: 2–11.
20. Gureje O, Von Korff M, Simon GE, Gater R. Persistent pain and well-being: a World Health Organization Study in Primary Care. *Journal of the American Medical Association.* 1998; **280**: 147–51.
21. Sandler RS, Stewart WF, Liberman JN *et al.* Abdominal pain, bloating, and diarrhea in the United States: prevalence and impact. *Digestive Diseases and Sciences.* 2000; **45**: 1166–71.
22. Reyes-Gibby CC, Aday L, Cleeland C. Impact of pain on self-rated health in the community-dwelling older adults. *Pain.* 2002; **95**: 75–82.
23. Magni G, Rigatti-Luchini S, Fracca F, Merskey H. Suicidality in chronic abdominal pain: an analysis of the Hispanic Health and Nutrition Examination Survey (HHANES). *Pain.* 1998; **76**: 137–44.
24. Magni G, Caldieron C, Rigatti-Luchini S, Merskey H. Chronic musculoskeletal pain and depressive symptoms in the general population. An analysis of the 1st National Health and Nutrition Examination Survey data. *Pain.* 1990; **43**: 299–307.
25. Magni G, Moreschi C, Rigatti-Luchini S, Merskey H. Prospective study on the relationship between depressive symptoms and chronic musculoskeletal pain. *Pain.* 1994; **56**: 289–97.
26. Turk DC, Okifuji A, Scharff L. Chronic pain and depression: role of perceived impact and perceived control in different age cohorts. *Pain.* 1995; **61**: 93–101.
27. McWilliams LA, Goodwin RD, Cox BJ. Depression and anxiety associated with three pain conditions: results from a nationally representative sample. *Pain.* 2004; **111**: 77–83.
28. Ohayon MM. Specific characteristics of the pain/depression association in the general population. *Journal of Clinical Psychiatry.* 2004; **65**: 5–9.
29. Onder G, Landi F, Gambassi G *et al.* Association between pain and depression among older adults in Europe: results from the Aged in Home Care (AdHOC) project: a cross-sectional study. *Journal of Clinical Psychiatry.* 2005; **66**: 982–8.
30. Stewart WF, Ricci JA, Chee E *et al.* Lost productive time and cost due to common pain conditions in the US workforce. *Journal of the American Medical Association.* 2003; **290**: 2443–54.
31. Sleed M, Eccleston C, Beecham J *et al.* The economic impact of chronic pain in adolescence: methodological considerations and a preliminary costs-of-illness study. *Pain.* 2005; **119**: 183–90.
32. Crook J, Rideout E, Browne G. The prevalence of pain complaints in a general-population. *Pain.* 1984; **18**: 299–314.
33. Helme RD, Gibson SJ. The epidemiology of pain in elderly people. *Clinics in Geriatric Medicine.* 2001; **17**: 417–31, v.
34. Ferrell BA, Ferrell BR, Osterweil D. Pain in the nursing home. *Journal of the American Geriatrics Society.* 1990; **38**: 409–14.
35. Weiner DK. Improving pain management for older adults: an urgent agenda for the educator, investigator, and practitioner. *Pain.* 2002; **97**: 1–4.

36. Bernabei R, Gambassi G, Lapane K *et al.* Management of pain in elderly patients with cancer. SAGE Study Group. Systematic Assessment of Geriatric Drug Use via Epidemiology. *Journal of the American Medical Association.* 1998; **279**: 1877–82.
37. Dao TT, Leresche L. Gender differences in pain. *Journal of Orofacial Pain.* 2000; **14**: 169–84.
38. Wiesenfeld-Hallin Z. Sex differences in pain perception. *Gender Medicine.* 2005; **2**: 137–45.
39. Fillingim RB, Gear RW. Sex differences in opioid analgesia: clinical and experimental findings. *European Journal of Pain.* 2004; **8**: 413–25.
40. Green CR, Anderson KO, Baker TA *et al.* The unequal burden of pain: confronting racial and ethnic disparities in pain. *Pain Medicine.* 2003; **4**: 277–94.
41. Green CR, Baker TA, Sato Y *et al.* Race and chronic pain: A comparative study of young black and white Americans presenting for management. *Journal of Pain.* 2003; **4**: 176–83.
42. Reyes-Gibby CC, Aday LA, Todd KH *et al.* Pain in aging community-dwelling adults in the United States: non-Hispanic whites, non-Hispanic blacks, and Hispanics. *Journal of Pain.* 2007; **8**: 75–84.
43. Aday LA. Access to what? For whom? *Health Managenent Quarterly.* 1990; **12**: 18–22.
44. Aday LA. Equity, accessibility, and ethical issues: is the U.S. health care reform debate asking the right questions? *American Behavioral Scientist.* 1993; **36**: 724–40.
45. Anonymous. Transforming healthcare: IOM panel discusses vision and reality after crossing the quality chasm. *Quality Letter for Healthcare Leaders.* 2004; **16**: 9–12, 1.

* 46. Rothman KJ, Greenland S. *Modern epidemiology.* Philadelphia: Lippincott-Raven, 1998.

* 47. Selvin S. *Statistical analysis of epidemiologic data*, 2nd edn. New York: Oxford University Press, 1996.

48. Hartvigsen J, Christensen K. Active lifestyle protects against incident low back pain in seniors: a population-based 2-year prospective study of 1387 Danish twins aged 70–100 years. *Spine.* 2007; **32**: 76–81.
49. Kopec JA, Sayre EC. Work-related psychosocial factors and chronic pain: a prospective cohort study in Canadian workers. *Journal of Occupational and Environmental Medicine.* 2004; **46**: 1263–71.
50. Wacholder S, Silverman DT, McLaughlin JK, Mandel JS. Selection of controls in case-control studies. III. Design options. *American Journal of Epidemiology.* 1992; **135**: 1042–50.
51. Wacholder S, Silverman DT, McLaughlin JK, Mandel JS. Selection of controls in case-control studies. II. Types of controls. *American Journal of Epidemiology.* 1992; **135**: 1029–41.
52. Wacholder S, McLaughlin JK, Silverman DT, Mandel JS. Selection of controls in case-control studies. I. Principles. *American Journal of Epidemiology.* 1992; **135**: 1019–28.
53. Zubieta JK, Heitzeg MM, Smith YR *et al.* COMT val158met genotype affects mu-opioid neurotransmitter responses to a pain stressor. *Science.* 2003; **299**: 1240–3.
54. Kim H, Lee H, Rowan J *et al.* Genetic polymorphisms in monoamine neurotransmitter systems show only weak association with acute post-surgical pain in humans. *Molecular Pain.* 2006; **2**: 24.
55. Diatchenko L, Slade GD, Nackley AG *et al.* Genetic basis for individual variations in pain perception and the development of a chronic pain condition. *Human Molecular Genetics.* 2005; **14**: 135–43.
56. Rakvag TT, Klepstad P, Baar C *et al.* The Val158Met polymorphism of the human catechol-O-methyltransferase (COMT) gene may influence morphine requirements in cancer pain patients. *Pain.* 2005; **116**: 73–8.
57. Reyes-Gibby CC, Shete S, Rakvag T *et al.* Exploring joint effects of genes and the clinical efficacy of morphine for cancer pain: OPRM1 and COMT gene. *Pain.* 2007; **130**: 25–30.
58. Wu X, Gu J, Grossman HB *et al.* Bladder cancer predisposition: a multigenic approach to DNA-repair and cell-cycle-control genes. *American Journal of Human Genetics.* 2006; **78**: 464–79.

* 59. Millstein J, Conti DV, Gilliland FD, Gauderman WJ. A testing framework for identifying susceptibility genes in the presence of epistasis. *American Journal of Human Genetics.* 2006; **78**: 15–27.

* 60. Ritchie MD, Hahn LW, Moore JH. Power of multifactor dimensionality reduction for detecting gene-gene interactions in the presence of genotyping error, missing data, phenocopy, and genetic heterogeneity. *Genetic Epidemiology.* 2003; **24**: 150–7.

61. Chatterjee N, Kalaylioglu Z, Moslehi R *et al.* Powerful multilocus tests of genetic association in the presence of gene-gene and gene-environment interactions. *American Journal of Human Genetics.* 2006; **79**: 1002–16.

* 62. Benjamini Y, Hochberg Y. Controlling the false discovery rate – a practical and powerful approach to multiple testing. *Journal of the Royal Statistical Society Series B – Methodological.* 1995; **57**: 289–300.

63. Westfall PH, Young SS. *Resampling-based multiple testing: examples and methods for p-value adjustment.* New York: John Wiley and Sons, 1993.
64. Storey JD. A direct approach to false discovery rates. *Journal of the Royal Statistical Society Series B – Statistical Methodology.* 2002; **64**: 479–98.

* 65. Storey JD, Tibshirani R. Statistical significance for genomewide studies. *Proceedings of the National Academy of Sciences of the United States of America.* 2003; **100**: 9440–5.

6

The economics of chronic pain

CERI J PHILLIPS

KEY LEARNING POINTS

- There will never be sufficient resources to address completely the problems posed by chronic pain.
- Health economics offers a mode of thinking which can assist in arriving at possible solutions to the often contentious problems in dealing with pain and its management, based on the concepts of effectiveness, efficiency, and equity.
- Economic impact of pain and its management need to be considered.
- Health economic evaluation enables decision-makers to assess the additional benefits generated from an intervention in relation to the additional costs that are incurred in its provision.
- High-quality relevant evidence and health economics techniques and approaches are essential components in developing a broader, strategic, whole systems agenda in pain management.
- Together they can provide the tools which decision-makers can utilize in the drive for reductions in pain and better health and healthcare for our respective communities and societies.

THE PAIN PROBLEM

Pain represents a major clinical, social, and economic problem and one which has challenged generations of healthcare professionals across many continents as they attempt to provide relief to reduce the suffering caused by pain. The advent of modern anesthetics and analgesics has meant that the effects of pain can be ameliorated, but even in hospital settings in recent years, nearly nine out of every ten patients have experienced pain levels considered to be excessive.[1, 2] This proportion is clearly unacceptable and represents a challenge to those involved in the commissioning and provision of services. It has been argued that "pain relief should not be seen as someone else's responsibility or simply dismissed because in the end the pain and the patient go away. Freedom from pain is important to patients. In 1846 the first anesthetic provided pain free surgery. One hundred and fifty years later, patients should not have to endure unrelieved pain anywhere in the hospital."[3] However, for many patients pain is more or less a permanent feature of their lives and extends well beyond the acute phase. Pain has a profound impact on their quality of life, and for them, it is the management of their pain that is important, so that suffering is minimized for as much of the time as possible. It has been recognized that chronic pain is one of the most widespread and difficult problems the medical community has to face,[4] with other symptoms, such as depression, anxiety, physical dysfunction, and social isolation, often presenting alongside.[5]

The epidemiology of chronic pain has been addressed in Chapter 5, Epidemiology of chronic pain: classical to molecular approaches to understanding the epidemiology of pain. While many attempts have been made to estimate the prevalence of chronic pain,[6, 7, 8, 9, 10, 11, 12, 13, 14, 15, 16, 17] the range of estimates bears testimony to the difficulties involved in defining the condition and the difference in approaches and methodologies employed to determine the extent of chronic pain across different population groups. Moreover, the impact of chronic pain is expected to increase dramatically as the effects of population ageing are manifest, while changes in lifestyle factors are also predicted to further increase the burden, as increased obesity and lack of physical activity resulting from the "increased urbanization and motorization of the developing world" will increase the prevalence of conditions associated with chronic pain.[16]

The prevalence and impact of chronic pain have also led to calls for it to be regarded as a disease entity in its own right,[18, 19] with a consensus emerging that failure to secure appropriate management strategies for pain is unethical and may be susceptible to legal and professional action.[18]

THE ECONOMIC PROBLEM

The fundamental economic problem confronting us all is that while we have insatiable wants and desires, we only have limited resources (time, energy, expertise, and money) at our disposal to satisfy them. Economics is founded on the premise that there will never be sufficient resources to completely satisfy human desires and the use of resources in one activity means that they cannot be used elsewhere.[20] How society's scarce resources are, could, or should be allocated among the infinite variety of competing activities provide the rationale for an economic perspective in setting priorities. The extent of the gap which exists between the demand for commodities and the level of resources available to meet them continues to frustrate politicians, professionals, and policymakers alike, and the range of economic systems which have existed and evolved over time have all attempted to address the basic economic problem of allocating resources in such a way as to maximize the benefits for society. This situation has become particularly evident in health care and has been compounded by factors such as the increasing expectations of the population as to what can be delivered by healthcare services, the continuing advancements in health technology and medical science, and the increasing health needs and demands of an ageing population.

However, it should be remembered that more does not necessarily mean better health care, and diverting additional resources into facilities and services will not automatically generate an improvement in the health of the population. It is far too simplistic to argue that in order to improve the health of the nation and reduce inequalities, additional resources need to be channeled into healthcare services. The USA spends over 2.5 times the average health expenditure of the other 29 OECD countries (Organisation for Economic Cooperation and Development) and yet is one of the least healthy of these nations.[21] The issue of whether health care and the availability of healthcare facilities are the most important determinants in securing good health for society has been widely challenged,[22, 23, 24, 25] and it has been shown that there is a level of healthcare expenditure, where maximum benefits are produced, and beyond which extra health gains cease and patients may actually be harmed.[26, 27]

Another facet to consider is whether the distribution of any additional resources provided for healthcare services could be regarded as being fair. An increase of resources may simply reinforce existing inequalities and inequities between groups within society, and do nothing to reduce differences between them in terms of life expectancy, health status, or access to treatments and facilities.

The two concepts of "efficiency" and "equity" are fundamental in economics, and together they combine to form, what has been termed, the social welfare function. In constructing policy decisions, there is a broad consensus that both of these aspects of social welfare should be considered in the location, method, and degree of government intervention in health care and there is general agreement on the need for a trade-off between achieving an efficient allocation of resources and ensuring that the resulting allocation is equitable.

Efficiency and equity

The term "efficiency" is defined as "maximizing well-being at the least cost to society."[26] The concept of efficiency embraces inputs (costs) and outputs and/or outcomes (benefits) and the relationship between them, with a society being judged in efficiency terms by the extent to which it maximizes the benefits for its population, given the resources at its disposal. However, a move towards efficiency may well result in a redistribution of resources in favor of the well-off, which may not be acceptable on grounds of fairness and equity. "Equity" is inextricably linked with notions of fairness and justice, with a healthcare intervention regarded as equitable if "similar outcomes were achieved for people with similar needs," but inequitable and unjust if "similar services were provided for people with different needs."[28, 29]

In setting the economic objectives of healthcare systems, both efficiency and equity considerations are vital components and must be given serious consideration. However, it is inevitable that in seeking to achieve a more equitable allocation of resources, a level of efficiency will have to be sacrificed, or, in attempting to move to a more efficient healthcare system, inequalities in provision or access to services may have to be compromised.

Health economics or the economics of health?

The two concepts of efficiency and equity lie at the heart of the discipline of health economics, described as the discipline of economics applied to the topic of health,[30] or as "a logical and explicit framework to aid healthcare workers, decision-makers, governments, or society at large, to make choices on how best to use resources."[31] It may be argued that health systems have been victims of their own success. Contrary to what might have been expected, as the health of communities has improved, the demands placed on healthcare services have also increased. However, as the nature of healthcare problems experienced has changed, the costs of developing treatment and care programs to deal with such problems have also followed an upward trend. The level of resources available to fund such services has not increased to the same extent, and we are therefore left with the dilemma of how to allocate limited resources to meet the demands placed on the health services and maximize the healthcare benefit to society.

Obviously, additional resources would help, but the gap between demand and supply would still remain. In addition, the question has to be asked as to which area(s) of health care additional funds should be allocated. Similarly, decisions on where additional resources should be located need to be made with information relating to the effectiveness of interventions, the competence of healthcare professionals and the safety of healthcare facilities.

Healthcare professionals are increasingly being exposed to extremely powerful and emotive choices, and while health economics is unable to provide the solution to such complex and difficult issues, it does offer a mode of thinking which can assist in arriving at possible solutions (notice the use of the term "assist" here – health economics cannot by itself offer the solutions, it has to be part of a wide-ranging approach to decision-making) to these often contentious problems. It aims to identify which package or bundle of services would provide the maximum healthcare benefit for society within the envelope of resources available.

THE ECONOMIC IMPACT OF PAIN

The extent of chronic pain poses a significant economic burden for patients, their families, health services, and societies. Cost of illness studies in pain tend to distinguish between direct costs and productivity or indirect costs, where direct costs represent the costs to the health services of patients suffering chronic pain (direct medical costs) and costs to the patients themselves in terms of travel costs and out-of-pocket expenses. Productivity costs are those which occur outside the healthcare sector and relate to losses of production, due to absenteeism and reduced productivity, plus those incurred through the informal care process – either as a result of a carer giving up paid employment or sacrificing leisure time to provide care, which would otherwise have been provided by formal care agencies.

These studies are useful as reference points for subsequent economic analyses,[32] but rely heavily on estimates and underlying assumptions and should be treated with caution.[33] In addition, there are theoretical debates about the most appropriate method for estimating productivity and indirect costs.[33] The human capital approach considers the value of potentially lost production resulting from a disease in terms of absenteeism, reduced productivity, and disability or premature death at a specific age until the age of retirement. The alternative, friction cost method, assumes that production losses are confined to the period needed to replace the "sick" worker.[34] The differences in results can be highly significant. For example, the indirect nonmedical costs of neck pain in the Netherlands in 1996 were estimated at US$ 530 million, using the human capital approach and US$ 96 million using the friction cost method.[35] Similarly, the indirect cost of back pain in the UK in 1998 was estimated at £11 billion (US$ 20 billion) using the human capital approach and £5 billion (US$ 9 billion) using the friction cost method.[36]

Direct costs of pain management

In assessing the direct costs of pain management, it is conventional to categorize the components. For example, a German study estimated that the cost of back pain amounted to 10 billion DM (US$ 5 billion) each year, with 35 percent due to physician visits, 22 percent of costs accounted for by medication, 21 percent by rehabilitation, 17 percent physiotherapy, and 5 percent hospital costs.[37] However, it is also worth noting that differences in estimates can occur due to what is included in the cost profile. For example, one US study estimated that total healthcare expenditure on back pain patients amounted to US$ 17.7 billion,[38] whereas another study suggested that expenditure was US$ 105.4 billion.[39] The difference was mainly due to the inclusion of all healthcare costs in patients with back pain in the latter study compared to the inclusion of only back care related expenditure in the former.

It is also possible to glean an indication by accessing published statistics. For example, in England during 2005, there were over 66 million prescriptions for analgesics (British National Formulary categories 4.7 – analgesics – and 10.1.1 – nonsteroidal anti-inflammatory drugs (NSAIDs)) aside from over-the-counter purchases, at a net ingredient cost of £510 million (US$ 940 million).

The vast majority of these were for nonopioids (34 million prescriptions and cost of £120 million (US$ 220 million)) and NSAIDs (18 million prescriptions and cost of £150 million (US$ 280 million)).[40] However, a significant number of people with chronic pain may not actually consult anyone about their condition or choose to self-medicate. A survey of nearly 6000 people across Europe found that up to 27 percent of respondents had never sought medical help for their pain, and at least 38 percent of this group were in constant or daily pain.[41] The extent to which people took nonprescription drugs varied between 23 and 59 percent,[41] while a conservative estimate of over-the-counter medication relating to back pain amounted to £24 million (US$ 44 million).[42]

It has been estimated that primary care management of patients with chronic pain accounts for 4.6 million appointments per year in the UK, equivalent to 793 whole-time GPs, at a total cost of around £69 million (US$ 128 million).[43] The study examined the treatment regimens used in patient management and found that poor efficacy was the trigger for almost as many consultations as poor tolerability. A study conducted in Denmark highlighted that considerably higher resource utilization use was observed in the pain population in both primary and secondary healthcare sectors, compared with a no-pain control group.[44, 45] An Australian study showed that chronic pain results in increased use of healthcare services, with a direct relationship between levels of pain disability and resource utilization.[19]

The economic impact associated with chronic pain is also evident in younger age groups. A study of 52 adolescents and their families, who had been suffering from pain for nearly five years, completed a modified version of the client service receipt inventory to generate the costs associated with chronic pain.[46] The direct costs, which also included additional educational services (such as home tutoring and educational social workers) amounted to £4400 (US$ 8100) on average per adolescent/year, but with considerable variation across the sample group and conditions, with those in the pain management group having a mean direct cost of £7900 (US$ 14 600), while those in the rheumatology group had a mean of £2400 (US$ 4400). While the authors rightly argue that care should be exercised in the interpretation of their findings, and highlight that the costs recorded for their patient group are different from adult and general populations, they also advocated that effective treatments are needed in adolescence "to slow down the escalation of costs over time".[46]

What is also apparent is that despite these high levels of resource utilization there remains what has been called the "crisis of inadequately treated pain",[47] with many misconceptions and ignorance among professionals regarding pain and its treatment[18] and many patients either not being treated or receiving suboptimal care.[10] One of the disturbing features is the discrepancy between professional and patient perspectives, as evidenced in a telephone survey of nearly 6000 patients with chronic pain and 1500 primary care physicians. The survey, conducted in eight European countries, showed that physicians generally believed that patients were well managed. However, it was also shown that up to 27 percent of people with pain did not seek medical help and of those who did, there were major flaws in their treatment and overall management.[41] Another study showed that 40 percent of chronic pain patients were not satisfied with the treatment offered,[48] similar to the percentage of patients across Europe who were not satisfied with their treatment.[10]

Productivity and indirect costs associated with pain

While costly, the direct costs of pain management are minor in comparison with the impact of pain on the economy,[49] with a Danish study estimating that 1 million working days were lost annually as a result of chronic pain.[50] As well as its impact on absenteeism, pain has a major impact on worker productivity, accounting for 85 percent of the total lower back pain costs per patient.[51] It has been estimated that common pain conditions in the USA result in lost productivity amounting to US$ 61 billion per year, of which 77 percent was explained by reduced performance – presenteeism – and not work absence.[52] An Australian study estimated that while the number of absent workdays was 9.9 million annually, reduced effectiveness workdays was estimated at 36.5 million per year, which elevated the productivity costs from AU$ 1.4 billion (US$ 1.1 billion), resulting from absenteeism, to AU$ 5.1 (US$ 3.8 billion) when both absenteeism and presenteeism were included.[53] As well as the impact on absenteeism and presenteeism, the odds of leaving one's job because of ill health have been shown to be seven times higher among people with chronic pain problems than "normals".[48]

However, while the economic impact of chronic pain is substantial and imposes a greater economic burden than many other diseases,[36] decision-makers and policy-makers have tended to concentrate attention on a very minor component of the cost burden, namely prescription costs, because they are easy to measure and therefore an obvious target for restrictions.[54] The acquisition costs of medication are but one very small and insignificant part of a complex and expensive jigsaw, and attempts to focus attention and energies on restricting expenditure in this one area fail to recognize the wide-reaching implications of pain management. Patients who can be safely transferred from intensive care settings to normal ward settings, patients who can be safely discharged home from hospital, and patients who do not place demands on doctors' time can release scarce resources for the use of other patients and return to normal functioning sooner. People whose pain can be effectively managed are less likely to be on long-term sickness absence and incapacity benefit. They are likely to be more productive and have fewer absences from school and further education. Investment in effective interventions and programs which deliver relief from pain and suffering and reductions in disability levels will generate economic and social returns that more than repay the original investment.[55] In order to develop such a mode of thinking it is essential that "policy-makers are fully aware of all aspects associated with the costs of pain and its management."[5]

One such example of this limited economic perspective in pain management is the iatrogenic costs associated with NSAIDs, which often result in costly side effects. These iatrogenic costs have been estimated at between £32 and £70 (US$ 58 and US$ 127) for each patient prescribed an NSAID in the UK, and the total effect on the National Health Service in the UK was estimated to be between £166 million (US$ 305 million) and £367 million (US$ 675 million) per year.[56] In Sweden, for example, estimates of NSAID-induced gastric side effects range from SEK320 million to SEK589 million (US$ 35 million to US$ 64 million);[57] in the Netherlands, they range between €39 million and €98 million (US$ 39 million to US$ 97 million);[58] and in Quebec (Canada), approximately one Canadian dollar (US$ 0.66) would be added to patient costs for every day a patient was on NSAID therapy.[59]

Impact of pain on quality of life

Estimates of the economic burden associated with pain fail to do justice to the extent of suffering and reduced quality of life experienced by patients and warrants pain relief being regarded as a universal human right.[18] Chronic pain, along with musculoskeletal disorders, has been shown to be associated with some of the poorest quality-of-life states.[60, 61, 62, 63] In patients referred to a Danish multidisciplinary pain center, the severity of impairment was equal to or lower than patients with cardiopulmonary diseases and major depression, and their Psychological General Well-being Scale scores were lower than those with hypertension and gastrointestinal problems, while they also displayed high levels of anxiety and depression, as measured by the Hospital Anxiety and Depression Scale.[63] In a study of over 600 patients attending a chronic pain clinic in Sydney, Australia, there were greatly reduced SF-36 domain scores between clinic patients and Australian norm values, as shown in **Table 6.1**.[61] Relatively low SF-12 scores were demonstrated in a European study on chronic musculoskeletal pain, which also highlighted that up to 57 percent of respondents were in constant pain and up to 22 percent were in daily pain.[41]

Focusing on the burden and impact of chronic pain, and allocating additional resources to deal with the problem, does not necessarily result in a more efficient, or indeed equitable, allocation of resources. In order to move in such a direction it is necessary to employ the techniques of economic evaluation.

Table 6.1 SF-36 scores in pain clinic attendees compared with norms.

SF-36 domain	Pain clinic	Australian norm
General health	48.5	71.6
Physical functioning	37.1	82.6
Role physical	12.7	79.9
Bodily pain	36.1	76.8
Vitality	40.7	64.5
Social functioning	41.4	85.0
Emotional health	36.9	82.9
Mental health	53.5	75.9

Source: Data reprinted with permission from Ref. 61.

THE ROLE OF ECONOMIC EVALUATION

Economic evaluation has been defined as "a comparative analysis of two or more alternatives in terms of their costs and consequences."[64] From this definition it can be seen that evaluation involves a comparison between alternatives, which may include "do nothing," while the evaluation includes both the direct costs (see above under Direct costs of pain management) and indirect costs (see above under Productivity and indirect costs associated with pain) incurred – depending upon the perspective employed – and the benefits derived from each of the alternatives. The process and techniques of economic evaluation are well documented and it is suggested that interested readers consult some of these sources.[20, 26, 29, 30, 31, 32, 64]

The nature and categorization of costs and benefits have already been highlighted, but in deciding which costs and benefits to include in the evaluation, it is the perspective employed in the evaluation that will determine this – a narrow health service perspective will not include patients' costs, productivity costs, and intangibles, whereas a societal perspective will include all costs, and wherever possible measured and valued. In reality, this would not be possible, but the decision-maker needs to be informed how the analysis has dealt with costs and benefits not specifically included in the calculations in determining cost effectiveness or cost benefit.

The valuation of costs and benefits also needs to reflect when costs are incurred and when benefits are realized. Individuals and societies are not indifferent to timing – preferring to delay costs as long as possible and to receive benefits as soon as possible. Therefore, costs and benefits which occur today are valued more highly than those which occur in the future, and the current value of any cost or benefit is lower the further in the future that it arises. In order to allow for this, future costs and benefits are subjected to discounting. The approach is quite simple using the formula:

$$PV = K \times (1/(1+r)^n)$$

where PV is the present value, K is the nominal value of the cost or benefit, r is the discount rate, and n is the number of years in the future the cost or benefit arises. If we expect to receive a benefit of £10,000 in five years' time, the present value, based on a discount rate of 5 percent, is equivalent to £7835.

In addition, when a new treatment or service is being considered it is unlikely that it will replace all existing and established therapies and services. Instead, some patients are switched, while others will remain on existing treatments and services. The issue therefore is what additional benefits are gained from the additional costs of the new therapy? This approach is termed "incremental analysis," where the difference in costs between the alternatives is divided by the difference in benefits. This provides a much more focused assessment of the impact of the new technology in context, rather than providing data relating to the total costs and benefits or the average cost and benefit generated by the new technology. The incremental cost–effectiveness ratio (ICER) (difference in costs divided by the difference in benefits) is used to address this issue.

Techniques of economic evaluation

Under the umbrella of economic evaluation there are five techniques available, depending on how the consequences of healthcare interventions and programmes are measured and valued and, as already stated, interested readers are invited to consult the array of available sources.

COST–EFFECTIVENESS ANALYSIS

Cost–effectiveness analysis is used when outcomes are one-dimensional and measured in terms of health effect, such as reduction in pain score. When survival is the key measure of outcome, cost–effectiveness would assess the cost per life year gained from each of the alternatives with the lowest cost–effectiveness ratio indicating the best course of action. When the outcomes generated by the alternatives are equal, it is possible to use cost–minimization analysis, where the choice of the best alternative is made purely on the basis of cost. However, in order for cost–minimization analysis to be used, the equivalence of all outcomes from the alternatives must be unequivocal, which is rarely seen in practice.

COST–BENEFIT ANALYSIS

Cost–benefit analysis enables the notion of efficiency to be viewed from a higher level, that of allocative efficiency, in that it enables judgments to be made about the relative value of pursuing one objective (e.g. full restoration of a person to employment) as opposed to another (e.g. ability to pursue some aspects of normal functioning). Cost–effectiveness analysis, on the other hand, can only provide an indication of technical efficiency, since it provides an assessment of different ways of fulfilling the same objective (for example, securing pain relief). However, cost–benefit analysis is reliant on being able to place monetary values on the identified costs and benefits. This is possible where, for example, people are willing to pay for a reduction in pain. Methods of arriving at indicators of willingness-to-pay can be arrived at by asking people directly through, for example, questionnaires. One such method is the contingent valuation approach, which asks people the maximum amount they would be prepared to pay for the benefit. An alternative to the questionnaire approach is to employ proxy values; for example, the price people would be prepared to pay for surgery in a private hospital would be an indicator of how much they were willing to pay to avoid having to join a waiting list. However, there are many issues relating to the translation of health outcomes into a monetary measure and thus cost–benefit analysis is not widely used when undertaking health economic evaluations.

QUALITY ADJUSTED LIFE YEARS

An alternative measure of value to that of a monetary approach is one of utility, where quality of life adjustments are made to a given state of outcomes, whilst simultaneously providing a common denominator for comparison of costs and outcomes in different healthcare programs. The common denominator, usually expressed as quality adjusted life years (QALYs) is arrived at by adjusting the duration of the outcome (e.g. life expectancy) by the utility value of the resulting health status. The basis of using utility effects is based on the notion that outcomes from treatments and other health-influencing activities have two basic components, quantity and quality of life. Life expectancy is a traditional measure with few problems of comparison. However, attempts to measure and value quality of life have a more recent history, with a number of approaches and instruments being utilized. Particular effort has gone into researching ways in which an overall health index might be constructed which would locate a specific health state on a continuum between 0 (worst possible health state) and 1 (perfect health). The QALY therefore takes one year of perfect-health life expectancy to be worth 1, but regards one year of less than perfect-health life expectancy as less than 1. QALYs are discussed and described elsewhere,[20, 64, 65, 66] but the comparison between healthcare programs and interventions in terms of QALYs gained is depicted in **Figure 6.1**.

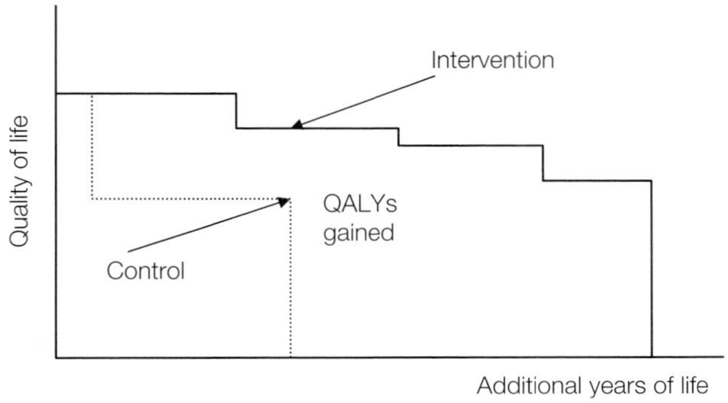

Figure 6.1 Quality adjusted life years gained.

COST–UTILITY ANALYSIS

When outcomes are measured in terms of QALYs, the technique used is that of cost–utility analysis. The beauty of cost–utility analysis is that it enables comparisons to be made across different areas of health care – so that the cost per QALY of a pain management program can be compared with those designed to treat people in advanced stages of cancer. While they provide an indication of the benefits gained from a variety of medical procedures, in terms of quality of life and survival for patients, they are far from perfect as a measure of outcome. However, their use means that decisions are made explicitly and not based on political pressures and power or the quest for technological advancement. To restrict decision-making to doctors, or for that matter administrators, is to result in situations where most resources go to those who shout the loudest or to those who pluck the heartstrings the hardest. Widening the decision-making process is a move in the right direction and the utilization of QALYs (despite their limitations) is a means whereby the benefits generated by the healthcare system can be included in the process, thereby enabling better decisions to be made.

COST–CONSEQUENCES ANALYSIS

When the outcomes are multidimensional – for example, changes in pain scores, return to normal functioning, etc. – the technique employed is that of cost–consequences analysis, where the outcomes are quantified and related to the costs for each of the alternative courses of action. It is this approach which is beginning to find increasing support among health economists, as it does not restrict the outcomes generated from healthcare interventions and programs to a single measure, such as QALY. It is easier to understand and enables decision-makers (on behalf of society) to impute their own specific, local values to these costs and consequences, and incorporate other aspects in the portfolio of information with which to inform the decision-making process.[67]

SENSITIVITY ANALYSIS

It should always be borne in mind that economic evaluation is not an exact science and findings from such studies should be treated with caution. Uncertainty is a fact of life and no economic evaluation can do anything other than reach a conclusion on the basis of the best (most informed) assumptions possible. In undertaking economic evaluations there are four sources of potential uncertainty:

1. methodological arising from different approaches and methods employed;
2. potential variation in the estimates of the parameters used in the evaluation;
3. extrapolation from observed events over time or from intermediate to final health outcomes;
4. generalizability and transferability of results.

It is important, therefore, to investigate how sensitive the findings of an evaluation are to changes in the assumptions used in the study and variations in the parameter estimates. Sensitivity analysis in such cases involves rerunning the analysis with the assumptions changed and asking "what if"-type questions. A number of approaches have been employed to estimate the effect of uncertainty, but it is not the intention to delve into these techniques here, and interested readers are invited to consult relevant sources.[20, 26, 29, 30, 31, 32, 64, 68]

ROLE OF ECONOMICS IN DEVELOPING STRATEGIES FOR MANAGING PATIENTS WITH CHRONIC PAIN

The burden of suffering pain imposes on individuals and the enormous costs, which society has to bear as a result, demonstrate that policy-makers, commissioners, and healthcare decision-makers should adopt a broad, strategic, and coherent perspective in determining issues relating to service provision and resource allocation. Fragmented, budgetary-based interventions and programs based on at best inadequate evidence do little to alleviate the problems associated with chronic pain and deprive patients of those services that would have a positive impact. Differentials between the demands placed on health services for treatments for pain relief, and other aspects of health care and the resources available to meet such needs, continue to be major headaches for those involved in policy-making, decision-making, commissioning services, and the provision and delivery of healthcare services. It has therefore been advocated that decisions relating to patient management are made with regard to "the three Es" – effectiveness, efficiency, and equity.[55]

Effectiveness

The evidence base for the effectiveness of interventions and management strategies in chronic pain is large,[69, 70] although questions relating to the quality of studies and their relevance for clinical practice and economic evaluation remain.[71] For example, an epidemiological survey of over 10,000 individuals concluded that "opioid treatment of long-term/chronic noncancer pain does not seem to fulfil any of the key outcome opioid treatment goals: pain relief, improved quality of life, and improved functional capacity."[44] The propensity to bolt on economic evaluations to clinical studies and to model the economic impact of interventions following on from randomized controlled trials, without taking into consideration some of the broader issues and factors from the complex environment that impinge on the overall impact of treatments and therapies, has been very noticeable in the last few years, as the focus has switched more to the assessment and appraisal of healthcare technologies. As a result, it may be more appropriate to rename cost–effectiveness studies as cost–efficacy studies and, while valiant efforts are being made to deal with the effect of uncertainty so as to aid the decision-making process, the fact remains that the everyday world of health care is very different from the quasi-laboratory conditions under which clinical studies are undertaken and, irrespective of the number of simulations of the available data, it is impossible to capture all possible scenarios and situations that might arise in the real world of clinical practice. The nature and extent of adverse events associated with some interventions have also resulted in considerable debate and discussion as to what constitutes effectiveness when the issues of efficacy and safety are combined. For example, a systematic review of over 5000 patients confirmed that most patients will experience at least one adverse event resulting from opioid use in chronic nonmalignant pain, and that substantial minorities will experience common adverse events of dry mouth, nausea, and constipation, and will not continue treatment because of intolerable adverse events.[72]

In relation to strategies for the management of chronic pain patients, the evidence base for their effectiveness is also increasing, although again the issue of what works, where, and when remains inconclusive. For example, a recent meta-analysis of psychological treatments of pain in children claimed that "there is, at present, no evidence for the effectiveness of psychological therapies in attenuating pain in conditions other than headache,"[73] while reviews of multidisciplinary pain treatments in adults have been more circumspect due to the quality of studies in low back pain[74] or concluded that there is very little evidence for effectiveness in neck and shoulder pain.[75]

Efficiency

The notion of efficiency has been discussed in general terms above, while in terms of pain management, there are three factors to consider in assessing the relative efficiency of interventions and programs, namely:

- maximizing the reduction in pain;
- minimizing the overall cost;
- minimizing the impact of adverse events.

It is essential to realize that the cost of treatment is not simply the costs of drugs or medical and nursing time, but the total costs of providing the treatment.[55] As shown above under The economic impact of pain, the costs of dealing with adverse events are not insubstantial, and by merely focusing attention on acquisition costs, decision-makers are only considering the tip of the iceberg and neglecting the "under the water" costs of dealing with adverse events, medical errors, and negligence claims, in addition to ineffective treatments and complementary medical examinations undertaken.[76] Similarly, it has been argued that less emphasis on technological solutions and a shift towards the biopsychosocial model would be an efficient use of limited resources in pain management – "every study published shows that aggressive, multidisciplinary pain management for the most disabled group of chronic patients will produce significant cost savings, to say nothing of the human suffering that will be alleviated."[77] However, even this claim can be called into question, as a systematic review of the effectiveness of multidisciplinary pain treatment of chronic nonmalignant pain patients in terms of economic outcomes, has concluded that "due to serious methodological problems in study designs and outcome measures, it is not possible to draw conclusions on clinical or economical effectiveness."[78]

Equity

The availability and accessibility of good quality services for all patients is highly desirable and should form part of the decision-making process. It has been argued that, in selected populations, patients managed through multidisciplinary programs have lower costs, return to work more frequently, and experience greater pain control than those who are managed with more traditional methods.[79] However, the availability of such facilities is sketchy and some populations have "no local access to services for patients with long-lasting pain"[2] – a situation likely to deteriorate, as demographic factors intensify the demand for chronic pain services for the foreseeable future.[80]

The patient perspective is extremely important in terms of trying to achieve some degree of equity. Pain management programs were regarded as relatively high priority in a survey of nearly 3500 patients in Scotland, undertaken to assess the feasibility of using patients' perceptions of need for primary healthcare services to develop priorities, although the authors highlighted the fact that the area had received marginal attention in terms of development.[81] It has been strongly advocated that society has an obligation to reduce levels of pain and restore normal functioning, based upon both moral principles and economic reality,[78] with the ethical dimension[18] being a powerful addition to the other three Es discussed earlier in this section.

CONCLUSIONS

Technological advancements, developments in medical science, and increasing expectations of communities as to what is available from healthcare providers continue to focus attention on the healthcare dilemma. Irrespective of funding levels, choices always have to be made as to where resources are allocated. In making such choices, decision-makers need to establish an explicit set of priorities while attitudes among professionals and societies need to be changed. The on-going development of evidence-based practice, the removal of interventions and services that provide no benefit, the recognition that resources are finite and choices have to be made, and an awareness of the need for fairness in resource allocation and service provision, are major steps along the road towards better health care, as well as addressing the issue of how much additional resources should be put into healthcare services. Although the evidence base on which to conduct economic analyses in the area of pain management is suboptimal and there are technical problems surrounding economic approaches to priority setting, these should not be allowed to detract from the fact that economic evaluation provides a rational framework within which other issues and approaches can be embraced and priorities established to move towards better health care.

Better health care does not necessarily require additional resources. Whole systems thinking, based on good quality relevant evidence rather than an aggregation of narrow, budgetary-focused organizations pursuing their own agendas without regard for the wider perspective, would have a major positive impact on the management of patients with chronic pain. More work is needed to develop a broader, strategic, whole systems agenda in pain management. High quality relevant evidence and health economics techniques and approaches are essential components of this particular agenda. Together they can provide the tools which decision-makers can utilize in the drive for reductions in pain and better health and health care for our respective communities and societies.

REFERENCES

1. Bruster S, Jarman B, Bosanquet N *et al.* National survey of hospital patients. *British Medical Journal.* 1994; **309**: 1542–6.
2. Audit Commission. *Anaesthesia under examination.* London: Audit Commission, 1997.
3. McQuay HJ, Moore RA, Justins D. Treating acute pain in hospital. *British Medical Journal.* 1997; **314**: 1531–5.
4. Latham J, Davis BD. The socio-economic impact of chronic pain. *Disability and Rehabilitation.* 1994; **16**: 39–44.
5. Rudy TE, Kerns RD, Turk DC. Chronic pain and depression: toward a cognitive behavioural model. *Pain.* 1988; **35**: 129–40.
6. Clark JD. Chronic pain prevalence and analgesic prescribing in a general medical population. *Journal of Pain and Symptom Management.* 2002; **23**: 131–7.
7. Blyth FM, March LM, Brnabic AJ *et al.* Chronic pain in Australia: a prevalence study. *Pain.* 2001; **89**: 127–34.
8. Verhaak PFM, Kerssens JJ, Dekker J *et al.* Prevalence of chronic benign pain disorder among adults: a review of the literature. *Pain.* 1998; **77**: 231–9.
9. Ospina M, Harstall C. *Prevalence of chronic pain: an overview.* Report, HTA 29. Edmonton: Alberta Heritage Foundation for Medical Research, 2002.
10. ∗ Breivik H, Collett B, Ventafridda V *et al.* Survey of chronic pain in Europe: prevalence, impact on daily life, and treatment. *European Journal of Pain.* 2006; **10**: 287–333.
11. Crook J, Rideout E, Browne G. The prevalence of pain complaints in a general population. *Pain.* 1984; **18**: 299–314.
12. Van Korff M, Wagner EH, Dworkin SF *et al.* Chronic pain and use of ambulatory healthcare. *Psychosomatic Medicine.* 1991; **53**: 61–79.
13. ∗ Elliott AM, Smith BH, Penny KI *et al.* The epidemiology of chronic pain in the community. *Lancet.* 1999; **354**: 1248–52.
14. ∗ Elliott AM, Smith BH, Hannaford PC *et al.* The course of chronic pain in the community: results of a 4-year follow-up study. *Pain.* 2002; **99**: 299–307.
15. White KP, Harth M. The occurrence and impact of generalised pain. *Baillière's Clinical Rheumatology.* 1999; **13**: 379–89.
16. Woolf AD, Pfleger B. Burden of major musculoskeletal conditions. *Bulletin of the World Health Organization.* 2003; **81**: 646–56.
17. Perquin C, Hazebroek-Kampscheur A, Hunfield J *et al.* Pain in children and adolescents: a common experience. *Pain.* 2000; **87**: 51–8.
18. ∗ Cousins MJ. Pain relief: a universal human right. *Pain.* 2004; **112**: 1–4.
19. Blyth FM, March LM, Brnabic AJM, Cousins MJ. Chronic pain and frequent use of healthcare. *Pain.* 2004; **111**: 51–8.
20. ∗ Phillips CJ. *Health Economics: an introduction for healthcare professionals.* Oxford: BMJ Books Blackwells, 2005.
21. Gould E. Healthcare: US spends more, gets less. Economic Policy Institute snapshots. Washington, DC: Economic Policy Institute. Last updated October 2004, cited February 2008. Available from: www.epinet.org/content.cfm/webfeatures_snapshots_10202004

22. Edwards RT. Paradigms and research programmes: is it time to move from healthcare economics to health economics. *Health Economics.* 2001; **10**: 635–49.
23. Evans RG, Barer ML, Marmor TRE (eds). *Why are some people healthy and other are not? The determinants of health of populations.* New York: Aldine de Gruyter, 1994.
24. Moore A. Waste in the NHS: the problem, its size and how we can tackle it, Oxford: Bandolier Extra. Last updated October 2000, cited February 2008. Available from: www.jr2.ox.ac.uk/bandolier/Extraforbando/Waste.pdf.
25. Borowitz M, Sheldon T. Controlling healthcare: from economic interventions to micro-clinical regulation. *Health Economics.* 1993; **2**: 201–04.
26. Mitton G, Donaldson C. *Priority setting toolkit: a guide to the use of economics in healthcare decision making.* London: BMJ Books, 2004.
27. Mallenson A. *Whiplash and other useful illnesses.* Montreal: McGill-Queen's University Press, 2002.
28. Palfrey C, Thomas P, Phillips CJ. *Effective healthcare management: an evaluative approach.* Oxford: Blackwell, 2004.
29. Phillips CJ, Palfrey CF, Thomas P. *Evaluating health and social care.* Basingstoke: Macmillan, 1994.
30. Mooney G. *Economics, medicine and health care.* London: Harvester Wheatsheaf, 1992.
31. Jefferson T, Demicheli V, Mugford M. *Elementary economic evaluation in healthcare.* London: BMJ Books, 2000.
32. Kobelt G. *Health Economics: an introduction to economic evalaution.* London: Office of Health Economics, 2002.
33. Drummond MF. Cost-of-illness studies: a major headache? *Pharmacoeconomics.* 1992; **2**: 1–4.
34. Koopmanschap MA, Rutten FFH, van Ineveld BM, van Roijen L. The friction cost method for measuring indirect costs of disease. *Journal of Health Economics.* 1995; **14**: 171–89.
35. Borghouts JAJ, Koes BW, Vondeling H, Bouter LM. Cost-of-illness of neck pain in The Netherlands in 1996. *Pain.* 1999; **80**: 629–36.
* 36. Maniadakis N, Gray A. The economic burden of back pain in the UK. *Pain.* 2000; **84**: 95–103.
37. Bolten W, Kempel-Waibel A, Pforringer W. Analysis of the cost of illness in backache. *Medizinische Klinik.* 1998; **93**: 388–93.
38. Mychaskiw MA, Thomas J. Direct costs of back pain in the United States: A national estimate. *Value in Health.* 2002; **5**: 508.
39. van der Roer N, Goosens ME, Evers SM, van Tulder MW. What is the most cost effective treatment for patients with low back pain? A systematic review. *Best Practice and Research. Clinical Rheumatology.* 2005; **19**: 671–84.
40. Department of Health. Prescription cost analysis for England 2005. Last updated April 2006, cited February 2008. Leeds: The Information Centre. Available from: www.ic.nhs.uk/statistics-and-data-collections/primary-care/prescribing/prescription-cost-analysis-2005
* 41. Woolf AD, Zeidler H, Hagland U *et al.* Musculoskeletal pain in Europe: its impact and a comparison of population and medical perceptions of treatment in eight European countries. *Annals of the Rheumatic Diseases.* 2004; **63**: 342–7.
42. Walsh K, Cruddas M, Coggon D. Low back pain in eight areas of Britain. *Journal of Epidemiology and Community Health.* 1993; **46**: 227-30.
43. Belsey J. Primary care workload in the management of chronic pain: A retrospective cohort study using a GP database to identify resource implications for UK primary care. *Journal of Medical Economics.* 2002; **5**: 39–52.
44. Eriksen J, Sjogren P, Bruera E *et al.* Critical issues on opioids in chronic non-cancer pain: An epidemiological study. *Pain.* 2006; **125**: 172–9.
45. Eriksen J, Sjogren P, Ekholm O, Rasmussen NK. Healthcare utilisation among individuals reporting long-term pain: an epidemiological study based on Danish National Health Surveys. *European Journal of Pain.* 2004; **8**: 517–23.
46. Sleed M, Eccleston C, Beecham J *et al.* The economic impact of chronic pain in adolescence: methodological considerations and a preliminary cost-of-illness study. *Pain.* 2005; **119**: 183–90.
47. Fishman SM, Gallagher RM, Carr DB, Sullivan LW. The case for pain medicine. *Pain Medicine.* 2004; **5**: 281–6.
48. Eriksen J, Jensen MK, Sjogren P *et al.* Epidemiology of chronic non-malignant pain in Denmark. *Pain.* 2003; **106**: 221–8.
49. Parthan A, Evans CJ, Le K. Chronic back pain: epidemiology, economic burden and patient-reported outcomes in the USA. *Expert Review of Pharmacoeconomics and Outcomes Research.* 2006; **6**: 359–69.
50. Eriksen J, Sjogren P. Epidemiological factors relating to long-term/chronic non-cancer pain in Denmark. *Ugeskrift for Laeger.* 2006; **168**: 1947–50.
51. Ekman M, Jonhagen S, Hunsche E, Jonsson L. Burden of illness of chronic back pain in Sweden: a cross-sectional, retrospective study in primary care setting. *Spine.* 2005; **30**: 1777–85.
* 52. Stewart WF, Ricci JA, Chee E *et al.* Lost productive time and cost due to common pain conditions in the US workforce. *Journal of the American Medical Association.* 2003; **290**: 2443–54.
53. Van Leeuwen MT, Blyth FM, March LM *et al.* Chronic pain and reduced work effectiveness: the hidden cost to Australian employers. *European Journal of Pain.* 2006; **10**: 161–6.
54. Smith I. Cost considerations in the use of anaesthetic drugs. *Pharmacoeconomics.* 2001; **19**: 469–81.
* 55. Phillips CJ. The real cost of pain management. *Anaesthesia.* 2001; **56**: 1031–3.
56. Moore RA, Phillips CJ. Cost of NSAID adverse effects to the UK National Health Service. *Journal of Medical Economics.* 1999; **2**: 45–55.
57. Jonsson B, Haglund U. Economic burden of NSAID-induced gastropathy in Sweden. *Scandinavian Journal of Gastroenterology.* 2001; **36**: 775–9.

58. Herings RM, Klungel OH. An epidemiological approach to assess the economic burden of NSAID-induced gastrointestinal events in The Netherlands. *Pharmacoeconomics*. 2001; **19**: 655–65.
59. Rahme E, Joseph L, Kong SX *et al.* Gastrointestinal healthcare resource use and costs associated with nonsteroidal anti-inflammatory drugs versus acetaminophen: retrospective cohort study of an elderly population. *Arthritis and Rheumatism*. 2000; **43**: 917–24.
* 60. Sprangers MAG, de Regt EB, Andries F *et al.* Which chronic conditions are associated with a better or poorer quality of life? *Journal of Clinical Epidemiology*. 2000; **53**: 895–7.
61. Kerr S, Fairbrother G, Crawford M *et al.* Patient characteristics and quality of life among a sample of Australian chronic pain clinic attendees. *Internal Medicine Journal*. 2004; **34**: 403–09.
62. Ellliott TE, Renier CM, Palcher JA. Chronic pain, depression and quality of life: correlations and predictive value of the SF-36. *Pain Medicine*. 2003; **4**: 331–9.
63. Becker N, Thomsens AB, Olsen AK *et al.* Pain epidemiology and health related quality of life in chronic non-malignant pain patients referred to a Danish multidisciplinary pain center. *Pain*. 1997; **73**: 393–400.
* 64. Drummond MF, O'Brien B, Stoddart GL *et al. Methods for the economic evaluation of healthcare programmes*. Oxford: Oxford Medical Publications, 1997.
* 65. Phillips CJ, Thompson G. What is a QALY? London: Hayward Medical Communications. Last updated May 2001, cited February 2008. Available from: www.jr2.ox.ac.uk/bandolier/painres/download/whatis/QALY.pdf.
66. Moore A, McQuay H. *Bandolier's little book of making sense of the medical evidence*. Oxford: Oxford University Press, 2006.
* 67. Coast J. Is economic evaluation in touch with society's health values? *British Medical Journal*. 2004; **329**: 1233–6.
68. Briggs A. Handling uncertainty in economic evaluation and presenting the results. In: Drummond M, Towse A (eds). *Economic evaluation in healthcare: merging theory with practice*. Oxford: Office of Health Economics and Oxford Medical Publications, 2001: 172–214.
* 69. McQuay HJ, Moore RA. *An evidence based resource for pain relief*. Oxford University Press: Oxford, 1998.
* 70. Moore A, Edwards J, Barden J, McQuay H. *Bandolier's little book of pain*. Oxford: Oxford University Press, 2003.
71. Moore RA. Pain and systematic reviews. *Acta Anaesthesiologica Scandinavica*. 2001; **45**: 1136–9.
72. Moore RA, McQuay HJ. Prevalence of opioid adverse events in chronic non-malignant pain: systematic review of randomised trials of oral opioids. *Arthritis Research and Therapy*. 2005; **7**: R1046–51.
73. Eccleston C, Yorke L, Morley S *et al.* Psychological therapies for the management of chronic and recurrent pain in children and adolescents. *Cochrane Database of Systematic Reviews*. 2003; **CD003968**.
74. Karjalainen K, Malmivara A, van Tulder M *et al.* Multidisciplinary biopsychological rehabilitation for subacute low back pain among working age adults. *Cochrane Database of Systematic Reviews*. 2003; **CD002193**.
75. Karjalainen K, Malmivara A, van Tulder M *et al.* Multidisciplinary biopsychological rehabilitation for neck and shoulder pain among working age adults. *Cochrane Database of Systematic Reviews*. 2003; **CD002194**.
76. Phillips CJ. And all because the doctor prescribed an NSAID: expenditure on PPIs and joined-up thinking in prescribing. *British Journal of Healthcare Management*. 2002; **8**: 272–5.
77. Loeser JD. Economic implications of pain management. *Acta Anaesthesiologica Scandinavica*. 1999; **43**: 957–9.
78. Thomsen AB, Sørensen J, Sjøgren P *et al.* Economic evaluation of multidisciplinary pain management in chronic pain patients: a qualitative systematic review. *Journal of Pain and Symptom Management*. 2001; **22**: 688–98.
79. Guzmán J, Esmail R, Karjalainen K *et al.* Multidisciplinary rehabilitation for chronic low back pain: systematic review. *British Medical Journal*. 2001; **322**: 1511–16.
80. McQuay HJ, Moore RA, Eccleston C *et al.* Systematic review of outpatient services for chronic patient control. *Health Technology Assessment*. 1997; **1**: i–iv.
81. Hopton JL, Dlugolecka M. Patients' perceptions of need for primary healthcare services: useful for priority setting? *British Medical Journal*. 1995; **310**: 1237–40.

7

The challenges of pain and suffering

DAVID B MORRIS AND PETER R WILSON

KEY LEARNING POINTS

- The International Association for the Study of Pain (IASP) definition of pain is valid, but flexible.
- Suffering has physical, psychological, legal, and ethical dimensions.
- Biology and culture both affect an individual's and society's response to injury or harm.
- Narrative is the most important component of pain expression.

INTRODUCTION

> The work which you are accomplishing is immensely important for the good of humanity, as you seek the ever more effective control of physical pain and of the oppression of mind and spirit that physical pain so often brings with it.
>
> Pope John Paul II (26 July 1987)[1]

Pain medicine arose during the last half of the twentieth century and accompanied the rise of new clinics and treatment centers devoted specifically to pain. Change accelerated after Ronald Melzack and Patrick Wall published their landmark gate-control theory of pain in 1965,[2] which was rapidly absorbed into mainstream biomedical thinking despite unresolved questions that eventually led Melzack to look beyond spinal gates.[3] Organizational developments kept pace. In 1973, John Bonica invited some 300 participants to a conference outside Seattle, where they discussed founding a worldwide medical–scientific association focused on pain (discussed in Ref. 4). Soon, several agencies within the US National Institutes of Health assigned priority to pain research and control, creating incentives, and guidelines for progress, and many academic medical centers responded by setting up pain teams. Public health systems and private insurers debated who would pay, how much, and for what. Multinational corporations invested huge sums to market powerful over-the-counter and prescription analgesics. Pain was big business. As the twenty-first century began, the organization that emerged from the now famous Seattle–Issaquah Conference – the International Association for the Study of Pain – had an impressive 6900 individual members in 106 countries (www.iasp-pain.org).

The proliferation of specialized journals and annual meetings on pain, together with new technologies for research and communication, maintains a fast pace of change. In 1991, for example, Melzack criticized the lack of serious interest in cortical dimensions of pain. "What happens in the brain after cortical activation," he observed, "is a question most people want to avoid."[5] The same year saw publication of the first studies that use positron emission tomography (PET) to examine the human brain, showing activation in the anterior cingulate cortex of subjects exposed to acutely painful heat.[6, 7] Almost instantly, brain imaging contributed remarkable new insights to pain research.[8] The mere expectation of pain, as magnetic resonance images (MRI) show, corresponds to activation of a specific area within the human brain.[9] A 2007 topical review described a possible direction of pain research – developing treatment methods based on "objective" functional MRI data rather than traditional subjective (50 percent improvement) methods."[10] As in other fields of science and medicine, one formidable challenge is simply to keep up with the speed and trajectory of change.

The challenges extend in many directions, especially as researchers examine pain processes at the cellular level. In tissue cultures from newborn rats, for example, specific neurons from the sympathetic nervous system grow axons that make contact with sensory neurons, which suggests possibilities of interaction between the two separate pain systems.[11] Advances in genetics have opened up fruitful areas of pain research that were unknown 50 years ago. We recently learned that certain strains of mice possess genetic variance in nociception and in morphine-induced analgesia.[12] Strains of rats possess a congenital hypersensitivity that makes them, in effect, prone to pain.[13] Despite the disclaimers about animal models, we will soon see huge advances in understanding genetic components of the human pain process, even as advances in pharmacology reveal how pain-killers ranging from nonsteroidal anti-inflammatory drugs (NSAIDs) to opioids operate with different effects on multiple sites within the nervous system, permitting better use of drugs in combination.[14, 15] Optimists believe that this accumulating knowledge will ultimately lead to the full-scale control or eradication of pain. Perhaps governments will lock away a few last pains for research purposes in case of national emergencies.

Unfortunately, pain is not likely to surrender its power during our lifetimes, and suffering is an ineradicable part of the human condition. Indeed, as social services and medical systems focus on pain, they find more pain that needs relief. Among adults, the prevalence of chronic benign pain – in which a nociceptive substrate is difficult to find – ranges between 2 and 40 percent of the population, depending on the study.[16] In the Netherlands, the cost of back pain alone equals 1.7 percent of the gross national product and lost work as a result of back pain costs the Netherlands on average $1.5 million per hour.[17, 18] In the USA, the rate of disability claims associated with low back pain has increased over the rate of population growth by 1400 percent.[19] Such massive costs and complex clinical dilemmas help to explain why an IASP Task Force in 1995 recommended that nonspecific low back pain be reconceived not as a medical condition but as "activity intolerance."[20] The controversial recommendation – linking low back pain, jobs, and disability insurance – stands as a reminder that neither pain nor suffering can be wholly reduced to a universal biology of nerves, neurotransmitters, and brain states. The administrative consequences appear to be insurmountable in the USA. In May 2007, the Social Security Administration reported that there were 738,000 disability cases waiting to be heard on appeal (denial) by Administrative Law Judges (ALJ), with an average waiting time of 505 days (www.ssa.gov/legislation/testimony_052307.htm). In the following text, pain and suffering in their implicit complications pose four specific challenges that are indirectly but firmly related to treatment: how to define them, how to classify them, how to understand them, and how to confront the implicit ethical dilemmas they encompass.

PAIN AND SUFFERING: WHAT ARE THEY?

Scientific and medical definitions are tools. Even when we recognize them as imperfect or provisional, awaiting replacement by an improved version, they perform work that cannot be accomplished by less precise instruments. It was thus a serious matter when in 1979 the subcommittee on taxonomy appointed by the newly formed IASP published its now familiar definition of pain as "an unpleasant sensory and emotional experience associated with actual or potential tissue damage, or described in terms of such damage."[21] This brief definition – reaffirmed in a 1994 second edition[22] – has made it possible for researchers and clinicians working in many different countries, in various languages, and in far-flung disciplines to possess at least a basic mutual understanding of what they mean (and, equally important, do not mean) by the all-purpose, ragtag, everyday English word "pain."

The IASP definition recognizes that tissue damage remains for most people – patients especially – the gold standard for pain. It also recognizes, however, that pain may occur when tissue damage is not present. The IASP definition even allows that tissue damage sometimes simply generates the language we apply to various unpleasant or traumatic sensory and emotional experiences. The extended note accompanying the IASP definition states clearly that pain is not equivalent to nociception, the process by which a signal of tissue injury is transmitted through the nervous system: "Activity induced in the nociceptor and nociceptive pathways by a noxious stimulus," the IASP authors insist, "is not pain, which is always a psychological state ...." As a psychological state, pain is irreducible to objective signs. The extended annotation begins with the blunt and unequivocal statement that "pain is always subjective."

It is fascinating how much matter for controversy has been packed into the brief IASP definition of pain. The definition and its supporting annotations gently but surely dissolve any necessary connection between pain and tissue damage. Extensive tissue damage may occur without pain, as Henry K Beecher showed in his classic study of soldiers wounded in the Second World War.[23, 24] Pain may also occur in the total absence of tissue damage, as researchers recently confirmed.[25] Most important, with a daring that merits repetition, the IASP definition recognizes that pain is always a subjective, psychological state. No purely pathophysiological model of pain can encompass such recognitions. At the same time, the task force authors also state in the annotation what is surely true: that pain, despite its psychological and subjective nature, "most often has a proximate physical cause." In short, the IASP definition proves to be concise, flexible, and accurate. It has served the community of pain medicine very well. Naturally, there are voices today arguing that we should get rid of it.

Recent objections to the IASP definition emphasize two claims: it is Cartesian and it neglects the ethical dimensions of pain. Cartesian today is often a synonym for wrong. As the best-known proponent of mind/body dualism, Descartes has erroneously been identified as the precursor or progenitor of any theory that separates body from mind. Complaints that the IASP definition of pain is Cartesian, however, ignores several facts. The definition implies no such thing. It implies, on the contrary, that minds as well as bodies are necessarily involved in the experience of pain, an experience that is multidimensional, not the straightforward projection of sensory impulses that Descartes had described. Moreover, Descartes did not separate body from mind as neatly as his modern critics assume.[26] The bodily mechanism responsible for pain in humans was ineffectual when disengaged from the mind or soul, which is why Descartes could argue that animals (soulless, by definition) do not feel pain. We should stop referring to all medical mind/body dualisms as Cartesian: most are not the direct legacy of Descartes but flow from nineteenth century positivist science.[27] True, Descartes sees the mind as a passive receiver of sensory impulses, not as an active participant in the pain process. This justifiable criticism of Descartes, however, does not underwrite unjustified criticism of the IASP definition. Mind–body interrelations are indispensable in any definition that views pain as "always psychological," since even painful psychological states distinct from nociception require our personal and cultural histories of tissue damage in order to generate the language in which such psychological states are described and perceived.

A second criticism of the IASP definition is that it ignores ethical concerns implicit in pain and thus indirectly sustains or promotes unethical practices. One critic observes that the definition fails to highlight pain among disempowered and neglected minorities, such as women, blacks, children, and the elderly.[28] Certainly, we need to pay increased attention to pain in minority or marginalized groups, and a vigorous biomedical literature is beginning to address this lapse. The IASP definition, however, neither supports nor promotes social injustice: reform must find more effective and appropriate expressions. It is equally short-sighted to claim, as another critic observes, that the IASP definition makes pain dependent upon "full linguistic competence," ignoring pain in neonates and other nonverbal individuals,[29] for example, and in animals.[30] Animal pain is not identical to human pain, and the IASP definition deals with pain in humans. More important, the IASP account treats linguistic competence not as a philosophical prerequisite for pain, but as a clinical resource. Its most radical implication lies in valuing the patient's subjective self-report – still too often devalued or dismissed by doctors unable to find an objectively verifiable lesion. We know that self-reports are imperfect, influenced by variables such as memory, mood, and the questions posed to patients or research subjects.[31] Like objective data, they must be evaluated within the context of a full medical record. The IASP definition, however, makes it clinically irresponsible to dismiss the patient's subjective account of pain, accounts that today go beyond verbal reports to include visual analog scales, drawings, and even electronic diaries that record numerical estimates of pain intensity.

One can criticize the IASP definition on various grounds – such as a circularity in defining pain as "unpleasant" – but pain is a complex state, resistant to language, and the IASP definition provides a solid, workable, valuable tool. It was created specifically, as subcommittee chair Harold Merskey writes, "for use in clinical practice."[22] Nobody ever claimed it was perfect or eternal. Moreover, a definition is exactly the wrong place to address serious ethical issues (some of which will be addressed below under The ethics of pain and suffering: narrative analysis). The burden lies on critics to provide a better tool capable of achieving widespread use. They should also come clean about what submerged medical, social, or philosophical agendas their own new definitions advance. A workable definition of pain need not be – and should not be – a theory of pain. We still lack a fully agreed-upon theory of pain that accounts for all the multiple combinations of causes and effects in numerous different diseases, syndromes, and cries for help. Thanks to the IASP definition, researchers and clinicians, even if they cannot always explain or treat it, mostly agree on what they do and do not mean by pain. General agreement disappears when we turn from pain to suffering.

There is no consensus about whether suffering falls within the boundaries of pain medicine – or even within medicine – but the medical neglect of suffering is palpable. Suffering rarely gets an entry in medical textbooks, and only a few authors with medical training discuss it directly.[32, 33] In a practical sense, health professionals confront the problems of suffering every day – as suffering emerges during the course of illnesses that range from cancer and depression to Alzheimer's disease. This practical, everyday approach, however, fails to tell us what suffering is – and suffering as a distinctive state (a state that transcends specific illnesses) tends to be ignored. Paradoxically, the demands of everyday patient care often manage to insulate biomedicine from any real contact with suffering, which may be regarded as a nonmedical consequence of illness and thus reassigned to pastoral care, a discipline where suffering is taken seriously.[34] The standard institutional separation between theologians and physicians only deepens medical unawareness of suffering. Despite some welcome signs of change, the stark question remains as to whether pain medicine will come to view suffering – at least suffering directly related to pain – as a condition that demands serious thought and effective responses. If so, we must begin (as the IASP did with pain) to define what we mean by suffering.

Suffering is sometimes employed as a synonym for pain – as if pain were the cause, suffering the effect, and their linguistic relation interchangeable[35] – but they are theoretically distinct. A broken bone may bring pain without suffering; a broken heart may bring suffering without pain. Suffering and pain thus cannot be exactly identical or synonymous. This theoretical difference, however, often collapses in practice, where suffering and pain may occur together in ways that not only undermine hypothetical distinctness, but also alter their relationship. The special complications that mark the unstable relations between pain and suffering have received attention from psychologist C Richard Chapman and pain specialist Jonathan Gavrin.[36] They define suffering as "threat or damage to the integrity of the self" – following physician and bioethicist Eric J Cassell[32] – and they specify that the threat or damage entails "a disparity between what one expects of one's self and what one does or is." Persistent pain, they observe, often causes "serious disruption" of a human life, and such disruption may constitute a crisis of identity that is experienced as suffering and perpetuated by physiological processes similar to the maladaptive stress response. Chapman and Gavrin do not set out to propose a solution to the problem of suffering, but they assert that physicians who understand suffering can learn how to prevent the predictable damage to the self that often accompanies persistent pain.

The medical discussion of suffering is at such an early stage that any account must remain incomplete, valuable especially for the questions it raises. Chapman and Gavrin offer an appropriately complex account of human self-hood in its neurological, behavioral, cognitive, and developmental aspects. Such complexity, however, also raises questions about whether most selves ever manage to possess a wholeness or harmony that would constitute the "integrity" presumed lost in suffering. Sociologists write about normative human identity today as characterized by a "destabilization" in which selves are not understandable as private inner cores but rather as a fluid *mélange* of public roles, performances, and appearances.[37, 38] In private communication, Chapman emphasizes his view that the self is "not so much an entity as a process of constant redefinition in reaction to a changing world." He describes the loss of integrity as a failure of "coherence," noting that "awareness of incoherence within one's self is a powerful negative experience." He observes that there is perhaps no more powerful source of human incoherence than the failure or loss of the relationships that bind us to others, including not only family and loved ones, but also peoples, nations, deities, or even cherished abstract versions of otherness, such as justice and freedom. Suffering understood as an experience of radical incoherence may prove ultimately to be a more useful concept than self-hood regarded as the possession of integrity, wholeness, or harmony. Unfortunately, a review of the pain literature by Fishbain *et al.*[38] showed that personality states were influenced both by personality trait and the presence of chronic pain. They cautioned that post-pain personality profiles were not necessarily indicative of pre-pain personality. Relief of the pain might restore the pre-pain status and integrity.

The compound term "pain and suffering" has certain legal connotations currently being explored by legal scholars, the judiciary, legislators, and juries. One goal is to define and to rationalize approaches so that "deserving" supplicants are not penalized and "undeserving" litigants do not "win the lottery." There is no assumption that such payments, which make up about 50 percent of total tort awards, should not occur.[39, 40] The question rather is when and how, within specific legal and insurance systems, to provide just compensation that take into account the difficulties inherent in quantifying – let alone in identifying – suffering and pain.

The work of Chapman and Gavrin invites us to ask why some pain patients suffer when others who face serious disruption of their lives seem to prosper under adversity? Suffering, in the view of some social scientists, is not only an individual experience, but also a cultural practice that certain societies or subcultures or ethnic groups code quite differently.[41] The differences in individual responses to disruption may reflect different ways of "coding" adversity that are learned from families or cultures. We might also understand more about suffering from studies in "learned helplessness."[42] Suffering is by definition a state of helplessness, as few people would choose to suffer if they could avoid it. The helplessness typical of suffering, however, is also learned and reinforced by repeated failures to find aid. The repeated failure of efforts to find assistance is not the same as suffering conceived as a state of helpless passivity. In an analysis of how suffering is learned, the therapeutic value lies in active interventions designed to break the self-reinforcing cycle of helplessness – as demonstrated in feminist responses to battered women, for example – through specific techniques designed to empower the disempowered.[43] Responses to the helplessness intrinsic to suffering allow sufferers to recognize the (limited) power they do not know they possess, which creates a basis for small steps forward.[44] From this perspective, suicide is less a product of suffering than suffering transformed to a state in which helplessness is absolute, immutable, and toxic.

A clinical definition of suffering, in addition to acknowledging threats to the self from incoherence and helplessness, will need to account for an elusive quality within suffering that resists any probe that seeks to lay it bare to objective analysis. Pope John Paul II acknowledged this elusiveness when he wrote about the "oppression of mind and spirit" that often accompanies pain. Suffering encompasses, like pain, an irreducible subjective dimension, but it is distinctive in shattering the norms of life in which even pain can be understandable and thus bearable. For contemporary philosopher Emanuel Levinas, suffering is "the *impasse* of life and being"; what he calls "the explosion and most profound articulation of absurdity."[45] We must not expect a crystal clear account of suffering when it constitutes an experience that plunges our most basic assumptions about life into utter chaos and absurdity. Suffering is like a text that suddenly plunges into an unknown language – or outside language. We do not so much know suffering (in ourselves or in others) as much as suffer or witness it. Yet, granted this resistance to understanding, a new challenge is emerging in connections between pain medicine and palliative care.[46] When cure is impossible, palliative care focuses on the alleviation of symptoms and on the relief of suffering.[47] Fear of pain is a regular source of suffering, especially among patients who fear dying in pain, and pain medicine is thus an indispensable resource for assisting hospices in the effort to relieve suffering at the end of life.[48] McNamara indicated that the "good death" – often an explicit goal in the original hospice movement – has become an increasingly inappropriate objective in the current climate that emphasizes patient autonomy and consumer choice. Without good pain relief, patients cannot think about preparing for death. The focus at end of life is thus shifting from the question of dying well to living well (until death). Patients must be given options to accept or refuse any treatment, including life-prolonging interventions or even interventions to relieve pain. The question of pain at the end of life is complex. Living wills and other medical power-of-attorney instruments typically request terminal pain relief, even at the cost of awareness, but also DNR/DNI (do not resuscitate, do not intubate) in cardiac or respiratory arrest. Some contend that protagonists of euthanasia and of physician-assisted suicide have taken arguments for patient autonomy to an inappropriate extreme.[49] The treatment of pain and suffering at the end of life remains an issue about which patients, families, and caregivers need to establish clear lines of communication that acknowledge emotional distress, ethical controversy, and cultural or personal differences.

CLASSIFICATION EXCESS: THE MULTIPLICITY OF PAIN AND SUFFERING

Pain and suffering are especially resistant to definition because they are plural concepts. The history of pain is a record of pain's multiple *re*-inventions.[50] The English word "pain" refers to innumerable different experiences linked together not by a common essence (or by an immutable shared core) but by what philosopher Ludwig Wittgenstein calls "family resemblances" (cited in Ref. 51). Pain (an abstract concept) exists only through concrete, multiple, and very distinctive pains. Even if we exclude metaphorical applications of pain to unhappiness and disappointment, as when coaches talk about the agony of defeat, it is now clear that the pain of migraine differs from cancer pain, that cancer pain differs from the pain of arthritis, that arthritis pain differs from the pain of fibromyalgia. Such differences go beyond variations in the quality, length, and intensity of sensation. They may correspond to distinctive biological processes and to particular experiences. As neuroscientist Tony Yaksh said in 1992, "At this moment, we're becoming just barely sufficiently sophisticated to say that all pain is not the same, and therefore to know why some analgesics may be very effective in some pain states and less effective in others. We need to learn the precise nature and mechanism of all the pain producers" (cited in Ref. 52).

The invention of pain medicine rests upon an awareness that pain is never a simple unity. The centers and clinics emerging in the late 1960s and the 1970s were mostly committed to a bedrock distinction between acute and chronic pain. The distinction is not trouble free, but the basic principle won rapid acceptance. Chronic pain differs in kind – not in degree – from acute pain, and neither holds its traditional status as a symptom. Ronald Dubner, another neuroscientist who focused on pain, summed up changes that constitute a thorough challenge to traditional biomedical thinking. "We know now that pain is not merely a passive symptom of disease," he stated in 1992, "but an aggressive disease in itself, producing changes in the brain that underlie the pathology of persistent or chronic pain" (cited in Ref. 52). Soon it became necessary to abandon even the ancient medical truism that nobody ever died from pain. Psychologist John Liebeskind showed in laboratory animals that pain depresses the immune system and destroys cancer-fighting cells. As the title of his seminal essay puts it bluntly, "Pain *can* kill."[53]

The specific syndromes discussed in the IASP *Classification of chronic pain* tabulate almost as many kinds of pain as there are strains of roses, from the steady sharp or throbbing ache of gout to the sudden severe stab of trigeminal neuralgia.[22] There is visceral pain in the neck, chest pain, vascular disease of the limbs, abdominal pain of neurological origin, pain in the bladder and rectum, lumbar spine syndromes, pain syndromes of the hip and thigh, musculoskeletal syndromes of the leg, and multiple pains of the foot, as well as burns to the skin, arthritis in the joints, nerve damage, and lesions to the central nervous system (called central pain). There is stiff man syndrome, sickle cell arthropathy, and the pain of acquired immunodeficiency syndrome (AIDS). No single sensory process underlies all these diverse forms of affliction, but the last place where most patients would expect to find a common source for their pains is in a region devoid of sensory neurons. This, however, is exactly the paradox that neurosurgeon John Loeser confronts us with. "The brain," he writes, "is the organ responsible for all pain. All sensory input, including nociception, can be altered by conscious or unconscious mental activity."[54] The brain is also the putative generator of the placebo and nocebo effects (see Chapter 41, Placebo and nocebo in the *Practice and Procedures* volume of this series). The cerebral location of these effects is not yet known, but it is reasonable to suppose that they are related to the reward–aversion curcuitry. Study of reward–aversion functions is a fruitful area of basic reseach.[55] Pain is typically aversive, and analgesia (particularly via opioids) seems to be rewarding. These circuits are not pure as other functions are also subserved. Pain and pain relief are thus possibly entangled with such reward–aversion functions as probability assessment, reward–intensity evaluation, motivationally salient stimuli, and cognitive/emotional outcome prediction.

The brain, as the organ responsible for all pain, holds a dual function. One function is biological and internal. The brain is crucial not only to the cortical activities that process nociceptive impulses from the periphery, but also to painful experiences generated in the absence of nociceptive input. You do not need a leg to feel pain in your leg – as patients with phantom limbs know, all you need is a working brain. The other function of the brain connects us with the external, interpersonal world of human culture. In effect, the brain is a natural interface between culture and biology. Your pain and my pain (even when evoked by nearly identical tissue damage) may differ significantly owing to variations in our social backgrounds and personal histories, including differences in our individual memories, beliefs, and emotional states.

The multiplicity of pain and suffering has no clear limit because our brains situate us within an open-ended matrix of biology and culture.[56] Gender, for example, plays a significant role in pain. The relationship between gender and pain is complex, since identifiable patterns change with different medical conditions and across the life cycle.[57] Men and women, however, show quantitative differences in sensitivity to pain and to analgesia that suggest differences in neural processing. Women also compose the majority of chronic pain patients, although it is unclear whether women face greater risk of pain or merely use healthcare services more often.[58] Women are certainly more likely to experience a variety of recurrent pains, to report more severe levels of pain, more frequent pain, and pain of longer duration.[59] While good evidence suggests that females exhibit greater sensitivity to noxious stimuli than do males, other studies suggest that women are better at coping with discomfort and that they complain less over time.[60] Biological differences are important in this gender-influenced pain. Kappa opioids work twice as well for women as for men.[61] Migraine affects about 6 percent of men and 15–18 percent of women.[62] (The diminished frequency of migraines during pregnancy suggests a link with estrogen.) A significant implication of this research on gender differences in pain is that we should also expect gender differences in suffering. Women are overrepresented among battered spouses, whose suffering often combines physical injury with emotional trauma. A woman's position as caregiver in dysfunctional or chaotic families also suggests that suffering may be inflected by the social distribution of gender roles. Social beliefs about gender certainly affect clinical decisions regarding pain treatment.[63] We should expect that suffering too, both inside and outside medical contexts, will reveal significant biocultural differences associated with gender.

The multidimensional quality of pain and suffering – situated within cultures, as well as within nervous systems – implies a need to resist the temptation to eliminate from research and from treatment all the messy local variations that come with living in societies. Low back pain is simply not the same experience in the USA as it is in Japan. In one study, Japanese patients proved significantly less impaired in psychological, social, vocational, and avocational function.[64] Research comparing ten American cancer patients with ten cancer patients from India found significant differences in quality of life and in the meaning of the pain experience.[65] Indian patients, who sought medical assistance only after their pain became intolerable, saw their suffering as the fulfillment of a "higher good," whereas American patients interpreted their own suffering as a form of "punishment." The authors of a review article focusing on numerous cross-cultural investigations conclude that more such studies are needed to explore the diverse "social and psychological variables that govern pain perceptions, beliefs, and reactions."[66] The culture-inflected character of pain is well illustrated in the reflections, commentaries, and essays collected in the Canadian–American anthology *When pain strikes*, with its self-conscious resolve to speak from and to the condition known as postmodernity.[67] In one sign of postmodern change, researchers are increasingly interested in relations between the religion/spirituality dyad and the trio of physical health, mental health, and pain.[68] One study of predominantly white, Christian, mid-western patients with chronic musculoskeletal pain produced some surprising information. Pain patients' religious and spiritual beliefs appeared different from the beliefs of a healthy population. Private religious practices, such as prayer and meditation, were inversely related to physical health outcomes. Patients experiencing worse physical health were more likely than less-challenged patients to engage in private religious activities, perhaps as a coping mechanism. The longer time that patients had been living with pain, the less "forgiving" they were, and the less support they received from their church community. Such patients tend to lose hope, become bitter, grow angry at themselves, at society, and at God. Forgiveness, negative religious coping, daily spiritual experiences, religious support, and self-rankings of religious/spiritual intensity significantly predicted mental health status.

Suffering and pain are persistent features of human life, but they are not timeless or placeless states. They can involve specific churches and local communities, as well as widely shared genes and neurons. We cannot fully understand them apart from an awareness of how the human brain situates us inescapably within the modifying environments of a particular time and place, and culture.

UNDERSTANDING: THE MATRIX OF BIOLOGY AND CULTURE

Human pain is always a biocultural condition – a composite experience requiring a biology of brain states and of neural processes negotiated within a social space where individuals interact with the surrounding culture, including the culture of medicine. One major challenge is to understand how the biological processes associated with pain are influenced directly and indirectly by individual beliefs, social institutions, and cultural forces. We continue to learn about the neuroanatomy of the human pain system and its modulating pathways.[69] It remains unclear, however, how this complex neuroanatomy is set in motion or modified by thoughts and emotions, which are influenced in turn by external and interpersonal forces, such as medical systems, disability insurance, religious beliefs, and cultural attitudes. There is also a crucial role in human pain played by human consciousness. We know more about what disability insurance and religious beliefs contribute to pain than about the slippery contributions of human consciousness.

The importance of psychosocial factors in pain has been demonstrated recently in numerous articles and books. Psychologists Dennis Turk and Robert Gatchell contend that post-1960 attention to the cognitive and behavioral psychology of pain constitutes nothing less than a "revolution," and they argue for the continuing relevance of a clinical model that recognizes the mutual interdependence of biological and psychosocial processes.[70] One fascinating illustration of this mutual interdependence concerns the role of memory in pain. A patient's recollection of pain is most closely related to the intensity of pain during the inciting episode, and severe pain that persists for more than a few hours creates changes in the structure and function of somatosensory and pain pathways.[71] The memory of severe pain thus differs from other, more casual memories, both at the cortical level and at the level of altered sensory neurons. Preemptive analgesia now commonly prescribed for postoperative patients not only prevents short-term discomfort, but also avoids long-term complications that can accompany the memory of pain.

Beliefs about pain illustrate a broader interdependence between biology and culture, i.e. human pain implies continuous processes of conscious and nonconscious interpretation.[72, 73] (Nonconscious interpretation occurs, for example, when we process traffic signals without awareness.) Meaning helps to constitute pain, even if only in the nonconscious acknowledgment that a scratch is usually meaningless. We cannot name or discuss pain except by employing a language that exists only at a specific moment in its historical development and inevitably colors our understanding.[74] Pain thus always comes already interpreted by the social world we inhabit. Meanings not only encompass articulate beliefs, such as the conviction that pain is a punishment, but in less obvious ways, they also interpenetrate our inarticulate attitudes, unexpressed emotions, habitual behavior, and even nonconscious knowledge. Pain-killing drugs may temporarily circumvent conscious meaning-making processes, but meaning does not therefore go away. A patient's knowledge of drugs – like the equally widespread fear of opioids – is not innate, but requires extensive, if largely nonconscious, cultural learning. In difficult cases of chronic pain, patients' beliefs and attitudes may impede, complicate, or entirely undermine treatment.

Recent research into pain beliefs challenges the entrenched opinion (still popular among patients) that pain is an electrochemical impulse triggered by tissue damage. Nociception is neither a necessary nor a sufficient condition for pain. Beliefs that help to shape the experience of pain include our convictions about cause, control, duration, outcome, and blame.[75, 76] Such beliefs affect not only chronic pain, but also acute and postoperative pain.[67] Furthermore, emotion is an intrinsic part of the pain experience – saturated with and shaped by cognitive processes – rather than a mere reaction to pain.[77, 78] Many beliefs about pain are directly linked to strong emotions: anger toward a negligent employer, fear of catastrophe, hope for financial gain, love for a spouse. Specific pain beliefs can predict pain intensity.[79] Beliefs also influence the ability to cope with pain. Researchers have found that patients function better when they believe they have some control over their pain, when they believe in the value of medical services, when they believe that family members care for them, and when they believe that they are not severely disabled.[80] A study of 100 patients showed that specific pain beliefs correlate directly with treatment outcomes.[81] Such research has clear implications for clinical practice, where the interdependence between culture and biology challenges us to consider new approaches to the ethics of pain and suffering.

THE ETHICS OF PAIN AND SUFFERING: NARRATIVE ANALYSIS

"Man by his very nature," wrote Cicely Saunders in 1962, "finds that he has to question the pain he endures and seek meaning in it."[82] For patients, the drive to find meaning in pain often takes the form of narrative – from extended personal stories to compressed beliefs. The belief that all pain and suffering is sent or sanctioned by God, for example, constitutes a compressed mininarrative that regularly occurs within larger accounts of divine providence throughout world religions. Although medicine officially distrusts narrative as mere anecdotal evidence far inferior to science or fact, medical education and practice are bursting with narrative, whether in formal case studies and patient histories or in casual tales swapped around the water cooler.[83] In 1999, the *British Medical Journal*, defying the culturally coded devaluation of narrative as no more than entertainment, ran a five-part series entitled "narrative-based medicine." The title, evoking a deliberate contrast with "evidence-based medicine," expresses a conviction that narrative in medical contexts constitutes useful (if limited) evidence and a valuable (if selective) tool that might complement traditional biomedical practices. The British Medical Journal Press republished the articles along with additional contributions in a book-length study (*Narrative-based medicine: dialogue and discourse in clinical practice*) that includes an essay by Sir Richard Bayliss entitled "Pain narratives."[84]

What are pain narratives and how might they help clinicians address urgent issues of bioethics? Pain, we might say, is the ancient antagonist of which the brain must perpetually make sense, and one way we make sense of pain is through narrative. Moreover, individual narratives are never wholly unique, but share basic features with other stories circulating inside a culture. We understand any text ultimately because we have learned the narrative conventions that govern it, from case studies to *Star Wars*. Furthermore, we inhabit cultures that surround us with prepackaged narratives. Country music specializes in miniature erotic narratives of pain and suffering, as do standard rock anthems such as John Mellancamp's *Hurts So Good*. (In edgier performance narratives, the American rock band Genitorturers draws spectators on stage at live concerts to have needles jammed into their groins.) Popular culture is awash with pain narratives. Televised talk-shows have added the newest variant with their tales of nonstop victimization. We all live out our lives, as philosopher Alasdair MacIntyre tells us, in terms of narrative.[85] It is rash to believe that the pain narratives circulating within popular culture have no impact on how people live. The study of pain beliefs shows the damage that ensues when patients anxiously imagine catastrophic outcomes. The challenge is to study the harmful or helpful consequences of pain beliefs that are enfolded within more fully developed social and personal narratives. Such research holds implications not only for medical treatment, but also for medical ethics.

One helpful approach to narratives of pain and suffering comes from sociologist Arthur W Frank in *The wounded storyteller: body, illness, and ethics.*[86] Frank offers a typology of four narrative structures that reappear when contemporary patients write about their illnesses. It would be useful for pain specialists to recognize instantly, almost as a diagnostic category, what Frank identifies as the recurrent type of "chaos" narrative. It would also be useful to develop an extended typology of the narratives that patients bring to a pain center. We know that chronic pain often constitutes a threat to individual identity.[87] If individual identity is inseparable from the tacit narratives of self-hood that we construct or accept, then the dilemmas of chronic pain and suffering include an inescapable narrative dimension. Frank argues that the self cannot be reconstructed in healing without the reconstruction of a new personal narrative. The Greek term *ethos* originally referred to a person's settled disposition or character, and the narrative reconstruction of a human life, in healing, is a profoundly ethical matter.

The skills developed through narrative are relevant enough to medical education to fit comfortably within the prevailing language of competencies.[88] Some narrative competencies are especially relevant to pain, including the basic clinical act of listening. As a low-technology virtue that everyone praises but few take seriously, listening is a skill that needs to be relearned inside medical contexts for professional purposes, much as a competitive swimmer must relearn how to breathe. One famous study showed that doctors listened on average for just 18 seconds before interrupting patients in order to take control.[89] Later studies indicate that the situation is not quite so one-sided, but listening is a skill that, for various reasons, comes hard in medical settings.[90] If a health maintenance organization (HMO) requires physicians to spend on average no more than seven minutes per patient, listening to pain narratives may seem an unaffordable luxury. A sounder approach, however, might regard skilled listening to patients as necessary for accurate medical understanding. Accurate medical understanding would thus require skills in listening. Failure to obtain skills necessary for medical practice is not merely unprofessional but unethical.

Skills in listening to patient narratives are sometimes crucial to pain medicine. For example, pain entails special problems for the elderly, who may suffer serious side effects from medications or hold erroneous pain beliefs that make any treatment less effective. The IASP study *Pain in the elderly* recommends exploring nondrug therapies.[91] The practice of skilled listening to patient narratives, like the practice of writing in narrative form for patients, can have therapeutic value. Narrative can help pain specialists learn how to listen and what to listen for. Speech and story are never wholly transparent. As bioethicist Tod Chambers writes, "Every telling of a story – real or imagined – encompasses a series of choices about what will be revealed, what will be privileged, and what will be concealed: there are no artless narrations."[92] There is no need to pump up claims for skilled listening or for the uses of narrative. They are not the answer to pain. However, nothing else is either, including morphine. Skilled listening is one more useful tool in a multidisciplinary approach to the multiple dimensions of pain, and research with hospice patients has demonstrated, at least in selected circumstances, the value of narrative-based therapies such as structured life review.[93]

Narrative helps to illuminate the ethical issues always implicit in pain. The mere act of paying attention, so basic to the reception of narrative, is a moral as well as cognitive state: in turning a deaf ear, we demonstrate how little we value the speaker. Narrative also helps us to recognize and respond to the ethical significance of unnoticed, everyday acts, such as the pain treatment accorded to ethnic minorities. Moreover, because narrative is among the ancient and enduring forms of moral knowledge, from *Aesop's Fables* to *Schindler's list*, it provides a resource for exploring the ways in which pain and suffering make a claim on us as moral beings. A cry of pain places us always, implicitly, under an ethical obligation. Its inevitable subjectivity is not impenetrable, but belongs to social, interpersonal codes as instantly comprehensible as SOS. We may not be able personally to answer every SOS, but it is self-deception to pretend that we do not know what it means or what response it asks from us. Narrative is a resource for developing skills in the recognition and interpretation of ethical dilemmas intrinsic to pain. Even an unresolved dilemma, if we recognize it for what it is, at least invites future resolution. An unrecognized ethical dilemma in medical settings, especially a dilemma that centers on pain and suffering, is a potentially harmful form of ignorance.

The medical undertreatment of pain has been well documented for over 20 years.[94] Its ethical implications, however, are not often recognized or addressed.[95] One prominent study, for example, shows that 50 percent of hospitalized dying patients in the USA spent at least half their time (according to family members) in moderate to severe pain.[96] The method that researchers employed to redress this undertreatment of pain in dying patients centered on staff education, not on ethics and certainly not on narrative, and it yielded no improvement. As an alternative method for recognizing and addressing the ethical implications of undertreatment for pain, narrative can hardly do worse. Consider the 1999 *New York Times* story about Mrs Ozzie Chavez.[97] Mrs Chavez, a California Medicaid patient, was refused proper anesthesia in childbirth because she had not paid an additional (illegal) fee required by the anesthesiologist. "The anesthesiologist wouldn't even come into the room until she got her money," Mrs Chavez was reported saying. "I was lying there having contractions, and they wouldn't give me an epidural. I felt like an animal."

Narrative will not get us to the bottom of the story – to expose the truth about what really happened in Mrs Chavez's room – but it helps us to unfold the ethical implications of the patient's experience. It illustrates too how the ethical implications of everyday acts often go unnoticed in our emphasis on megawatt, headline-grabbing, life-and-death bioethical issues.[98] When this story ran in the newsletter of the American Society of Anesthesiologists, it evoked the following commentary from one doctor: "Poor people can't expect to drive a Rolls Royce, so why should they expect to receive the Cadillac of analgesics for free." As if to head off a looming public relations disaster, the president of the American Society of Anesthesiologists, John B Neeld Jr, vaulted directly to first principles. "It is unethical," he said, "to withhold services because of reimbursement." End of story?

A narrative on bioethics would not consider the story to have finished when one character, no matter how eminent, denounces the behavior of another character as unethical. Just as there are no artless narrations, narrative theory reminds us to consider what is unsaid or even unsayable. Neeld, for example, does not mention (is it unsayable?) that medical services are withheld every day in America because of inability to pay. Nor is the USA alone in withholding services. Furthermore, as in the dilemma of hospitalized dying patients, medical services for pain are routinely withheld for causes apparently unconnected with cost.[27] These causes – reflected in what William Breitbart has called the "dramatically undertreated" pain of AIDS patients[74] – express bias, as well as economics. Sex and race, as one (disputed) study shows, affect a medical decision as seemingly neutral as recommendations for cardiac catheterization.[99] Sickle cell pain, with its predominant impact on people of African heritage, is not untroubled by issues of race. Within this cultural mix, as it applies to Mrs Chavez, we must consider the substandard payment policies of certain government agencies. Finally, in a narrative analysis which assumes that language matters, we should note that Mrs Chavez did not say she felt pain. She said she felt like an animal. Pain for Mrs Chavez evokes a down-to-earth ethics of respect and degradation. Narrative analysis does not say who is right or wrong, but it helps us to understand and to unfold the ethical implications of neglected everyday acts.

One benefit of a renewed attention to narrative would be an emphasis on the ethical – rather than on the strictly regulatory – aspects of undertreatment. Of course, we need effective institutional guidelines and review processes in place to combat the long-standing neglect and medical myths that prevent patients from receiving adequate pain medication.[100] We need political action to combat the negative influence that licensing boards, disciplinary groups, and drug enforcement agencies exert on the medical use of opioid analgesics.[101] Such pragmatic changes, however, are not enough. The distinguished philosopher of medicine Edmund D Pellegrino has recently insisted in a discussion of emerging ethical issues in palliative care that – given the availability of effective medications – not to relieve pain optimally is "tantamount to ethical and legal malpractice."[102] Serious inquiry into the ethics of undertreatment may avoid a deluge of legal challenges.

We lack medications to relieve suffering that are as effective as opioids in relieving pain. There is, however, an equally serious issue to face. The best medical approach to suffering is not always aggressive action. Although medicine prefers action and thrives on problem-solving, sometimes little or nothing can be done. Surgeon Sherwin B Nuland writes, "The diagnosis of disease and the quest for overcoming it with his intellect are the challenges that motivate every specialist who is any good at what he does. He is fascinated with pathology. When faced by the certainty of his own impotence to treat it, the would-be healer too often turns away."[103] This is unfortunate, but not surprising. When medical practice becomes preeminently an arena of action, inaction is usually misinterpreted as failure. Yet sometimes suffering will run its terrible course regardless of any intervention. In such cases, there is great value in openly discussing the role of witness.

An almost inescapable logic drives professional disciplines to remove human experience from its flow in everyday local worlds and to reshape it in accordance with the needs of the profession that addresses it.[104] This logic proves dangerous when it comes to the experience of suffering. Therefore, as a complement to the preferred medical stance of active, even heroic, practice, it is important to consider the role of witness. *Witness* comes from an Old English verb meaning "to know." The witness is someone who knows first hand, and such knowing is not a passive possession, mere looking or seeing, as opposed to practice. Witnessing is an action. The witness is one who – in the medical term derived from a Latin root that means "to bend to, to notice" – "attends," and such vigilant attending requires far more than physical presence. The witness cannot erase suffering, prevent tragedy, or defeat death. When suffering is inescapable, however, the active role of witnessing opens up possibilities that can in part offset or redeem sheer loss. The decision to be present, as witness, is an ethical choice. Moreover, the presence of the witness can comfort the person who suffers, and there is no higher act, inside or outside medicine, that we are called upon to perform. However, inability to witness during the dying process or at the death itself must not be regarded as weakness of character, lack of moral fiber, or paucity of empathy. The emotions may simply be too powerful for an ordinary person to withstand. Unfortunately, this inability can also produce life-long guilt and recriminations in the survivor, movingly expressed by a son:

> Nancy died during visiting time.
> Whose hands held her? Were they mine?
> Did I stay to rage against the dark
> To hear the last beat of her heart?
> Did I quench my fears, did I stand fast?
> Did I stay with her until the last?
> Did I comfort her as best I could?
> Did I cry for her as a loving son should?
> Did I hold her hand as she died?
> I said I did, but I lied
> Just to myself at first, to dull the pain,
> Ease the guilt, erase the shame.
> The more the lie soothed and seduced
> The more I believed it to be the truth.
> Told others the tale, believed it myself,
> How I was there until her very last breath.
> In my mind how fine the picture had become –
> Dying mother, dutiful sorrowing son.
> But the truth, oh the truth, screams to be heard.
> No more lies, no more lies, no more lies. I was not there.
> I could not, I would not, stay,
> So I ran – I ran away
> You're hard and you're cruel, Jimmy Dancer,
> You just don't take life, but dignity as well.

Eric Bogle, *Jimmy Dancer,*

Jimmy Dancer – rhyming slang for cancer.

REFERENCES

1. Pope John Paul II. Letter handed to John Bonica on the occasion of the Fifth World Congress on Pain. In: Benedetti C, Chapman CR, Giron G (eds). *Opioid analgesia: recent advances in systemic administration.* Advances in Pain Research and Therapy 14. New York, NY: Raven Press, 1990.
2. Melzack R, Wall PD. Pain mechanisms: a new theory. *Science.* 1965; **150**: 971–9.
3. Melzack R. Gate control theory: on the evolution of pain concepts. *Pain Forum.* 1996; **5**: 128–38.
4. Baszanger I. *Inventing pain medicine: from the laboratory to the clinic.*. New Brunswick, NJ: Rutgers University Press, 1998; first published in French in 1995.
5. Melzack R. Central pain syndromes and theories of pain. In: Casey KL (ed.). *Pain and central nervous system disease: the central pain syndromes.* New York: Raven Press, 1991: 59–64.

6. Jones AKP, Brown WD, Friston KJ *et al.* Cortical and subcortical localization of response to pain in man using positron emission tomography. *Proceedings of the Royal Society of London. Series B.* 1991; **244**: 39–44.
7. Talbot JD, Marrett S, Evans AC *et al.* Multiple representations of pain in human cerebral cortex. *Science.* 1991; **251**: 1355–8.
8. Derbyshire SWG. Imaging the brain in pain. *American Pain Society Bulletin.* 1999; **9**: 7–9.
* 9. Apkarian AV, Bushnell MC, Treede RD *et al.* Human brain mechanisms of pain perception and regulation in health and disease. *European Journal of Pain.* 2005; **9**: 463–84.
10. Chizh BA, Hobson AR. Using objective markers and imaging in the development of novel treatments of chronic pain. *Expert Review of Neurotherapeutics.* 2007; **7**: 443–7.
11. Belenky M, Devor M. Association of postganglionic sympathetic neurons with primary afferents in sympathetic-sensory co-cultures. *Journal of Neurocytology.* 1997; **26**: 715–31.
12. Elmer GI, Pieper JO, Negus SS, Woods JH. Genetic variance in nociception and its relationship to the potency of morphine-induced analgesia in thermal and chemical tests. *Pain.* 1998; **75**: 129–40.
13. Devor M, Raber P. Heritability of symptoms in an experimental model of neuropathic pain. *Pain.* 1990; **42**: 51–67.
* 14. Devor M. Sodium channels and mechanisms of neuropathic pain. *Journal of Pain.* 2006; **7** (Suppl. 1): S1–S12.
* 15. Yaksh TL. Calcium channels as therapeutic targets in neuropathic pain. *Journal of Pain.* 2006; **7** (Suppl. 1): S13–S30.
16. Verhaak PFM, Kerssens JJ, Dekker J *et al.* Prevalence of chronic benign pain disorder among adults: a review of the literature. *Pain.* 1998; **77**: 231–9.
17. van Tulder MW, Koes BW, Bouter LM. A cost-of-illness study of back pain in The Netherlands. *Pain.* 1995; **62**: 233–40.
18. Linton SJ. The socioeconomic impact of chronic back pain: is anyone benefiting? *Pain.* 1998; **75**: 163–8.
19. Robertson JT. The rape of the spine. *Surgical Neurology.* 1993; **39**: 5–12.
20. Fordyce WE (ed.). *Back pain in the workplace: management of disability in nonspecific conditions.* Seattle, WA: IASP Press, 1995.
21. Pain terms: a list with definitions and notes on usage. *Pain.* 1979; **6**: 249–52.
* 22. Merskey H, Bogduk N (eds). *Classification of chronic pain: descriptions of chronic pain syndromes and definitions of pain terms*, 2nd edn. Seattle, WA: IASP Press, 1994.
23. Beecher HK. Pain in men wounded in battle. *Bulletin. United States. Army Medical Dept.* 1946; **5**: 445–54.
24. Blank JW. Pain in men wounded in battle: Beecher revisited. *IASP Newsletter.* 1994: 2–4.
25. Bayer TL, Baer PE, Early C. Situational and psychophysiological factors in psychologically induced pain. *Pain.* 1991; **44**: 45–50.
26. Duncan G. Mind-body dualism and the biopsychosocial model of pain: what did Descartes really say? *Journal of Medicine and Philosophy.* 2000; **25**: 485–513.
27. Sullivan M. In what sense is contemporary medicine dualistic? *Culture, Medicine and Psychiatry.* 1986; **10**: 331–50.
28. Cunningham N. Primary requirements for an ethical definition of pain. *Pain Forum.* 1999; **8**: 93–9.
29. Herr K, Coyne PJ, Key T *et al.* Pain assessment in the nonverbal patient: position statement with clinical practice recommendations. *Pain Management Nursing.* 2006; **7**: 44–52.
30. Rollin BE. Some conceptual and ethical concerns about current views of pain. *Pain Forum.* 1999; **8**: 78–83.
31. Jensen MP. Validity of self-report and observation measures. In: Jensen TS, Turner JA, Wiesenfeld-Hallin Z (eds). *Proceedings of the 8th World Congress on Pain. Progress in Pain Research and Management*, Vol. 8. Seattle, WA: IASP Press, 1997: 637–61.
* 32. Cassell EJ. *The nature of suffering and the goals of medicine.* New York, NY: Oxford University Press, 1991.
33. Kleinman A. *The illness narratives: suffering, healing, and the human condition.* New York, NY: Basic Books, 1988.
34. Bowker J. *Problems of suffering in religions of the world.* Cambridge: Cambridge University Press, 1970.
35. Wall PA. *Pain: the science of suffering.* London: Weidenfeld, 1999.
* 36. Chapman CR, Gavrin J. Suffering: the contributions of persistent pain. *Lancet.* 1999; **353**: 2233–7.
37. *The Hedgehog Review: Critical Reflections on Contemporary Culture.* 1999; **1**: 5–102; the entire issue is devoted to sociological reflections on "identity."
38. Fishbain DA, Cole B, Cutler RB *et al.* Chronic pain and measurement of personality: do states influence traits? *Pain Medicine.* 2006; **7**: 509–29.
39. Avraham R. Putting a price on pain-and-suffering damages: a critique of the current approaches and a preliminary proposal for change. *Northwestern University Law Review.* 2006; **100**: 87–120.
40. Avraham R. Should pain-and-suffering damages be abolished from tort law? More experimental evidence. *Univeristy of Toronto Law Journal.* 2005; **55**: 941–79.
41. Kleinman A, Das V, Lock M (eds). *Social suffering.* Berkeley, CA: University of California Press, 1997.
42. Peterson C, Maier SF, Seligman MEP. *Learned helplessness: a theory for the age of personal control.* New York: Oxford University Press, 1993.
43. Ferrell B. Ethical perspectives on pain and suffering. *Pain Management Nursing.* 2005; **6**: 83–90.
44. Candib LM. Power-in-relation. In: *Medicine and the family: a feminist perspective.* New York: Basic Books, 1995: 240–53.
45. Levinas E. Useless suffering. In: Bernasconi R, Wood D (eds). *The provocation of Levinas: rethinking the other.*

London: Routledge, 1988: 156–67; first published in French in 1982 and translated by R Cohen.

46. Portenoy RK. Palliative care: an opportunity for pain specialists. *American Pain Society Bulletin*. 1999; **9**: 2–5.
47. Gawande A. A queasy feeling: why can't we cure nausea? *The New Yorker*. 1999: 34–41.
48. McNamara B. Good enough death: autonomy and choice in Australian palliative care. *Social Science and Medicine*. 2004; **58**: 929–38.
49. Hendin H. The Dutch experience. In: Foley K, Hendin H (eds). *The case against assisted suicide: for the right to end-of-life care*. Bethesda, MD: Johns Hopkins Press, 2002.
50. Rey R. *The history of pain*. Wallace LE, Cadden JA, Cadden SW (trans). Cambridge, MA: Harvard University Press, 1993; first published in French in 1993.
51. Sullivan MD. Pain in language: from sentience to sapience. *Pain Forum*. 1995; **4**: 3–14.
52. Goldsmith MF. Pain speaking – and anesthesiologists answer. *Journal of the American Medical Association*. 1992; **267**: 1578–9.
53. Liebeskind JC. Pain can kill. *Pain*. 1991; **44**: 3–4.
54. Loeser JD. What is chronic pain? *Theoretical Medicine*. 1991; **12**: 213–25.
55. Borsook D, Becerra L, Carlezon WA *et al.* Reward-aversion circuitry in analgesia and pain: implications for psychiatric disorders. *European Journal of Pain*. 2007; **11**: 7–20.
56. Kirmayer LJ, Looper KJ. Abnormal illness behaviour: physiological, psychological and social dimensions for coping with distress. *Current Opinion in Psychiatry*. 2006; **19**: 54–60.
57. LeResche L. Gender considerations in the epidemiology of chronic pain. In: Crombie IK, Croft PR, Linton SJ *et al.* (eds), *Epidemiology of pain*. Seattle, WA: IASP Press, 1999: 43–52.
58. Weir R, Browne G, Tunks E *et al.* Gender differences in psychosocial adjustment to chronic pain and expenditures for health care services used. *Clinical Journal of Pain*. 1996; **12**: 277–90.
59. ∗ Unruh AM. Gender variations in clinical pain experience. *Pain*. 1996; **65**: 123–67.
60. Fillingim RB, Maixner W. Gender differences in the responses to noxious stimuli. *Pain Forum*. 1995; **4**: 209–21.
61. Gear RW, Miaskowski C, Gordon NC *et al.* Kappa-opioids produce significantly greater analgesia in women than in men. *Nature Medicine*. 1996; **2**: 1248–50.
62. Lipton RB, Stewart WF. Prevalence and impact of migraine. *Neurologic Clinics*. 1997; **15**: 1–13.
63. Berkley KJK, Zalcman SS, Simon VR. Sex and gender differences in pain and inflammation: a rapidly maturing field. *American Journal of Physiology. Regulatory, Integrative and Comparative Physiology*. 2006; **291**: R241–2446.
64. Brena SF, Sanders SH, Motoyama H. American and Japanese low back pain patients: cross-cultural similarities and differences. *Clinical Journal of Pain*. 1990; **6**: 113–24.
65. Kodiath MF, Kodiath A. A comparative study of patients who experience chronic malignant pain in India and the United States. *Cancer Nursing*. 1995; **18**: 189–96.
66. Moore R, Brodsgaard I. Cross-cultural investigations of pain. In: Crombie IK, Croft PR, Linton SJ *et al.* (eds). *Epidemiology of pain*. Seattle, WA: IASP Press, 1999: 53–80.
67. Burns B, Busby C, Sawchuk K (eds). *When Pain Strikes*. Minneapolis, MN: University of Minnesota Press, 1999.
68. Rippentropp AE, Altmaier EM, Chen JJ, Keffala VJ. The relationship between religion/spirituality and physical health, mental health, and pain in a chronic pain populations. *Pain*. 2005; **116**: 311–21.
69. Willis WD, Westkund KN. Neuroanatomy of the pain system and of the pathways that modulate pain. *Journal of Clinical Neurophysiology*. 1997; **14**: 2–31.
70. Gatchell RJ, Turk DC (eds). *Psychosocial factors in pain: critical perspectives*. New York: Guilford Press, 1999.
71. Bagley CA, Ohara S, Lawson HC *et al.* Psychophysics of CNS pain-related activity: binary and analog channels and memory encoding. *Neuroscientist*. 2006; **12**: 29–42.
72. Morris DB. *The culture of pain*. Berkeley, CA: University of California Press, 1991.
73. Morris DB. *Illness and culture in the postmodern age*. Berkeley, CA: University of California Press, 1998.
74. Stephenson J. Experts say AIDS pain "dramatically undertreated". *Journal of the American Medical Association*. 1996; **276**: 1369–70.
75. Williams DA, Thorn BE. An empirical assessment of pain beliefs. *Pain*. 1989; **36**: 351–8.
76. ∗ Wachholtz AB, Pearce MJ, Koenig H. Exploring the relationship between spirituality, coping and pain. *Journal of Behavioral Medicine*. 2007; **30**: 311–18.
77. Bromm B. Consciousness, pain, and cortical activity. In: Bromm B, Desmedt JD (eds). *Pain and the brain: from nociception to cognition*. Advances in Pain Research and Therapy 22. New York: Raven Press, 1995: 35–59.
78. Chapman CR. The affective dimension of pain: a model. In: Bromm B, Desmedt JD (eds). *Pain and the brain: from nociception to cognition*. Advances in Pain Research and Therapy 22. New York: Raven Press, 1995: 283–301.
79. Williams DA, Keefe FJ. Pain beliefs and the use of cognitive-behavioral coping strategies. *Pain*. 1991; **46**: 185–90.
80. Jensen MP, Karoly P. Pain-specific beliefs, perceived symptom severity, and adjustment to chronic pain. *Clinical Journal of Pain*. 1992; **8**: 123–30.
81. Shutty Jr MS, DeGood DE, Tuttle DH. Chronic pain patients' beliefs about their pain and treatment outcomes. *Archives of Physical Medicine and Rehabilitation*. 1990; **71**: 128–32.
82. Saunders C. And from sudden death .... *Nursing Times*. 1962: 1045–6.

83. Hunter KM. *Doctors' stories: the narrative structure of medical knowledge*. Princeton, NJ: Princeton University Press, 1991.
84. Bayliss R. Pain narratives. In: Greenhalgh T, Hurwitz B (eds). *Narrative based medicine: dialogue and discourse in clinical practice*. London: British Medical Journal Press, 1998: 75–82.
85. MacIntyre A. *After virtue: a study in moral theory.* Notre Dame, IN: University of Notre Dame Press, 1981.
86. Frank AW. *The wounded storyteller: body, illness, and ethics*. Chicago, IL: University of Chicago Press, 1995.
87. Eccleston C, Williams ACdeC, Rogers WS. Patients' and professionals' understandings of the causes of chronic pain: blame, responsibility and identity protection. *Social Science and Medicine*. 1997; **45**: 699–709.
88. Hunter KM, Charon R, Coulehan JL. The study of literature in medical education. *Academic Medicine*. 1995; **70**: 787–94.
89. Beckman HB, Frankel RM. The effect of physician behavior on the collection of data. *Annals of Internal Medicine*. 1984; **101**: 692–6.
90. Lown B. *The lost art of healing*. Boston, MA: Houghton-Mifflin, 1996.
91. Ferrell BR, Ferrell BA (eds). *Pain in the elderly.* Seattle, WA: IASP Press, 1996.
92. Chambers T. From the ethicist's point of view: the literary nature of ethical inquiry. *Hastings Center Report*. 1996; **26**: 25–33.
93. Haight BK. The therapeutic role of a structured life review process in homebound elderly subjects. *Journal of Gerontology.* 1988; **43**: 40–4.
94. American Pain Society Quality of Care Committee. Quality improvement guidelines for the treatment of acute pain and cancer pain. *Journal of the American Medical Association*. 1995; **274**: 1874–80.
95. Rich BA. A legacy of silence: bioethics and the culture of pain. *Journal of Medical Humanities*. 1997; **18**: 233–59.
96. SUPPORT Principal Investigators. A controlled trial to improve care for seriously ill hospitalized patients. *Journal of the American Medical Association*. 1995; **274**: 1591–8.
97. Pear R. Mothers on Medicaid overcharged for pain relief. *New York Times*. 1999. Available from: http://archives/nytimes.com/archives.
98. Komasaroff PA. From bioethics to microethics: ethical debate and clinical medicine. In: Komasaroff PA (ed.). *Troubled bodies: critical perspectives on postmodernism, medical ethics, and the body.* Durham, NC: Duke University Press, 1995: 62–86.
99. Schulman KA, Berlin JA, Harless W *et al.* The effect of race and sex on physicians' recommendations for cardiac catheterization. *New England Journal of Medicine*. 1999; **340**: 618–26 (see also erratum in *New England Journal of Medicine*. 1999; **340**: 1130 and critical responses in *New England Journal of Medicine*. 1999; **341**: 285–7).
100. Hill Jr CS. When will adequate pain treatment be the norm? *Journal of the American Medical Association*. 1995; **274**: 1881–2.
101. Hill Jr CS. The negative influence of licensing and disciplinary boards and drug enforcement agencies on pain treatment with opioid analgesics. *Journal of Pharmaceutical Care in Pain and Symptom Control*. 1993; **1**: 43–62.
102. Pellegrino ED. Emerging ethical issues in palliative care. *Journal of the American Medical Association*. 1998; **279**: 1521–2.
103. Nuland SB. *How we die: reflections on life's final chapter.* New York, NY: Alfred A Knopf, 1994.
104. Kleinman A, Kleinman J. Suffering and its professional transformation: toward an ethnography of interpersonal experience. *Culture, Medicine and Psychiatry.* 1991; **15**: 275–301.

8

Pain in society: ethical and legal perspectives

BEN A RICH

KEY LEARNING POINTS

- The commonly identified barriers to pain relief are not merely clinical in nature, but have important ethical dimensions.
- Particularly in the United States, the ethical implications of undertreated pain have influenced the outcome of civil suits against healthcare institutions and professionals.
- In the United States, physicians may be vulnerable to criminal prosecution for drug trafficking if their prescribing of controlled substances is determined not to have been a good faith effort to stay within the bounds of acceptable medical practice.
- Drug control laws and governmental regulations have created a hostile environment in which to care for patients with chronic pain.
- Recent reform initiatives seek to establish a balance in law and public policy between the need to prevent drug diversion and trafficking and the need to insure that opioid analgesics are available to patients who would benefit from them.

INTRODUCTION

There are many perspectives from which one might consider the interrelationship between pain and society, i.e. the impact that a particular configuration of social norms, customs, and experiences has on an individual's particularized experience of pain and search for relief. Excellent studies have been conducted on ethnic and racial influences on pain.[1, 2, 3, 4] The role of religion in shaping a person's perceptions of, and responses to, pain is also especially important, as we shall consider later in this chapter (see below under Pain, suffering, and other semantic points) when the search for meaning begins.[5] As David Morris has astutely observed, "The dismissive or contradictory attitudes that most people – not just health professionals – hold toward pain seem rooted not in biology but in culture."[6] These "dismissive or contradictory attitudes" range from the trivial sloganeering of the health club set – "no pain, no gain" – to the quasi-religious notion that the stoical, if not heroic, bearing of pain and suffering does not merely build character but tests one's ultimate spiritual mettle.

While it is certainly unwise to minimize the extent to which these cultural elements shape our encounters with pain – our own and that of others – it is a topic that has been brilliantly and comprehensively considered elsewhere and is far beyond the scope which this chapter affords.[7] What has only begun to be considered, and as yet very tentatively, are the ethical and legal dimensions and implications of pain, and, more particularly, of modern medicine's legacy of undertreated pain. Heretofore, the ethical and legal aspects of pain management were considered, if at all, in an extremely simplistic fashion that typically proceeded in the following manner:

- opioid analgesics, the most effective method of treating many types of severe pain, are powerful and dangerous drugs that must be rigidly regulated and utilized infrequently at the smallest possible dosage;
- laws and regulations governing the licit use of opioids by healthcare professionals had, as their primary objective, the prevention of drug diversion and addiction;
- the traditional medical aphorism – *primum non nocere* (first do no harm) – has been integrated with an exaggeration of the risks and adverse side effects of opioid analgesics and a significant underestimation of the risks and adverse side effects of severe, persistent pain to produce an ethic of undertreatment.

Neither the ethical nor the legal propriety of this philosophy of patient care was ever challenged by the prevailing norms of western medicine. This "therapeutic" approach to patients with severe and persistent pain, when carefully considered, turns out to be grounded upon a mountain of myth, misunderstanding, misinformation, and flawed ethical analysis.

This chapter will, in large part, be devoted to an examination of the weaknesses of the traditional view. There will also be an exploration of an alternative view that appears to comport much better to medicine's core values and fundamental goals, which have always placed the relief of suffering on an equal level with the prevention and the cure of maladies. Before undertaking this examination, however, a few preliminary matters warrant brief consideration.

PAIN, SUFFERING, AND OTHER SEMANTIC POINTS

The subject matter of this volume is chronic pain, as distinguished from acute pain and pain associated with terminal illness. Pain is, of course, distinguishable in a number of important ways from suffering. It is virtually axiomatic that pain can exist in the absence of suffering and that the opposite is equally true. There have been efforts, ultimately misguided, to characterize pain as physical and suffering as mental. Such characterizations have given rise to what David Morris refers to as the "myth of two pains."[7] Unfortunately, the myth has also engendered the tendency among health professionals to label physical pain, i.e. that which can be directly and objectively related to an identifiable lesion, as "real," and all other reported pain, consequently, as "in one's head" and unreal. As we shall see, the regulatory climate, particularly in the USA, has encouraged medicine's search for an identifiable physiologic cause that would legitimize the pain reported by the patient and justify a physician in the prescribing of controlled substances for pain relief. This approach can have horrendous consequences for the victims of chronic pain syndromes, which, as has been pointed out, "are almost by definition conditions in which the degree of pathology does not seem to explain the severity of the perceived pain or the limitations in bodily functioning the pain produces."[8] When physicians intentionally withhold or reduce readily available palliative measures from their patients with chronic pain, there is added to the baseline level of suffering an incremental level of iatrogenic suffering which may be exacerbated even further to the extent that the physician calls into question the patient's veracity or suggests that the patient is derelict in some unacknowledged yet presumed duty to bear affliction.

Eric Cassell, who has written extensively on the physician's responsibility to relieve suffering, observes that, "While pain and suffering are not synonymous, physical pain remains a major cause of human suffering and is the primary image formed by people when they think about suffering."[9] Moderate to severe, persistent, nonmalignant pain can produce significant suffering, and at some point in the chronicity of the condition efforts to make precise semantic distinctions between pain and suffering, and the extent to which one is physical and the other is mental, become not merely absurd, but unintelligible. Cassell cuts to the shallow core of the effort to impart some meaningful distinction between physical and mental pain or suffering when he states, "bodies do not suffer, persons suffer." Implicit in this observation is the incontrovertible fact that people, and hence patients, are not merely bodies. To the extent that I use the terms pain and suffering interchangeably in this chapter, as to some extent I do when I address the physician's responsibility to relieve suffering, I will be referring specifically to the suffering that is produced by severe and persistent pain.

Another term has entered, and to some degree further complicated, the nomenclature: intractable pain. During the last 15 years, a number of state legislatures in the United States passed "Intractable Pain Treatment Acts." In such legislation, the term "intractable," which is most commonly defined as uncontrollable, is applied to chronic nonmalignant pain that arises from an underlying condition that is resistant to diagnosis or cure. The purpose of these statutes was ostensibly to legitimize the use of opioid analgesics in the care of such patients. However, the actual experience after their enactment may provide a glaring example of the law of unintended consequences. Many of these statutes strongly suggest that opioids will only be considered appropriate for the management of chronic pain after the clinician has painstakingly documented that all other approaches to pain management have failed. Few clinicians can be expected to demonstrate the expertise, patience, and determination such an approach would require.[10]

THE PHYSICIAN'S DUTY TO RELIEVE SUFFERING

Historically, western medicine has recognized two transcendent goals:

1. the diagnosis and treatment of disease;
2. the relief of pain and suffering.

Before the modern era, physicians could diagnose many more conditions than they could cure. Consequently, the duty to relieve pain and suffering, i.e. to provide care and comfort when cure was not an option, was commensurate with the duty to effectuate a cure. With the advent of modern medicine, and its remarkable advances in curative measures, the importance of relieving pain and suffering, at least when separate and distinct from treatment of an underlying disease, seems to have diminished drastically. Indeed, Eric Cassell begins the preface to his book on the relationship between suffering and medicine with the following remarkable statement: "The test of a system of medicine should be its adequacy in the face of suffering; this book starts from the premise that modern medicine fails that test."[11] The contemporary model of both medical education and medical practice is the "curative" model, and it is so designated to distinguish it from what is now characterized as its polar opposite – the palliative model.[12] The focus of the curative model of medicine is the reversal of a disease process. The focus of the palliative model is the care and comfort of the patient through a compassionate response to each individual's unique experience of illness (**Table 8.1**).

Unquestionably, the prevailing model of medical education, and hence, unsurprisingly, of medical practice, is the curative model. The curative model is not merely an aspect of the current culture of medicine, it is also the defining attribute of that culture. It is this attribute which explains why the profession has accepted, virtually without question or qualm, the marginalization of the relief of suffering as a fundamental goal and core value of medicine.

Table 8.1 Characteristics of the curative and palliative models of medicine.

Curative model	Palliative model
Objective	Subjective
Scientific	Humanistic
Rational	Empathic
Impersonal	Personal
Reductionist	Holistic

Such a stark dichotomy might seem to be more of a caricature than a realistic portrait were it not for the data produced by studies such as the Study to Understand Prognosis, Preferences for Outcomes, and Risks of Treatment (SUPPORT), which found among other things that half of the gravely ill patients in intensive care units (ICUs) at major academic medical centers in the USA in the 1990s were in moderate to severe pain in the last three days of their lives.[13] SUPPORT simply reconfirmed the persistence of one aspect of a general phenomenon of undertreated pain of all types that has pervaded the medical literature for over 20 years.[14] The primary locus of curative medicine is the tertiary care hospital; the primary locus of palliative medicine is the hospice. When one abandons the hope of a cure, one accepts the tender mercies of hospice. While one continues to strive for a cure or remediation of a disease, which is presumably why one becomes a patient in academic medical centers such as those participating in SUPPORT, one accepts the pain and suffering that attend many of modern medicine's interventions.

The hegemony of the curative model in modern medical education and medical practice has, it can be argued, displaced the relief of pain and suffering from its traditional status as a fundamental goal and core value of medicine. Strict adherence to this model also creates an inhospitable environment for the care of patients with chronic illness, which by definition is refractory to cure and can only be managed competently so as to minimize the symptoms and life-limiting effects of the disease.

In 1996, an International Project of the Hastings Center, entitled The Goals of Medicine – Setting New Priorities, issued its report. The goals of medicine identified by this distinguished panel of physicians are the following:[15]

- the prevention of disease and injury and promotion and maintenance of health;
- the relief of pain and suffering caused by maladies;
- the care and cure of those with a malady, and the care of those who cannot be cured;
- the avoidance of premature death and the pursuit of a peaceful death.

Perhaps the most striking aspect of these goals, in contrast to the hegemony of the curative model, is the remarkable balance between the curative and palliative aspects of medicine. With regard to the relief of pain and suffering in particular, the special report emphasizes that this is by no means a new goal, but rather one of "the most ancient duties of the physician and a traditional goal of medicine." Nevertheless, the report goes on to say that, for a host of reasons, the goal remains largely unfulfilled. While in many underdeveloped countries access to state-of-the-art medications and advanced nonpharmacologic treatment modalities is an important part of the problem, in developed countries even affluent patients encounter formidable barriers to pain relief, barriers which are sociopolitical rather than economic or technological. Moreover, if there is one type of pain that is more frequently or consistently unrelieved than others, it is chronic nonmalignant pain.[16] A rigorous ethical analysis of the phenomenon of undertreated pain requires a detailed examination of these barriers, particularly if they are offered, as they often are, not merely as reasons why physicians undertreat pain, but as excuses for such practice. First, however, we should briefly note the pervasiveness of the problem of undertreated pain.

THE INTERNATIONAL SCOPE OF UNDERTREATED PAIN

The international literature examining the phenomenon of undertreated pain is dominated by studies that focus on cancer pain. There is, nonetheless, reason to believe that such findings may indicate the magnitude of the problem of undertreated chronic nonmalignant pain as well. An aggressive approach to pain management, including the use of large, sustained doses of the strongest opioid analgesics, has been advocated by pain management experts when necessary to achieve optimal pain relief for patients with cancer or other conditions in their terminal phase.[17] Quite to the contrary, with regard to the treatment of patients with chronic nonmalignant pain, it has been axiomatic that the long-term use of opioids is inappropriate.[18] Thus, many patients who fail to achieve adequate relief from nonopioid therapies are admonished to live with their pain.

Recent studies indicate that opiophobia among healthcare professionals is not strictly an American phenomenon, but is widespread in European countries as well.[19] In Germany, for example, it was noted that 98 percent of cancer patients never received a strong opioid for pain.[20] In France, 51 percent of cancer patients received inadequate pain relief, and 30 percent of the patients who reported pain were not receiving any drugs for pain relief.[21] While there are differences among nations in the regulation of physician-prescribing practices, drug availability, and educational requirements for professionals with prescribing authority, studies of physicians' attitudes about pain management in a wide variety of countries reveal common barriers to adequate pain control.[22] While any particular barrier may be more of a factor in the undertreatment of pain in one country than another, the frequency with which physicians identify these barriers in each country surveyed strongly suggests that they have achieved a status and exert an influence that transcends political and cultural boundaries.

Although a disproportionate amount of the available data, both regarding the situation in the United States and elsewhere in the world, pertains to opioid availability and use in the care of patients with cancer, the implications of such data for the treatment of chronic nonmalignant pain is inescapable. The 1961 Single Convention on Narcotic Drugs, as amended by the 1972 Protocol, is the international treaty regulating the availability of opioids. The preamble of this treaty recognizes that "the medical use of narcotic drugs continues to be indispensable for the relief of pain." Of course, the treaty also states that "addiction to narcotic drugs constitutes a serious evil." Thus, the treaty, just as with national drug regulation laws, purports to at one and the same time prevent the abuse of opioids while assuring that they will be available for legitimate medical use.[23] The World Health Organization (WHO) has urged, with varying degrees of success, that individual countries fashion their regulatory requirements for physicians, nurses, and pharmacists to dispense opioids to patients so as to recognize that "decisions concerning the type of drug to be used, the amount of the prescription and the duration of therapy are best made by medical professionals on the basis of the individual needs of each patient, and not by regulation."[24]

The International Narcotics Control Board (INCB), created by the 1961 Single Convention, compiles statistical data supplied by national governments and publishes an annual report that provides a comprehensive survey of the world drug situation. A 1995 study by the INCB on the availability of opioids for pain management worldwide noted that in many countries opioids are unavailable for medical needs.[25] Remarkably, the study revealed that only 48 percent of the governments reported that morphine in any form was available in all cancer treatment facilities. In addition to periodic shortages in the availability of opioids that were attributed to insufficient importation, distribution delays, and health system administrative problems, the perennial obstacles of physician concerns about addiction and fears of legal sanctions for prescribing opioids were also offered as partial explanations.[26]

THE BARRIERS TO EFFECTIVE PAIN RELIEF

Certain barriers to effective pain relief are so consistently cited in the literature that there would appear to be no genuine dispute about either their existence or their nature. Here are the usual suspects that are rounded up by the advocates of improved pain management practices:

- the failure of clinicians (primarily physicians and nurses) to identify pain relief as a priority in patient care;
- insufficient knowledge among clinicians about the assessment and management of pain;
- clinicians' fear of regulatory scrutiny of the prescribing and administering of opioid analgesics;
- the failure of healthcare institutions and organizations to hold clinicians accountable for effective pain relief.

Other barriers are mentioned with varying degrees of frequency that do not implicate physicians quite so directly, e.g. patient and family concerns about addiction, tolerance, and side effects, absence of certain narcotics from formularies, and reimbursement problems with pain therapies. However, patients and families must look to physicians for accurate information about opioid analgesics, and formulary and reimbursement issues came about long after the other barriers had been recognized and copiously documented.

There is important information in the use of the term "barrier" to explain the phenomenon of undertreated pain. It suggests that, but for the existence of these barriers, physicians would consistently provide optimal pain relief to their patients. Indeed, these barriers are sometimes described as though they were artifacts of nature, as formidable and immutable as a mountain range. The fact of the matter is, of course, that these barriers are the product of cultural beliefs, attitudes, and prejudices. We have created them, and, if necessary or appropriate, we can remove them. The fact that they have been with us for at least the last 50 years suggests that there is something less than a strong consensus and a concerted effort to bring them down. Perhaps, in scrutinizing each more carefully, we can gain some understanding as to why that might be so.[27]

The failure of clinicians to identify pain relief as a priority in patient care

Accepting as we (at least tacitly) do, the professional obligation of physicians to relieve human suffering, including that which is engendered by severe, persistent pain, this well-recognized failure of healthcare professionals to make it a priority in their care of patients verges on the inexplicable. There is a "chicken and egg" conundrum about the first two barriers to effective pain management. Do clinicians fail to identify pain relief as a priority because they have not been taught how to provide it? Or is it rather the case that medical schools and residency training programs do not emphasize training in pain management because clinicians, including medical educators, do not consider pain relief to be a priority in patient care? There may be a synergy between the forces that have erected these two barriers that confounds the search for a satisfactory answer to these questions.

Some insight into the problem can be gained by noting that it appears to have been exacerbated by the advent of modern, scientifically based, high-technology medicine that has shaped what we have previously noted to be the curative model of medical practice. As the term suggests, the curative model focuses primarily, if not exclusively, upon the goal of cure, i.e. the eradication or radical reversal of a disease process. Particularly to the extent that curative interventions themselves cause pain, discomfort, temporary dysfunction, or risk of death, the relief of pain and suffering can be interpreted as a conflicting goal, and hence one that must be abandoned during the pursuit of a cure. One commentator suggests that the pain experienced by the patient is subjected to two kinds of forgetting: one psychologic and the other conceptual.[28] The psychologic component arises from a need of the clinician to distance him- or herself from the patient's pain, as well as to convince the patient that the pain is not really as bad as it seems, or that it is a regrettable byproduct of the necessary means to a desirable clinical outcome. The conceptual component treats pain as a symptom of the underlying disease process, something to be observed but not managed or eliminated. This is particularly the case given the widely held (mis)perception that relieving pain impedes the process of cure. The patient's reports of pain are noted, if at all, as information about the progression of the disease, not as cries of distress giving rise to a duty to provide relief. To the extent that this perspective is accurate, it may call into question the ultimate effectiveness of one proposal by pain specialists to improve pain management in the inpatient setting – charting pain as the "fifth vital sign."[29] The implicit assumption is that pain is more likely to be treated if it is measured and recorded. However, if pain continues to be conceptualized as nothing more than an indicator of the progression of disease, noting its presence and severity in the chart will not necessarily result in interventions to relieve it. For insight into why that might be the case, we need to explore further the nature of the prevailing model of medical practice.

It has been persuasively argued that the pervasiveness and the overemphasis of the curative model in medical education not only results in a particular style of medical practice but also engenders a set of assumptions, attitudes, and values which are inherent in the model.[12] Among these are the focus on the disease process rather than the patient's experience of illness. Such a focus privileges the objective and scientifically verifiable, and discounts the subjective and unverifiable. This focus, of course, has significant implications for the care of patients with chronic, nonmalignant pain. The implicit message of the curative model is that there is no compelling need to know the patient as a person as long as the professional has a firm grasp upon the pathophysiology of their disease and an interventional strategy for reversing it. While the curative model may not pose any significant problems for patients whose pain is of the acute variety and limited in its severity and duration, it has itself been the cause of considerable unnecessary suffering for patients with chronic malignant or nonmalignant pain. The predominance of the curative model of medical education and its obsession with the pathophysiology of disease rather than the patient's subjective experience of illness is "disastrous," according to Arthur Kleinman, to the care of the chronically ill.[30] Indeed, the curative model, in conjunction with rampant opiophobia and an ethic of undertreatment of pain, has resulted in numerous instances of pseudoaddiction among chronic pain patients. Pseudoaddiction is an iatrogenic condition caused by the failure of physicians to provide adequate pain relief that forces the patient to employ (legitimate) drug-seeking behaviors to obtain analgesics they are entitled to.

Kleinman's work with chronic pain patients, as physician, psychiatrist, and medical anthropologist, provides a number of important maxims for those who seek to provide compassionate care to such individuals.

- One of the core tasks in the effective clinical care of the chronically ill is to affirm the patient's experience of illness as constituted by their explanatory models and to use those models in the development of an acceptable therapeutic approach.
- Chronic illness is as distinctive as the lived experience of different individuals because in the end it is the lived experience of different individuals.
- One half of all patients with chronic pain syndrome, like many others afflicted with chronic illness, meet the official criteria for major depressive disorder. More than anything else, the depressive mood represents demoralization from the life of pain and the persistent questioning by others, including healthcare professionals, of the authenticity of the patient's experience of pain.
- The science of pain medicine must include social science interpretations together with biomedical explanations. It must bring to bear knowledge of the economic, political, and social psychologic sides of pain.

The maxims I have gleaned from Kleinman's work describe what he characterizes as a "meaning-centered" model of chronic illness that he deems essential to the compassionate and effective care of such patients. It is a biocultural model that places the emphasis upon the patient's illness experience, as does the palliative model, and in doing so stands in stark contrast to the biomedical model whose exclusive focus is the disease process – its diagnosis and its cure or remediation.[31] While it may be much too simplistic to suggest that restoring some proportionality between the curative and palliative (or biomedical and biocultural) models of medicine in the education and training of physicians would eliminate this and related barriers to effective pain relief, it is also the case that it is naive and unrealistic to suggest that continuing professional education programs on pain management alone can overcome the assumptions, attitudes, and values that have been instilled in physicians by the curative model of medical education. Physician practice styles and patterns are acquired early and thereafter are highly resistant to change. Part of the solution goes not only to the substantive content of medical education but also to the venue. While most physicians practice in settings that would be hospitable to a balance between the curative and palliative approach to patient care, by far most medical education and residency training takes place in the acute, tertiary care setting where the hegemony of the curative model is most complete.[32]

Insufficient knowledge among physicians about pain assessment and management

Critics of medical education in the area of pain – its causes, assessment, and treatment – suggest that the typical medical school curriculum seems almost purposely designed to keep physicians in the dark about pain. In a 1989 interview, John J Bonica, generally regarded as the founder of the movement toward specialized pain clinics, observed, "No medical school has a pain curriculum."[33] Over 15 years earlier, a study of hospital inpatients revealed significant undertreatment of pain based in part on marked knowledge deficits on the part of physicians with regard to effective dose range, duration of action, and risks of addiction for narcotic analgesics.[14] At the conclusion of the study, the authors called for a major educational initiative, beginning in medical school, to improve the knowledge and skills of physicians in the use of narcotic analgesics for the management of pain. Interestingly, in addition to basic medical information, the authors suggested that any program of instruction must take into account the fact that for many physicians these drugs "have a special emotional significance that interferes with their rational use." The term which has been coined to describe this phenomenon is "opiophobia."[34] Like other, more generally recognized phobias, opiophobia cannot be cured or even effectively controlled by classroom education about the groundless nature of the fears. It is a behavior that is modelled and reinforced throughout all levels of medical education, from student clerkships to internship and residency.

The pharmacologist who coined the term "opiophobia" indicates that, after closely observing the opioid analgesic prescribing patterns of physicians in the United States, it would be tempting, but technically incorrect, to declare that "American physicians know nothing of the treatment of severe pain with narcotic opioids." They have learned well, as they progressed through their medical education, the prescribing patterns that are customary. Those patterns, however, are inconsistent with the best current medical knowledge. Indeed, they suggest that the patterns and practices that are at the root of undertreated pain have nothing to do with medical science whatsoever. For example, the belief that chronic pain patients managed with opioids are likely to become addicted (as opposed to physiologically dependent) runs directly counter to the best clinical data, which indicate that the risk of iatrogenic addiction for pain patients is less than 0.01 percent.[35] Similarly, the widespread fear of severe, perhaps even fatal, episodes of respiratory depression runs directly counter to numerous reports in the medical literature. Although many of these reports pertain to cancer patients, the salient point made therein is that it is only the opioid-naive patient who is at serious risk of respiratory depression.[36] A patient with moderate to severe chronic pain, regardless of whether it is caused by malignancy, whose analgesic level has been titrated upward appropriately, is not at serious risk.

It would be a mistake, however, to assume that opiophobia is entirely an American phenomenon, one secondary to such unique aspects of American culture and social history as the puritan heritage, the "noble" experiment of prohibition, or the contemporary "war on drugs." Restrictive prescribing laws are common in many European countries, both reflecting and sustaining an international opiophobia among healthcare professionals as well as patients.[20] In 2004, the International Narcotics Control Board Annual Report identified three reasons for the continued inadequate use of opioid analgesics:

1. unnecessarily strict rules and regulations governing their use;
2. negative perceptions about controlled drugs among medical professionals and patients; and
3. lack of economic means and resources.[37]

The role played by overly strict rules and regulations will be considered below under Fear of regulatory scrutiny of opioid-prescribing practices. The negative perception of opioids is one that appears to be not merely sociocultural in nature, encompassing both lay persons and healthcare professionals, but also linguistic. A recent European white paper offered several vivid examples. In Austria, narcotics are referred to as *Suchtmittel*, the literal translation of which is "the means to make you addicted." In Germany, narcotics are referred to as *Betaubungsmittle*, or the means to "knock you out."[38]

It is extremely difficult to measure the extent to which opiophobia is a product of overzealous regulatory measures (such as a declared "war on drugs" in the United States) to deter and detect drug diversion rather than the persistence of myths and misinformation about the risks and benefits of opioid analgesics. Nevertheless, it is a lamentable fact that the rhetoric and *modus operandi* of the regulators in their efforts to prevent or punish the diversion of or trafficking in narcotics has made physicians conscripts and pain patients noncombatant casualties, and has inflicted grave collateral damage on one of medicine's core values – the duty to relieve suffering. Recently published follow-up studies strongly suggest that state medical licencing board members, who play a pivotal role in the regulation of physician prescribing of opioid analgesics, have been particularly resistant to reeducation on such issues as the nature of addiction and the appropriateness of opioids in the management of some patients with chronic nonmalignant pain.[39] We will consider this issue below under Fear of regulatory scrutiny of opioid-prescribing practices.

In concluding our analysis of this particular barrier to effective pain management, I wish to introduce a concept which I characterize as "the culpability of cultivated ignorance." As we have seen in this brief survey, it has been known and identified as a problem for decades that medical school and residency training program curricula are woefully inadequate with regard to the assessment and management of all types of pain. Yet these institutions have failed or refused to reform themselves. It surely cannot be because pain has not been shown to be a pervasive problem frequently encountered by most physicians in their practice. The continuing absence of a significant pain component in medical education and training is indefensible, and the calling to account of these institutions by society for the persistence of such curricular deficits and their negative impact on patient care is long overdue.

A pain curriculum in medical school that is worth the effort it would take to implement would need to be comprehensive. It must begin in the lecture hall and continue through the role modelling and mentoring by a faculty of senior medical students, interns, and residents. The custom and practice in the institutions where young physicians are enculturated must be consistently based on the latest scientific knowledge and outcome studies of pain treatment modalities, something that the prevailing practice of physicians in most countries presently does not provide.

What is equally troublesome, however, from an ethical standpoint, is the continuing reliance by practicing physicians upon these curricular deficits as an excuse for why they fail to possess state-of-the-art knowledge and skill in pain assessment and management. While deficiencies in their professional education and training may provide an explanation for substandard care of patients with pain, they do not constitute an excuse. Entering a profession entails the acceptance of a responsibility to engage in lifelong learning and the continuing development and refinement of the knowledge and skills essential to the competent practice of that profession. The law can and will hold people responsible not only for applying their knowledge and skills in a prudent manner, but also for a failure to possess the knowledge and skills necessary to adequately engage in their profession or calling.

Fear of regulatory scrutiny of opioid-prescribing practices

There is an ongoing debate between the regulators and the regulated about the extent to which the regulations, and/or the manner of their enforcement, do or should have a chilling effect upon the quality of pain relief provided by healthcare professionals. Physicians in the United States recount horrific tales of armed Drug Enforcement Administration (DEA) agents descending upon physicians' offices in response to a report, often by a local pharmacist, of excessive prescribing practices.[40] Similarly, state medical licensing boards have been known to harshly discipline physicians for deviating from the customary practice of underprescribing opioid analgesics, or for prescribing them at all in the care of patients with chronic, nonmalignant pain. Later in this section, we will consider one such case in detail because it illustrates both the attitudes of many licensing board members and the reason why physician fears of regulatory scrutiny and disciplinary action have some foundation in fact.

The DEA is the federal agency primarily responsible for enforcement of the Controlled Substances Act (CSA). It was this legislation, passed by Congress in 1970, that established the five schedules of controlled substances. Schedule II drugs include morphine and other strong opioid analgesics such as fentanyl and oxycodone. The legislative history of the CSA makes it abundantly clear that its purpose was to deter and punish the diversion of controlled substances from legitimate medical purposes and narcotics trafficking, and not to insinuate the federal government or its law enforcement agencies into the legitimate prescribing practices of physicians. In response to charges that the DEA has attempted to become the arbiter of what constitutes the legitimate prescribing of controlled substances, and in doing so intimidating physicians into withholding controlled substances from patients who need them, the DEA notes that its *Physicians' manual* explicitly acknowledges that opioid analgesics can and should be considered one of the primary means of controlling many types of moderate to severe pain, including chronic nonmalignant pain. Such an official pronouncement, the DEA insists, should provide physicians with all of the reassurance they can legitimately demand that the DEA does not stand between them and proper treatment of their patients' pain problems.

Despite the pervasive view among healthcare professionals in the United States that the policies and practices of the DEA have had a chilling effect on the willingness of professionals to prescribe opioid analgesics for their patients even when clinically indicated, the DEA remains in denial, going so far as to post on its website in October of 2003 a press release entitled "The Myth of the Chilling Effect." The thrust of the statement was that "doctors operating within the bounds of accepted medical practice have nothing to fear from the DEA."[41] The purported justification for the "have no fear" message was that only a small percentage (less than 0.10) of all physicians registered by the DEA were investigated or prosecuted in 2003. What the DEA, and other governmental agencies with jurisdiction over prescription drugs fail to recognize is that "perception is reality," for healthcare professionals, as well as the lay public.

A recently published report on the use of opioids in Europe for the management of chronic pain notes, "In every country in Europe prescriptions for strong opioids must be filled in differently from those for other medicines."[38] In quite a few countries, including France, Germany, Italy, Spain, and many in Scandinavia, separate prescription forms must be used for strong opioids. Triplicate forms, an experiment that was undertaken by a number of states in the United States but subsequently abandoned, are required in Austria, Germany, Portugal, Italy, and Switzerland. Studies conducted in the United States revealed that immediately following the adoption of triplicate prescription form requirements for particular types of narcotics, the number of those drugs prescribed in subsequent years decreased substantially. Furthermore, there was an increase in the prescribing of less effective medications that did not require the triplicate form.[42] Such data strongly support the proposition that some narcotic diversion control measures do influence physician-prescribing practices in ways that have a negative impact on patient care. Below under The pursuit of balance in drug control law and public policy, we will consider ongoing efforts in the United States, Europe, and elsewhere to modify law and policy so as to provide some measure of balance between the goals of reducing drug diversion and addiction on the one hand, while promoting effective pain and symptom management on the other.

A number of state medical licensing boards, sometimes but not always through the prodding of state legislative initiatives, have begun to issue guidelines or policies with regard to the use of opioid analgesics for the management of chronic pain, especially chronic nonmalignant pain. Rarely do such boards acknowledge that their prior practices in any way justified the undertreatment of pain. Nevertheless, they offer these guidelines as further assurances to physicians that they certainly can no longer point to medical board policies and practices as justification for undertreating pain.[43]

In the United States, the Federation of State Medical Licensing Boards adopted "Model Guidelines for the Use of Controlled Substances for the Treatment of Pain" in 1998. The introduction to these model guidelines declared that pain management should be a priority in patient care, and strongly encouraged each state medical licensing board to adopt similar guidelines. Such guidelines accomplish several important goals. First, they make an important public policy statement that licensing boards expect physicians to provide effective pain relief to their patients. Second, they provide general guidelines for the physician to follow in order to document, among other things, that the opioid analgesics prescribed for a particular patient are medically indicated, properly monitored, and demonstrably improve the patient's level of function and/or quality of life. Third, they often incorporate by specific reference the significantly more comprehensive clinical practice guidelines for acute and cancer pain management of the Agency for Health Care Policy and Research. In 2004, the federation issued an expanded document, in the process recharacterizing it as a "'Model policy' to better reflect the practical use of the document." From the perspective of pain patients, the document is significantly strengthened by the provision indicating that "inappropriate treatment of pain includes nontreatment, undertreatment, overtreatment, and continued use of ineffective treatments."[44] The precise legal status of such a policy, even when formally adopted by a particular jurisdiction, remains uncertain, particularly with the disclaimer that the policy "is not intended to establish clinical practice guidelines." However, it will become increasingly difficult for physicians who depart frequently and materially from the best practices delineated by such policies to justify their approach, especially when the outcome is the unnecessary pain and suffering of their patients. We will consider court cases that may shed further light on the legal implications of substandard pain management practice below under Pain and the courts.

Another question that at this time has not been definitively answered is whether such guidelines will actually be utilized by state medical licensing boards to discipline physicians who deviate from such statements of accepted practice by underprescribing opioid analgesics for their patients with pain. In 1998, the California Medical Board declined to take any disciplinary action against a physician who it found to have provided inadequate pain management to a patient dying of cancer. In 2001, a jury awarded a sizeable judgment to the family of that patient in a lawsuit charging the attending physician with elder abuse.[45] This is one of two cases we will consider below under Pain and the courts. In 1999, the Oregon Board of Medical Examiners became the first to actually take disciplinary action against a physician for undertreating the pain of his patients.[46]

Those who support the Oregon Board do so, at least in part, on the grounds that such actions are the only way to send a clear message to practicing physicians, and indirectly to their patients, that both overprescribing and underprescribing of opioid analgesics constitute unprofessional practice for which there will be genuine accountability. In 2003, the Medical Board of California undertook two measures that strongly suggested a new approach to the subject of pain management. First, it issued updated guidelines on pain management, further emphasizing the significance of pain relief in sound patient care. Second, it initiated disciplinary action against a physician for alleged inadequacies in knowledge related to his treatment of a nursing home patient who was dying of mesothelioma. In a stipulated decision the following year, the physician in question agreed to remedial and punitive measures imposed by the Board.[47] In all other jurisdictions at the present time, the message implicit in licensing board conduct is that, while providing appropriate pain relief is commendable, drug diversion and "overprescribing" will actually place the physician at risk of disciplinary action.

Recent studies reveal that many members of state licensing boards in the USA are ill-equipped by training or experience to evaluate the quality of pain management provided by their licensees.[39] Furthermore, some recent disciplinary actions against physicians who used opioid analgesics for patients with severe, chronic nonmalignant pain suggest that medical boards do not even recognize a need to compensate for their lack of expertise by relying on specialists in the field. A case in point is a disciplinary action by the Florida Medical Licensing Board that was reversed by an appellate court.[48] Katherine Hoover, a board-certified internal medicine physician, was charged with "inappropriately and excessively" prescribing Schedule II narcotics to seven chronic pain patients. The agency's case against Dr Hoover consisted of the testimony of two physicians whom it recognized as experts. Neither of the agency's witnesses had examined any portion of the medical records of any of the seven patients in question. Furthermore, neither of the agency's witnesses specialized in the care of patients with chronic pain. In fact, both testified that they referred all such patients to pain management clinics. The sole basis for the opinions which they offered with regard to the appropriateness of Dr Hoover's care of the seven patients was a review of the computer printouts from the pharmacies which had filled the prescriptions written by Dr Hoover. On that basis alone, they opined, and the agency ultimately determined, that Dr Hoover had prescribed amounts of opioid analgesics that were "excessive, perhaps lethal." It did not seem to influence the agency's assessment of this testimony that none of these seven patients had suffered any adverse effects from these so-called "lethal doses" prescribed by Dr Hoover. In deciding to discipline Dr Hoover for her prescribing practices, the board disregarded the findings and conclusions of the hearing officer, who had determined that the evidence submitted by Dr Hoover's experts persuasively demonstrated that her care of the patients under consideration was appropriate.

Dr Hoover appealed the adverse ruling by the Board of Medicine to an appellate court, which held that the board's actions in disregarding the recommendations of the hearing officer were not supported by clear and convincing evidence. Still more disconcerting, however, was the appellate court's references in its written opinion to previous cases in which the board had disregarded the findings and conclusions of hearing officers as to the weight of the evidence, and forged ahead with disciplinary action against the physician for "overprescribing" Schedule II narcotics. In each of those cases, an appellate court of the State of Florida had chastised the board for taking disciplinary action against a physician on the basis of sparse and inadequate evidence.

What is particularly revealing about the board's missionary zeal in policing the prescribing practices of physicians who treat patients with chronic pain, which the court in *Hoover* described as "draconian," is that they continued unabated despite the fact that the Florida legislature had recently enacted an intractable pain statute specifically intended to encourage physicians to provide state-of-the-art care for such patients. Because the statute was not technically applicable to the Hoover case owing to the chronology of events, the board completely disregarded its policy implications. Such intransigence in the face of a clear public policy mandate does not serve to reassure clinicians that state medical licensing boards have embarked upon a new and more enlightened view of the role of opioid analgesics in the care of patients with chronic pain.

One might be tempted to conclude that the philosophy underlying the regulatory strategies of medical licensing boards appears to be that patients who require large, sustained doses of Schedule II narcotics to manage their pain are better off enduring the pain than relying on opioid analgesics for relief. However, as the approach of the board in the Hoover case demonstrates, the welfare of the patients was not really a genuine concern of the board. If it had been, some attention might have been paid to the patient records, and to patient testimony about the actual outcomes of Dr Hoover's treatment of their chronic pain, rather than exclusively focusing on pharmacy computer printouts. What we find, instead, is an unreflective, essentially reactionary approach to prescribing practices that are tailored to the needs of the patient rather than to some antiquated and scientifically unsubstantiated set of algorithms that has heretofore defined "good medical practice" with regard to the prescribing of opioid analgesics. Consequently, from an ethical perspective, licensing boards cannot justify their policies by reference to the ancient medical aphorism *primum non nocere*.

There are additional ethical considerations related to this particular barrier to effective pain management. The typical medical board, after all, is not composed of government bureaucrats or the lay public, but rather of practicing physicians. Presumably, they reflect the knowledge, attitudes, and beliefs of their profession. Indeed, one of the perennial concerns about and critiques of such boards is that they are simply a means by which the profession looks out for itself and perpetuates its own values and agenda. Regardless of whether and to what extent that may be true, it is nonetheless the case that organized medicine has yet to initiate any concerted effort to persuade all professional licensing boards to embrace a more scientifically based and patient-friendly approach to their oversight of physician prescribing practices. Instead, the typical physician has allowed opiophobic attitudes of medical licensing boards to establish and maintain a standard, and indeed an ethic of underprescribing. So long as such a standard and ethic prevail, exceptional physicians like Katherine Hoover, who have the moral courage to take on their board when necessary to the welfare of their patients, must become martyrs to the cause of pain relief for their patients.

The failure of healthcare institutions to hold clinicians accountable for pain relief

Traditionally, healthcare institutions have been dominated by their organized medical staff, at least with regard to determinations of what constitutes appropriate patient care. It logically follows that if effective pain management is not a priority of the medical staff, neither will it be an institutional priority of the hospital, long-term care facility, or clinic. The notable exception that proves the general rule is hospice. Since the defining role and mission of hospice is to provide palliative care to dying patients, only physicians who share that priority tend to associate themselves with it. However, even hospices and their physicians sometimes fail to make the relief of a patient's pain the cardinal principle of care.[49]

Decades ago, a seminal study of the institutional response (or lack thereof) of hospitals and their medical and nursing staffs framed the issue as the "politics of pain management."[50] The modern hospital is preeminently an acute care facility, typically consisting of an emergency room, diagnostic facilities, surgical suites, one or more intensive care units, and other units where generally short-term therapeutic measures are undertaken. Pain in such settings, as previously noted, is viewed as an important diagnostic tool, a symptom of some more serious underlying condition that must be diagnosed and hopefully cured. Eliminating or significantly mitigating the pain would be (or so it has been assumed) counterproductive to the diagnostic and therapeutic agenda. Similarly, patients who have recently undergone a procedure are monitored closely for complications, one indication of which is pain. Patients who are receiving optimal pain control will be at risk of unnoticed problems. Finally, many of the interventions that are indicated in the pursuit of diagnosis or cure themselves cause pain, only some of which may be alleviated without in some manner compromising its ultimate success.

Anecdotal evidence abounds, and has found its way into plays, motion pictures, and television, of patients and families who are subjected to considerable distress (physical and emotional) by healthcare professionals who scrupulously titrate pain medications and rigidly adhere to dosages and administration schedules. Complaints of severe pain are met with the staff response that another administration of the prescribed form of pain relief is not due yet, and the patient is then admonished not to complain because everything that can be done has been done. Particularly influential in the care of hospitalized patients are anticipated pain trajectories. When a patient demonstrates an unexpected pain trajectory, particularly one where the pain persists beyond the paradigm or is reported to be more severe than that which is usually reported, the staff may not be organizationally or emotionally equipped to respond appropriately.[50] A not uncommon response of the staff in such situations is to question the accuracy of the patient's complaints of pain, or to dismiss the patient as histrionic or attention-seeking. If the complaints persist, and focus on the need for more pain medication, the patient is at risk for being labelled a drug-seeker or even an addict. Such labelling constitutes the ultimate means of discrediting the patient's complaints, which at bottom constitute a charge that the staff has failed in one of its fundamental responsibilities – to relieve patient suffering.

The study to which we have been referring concludes that "staff is not really accountable ... for the actions it takes in regard to the patient in pain." Furthermore, the prognosis for any demonstrable improvement was grim:[50]

> Genuine accountability concerning pain work could only be instituted if the major authorities on given wards or clinics understood the importance of that accountability and its implications for patient care. They would then need to convert that understanding into a commitment that would bring about necessary changes in written and verbal communication systems. This kind of understanding and commitment can probably come about only after considerable nationwide discussion, such as now is taking place about terminal care, but that kind of discussion seems to lie far in the future.

Ironically, phase II of the SUPPORT study undertook precisely such an intervention designed to improve written and verbal communication on wards or clinics with the aim of improving the care of seriously ill patients. The intervention was a notorious failure, and the failure was attributed in significant part to the prevailing culture of medicine, which is driven by the therapeutic rather than the palliative model of care.

Realistically, boards that regulate healthcare professionals cannot be a patient's first line of defense against substandard medical care. Neither can medical malpractice litigation serve this function. That role and responsibility falls upon the institutions and organizations in which patient care is most commonly provided: the hospital and its clinics, ambulatory care centers, and long-term care facilities. Their tolerance of healthcare professionals who are unable or unwilling to provide appropriate pain relief to patients is an abrogation of their social and moral responsibility. For example, several of the patients whose inappropriate pain management served as the basis of the Oregon Board of Medical Examiner's ground-breaking disciplinary action against Dr Paul Bilder were receiving their treatment at the same institution. Yet there is no indication that any of the standing committees of the hospital responsible for the monitoring of the quality of patient care, e.g. quality assurance or medical staff credentials, had undertaken any measures to protect future patients from similar instances of unnecessary suffering. Hence, a period of five years and a total of six patients had to accrue before the medical board was in a position to initiate corrective action.

Within the last few years, a more concerted effort has been initiated by some leaders in the field, particularly nurses, to institutionalize good pain management and to institute mechanisms for holding the staff accountable for providing it.[51] However, what holds the greatest promise for actually bringing about systematic changes in the way in which pain is managed in most healthcare institutions are the new standards that have been promulgated and implemented by the Joint Commission for the Accreditation of Health Care Organizations (JCAHO).[52] In order to comply with these standards, institutions must do the following:[53]

- recognize the right of patients to appropriate assessment and management of their pain;
- identify patients with pain in an initial screening assessment;
- when pain is identified, perform a more comprehensive pain assessment;
- record the results of the assessment in a way that facilitates regular reassessment and follow up;
- educate relevant providers in pain assessment and management;
- determine and assure staff competency in pain assessment and management;
- address pain assessment and management in the orientation of all new staff;
- establish policies and procedures that support appropriate prescription or ordering of effective pain medications;
- ensure that pain does not interfere with participation in rehabilitation;
- educate patients and their families about the importance of effective pain management;
- address patient needs for symptom management in the discharge planning process;
- collect data to monitor the appropriateness and effectiveness of pain management.

The expedited introduction of these standards into the JCAHO institutional survey process is a strong indication of the perceived need to bring healthcare organizations promptly into compliance. Because of the importance that is attached to the JCAHO survey process, these standards create a realistic expectation that we may be in the process of moving from mere rhetoric to genuine reform of pain management practises in the United States. A final important note about the JCAHO standards is that they do not undertake to emphasize distinctions among acute, cancer, and chronic nonmalignant pain. Accredited institutions, through their professional staffs, are to be held accountable for appropriate management of all types of pain.

PAIN AND THE COURTS

A discussion of pain in society, at least one that deals in part with the situation in the United States, would not be complete without a review of important legal cases. That is because the United States, particularly in the last 50 years, has been characterized as the most litigious society in history.[54] While there are also those who argue that the data do not support such a sweeping statement, there is little doubt that healthcare professionals fear not only that regulatory scrutiny of their prescribing practices may lead not only to disciplinary actions by administrative agencies, but also to civil or even criminal actions. In the last 15 years a number of high profile cases have confirmed the role of law in explicating societal norms and professional standards in pain management. While a disproportionate number of the civil actions have related to the care of dying patients, recent criminal prosecutions, particularly by the federal government, have focused on physicians with a substantial number of chronic pain patients.

We begin with the 1997 Supreme Court decisions in *Washington v. Glucksberg*[55] and *Vacco v. Quill*.[56] These two cases challenged the constitutionality of statutes prohibiting physician-assisted suicide in Washington and New York, respectively. The justices ruled 9–0 that there is no constitutional right to physician-assisted suicide, even when such a right is narrowly circumscribed to include only competent patients with a terminal condition who are in great pain and repeatedly request such assistance. However, five of the nine justices wrote or joined in concurring opinions that have been interpreted as recognizing that such patients may well have a constitutional right to effective pain relief, such that any law creating an undue burden on access to such care would be unconstitutional.[57] Because the issue of pain management for such patients was arguably tangential to the issue before the court for decision, the fact that these justices were moved to write these opinions is a strong indication of the seriousness they attach to the provision of appropriate relief to patients with severe, persistent pain.

In 1991, and again in 2001, juries rendered large damage awards to the families of elderly patients whose pain associated with a terminal illness was undertreated. What distinguishes these cases – the first was in rural, northeastern North Carolina and was brought against a nurse and the nursing home that employed her; the second was in the Bay Area of northern California and was brought against a physician and an acute care hospital – is less significant than what they have in common. Both cases involved the failure or refusal to provide appropriate doses of opioid analgesics, such as morphine to control the pain associated with terminal cancer. The defendants in both cases denied that the care provided was below that which is usually or customarily provided to such patients, and both challenged the plaintiffs' contention that the patient suffered severely and unnecessarily. At both trials, expert witnesses for the plaintiffs testified that the patient's suffering was unnecessary and was proximately caused by the defendant's failure to meet a recognized standard of care for the management of pain for patients in the terminal phase of an illness in which significant pain should be anticipated and promptly and effectively addressed.

In the first case, *Estate of Henry James v. Hillhaven Corp.*,[58] the jury awarded the plaintiff $7.5 million in compensatory damages and $7.5 million in punitive damages. The case was never reviewed by an appellate court because the parties settled for an undisclosed amount following the trial. In the second case, *Bergman v. Wing Chin, MD, and Eden Medical Center*,[59] the jury found that the defendant Chin's care constituted elder abuse and awarded $1.5 million in compensatory damages to the patient's family. Eden Medical Center settled with the patient's family prior to trial. In neither case had state authorities taken any disciplinary action against the institutions or individuals involved.

These jury verdicts provide compelling evidence of an observation by Eric Cassell many years ago: "The relief of suffering, it would appear, is considered one of the primary ends of medicine by patients and lay persons, but not by the medical profession."[60] As we reflect upon pain and society, and particularly its ethical and legal dimensions, we must be concerned about this continuing and significant disparity between lay and professional opinion about the duty of healthcare professionals to relieve suffering and the seriousness that should be attached to a failure to fulfill that duty. Juries are, in a sense, the conscience of the community, and when they award millions of dollars in damages for the failure to properly manage pain, they are sending a clear message to the health professions that a custom and practice of undertreating pain is unacceptable and will not be tolerated.

A civil action, filed in the state of California in 2002 and settled the following year, suggests that important changes in perceptions and attitudes about the significance of undertreated pain have taken place in a relatively short period of time. The case challenged the quality of palliative care provided to Lester Tomlinson, an elderly man diagnosed with advanced mesothelioma. First in an acute care hospital, and subsequently in a skilled nursing facility (SNF), his family alleged that he received woefully inadequate relief for his pain in what proved to be the last month of his life. Following his death, a complaint was filed with the Medical Board of California against the physician responsible for Mr Tomlinson's care at the SNF and with the state agency responsible for oversight of long-term care facilities. Separately, an elder abuse civil suit was filed against the acute care hospital, the SNF, and several physicians alleging grossly negligent (reckless) or complete failure to manage Mr Tomlinson's pain in both facilities.[61] This claim was settled as to all defendants prior to the scheduled trial date in April 2003. The Medical Board pursued disciplinary action against the nursing home physician, and a settlement agreement involving a public reprimand, 40 hours of continuing medical education, and reassessment was entered into later that year. The SNF was cited by the regulatory agency for multiple deficiencies related to Mr Tomlinson's pain and symptom management, and numerous corrective actions were required.[62] Clearly, the defendants and their attorneys, as well as the regulatory agencies, took a much more serious view of the implications of undertreated pain than their counterparts had in the *Bergman* case only a few years earlier.

In the last several years, the DEA and the US Department of Justice have vigorously pursued criminal prosecutions against a small number of physicians whose practices primarily involved chronic pain patients. We will consider one in particular, which resulted in a conviction and long prison sentence for the defendant physician. William Hurwitz, MD, treated a large number of chronic pain patients in his northern Virginia medical practice. Some came from long distances because they could not receive the relief they needed in their own communities. Dr Hurwitz had actually been the subject of prior disciplinary measures by the Virginia Medical Board, and at all times pertinent to the federal prosecution he was monitored by the state entity.

Dr Hurwitz was convicted by a federal district court jury of 50 counts of distributing and conspiring to distribute controlled substances, for which he was sentenced to 25 years in prison. The thrust of the prosecution's case was that the doses of narcotics that Dr Hurwitz prescribed to his chronic pain patients were so excessively high that they were "outside the bounds of medical practice." Once categorized in this way, Dr Hurwitz was (in the words of the DEA administrator) "no different from a cocaine or heroin dealer peddling poison on the street."[63] One of the key arguments on the appeal of Dr Hurwitz's conviction was that in violation of the precedent established by the US Supreme Court in other criminal prosecutions under the Controlled Substances Act, the trial judge precluded the jury from considering evidence that the prescriptions in question were written in a good faith effort to care for these patients, and not for the purpose of drug trafficking.[64] Other factors used by the prosecution in the Hurwitz case in pursuit of a conviction were that some of his patients were known by him to be addicted, and others sold the drugs they obtained from him. Dr Hurwitz argued on appeal that neither of these factors necessarily makes his prescribing criminal, since those addicted to drugs are still entitled to pain relief, and unless a physician knew, or in the reasonable exercise of professional judgment should have known, that a patient was selling prescriptions, the physician cannot be held criminally responsible for the patient's conduct.

A number of prominent experts in the field of pain medicine, as well as the American Academy of Pain Medicine, submitted *amicus curiae* (friend of the court) briefs to the appellate court in support of Dr Hurwitz. The briefs do not constitute a blanket endorsement of his chronic pain management practices, but rather argue that at worst he may have in some instances departed from the prevailing standard of care. Departing from the standard of care does not remove a physician's conduct from "the bounds of medical practice" and hence make it subject to criminal prosecution. The reason is that the federal Controlled Substances Act has consistently been interpreted so as to insulate from liability clinicians who prescribe controlled substances for "a legitimate medical purpose in the usual course of professional practice."[65] The critical issue becomes that of good faith. As the very court reviewing the Hurwitz appeal stated in a previous criminal prosecution of a physician under the Controlled Substances Act, "[If] [a] doctor dispenses a drug in good faith in medically treating a patient, then the doctor has dispensed the drug for a legitimate medical purpose in the usual course of medical practice."[66] The trial court refused to provide a jury instruction on the issue of good faith and provided no guidance on how to define "the bounds of medical practice."[67]

In August 2006, the Fourth Circuit Court of Appeals overturned the conviction of Dr Hurwitz on the grounds that the trial court had committed reversible error in its refusal to instruct the jury that it could consider the defense of good faith to the charges of drug trafficking. The court went on to explain that the good faith standard to be applied at any subsequent retrial of the case would be an objective rather than a subjective one. In other words, the critical question for the jury is whether a reasonable physician in the same or similar circumstances would have a good faith basis for believing she was acting consistent with the generally recognized and accepted standard of medical practice?[68]

The pursuit of balance in drug control law and public policy

Beginning just before the year 2000, a major public policy initiative focused on pain relief and drug control law began. The central or governing principle of the initiative was "balance," which was characterized as "the dual imperative of governments to establish a system of controls to prevent abuse, trafficking, and diversion of narcotic drugs while, at the same time, ensuring their medical availability."[69] Inherent in the initiative appeared to be a genuine concern that there was currently, and had been for some time, an imbalance produced by a disproportionate emphasis on preventing or punishing drug diversion and a lack of emphasis on access to opioids for pain relief. The evaluation guide was intended to provide a tool with which to measure the level of imbalance in a jurisdiction's laws and policies. It identified eight criteria for provisions that may tend to enhance pain management, e.g. prescription amount alone is recognized as insufficient to determine the legitimacy of prescribing, and nine criteria for provisions that may tend to impede pain management, e.g. medical use of opioids is implied to be outside legitimate professional practice. In the United States, the University of Wisconsin Pain and Policy Studies Group conducted evaluations of the states in 2000 and 2003 and grades were assigned on a scale of A–F. In neither year did any state receive either an "A" or an "F," with "C" being average.[70] In the three years between the two evaluations, 14 states improved their grades, 36 remained the same, and one (Ohio) had a negative change.

During the same period, the Pain and Policy Studies Group collaborated with the WHO to prepare a similar guide that was international in scope.[71] The stated purpose of this document was to enable governments "to determine whether their national drug control policies have established the legal and administrative framework to ensure the medical availability of opioid analgesics, according to international treaties and the recommendations of the International Narcotics Control Board (INCB) and the World Health Organization (WHO)." The INCB had implicitly endorsed the principle of balance in public policy in an earlier report when it stated: "…an efficient national drug control regime must involve not only a programme to prevent illicit trafficking and diversion, but also a programme to ensure the adequate availability of narcotic drugs for medical and scientific purposes."[72] The INCB officially endorsed the WHO guidelines for policy assessment in 2001, and in 2005 reiterated its request that individual nations examine the extent to which their laws and regulations allow the medical use of opioids and develop plans for addressing problems revealed by such an examination.[73]

Rumania has become the first country to initiate a government-sponsored program to conduct a comprehensive assessment of drug control policy to address regulatory barriers and improve access to opioids by collaborating with the Pain and Policy Studies Group on recommendations for changing the country's regulatory policies for opioids.[74] However, perhaps prompted to some extent by the WHO report and previous statements by the INCB, Italy eliminated a complex triplicate prescription form for opioids. The question that remains open, even when governmental policies are made more conducive to good pain management, is the extent to which clinicians will change their traditionally ultraconservative approach to opioid analgesics, which has been shaped for so long by the history of unbalanced policies focused on drug diversion.

CONCLUSIONS

Opiophobia and an ethic of undertreating pain are aspects of clinical practice that are international in scope and negatively impact all patients with pain. While physicians who regularly care for such patients continue to be at risk of close, even chilling regulatory scrutiny, and in rare cases even criminal prosecution, they now have available an unprecedented number of nationally and internationally recognized policy statements, guidelines, texts, and scientific journal articles supporting in the strongest of terms the prompt, effective, and diligent approach to pain management, with opioid analgesics as the often indispensable weapon against severe chronic pain. Clinically appropriate utilization of state-of-the-art pain management techniques, careful monitoring of patients, and scrupulous and thorough documentation should in most instances insure that healthcare professionals will not be at an unreasonable risk of adverse action when they provide their patients with the kind of sensitive, skillful, and compassionate care that they have a right to expect and that is consistent with the most ancient goal and core values of medicine – the relief of suffering.

REFERENCES

1. Zborowski M. *People in pain.* San Francisco, CA: Jossey-Bass, 1969.
2. Lipton JA, Marbach JJ. Ethnicity and the pain experience. *Social Science and Medicine.* 1984; **19**: 1279–98.
3. Bates MS, Edwards W, Anderson K. Ethno-cultural influences on chronic pain perception. *Pain.* 1993; **52**: 101–12.
4. Edwards RR, Moric M, Husfeldt B *et al.* Ethnic similarities and differences in the chronic pain experience: a comparison of African American Hispanic and white patients. *Pain Medicine.* 2005; **6**: 88–98.
5. Caton D. The secularization of pain. *Anesthesiology.* 1985; **62**: 493–501.
6. Morris DB. What we make of pain. *Wilson Quarterly.* 1994; **18**: 8–26.
7. * Morris DB. *The culture of pain.* Berkeley, CA: University of California Press, 1991.
8. Kleinman A. *The illness narratives: suffering, healing and the human condition.* New York: Basic Books, 1988.
9. * Cassel EJ. *The nature of suffering and the goals of medicine.* New York: Oxford University Press, 1991: 32.
10. Joranson DE. Intractable pain treatment laws and regulations. *American Pain Society Bulletin.* 1995; **5**: 1–3, 15-17.
11. Cassel EJ. *The nature of suffering and the goals of medicine.* New York: Oxford University Press, 1991.
12. Fox E. Predominance of the curative model of medical care – a residual problem. *Journal of the American Medical Association.* 1997; **278**: 761–3.
13. The SUPPORT Principal Investigators. A controlled trial to improve care for seriously ill hospitalized patients. *Journal of the American Medical Association.* 1995; **274**: 1591–8.
14. Marks RM, Sachar EJ. Undertreatment of medical inpatients with narcotic analgesics. *Annals of Internal Medicine.* 1973; **78**: 173–81.

15. The International Project Special Report. The goals of medicine: setting new priorities. *Hastings Center Report.* 1996; (Special supplement): 1–27.
16. Brena S. *Chronic pain: America's hidden epidemic.* New York: Atheneum/SMI, 1978.
17. World Health Organization. *Cancer pain relief and palliative care.* Geneva: World Health Organization, 1990.
* 18. Turk DC, Brody MC, Okifuji EA. Physicians' attitudes and practices regarding the long-term prescribing of opioids for non-cancer pain. *Pain.* 1994; **59**: 201–8.
19. Zenz M, Willweber-Strumpf A. Opiophobia and cancer pain in Europe. *Lancet.* 1993; **341**: 1075–6.
20. Zenz M, Zenz T, Tryba M, Strumpf M. Severe undertreatment of cancer pain. *Journal of Pain and Symptom Management.* 1995; **10**: 187–91.
21. Larue F, Colleau SM, Brasseur L, Cleeland CS. Multicentre study of cancer pain and its treatment in France. *British Medical Journal.* 1995; **310**: 1034–7.
* 22. Larue F, Colleau SM, Fontaine A, Brasseur L. Oncologists and primary care physicians' attitudes toward pain control and morphine prescribing in France. *Cancer.* 1995; **76**: 2375–82.
23. United Nations. *Single convention on narcotic drugs, 1961 (as amended by the 1972 Protocol).* New York: United Nations, 1977.
24. World Health Organization. *Cancer pain relief,* 2nd edn. Geneva: World Health Organization, 1996.
25. International Narcotics Control Board. *Availability of opiates for medical needs.* New York: United Nations, 1996.
26. Selva C. International control of opioids for medical use. *European Journal of Palliative Care.* 1997; **4**: 194–8.
* 27. Joranson DE, Cleeland CS, Weissman DH. Opioids for chronic cancer and non-cancer pain: a survey of state medical board members. *Federation Bulletin.* 1992; **79**: 15–49.
28. Ruddick W. Do doctors undertreat pain? *Bioethics.* 1997; **11**: 244–6.
29. Foley K. Pain relief into practice: rhetoric without reform. *Journal of Clinical Oncology.* 1995; **13**: 2149–51.
30. Kleinman A. *The illness narratives: suffering, healing and the human condition.* New York: Basic Books, 1988: 254.
31. Morris DB. *Illness and culture in the postmodern age.* Berkeley, CA: University of California Press, 1998: Chapter 4.
32. Billings JA, Block S. Palliative care in undergraduate medical education: status report of future directions. *Journal of the American Medical Association.* 1997; **278**: 733–8.
33. Weiner RS. An interview with John J. Bonica, MD. *Pain Practice.* 1989; **1**: 2.
* 34. Morgan JP. American opiophobia: customary underutilization of opioid analgesics. *Advances in Alcohol and Substance Abuse.* 1985; **5**: 163–73.
35. Porter J, Jick H. Addiction rare in patients treated with narcotics. *New England Journal of Medicine.* 1980; **302**: 123.
36. Walsh TD. Opiates and respiratory function in advanced cancer. *Recent Results in Cancer Research.* 1984; **89**: 115–17.
* 37. International Narcotics Control Board. *Annual report.* Vienna: International Narcotics Control Board, 2004.
38. Opioids and Pain European Network of Minds. The White Paper on opioids and pain: a pan-European challenge, June 2005.
* 39. Gilson AM, Joranson DE. Controlled substances and pain management: changes in knowledge and attitudes of state medical regulators. *Journal of Pain and Symptom Management.* 2001; **21**: 227–37.
40. McKinney M, Fintor L. News: how physicians handle drug investigations. *Journal of the National Cancer Institute.* 1991; **83**: 1282–4.
41. Drug Enforcement Association. The myth of the chilling effect. Press release, 30 October 2003.
42. Weintraub M, Singh S, Byrne L *et al.* Consequences of the 1989 New York State Triplicate Benzodiazepine Prescription Regulations. *Journal of the American Medical Association.* 1991; **266**: 2392–7.
43. Pain and Policy Studies Group. US Pain Policy Resources. Madison, WI, USA: Pain and Policy Studies Group. Cited December 2007. Available from: www.medsch.wisc.edu/painpolicy/states.htm.
44. Federation of State Medical Boards of the United States, Inc. Model policy for the use of controlled substances for the treatment of pain. Dallas, TX, USA: Federation of State Medical Boards, last updated 2004; cited December 2007. Available from: www.fsmb.org/pdf/2004_grpol_Controlled_Substances.pdf.
45. *Bergman* v. *Chin*, No. H205732-1 (Cal. App. Dept. Sup. Ct. 1999).
46. Barnett EH. Case marks big shift in pain policy. The Oregonian September 2, 1999. Available from: www.oregonlive.com:80/news/99/09/st090201-html.
47. In the Matter of Eugene B. Whitney, MD. Accusation and stipulated decision. Medical Board of California, 2003.
48. *Hoover* v. *Agency for Health Care Administration*, 676 So. 2d 1380 (Fla. Dist. Ct. App. 1996).
49. Webb M. *The good death.* New York: Bantam Books, 1997: 63–71.
50. Fagerhaugh S, Strauss A. *Politics of pain management: staff–patient interaction.* Menlo Park, CA: Addison-Wesley, 1977: 22–27.
51. Ferrell BR, Dean GE, Grant M. An institutional commitment to pain management. *American Pain Society Bulletin.* 1994; 16.
52. Joint Commission for the Accreditation of Health Care Organizations. *Accreditation manual.* Chicago, IL: JCAHO, 2000.
53. Berry PH, Dahl JL. Making pain assessment and management a healthcare system priority through the new JCAHO pain standards. *Journal of Pharmaceutical Care in Pain and Symptom Control.* 2000; **8**: 5–20.
54. Lieberman JK. *The litigious society.* New York: Basic Books, 1981.

55. *Washington* v. *Glucksberg*, 521 US 702 [1997].
56. *Vacco* v. *Quill*, 521 US 793 [1997].
57. Burt R. The supreme court speaks: not assisted suicide but a constitutional right to palliative care. *New England Journal of Medicine*. 1997; **337**: 1234–6.
58. *Estate of Henry James* v. *Hillhaven Corp.*, No. 89 CVS 64 (N.C. Super. Ct. Jan 15, 1991).
59. *Bergman* v. *Chin*, No. H205732-1 (Cal. App. Dep't. Super. Ct. Feb. 16, 1999).
60. Cassell EJ. The nature of suffering and the goals of medicine. *New England Journal of Medicine*. 1982; **306**: 639–45.
61. *Rosa Tomlinson et al.* v. *Bayberry Care Center et al.*, Contra Costa County Superior Court, No. C-02-00120.
62. Tucker KL. Medico-legal case report and commentary: inadequate pain management in the context of terminal cancer, the case of Lester Tomlinson. *Pain Medicine*. 2004; **5**: 214–17.
63. Tandy K. DEA Administrator Karen Tandy's remarks on Hurwitz sentencing. USA: Drug Enforcement Administration, last updated: April 14, 2005; cited December 2007. Available from: www.dea.gov/pubs/pressrel/pr041405b.html.
64. Brief of Appellant William Eliot Hurwitz, United States Court of Appeals for the Fourth Circuit, Case No. 05-4474.
65. 21 Code of Federal Regulations §1306.04, Purpose of issue of prescription.
66. *United States* v. *Tran Trong Cuong*, 18 F.3d 1132, 138 (4th Cir. 1994).
67. Brief for Amicus Curiae the American Academy of Pain Medicine in Support of Appellant and for Reversal, United States Court of Appeals for the Fourth Circuit, September 2, 2005.
68. *United States of America* v. *William Hurwitz*, No. 05-4474, U.S. Ct. App. 4th Cir. Aug. 22, 2006.
* 69. University of Wisconsin Pain and Policy Studies Group. Achieving balance in federal and state pain policy: a guide to evaluation. Madison, WI: Pain and Policy Studies Group, University of Wisconsin Comprehensive Cancer Center, 2007. Available from: www.painpolicy.wisc.edu/Achieving_Balance/EG2007.pdf.
70. University of Wisconsin Pain and Policy Studies Group. Achieving balance in state pain policy – a progress report card. Madison, WI: University of Wisconsin Comprehensive Cancer Center, September 2003.
71. World Health Organization. Narcotic and psychotropic drugs: achieving balance in national opioids control policy – guidelines for assessment. Geneva: World Health Organization, 2000.
72. International Narcotics Control Board. Availability of opiates for medical needs. Report of the International Narcotics Control Board for 1995. New York: United Nations, 1996.
* 73. International Narcotics Control Board. Report of the International Narcotics Control Board for 2004. New York: United Nations, 2005.
74. Mosoiu D, Ryan KM, Joranson DE, Garthwaite JP. Reform of drug control policy for palliative care in Romania. *Lancet*. 2006; **367**: 2110–17.

9

Chronic pain, impairment, and disability

ROBERT J GATCHEL AND NANCY D KISHINO

KEY LEARNING POINTS

- Chronic pain, impairment, and disability, rather than being actual entities, are constructs that can only be inferred in order to account for some form of behavior or phenomenon of interest.
- There is often a discordance or low degree of correlation among levels of chronic pain, impairment, and disability.
- What makes the operational definition and use of these three constructs difficult is that there are three broad categories of measures that can be used to operationally define them – physical, psychosocial, and overt behavior/function – that are, in turn, not always correlated highly with one another. The scientific literature is replete with many different measurement techniques and tests of these three constructs. However, the literature is beginning to demonstrate which specific measures appear to be the most reliable and valid.
- Pain is now considered as the fifth vital sign (added to pulse, blood pressure, core temperature, and respiration). The biopsychosocial perspective is currently recognized as the most comprehensive and heuristic approach to the assessment and treatment of this experiential state.
- Impairment has been traditionally a medical term, defined as a significant loss, or loss of use, of a body structure or function in an individual with a health condition, disorder, or disease, which can be objectively measured. Because chronic pain has a major subjective component to it, it has created a major problem in the area of objective impairment evaluation.
- Disability is more an administrative term that refers to a diminished capacity or inability to perform certain activities of daily living as a result of loss of function due to impairment.

OVERVIEW

It is now recognized that the most comprehensive and heuristic approach to the evaluation/management of medical conditions, especially those involving pain, is the biopsychosocial perspective.[1,2,3] This biopsychosocial model focuses on the complex interaction among biological, psychological, and medicolegal variables that patients encounter when dealing with a persisting, distressing medical condition. Such an interaction may perpetuate, and even worsen, the clinical presentation. It also accounts for the likelihood that patients' lives are adversely affected in a variety of ways by their medical condition, thus requiring a more comprehensive assessment and treatment approach designed to address all aspects of required care, both biological as well as psychosocial. This approach is in striking contrast with the outdated, overly simplistic biomedical reductionist approach which erroneously assumed that most medical disorders could be broken down into distinct, independent physical and psychosocial components. Indeed, one study highlighted how individuals differed significantly in the frequency they report physical symptoms, and their tendency to visit physicians when experiencing identical symptoms, and in their responses to the same treatment.[4] Often, the nature of a patient's response to treatment has little to do with his or her objective physical condition.

Another important aspect of the biopsychosocial model that deserves independent mention is in the area of compensation injuries (e.g. workers' compensation, short-/long-term disability, personal injury litigation, etc.). It has long been known that objective societal outcomes, such as return to work, future healthcare utilization, and recurrent injury rates, are considerably lower than in the general population for similar injuries, independent of the severity of injury or treatment.[1] For example, a large meta-analysis demonstrated return-to-work rates for spinal fusion surgery to be as low as 16 percent in workers' compensation populations.[5] It has become clear that financial secondary gain is closely related to patient behaviors when compensation is being provided for illness. Compensated illness is a frequent finding in almost all industrialized countries.

The above is simply a preamble to our subsequent discussion of the complexities involved in the evaluation of pain, impairment, and disability. In an earlier review of such complexities, Robinson *et al.*[6] began their discourse with a quotation concerning back injuries (made almost 100 years ago) about how such assessment is rife with problems:

> Back injuries have a bad reputation. The workman looks upon them with apprehension, the insurance company with doubt, the medical examiner with suspicion, the lawyer with uncertainty ... The medical examiner is faced with the difficulty of estimating the true value of the subjective symptoms in the comparative absence of physical signs. His suspicion is born of the frequent disparity between these two.
>
> McKendrick, 1916: p. v.[7]

Robinson and colleagues[6] then went on to discuss how they confronted this complex problem as contributors to the American Medical Association's *Guides to the evaluation of permanent disability, 5th edn.*[8]

With the above in mind, it should also be noted that, when discussing constructs such as chronic pain, impairment, and disability, rather than being actual entities, these are constructs that can only be inferred in order to account for some form of behavior or phenomenon of interest. For example, chronic pain is usually viewed as a mediator (i.e. an unobservable inferred construct) which is hypothesized to account for certain observable behaviors such as differences in activities of daily living or work ability among individuals. Of course, if one uses a construct to explain some form of behavior or phenomenon, it is essential that one develop a precise operational definition and employ objective referents as measures of the construct. As will be discussed in this chapter, this is no easy task.

As previously highlighted by Gatchel,[1] it is extremely important to be aware of the important distinctions among the constructs of pain, impairment, and disability. This is due to the fact that there is often a discordance or low degree of correlation among levels of chronic pain, impairment, and disability. For example, in an early influential report by Waddell,[9] the problem of discordance in the evaluation of chronic low back pain was noted (see **Figure 9.1**). Although correlations were found among these three constructs, there was not perfect overlap among these phenomena. Although they are all logically and clinically related to one another, there is usually not a 1:1:1 relation among them. Waddell[9] found correlations among them to be in the range of only about 0.6. Also, what makes these imperfect correlations even more complex is the wide range of individual differences in such concordance from one individual to the next.[10] Healthcare professionals, therefore, need to be aware of the varying relationships among these constructs during the evaluation of patients. For example, one patient may display very little medical impairment that can be objectively evaluated, although he/she may verbally report a great amount of pain. Ratings of disability may perhaps fall somewhere in between the two in terms of severity. In stark contrast, another patient with a seemingly

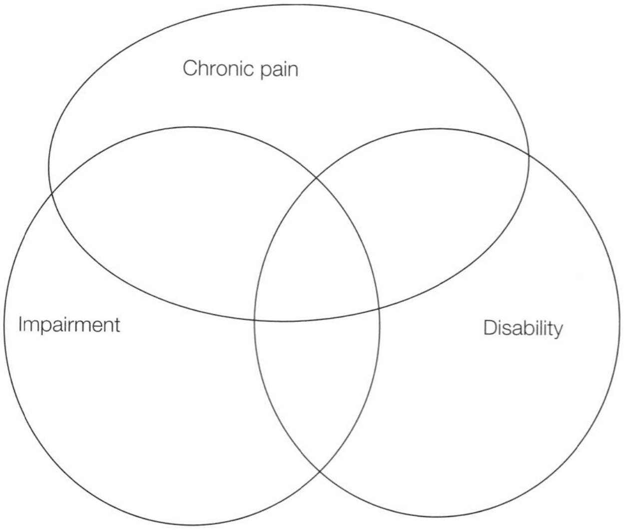

Figure 9.1 Diagram demonstrating low concordance among chronic pain, impairment, and disability.

comparable injury may report very little pain, but may display a great deal of impairment and disability.

Obviously, clinicians need to be aware of the operational definitions of these above three constructs or phenomena because they are fundamentally different. Also, it is important to assess all three in specific diagnostic situations wherever possible, with the expectation that there may be complex interactions among them that may differ from one patient to the next, as well as from one assessment time period to the next. These three constructs have been discussed in the medical impairment and disability evaluation literature.[1, 11, 12]

Chronic pain (i.e. pain lasting for greater than three months) is a biopsychosocial concept based primarily on an experiential or subjective evaluation.[13] The construct of pain is frequently used to infer the presence of some biopsychosocial mechanisms that prompts patients' complaints and inhibition of normal functioning and behavior. The International Association for the Study of Pain defines pain as "an unpleasant sensory and emotional experience associated with actual or potential tissue damage or described in terms of such damage."[14] As will be discussed, chronic pain is often difficult to quantify in a totally objective and reliable manner. Impairment is a medical term which is used to refer to an alteration of an individual's usual health status (i.e. some anatomical or pathophysiological abnormality) that is evaluated by medical methods. The evaluation of impairment is conducted to determine some inferred pathophysiology or anatomical dysfunction that is assumed to have a negative impact on a patient's current health status or behavior. Unfortunately, however, such impairment evaluation relies upon methods that are often not totally reliable, and that are often subject to examiner bias. Finally, disability is more of an administrative term that refers to a diminished capacity or inability to perform certain activities of everyday living as a result of loss of function, due to impairment. Again, though, disability evaluations are not totally reliable and are also subject to various examiner and patient response biases.

THE MEASUREMENT OF CHRONIC PAIN, IMPAIRMENT, AND DISABILITY

In addition to the aforementioned fact that there are often complex interactions among chronic pain, impairment, and disability, what makes this issue even more complicated is that there are three broad categories of measures – physical, psychosocial, and overt behavior/function – that have all been used to assess patients.[1] Again, however, these three major category measurements (or biopsychosocial referents) often do not display high concordance with one another when measuring a construct such as chronic pain, or impairment, or disability. Therefore, this creates a second layer of complexity. For example, if one uses a self-report measure (e.g. a visual analog rating scale) as a primary index of a construct such as pain, and compares it to the overt behavior/function measure (e.g. total distance walked during a certain amount of time) of this same pain construct, direct overlap or perfect correlation cannot be automatically expected. Moreover, two different self-report indices (e.g. a visual analog rating scale versus the McGill Pain Questionnaire) or behavior/function indices (e.g. total distance walked during a certain time period versus lifting performance) of this same pain construct may not be as highly correlated as one would expect. What has plagued the evaluation arena in general has been the lack of agreement in the wide variation in measures used to document constructs, such as chronic pain, impairment, and disability, as well as changes in these measures. Thus, the literature is replete with many different measurement techniques and tests of a construct, such as chronic pain.[10, 15] It is beyond the scope of the present chapter to review these complexities comprehensively. The scientific literature, though, is beginning to demonstrate which specific measures appear to be the most reliable and valid.[1, 15]

Chronic pain

Several important organizations in the United States have now developed new standards for the evaluation of pain. For example, the Joint Commission on Accreditation of Healthcare Organizations (JCAHO)[16] requires that healthcare professionals consider pain to be a fifth vital sign (added to pulse, blood pressure, core temperature, and respiration) when evaluating patients. As reviewed by Gatchel and Oordt,[2] the JCAHO guidelines require that pain severity be documented using a pain scale. Moreover, the following also need to be assessed:

- the patients' own words describing their pain;
- the location of the pain and its duration, as well as aggravating or alleviating factors;
- present pain management regimen and its effectiveness;
- effects of pain;
- patients' pain goals;
- a physical examination.

As noted by Gatchel,[1] it is now recognized that the most comprehensive and heuristic approach to the assessment and treatment of chronic pain is the biopsychosocial perspective. This biopsychosocial model focuses on the complex interaction among biological, psychological, and medicolegal variables that patients encounter when dealing with a persisting, distressing, chronic pain condition. Such an interaction may perpetuate, and even worsen, the clinical presentation. It accounts for the likelihood that patients' lives are adversely affected in a variety of ways by their chronic pain condition, thus requiring a comprehensive assessment and treatment approach designed to address all aspects of required care, both biological as well as psychosocial. As noted earlier, this approach is in stark contrast with the outdated, overly simplistic biomedical reductionist approach which mistakenly assumed that most pain disorders could be broken down into distinct, independent physical and psychosocial components. There is often an absence of a documentable association between pain and a pathophysiologic process in the organ or body part from which the pain is perceived as emanating.

Each individual will experience a chronic pain condition uniquely. The complexity of such conditions is especially evident when it persists over time, as a range of psychological, social, and economic factors can interact with physical pathology to modulate a patient's report of discomfort and disability associated with the chronic pain. It is therefore essential to comprehensively evaluate all these major components for each individual in order to subsequently tailor a unique treatment program to account for his or her specific needs.

What are some of the commonly used measures of chronic pain? A visual analog scale (VAS) has traditionally been one of the most widely used self-report measures of pain. For example, the Million VAS (MVAS) is a 15-item measure designed to assess pain, disability, and physical functioning, and it is useful primarily for patients with chronic low back pain disorders.[17] It provides a simple, easy-to-understand format for patients. In a recent study,[18] MVAS scores were used to categorize patients into one of six groups: no reported pain/disability (score of 0); mild pain/disability (score of 1–40); moderate pain/disability (score of 41–70); severe pain/disability (score of 71–100); very severe pain/disability (score of 101–130); and extreme pain/disability (score of 131–150). Using this categorical method, it was found that this measurement was related to several important outcomes, such as treatment dropout rate and level of depression, as well as one-year socioeconomic outcomes (such as return-to-work rate, work retention, post-rehabilitation surgeries, etc.). Such results indicate that the use of the MVAS scores as categorical indices is effective in predicting treatment outcomes in patients with chronically disabling spinal disorders. Of course, a more general VAS instrument can be used for types of pain other than low back pain.

In fact, a recent measure developed by Anagnostis *et al.*[19] evaluates functional status due to pain and disability – the Pain Disability Questionnaire (PDQ). The PDQ yields a total functional pain and disability score ranging from 0 to 150. The focus of the PDQ, much like other health inventories, is primarily on pain, disability, and function. Unlike most other measures, though, the PDQ is also designed for the full array of chronic pain disorders, rather than purely one type of pain, such as low back pain. Psychosocial variables, which recent studies have shown play an integral part in the development and maintenance of chronic pain and disability, form an important core of the PDQ. The psychometric properties of the PDQ are excellent, demonstrating stronger reliability, responsiveness, and validity relative to many other existing measures of functional status, such as the Oswestry, the MVAS, and the SF-36 instruments. A factor analysis of the PDQ revealed two independent factors that can be evaluated: a functional status component and a psychosocial component. Analyses demonstrated each of these two components to be valid in assessing their theorized constructs.

Of course, one of the most widely used self-report measures is the Medical Outcomes Study 36-Item Short Form (SF-36), which was developed for various uses in clinical practice and research.[20] It is a good global index of patient functioning and measures the functional status of the whole patient. The SF-36 has eight scales that measure health concepts: physical function, role limitation because of physical health problems, bodily pain, social functioning, general mental health, role limitation because of emotional problems, vitality, and general health perception. There are also two global summary or component scales: a physical component summary scale and a mental component summary scale. Lower scores on the mental component scale are usually a good index of potential emotional distress; low scores on the physical component scale are usually a good index of potential physical function limitations. The advantages of the SF-36 are that it is brief (taking approximately 10–20 minutes to complete), and it divides health into distinct physical, social, and mental components. An even shorter form, the SF-12, is now available. One shortcoming, though, is that the actual clinical usefulness of the SF-36 with individual patients is not well established because of these test's psychometric properties. However, it can be used to monitor overall group changes.

In addition to the above, there are many other measures of chronic pain that can be used. The reader is referred to Turk and Melzack[10] and Gatchel[1] for a comprehensive review of these various measures.

Many of the above measures used for assessing chronic pain are often also used to measure degree of self-reported disability (see below under Disability). Indeed, for example, the PDQ was developed specifically for evaluating self-reported pain, as well as disability. Such questionnaires were designed to assess a patient's degree of functional status, disability, as well as pain that would interfere in activities of daily living. There are also other self-report measures that evaluate more specific on-the-job disability limitations and work performance. For example, the Work Limitations Questionnaire (WLQ) scale developed by Lerner and colleagues[21] assesses limitations in handling work-time demands, work-physical demands, mental-interpersonal demands at work, and output demands. The full instrument is 25 items, divided into four scales. Each WLQ scale score is interpreted as the percentage of time in the previous two weeks that a person was limited in performing a specific class of job demands. Scores are the means of nonmissing responses and converted to a range of 0 (no limitations) to 100 (limited all the time). An algorithm is available from the developer to convert these percentages to projected economic losses in a cross-sectional study of a general working population. The psychometric properties of this instrument are good.

Another instrument developed to measure human performance indices of disability is the Spinal Function Sort (SFS), which is a 50-item, paper-and-pencil, self-report questionnaire that assesses ability to perform physical tasks.[22] This instrument is used to identify functional consequences of disability and medical intervention. On the SFS, the evaluee ranks ability to perform 50 common physical tasks depicted by drawings and text captions on a six-point scale. The "rating of perceived capacity" is an estimate of work capacity in terms of the United States Department of Labor Physical Demands Characteristics System for people who have experienced soft tissue musculoskeletal injury. It is administered as a stand-alone evaluation or as part of a more comprehensive functional capacity evaluation. Again, the reader is referred to Turk and Melzack[10] and Gatchel[1] for fuller descriptions of a variety of other evaluations such as these.

Disability

Robinson[23] and Gatchel[1] provided a comprehensive overview of the complexities involved in the assessment of disability of a patient with a painful condition. Such assessment is usually based on subjective self-report measures of restrictions of activities of daily living, such as walking, work, and recreational activities, sleep, sex, and so on. A fundamental goal of such a disability evaluation is usually to ascertain whether a patient can or cannot work. A comprehensive review of such measures has been presented by Gatchel.[24] However, again, such a determination is quite difficult in evaluating painful conditions because of the misguided assumption that impairment can be precisely and objectively measured and is closely linked to "mechanical failure" of an organ or body part. Often, chronic pain patients will report activity restrictions that cannot be fully understood in terms of a specific "mechanical failure." As discussed, there is often a low concordance between subjective reports of pain and objective data of impairment. Thus, this will introduce vagaries into the disability evaluation process. One disability evaluator may tend to ignore the patient's subjective reports of pain and disability, and rely more heavily on any objective evidence of mechanical dysfunction that is available. Another evaluator may rely more exclusively on the subjective appraisals and activity restrictions reported by the patient, regardless of whether they can be objectively quantified in terms of any measurable mechanical failure or dysfunction. Another evaluator may attempt to develop a composite of both the subjective and objective measures. Unfortunately, as noted by Robinson[23] and Dembe,[11] there is currently no totally agreed upon disability evaluation system that can be used. Thus, disability agencies across different states will be quite different in the methods used. It should also be remembered that across the different states, there is no one workers' compensation system; each state's workers' compensation is specific for that state. Therefore, disability evaluations in Texas may be quite different from those in California or Connecticut. Nevertheless, in terms of a disability evaluation, physicians are usually required to address the following areas: assessment and diagnosis, impairment, ability to work, and a need for further treatment. Again, Robinson[23] has provided examples of the questions that are usually asked by disability agencies when conducting such evaluations.

Impairment

The American Medical Association's *Guides to the evaluation of permanent impairment*[8] defines impairment as "A significant deviation, loss, or loss of use, of any body structure or body function in an individual with a health condition, disorder, or disease." As traditionally viewed, such impairments are considered as biomedical abnormalities that can be evaluated at the level of organs or body parts. Also, it has been assumed that impairments can be assessed on the basis of objective medical data, and not on the basis of patient self-report. For example, cardiac impairment can be assessed by the physician on the basis of ventricular ejection function. An impairment rating can then be given based on a "consensus-derived" percentage estimation of loss (reflecting the severity of impairment for a given health condition), and the degree of associated limitations caused by the loss, as reflected by diminution of activities of daily living.

Unfortunately, the major limitation of such a biomedical approach to evaluating impairment in a phenomenon such as chronic pain is the fact that a unique underlying pathophysiology or nociception directly linked to pain frequently cannot be unequivocally delineated. Thus, traditionally, there has been the misguided assumption that impairment can be precisely and objectively measured, and that it is closely linked to some "mechanical or biomedical failure" of an organ or body part. However, as we have discussed, one of the key components of constructs, such as pain and impairment, are their potential subjectivity. The assessment of such subjective factors will require an examiner to interpret the communications of pain by the patient, and to then use such communications to infer the patient's experiences. In addition, no matter what the level of accuracy or sophistication of a medical test used in collecting physiologic measures, it is always the case that human interpretation ultimately must be used in the understanding of the resulting findings. Moreover, as highlighted earlier, ratings of impairment are often not highly correlated with overt behavior/function or physiologic concomitants of the same chronic pain phenomenon. Because of such concordance issues, there is still a great deal of controversy with the *Guides to the evaluation of permanent impairment* as to how to provide an impairment rating for chronic pain. These guides strive to base any impairment rating on objective factors whenever possible (as in our example of ventricular ejection function for cardiac impairment). This basic principle is violated when one needs to include subjective factors, such as experiential self-report, in attempting to rate the impairment associated with chronic pain. Indeed, there are fundamental conceptual problems when pain is inferred as a cause of impairment, primarily due to the subjectivity of pain and the need to assess pain-related impairment at the level of the "whole person," rather than at the level of specific organs or body parts. Moreover, impairment ratings based solely on objective factors are likely to fail to capture the "full burden of illness" of the disorder (factors such as emotional distress, fatigue, etc.). To this day, such a violation is viewed as a fundamental deviation from the major purpose of the guides. Why the basic logic of the guides (i.e. objective evaluation) should be compromised in order to provide an impairment rating for chronic pain remains a major conundrum in the field of impairment evaluation within the American Medical Association.

Nevertheless, in spite of the aforementioned limitations/issues in evaluating impairment, for lack of a better approach to help partially document impairment, the functional capacity evaluation (FCE) has been used as a favorite tool for assessing the extent of a patient's impairment. The FCE is composed of a series of test methods that assess individual components of overall human performance. They include measures of range of motion, functional strength, endurance, and dexterity using standardized tasks. Unfortunately, test methods may take many forms across vendors or facilities. However, they should include (based on a match with the individual's job requirements), a battery of assessments that include standing, walking, sitting, lifting, carrying, pushing, pulling, climbing, balancing, stooping, kneeling, crouching, crawling, reaching, handling, fingering, and feeling. Of course, critical to all issues relating to appropriate use of an FCE is the use of consistent instructions for testing, as well as a standardized test battery. Unfortunately, there are often vagaries from one facility to another, which create difficulties in making comparisons across facilities and patients. This is an area that requires a great deal of additional scientific research in order to standardize the most valid and reliable FCE battery.

CONCLUSIONS

Chronic pain is best viewed as a biopsychosocial process involving the often complex interaction among physical and psychosocial factors that make the experience of pain unique from one individual to the next. Impairment is more a medical term used to refer to an alteration of the patient's usual health status (i.e. some anatomical or pathological abnormality) that is evaluated by medical means. Finally, disability is more an administrative term that refers to the diminished capacity or inability to perform certain activities of daily living due to a medical impairment. In any discussion of these three constructs, one must be aware of the issue of discordance or low correlation among them. For example, in an early report highlighting this problem of discordance in the evaluation of chronic low back pain, Waddell[9] demonstrated that, although correlations are found among these three constructs, there is often not perfect overlap among them. Thus, one needs to be able to ascertain the relative contributions of all three constructs in order to assess the impact on the whole person, with the expectation that such contributions will differ from one patient to the next.

Another significant factor that makes the operational definition and use of these above three constructs even more difficult is the fact that there are three broad categories of measures that can be used to operationally define them – physical, psychosocial, and overt behaviors/function. These categories, in turn, are also not always highly correlated with one another. Fortunately, the scientific literature is beginning to demonstrate which specific measures appear to be the most reliable and valid for the purposes of operationally defining chronic pain, impairment, and disability. Clinicians will need to be aware of the above complexities and best definitions of these three different constructs. They will need to constantly remain up to date in terms of what assessment/evaluation methods have the best psychometric properties and validity.

Finally, the basic scientific fact must now be recognized that any attempt to operationally define chronic pain, disability, or impairment by using only objective indicators, without the inclusion of subjective indices, is doomed to failure. With the advent and empirical support of the heuristic biopsychosocial perspective of illness during the last decade, a great deal of additional research must be directed at more validly assessing these constructs, as well as their unique interactions that may differ from one patient to the next.

ACKNOWLEDGMENTS

The writing of this chapter was supported in part by grant Nos 2R01 DE 010713, 3R01 MH 046452, and K05 MH

071892 from the National Institutes of Health, and grant No. DAMD17-03-0055 from the Department of Defense.

REFERENCES

* 1. Gatchel RJ. *Clinical essentials of pain management.* Washington, DC: American Psychological Association, 2005.
2. Gatchel RJ, Oordt MS. *Clinical health psychology and primary care: practical advice and clinical guidance for successful collaboration.* Washington, DC: American Psychological Association, 2003: 263.
* 3. Turk DC, Monarch ES. Biopsychosocial perspective on chronic pain. In: Turk DC, Gatchel RJ (eds). *Psychological approaches to pain management: a practitioner's handbook*, 2nd edn. New York: Guilford, 2002: 3–29.
* 4. Gatchel RJ, Kishino ND, Strezak A. The importance of outcome assessment in orthopaedics: An overview. In: Spivak JM, Connolly PJ (eds). *Orthopaedic knowledge update: spine.* Chicago, IL: American Academy of Orthopaedic Surgeons, 2006, 95–102.
5. Turner JA, Ersek M, Herron L *et al.* Patient outcomes after lumbar spinal fusions. *Journal of the American Medical Association.* 1992; **268**: 907–11.
* 6. Robinson JP, Turk DC, Loeser JD. Pain, impairment, and disability in the AMA guidelines. *Journal of Law, Medicine and Ethics.* 2004; **32**: 315–26.
7. McKendrick A. *Back injuries and their significance.* Edinburgh: E&S Livingstone, 1916.
* 8. American Medical Association. *Guides to the evaluation of permanent impairment*, 5th edn. Chicago, IL: American Medical Association, 2001.
* 9. Waddell G. Clinical assessment of lumbar impairment. *Clinical Orthopedic Related Research.* 1987; **221**: 110–20.
* 10. Turk DC, Melzack R. *Handbook of pain assessment*, 2nd edn. New York: Guilford, 2001.
11. Dembe AE. Pain, function, impairment and disability: Implications for workers' compensation and other disability insurance systems. In: Mayer TG, Gatchel RJ, Polatin PB (eds). *Occupational musculoskeletal disorders: function, outcomes and evidence.* Philadelphia: Lippincott Williams & Wilkins, 2000, 563–76.
* 12. Gatchel RJ. Psychological disorders and chronic pain: Cause and effect relationships. In: Gatchel RJ, Turk DC (eds). *Psychological approaches to pain management: a practitioner's handbook.* New York: Guilford, 1996: 33–52.
13. Gatchel RJ. Comorbidity of chronic mental and physical health disorders: The biopsychosocial perspective. *American Psychologist.* 2004; **59**: 792–805.
14. Merskey H, Bogduk N (eds). *Classification of chronic pain: Descriptions of chronic pain syndromes and definitions of pain terms.* (Report of the Task Force on Taxonomy of the International Association for the Study of Pain), 2nd edn. Seattle, WA: IASP Press, 1994.
* 15. Gatchel RJ, Okifuji A. Evidence-based scientific data documenting the treatment- and cost-effectiveness of comprehensive pain programs for chronic nonmalignant pain. *Journal of Pain.* 2006; **7**: 779–93.
* 16. Joint Commission on Accreditation of Healthcare Organizations. *Pain assessment and management: an organizational approach.* Oakbrook, IL: Joint Commission on Accreditation of Healthcare Organizations, 2000.
17. Million S, Hall W, Haavik NK *et al.* Assessment of the progress of the back-pain patient. 1981 Volvo Award in Clinical Science. *Spine.* 1982; **7**: 204–12.
18. Anagnostis C, Mayer TG, Gatchel RJ, Proctor T. The Million Visual Analog Scale: Its utility for predicting tertiary rehabilitation outcomes. *Spine.* 2003; **28**: 1–10.
19. Anagnostis C, Gatchel RJ, Mayer TG. The pain disability questionnaire (PDQ); A new psychometrically sound measure for chronic musculoskeletal disorders. *Spine.* 2004; **29**: 2290–302.
20. Ware JE, Snow KK, Kosinski M, Gandek B. *SF-36 health survey: manual and interpretation guide.* Boston: The Health Institute, New England Medical Center, 1993.
21. Lerner D, Amick BC, Rogers WH *et al.* The Work Limitations Questionnaire. *Medical Care.* 2001; **39**: 72–85.
22. Matheson L, Matheson M, Grant J. Development of a measure of perceived functional ability. *Journal of Occupational Rehabilitation.* 1993; **3**: 15–30.
* 23. Robinson RC. Disability evaluation in painful conditions. In: Turk DC, Melzack R (eds). *Handbook of pain assessment*, 2nd edn. New York: Guilford, 2001.
* 24. Gatchel RJ. *Compendium of outcome instruments for assessment and research of spinal disorders*, 2nd edn. La Grange, IL: North American Spine Society, 2006.

10

The psychological assessment of pain in patients with chronic pain

ALLEN H LEBOVITS

KEY LEARNING POINTS

- The evaluation of pain in the chronic pain patient must be multidisciplinary.
- The objectives of the psychological evaluation are not to determine whether the patient's pain is "real" or "imagined," but rather is multifactorial.
- The standard evaluation protocol of most pain centers is the pain questionnaire, the clinical interview, pain assessment measures, and a psychological evaluation.
- One of the more common uses of the psychological evaluation has been to determine the appropriateness of a potential candidate for chronic opioid therapy, implantation of a spinal cord stimulator or implantable pump.
- As important as the psychological assessment of the chronic pain patient is in general, it takes on added significance with the patient who presents with a history of past or present substance abuse.
- One of the controversial issues in chronic pain management today is whether every chronic pain patient who is being treated should first receive a psychological evaluation.
- Better, more individualized assessment of pain patients, particularly those with comorbid psychiatric issues, will lead to more effective treatment of this very difficult to treat population.

INTRODUCTION

The multidisciplinary evaluation and treatment approach is widely practiced today and considered to be the standard of care.[1] The psychological evaluation and assessment of chronic pain patients has evolved from unidimensional to multidimensional models and the utility of these approaches has increased exponentially.[2] As its sophistication has increased so has its distance from the standard mental health intake assessment.

The inadequate assessment of the pain patient is based on a surprising lack of knowledge and misunderstanding about chronic pain issues. In a survey of pain knowledge and attitudes of nearly 700 healthcare providers in three hospitals, Lebovits *et al.*[3] found a correct response rate of only 56 percent, with the addiction knowledge-related items responded to least correctly. Seventy-two percent of providers agreed incorrectly with the item "25 percent of patients receiving narcotics around the clock become addicted," when, in fact, the prevalence rate of opioid addiction in patients with chronic pain, is much lower than the prevalence of substance use disorders in the population at large. The unwarranted fear of addiction is a misunderstood concept in pain management that can lead to the undertreatment of pain, a problem that has been well-documented in AIDS and cancer patients.[4, 5] [III], [6][III], [7][III]

There is an ethical imperative for all pain specialists to assess the pain patient as a whole person, including all their biological, social, and psychological dimensions.[8] Evaluating chronic pain patients with a unimodal strictly medical approach is not in the patient's best interests. Radiologic findings are not reliable indices of pain; significant spinal abnormalities are often found in patients who do not experience pain.[9] The unimodal medical pain evaluation without a psychological evaluation can lead to iatrogenic effects, such as failed surgical interventions and pharmacologic disasters with attendant side effects and exacerbation of pain. Not appreciating the psychopathology of some pain patients, such as somatization, often results in repeated medical interventions that lead, in turn, to medical and psychological morbidity. The interdisciplinary evaluation of these patients, requiring collaboration among healthcare professionals is essential.[1, 10][II], [11] The well-meaning clinician who has not done a thorough psychological evaluation can soon find himself/herself with an increasingly difficult to manage patient on increasingly high doses of opioids with unremitting pain.

OBJECTIVES OF PSYCHOLOGICAL EVALUATIONS

The objectives of the psychological evaluation of the patient with chronic pain are not to determine whether the patient's pain is real or imagined (all pain is "real") but rather:

- to determine the degree of psychological adaptation to chronic pain which includes mood state, coping skills, effect on family, and particularly level of physical functioning;
- to evaluate the patient's premorbid psychological state and personality factors and its effect on onset and etiology of pain;
- to establish the role of psychological factors in the etiology, maintenance, and exacerbation of pain;
- to formulate a DSM-IV diagnosis;
- to devise a treatment plan in conjunction with the patient and the rest of the multidisciplinary team;
- to predict outcome of invasive medical procedures, such as surgical implantation of spinal cord stimulators or continuous infusion pumps;
- to determine which psychological and medical interventions would be most appropriate for which patients;
- to identify environmental reinforcers of chronic pain and illness behaviors, such as family, litigation status, and disability insurance status;
- to evaluate the likelihood of the development of chronic pain-related disability.

STANDARD PAIN CENTER EVALUATION PROTOCOL

A common procedure in many multidisciplinary pain centers is to mail a background and demographic questionnaire before the patient's first visit to either mail back prior to their visit or bring with them at their first visit. This allows for prior review of data which can save time for the clinician and can begin to frame the clinical interview. It also serves as a very valuable educational lesson for the patient, structuring their thoughts in a certain direction, such as relating pain to various factors and, most significantly, introducing the concept of the relationship between psychological factors and pain. This is an important therapeutic principle that many patients have a great deal of defensiveness about. Unless this can be overcome, psychological interventions will not succeed. The standard evaluation protocol of most pain centers is the pain questionnaire, the clinical interview, pain assessment measures, physical examination, and a psychological evaluation. Many patients perceive the careful detailed analysis of their pain and related factors as an understanding and willingness to listen to them. This gains their respect and cooperation, and is often something previous healthcare personnel may have been reluctant to do.

Pain center pain questionnaire

The pain center pain questionnaire is a structured questionnaire, with open-ended questions kept to a minimum, which facilitates data entry and speeds up the time it takes to complete the questionnaire. The questionnaire should be designed to yield objective clinical outcome measures, as suggested by the criteria of the Commission on Accreditation of Rehabilitation Facilities (see Chapter 49, Comprehensive pain rehabilitation programs: a North American reappraisal in the *Practice and Procedures* volume of this series). **Table 10.1** shows the content of most questionnaires.

Structured clinical interview

A structured clinical interview is typically performed as part of any comprehensive psychological evaluation and

Table 10.1 Contents of a pain questionnaire.

Category	Detail
Demographic characteristics	Age, marital status, ethnicity, occupation, and educational level
Pain characteristics	Location, intensity (typically evaluated on a 0–10 rating scale regarding least, average, and worst severity), duration, sensory and affective descriptors, what makes the pain better and worse, and interference with sleep
Circumstances of onset of pain	Date, traumatic onset versus insidious onset
Review of previous medical history	Previous pain interventions and their efficacy, prior hospitalizations for pain, current and past medication use, litigation and compensation status
Social environment	Interference of pain in marriage, sexual ability, and social/recreational activities
Functional status	Current employment status, interference of pain on activity levels, working ability, number of hours spent resting during the day because of the pain, number of blocks able to walk, ability to perform household chores, such as laundry, meal preparation, cleaning, shopping, child care, and financial management

assessment of chronic pain patients. It represents a good opportunity to review the data obtained on the pain questionnaire, which often may be incomplete or inconsistent. It is an even better opportunity to observe the patient and his/her subjective experience of pain, as well as any illness behavior (facial expressions, frequent posture change, and guarding/bracing). It is an excellent idea to evaluate the patient together with their significant other and their interactions with each other and the interviewer. This facilitates evaluation of the response of the significant other to the patient's pain – whether it is a solicitous, punishing, or distracting response,[12] and can be a valuable educational tool for the patient, significant other, and interviewer.

The clinical interview is ideally suited to review the patient's pain complaints, onset of pain and relationship to trauma, prior medical and psychiatric history, prior alcohol and drug usage. It also reviews current marital and family environment, current functional level, disability status, motivational level to return to work, primary, secondary and tertiary gain issues, ability to sleep, and utilization of coping skills. Coping strategies that lead to less pain are the active ones, such as staying busy and distraction. The bad coping strategies that lead to more pain are the passive ones – restricting activities, dependency, wishful thinking, and catastrophizing (seeing everything in a negative light). An additional area of investigation of the clinical interview, particularly with women presenting with chronic pelvic pain, is a history of childhood physical, emotional, or sexual abuse. Studies have shown a high rate of incidence of childhood abuse appearing later in adulthood as physical pain.

Patients with chronic pain often have a traumatic onset etiology. A significant number of patients seen by chronic pain specialists may therefore experience considerable amounts of psychological distress and some may have posttraumatic stress disorder (PTSD). PTSD has been estimated to occur in about 10 percent of chronic pain patients. When patients with pain as a result of an accident are referred for psychological treatment, the reported PTSD rates increases from 50 to 100 percent. The failure to diagnose and treat PTSD properly in chronic pain patients can lead to minimal or inadequate pain relief. A useful assessment measure for patients with chronic pain and trauma is the Posttraumatic Chronic Pain Test (PCPT).[13] The PCPT contains six true-false items that evaluate the presence of PTSD related to the accident that caused the patient's pain.

The clinical interview also affords the opportunity to evaluate the patient's beliefs and cognitions about their pain. However, the primary utility of the clinical interview is to formulate a diagnosis in conjunction with the standardized questionnaires. Particular diagnostic categories carefully evaluated for include levels of depression and anxiety, PTSD, and somatization disorders. This facilitates the design of a comprehensive treatment plan, devised together with the patient as well as the rest of the multidisciplinary team.

Pain assessment measures

The third important aspect of all pain evaluation protocols is the assessment of the intensity and quality of pain. Verbal, numerical, and visual analog scales are commonly used to assess the intensity of pain. Verbal rating scales consist of a list of adjectives that describe different levels of pain intensity. The patient is asked to choose the adjective, from as few as four to over ten depending on the scale used, that best describes his or her pain. Verbal rating scales are easy to administer, score, and understand, but are less sensitive than visual analog scales because of fewer response categories which may miss small changes in pain intensity.[14] They assume fluency in communicating in a particular language and are not appropriate for preverbal patients or patients with cognitive impairments.

Numerical rating scales are based on asking pain patients to rate their pain from 0 to 10 or 0 to 100, with the anchor descriptors of "no pain" and "worst imaginable pain." Numerical rating scales are easy to administer, score, and understand, and have demonstrated their validity as pain intensity measures.[15]

Visual analog scales usually are 10-cm lines, with defined anchors at the ends of the line ranging from "no pain" to "worst pain imaginable." The patient is required to make a mark along the line that best reflects their pain intensity. Scoring is accomplished by measuring the distance from the left end of the scale to the mark. Although there is demonstrated validity with this technique, both very young and older patients have difficulty with this method,[15] and photocopied versions change the length of the line.[14] Visual analog scales are effective, however, with an older pediatric population.[16][III]

In the pediatric setting, age-appropriate pain intensity measures have been devised for the different developmental stages of the child. The Poker Chip Tool[17] requires that the four- to eight-year-old chooses one to four poker chips, representing the "pieces of hurt" experienced. Various faces scales have also been devised for young children, with each face being assigned a numerical value reflecting its order within a series of facial expressions. Excellent psychometric properties have been demonstrated.[18]

One of the most commonly used pain assessment measures is the McGill Pain Questionnaire (MPQ).[19] When it first appeared, it differed significantly from standard pain intensity measures, in that it offered, for the first time, a multidimensional assessment of pain – evaluating the sensory, affective, and evaluative dimensions of pain. Patients are asked to choose an adjective from each of 20 subclasses of adjective groupings. Each word is associated with a specific score. Pain-rating indices are calculated for the total score, as well as for each dimension. The MPQ is useful in differentiating psychiatric patients from those who do not have a psychiatric disturbance, and particularly in its ability to discriminate between patients who have different kinds of pain. For example, postherpetic neuralgia (PHN) is often described using the adjectives "tender, burning, throbbing, stabbing, shooting, sharp," which correlate with the three different types of pain experienced with PHN:

1. steady throbbing or burning pain;
2. an intermittent sharp or shooting pain;
3. allodynia (tender), (pain in response to a stimulus that does not normally provoke pain).

Confirmatory factor analyses of the MPQ have shed some doubt on the original three subscales of the test.[20] Holroyd *et al.*,[21] conducting a multicenter evaluation of the MPQ with 1700 chronic pain patients, showed that a factor analysis revealed a four-factor model instead of three factors: one affective, one evaluative, and two sensory factors. Furthermore, examination of the relationships between the MPQ and the Minnesota Multiphasic Personality Inventory (MMPI) failed to provide evidence of the discriminant validity of the MPQ subscales. They concluded that the utility of the three scale scores in clinical decision-making remains unstandardized and the value in diagnosis or in forming useful subgroups of patients remains unclear.

Administration of the test needs to be carefully monitored, to make sure that no more than one word is selected from each subclass and to ensure that the patient understands each word. Patients for whom English is not their first language have particular difficulty with this test, although foreign language versions are available. The short form (SF-MPQ) has gained in popularity due to its brevity and good reliability.[22] The SF-MPQ consists of 15 representative words from the sensory and affective categories of the original MPQ as well as an additional word "splitting" because it is a discriminant word for dental pain. The SF-MPQ is sensitive to clinical changes from therapeutic interventions.[23][II]

MEASURES OF PSYCHOLOGICAL STATUS

Because of the close interplay of psychological factors, stress, and emotional reactions with the etiology, maintenance, and exacerbation of pain, measures of psychological status have become part of the standard pain center evaluation protocol. Measures of psychological symptomatology, as well as specific pain coping measures, are widely used.

Beck Depression Inventory

The Beck Depression Inventory (BDI)[24][III] is one of the most widely used tests with chronic pain patients because it is a relatively quick measure of depression, a mood state closely interlinked with chronic pain.[25] The most prevalent psychological characteristic of chronic pain patients is depression. Depression and chronic pain occur together so frequently it is often difficult to determine whether the depression is a precipitant of the pain or a consequence of living with intractable pain. Levels of depression can range from minor mood state disturbances to major clinical depressions with active suicidal ideation. In an unpublished study, the author has found that 25 percent of 821 chronic pain patients score in the moderate to severe range of depression on the BDI. The BDI is a 21-item questionnaire requiring the patient to endorse various symptoms of depression that produces a total score of depression ranging from 0 to 63. Scores above 10 reflect minor depressive states, while above 17, are indicative of a moderate to severe state. The BDI is easy to administer and score. The item on suicidal ideation is helpful in assessing suicidality in chronic pain patients. The BDI is predictive of many aspects of patient functioning.[26] Comparing the BDI to another measure of depression, the CES-D, Geisser *et al.*[27] found that both the BDI and the CES-D discriminated significantly between chronic pain patients who were depressed versus those who were not. One of the criticisms of the use of an instrument such as the BDI is that some of the physical "vegetative" items such as sleeplessness, which can be endorsed because of pain, can artificially elevate BDI scores for pain patients. Geisser *et al.*[27] found, however, that removal of these somatic items did not improve its accuracy.

Spielberger State-Trait Anxiety Inventory

The Spielberger State-Trait Anxiety Inventory (STAI)[28] is the most widely used measure of anxiety, a construct that is not used as extensively as depression is with chronic pain patients, but nevertheless a very important one with pain patients. The STAI is a 40-item inventory that assesses "trait" anxiety, a characterological, stable dimension of anxiety that is relatively consistent over time, as well as "state" anxiety, transitory feelings of anxiety usually in response to specific situations. Patients are asked to rate statements on a four-point scale regarding how they feel right now (state anxiety) and how they feel generally (trait anxiety).

Minnesota Multiphasic Personality Inventory

The Minnesota Multiphasic Personality Inventory (MMPI, MMPI-2),[29] one of the most widely used and researched tests of all time, is used quite extensively with chronic pain patients. **Figure 10.1** shows that the use of the MMPI for pain is quite extensive, as evidenced by citations in the literature on the use of MMPI with pain

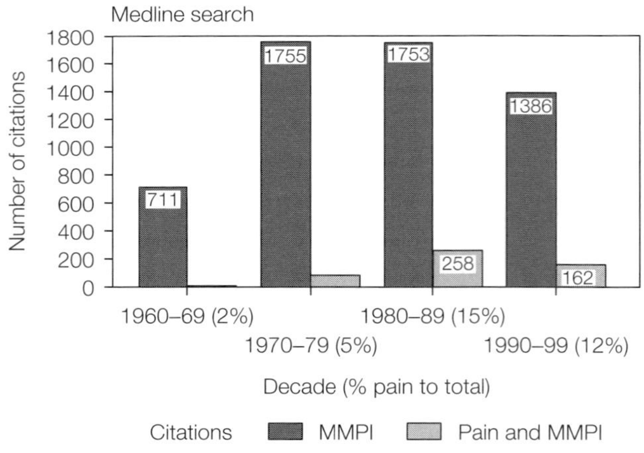

Figure 10.1 Pain and the Minnesota Multiphasic Personality Inventory (MMPI) by decade.

patients, with the most recent decade of data indicating that 12 percent of all MMPI citations are pain related. The MMPI is a 566-question, true-false test that evaluates the presence of psychopathology through three validity scales (the degree to which respondents may be trying to distort their true persona), and clinical scales, ten of which are most commonly used: hypochondriasis, depression, hysteria, psychopathic deviance (history of antisocial behavior and nonconformance), paranoia, psychasthenia (obsessive-compulsive tendencies as well as anxiety), schizophrenia, hypomania, masculinity-femininity, and social introversion. Two additional scales used with chronic pain patients are the Low Back Pain Scale and the Dorsal Scale. Careful examination of the pattern or "profile" of scale scores, particularly those above a T score of 70, enables the experienced clinician to evaluate the degree of psychological distress experienced by the patient and enables the prediction of behaviors, as well as treatment compliance and responsiveness.

The most common profile of chronic pain patients is the "conversion V": elevations of the hypochondriasis, depression, and hysteria scales. Individuals whose profiles reflect greater psychopathology tend to display more severe pain symptoms.[30] Problems with utilization of the MMPI with chronic pain patients are its length (over two hours to complete it), and its strong orientation to psychopathology (which suggests to pain patients that they are being perceived as "crazy" and their pain is in their head). A criticism that has been directed at the use of the MMPI with chronic pain patients is that there is an overlap of symptoms of chronic pain with MMPI items which can lead to erroneous estimates of psychopathology.[30] For example, five items on the MMPI reflect the presence and severity of rheumatoid arthritis. These items code on scales 1, 2, and 3 (hypochondriasis, depression, and hysteria). Responses to these items reflected disease activity rather than emotional distress.

The MMPI-2, the recent revision of the MMPI, has reduced some of the psychiatric bias, and has also updated the normative samples. While some pain centers administer the MMPI or MMPI-2 as part of the standard evaluation protocol, some pain centers reserve it for patients with suspected major psychopathology or treatment refractory patients.

Symptom Checklist 90-Revised

The Symptom Checklist 90-Revised (SCL-90R)[31] is a commonly used assessment of psychological symptom patterns that is also used, on a more limited basis, with chronic pain patients. Patients indicate the degree to which they are bothered by 90 symptoms on a five-point scale ranging from "not at all" to "extremely," which yield nine "symptom dimensions": somatization, obsessive-compulsive, interpersonal sensitivity, depression, anxiety, hostility, phobic anxiety, paranoid ideation, and psychoticism. There are also three general measures of distress: global severity index, positive symptom distress index, and positive symptom total. The SCL-90R is easier to administer than the MMPI, and is considered to be a state-oriented measure sensitive to treatment changes.[32]

The Brief Symptom Inventory (BSI) is the short version of the SCL-90R, that consists of only 53 items utilizing the same rating scale, and yielding the same symptom patterns and global indices as the SCL-90R. Correlations between the BSI and the SCL-90R are 0.92 and higher for each of the scales. If testing time is an issue with the patient, as it often is in a multidisciplinary center, then the BSI may be a more suitable instrument to use than the SCL-90R.

Multidimensional Pain Inventory

Multidimensional Pain Inventory (MPI),[12] originally derived from the West Haven-Yale Multidimensional Pain Inventory (WHYMPI),[33] is a specific self-report pain measure, based on a cognitive-behavioral approach, that evaluates subjective, behavioral, and psychophysiological indices. The first section assesses:

- perceived interference of pain in daily activities;
- support experienced from significant others;
- pain severity and level of suffering;
- perceived self-control over life and life's problems;
- affective distress.

The second section is unique in that it evaluates the patient's perception regarding the responses of his/her significant other to his/her pain and assesses:

- the degree to which the patient's pain behavior is reacted to with irritation, frustration, or anger by the significant other (punishing responses);
- the frequency with which the significant other responds to pain behavior with encouragement (soliciting responses);
- the level of distracting responses that the significant other uses in response to pain behavior (distracting responses).

The third section assesses the frequency with which the patient participates in five categories of activity, as follows:

1. household chores;
2. outdoor work;
3. activities away from home;
4. social activities;
5. general activity level.

The MPI is easily administered, has face validity for the patient (the relationship to pain is obvious), and is a multidimensional tool that is unique in its assessment of environmental contingencies.

Coping Strategies Questionnaire

The Coping Strategies Questionnaire (CSQ)[34][V] is a specific pain measure, designed to evaluate how pain patients cope with their pain. Patients respond to 48 items on a seven-point Likert type scale. The results indicate:

- six cognitive coping strategies: (1) diverting attention; (2) reinterpreting pain sensations; (3) calming self statements; (4) ignoring pain sensations; (5) praying and hoping; (6) catastrophizing; and
- two behavioral coping strategies: (1) increasing behavioral activity; (2) increasing pain behaviors.

These are combined into three general coping measures: (1) cognitive coping and suppression; (2) helplessness; (3) diverting attention and praying. The three general measures are predictive of other pain-related variables as well as mood state. The CSQ has been revised, retaining only 27 of the 48 original items.[35] The original "catastrophizing" and "diverting attention" subscales were most robust. Although the original six cognitive factors were retained, the behavioral factors were not replicated.

Generally speaking, the literature has identified the adaptive coping strategies associated with less pain as the active coping strategies of staying busy, ignoring pain, and distraction. Maladaptive coping strategies, associated with increased pain, include catastrophizing, as well as the passive coping strategies such as restricting activities, wishful thinking, and depending on others.

PREDICTORS OF OUTCOME OF INVASIVE PROCEDURES AND OF DISABILITY

Pain management has become more technologically sophisticated and aggressive (and expensive!) in its approach. One of the more common contemporary uses of the psychological evaluation has been to determine the appropriateness of a potential candidate for implantation of a spinal cord stimulator (SCS) or drug delivery system. This is usually based on a set of predetermined, empiric psychosocial characteristics. Nelson and colleagues,[36] conducting a meta-analysis of the literature on this topic, concluded that patients should be excluded from implantable spinal cord stimulators if they had evidence of:

- active psychosis;
- suicidality;
- untreated major depression;
- somatization disorder;
- alcohol or drug dependency;
- compensation/litigation disincentive to recovery;

- lack of social supports;
- cognitive deficits.

Additional considerations for exclusion include:

- unusual pain ratings or pain drawings;
- personality disorders;
- physical incongruence;
- a high elevation on the Depression scale of the MMPI;
- elevations on four or more MMPI scales.

Doleys *et al.*,[37] however, were not as optimistic about the predictability of these factors. They concluded that there were no definitive multicenter studies that could identify any statistically significant psychological factor or combination of factors that predict outcome. They did indicate that the psychological evaluation is useful if not necessary, but caution about interpreting test data. One of the limiting factors in evaluating the data in these studies is that the definition of SCS success is not standard. One predictive factor they did identify is that serious personality disorder patients are not likely to improve.

Under some circumstances, the MMPI has also been shown to be a very powerful predictor of the success of lumbar surgery. In one study, six MMPI scales administered preoperatively were predictive of surgical outcome in a herniation but not stenosis group.[38] In another study, 84 patients evaluated before lumbar discectomy with an objective evaluation system (neurological signs, sciatic-tension signs, MMPI, and lumbar myelography) accurately predicted treatment outcome one year later (accounting for 40 percent of the variance).[39][IV] The MMPI was the most powerful predictor of treatment outcome.

Similar to the prediction of success with implantable pumps and stimulators, Block and Callewart[40] have developed a presurgical scoring card that predicts surgical success based on three groups of factors.

1. Medical: chronicity of condition, previous spine surgery, smoking, and/or obesity.
2. Psychological interview: litigation, workers' compensation, job dissatisfaction, heavy lifting job, substance abuse, family reinforcers of pain, marital dissatisfaction, abuse, and/or a preinjury psychiatric history.
3. Psychological Testing: elevations on these five MMPI scales (Hs, D, Hy, Pd, Pt), as well as choosing poor coping strategies on the Coping Strategies Questionnaire.

Unresolved traumatic stress can help maintain chronic pain for many years or actually activate physical pain many years later. In a study of 100 spinal surgery patients, of patients who recalled no developmental traumas (physical, sexual, or emotional abuse, or alcohol/drug abuse in caregiver, or abandonment), 95 percent had a successful postsurgical outcome.[41] Only 15 percent of patients who recalled three or more of these traumas/risk factors had a successful postsurgical outcome. Thus, childhood traumas were significantly predictive of surgical success many years later. The authors of this study theorized that for those patients with a history of abuse, surgery is another traumatic event that reactivates the childhood template of abuse. Patients who can be consoled are likely to improve; those who have been psychologically traumatized and are not readily consolable may not improve.

As disability claims are increasing in alarming rapidity, another purpose of the psychological evaluation has arisen: the prediction of the development of disability. Gatchel *et al.*[42] conducted a prospective study of 504 acute low back pain patients to identify work status one year later. A logistic regression analysis identified 91 percent of patients' work status one year later. Patients were more likely not to be at work if they were female, had workers' compensation injuries, scored high on self-reported pain and disablity, and scored high on the "hysteria" scale of the MMPI.

THE PAIN PATIENT WITH A SUSPECTED SUBSTANCE ABUSE PROBLEM

Among the most difficult to manage and treat populations of chronic pain patients are the patients who present with a current or past history of addiction to illicit substances, alcohol, or prescription drugs.[43] Pain patients who are perceived to have addictive disorders are often undertreated. The unwarranted fear of addiction is a misunderstood concept in pain management that can lead to the undertreatment of pain. The increasingly accepted management of chronic nonmalignant pain with opioid therapy underscores the importance of understanding the nature of opioid addiction. As important as the psychological assessment of the chronic pain patient is in general, it takes on added significance with the patient who presents with a history of past or present substance abuse. Observation, history, monitoring, and being aware of the "red flags" are very important in the specific assessment of the chronic pain patient with suspected abuse.

Specific substance abuse/addiction measures that can be of help include the Drug Abuse Screening Test (DAST-20),[44] CAGE-AID,[45] and the Cyr-Wartman Screen.[46] Passik *et al.*[47] has recently developed the Pain Assessment and Documentation Tool (PADT),[47] a 41-item tool that assesses four domains: analgesia, activities of daily living, adverse events, and potential aberrant drug-related behavior. The PADT has been formatted for use as a chart note designed to assist clinicians in assessing and documenting these for main outcome domains during long-term opioid use.

A new score by Belgrade *et al.*[48][V] attempts to predict risk and outcome of chronic opioid prescribing. This score is derived from four factors:

1. diagnosis;
2. intractability;
3. risk (psychological, chemical health, reliability, social support);
4. efficacy.

This score was developed at the request of the Minnesota Board of Medical Practice (www.state.mn.us/portal/mn/jsp/home.do?agency=BMP), which has information about the management of chronic pain and prescribing rules.

Pain specialists need to educate themselves about standards of care in addictive disease and substance abuse disorders, as well as be knowledgeable about prescribing and practice laws.

SHOULD EVERY CHRONIC PAIN PATIENT BE ASSESSED PSYCHOLOGICALLY?

One of the controversial issues in chronic pain management today is whether every chronic pain patient who is being treated should first receive a psychological evaluation. The arguments against this are practical in nature; there are increased costs associated with this as well as limited resources (access to mental health professionals with pain expertise may be quite limited). Additionally, the fear of communicating to the patient that their "pain is in their head," as well as resistance on the part of referring doctors (particularly in settings where referrals are made for specific procedures to be done) are all very practical and significant considerations.

The other side of the argument, however, is based on clinical experience as well as research. Almost all practicing pain management specialists today would agree that there is a high incidence of comorbid psychopathology associated with chronic pain, such as depression and posttraumatic stress disorder. Treating the emotional disorder often helps the pain disorder quite significantly, while not treating the psychiatric disorder hampers improvement of the physical pain, regardless of the medical intervention. Additionally, and quite powerfully, there is a growing body of literature showing that most predictors of treatment success with interventional procedures are psychological, while most predictors of treatment failures are also psychological.

CONCLUSIONS

While there are many excellent psychological assessment tools to choose from in assisting the clinician in diagnosing and treating the patient with chronic pain, there is no substitute for listening to the patient and his or her story. Patients appreciate being listened to, rather than being dismissed as having imaginary pain. One important question to keep in mind when listening to their stories is how have their lives changed as a result of their pain. Invariably, the more their lives have changed, the greater the suffering and emotional distress. One needs to read between the lines, however, in evaluating the pain patient. One needs to be the Lieutenant Columbo of clinicians, rather than always sticking to the facts, as Sergeant Joe Friday did. The experienced clinician can thus take his or her pain questionnaire, clinical interview and examination, and psychological assessment measures, and apply them together with sound clinical judgment in formulating a diagnosis and treatment plan that is individually geared to that patient.

Although the treatment of a patient with chronic pain mandates a comprehensive evaluation of the medical, as well as psychological, contributors to the etiology, maintenance, and exacerbation of pain, evaluating and treating chronic pain patients with a unimodal, strictly medical approach still occurs. Therefore, the Commission on Accreditation of Rehabilitation Facilities (CARF) accredits chronic pain programs that are interdisciplinary in both their evaluation and treatment of patients, and require, as part of the core pain team, a psychologist or psychiatrist. Multidisciplinary approaches that include a psychological component lower levels of psychological interference and increase rates of return to work.[49]

As the state of chronic pain management moves rapidly towards increasingly invasive "high-tech" procedures, partly as a response to economic pressures on pain management centers, the psychological evaluation of every chronic pain patient has become increasingly essential so that:

- patients are carefully screened to determine (or predict) their suitability for such a procedure;
- more conservative, less costly treatments, such as cognitive-behavioral methods, can first be implemented within a multidisciplinary approach.

Pain specialists need to educate themselves about standards of care in pain management, as well as be knowledgable about prescribing and practice laws. Although the evaluation and management of the patient with unremitting pain is very complex, it needs to be undertaken in a sensitive and nonjudgmental manner, with comprehensive knowledge of the relevant issues. Nowhere is this more essential than with the chronic pain patient. Better, more individualized assessment of pain patients, particularly those with comorbid psychiatric issues, can only lead to more effective treatment of this very difficult to treat population. To paraphrase Sir William Osler, it is not the type of disease that a patient has that is as important as the type of patient that has the disease. Nowhere in medicine is this more true than with the patient with chronic pain.

REFERENCES

1. Meldrum ML. Brief history of multidisciplinary management of chronic pain, 1900–2000. In: Schatman ME, Campbell A (eds). *Chronic pain management: Guidelines for multidisciplinary program development.* New York: Informa Healthcare, 2007: 1–13.
2. Lebovits AH. The psychological assessment of chronic pain patients. *Current Review of Pain.* 2000; **4**: 122–6.
3. Lebovits AH, Florence I, Bathina R *et al.* Pain knowledge and attitudes of health care providers: Practice characteristic differences. *Clinical Journal of Pain.* 1997; **13**: 237–43.
4. Lebovits AH, Lefkowitz M, McCarthy D *et al.* The prevalence and management of pain in patients with AIDS: A review of 134 cases. *Clinical Journal of Pain.* 1989; **5**: 245–8.
5. Lebovits AH, Smith G, Maignan M, Lefkowitz M. Pain in hospitalized patients with AIDS: Analgesic and psychotropic medications. *Clinical Journal of Pain.* 1994; **10**: 156–61.
6. Lebovits AH. Psychological interventions with patients who have cancer pain. In: de Leon-Casasola OA (ed.). *Cancer pain: pharmacologic, interventional, and palliative care approaches.* Philadelphia, PA: Elsevier Science, 2006: 361–8.
7. Cleeland C, Gonin R, Hatfield A *et al.* Pain and its treatment in outpatients with metastatic cancer. *New England Journal of Medicine.* 1994; **330**: 592–6.
8. AAPM Council on Ethics. Ethics charter from American Academy of Pain Medicine. *Pain Medicine.* 2005; **6**: 203–12.
9. * Jensen MC, Brant-Zawadzki MN, Obuchowski N *et al.* Magnetic resonance imaging of the lumbar spine in people without back pain. *New England Journal of Medicine.* 1994; **331**: 69–73.
10. Okifuji A. Interdisciplinary pain management with pain patients: Evidence for its effectiveness. *Seminars in Pain Medicine.* 2003; **1**: 110–19.
11. Stanos SP. Developing an interdisciplinary multidisciplinary chronic pain management program: Nuts and bolts. In: Schatman ME, Campbell A (eds). *Chronic pain management: guidelines for multidisciplinary program development.* New York: Informa Healthcare, 2007: 151–72.
12. Turk DC, Rudy TE. Toward an empirically derived taxonomy of chronic pain patients: integration of psychological assessment data. *Journal of Consulting and Clinical Psychology.* 1988; **56**: 233–8.
13. Muse M, Frigola G. Development of a quick screening instrument for detecting posttraumatic stress disorder in the chronic pain patient: construction of the Posttraumatic Chronic Pain Test (PCPT). *Clinical Journal of Pain.* 1986; **2**: 151–3.
14. Jenson MP, Karoly P. Self-report scales and procedures for assessing pain in adults. In: Turk DC, Melzack R (eds). *Handbook of pain assessment*, 2nd edn. New York: Guilford Press, 2001: 15–34.
15. Jensen MP, Karoly P, Braver S. The measurement of clinical pain intensity. *Pain.* 1986; **27**: 117–26.
16. Varni JW, Jay SM, Masek BJ, Thompson KL. Cognitive-behavioral assessment and management of pediatric pain. In: Holzman AD, Turk DC (eds). *Pain management: a handbook of psychological treatment approaches.* New York: Pergamon Press, 1986: 168–92.
17. Hester NK, Foster R, Kristensen K. Measurement of pain in children: generalizability and validity of the pain ladder and the poker chip tool. In: Tyler DC, Krane EJ (eds). *Advances in pain research and therapy: pediatric pain.* New York: Raven Press, 1990: 79–84.
18. Bieri D, Reeve RA, Champion GD *et al.* The Faces Pain Scale for the self-assessment of the severity of pain experienced by children: development, initial validation, and preliminary investigation for ratio scale properties. *Pain.* 1990; **41**: 139–50.
19. Melzack R. The McGill Pain Questionnaire: major properties and scoring methods. *Pain.* 1975; **1**: 277–99.
20. Turk DC, Rudy TE, Salovey P. The McGill Pain Questionnaire reconsidered: confirming the factor structure and examining appropriate uses. *Pain.* 1985; **21**: 385–97.
21. Holroyd KA, Holm JE, Keefe FJ *et al.* A multi-center evaluation of the McGill Pain Questionnaire: results from more than 1700 chronic pain patients. *Pain.* 1992; **48**: 301–11.
22. Melzack R. The short-form McGill Pain Questionnaire. *Pain.* 1987; **30**: 191–7.
23. Backonja M, Beydoun A, Edwards KR *et al.* Gabapentin for the symptomatic treatment of painful peripheral neuropathy in patients with diabetes mellitus: a randomized controlled trial. *Journal of the American Medical Association.* 1998; **280**: 1831–6.
24. Beck AT, Rush AJ, Shaw BF, Emery G. *Cognitive therapy of depression.* New York: Guilford, 1979.
25. Fernandez E. *Anxiety, depression, and anger in pain: Research findings and clinical options.* San Antonio, TX: Advanced Psychological Resources, 2002.
26. Dworkin RH, Turk DC, Farrar JT. Core outcome measures for chronic pain clinical trials: IMMPACT recommendations. *Pain.* 2005; **113**: 9–19.
27. Geisser ME, Roth RS, Robinson ME. Assessing depression among persons with chronic pain using the Center for Epidemiological Studies-Depression Scale and the Beck Depression Inventory: a comparative analysis. *Clinical Journal of Pain.* 1997; **13**: 163–70.
28. Spielberger CD. *Manual for the State-Trait Anxiety Inventory.* Palo Alto, CA: Consulting Psychologists Press, 1983.
29. Butcher NB, Dahlstrom WG, Graham JR *et al. MMPI-2, manual for administration and scoring.* Minneapolis: University of Minnesota Press, 1989.
30. Bradley LA. McKendree-Smith. Assessment of psychological status using interviews and self-report instruments. In: Turk DC, Melzack R (eds). *Handbook of*

pain assessment, 2nd edn. New York: Guilford Press, 2001: 292–319.
31. Derogatis LR. *The SCL-90R: Administration scoring and procedures manual I.* Baltimore, MD: Clinical Psychometrics Research, 1977.
32. Lynch NT, Lyman DR. Psychological assessment in chronic pain syndrome. In: Lefkowitz M, Lebovits AH, Wlody D, Rubin S (eds). *A practical approach to pain management.* Boston: Little Brown, 1996: 115–23.
33. Kerns RD, Turk DC, Rudy TE. The West Haven-Yale Multidimensional Pain Inventory (WHYMPI). *Pain.* 1985; **23**: 345–56.
34. Rosenstiel AK, Keefe FJ. The use of coping strategies in chronic low back pain patients: relationship to patient characteristics and current adjustment. *Pain.* 1983; **17**: 33–44.
35. Riley JL, Robinson ME. CSQ: Five factors or fiction? *Clinical Journal of Pain.* 1997; **13**: 156–62.
* 36. Nelson DV, Kennington M, Novy DM *et al.* Psychological selection criteria for implantable spinal cord stimulators. *Pain Forum.* 1996; **5**: 93–103.
37. Doleys DM, Klapow JC, Hammer M. Psychological evaluation in spinal cord stimulation therapy. *Pain Reviews.* 1997; **4**: 189–207.
38. Herron LD, Turner J, Clancy S *et al.* The differential utility of the Minnesota Multiphasic Personality Inventory. A predictor of outcome in lumbar laminectomy for disc herniation versus spinal stenosis. *Spine.* 1986; **11**: 847–9.
39. Spengler DM, Tillete EA, Battie M *et al.* Elective discectomy for herniation of a lumbar disc. Additional experience with an objective method. *Journal of Bone and Joint Surgery.* 1990; **72**: 230–7.
40. Block AR, Callewart C. Surgery for chronic spine pain: procedures for patient selection and outcome enhancement. In: Block AR, Kremer EF, Fernandez E (eds). *Handbook of pain syndromes.* Mahwah, NJ: Erlbaum, 1999: 191–212.
41. Schofferman J, Anderson D, Hines R *et al.* Childhood psychological trauma correlates with unsuccessful lumbar spines surgery. *Spine.* 1992; **17**: S138–44.
* 42. Gatchel RJ, Polatin PB, Mayer TG. The dominant role of psychosocial risk factors in the development of chronic low back pain disability. *Spine.* 1995; **20**: 2702–09.
43. Lebovits AH. The psychological assessment of the chronic pain patient with a suspected substance abuse disorder. *Techniques in Regional Anesthesia and Pain Management.* 2005; **9**: 195–9.
44. Skinner HA. The drug abuse screening test. *Addictive Behaviors.* 1982; **4**: 363–71.
45. Brown RL, Leonard T, Saunders LA. The prevalence and detection of substance use disorders among inpatients ages 18–49: An opportunity for prevention. *Preventive Medicine.* 1998; **27**: 101–10.
46. Cyr M, Wartman A. The effectiveness of routine screening questions in the detection of alcoholism. *Journal of the American Medical Association.* 1984; **259**: 51–4.
47. Passik S, Kirsh K, Whitcomb L *et al.* A new tool to assess and document pain outcomes in chronic pain patients receiving opioid therapy. *Clinical Therapeutics.* 2004; **26**: 552–61.
48. Belgrade MJ, Schamber CD, Lindgren BR. The DIRE score: predicting outcomes of opioid prescribing for chronic pain. *Journal of Pain.* 2006; **7**: 671–81.
49. Hoffman BM, Papas RK, Chatkoff DK *et al.* Meta-analysis of psychological interventions for chronic low back pain. *Health Psychology.* 2007; **26**: 1–9.

11

Assessment of the patient with neuropathic pain

HANNE GOTTRUP AND TROELS S JENSEN

KEY LEARNING POINTS

- Assessment of neuropathic pain involves a series of systematic steps (history of pain distribution and intensity of pain, sensory testing, neurological and physical examination).
- Loss of spinothalamic functions (cold, warmth, pinprick) appears to be crucial in neuropathic pain.
- An essential part of neuropathic pain is a partial or complete loss of afferent sensory function and the paradoxical presence of certain hyperphenomena.
- Allodynia and hyperalgesia are key features in neuropathic pain, although anesthesia dolorosa may be present.
- Sensory abnormalities can be examined by simple bedside tests or by more sophisticated laboratory and experimental techniques.
- Careful sensory, motor, and autonomic examination plays an important role in diagnosing neuropathic pain.

INTRODUCTION

The main function of the nociceptive system is an important protective role by alerting the individual to the threat of tissue damage. Following disruption of the somatosensory system, the expected result is loss of sensation with possible analgesia in the involved area.[1, 2, 3, 4, 5] On rare occasions, however, this loss of sensation presents itself with a paradox: pain in the hypoesthetic area. This type of pain, termed "neuropathic pain," is important for several reasons: the pain is often severe and long-lasting, it is often resistant to treatment with current analgesics, and the best available treatments produce only moderate to good pain relief in less than one-third of the patients. In addition, neuropathic pains in practice may be difficult to distinguish and diagnose, with a risk of both false-positive and false-negative diagnoses (see below under Classification of neuropathic pain).

Neuropathic pain is not a single entity; it includes heterogeneous conditions that differ not only in etiology, but also in location of the underlying pathology.[6][I], [7, 8, 9][I] Different disorders such as diabetes, herpes zoster, immune deficiencies, and malignant, traumatic and ischemic conditions may all give rise to the same type of pain, but by different mechanisms. The anatomical sites of lesions causing neuropathic pain are multiple: they can be located at any level from the peripheral receptor to the highest cortical centers, the most common being:[1, 3, 4]

- peripheral nerves;
- major nerve plexuses;
- dorsal nerve roots;
- spinal cord;
- the thalamus.

In spite of the diverse etiology and topography, the cli nical picture is surprisingly similar in many cases, suggesting that these disorders share common pathophysiological mechanisms.[3, 10]

Recent studies have shown a cascade of temporally related biological changes following damage to the nervous system. This cascade eventually results in a sensitization of neural elements involved in the processing of noxious information.[5, 8, 10, 11, 12, 13, 14] Although the significance of these molecular changes following nerve damage is still being explored, they may represent a link between different neuropathic conditions. Hence, understanding of the dynamic events following nerve damage may be a key to understanding this hyperexcitability and how to treat it.

A major contribution to this new information has been the demonstration of changes in the nervous system following sustained noxious input different from the normal processing of noxious information. This plasticity of the nervous system is displayed at many levels of the neuraxis from the peripheral nociceptor to the spinal cord and even to the cortex of the brain.[5, 8, 15, 16] This chapter reviews the etiology of the symptoms of neuropathic pain conditions and examines how these conditions can be diagnosed both at the bedside and in the laboratory using more sophisticated experimental techniques.

In the evaluation of a patient with a suspected neuropathic pain disorder, it is important to assess and classify the condition on the basis of:

- the underlying disorder;
- the anatomical location;
- the characteristics of the pain;
- the pain intensity;
- the associated features; and
- the possible mechanisms involved.

It is important to emphasize that the evaluation of neuropathic pain is often complicated and time-consuming, often requiring the use of laboratory techniques.[17, 18, 19, 20]

CLASSIFICATION OF NEUROPATHIC PAIN

Neuropathic pain has usually been classified on the basis of the underlying etiology, e.g. peripheral diabetic neuropathy, postherpetic neuralgia, nerve damage due to injury, spinal or brain lesions following infarction, or multiple sclerotic plaques. Neuropathic pain can also be defined on the basis of the location of the lesion: in the peripheral nerves, in the spinal roots, in the spinal cord, or in the brain. **Table 11.1** presents a commonly used scheme for classifying neuropathic pain on the basis of either etiology or anatomy. More recently, a mechanism-based approach for classifying and analyzing neuropathic pain has been proposed as a mode to link treatment strategies and pathophysiological mechanisms.[8, 20] An attempt has been made to elucidate the various mechanisms that may be involved in the particular pain felt by a patient and link such a mechanism to a rational type of treatment. It is beyond the scope of this chapter to present a detailed description of current mechanisms, some of which are still hypothetical.[5, 12, 13, 14] Briefly, however, these mechanisms include:

- pathological activity of sensitized nociceptors with recruitment of silent nociceptors and ectopic activity in spinal ganglion cells. The increased afferent neuronal barrage causes sensitization of the dorsal horn neurons:
- a severe loss of small fiber input may also give rise to central sensitization due to a spinal reorganization from sprouting of large myelinated fibers into superficial "nociceptive" laminae in the dorsal horn;
- inflammation along nerve trunks, producing ectopic activity and therefore representing a source for central sensitization;
- increased sympathetic activity, producing further sensitization of nociceptors;
- altered brain processing due to plastic changes with recruitment of new brain areas not usually involved in pain. This may lead to changed modulation of input.

Because of the direct connections between the peripheral, autonomic, and central nervous systems (CNSs), and because of the considerable plasticity in the nociceptive and connected systems, different mechanisms may be

Table 11.1 Classification of neuropathic pain according to location and cause.

Peripheral	Spinal	Brain
Neuropathies	Multiple sclerosis	Stroke
Herpes zoster	Spinal cord injury	Multiple sclerosis
Nerve injuries	Arachnoiditis	Neoplasms
Amputations	Neoplasms	Syringomyelia
Plexopathies	Syringomyelia	Parkinson's disease?
Radiculopathies	Spinal stroke	Epilepsy?
Avulsions		
Neoplasms		
Trigeminal neuralgia		

involved within each patient. One mechanism may account for several etiologically different conditions and be the source of different symptoms. For example, a diabetic patient may have continuous pain, touch-evoked pain, paroxysms, and nonpainful paresthesiae and dysesthesiae. In such cases, several mechanisms can be involved, such as tissue injury due to ischemia, sensitization of peripheral receptors, ectopic activity in sprouting regenerating fibers, phenotypic changes in dorsal root ganglion (DRG) cells, and spinal reorganization.[1, 2, 3, 4, 5, 11, 17, 18, 19, 21, 22, 23]

An additional approach to classifying pain involves the use of specific pharmacological agents.[6][I], [7][I], [9, 19][I] The pain-generating mechanisms may be pharmacologically distinguishable in the individual patient.[24][II], [25][II] However, the possibility of predicting the therapeutic outcome of pharmacological treatment from clinical symptoms and signs is still difficult and disappointing.[26][II], [27][II], [28][II]

Although a mechanism-based classification is an attractive approach, it is not known at present whether this provides a reliable, reproducible method for classifying neuropathic pain. However, it will be of interest to determine the possible additional clarification provided by a hierarchical structured system that classifies pain on the basis of: (1) symptoms; (2) symptoms plus signs; (3) symptoms plus signs plus mechanisms; and (4) symptoms plus signs plus mechanisms plus pharmacological analysis. However, a considerable overlap between symptoms and signs was found in a large group of patients with increasing clinical suspicion of neuropathic pain. Superficial ongoing pain intensity, brush-evoked allodynia, and cold-provoked pain intensity was higher in patients more likely to have neuropathic pain.[29]

ONGOING AND EVOKED PAIN

From a clinical point of view, it is often helpful to distinguish between stimulus-independent and stimulus-dependent types of pains (**Table 11.2**).

Table 11.2 Recording of various parameters in neuropathic pain.

Stimulus independent	Stimulus dependent
Pain character	Stimulus type(s)
Pain duration	Pain character
Pain intensity of different pain types	Pain intensity evoked by different stimuli
Pain unpleasantness	Pain radiation
Pain radiation	Pain aftersensation
Pain distribution	Pain summation
Pain area	Pain area

Stimulus-independent pains

Stimulus-independent pains are spontaneous and may be continuous or paroxysmal. Their characteristics differ, but can be shooting, shock-like, aching, cramping, crushing, smarting, or burning. Episodic, paroxysmal types of pain can be brief and shooting, electric, shock-like, or stabbing in their character. In its most typical form, paroxysmal pain is seen in tic douloureux, in entrapment neuropathies, in amputees, and in luetic diseases. For example, in tabes dorsalis, shooting pains are described often in the form of transverse lightning pains in the legs and are provoked by emotional stress. Shooting pains can also occur in cases with a nerve compression (e.g. slipped disk, vertebral compression, neoplastic nerve compression, and entrapment syndromes).[4, 30]

The mechanism underlying these pains is assumed to reflect an increased discharge in sensitized C-nociceptors, but occasionally the pains may reflect increased activity in sensitized receptors associated with large myelinated A-fibers, giving a sensation of burning or dysesthesia.[31]

Stimulus-dependent pains

Stimulus-evoked pains are classified according to the stimulus type that provokes them: mechanical, thermal, or chemical.[1, 11, 17, 18, 19, 21, 32, 33]

Several of these phenomena can be present in some patients. In other patients, only one type of hyperalgesia may be present. For example, patients with nerve injury pain or amputation may have trigger points on mechanical stimulation, but with entirely normal thermal sensation. In some patients with peripheral neuropathy or complex regional pain syndrome, cold allodynia may be the only abnormality present. Therefore, a series of stimuli have to be used to document or exclude abnormality. The evoked pains are usually brief, lasting only for the period of stimulation, but sometimes the evoked pain can persist even after cessation of stimulation, causing aftersensations (see below under Wind up-like pain and aftersensations), which can last for hours. These aftersensations can therefore be difficult to distinguish from spontaneous pain.

FINDINGS IN NEUROPATHIC PAIN

Sensory deficit and pain

An essential part of neuropathic pain is partial or complete loss of afferent sensory function and the paradoxical presence of certain hyperphenomena (see below under Laboratory and experimental examination) in the painful area. There may be considerable variations in the sensory findings in different patients. Some patients may have obvious sensory deficits at bedside tests, whereas in others it may be subtle and difficult to detect with bedside methods, but quantitative measures can usually reveal minor changes.[19, 34, 35] The sensory loss may involve all sensory abnormalities, but a loss of spinothalamic functions (cold, warmth, pinprick) appears to be crucial and the possibility that such spinothalamic loss is a requirement has been raised.[36] For example, in poststroke pain, large-scale studies have suggested that sensory deficit is a necessary, albeit insufficient, condition for the occurrence of pain.[37, 38] Sensory loss and cutaneous hypersensitivity are also characteristic features in central pain following spinal cord injury.[39, 40] It remains to be seen whether similar patterns also occur in other neuropathic pain states.

Allodynia and hyperalgesia

Hyperalgesia (the lowering of the pain threshold and an increased response to noxious stimuli) and allodynia (the evocation of pain by non-noxious stimuli) are typical elements of neuropathic pain.

Three types of mechanical hyperalgesia can be distinguished:

1. **static hyperalgesia**: gentle pressure on skin evokes pain;
2. **punctate hyperalgesia**: punctate stimuli such as pinprick-evoked pain;
3. **dynamic hyperalgesia**: light brush evokes a sensation of pain.

For thermal stimuli, both cold and heat can evoke abnormal pain:

- **cold hyperalgesia**: cold stimuli evoke a sensation of pain (the underlying mechanism is unclear, but cortical reorganization due to a loss of cold Aδ-fibers is one possibility);
- **heat hyperalgesia**: warm and heat stimuli-evoke pain (sensitization of C-nociceptors and a corresponding sensitization of second-order neurons).

The dynamic mechanical-type allodynia is mediated by Aβ-fibers, whereas the static high-threshold type of hyperalgesia, which is evoked by blunt pressure, appears to be mediated by sensitized C-nociceptors.[41, 42] The static type of hyperalgesia would also be expected to be associated with thermal hyperalgesia; however, this is not always the case.[34] Punctate hyperalgesia evoked by pinprick stimuli, usually a stiff von Frey hair, is mediated by sensitized Aδ-nociceptors. While certain types of hyperalgesia reflect sensitization of receptors, allodynia is always a central phenomenon mediated by large myelinated fibers.[18]

Allodynia is considered to be exclusively a cutaneous disorder, but recent findings suggest that it can be a manifestation of deep tissue pathology. For example, in poststroke pain, which is a central neuropathic disorder, deep pain may be associated with a lowering of pain threshold to mechanical pressure and with an exaggerated response to a challenge of 0.5 mL 9 percent hypertonic saline i.m. into the painful deep tissue (unpublished observations). In patients with sciatica or Guillain–Barré syndrome, proximal limb pain is often accompanied by soreness on palpation. Allodynia can usually be separated from the tenderness seen in musculoskeletal pain conditions. In patients with allodynia, a firm pressure in the allodynic area can sometimes relieve their pain. These findings indicate that at the receptor level separate mechanisms are involved, e.g. touch allodynia is elicited by rapidly adapting mechanoreceptors, while the pressure-induced pain relief may be related to the recruitment of slowly adapting mechanoreceptors in addition to other deeply located receptors.

When present, allodynia or hyperalgesia can be quantified by measuring intensity, threshold for elicitation, duration, and area of allodynia.[43] The evocation of pain by a stimulus implies that a complete abolition of afferent information does not give rise to allodynia. Nevertheless, on occasions, in spite of a complete injury, abnormal sensations may develop subsequently and present as anesthesia dolorosa in the deafferented body part. This phenomenon can probably be ascribed to spontaneous firing in nerve sprouts, to alteration in peripheral innervation territory, to an expansion of receptive fields of sensitized central neurons that have lost their normal innervation, or to a combination of such mechanisms. Hyperalgesia can be provoked in normal subjects following blockade of large-diameter afferent fibers. Pinprick or cold is now perceived as burning or squeezing pain, suggesting that afferent fibers under normal conditions exert an inhibitory input on dorsal horn neuronal activity. In neuropathic pain, this inhibition may be disrupted. The chemical mediators of this inhibition are unknown, but γ-aminobutyric acid (GABA) and glycine are likely candidates.

Hyperpathia

Hyperpathia is a variant of hyperalgesia and allodynia and it is the archetypal disorder in neuropathic pain whenever there is axonal loss. In these cases, an explosive pain response is suddenly evoked from cutaneous areas with an increased sensory detection threshold when the stimulus intensity exceeds that sensory threshold.[3, 18, 35] Hyperpathia is a reflection of peripheral or central deafferentation leading to an elevation of threshold on one hand and a central hyperexcitability on the other, as a result of lost or abnormal input from afferents.

Paroxysms

Some patients complain of shooting, electric shock-like, or stabbing pain that occurs spontaneously or, more often, following stimulation. These types of pain are termed "paroxysms" and can be elicited by an innocuous tactile stimulus or by blunt pressure. In their most typical form, paroxysms are seen in tic douloureux, where they dominate the clinical picture; it is characteristic that non-noxious tactile inputs elicit these paroxysms, while noxious stimuli fail to do so.

Paresthesiae

Paresthesiae are abnormal but nonpainful sensations which can be spontaneous or evoked. They are often described as "pins and needles" and are assumed to reflect spontaneous bursts of activity in Aβ-fibers.

Dysesthesiae

Dysesthesiae is defined as abnormal, unpleasant, but not necessarily painful sensations, which can be spontaneous or provoked by external stimuli. These are probably due to sensitization of the C-nociceptors and it is unlikely that there is any qualitative difference between evoked dysesthesiae and evoked hyperalgesia.

Referred pain and abnormal pain radiation

In neuropathic pain, an abnormal spread of pain can be seen following both peripheral and central lesions. In painful myelopathic disorders, patients may experience a circular spreading sensation following single punctate stimulation, with a relationship between the spread of the pain and the intensity of the perceived pain. Similarly, there is a relationship between the magnitude of deep muscle pain and the area of referred cutaneous pain from such deep structures.[44, 45, 46, 47] While referral generally is described from deep to cutaneous structures, the reverse is far less common. Referral can be seen following skin sensitization, e.g. in capsaicin-induced hyperalgesia.[48] There is a link between pain intensity, pain radiation, and pain referral. The magnitude of pain from, for example, deep tissue is proportional to the extent of referral in cutaneous tissue both experimentally and clinically.[44, 45, 46, 47] Similarly, in experimental pain induced by intradermal capsaicin the spread increases with increasing pain intensity.[49]

Experimental studies in humans and animals[50] have shown that such abnormal radiation may be related to changes in spinal wide dynamic range (WDR) neurons encoding noxious information. WDR cells are in part characterized by small receptive zones that can be excited by non-noxious stimuli (touch, gentle pressure) surrounded by a much larger zone from which noxious stimuli (pinch, firm pressure, temperature $>45°C$) can evoke neuronal discharges. These large receptive field zones are overlapping, extend over several dermatomes, and their receptive fields are a reflection of synaptic propriospinal interconnections in the spinal dorsal horn that extend over several segments. Therefore, a noxious stimulus will, in contrast to a non-noxious stimulus, activate several WDR neurons, and increasing the stimulus intensity will result in activation of further WDR neurons in a rostrocaudal distribution manner. Since increasing stimulus intensity has the effect of recruiting more dorsal horn neurons, the degree of radiation and referral is likely to be a reflection of a progressive recruitment of WDR neurons spreading along the spinal cord. A similar mechanism may be involved in the sensory abnormalities seen in patients with nerve injury and in the extensive spread of sensory dysfunction to the contralateral side, as well as proximally and distally to the lesion.

Wind up-like pain and aftersensations

Wind up-like pain or abnormal temporal summation, is the clinical equivalent to increasing neuronal activity following repetitive C-fiber stimulation of more than 0.3 Hz.[51, 52] In humans, such pains may be evoked by either repetitive noxious or non-noxious stimulation from normal or hyperalgesic cutaneous areas, respectively. When repetitive low-threshold stimuli, which exclusively activate Aβ-fibers, are applied at intervals of less than three seconds, they give rise to pain, which means that these stimuli have gained access to central wind up mechanisms that are normally reserved for nociceptors and C-fiber input. Wind up-like pain can be produced by a variety of stimuli, including mechanical, thermal, and electrical types, and can be elicited not only from skin but also from other tissues, e.g. muscle.[52] It is now clear that abnormal temporal summation with wind up-like phenomena is a characteristic feature of many chronic pain conditions, including neuropathic pain[21, 30, 38, 53, 54, 55] and that this can be blocked or attenuated by compounds that affect wind up.[25][II], [56, 57, 58][II], [59][II], [60][II], [61][II], Aftersensation, which is the persistence of pain long after a painful stimulus has stopped, are another characteristic feature of neuropathic pain.[35] Examples of such aftersensations include repetitive paroxysms following short-lasting stimulation of trigger points in trigeminal neuralgia, persistence burning sensation in postherpetic neuralgia after light touch, and long-lasting exaggeration of pain after exercise. Aftersensations correlate with existing evoked pain both experimentally and in neuropathic pain patients, suggesting that they are mediated by a common mechanism.[62] Because of the strong relationship between wind up-like pain and aftersensations, it is thought that both of these phenomena may reflect neuronal discharges in WDR neurons.

ASSESSMENT OF NEUROPATHIC PAIN

History

The examination of a patient with suspected neuropathic pain begins with the history. Patients may describe the quality of their pains in a variety of ways: they may complain of unpleasant pricking or sticking sensations in parts of the body. They may have a burning, scalding, aching, or deep sore pain. Many patients with neuropathic pain suffer from allodynia following exposure to nonpainful cold. In such cases, patients may describe their pain in a paradoxical manner as burning hot or ice-burning or as if holding a snowball in the hand. Some patients with central pain complain of pain evoked by movement in which the movement itself elicits a tightening, squeezing, or burning sensation in the skin. At other times, the pain is one of paroxysms with stabbing, shooting, lancinating types of pain. Paroxysms last seconds, but can be repeated with ultrashort intervals, giving a false impression of continuous types of pains.

An important point concerns the possible classification of pain just on the basis of symptoms, but a considerable overlap has been seen with the clinical presentation of patients with a high suspicion of having neuropathic pain and patients unlikely to have neuropathic pain.[29] Galer and Jensen[63] have presented a neuropathic pain scale in which presumed common symptoms encountered in neuropathic pain are recorded and scored as: intense, sharp, hot, dull, cold, or itchy skin sensitivity. This test has shown validity in normal volunteers and in response to treatment. The Leeds Assessment of Neuropathic Symptoms and Signs (LANSS) pain scale assesses neuropathic symptoms and signs[64] and it seems to at least some degree be possible to distinguish neuropathic pain patients from other chronic pain patients by using those scales.[65, 66]

Distribution of sensory abnormalities on a map

Plotting the distribution of various types of pain on a template body map is an important initial step in pain assessment. The area in which pain is felt can be quantified and any temporal variation in the size of that area over time as a result of, for example, therapy or the natural history of the disease can be measured. Such procedures are useful, e.g. when recording the effects of drugs. Automated drawing systems have been proposed, and may eventually be of value for more accurate measurements.

Clinical examination

All patients should have a general physical and neurological examination. Sensory abnormalities can be specifically assessed and quantified using simple bedside equipment (**Figure 11.1**). A bedside sensory examination most commonly includes examination of pinprick, touch, cold, heat, and vibration sensation. Touch is examined by gently touching the involved skin area with a cotton swab. It is important to distinguish between dynamic stimuli in which the area is stroked and a static stimulus in which

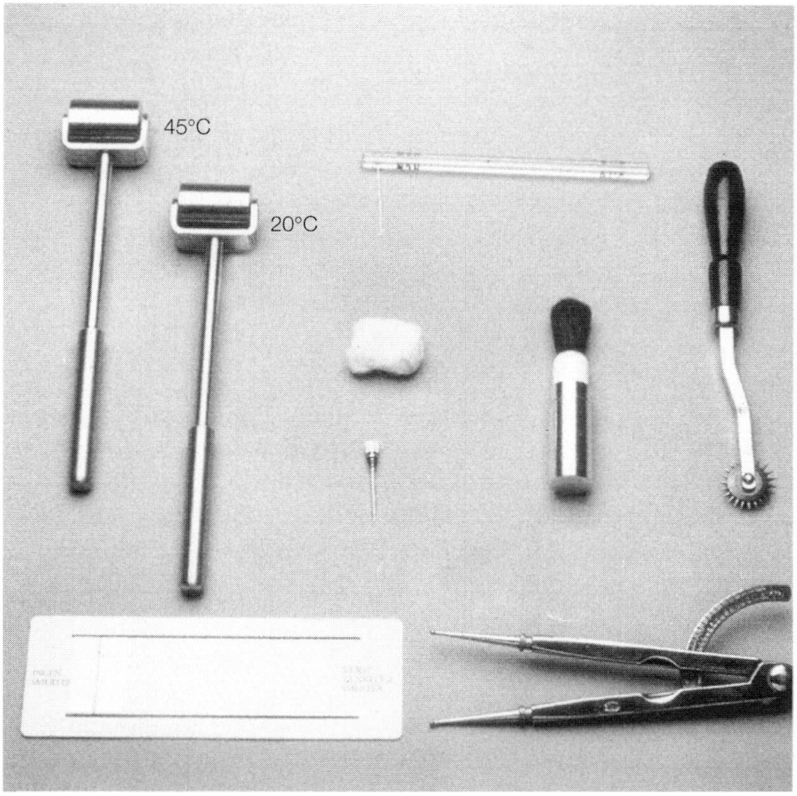

Figure 11.1 Bedside equipment for analyzing sensory function in humans: metal thermorollers (kept at specific temperatures), von Frey hair, cotton wool, brush, pinprick roller, two-point discriminator, and a visual analog scale (VAS) meter.

the skin is exposed to a static, i.e. a nondynamic, stimulus. Cold and warm sensations are recorded by measuring the response to a specific cold or warm thermal stimulus, e.g. thermorollers maintained at 20 and 40°C, respectively. Cold sensation can also be assessed by the response to a drop of acetone on the skin. Vibration is assessed by a tuning fork placed at strategic points (malleoli, interphalangeal joints). At present, there is no consensus about the site where such activity should be measured, but it is generally agreed that this is best performed in the area with maximal abnormality using the unaffected contralateral mirror image skin area as control. However, this needs to be qualified by understanding that some studies have described contralateral segmental sensory abnormalities following a unilateral nerve or root lesion. An examination of the mirror image area of a nerve injury may therefore not represent a true control, but without a body of validated "normal values" for the various psychophysical modalities this appears to be the best option at present. For all types of stimuli, the response can be graded simply as:[67]

- normal;
- decreased (−1 to 4];
- increased (+1 to 4).

If the response is hyperesthetic, it is classified as dysesthetic (unpleasant abnormal sensation to a stimulus), hyperalgesic (increased response to a normally painful stimulus), or allodynic (pain evoked by a normally nonpainful stimulus). A correlation between spontaneous pain and sensory response in the painful area suggests that the two phenomena are reflections of the same mechanism: a central sensitization of dorsal horn neurons.[31, 41]

An essential point concerns the detailed description of what the sensory abnormalities reflect: does the distribution correspond to the innervation territory of a sensory nerve, to fascicles, to roots, to cord segment, or to a cerebral structure? This is not always an easy task and may require detailed neurological knowledge. However, this is important because a distinction has to be made between the sensory abnormalities seen in, for example, somatization disorders and those seen in diseases of the nerves or CNS.

LABORATORY AND EXPERIMENTAL EXAMINATION

More detailed and accurate testing can be carried out using various methods. These include mechanical, thermal, and chemical tools, and the practical aspects of these methods of quantitative sensory testing are discussed in Chapter 4, Sensory testing and clinical neurophysiology in the *Practice and Procedures* volume of this series.

Mechanical stimuli

Von Frey hairs and blunt pressure are the standard tools for mechanical testing in the experimental laboratory. Von Frey hairs bend at different forces, permitting both a stimulus-dependent (threshold to detection and threshold to pain perception) and a response-dependent (evoked sensation to a particular stimulus) pain assessment. This can be performed for single and for repetitive pinprick stimuli. For a dynamic brush, camel hair paintbrushes can be used.

Determination of the area of abnormality may also be a useful outcome measure because such an area of cutaneous abnormality probably reflects the expansion of receptive fields of sensitized dorsal horn neurons.[1, 30]

Thermal stimuli

Thermal testing is often carried out using probes or thermodes and several instruments are commercially available. Lasers, with argon or CO_2 stimuli, have also been used. The size and duration of the thermal stimulus seem to be important because temporal and spatial summation is pronounced for C-fibers, but is only weak for Aδ-fibers. While short-lasting heat stimuli on small areas normally evoke a pinprick sensation (indicating Aδ-fiber activation), heat stimuli of long duration on larger areas give rise to a burning sensation (indicating C-fiber activation). To what extent this observation is also present in neuropathic skin is unclear.

Chemical stimuli

Chemical stimuli can be used to determine the threshold of the evoked response. Capsaicin, the pungent ingredient of hot chili peppers, can be applied either topically or intradermally. It has been widely used in normal volunteers to show that an area of primary and secondary hyperalgesia develops as a result of an explosive discharge from activated C-nociceptors by stimulating VR-1 receptors.[32, 49, 68][II], [69, 70][II] A similar approach has been used in patients with postherpetic neuralgia to test C-fiber activity and to assess the degree of surviving sensitized C-nociceptors compared with the degree of deafferentation.[71] It remains to be seen whether this technique can differentiate between peripheral and central sensitization.

Many patients with neuropathic pain demonstrate a paradoxical sensibility with an increased detection threshold to thermal (cold and heat) stimuli and a reduced pain threshold to the same stimuli. Such a response pattern reflects both a loss of afferent fibers/disturbance of central pathways and a sensitization of peripheral receptors/central neurons along the somatosensory pathway.[1, 3, 4, 17, 18, 19, 34, 72, 73, 74, 75, 76, 77]

Alterations in the spatial and temporal characteristics of these stimuli may add another dimension to the pain experience, e.g. the presence of spatial and temporal summation. In addition to the above psychophysical measures, various physiological examinations can be used in the analysis of neuropathic pain. These include microneurographic recordings, electromyogram (EMG) activity, brain imaging techniques, evoked potentials, and measurement of "pain substances" in body fluids. There is at present insufficient information to determine the most useful pain correlate, but in time it is possible that some of these experimental techniques may be added to the portfolio of measures used in the routine clinical assessment of neuropathic pain and may even permit a further elucidation of the underlying mechanisms in neuropathic pain.

For sensory modality (mechanical, thermal, chemical, electrical), it is possible to determine threshold, summation threshold, response function, and area of abnormality (**Table 11.3**).

Assessment of sympathetic activity

Sympathetic hyperactivity may be present in some peripheral neuropathic pain states as part of complex regional pain syndrome (CRPS; formerly known as causalgia or reflex sympathetic dystrophy; see Chapter 27, Complex regional pain syndromes). The clinical aspects of sympathetic hyperactivity include a perception of burning-type pain soon (hours or days) after injury together with the demonstration of swelling, smooth glossy skin, and vasomotor instability. A characteristic localized osteoporosis may be observed in the extremities (Sudeck's atrophy) later on. These features may exist alone or in combination. Sweating may be affected, producing either wet or dry skin. Similarly, the skin may be cooler or warmer, depending on the degree of cutaneous vasoconstriction. In patients suspected of sympathetic dysfunction, tests can be useful to document the degree of sympathetic involvement. These include sweat testing, galvanic skin resistance, plethysmography, skin blood flow measurement (laser Doppler test, thermography), and cutaneous histamine response. Diagnostic sympathetic blocks may also be used to determine the possible involvement of the sympathetic nervous system in a particular pain condition.[77] There is at present no single test that can be used to exclude sympathetically maintained pain and there are no known symptoms that predict it.[74]

OUTCOME MEASURES

In the evaluation of a pharmacological or non-pharmacological intervention, therapeutic success is often equated with pain reduction. As a result, many clinicians limit themselves to the measurement of pain and pain relief, thereby overlooking other important aspects of the therapeutic outcome, such as functional improvement or improvement in quality of life. In order to assess mechanisms, it is important that the measures used in experimental research reflect the pain measures used in humans.[78, 79] These are discussed in more detail in Chapter 14, Outcome measurement in chronic pain, and in Part I, Principles of measurement and diagnosis, in the *Practice and Procedures* volume, and only the elements immediately relevant to the patient suffering from neuropathic pain will be discussed here.

Clinical pain measures

Pain measures can be divided into the recording of spontaneous pain and recording of evoked pains to different stimuli. For this purpose, visual analog scaling as well as multidimensional descriptor (e.g. the McGill Pain Questionnaire) and cross-modality matching scales have been used. Specific measures may be important in assessment in different pain conditions. For example, in neuropathic pain allodynia, wind up-like pain, after sensations, pain radiations, and area of hypersensitivity (e.g. allodynia) may be relevant. Recording of pain intensity is still the most frequently assessed dimension of therapeutic outcome. The visual analog scale (VAS), verbal category scales, and numerical rating scales are the

Table 11.3 Stimulus and response measures in neuropathic pain patients.

Stimulus modality	Threshold	Summation	Stimulus response	Area of abnormality
Touch	Detection	Touch-evoked allodynia	+	+
von Frey hair	Detection Pain	Repetitive stimulation >2 Hz	+	+
Thermal	Detection Pain	Repetitive stimulation	+	+
Mechanical pressure	Pain	Repetitive stimulation	+	+
Capsaicin	Pain	Repetitive stimulation	+	+
Electrical stimuli	Detection Pain	Repetitive stimulation	+	+ (Referred pain)

most commonly used scales. An example of a numerical rating scale is the 11-point Likert rating scale, whereby the subject is asked to rate his pain by giving a number between 0 (no pain) and 10 (most intense pain). Another widely used category scale is the four-point intensity scale (none, mild, moderate, and severe pain). However, this scale usually does not have sufficient levels to describe the effects of treatment accurately. Improved category scales with more descriptors are available. Pain intensity does fluctuate over time in many clinical pain conditions. In these cases, it may be necessary to rate the percentage of time that the patient's pain falls within certain intensity categories. A slightly different approach has been taken in the Brief Pain Inventory (BPI) of Wisconsin, which involves measurement of the pain intensity when it is at its worst, when it is at its least, and the average pain intensity.

A unidimensional recording of pain intensity or pain relief may overlook other important aspects of a therapeutic outcome, such as functional improvement or improvement in quality of life. Certain therapies which reduce pain intensity may be associated with side effects that diminished quality of life. If pain intensity or relief measures are used in isolation in this situation, then a falsely optimistic view of the effect of that therapy may be formed by the clinician.

In neuropathic pain, it is not sufficient to record one single pain condition; the various other neuropathic phenomena such as paroxysms, spontaneous ongoing pain, wind up-like pain, touch-evoked pain, and cold allodynia are equally important. Each pain component in a particular neuropathic pain condition may have its own magnitude and each may be influenced separately by a particular drug.

Whereas pain intensity scales focus on the present pain experience, pain relief scores rely on the patient's memory of pain. Since patients tend to overestimate their past pain, the use of pain relief scores may lead to an overestimation of the effects of the treatment, certainly in cases of prolonged follow up. On the other hand, it has been suggested that pain relief category scales are more sensitive to small reductions in pain. A neuropathic pain scale (NPS) and the LANSS pain scale have been recently introduced and validated.[63, 64] It seems to be possible, at least to some degree, to identify patients in whom neuropathic mechanisms dominate their pain.[65, 66]

ASSESSMENT OF QUALITY OF LIFE AND HEALTH STATUS

An increasing number of clinical trials include measures of quality of life in the evaluation of the treatment of chronic pain. These measures have become an important indicator of treatment success. Among the measures of quality of life, the Sickness Impact Profile (SIP), the SIP Roland, the West Haven–Yale Multidimensional Pain Inventory, the Nottingham Health Profile, and the SF-36 have been validated (for further details of pain measures, see Chapter 3, Selecting and applying pain measures in the *Practice and Procedures* volume of this series).

TREATMENT AS A TOOL TO ASSESS NEUROPATHIC PAIN

Specific treatments have been designed and tried for different pain conditions, including neuropathic pain. They will be described in detail in other chapters. These treatments, which currently include tricyclic antidepressants, sodium channel blockers (such as carbamazepine and lamotrigine), gabapentin and pregabalin, opioids, and *N*-methyl-D-aspartic acid (NMDA) channel blockers have specific targets for their mode of action. It has been suggested that this may help to unravel the mechanisms of neuropathic pain based on the specific action of these drugs. Previous studies have shown that such drugs may have an action not only on pain intensity, but also on specific aspects of pain, such as evoked pain. Studies have shown that in patients with neuropathic pain due to nerve injury and amputation, NMDA receptor antagonists can block both pain and evoked pain produced by touch stimuli, indicating that these phenomena are probably produced by the same mechanism, i.e. a central sensitization mediated by excess activity at NMDA receptor channels. An additional example would be the joint blockade of pain by sodium channel-blocking agents and NMDA receptor-blocking drugs, suggesting that at least two different mechanisms may operate in concert.

The introduction of the concept of number needed to treat (NNT) from systematic reviews has made it possible to compare the efficacy (NNT) and side-effect profile (NNH; number needed to harm) for a particular therapy in different pain conditions[80] and thus to determine whether a drug with a known mechanism of action is effective in specific neuropathic pain conditions. In theory, this could enable the determination of the pain mechanisms involved for certain types of neuropathic pains. The same principle could also be applied using separate drugs for the same pathological condition to determine whether distinct or identical mechanisms may be in operation.[6][I], [7][I] For example, a sodium channel blocker and an NMDA receptor antagonist modulate spontaneous pain, wind up-like pain, and touch-evoked pain in a different way in individual neuropathic pain patients which proposed that separate molecular mechanisms are involved in individual patients.[25][II]

POSSIBLE RELATIONSHIP BETWEEN SYMPTOMS, FINDINGS, AND MECHANISMS

There are as yet no obvious relationships between the symptoms in neuropathic pain, the stimulus that evokes these symptoms, and the possible mechanisms associated with that pain.

Table 11.4 summarizes symptoms, stimuli, clinical presentation, mechanisms, and the response to

Table 11.4 Symptoms and findings in neuropathic pain.

Symptom/finding	Stimulus	Clinical presentation	Mechanism	Pharmacological blockade
Static hyperalgesia	Gentle mechanical pressure	In area of injury (primary hyperalgesic zone)	Sensitized C-nociceptors	Systemic and topical lidocaine, opioids
Punctate hyperalgesia	Pinprick stimuli	In area of injury and outside (primary and secondary zone)	Sensitized A^{TM}-nociceptors and central sensitization	Systemic and topical lidocaine, opioids?
Dynamic hyperalgesia	Light brush stimuli	In area of injury and outside (primary and secondary zone)	1. Central sensitization due to increased input 2. Central sensitization due to loss of input	Systemic NMDA antagonists and systemically; opioids?
Cold hyperalgesia	Cool stimuli (acetone, alcohol)	Nerve injuries, neuropathies, and central pain	Central disinhibition because of loss of input	None?
Heat hyperalgesia	Radiating heat	In area of injury (primary hyperalgesia)	Sensitized C-nociceptors	Systemic and topical lidocaine, opioids
Wind up-like pain	Light brush or pin prick >3 Hz	Evoked pain by repetitive stimulation on and surrounding injury	Central sensitization due to increased input	Systemic NMDA antagonists and lidocaine systemically
Chemical hyperalgesia	Topical capsaicin or histamine	Evoked pain/itch or vasodilatation	Sensitized mechanoinsensitive VR1/histamine receptors	Topical lidocaine
Aftersensations	Any stimulus	Inside and outside injury zone	Central sensitization	?
Sympathetically maintained	Sympathetic stimulation or blockade	Present in nerve injuries	Sympathetic hyperactivity	Stimulation: norepinephrine Blockade: stellate block

NMDA, *N*-methyl-D-aspartic acid; VRI, vanilloid receptor subtype 1.

pharmacological blockade for various types of stimuli/findings. It is important to bear in mind that mechanisms can rarely be determined with certainty for neuropathic pain. We are only able to record the symptoms and findings, and, on the basis of any tests carried out, proposed mechanisms of the pain can be delineated.

CONCLUSIONS

Assessment of neuropathic pain involves a series of systematic steps, which include past and present history, a detailed description of pain distribution, quality and intensity of pain, and a neurological examination with the emphasis on sensory testing. The sensory examination often needs to be supported by neurophysiological testing and quantitative sensory analysis. It has now become clear that neuroplastic changes in the nervous system play a significant role in the development and maintenance of chronic neuropathic pain with interaction between peripheral and central mechanisms. There is still a wide gap between our preclinical knowledge of pain mechanisms and the translation of such knowledge into daily clinical practice.

The lack of standardized criteria for pain assessment and no systematic examination of patients have made it difficult to close the gap in our knowledge. A better understanding of neuropathic pain mechanisms and their clinical manifestations is a prerequisite for designing a rationally founded treatment.

REFERENCES

* 1. McMahon SB, Koltzenburg M (eds). Section 7: Clinical states: neuropathic pain. *Wall and Melzack's Textbook of pain*, 5th edn. Philadelphia: Elsevier, 2006: 903–1084.

2. Bennett GJ. Animal models of neuropathic pain. In: Gebhart GB, Hammond DL, Jensen TS (eds). *Progress in pain research and management*, vol. 2. Seattle, WA: IASP Press, 1994: 495–510.

3. Jensen TS. Mechanisms of neuropathic pain. In: Campbell JN (ed.). *Pain 1996: an updated review.* Seattle, WA: IASP Press, 1996: 77–86.

4. Fields HL. *Pain syndromes in neurology.* London: Butterworths, 1990: 286.

∗ 5. Woolf CJ, Salter MW. Neuronal plasticity: increasing the gain in pain. *Science*. 2000; **288**: 1765–8.

∗ 6. Sindrup SH, Jensen TS. Efficacy of pharmacological treatments of neuropathic pain: an update and effect related to mechanism of drug action. *Pain*. 1999; **83**: 389–400.

∗ 7. Sindrup SH, Jensen TS. Pharmacologic treatment of pain in polyneuropathies. *Neurology*. 2000; **55**: 915–20.

8. Woolf CJ, Bennett GJ, Doherty M *et al*. Towards a mechanism-based classification of pain? *Pain*. 1998; **77**: 227–9.

∗ 9. Finnerup NB, Otto M, McQuay HJ *et al*. Algorithm for neuropathic pain treatment: an evidence based proposal. *Pain*. 2005; **118**: 289–305.

∗ 10. Dubner R, Ren K. Endogenous mechanisms of sensory modulation. *Pain*. 1999; **6** (Suppl.): 45–53.

∗ 11. Woolf CJ, Mannion RJ. Neuropathic pain: aetiology, symptoms, mechanisms, and management. *Lancet*. 1999; **353**: 1959–64.

∗ 12. Besson JM. The neurobiology of pain. *Lancet*. 1999; **353**: 1610–15.

∗ 13. Kieffer BL. Opioid receptors: from genes to mice. *Journal of Pain*. 2000; **1**: 45–50.

∗ 14. Wood JN, Heath MJS. Molecules that specify modality: mechanisms of nociception. *Journal of Pain*. 2000; **1**: 19–25.

15. Davis KD, Kiss ZH, Luo L *et al*. Phantom sensations generated by thalamic microstimulation. *Nature*. 1998; **391**: 385–7.

16. Flor H, Elbert T, Mühlnickel W *et al*. Cortical reorganisation and phantom phenomena in congenital and traumatic upper-extremity amputees. *Experimental Brain Research*. 1998; **119**: 205–12.

∗ 17. Lindblom U. Assessment of abnormal evoked pain in neurological pain patients and its relation to spontaneous pain: a descriptive and conceptual model with some analytical results. *Advances in Pain Research and Therapy*. 1985; **9**: 409–23.

18. Hansson P, Lindblom U. Hyperalgesia assessed with quantitative sensory testing in patients with neurogenic pain. In: Willis Jr WD (ed.). *Hyperalgesia and allodynia*. New York, NY: Raven Press, 1992: 335–43.

19. Jensen TS, Gottrup H, Bach FW, Sindrup SH. The clinical picture of neuropathic pain. *European Journal of Pharmacology*. 2001; **429**: 1–11.

20. Woolf CJ, Decosterd I. Implications of recent advances in understanding of pain pathophysiology for assessment of pain in patients. *Pain Supplement*. 1999; **6**: 141–7.

21. Koltzenburg M. Painful neuropathies. *Current Opinion in Neurology*. 1998; **11**: 515–21.

22. Terrence CF, Jensen TS. Trigeminal neuralgia and other facial neuralgias. In: Olesen J, Tfelt-Hansen P, Welch KMA (eds). *The headaches*, 2nd edn. New York, NY: Raven Press, 1999: 929–38.

23. Nordenbos W. *Pain*. Amsterdam: Elsevier, 1959: 68–80.

24. Raja SN, Haythornthwaite JA, Pappagallo M *et al*. Opioids versus antidepressant in postherpetic neuralgia: A randomised, placebo-controlled trial. *Neurology*. 2002; **59**: 1015–21.

25. Gottrup H, Bach FW, Juhl G, Jensen TS. Differential effect of ketamine and lidocaine on spontaneous pain and mechanically evoked pain in patients with nerve injury. *Anesthesiology*. 2006; **104**: 527–36.

26. Rasmussen PV, Sindrup SH, Jensen TS, Bach FW. Therapeutic outcome in neuropathic pain: relationship to evidence of nervous system lesion. *European Journal of Neurology*. 2004; **11**: 545–53.

27. Finnerup NB, Biering-Soernsen F, Jahannesen IL *et al*. Intravenous lidocaine relieves spinal cord injury pain: a randomized controlled trial. *Anesthesiology*. 2005; **102**: 1023–30.

28. Attal N, Rouaud J, Brasseur L *et al*. Systemic lidocaine in pain due to peripheral nerve injury and predictor response. *Neurology*. 2004; **62**: 218–25.

∗ 29. Rasmussen PV, Sindrup SH, Jensen TS, Bach FW. Symptoms and signs in patients with suspected neuropathic pain. *Pain*. 2004; **110**: 461–9.

30. Gracely RH, Lynch SA, Bennett GJ. Painful neuropathy: altered central processing, maintained dynamically by peripheral input. *Pain*. 1992; **51**: 175–94.

31. Koltzenburg M. Stability and plasticity of nociceptor function and their relationship to provoked and ongoing pain. *Seminars in Neurosciences*. 1995; **7**: 199–210.

∗ 32. Kilo S, Schmelz M, Koltzenburg M, Handwerker HO. Different patterns of hyperalgesia induced by experimental inflammation in human skin. *Brain*. 1994; **117**: 385–96.

33. Koltzenburg M, Lundberg LER, Torebjörk HE. Dynamic and static components of mechanical hyperalgesia in human hairy skin. *Pain*. 1992; **51**: 207–19.

34. Lindblom U, Verillo RT. Sensory functions in chronic neuralgia. *Journal of Neurology, Neurosurgery, and Psychiatry*. 1979; **42**: 422–35.

35. Lindblom U. Analysis of abnormal touch, pain and temperature sensation in patients. In: Boivie J, Hansson P, Lindblom U (eds). *Touch, temperature and pain in health and disease: mechanisms and assessment. Progress in Pain Research and Management*, vol. 3. Seattle, WA: IASP Press, 1994: 63–84.

36. Jensen TS, Lenz FA. Central post-stroke pain: a challenge for the scientist and the clinician. *Pain*. 1995; **61**: 161–4.

37. Boivie J. Central pain. In: Wall PD, Melzack R (eds). *Textbook of pain*, 3rd edn. Edinburgh: Churchill Livingstone, 1999: 871–902.

38. Vestergaard K, Nielsen J, Andersen G *et al*. Sensory abnormalities in consecutive, unselected patients with central post-stroke pain. *Pain*. 1995; **61**: 177–86.

39. Finnerup NB, Johannesen IL, Fuglsang-Frederiksen A *et al*. Sensory function in spinal cord injury patients with and without central pain. *Brain*. 2003; **126**: 57–70.

40. Finnerup NB, Johannesen IL, Bach FB, Jensen TS. Sensory function above lesion level in spinal cord injury patients with and without pain. *Somatosensory and Motor Research*. 2003; **20**: 71–76.

* 41. Koltzenburg M, Torebjörk HE, Wahren LK. Nociceptor modulated central sensitization causes mechanical hyperalgesia in acute chemogenic and chronic neuropathic pain. *Brain.* 1994; **117**: 579–91.
* 42. Ochoa JL, Yarnitsky D. Mechanical hyperalgesias in neuropathic pain patients: dynamic and static subtypes. *Annals of Neurology.* 1993; **33**: 465–72.
43. Jensen TS, Brennum J. The relation of thermally and mechanically evoked pain to pathological pain. In: Boivie J, Hansson P, Lindblom U (eds). *Touch, temperature and pain in health and disease: mechanisms and assessment. Progress in Pain Research and Management*, vol. 3. Seattle, WA: IASP Press, 1994: 373–88.
44. Graven-Nielsen T, Arendt-Nielsen L, Svensson P, Jensen TS. Stimulus–response functions in areas with experimentally induced referred muscle pain: a psychophysical study. *Brain Research.* 1997; **744**: 121–8.
45. Laursen RJ, Graven-Nielsen T, Jensen TS, Arendt-Nielsen L. Quantification of local and referred pain in humans induced by intramuscular electrical stimulation. *European Journal of Pain.* 1997; **1**: 105–13.
46. Graven-Nielsen T, Slot L, Svensson P *et al.* Quantification of deep and superficial sensibility in saline-induced muscle pain: a psychophysical study. *Somatosensory and Motor Research.* 1998; **15**: 46–53.
47. Laursen RJ, Graven-Nielsen T, Jensen TS, Arendt-Nielsen L. Referred pain is dependent on sensory input from the periphery: a psychophysical study. *European Journal of Pain.* 1997; **1**: 261–9.
48. Witting N, Svensson P, Gottrup H *et al.* Intramuscular and intradermal injection of capsaicin: a comparison of local and referred pain. *Pain.* 2000; **84**: 407–12.
* 49. LaMotte RH, Shain CN, Simone DA, Tsai EFP. Neurogenic hyperalgesia: psychophysical studies of underlying mechanisms. *Journal of Neurophysiology.* 1991; **66**: 190–211.
50. Dubner R. Neuronal plasticity in the spinal and medullary dorsal horns: a possible role in central pain mechanisms. In: Casey KL (ed.). *Pain and central nervous disease: the central pain syndromes.* New York: Raven Press, 1991: 143–55.
* 51. Mendell LM, Wall PD. Responses of single dorsal cord cells to peripheral cutaneous unmyelinated fibres. *Nature.* 1965; **206**: 97–9.
52. Arendt-Nielsen L, Graven-Nielsen T, Svensson P, Jensen TS. Temporal summation in muscles and referred pain areas: an experimental human study. *Muscle and Nerve.* 1997; **20**: 1311–13.
53. Bonica JJ. Clinical importance of hyperalgesia. In: Willis Jr WD (ed.). *Hyperalgesia and allodynia.* New York: Raven Press, 1992: 17–43.
* 54. Gottrup H, Nielsen J, Arendt-Nielsen L, Jensen TS. The relationship between sensory thresholds and mechanical hyperalgesia in nerve injury. *Pain.* 1998; **75**: 321–9.
55. Gottrup H, Andersen J, Arendt-Nielsen L, Jensen TS. Psychophysical examination in patients with postmastectomy pain. *Pain.* 2000; **87**: 275–84.
56. Dickenson AH, Sullivan AF. Evidence for a role of the NMDA receptor in the frequency dependent potentiation of rat dorsal horn nociceptive neurones following C fibre stimulation. *Neuropharmacology.* 1987; **26**: 1235–8.
* 57. Dickenson AH. A cure for wind-up: NMDA receptor antagonists as potential analgesics. *Trends in Pharmacological Sciences.* 1990; **11**: 307–09.
* 58. Attal N, Gaude V, Brasseur L *et al.* Intravenous lidocaine in central pain, a double-blind, placebo-controlled psychophysical study. *Neurology.* 2000; **1**: 564–74.
59. Eide PK, Jørum E, Stubhaug A *et al.* Relief of post-herpetic neuralgia with the *N*-methyl-D-aspartic receptor antagonist ketamine: a double-blind, cross-over comparison with morphine and placebo. *Pain.* 1994; **58**: 347–54.
60. Felsby S, Nielsen J, Arendt-Nielsen L, Jensen TS. NMDA receptor blockade in chronic neuropathic pain: a comparison of ketamine and magnesium chloride. *Pain.* 1996; **64**: 283–91.
61. Nikolajsen L, Hansen CL, Nielsen J *et al.* The effect of ketamine on phantom pain: a central neuropathic disorder maintained by peripheral input. *Pain.* 1996; **67**: 69–77.
* 62. Gottrup H, Kristensen AD, Bach FW, Jensen TS. Aftersensations in experimental and clinical hyperalgesia. *Pain.* 2003; **103**: 57–64.
63. Galer BS, Jensen MP. Development and preliminary validation of a pain measure specific to neuropathic pain: the neuropathic pain scale. *Neurology.* 1997; **48**: 332–8.
64. Bennett MI. The LANSS Pain Scale: The Leeds assessment of neuropathic symptoms and signs. *Pain.* 2001; **92**: 147–57.
65. Bennett MI, Smith BH, Torrance N, Potter J. The S-LANSS score for identifying pain of predominantly neuropathic origin: validation for use in clinical and postal research. *Journal of Pain.* 2005; **6**: 149–58.
66. Bennett MI, Smith BH, Torrance N, Lee AJ. Can pain be more or less neuropathic? Comparison of symptom assessment tools with ratings of certainty by clinicians. *Pain.* 2006; **122**: 289–94.
67. Andersen G, Vestergaard K, Ingeman-Nielsen M, Jensen TS. The incidence of central post-stroke pain. *Pain.* 1995; **61**: 187–93.
68. Gottrup H, Hansen PO, Arendt-Nielsen L, Jensen TS. Differential effects of systemically administered ketamine and lidocaine on dynamic and static hyperalgesia induced by intradermal capsaicin in humans. *British Journal of Anaesthesia.* 2000; **85**: 155–63.
69. Witting N, Svensson P, Arendt-Nielsen L, Jensen TS. Repetitive intradermal capsaicin: differential effect on pain and areas of allodynia and punctate hyperalgesia. *Somatosensory and Motor Research.* 2000; **17**: 5–12.
70. Gottrup H, Bach FW, Arendt-Nielsen L, Jensen TS. Peripheral lidocaine, but not ketamine inhibits capsaicin-induced hyperalgesia in humans. *British Journal of Anaesthesia.* 2000; **85**: 1–9.

71. Petersen KL, Fields HL, Brennum J *et al.* Capsaicin evoked pain and allodynia in post-herpetic neuralgia. *Pain.* 2000; **88**: 125–33.

72. Asbury AK, Fields HL. Pain due to peripheral nerve damage: an hypothesis. *Neurology.* 1984; **34**: 1587–90.

73. Baron R, Saguer M. Postherpetic neuralgia: are C-nociceptors involved in signalling and maintenance of tactile allodynia? *Brain.* 1993; **116**: 1477–96.

* 74. Rowbotham MC, Fields HL. The relationship of pain, allodynia and thermal sensation in post-herpetic neuralgia. *Brain.* 1996; **119**: 347–54.

75. Fields HL, Rowbotham M, Baron R. Postherpetic neuralgia: irritable nociceptors and deafferentation. *Neurobiology of Disease.* 1998; **5**: 209–27.

76. Baron R. Peripheral neuropathic pain: from mechanisms to symptoms. *Clinical Journal of Pain.* 2000; **16**: 12–20.

77. Löfström JB, Cousins MJ. Sympathetic neural blockade of upper and lower extremity. In: Cousins MJ, Bridenbaugh PO (eds). *Neural blockade in clinical anesthesia and management of pain.* Philadelphia, PA: JB Lippincott, 1988: 461–500.

78. Gracely RH. Studies of pain in normal man. In: Wall PD, Melzack R (eds). *Textbook of pain*, 3rd edn. Edinburgh: Churchill-Livingstone, 1994: 315–36.

79. Chapman CR, Casey KL, Dubner R *et al.* Pain measurement: an overview. *Pain.* 1985; **22**: 1–31.

* 80. McQuay HJ, Moore RA. *An evidence-based resource for pain relief.* Oxford: Oxford University Press, 1998.

12

Diagnostic procedures in chronic pain

NIKOLAI BOGDUK

KEY LEARNING POINTS

- Investigations for chronic pain are limited by what particular tests can and cannot show, and by the nature of conditions that cause chronic pain.
- Imaging tests are appropriate only for particular conditions: plain radiography for fractures; computed tomography (CT) for intracranial and visceral disorders. Magnetic resonance (MR) imaging is the best overall screening test for serious disorders.
- Nerve conduction studies have no application for the diagnosis of pain. Their utility is limited to confirming some forms of neuropathy.
- Diagnostic blocks are the most powerful tool by which to pinpoint the mechanism or the source of chronic pain, but in order to be valid, diagnostic blocks must be controlled.
- The conditions that cause chronic pain can be grouped into three classes.
- Various visceral disorders are ones diagnosed by other specialists.
- Some disorders have a known, detectable pathology. Various laboratory screening tests are indicated before imaging is undertaken.
- Spinal pain can be investigated using disk stimulation and controlled diagnostic blocks.
- The objective of diagnosis is to establish the source and cause of a patient's symptoms. Classically in medical practice, the diagnostic process has been divided into history, examination, and investigations. From the history and examination, the physician formulates a provisional diagnosis or a list of differential diagnoses. Thereafter, investigations constitute the definitive test, either, or both, to confirm a diagnosis and to exclude competing diagnoses.
- For disorders of the cardiovascular, respiratory, gastrointestinal, and other systems, diagnostic algorithms can be followed, in which various investigations have a well-defined role and proven utility. When this process is applied to pain medicine, however, difficulties arise. Conventional investigations have limitations in the pursuit of pain, and conditions that cause chronic pain typically do not express abnormalities in conventional tests.
- Responsible and efficient practice in pain medicine requires understanding of what investigations can and cannot show, and when they should and should not be used. This needs to be complemented by understanding the conditions that cause chronic pain, which investigations are inappropriate, and which are likely to be informative.

INVESTIGATIONS

Radiography

Plain radiography produces images based on the degree to which tissues of the body absorb x-rays. Muscles and viscera absorb x-rays weakly and, therefore, cast poor images on radiographs. Bone is essentially the only tissue demonstrated. Occasionally, plain radiographs might demonstrate displacements of soft-tissue shadows, which are indicative of effusion, abscess, or hematoma, but in practice, the utility of plain radiography is limited to demonstrating abnormalities of bone. These constitute deformities, anomalies, fractures, and major destructive disorders.

Deformities and congenital anomalies are often painless. Therefore, when evident in a patient with pain, they cannot summarily be invoked as the cause of pain. Some practitioners believe that deformities somehow alter the biomechanics of the affected part and, thereby, cause pain; but the nature of the alteration and the site at which nociception is generated have never been established.

For the pursuit of fractures in patients with trauma, various rules and guidelines have been developed for use in primary care and emergency medicine (**Table 12.1**, **Figure 12.1**).[1, 2, 3, 4, 5, 6] These rules emphasize that radiography should only be undertaken if the patient is elderly, or if they have signs indicative of a significant fracture. In the absence of such features, radiography is not indicated. The low positive likelihood ratios of the clinical criteria indicate that not all patients selected for radiography will necessarily have a fracture. However, the very low negative likelihood ratios indicate that virtually no patient who lacks the criteria will have a fracture, which would be missed if radiography were not undertaken. In patients with chronic pain, previously unrecognized fractures are very unlikely to be the cause of pain. Radiography, just in case the patient has a fracture, is not justified. In that context, the rules for acute pain serve as sensible initial guidelines for chronic pain.

Perhaps the most distracting property of plain radiography is that it demonstrates features that are not relevant to pain. Osteophytes and joint narrowing indicate changes in a joint, but do not necessarily implicate either a source or a cause of pain. It is in this regard that too much reliance has been placed on plain radiographs.

Degenerative changes in the vertebral column are normal accompaniments of age.[7, 8, 9, 10, 11, 12, 13, 14, 15] Essentially, they are equally common in symptomatic and asymptomatic individuals of the same age. They correlate poorly, if at all with pain.[9, 10, 11, 12, 13, 14, 15] Indeed, osteoarthritis of the cervical zygapophysial joints is ironically more common in individuals who do not have pain.[10] Degenerative changes, therefore, are not a surrogate for pain, and do not constitute a diagnosis.

The same applies for joints of the appendicular skeleton. Although osteoarthritis is the most common diagnosis for pain ostensibly stemming from joints, such as the hip and knee, the radiographic changes of osteoarthritis correlate imperfectly with pain.[16, 17] Indeed, this lack of correlation has led some authorities to consider that knee pain attributed to osteoarthritis may not always be due to osteoarthritis,[18, 19] and should be regarded as a problem of regional pain and disability.[18, 20] Osteoarthritis is essentially a clinical diagnosis. X-rays can demonstrate the bony architecture of the joint, but are not diagnostic in their own right.

For destructive lesions, such as infection and tumors of bone, plain radiographs are limited in their sensitivity to detect early lesions. The features that they show typically occur only when the disease is advanced. Plain radiographs, therefore, are an inappropriate screening test for these conditions. If they fail to detect a condition that is too early in its evolution, they provide a false sense of security. Other investigations are better suited as screening tests for serious diseases of bone.

Table 12.1 Various rules listing criteria that should be satisfied before undertaking radiography for painful injuries to joints of the lower limb.

Rule	Criteria	
Ottawa Ankle Rules	Pain in the zone of either malleolus, and tenderness at: the posterior edge of the lateral malleolus, or the posterior edge of the medial malleolus, or the base of the fifth metatarsal, or the navicular bone or inability to walk four steps	Sens = 1.00 Spec = 0.39 PLR = 1.6 NLR = 0.00
Ottawa Knee Rules[1, 2]	At least one of: age greater than 55 years isolated tenderness of patella tenderness head of fibula unable to flex 90° unable to bear weight two steps	Sens = 1.00 Spec = 0.49 PLR = 2.0 NLR = 0.00
Pittsburgh Knee Rules[3, 4]	At least one of: age greater than 51 or less than 11 years unable to bear weight four steps	Sens = 99% Spec = 60% PLR = 2.5 NLR = 0.02

NLR, negative likelihood ratio; PLR, positive likelihood ratio; Sens, sensitivity; Spec, specificity.

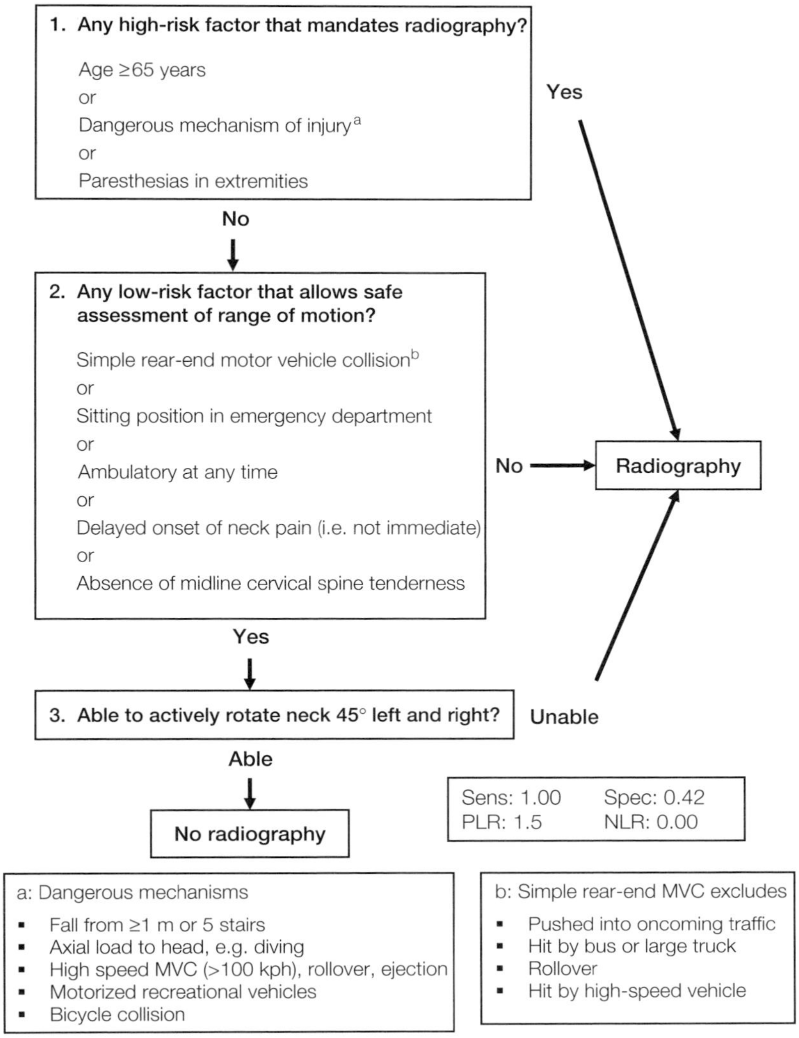

Figure 12.1 The Canadian C-spine rule for radiography after cervical spine trauma.[5] NLR, negative likelihood ratio; PLR, positive likelihood ratio; Sens, sensitivity; Spec, specificity.

Computed tomography

Computed tomography (CT) samples the x-ray density of body tissues along multiple meridians around the long axis of the target region. The information obtained is processed by a computer program that reconstructs views of the area of interest. Technological developments have reduced acquisition time, provide much higher resolution than in the past, and enable three-dimensional images to be reconstructed, which can be viewed from any perspective.

CT provides resolution of bone in exquisite detail. It is capable of reconstructing the exact morphology of fractures in three dimensions. Its high resolution allows even the smallest of fractures to be detected. CT is, therefore, the investigation of choice when there are strong clinical grounds for suspecting an occult fracture as the cause of pain. However, fractures are rare causes of chronic pain and CT should not be abused as a screening test for a condition that is highly unlikely to be present.

The cardinal virtue of CT is that it allows investigators to "see" inside body cavities, such as the chest, abdomen, skull, and head. In these regions, CT can demonstrate enlargement or displacement of soft-tissue structures, by tumors, infiltrations, infection, and inflammation. Hollow organs can be enhanced by injecting contrast medium into their lumina. Of particular relevance to pain medicine is the ability of CT to demonstrate intracranial pathology in patients with headache, and the relationship between spinal nerves and the vertebral column in patients with radicular pain.

Magnetic resonance imaging

MR imaging provides images of the tissues of the body based on proton density. The images are obtained by using a magnetic field to force protons to precess around a predetermined axis, and subsequently measuring the radiation emitted as the precession decays. Radiation is sampled along multiple meridians around the long axis of the region being investigated, and computer programs are used to reconstruct images in any selected plane, typically sagittal, coronal, and axial, through the region. By manipulating the rate of decay of precession, different properties of the tissues can be depicted. The terms T1 and T2 refer to the time constants of particular types of decay of precession. Images based on the T1 constant typically depict the location and shape of bones and other tissues. Images based on the T2 constant enhance the appearance of relatively unbound hydrogen within tissues (e.g. water) and reveal the internal structure of connective tissues, and the presence of edema.

MR imaging depicts bone in less detail than does CT, but its advantage over CT is its ability to reveal the internal architecture of soft tissues, notably that of the brain, and of fibrous connective tissues. Moreover, it demonstrates cerebrospinal fluid and flowing blood without the need for contrast medium. Particularly useful is the ability of MR imaging to resolve edema, and cellular infiltrates such as those of leukemia and spreading tumors like endometriosis. These properties give MR imaging high sensitivity and high specificity, not only for common lesions, but also for exotic and rare lesions not visible by any other means.

In relation to pain medicine, the high sensitivity of MR imaging makes it the most useful form of medical imaging for screening purposes to rule out unexpected conditions, or ones that cannot be detected by other means. In musculoskeletal medicine, MR imaging is the best way to detect osteonecrosis.[21] For this condition, MR imaging is both sensitive and specific, and is able to detect changes earlier than can plain radiography or CT. Because of its better resolution of nerves, and its ability to provide coronal and sagittal images, as well as axial images, MR imaging is the preferred means of investigating radiculopathy. Its ability to demonstrate the internal structure of intervertebral disks accords it a unique role in the investigation of chronic back pain. Its ability to resolve connective tissues makes it the premier means of assessing joints and periarticular structures.

Nevertheless, like other imaging procedures, MR imaging demonstrates many irrelevant and false-positive abnormalities. Disk bulges, disk herniations, degenerative changes, and even spinal cord impingement, occur in totally asymptomatic individuals, and with increasing frequency with age.[22, 23, 24, 25] They are not diagnostic of causes of pain. Similarly, tears of the rotator cuff and other lesions occur in totally asymptomatic subjects, and increasingly with age.[26, 27, 28] They are not diagnostic of the cause of shoulder pain.

Myelography

By instilling contrast medium into the dural sac, myelography demonstrates the location and shape of the subarachnoid space of the vertebral canal. It indirectly demonstrates lesions that encroach upon this space either internally or externally. Its role in this regard, however, has largely been supplanted by the advent of CT and MR imaging, for these other procedures provide images of the lesion itself, not just its effects on the subarachnoid space.

Some physicians believe myelography combined with CT to be the preferred method of investigating cervical radiculopathy, on the grounds that it provides better resolution of bony lesions than MR imaging.[29, 30] Other authorities contend that the preferred investigation is MR imaging coupled with plain radiographs.[31, 32, 33]

Ultrasound

Ultrasound images are derived by plotting the echoes of sound waves beamed at tissues. They depict the interface between tissues of different density. Accordingly, ultrasound is particularly useful for demonstrating hollow organs and cystic pathology. In that regard, it is particularly useful as a screening test for aortic aneurysms, gynecologic disorders, diverticulitis, urinary calculi, appendicitis, and incarcerated hernia.

Ultrasound depicts laminated structures well, such as muscles and tendons arranged in parallel layers. In such structures, it can reveal swelling, displacement, and discontinuities. It has, therefore, been applied in the pursuit of tendinitis, tendonopathy, and tears of tendons. However, technical artifacts are easily produced by ultrasound and can be misconstrued as lesions. Consequently, accurate use of ultrasound involves a steep learning curve. For this reason, authorities recommend that ultrasound be performed only by experienced operators.[34, 35] However, although this may secure reliability, it does not guarantee validity.

Compared to arthrography and operative findings, the sensitivity and specificity of ultrasound for the detection of rotator cuff tears range from 60 to 100 percent.[36] Missing, however, are data that show that such tears are the cause of pain, or that repairing such tears guarantees relief of pain. In orthopedic circles, it has been customary to assume that tears in the rotator cuff seen on ultrasound must be the cause of patients' shoulder pain. The validity of this assumption is fatally challenged when ultrasound demonstrates the same pathology in the contralateral, but asymptomatic, shoulder. Tears are not a surrogate diagnosis for shoulder pain.

In other regions of the body, ultrasound is used to demonstrate inflamed or swollen tendons in patients with soft-tissue pain. While demonstrating such lesions may be satisfying, it is arguably superfluous to do so. Tendonopathy is readily diagnosed simply on the basis of focal tenderness on clinical examination, and does not require ultrasound confirmation. Moreover, there is no demonstrated therapeutic utility in demonstrating tendonopathy, for there is no proven treatment. Exercises may be prescribed, and local anesthetic or corticosteroids can be injected without the necessity for ultrasound.

Perhaps where ultrasound is unarguably useful is in the detection of effusions in deep joints, such as the hip.

Moreover, it can be used to guide needles into the joint in order to aspirate it, or to inject local anesthetic or corticosteroids.

Bone scan

Bone scanning produces images of the distribution and accumulation of the radioactive isotope of technetium. Its particular virtue is the ability to demonstrate areas of hyperemia that occur in association with tumors, infections, osteonecrosis, and stress fractures. It is a highly sensitive test, in that it detects changes in blood flow, even very early in a disease; but because it cannot distinguish one cause of hyperemia from another, it lacks specificity. Because of its sensitivity, bone scan is a very useful screening test to rule in or to rule out internal abnormalities of bone, but its apparent utility should be gauged against that of MR imaging, which is just as sensitive but far more specific. For this reason, MR imaging is a better screening test for tumors, infections, and osteonecrosis.

The foremost application of bone scan in pain medicine lies in the detection of stress fractures, in patients with leg pain and foot pain precipitated by prolonged activity, and in athletes with back pain. Bone scanning is particularly useful for detecting a stressed pars interarticularis before it actually fractures. Doing so allows rest from the offending activity to be implemented with a good chance of averting fracture. The utility of bone scan once a fracture has occurred is more contentious. Classical teaching maintains that a positive bone scan would indicate a recent fracture, which would implicate the fracture as the source of pain. However, the relationships between bone scan, pars defect, and symptoms are imperfect. Although a positive scan is likely to be associated with pain, scans are negative in the majority of patients with pain.[37] In patients with a radiologically evident pars fracture, bone scans are just as likely to be negative as positive.[38, 39, 40]

Some centers and some individuals use bone scan as an ancillary investigation of complex regional pain syndromes. It is used to detect juxta-articular hyperemia, seemingly as a confirmation of the diagnosis, or perhaps to stage the disease.[41, 42, 43] As a diagnostic test, however, bone scan is redundant. In the first instance, complex regional pain syndrome is diagnosed on the basis of clinical features, and the correlation between clinical features and bone scan is weak to poor.[43] Although bone scan may be sensitive in the diagnosis of complex regional pain syndrome, it is not specific. In other words, bone scan is likely to be positive in patients in whom the diagnosis is clinically obvious; but a negative bone scan does not rule out the diagnosis in such instances. In the second instance, although it has been traditional to recognize stages of complex regional pain syndrome, this is an idealization; it is not borne out by factor analysis.[43, 44] There are too many exceptions to the desired pattern of staging. In the absence of a valid staging system for complex regional pain syndrome, there is no utility for bone scan to stage the condition.

Single photon emission computed tomography scan

Single photon emission computed tomography (SPECT) combines the virtues of bone scan and computed tomography. It provides axial views of areas of increased uptake of radioisotope. The utility of SPECT scanning in pain medicine, however, is far from demonstrated. For spinal disorders, interobserver agreement is poor,[45] and the observed abnormalities lack any correlation with pain. A systematic review cast doubts on the utility of SPECT,[46] and subsequent studies have not redressed its shortcomings.

Reports that SPECT scans can identify symptomatic lumbar zygapophysial joint lack foundation. None of the studies used controlled blocks of the purportedly symptomatic joints.[47, 48] When controlled blocks have been used, SPECT did not correlate with response to blocks.[49]

Nerve conduction studies

Nerve conduction studies determine the velocity of conduction and magnitude of evoked action potentials in peripheral nerves. Slowing of conduction across a selected segment of the nerve indicates compression or focal damage to the nerve at that segment. Decreased amplitude indicates loss of nerve fibers. Electromyography selectively tests alpha motor neurons. Loss of motor neurons is indicated by denervation fibrillation potentials in the muscles innervated, or by the presence of large and abnormal muscle action potentials.

Nerve conduction studies and electromyography are not tests of pain. They assess the integrity of large diameter sensory and motor fibers, and are useful for objectively establishing the presence of large fiber neuropathy. Any utility for the study of pain relies on the relationship between pain and impaired function in large diameter fibers. This relationship obtains in few conditions.

It is accepted that in patients with diabetic neuropathy, and other peripheral neuropathies, the pain experienced can be attributed to the neuropathy. Consequently, nerve conduction studies have a valid role to play in objectively establishing the presence and nature of the neuropathy.

Similarly, nerve conduction studies can objectively establish the presence of nerve compression in conditions such as carpal tunnel syndrome, tarsal tunnel syndrome, and ulnar nerve entrapment. Reciprocally, nerve conduction studies can exclude radial nerve entrapment as a differential diagnosis of lateral epicondylalgia of the elbow.[50] In these conditions, although the mechanism by which pain is produced is uncertain, there seems to be general agreement that objective evidence of nerve compression is critical to making the diagnosis.[51, 52, 53, 54] Caveats, however, apply.

Particularly with respect to the carpal tunnel, abnormal conduction velocities occur in asymptomatic individuals.[55, 56] Consequently, nerve conduction studies carry a substantial and annoying false-positive rate. Although only a minority of normal individuals exhibit abnormal conduction velocities, these individuals outnumber patients with pain ostensibly due to carpal tunnel syndrome. Consequently, in patients with suspected carpal tunnel syndrome, investigators cannot be certain whether the abnormal conduction velocities they detect are due to disease or are an incidental (false-positive) finding. Investigators may choose to believe that the positive findings confirm their diagnosis, but this is a self-serving decision, not one based on epidemiological probity. For this reason, eminent authorities have challenged the validity of contemporary criteria for the diagnosis of carpal tunnel syndrome.[57]

Although commonly used in the assessment of patients with radicular pain, nerve conduction studies and electromyography serve no useful purpose in this condition. They lack validity for any particular diagnosis. For the diagnosis of lumbar disk herniation, electromyography is confounded by too high a false-positive rate (**Table 12.2**).[58, 59, 60] For the identification of the segmental level involved, electromyography is confounded by variations in the segmental innervation of muscles. It does not assist in pinpointing the diagnosis to any greater extent than clinical examination (**Table 12.3**).

Review articles have highlighted the lack of sensitivity and specificity of nerve conduction studies in the evaluation of radicular pain, and underscore their lack of utility in this condition.[61, 62, 63, 64] More elaborate studies, such as H reflexes and somatosensory-evoked potentials, do not improve the situation.[61, 63, 64] The only justifiable application of nerve conduction studies in patients with radicular pain is when the clinical picture is not clearly one of radiculopathy, and when the physician is genuinely concerned that the condition may be a peripheral neuropathy.

Table 12.2 The correlation between electromyography (EMG) findings and presence of a lumbar disc herniation identified at surgery.

EMG	Disk herniation		Sens.	Spec.	LR
	Present	Absent			
Positive	126	14	0.78	0.30	1.1
Normal	35	6			

Based on the data of Knutsson.[58]
LR, likelihood ratio; Sens, sensitivity; Spec, specificity.

Table 12.3 The correlation between electromyography (EMG) findings and the anatomical level of a lumbar disk herniation identified at surgery.

EMG	Level affected		Sens.	Spec.	LR
	Correct	Wrong			
Positive	126	14		0.18	0.93
Normal	38	3	0.77		

Based on the data of Knutsson.[58]
LR, likelihood ratio; Sens, sensitivity; Spec, specificity.

Thermography

Thermography measures heat emission from the body surface and displays it photographically. The heat measured is that emanating from skin. Thermography does not measure heat from muscles. Any utility of thermography in the investigation of pain depends on the relationship between cutaneous blood flow and pain. Since there is no direct relationship, thermography does not measure or depict pain; it depicts only associated features that may or may not regularly occur with pain in various conditions.

Thermography correlates reasonably well with clinical examination and MR imaging findings in patients with radiculopathy.[65] However, it adds nothing to the diagnosis. The presence of radiculopathy is readily established by clinical examination and does not require corroboration by thermography. The causative lesion is demonstrated by CT or MR imaging.

Thermography can objectively and quantitatively determine temperature changes in limbs affected by complex regional pain syndromes.[66] Its use in these conditions is attractive, in that it seems to offer an objective diagnosis, but it is essentially superfluous. Temperature changes are only one of the lesser features of these conditions. The cardinal diagnostic criteria are inordinate pain, allodynia, and a history, at some time, of swelling and color changes, apart from temperature changes. The diagnosis can be made clinically without resort to thermography.

Moreover, it has been shown that thermographic changes correlate only weakly with clinical features; and the correlation is with temperature asymmetries on clinical examination.[43] Thermography is unlikely to be positive unless there are already evident temperature asymmetries clinically.

Complex regional pain syndrome

Apart from thermography and SPECT scanning, a variety of other tests have been advocated for the assessment of complex regional pain syndromes. These include quantitative sensory testing (QST), resting sweat output

(RSO), thermoregulatory sweat test (TST), quantitative sudomotor axon reflex testing (QSART), and sympathetic skin response (SSR). A comprehensive review found no compelling evidence of the utility of these investigations as diagnostic tests for complex regional pain syndrome.[67] For QST, the review concluded that the findings are not specific for the disease and do not deliver relevant additional diagnostic information. It considered RSO, TST, and QSART useful in the research setting, but they are difficult to conduct and have little clinical applicability. The SSR is still affected by differences in technique used, and cannot be recommended in routine diagnosis of complex regional pain syndrome (CRPS).

Neuropathies

Some painful neuropathies can be diagnosed on the basis of history, family history, clinical features, and features of the primary disease. These include Guillain–Barré neuropathy, rheumatoid vasculitis, systemic lupus erythematosis, sarcoidosis, leprosy, malignancy, and drug toxicity. They do not require special tests for diagnosis, or special tests are not available. Other painful neuropathies can be diagnosed by detecting characteristic metabolites in the serum or urine (**Table 12.4**).[68, 69] Some neuropathies may require biopsy for confirmation, and some can be diagnosed only by biopsy.

Sympathetic blocks

Blocks of the sympathetic nervous system used to be the mainstay for diagnosing reflex sympathetic dystrophy and causalgia. However, modern research has shown that these conditions, now embraced by the rubric – complex regional pain syndromes – do not necessarily involve the sympathetic nervous system. The diagnosis can be rendered on clinical grounds, without the use of sympathetic blocks. Blocks of sympathetic nerves have been relegated to testing whether or not the pain is sympathetically maintained.

Traditionally, sympathetic blocks have involved the injection of local anesthetic agents on to that section of the sympathetic trunk that innervates the affected region of the body. Such blocks interrupt conduction in sympathetic nerves, and relief of symptoms is taken to indicate that the symptoms are sympathetically mediated. Alternatives have been the use of intravenous injections of drugs that ostensibly block the terminal of sympathetic nerves in the periphery, or the action of their transmitter substances. The validity of these procedures has been challenged.

Table 12.4 Painful neuropathies and the laboratory tests for their diagnosis.

Neuropathy	Diagnostic test		
	Serum	Urine	Biopsy
Diabetic	Glucose Glucose tolerance	Glucose	
Alcohol	Liver function tests		
Vitamin deficiency	B_{12}		
Vasculitis	Antinuclear antibodies		Biopsy
Sjögren's disease	Sjögren antibodies		
AIDS	HIV antibodies		
Primary amyloid	Protein electrophoresis	Protein electrophoresis	Biopsy
Fabry's disease	δ-galactosidase Globotriasosylceramide	Globotriasosylceramide	
Uremic	Electrolytes Renal function tests		
Porphyric		δ-aminolevulinic acid Porphobilinogen	
Tangier's disease	Low cholesterol Low HDLs Low apoprotein		
Churg–Strauss	Eosinophilia		
Heavy metal	Arsenic, thallium		
Familial amyloid			Biopsy
Hereditary			Biopsy
Charcot–Marie–Tooth			Biopsy
Cryoglobulinemic			Biopsy

HDL, high-density lipoprotein.

Since their inception, stellate ganglion blocks have customarily been performed without controls. If a stellate ganglion block abolished the patient's pain, the response was assumed to be genuine and physiological. Indeed, so strongly established has been the faith in stellate ganglion blocks that they were excused challenge with controls. Textbooks that describe these blocks make no mention of the need for controls.[70, 71] The face validity and construct validity of the blocks is simply assumed. Only Bonica[72] briefly calls for the repetition of blocks with different agents in order to test the validity of the response.

The first controlled study of stellate ganglion blocks appeared some 50 years after their introduction into pain medicine. In patients with complex regional pain syndrome, Price *et al.*[73] injected the ganglion with either normal saline or local anesthetic. With either agent, just as many patients reported relief of pain immediately after the block. The only difference that emerged was that patients who received local anesthetic retained relief the following day; no patient who received normal saline was so relieved. Consequently, the immediate response to sympathetic blocks is not a valid criterion for sympathetically mediated pain. That criterion must be amended to prolong relief lasting to the following day.

Intravenous sympathetic blocks have not withstood challenge with placebo controls. Intravenous guanethidine does not have effects distinguishable from those of normal saline;[74, 75, 76, 77] nor does phentolamine.[78, 79, 80] This lack of specificity has led some authorities to suggest that the active component of intravenous sympathetic blocks is the application of the sphygmomanometer cuff.[77]

Diagnostic blocks

When the actual cause of a patient's pain cannot be established it might, nonetheless, be possible to establish its source. This can be done either by anesthetizing a suspected source directly, or by anesthetizing the nerves that mediate pain from that source. The attitude of pain physicians to such diagnostic blocks constitutes a fascinating exercise in pain politics and sociology.

In the assessment of patients with neuropathic pain, the use of diagnostic blocks is neither disputed nor frowned upon. In such patients, diagnostic blocks are used to determine if the pain is evoked by a peripheral source, such as a neuroma or ectopic discharges from an injured nerve. Failure to relieve neuropathic pain by peripheral blockade of nerves is taken as evidence of a more central mechanism for the pain. In this regard, diagnostic blocks are used not to make the diagnosis, but to determine the mechanism and source of pain.

Diagnostic blocks are also accepted procedures for the investigation of certain types of visceral pain, notably the pain of chronic pancreatitis. For these conditions, celiac plexus blocks or splanchnic nerve blocks are undertaken, usually as a prelude to neurolytic therapy. In this context, diagnostic blocks are undertaken as a prognostic exercise: as a test that neurolytic therapy might work.

Interestingly, there is no pressure or demand in the literature that diagnostic blocks for neuropathic pain or for visceral pain should be controlled; just as there has been no requirement that sympathetic blocks for complex regional pain syndromes be controlled. The same does not apply for diagnostic blocks for spinal pain.

Among the possible sources of low back pain are the lumbar zygapophysial joints and the sacroiliac joints. Among the sources of neck pain and headache are the cervical zygapophysial joints, the lateral atlantoaxial joints, and the atlantooccipital joints. For these joints, a variety of diagnostic blocks has been devised and implemented in some circles. Yet their use has met with acrimonious dissidence. Even though the validity of these blocks has been established in double-blind, controlled studies, they have been decried as amounting to no more than placebos.[81] The irony is that the same critics extol the virtues of sympathetic blocks, which lack double-blind, controlled studies.[81]

In the pursuit of neck pain, the atlantooccipital and lateral atlantoaxial joints can be anesthetized using intraarticular injections of local anesthetic agents.[82, 83, 84, 85, 86, 87] The cervical zygapophysial joints can be anesthetized using intraarticular blocks or blocks of the medial branches of the cervical dorsal rami.[88, 89, 90] These blocks have been shown to have face validity,[91] construct validity,[92, 93, 94] and therapeutic utility. When performed correctly, they block only the target nerve and not adjacent structures that feasibly might be an alternative source of pain.[91] When performed using appropriate controls, they reduce the rate of false-positive response.[92, 93, 94] When the response is positive, pain can be successfully relieved by a specific treatment (see below under Discussion).

In the pursuit of back pain, the sacroiliac joints can be anesthetized with intraarticular blocks,[95, 96, 97, 98, 99] and the lumbar zygapophysial joint can be anesthetized with intraarticular blocks or by blocks of the medial branches of the lumbar dorsal rami.[89, 99] Lumbar medial branch blocks have been shown to have face validity,[100] construct validity,[101, 102] and therapeutic utility. They selectively block only the target and do not spread to other structures, which might be alternative sources of pain, provided that correct techniques are used.[100] They protect normal volunteers from experimentally induced pain from the lumbar zygapophysial joints.[101] If used with appropriate controls, they reduce the rate of false-positive responses.[102] A positive response can be matched with a successful treatment (see below under Discussion).

No other blocks have been as thoroughly tested as diagnostic blocks of the zygapophysial joints. No other blocks have such a systematic and comprehensive literature covering studies in normal volunteers, face validity, construct validity, and predictive validity. That literature surpasses the literature on any of the more traditional blocks used in pain medicine. The reason for the bias against them remains unexplained.

Controls

Single, diagnostic blocks have unacceptably high false-positive rates. When these rates have been measured, they amount to between 25 and 41 percent.[102, 103, 104, 105] These high false-positive rates compromise the validity of any response. Without performing control blocks, the operator cannot tell if a positive response is true or false.

In practice, two types of control are available.[106] Pharmacologic controls require using different agents on the same target on separate occasions. Anatomic controls require applying the test to a different structure.

The ultimate pharmacologic control is a placebo block. However, this requires a sequence of three blocks.[106] On the first occasion, a local anesthetic must be used in order to establish, *prima facie*, that blocking the target nerve or structure does indeed relieve the patient's pain. Unless this is established, there is no point performing control blocks on a structure that is not the source of pain. The second block must be either a local anesthetic or normal saline, allocated randomly and in a double-blind fashion. The second block cannot routinely be the placebo, for an insightful patient would know that the second block is always the "dummy." Chance must be maintained. On the third occasion, the agent administered is the one not administered on the second occasion. Under these conditions, a positive response would be relief of pain on each occasion that a local anesthetic agent was used and no relief when normal saline was used.

There are no ethical objections to such a process, provided that the patient provides informed consent to undergo the sequence of tests. What is often prohibitive, however, is the number of procedures required.

A practical alternative is comparative local anesthetic blocks.[106] The patient undergoes the same block on separate occasions, but different local anesthetic agents are used. A concordant response is one in which the duration of relief is concordant with the expected duration of action of the agent used. The patient reports short-lasting relief when a short-acting agent is used (e.g. lidocaine) and long-lasting relief when a long-acting agent is used (e.g. bupivacaine). A discordant response is one in which the patient reports complete relief of pain following each block, but the duration of response is discordant with the expected duration of the agent used. Typically, this amounts to a prolonged response to lidocaine.

Validation studies, using placebo controls as the reference standard, have shown that concordant responses have only a 14 percent chance of being false-positive.[94] Reciprocally, that means an 86 percent chance of being true-positive. Discordant responses have a 35 percent chance of being false-positive, but a 65 percent chance of being true-positive. Whether an operator should accept concordant or discordant responses as constituting a positive response depends on the circumstances. If 65 percent diagnostic confidence is enough for practical purposes, a discordant response becomes acceptable. If greater diagnostic confidence is required, say before a destructive therapy based on the diagnosis, a concordant response may be preferable.[94]

For intraarticular blocks, pharmacologic controls cannot be used, because the normal duration of action of local anesthetic agents within joints is not known. Under these conditions, anatomic controls can be used. Under single-blind conditions, the operator targets an adjacent structure that is believed not to be the source of pain. Anatomic controls, however, are valid only if the target and control structures are both small and indistinguishably close to one another. If it is obvious to the patient that a different structure is being tested, the purpose of the control is defeated.

Disk stimulation

Disk stimulation is a test that involves provoking an intervertebral disk with injections of contrast medium into its nucleus pulposus. The test determines if stressing the disk in this way reproduces the patient's pain. A positive response implicates the disk as the source of the patient's pain.

Because disk stimulation relies on provoking a patient's pain, not relieving it, several measures need to be taken in order to secure the validity of the test. In general terms, these measures guard against a positive response being due to hyperalgesia.

In the first instance, disk stimulation requires anatomic controls. In order for the test to be positive, reproduction of pain upon testing one disk must be accompanied by no pain when adjacent disks are tested.

In the second instance, disk stimulation requires manometric controls. In a substantial proportion of normal individuals, a lumbar disk can be painful upon stimulation provided that the pressure of injection is sufficiently high.[107] A corollary to this phenomenon, however, is that below certain pressures of injection, normal disks have never been found to be painful.[107] Furthermore, when stimulation of normal disks does evoke pain, the pain is of low intensity. Consequently, in order for disk stimulation to be positive, the pressure of injection must be low (generally less than 40 psi), and the pain evoked must be of an intensity greater than five on a ten-point numerical pain rating scale.[107, 108]

If these precautions are not taken, lumbar disk stimulation can have an inordinately high false-positive rate.[109, 110] If anatomical and manometric controls are used, the false-positive rate can be kept to less than 10 percent.[107, 108]

Similar principles apply to cervical disk stimulation, but with certain modifications. In normal volunteers, cervical intervertebral can be made to hurt when stressed, but the evoked pain is typically of less intensity than that reported by patients.[111] Accordingly, for cervical disk stimulation to be positive, the evoked pain must be registered as greater than seven on a ten-point scale.[111, 112] Anatomical controls are mandatory, for it has been shown that it is uncommon for a single cervical disk to be painful; disks can be painful at two, three, and more levels.[113] Therefore, all cervical disks need to be studied, lest the result be confounded by sampling bias.[112] Furthermore, cervical disks can be false-positive when the patient has zygapophysial joint pain.[114] Therefore, cervical disk stimulation should only be performed once diagnostic blocks have excluded the zygapophysial joint as the source of pain.[112] Manometry of cervical disk stimulation has not been studied. Therefore, no manometric criteria for cervical disk stimulation have been developed or proposed.

APPLICATION

The *Classification of Chronic Pain* of the International Association for the Study of Pain[115] lists the common and rare chronic pain problems that pain physicians might encounter. For purposes of discussion, these conditions can be grouped into three categories: vascular and visceral diseases (**Table 12.5**), neurological, rheumatological, dental, and spinal diseases of known pathology (**Table 12.6**), and miscellaneous disorders for which no pathology is known (**Table 12.7**).

Vascular and visceral disorders

For vascular and visceral diseases (**Table 12.5**), the objective of investigations is to depict and define the lesion. Typically, these would involve imaging, such as ultrasound, MR imaging, or contrast studies for vessels and hollow viscera, direct visualization by endoscopy, biopsy, or organ-specific studies, such as electrocardiography, or disease-specific blood tests. The nature of these investigations and their application is not the province of pain medicine to dictate. They are determined by the medical specialties that conventionally deal with these problems.

Disorders of known pathology

The neurological conditions with known pathological causes (**Table 12.6**) are usually diagnosed on the basis of clinical features, and by and large do not require investigations. Peripheral neuropathies will be diagnosed clinically and by blood tests, but nerve conduction studies or nerve biopsy may be indicated if the diagnosis is in doubt. Syringomyelia will require MR imaging to determine the size and extent of the lesion. For Tolosa–Hunt syndrome, MR imaging is the best means of

Table 12.5 Visceral and vascular diseases associated with pain.

Diseases	
Angina pectoris	Carcinoma of the stomach
Myocardial infarction	Carcinoma of the pancreas
Pericarditis	Mesenteric ischemia
Aneurysm of the aorta	Crohn's disease
Cardiac failure	Diverticular disease
Postmastectomy pain	Carcinoma of the colon
Postthoracotomy pain	Porphyria
Internal mammary artery syndrome	Secondary dysmenorrhea
Ergotism	Endometriosis
Thromboangiitis obliterans	Parametritis
Chronic venous insufficiency	Salpingitis
Intermittent claudication	Retroversion of the uterus
Subphrenic abscess	Ovarian pain
Carcinoma of the esophagus	Carcinoma of thyroid
Herniated abdominal organs	Carcinoma of larynx
Esophageal motility disorders	Tuberculosis of larynx
Esophagitis	
Gallbladder	
Chronic gastric ulcer	
Chronic duodenal ulcer	

Table 12.6 Neurological, rheumatological, dental, and spinal diseases of known pathology that can cause pain.

Diseases	
Peripheral neuropathy	Rheumatoid arthritis
Guillain–Barré syndrome	Polymyalgia rheumatica
Stump pain	CPPD
Phantom pain	Gout
Central pain	Hemophilic arthropathy
Carpal tunnel syndrome	Tenosynovitis
Trigeminal neuralgia	Scleroderma
Postherpetic neuralgia	
Eagle's syndrome	Maxillary sinusitis
Tumors of the brachial plexus	Odontalgia
Chemical irritation of the brachial plexus	Dry socket
Avulsion of the brachial plexus	
Thoracic outlet syndrome	Spinal pain attributable to:
Syringomyelia	Fracture
Tolosa–Hunt syndrome	Infection
Temporal arteritis	Neoplasm
Low cerebrospinal fluid pressure headache	Metabolic bone disease
Postdural puncture headache	Arthritis

CPPD, calcium pyrophosphate deposition disease.

Table 12.7 Disorders associated with chronic pain for which no pathology is known.

Disorders	
Mittelschmerz	Acceleration–deceleration injury of the neck
Primary dysmenorrhea	Spinal pain of unknown origin
Irritable bowel syndrome	Gluteal syndromes
Recurrent abdominal pain in children	Piriformis syndrome
Acute tension headache	Spinal pain attributed to:
Chronic tension headache	Trigger point
Classic migraine	Muscle spasm
Common migraine	Segmental dysfunction
Cluster headache	Instability
	Spinal stenosis
Temporomandibular dysfunction	
Glossodynia and burning mouth	Discogenic pain
	Zygapophysial joint pain
Posttraumatic headache	Sacroiliac joint pain
Cervicogenic headache	
Occipital neuralgia	

confirming the presence of the lesion,[116, 117] but CT-guided needle biopsy may be required to establish the nature of the tissue.[118, 119] Temporal arteritis is diagnosed first by clinical features and a high erythrocyte sedimentation rate, but may require biopsy preceded by angiography to avoid skip lesions.

Rheumatologists will rely largely on clinical features and serology. Having diagnosed arthritis they will usually obtain plain films both to corroborate the diagnosis and to stage the severity of any joint destruction. No special investigations are required to determine the nature or cause of pain.

CT or MR imaging may be required to confirm a diagnosis of maxillary sinusitis. Chronic dental problems are diagnosed clinically, on the basis of history and examination, but imaging may be required to exclude underlying bone pathology.

For serious causes of spinal pain, a variety of screening tests are applicable, depending on the nature of the suspected pathology (**Table 12.8**). In all instances, testing should be predicated on the presence of clinical indicators. In the absence of clinical indicators, serious causes of spinal pain are extremely unlikely, and investigation is neither warranted nor indicated.

For infection, the patient should have features indicative of an infection, or should have a history of risk factors for infection. The latter encompass all manner of body penetrations that may be the source of inoculation, or suppressed immunity against infection. In the presence of such features, the first line of investigation is not routine imaging but serological tests (**Table 12.8**). Thereafter, MR imaging is the investigation of choice because of its high sensitivity and specificity for infection in and around the spine. For lack of sensitivity, plain radiography should not be used either to search for or to exclude spinal infection.

For suspected primary or secondary neoplastic disease of the spine, the clinical indicators are risk factors that raise the likelihood of cancer, and clinical features suggestive of neoplastic disease (**Table 12.8**). In the absence of such indicators, the likelihood that a patient has spinal pain due to neoplastic disease is virtually nil. In the presence of clinical indicators, or if cancer is nevertheless suspected, various laboratory tests are appropriate as first-line investigations (**Table 12.8**). Imaging is not indicated or warranted if laboratory tests are normal.

An explicit protocol has been advocated and tested for the investigation of patients in whom cancer is suspected.[120] It recommends the following:

- patients with a past history of cancer should be considered "high risk." In these patients an immediate erythrocyte sedimentation rate (ESR) and imaging is warranted; and a positive result on either test mandates further work up;
- patients under the age of 50 years, with no history of cancer, no weight loss, no signs of systemic illness, and who do not fail to improve, are considered "low risk." For these patients no laboratory tests or imaging are warranted;
- patients over 50 years, or those who fail to respond to treatment, or who have unexplained weight loss or signs of systemic illness constitute "intermediate risk." For these patients, an ESR is appropriate. If the ESR is <20 mm/hour, no further investigation is warranted. If the ESR is >20 mm/hour, imaging should be undertaken. If the imaging is normal, these patients should be closely monitored.

This protocol secures the detection of cancer without gratuitous use of unnecessary imaging. When first tested, this protocol considered plain radiography as the imaging investigation. A subsequent study promoted MR imaging or bone scan as the investigation of choice.[121] That study also showed that raising the threshold for imaging to an ESR of 50 increased the specificity of the protocol.

Aneurysms are an important differential diagnosis of spinal pain. The clinical indicators are the risk factors for aneurysm, and the absence of musculoskeletal signs consistent with a musculoskeletal source of pain. Aneurysms of the vertebral or internal carotid arteries can present with neck pain, and aortic aneurysms can present with back pain. Indeed, a pathology study reported that back pain was the most common presenting feature of patients who died of aortic aneurysm.[122] Magnetic resonance angiography is the preferred investigation for

Table 12.8 Clinical indicators and preferred investigations for possible serious causes of spinal pain.

Suspected pathology	Clinical indicators	Preferred test	
Infection	Fever Sweating Risk factors for infection (invasive medical procedure, injection, illicit drug use, trauma to skin or mucous membrane, immunosuppression, diabetes mellitus, alcoholism)	1st line 2nd line	ESR, FBC, CRP MR imaging
Tumor	Past history of malignancy Age greater than 50 Failure to improve Weight loss Pain not relieved by rest	All cases 1st line 2nd line Prostate Myeloma	 1: ESR, CRP 2: MR imaging PSA IEPG, serum protein electrophoresis
Aneurysm	Cardiovascular risk factors Anticoagulants Transient ischemic attacks Bruit History of torsion to neck No musculoskeletal signs	Vertebral, carotid Aorta	MRA Ultrasound

CRP, C-reactive protein; ESR, erythrocyte sedimentation rate; FBC, full blood count; IEPG, immunoelectrophoretogram; MRA, magnetic resonance angiography; MR imaging, magnetic resonance imaging; PSA, prostate-specific antigen.

cervical vascular disease. Ultrasound can be used for the abdominal aorta.

In patients with chronic spinal pain, fractures are most likely to have been detected during the early, acute phases of illness. Fractures, however, are uncommon causes of spinal pain. They should be considered in patients with a history of trauma, or following minor trauma in individuals with a risk factor for fracture, such as osteoporosis due to age or consumption of steroids. Even so, the prevalence of fractures is low. In emergency rooms, the prevalence of cervical fractures in patients presenting with suspected neck trauma is only about 3 percent.[123, 124, 125] In patients with neck pain, with no history of trauma, plain films typically reveal no abnormalities or only age-changes.[9, 126] In patients with back pain, with no history of trauma, the chances of an occult fracture being the cause of pain are essentially nil.[127]

Spinal pain due to arthritis does not refer to degenerative disc disease, it pertains to spinal pain due to rheumatoid arthritis or the spondylarthropathies. In these conditions, spinal pain does not occur in isolation; it occurs in the context of associated systemic features or arthropathy elsewhere in the body. As with other rheumatological diseases, the diagnosis is essentially clinical. Special investigations to determine the cause of pain are not required.

Metabolic diseases of bone, such as Paget's disease and primary hyperparathyroidism, are extremely rare causes of chronic spinal pain. For these conditions, laboratory tests, such as serum alkaline phosphatase levels and calcium levels, are the appropriate screening test.

Disorders of unknown pathology

The most troublesome conditions that befall a pain clinic are those for which no pathology is known (**Table 12.7**). For the visceral disorders, no special investigations are indicated once the condition has been established and other gynecological or gastrointestinal problems have been excluded. The various headaches are diagnosed by clinical features alone, and usually do not require further investigation. The investigation of temporomandibular dysfunction is highly controversial, and beyond the scope of this chapter. Options range from nothing to MR imaging and arthroscopy. No special investigations are known to be useful for burning mouth.

The remaining rubrics listed in **Table 12.7** concern the differential diagnosis of spinal pain. Some require and invite no investigations. Acceleration–deceleration injury of the neck is the formal rubric for whiplash – a diagnosis made on the basis of history alone. Similarly, spinal pain of unknown origin pertains to pain whose cause cannot be or has not been pursued. The gluteal and piriformis syndromes are diagnosed clinically, and do not require special investigations.

Although listed in the taxonomy,[115] spinal pain attributed to trigger point, muscle spasm, etc., are entities that effectively cannot be diagnosed. The reliability of examination for paraspinal trigger points is so poor that the entity defies validation.[128, 129] No reliable or valid tests are available for muscle spasm or segmental dysfunction. Although touted as a concept, instability remains undefined or undetectable by any conventional means. Whereas spinal stenosis can be demonstrated by CT of the lumbar spine, and whereas it is tenable as an explanation for claudication-like symptoms in the lower limbs, it is an inadequate explanation for any spinal pain suffered by patients with this condition.

The only entities for which investigations can be undertaken are discogenic pain, zygapophysial joint pain, and sacroiliac joint pain. Contrary to popular and traditional belief, these conditions account for the majority of patients with chronic spinal pain. Beliefs that chronic spinal pain cannot be, and should not be, investigated are predicated on the use, in the past, of tests to pinpoint the source or cause of pain that were never capable of doing so (e.g. plain radiography).

Chronic back pain

The disciplined investigation of chronic low back pain is predicated on the relative prevalence of various possible sources and causes of pain. In younger patients and in patients with a history of injury, the most common lesion is internal disk disruption. It accounts for at least 40 percent of cases.[130] Next most common is sacroiliac joint pain, which accounts for some 20 percent of cases.[96, 97] The prevalence of lumbar zygapophysial joint pain is not more than 15 percent,[131] and is probably less than 5 percent in these patients.[132, 133] In contrast, in elderly, uninjured patients, the prevalence of lumbar zygapophysial joint pain can be as high as 40 percent.[134]

These data influence the diagnostic strategy that might be assumed. The choice lies between pursuing discogenic pain or a source of pain in the synovial joints (**Figure 12.2**). The former would be indicated in younger injured patients and the latter in older patients with no history of trauma.

Another factor bears on this initial consideration. An MR image of the lumbar spine is an appropriate screening test before undertaking any invasive investigations for low back pain. Not only will it reveal any occult lesions not evident on or suspected from history, it also streamlines invasive investigations, preventing them from being undertaken arbitrarily or routinely.

If the MR image is absolutely normal and shows no changes in the intervertebral disks, the disks are unlikely to be the source of pain. Although disk stimulation may be positive in disks of normal appearance, this is an uncommon event (**Table 12.9**). Moreover, the available data are derived from studies conducted before contemporary manometric criteria were applied. Therefore, they may overstate the yield of disk stimulation in disks with normal appearance on MR imaging.

Consequently, in the interests of efficiency, the pursuit of discogenic pain should be avoided, in the first instance, in patients with pristine disks on MR imaging. Whether or not the disks should be investigated later is a practical and ethical question that can be considered once the diagnostic algorithm is otherwise exhausted. The pursuit of pain from the synovial joints is the option more likely to be productive in younger patients with normal disks, and in elderly patients with no evident source of pain.

DISK ALGORITHM

The MR image may show a high intensity zone (HIZ) in an annulus fibrosus. This sign should not be confused with fissure or unremarkable spots in the annulus. It consists of a bright signal, seen on carefully acquired T2-weighted images, with a brightness greater than that of the nucleus, and at least equivalent to that of the cerebrospinal fluid.[138, 139, 140, 141] When present in patients with back pain, it implicates the affected disk as the source of the patient's pain, with a positive likelihood ratio of 6.[138, 142] The sign is not common, being found in fewer than 30 percent of patients.[138, 139, 140, 141] However, when present, its high likelihood ratio renders it a diagnostic sign. For the diagnosis of internal disk disruption, a likelihood ratio of 6 converts the pretest likelihood of 40 percent to a diagnostic confidence of 80 percent. In that event, internal disk disruption can be diagnosed on the basis of MR imaging alone, and further investigation may not be necessary if all that is required is a diagnosis. Confirmation of discogenic pain by discography would be required only if destructive treatment is being entertained.

If the MR image does not show an HIZ, a critical consideration is if multiple disks are degraded. If that is the case, pursuit of discogenic pain is questionable, for if multiple disks are likely to be symptomatic there is no available, efficient treatment for multilevel disk disease.

If, however, only one or perhaps two, disks are abnormal, it is potentially profitable to establish a diagnosis of discogenic pain. This can be done by disk stimulation complemented by post-discography CT scanning.[108] Disk stimulation establishes if the disk is symptomatic. CT scanning established the internal morphology of the disk, and whether or not a fissure characteristic of internal disk disruption is present.

If disk stimulation is negative, investigating the sacroiliac and zygapophysial joint blocks should be considered (**Figure 12.2**). These may or may not be the source of pain despite the appearance of the disks on MR imaging, but having excluded the disks as the source of pain the chances are greater that the sacroiliac joint or the zygapophysial joints are the source of pain.

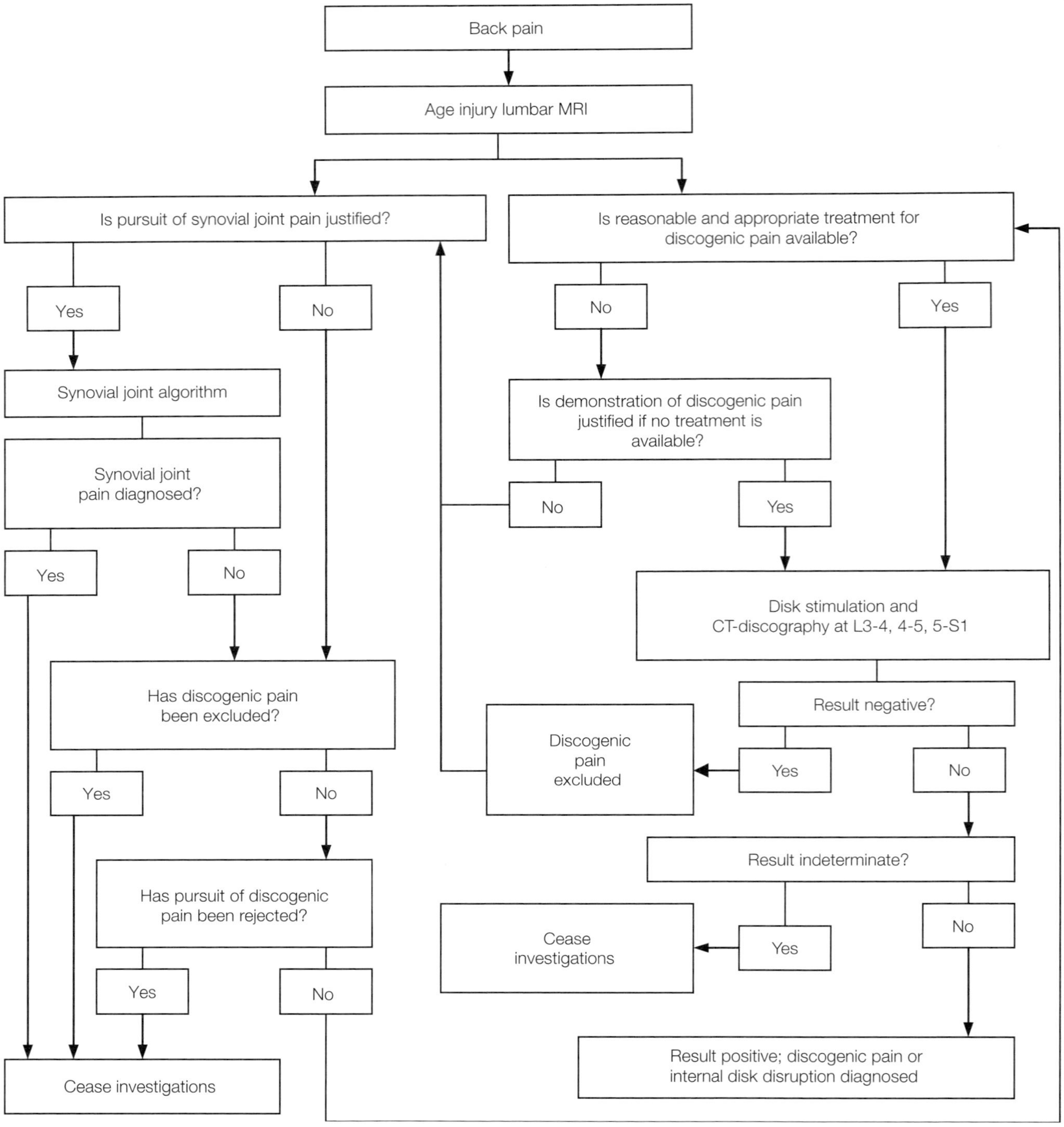

Figure 12.2 An algorithm for the investigation of low back pain.

SYNOVIAL JOINT ALGORITHM

If the synovial joint strategy is initiated, certain clinical decisions need to be taken before blocks are commenced (**Figure 12.3**). Rarely, if at all, have invasive tests been able to establish the source of pain in patients who have pain restricted to the midline, i.e. with no lateral radiation. Therefore, operators should carefully consider pursuing diagnostic blocks in such patients. Similarly, in patients with bilateral pain, operators should carefully consider if it is feasible and likely that the patient has bilateral sacroiliac joint pain. If not, it would be more efficient to pursue zygapophysial joint pain as the source, because these joints are far more likely to have suffered injuries bilaterally. Third, it is conspicuous from the research literature that sacroiliac joint pain does not project rostrally

Table 12.9 A contingency table correlating the results of magnetic resonance imaging against the results of provocation discography as the criterion standard for a symptomatic lumbar disk.

Magnetic resonance imaging	Disk stimulation	
	Symptomatic	Asymptomatic
Abnormal	201	152
Normal	50	234

Based on the pooled data of Osti and Fraser,[135] Horton and Daftari,[136] and Simmons *et al.*[137]
Sensitivity = 0.80; specificity = 0.60; positive predictive value = 0.57; negative predictive value = 0.82.

above L5.[96, 98] So, if the patient's pain is restricted to below this level, the sacroiliac joint becomes the more likely target. Conversely, if the pain extends above L5, the zygapophysial joints (or the disks) are the more likely source.

None of these clinical indicators is diagnostic of the source of pain in a positive sense; they do not predict that the chosen investigation will be positive. Their utility works in reverse. They render the competing source of pain as less likely, and serve to choose which investigation is less likely to be productive.

If the sacroiliac joint is selected as the target, this joint can be blocked using well-defined, established techniques.[95] If the response to a first block is negative, sacroiliac joint pain is excluded, and the investigations can turn to the zygapophysial joints (**Figure 12.4**). If the response to a first block is positive, that response is not diagnostic, because it could be false-positive. A control block must subsequently be performed. If the control block is negative, the diagnosis of sacroiliac joint pain is refuted, and the operator should carefully consider their next steps. They need to be confident that the placebo response to the first block was an isolated event, and not a sign that the patient is confused about their pain and its investigation. If the response to the control block is positive, a diagnosis of sacroiliac joint pain is established, and no further investigations are required.

A similar process applies to the investigation of zygapophysial joint pain. It is inefficient to investigate one joint at a time. The prevalence of zygapophysial joint pain is low, and the chances of negative responses are high. If joints are investigated one at a time, the chances are that multiple blocks will prove negative. This constitutes a waste of resources. It is more efficient to conduct a screening block, targeting multiple levels, in the first instance. If a screening block of multiple levels proves negative, further investigations are not warranted. Thereby, patients who do not have zygapophysial joint pain are identified with one test, and resources are not wasted performing multiple tests with negative results. The lower two segmental levels are the most commonly affected. So, the screening blocks should target these levels. Operators should have good cause to target joints at higher levels.

The appropriate procedure for screening blocks are medial branch blocks at L5, L4, and L3.[99] These are preferred over intraarticular blocks because they have been validated and are prognostic of the only proven treatment for lumbar zygapophysial joint pain, which is lumbar medial branch neurotomy.

If a patient proves negative to screening blocks, the operator needs to consider what next steps are justified. Sacroiliac joint blocks might be entertained, or investigations might cease.

If a patient has a positive response to screening blocks, further blocks should be undertaken in order to pinpoint the actual source of pain. For an accurate diagnosis, joints should be anesthetized one segment at a time, and the diagnosis confirmed by controlled blocks. Some operators elect to block multiple joints at a time, largely on the grounds that they are not reimbursed for multiple, sequential blocks. It should be recognized that this amounts to an idiosyncrasy of the reimbursement system, which does not reflect optimal practice.

If confirmatory blocks prove positive, a diagnosis of zygapophysial joint pain is established. If confirmatory blocks are negative, the operator should carefully consider if further investigations are justified.

Chronic neck pain

In order to rule out serious causes of pain, MR imaging of the cervical spine is the most appropriate screening test. Thereafter the possible sources of idiopathic pain are the muscles, ligaments, and joints of the cervical spine.

For muscles, there are no validated investigations. Some practitioners elect to inject tender points in cervical muscles, but usually as a form of treatment. No studies have validated intramuscular injections as a diagnostic test of neck pain.

Tears of the transverse ligament of the atlas, or of the alar ligaments, can occur after trauma, or in patients with upper cervical rheumatoid arthritis. No tests are available by which pain can be traced to these ligaments, but damage to them is manifest by upper cervical instability. Widening of the atlantoodontoid interval by more than 3 mm on flexion radiographs is evidence of impairment of the transverse ligament of the atlas. Rotation of the atlas to more than 56° on functional CT scans is evidence of tear of the contralateral alar ligament.[143] Functional MR imaging can demonstrate the lesion directly.[144] Such investigations are indicated in patients with upper neck pain and headache, with a history of trauma or rheumatoid arthritis, particularly in those patients in whom neck movement provokes nausea, and who themselves "feel" unstable.

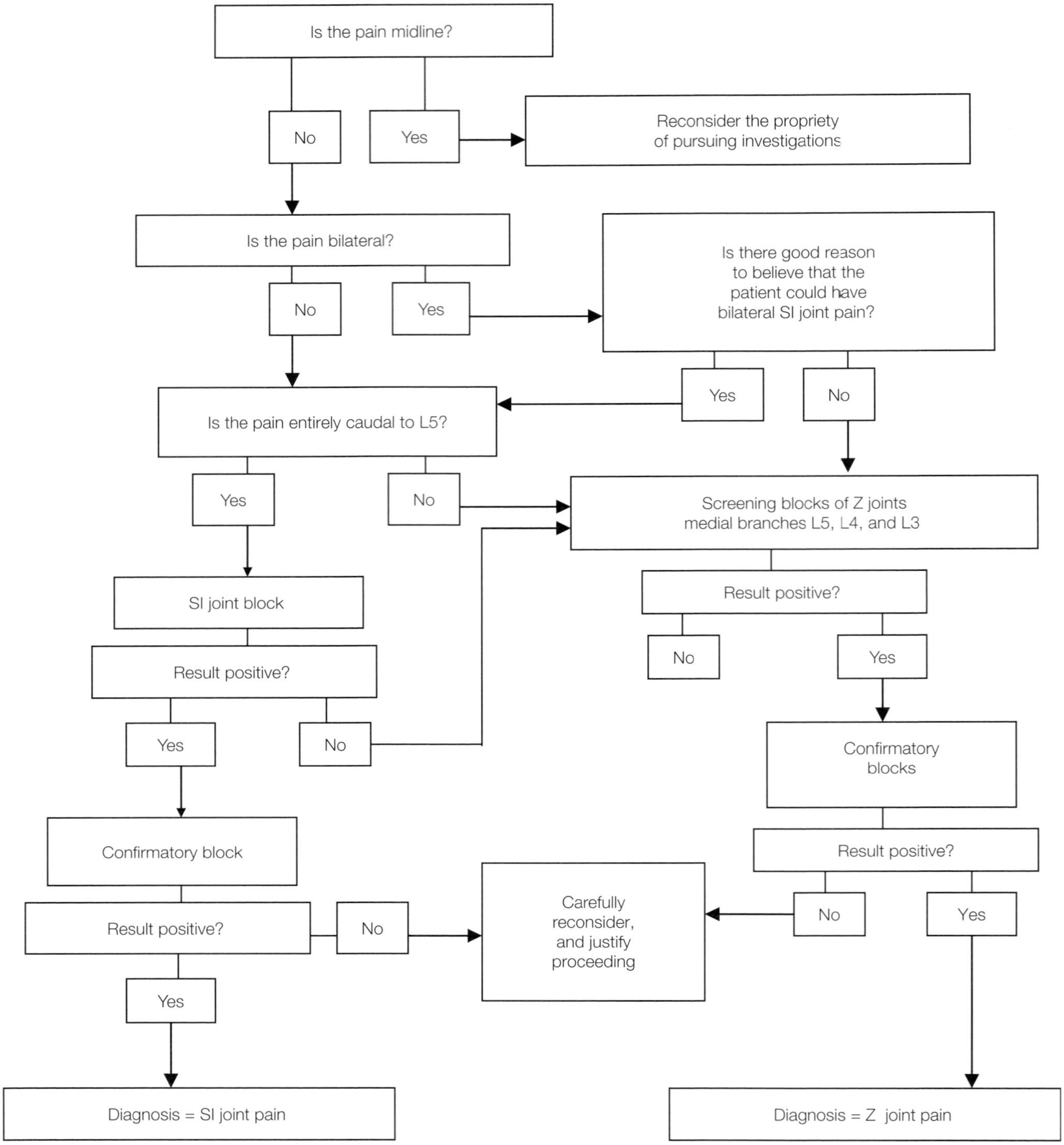

Figure 12.3 Algorithm for the investigation of the synovial joints of the lumbar and sacral region.

Disk stimulation can be undertaken in order to pursue sources of pain in the cervical disks, but this is a contentious issue. Some surgeons contend that finding the symptomatic disk indicates which level should be fused as treatment for the pain. However, no properly conducted outcome studies have yet vindicated this paradigm. Furthermore, the most comprehensive, available data indicate that surgery is indicated in only some 10 percent of cases with positive cervical disk stimulation.[113] In the remainder, too many disks at disparate levels prove positive and constitute a contraindication to surgery. In that regard, however, the diagnostic utility of cervical disk stimulation lies more in preventing surgery than in promoting it.

Moreover, cervical disk stimulation is false-positive in some 40 percent of cases, because the patient has zygapophysial joint pain at the affected segment.[114] Contemporary guidelines, therefore, recommend performing zygapophysial joint blocks before cervical disk stimulation.[112]

Multiple studies have shown that the cervical synovial joints are the most common source of chronic neck pain. Prevalence estimates range between 36 and 74 percent, with a representative value of 60 percent.[145, 146, 147, 148] These data justify, if not warrant, the pursuit of synovial joint pain for the diagnosis of chronic neck pain.

An algorithm can be followed to ensure optimal efficiency in the use of these blocks (**Figure 12.4**). Such an algorithm prevents blocks being performed arbitrarily. The algorithm is predicated on the prevalence of neck

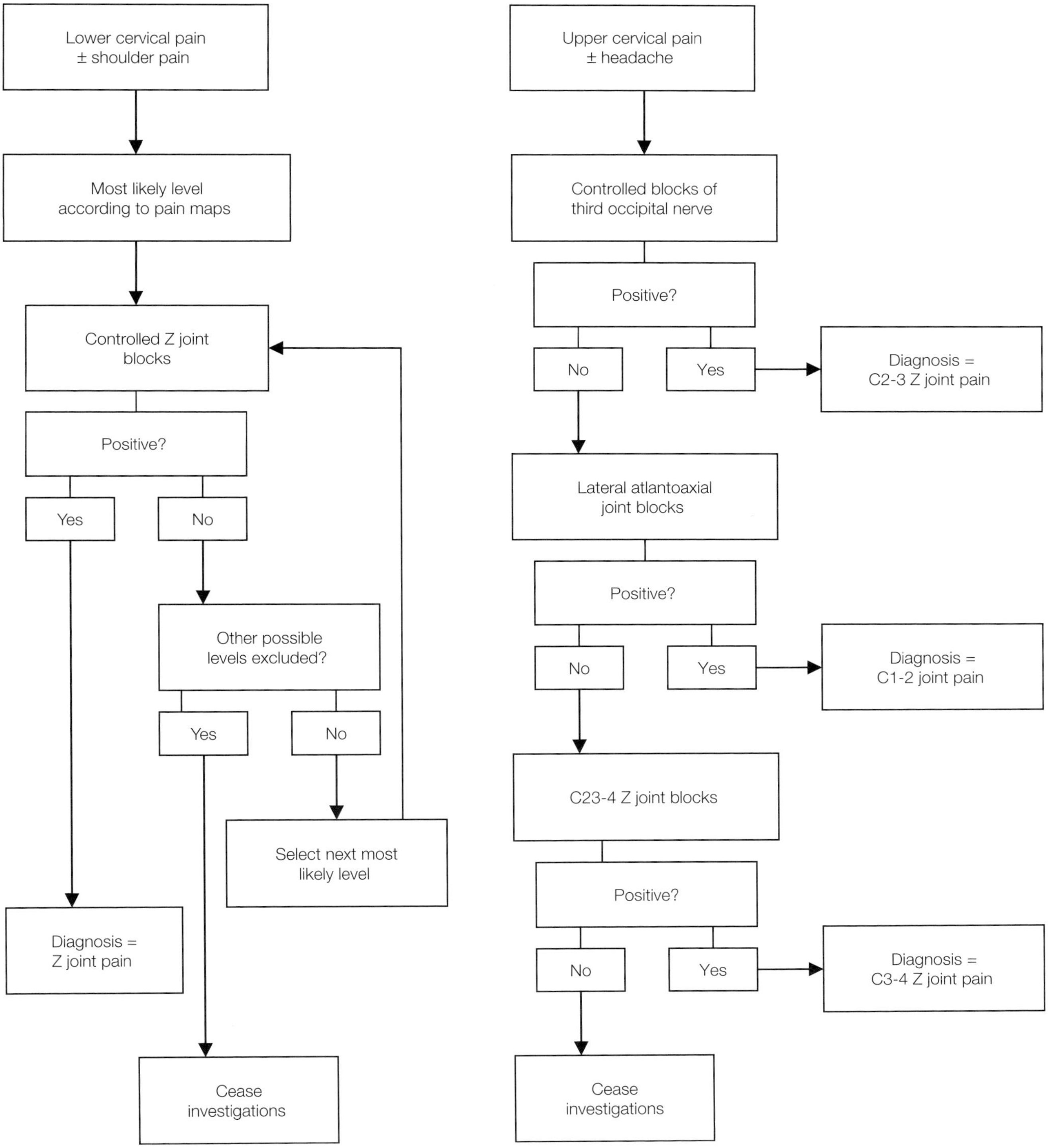

Figure 12.4 An algorithm for the investigation of neck pain, using diagnostic blocks.

pain stemming from the synovial joints, and on the recognition of pain patterns from these joints.

The first clinical step is to determine if the patient has upper cervical pain, with or without headache, or lower cervical pain, with or without referred pain to the shoulder girdle or upper limb. If a patient has both upper and lower cervical pain, their investigation can be staged, by addressing first either the lower or upper pain, and then the pain in the other distribution. This recommendation is predicated on the fact that lower cervical pain most often stems from the C5-6 or C6-7 joints, whereas upper cervical pain stems from the upper three segments.[149] When headache is the dominant symptom, the source of pain can nearly always be found in the upper synovial joints.[149] Rarely does headache stem from joints below C3-4, and when it does it is not the dominant symptom; lower neck pain is the cardinal complaint, and the headache appears only secondary.

Lower cervical pain can be investigated using cervical medial branch blocks to anesthetize the lower cervical zygapophysial joints. For the safe and accurate execution of this procedure, guidelines have been published.[90]

Pain maps[149, 150] can be used to select the most appropriate level at which to commence investigations (**Figure 12.5**). For pain that spreads over the supraspinous region of the scapula and into the deltoid region, C5-6 is the more likely source. For pain located more over the medial border of the scapula, C6-7 is the more likely source. Some patients can have pain stemming from both C5-6 and C6-7. Other publications provide instructions as to how to establish this diagnosis systematically and efficiently.[89, 90]

If controlled blocks at the first selected level are positive, the diagnosis of cervical zygapophysial joint pain is established. If the block is negative, the next most likely joint can be tested. Usually this will be the next joint above or below the first selected. If testing this second level with controlled blocks is positive, a diagnosis is established. If blocking the second level proves negative, investigations should cease. Careful consideration should be given before pursuing a third or more levels, for published experience has shown that the yield of positive responses of a third level is dwindling to small.

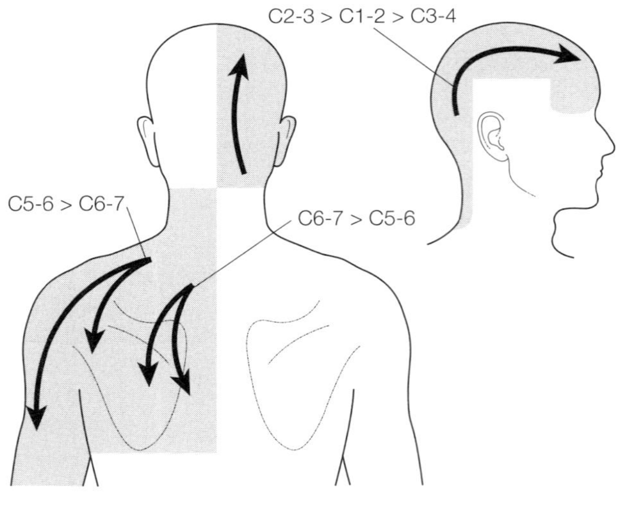

Figure 12.5 A map of the representative distribution of upper cervical and lower cervical pain, and the relative likelihoods of joints at the segments indicated being the source of pain.

For upper cervical pain and headache, the published data currently indicate that the C2-3 zygapophysial joint is the most likely source, followed by the lateral atlantoaxial joint. These pretest probabilities might change in the face of new data, but these are reigning likelihoods at present. C3-4 is an uncommon source of pain, and should be considered only after the first two levels have been excluded.

Accordingly, the algorithm (**Figure 12.4**) recommends that blocks be initiated at C2-3, using third occipital nerve blocks, for which guidelines have been published. If controlled blocks of the third occipital nerve prove positive, the diagnosis is established. If blocks are negative, the next investigation should be lateral atlantoaxial joint blocks. These require intraarticular placement of local anesthetic, because the nerve supply to this joint cannot be selectively anesthetized. If lateral atlantoaxial joint blocks prove positive, a diagnosis is established. If they are negative, the C3-4 joint should be investigated with medial branch blocks.

If blocks of these three joints prove negative, investigations should cease. Careful consideration should precede pursuing any other joints. Techniques are available by which to investigate the atlantooccipital joint, but no data are available as to how often these joints are a source of pain.

In patients with both upper and lower cervical pain, the most common diagnostic pattern is upper cervical pain stemming from C2-3 and lower cervical pain stemming from C5-6 or C6-7. In such patients, blocking C2-3 relieves their headache, but not their lower neck pain; blocking C5-6 or C6-7 relieves their lower neck pain, but not their upper neck pain and headache; while blocking C2-3 and C5-6 (or C6-7) simultaneously relieves all of their pain.

DISCUSSION

The utility of pursuing a diagnosis of spinal pain by invasive tests lies in two domains. It has diagnostic utility and can have therapeutic utility.

Diagnostic utility is an abstract concept. Establishing a diagnosis does not necessarily lead to a definitive treatment, but it nevertheless improves management. If a diagnosis is established, the patient has the satisfaction of knowing that their pain is real, and has a detectable source, even though it might not be treatable (at present). Establishing a diagnosis also provides closure. The patient may embark on a quest for treatment, but they no longer require further investigations for the sake of diagnosis.

Therapeutic utility is a more practical concept. It means that the diagnostic test leads to a valid treatment. For some spinal investigations therapeutic utility is still lacking. For others, there is a treatment that ensues.

Spinal fusion is still recommended, in some quarters, for patients with proven diskogenic pain, both in the cervical and in the lumbar spine. This remains a contentious issue, for there are no compelling data, to date, that fusion succeeds in relieving patients of their pain. Other options are being explored. This includes disk replacement and various intradiskal therapies. None is yet proven to the satisfaction of all critics, but patients might decide to avail themselves of these treatments in evolution.

Nor is there any proven treatment for sacroiliac joint pain. Arthrodesis is used by some surgeons, but convincing outcome data are lacking. Others have explored various ways of denervating the affected joint, but only preliminary data have appeared.

No conservative therapies have been validated for pain stemming from the atlantoaxial joints, but arthrodesis can be entertained. Fusing the joint provides long-term relief of pain.[151, 152]

For zygapophysial joint pain there are established treatments. Therefore, medial branch blocks for zygapophysial joint pain have therapeutic utility. For lumbar medial branch neurotomy, a controlled trial showed that the effect cannot be attributed to placebo.[152] An outcome study showed that, if patients are selected using controlled blocks, and if the correct technique is used, some 60 percent of patients maintain at least 80 percent relief of pain at 12 months, and some 80 percent of patients maintain at least 60 percent relief.[153] Since the treated nerves recover, pain can recur. In that event, repeating the treatment reinstates relief.[154]

Similar, but stronger data apply to cervical medial branch blocks. Pain that is completely relieved by controlled medial branch blocks can be relieved by cervical radiofrequency neurotomy. The efficacy of this procedure has been established in a placebo-controlled trial, complemented by long-term follow up.[155, 156, 157, 158] For lower cervical pain, the success rate is 70 percent for achieving complete relief of pain.[155, 156, 157] Third occipital neurotomy completely relieves headache stemming from the C2-3 joint in some 86 percent of cases.[158] If pain recurs, when the nerve recovers, relief can be reinstated by repeating the procedure.[156, 157, 158]

REFERENCES

1. Stiell IG, Greenberg GH, Wells GA *et al.* Prospective validation of a decision rule for the use of radiography in acute knee injuries. *Journal of the American Medical Association.* 1996; **278**: 611–5.

* 2. Stiell IG, Wells GA, Hoag RH *et al.* Implementation of the Ottawa Knee Rule for the use of radiography in acute knee injuries. *Journal of the American Medical Association.* 1997; **278**: 2075–9.

3. Seaberg DC, Yealy DM, Lukens T *et al.* Multicenter comparison of two clinical decision rules for the use of radiography in acute, high-risk knee injuries. *Annals of Emergency Medicine.* 1998; **32**: 8–13.

4. Seaberg DC, Jackson R. Clinical decision rule for knee radiographs. *American Journal of Emergency Medicine.* 1994; **12**: 541–3.

* 5. Stiell IG, Wells GA, Vandemheen KL *et al.* The Canadian C-spine rule for radiography in alert and stable trauma patients. *Journal of the American Medical Association.* 2001; **286**: 1841–8.

* 6. Stiell IG, Greenberg GH, McKnight RD *et al.* Decision rules for the use of radiography in acute ankle injuries. *Journal of the American Medical Association.* 1993; **269**: 1127–32.

7. Gore DR, Sepic SB, Gardner GM. Roentgenographic findings of the cervical spine in asymptomatic people. *Spine.* 1986; **11**: 521–4.

8. Elias F. Roentgen findings in the asymptomatic cervical spine. *New York State Journal of Medicine.* 1958; **58**: 3300–03.

* 9. Heller CA, Stanley P, Lewis-Jones B, Heller RF. Value of x ray examinations of the cervical spine. *British Medical Journal.* 1983; **287**: 1276–8.

10. Friedenberg ZB, Miller WT. Degenerative disc disease of the cervical spine. A comparative study of asymptomatic and symptomatic patients. *Journal of Bone and Joint Surgery.* 1963; **45**: 1171–8.

11. Torgerson WR, Dotter WE. Comparative roentgenographic study of the asymptomatic and symptomatic lumbar spine. *Journal of Bone and Joint Surgery.* 1976; **58**: 850–3.

12. Magora A, Schwartz A. Relation between the low back pain syndrome and x-ray findings. *Scandinavian Journal of Rehabilitation Medicine.* 1976; **8**: 115–26.

13. Fullenlove TM, Williams AJ. Comparative roentgen findings in symptomatic and asymptomatic backs. *Radiology.* 1957; **68**: 572–4.

14. Splithoff CA. Lumbosacral junction: Roentgenographic comparison of patients with and without backaches. *Journal of the American Medical Association.* 1953; **152**: 1610–3.

15. Witt I, Vestergaard A, Rosenklint A. A comparative analysis of x-ray findings of the lumbar spine in patients with and without lumbar pain. *Spine.* 1984; **9**: 298–300.

16. Lawrence JS, Bremner JM, Bier F. Osteo-arthrosis. Prevalence in the population and relationship between symptoms and x-ray changes. *Annals of the Rheumatic Diseases.* 1966; **25**: 1–24.

17. McAlindon TE. The knee. *Bailliere's Clinical Rheumatology.* 1999; **13**: 329–44.

18. Croft P. Diagnosing regional pain: the view from primary care. *Bailliere's Clinical Rheumatology.* 1999; **13**: 231–42.

19. Lane NE, Thompson JM. Management of osteoarthritis in the primary care setting: an evidence-based approach to treatment. *American Journal of Medicine*. 1997; **103**: 25S–30S.
20. Hadler NM. Knee pain is the malady – not osteoarthritis. *Annals of Internal Medicine*. 1992; **116**: 598–9.
21. Mont M, Hungerford DS. Non-traumatic avascular necrosis of the femoral head. *Journal of Bone and Joint Surgery*. 1995; **77**: 459–74.
* 22. Boden SD, Davis DO, Dina TS *et al*. Abnormal magnetic-resonance scans of the lumbar spine in asymptomatic subjects. *Journal of Bone and Joint Surgery*. 1990; **72**: 403–08.
23. Jensen MC, Bran-Zawadzki MN, Obucjowski N *et al*. Magnetic resonance imaging of the lumbar spine in people without back pain. *New England Journal of Medicine*. 1994; **331**: 69–73.
24. Boden SD, McCowin PR, Davis DG *et al*. Abnormal magnetic-resonance scans of the cervical spine in asymptomatic subjects: a prospective investigation. *Journal of Bone and Joint Surgery*. 1990; **72**: 1178–84.
25. Teresi LM, Lufkin RB, Reicher MA *et al*. Asymptomatic degenerative disk disease and spondylosis of the cervical spine: MR imaging. *Radiology*. 1987; **164**: 83–8.
* 26. Sher JS, Uribe JW, Posada A *et al*. Abnormal findings on magnetic resonance images of asymptomatic shoulders. *Journal of Bone and Joint Surgery*. 1995; **77**: 10–15.
27. Milgrom C, Schaffler M, Gilbert S, van Holsbeeck M. Rotator-cuff changes in asymptomatic adults. *Journal of Bone and Joint Surgery*. 1995; **77**: 296–8.
28. Chandnani V, Ho C, Gerharter J *et al*. MR findings in asymptomatic shoulders: a blind analysis using symptomatic shoulders as controls. *Clinical Imaging*. 1992; **16**: 25–30.
29. Modic MT, Masaryk TJ, Mulopulos GP *et al*. Cervical radiculopathy: prospective evaluation with surface coil MR imaging, CT with metrizamide, and metrizamide myelography. *Radiology*. 1986; **161**: 753–9.
30. Yousem DM, Atlas SW, Goldberg HI, Grossman RI. Degenerative narrowing of the cervical spine neural foraminal evaluation with high-resolution 3-DFT gradient echo MR imaging. *American Journal of Roentgenology*. 1991; **156**: 1229–36.
31. Kaiser JA, Holland BA. Imaging of the cervical spine. *Spine*. 1998; **23**: 2701–12.
32. Brown BM, Schwartz RH, Frank E, Blank NK. Preoperative evaluation of cervical radiculopathy and myelopathy by surface-coil MR imaging. *American Journal of Roentgenology*. 1988; **151**: 1205–12.
33. Hedberg MC, Drayer BP, Flom RA *et al*. Gradient echo (GRASS) MR imaging in cervical radiculopathy. *American Journal of Roentgenology*. 1988; **150**: 683–9.
34. Tyson LL. Imaging of the painful shoulder. *Current Problems in Diagnostic Radiology*. 1995; **24**: 110–40.
35. Norris TR, Green A. Imaging modalities in the evaluation of shoulder disorders. In: Matsen FA, Fu FH, Hawkins RJ (eds). *The shoulder: a balance of mobility and stability*. Rosement, IL: American Academy of Orthopaedic Surgeons, 1993: 353–67.
36. Stiles RG, Otte MT. Imaging of the shoulder. *Radiology*. 1993; **188**: 603–13.
37. Lowe J, Schachner E, Hirschberg E *et al*. Significance of bone scintigraphy in symptomatic spondylolysis. *Spine*. 1984; **9**: 653–5.
38. Elliot S, Huitson A, Wastie ML. Bone scintigraphy in the assessment of spondylolysis in patients attending a sports injury clinic. *Clinical Radiology*. 1988; **39**: 269–72.
39. Jackson DW, Wiltse LL, Dingeman RD, Hayes M. Stress reactions involving the pars interarticularis in young athletes. *American Journal of Sports Medicine*. 1981; **9**: 304–12.
40. Van den Oever M, Merrick MV, Scott JHS. Bone scintigraphy in symptomatic spondylolysis. *Journal of Bone and Joint Surgery*. 1987; **69B**: 453–6.
41. Mackinnon SE, Holder LE. The use of three-phase radio-nucleotide bone scanning in the diagnosis of reflex sympathetic dystrophy. *Journal of Hand Surgery*. 1984; **9**: 556–63.
42. Atkins RM, Tindale W, Bickerstaff D, Kanis JA. Quantitative bone scintigraphy in reflex sympathetic dystrophy. *British Journal of Rheumatology*. 1993; **32**: 41–5.
* 43. Harden RN, Bruehl S, Galer BS *et al*. Complex regional pain syndrome: are the IASP diagnostic criteria valid and sufficiently comprehensive? *Pain*. 1999; **83**: 211–9.
44. Harden RN, Bruehl SP. Diagnostic criteria: the statistical derivation of the four criterion factors. In: Wilson PR, Stanton-Hicks M, Harden RN (eds). *CRPS: Current diagnosis and therapy*. Progress in Pain Research and Management, Vol 32. Seattle: IASP Press, 2005: 45–58.
45. Mulconrey DS, Knight RQ, Bramble JD *et al*. Interobserver reliability in the interpretation of diagnostic lumbar MRI and nuclear imaging. *Spine Journal*. 2006; **6**: 177–84.
46. Littenberg B, Siegel A, Tosteson ANA, Mead T. Clinical efficacy of SPECT bone imaging for low back pain. *Journal of Nuclear Medicine*. 1995; **36**: 1707–13.
47. Pneumaticos SG, Chatziioannou SN, Hipp JA *et al*. Low back pain: prediction of short-term outcome of facet joint injection with bone scintigraphy. *Radiology*. 2006; **238**: 693–8.
48. Dolan AL, Ryan PJ, Arden NK *et al*. The value of SPECT scans in identifying back pain likely to benefit from facet joint injection. *British Journal of Rheumatology*. 1996; **35**: 1269–73.
49. Schwarzer AC, Scott AM, Wang S *et al*. The role of bone scintigraphy in chronic low back pain: comparison of SPECT and planar images and zygapophysial joint injection. *Australia and New Zeland Journal of Medicine*. 1992; **22**: 185.
50. von Rossum J, Brauma OJ, Kamphuisen HA, Onvlee GJ. Tennis elbow – a radial tunnel syndrome? *Journal of Bone and Joint Surgery*. 1978; **60B**: 197–8.
51. Rozmaryn LM. Carpal tunnel syndrome: a comprehensive review. *Current Opinion in Orthopedics*. 1997; **8**: 33–43.

52. Buch-Jaeger N, Foucher G. Correlation of clinical signs with nerve conduction tests in the diagnosis of carpal tunnel syndrome. *Journal of Hand Surgery.* 1994; **19B**: 720–4.
53. Nathan PA, Keniston RC, Myers LD, Meadows KD. Longitudinal study of median nerve sensory conduction in industry: relationship to age, gender, hand dominance, occupational hand use, and clinical diagnosis. *Journal of Hand Surgery.* 1992; **17**: 850–7.
54. Katz JN, Larson MG, Fossel AH, Liang MH. Validation of surveillance case definition of carpal tunnel syndrome. *American Journal of Public Health.* 1991; **81**: 189–93.
55. Atroshi I, Gummesson C, Johnsson R *et al.* Prevalence of carpal tunnel syndrome in a general population. *Journal of the American Medical Association.* 1999; **282**: 153–8.
56. Redmond MD, Rivner MH. False positive elecrodiagnostic tests in carpal tunnel syndrome. *Muscle and Nerve.* 1988; **11**: 511–7.
57. Hadler NM. Carpal tunnel syndrome, diagnostic conundrum. *Journal of Rheumatology.* 1997; **24**: 417–9.
58. Knutsson B. Comparative value of electromyographic myelographic and clinical-neurological examinations in diagnosis of lumbar root compression syndrome. *Acta Orthopaedica Scandinavica. Supplementum.* 1961; **49**: 1–135.
59. Tullberg T, Svanborg E, Isacsson J, Grane P. A preoperative and postoperative study of the accuracy and value of electrodiagnosis in patients with lumbosacral disc herniation. *Spine.* 1993; **18**: 837–42.
60. La Joie WJ. Nerve root compression: correlation of electromyographic, myelographic and surgical findings. *Archives of Physical Medicine and Rehabilitation.* 1972; **53**: 390–2.
∗ 61. Dvorak J. Neurophysiologic tests in diagnosis of nerve root compression caused by disc herniation. *Spine.* 1996; **21** (Suppl. 24S): 39S–44S.
∗ 62. Andersson GBJ, Brown MD, Dvorak J *et al.* Consensus summary on the diagnosis and treatment of lumbar disc herniation. *Spine.* 1996; **21** (Suppl. 24S): 75S–8S.
63. Dvorak J. Epidemiology, physical examination and neurodiagnostics. *Spine.* 1998; **23**: 2663–73.
64. Dumitru D, Dreyfuss P. Dermatomal/segmental somatosensory evoked potential evaluation of L5-/S1 unilateral/unilevel radiculopathies. *Muscle and Nerve.* 1996; **19**: 442–9.
65. Thomas D, McCullum D, Siahamis G, Langlois S. Infrared thermographic imaging, magnetic resonance imaging, CT scan and myelography in low back pain. *British Journal of Rheumatology.* 1990; **29**: 268–73.
66. Uematsu S, Hendler N, Hungerford D *et al.* Thermography and electrode-myography in the differential diagnosis of chronic pain syndromes and reflex sympathetic dystrophy. *Electromyography and Clinical Neurophysiology.* 1981; **21**: 165–82.
67. Rommel O, Häbler HJ, Schürmann MA. Laboratory tests for complex regional pain syndrome. In: Wilson P, Stanton-Hicks M, Harden RN (eds). *CRPS: Current diagnosis and therapy.* Progress in Pain Research and Management, Vol 32. Seattle: IASP Press, 2005: 139–59.
68. Sommer C, Lauria G. Painful small-fibre neuropathies. In: Cervero F, Jensen TS (eds). *Handbook of clinic neurology, vol. 81 (3rd series): Pain.* Elsevier, Amsterdam, 2005: 621–33.
69. Ginsberg L. Specific painful neuropathies. In: Cervero F, Jensen TS (eds). *Handbook of clinic neurology, volume 81 (3rd series): Pain.* Elsevier, Amsterdam, 2005: 635–52.
70. Lofstrom JB, Cousins MJ. Sympathetic neural blockade of upper and lower extremity. In: Cousins MJ, Bridenbaugh PO (eds). *Neural blockade in clinical anesthesia and management of pain*, 2nd edn. Philadelphia: Lippincott, 1988: 461–500.
71. Verril P. Sympathetic ganglion lesions. In: Wall PD, Melzack R (eds). *Textbook of pain*, 2nd edn. Edinburgh: Churchill Livingstone, 1989: 773–83.
72. Bonica JJ. Causalgia and other reflex sympathetic dystrophies. In: Bonica JJ (ed.). *The management of pain*, 2nd edn. Volume 1. Philadelphia: Lea and Febiger, 1990: 220–43.
∗ 73. Price DD, Long S, Wilsey B, Rafii A. Analysis of peak magnitude and duration of analgesia produced by local anesthetics injected into sympathetic ganglia of complex regional pain syndrome patients. *Clinical Journal of Pain.* 1998; **14**: 216–26.
74. Rocco AG, Kaul AF, Reisman RM *et al.* A comparison of regional intravenous guanethidine and reserpine in reflex sympathetic dystrophy: a controlled, randomized, double-blind cross-over study. *Clinical Journal of Pain.* 1989; **5**: 205–09.
75. Blanchard J, Ramamurthy S, Walsh N *et al.* Intravenous regional sympatholysis: a double-blind comparison of guanethidine, reserpine, and normal saline. *Journal of Pain and Symptom Management.* 1990; **5**: 357–61.
76. Ramamurthy S, Hoffman J, Group GS. Intravenous regional guanethidine in the treatment of reflex sympathetic dystrophy/causalgia: a randomized, double-blind study. *Anesthesia and Analgesia.* 1995; **81**: 718–23.
∗ 77. Jadad AR, Caroll D, Glynn CJ, McQuay HJ. Intravenous regional sympathetic blockade for pain relief in reflex sympathetic dystrophy: a systematic review and a randomized double-blind crossover study. *Journal of Pain and Symptom Management.* 1995; **10**: 13–20.
78. Fine PG, Roberts WJ, Gillete RG, Child TR. Slowly developing placebo responses confound tests of intravenous phentolamine to determine mechanisms underlying idiopathic chronic low back pain. *Pain.* 1994; **56**: 235–42.
79. Verdugo RJ, Ochoa JL. 'Sympathetically maintained pain'. I: Phentolamine block questions the concept. *Neurology.* 1994; **44**: 1003–10.
80. Verdugo RJ, Campero M, Ochoa JL. Phentolamine sympathetic block in painful polyneuropathies. II: Further questioning of the concept of 'sympathetically maintained pain'. *Neurology.* 1994; **44**: 1010–4.
81. Hogan QH, Abram SE. Diagnostic and prognostic neural blockade. In: Cousins MJ, Bridenbaugh PO (eds). *Neural*

blockade in clinical anesthesia and management of pain, 3rd edn. Philadelphia: Lippincott-Raven, 1998: 837–977.

82. Dreyfuss P, Michaelsen M, Fletcher D. Atlanto-occipital and lateral atlanto-axial joint pain patterns. *Spine*. 1994; **19**: 1125–31.
83. Busch E, Wilson PR. Atlanto-occipital and atlanto-axial injections in the treatment of headache and neck pain. *Regional Anesthesia*. 1989; **14** (Suppl. 2): 45.
84. McCormick CC. Arthrography of the atlanto-axial (C1-C2) joints: technique and results. *Journal of Interventional Radiology*. 1987; **2**: 9–13.
85. Dreyfuss P, Rogers J, Dreyer S, Fletcher D. Atlanto-occipital joint pain. A report of three cases and description of an intra-articular joint block technique. *Regional Anesthesiaesia*. 1994; **19**: 344–53.
*86. Aprill C, Axinn MJ, Bogduk N. Occipital headaches stemming from the lateral atlanto-axial (C1-2) joint. *Cephalalgia*. 2002; **22**: 15–22.
87. International Spine Intervention Society. Lateral atlanto-axial joint blocks. In: Bogduk N (ed.). *Practice guidelines for spinal diagnostic and treatment procedures*. San Francisco: International Spinal Intervention Society, 2004: 138–51.
*88. Bogduk N, Lord SM. Cervical zygapophysial joint pain. *Neurosurgery Quarterly*. 1998; **8**: 107–17.
89. Bogduk N. International Spinal Injection Society guidelines for the performance of spinal injection procedures. Part 1: zygapophysial joint blocks. *Clinical Journal of Pain*. 1997; **13**: 285–302.
90. International Spine Intervention Society. Cervical medial branch blocks. In: Bogduk N (ed.). *Practice guidelines for spinal diagnostic and treatment procedures*. San Francisco: International Spinal Intervention Society, 2004: 112–37.
91. Barnsley L, Bogduk N. Medial branch blocks are specific for the diagnosis of cervical zygapophysial joint pain. *Regional Anesthesia*. 1993; **18**: 343–50.
92. Barnsley L, Lord S, Wallis B, Bogduk N. False-positive rates of cervical zygapophysial joint blocks. *Clinical Journal of Pain*. 1993; **9**: 124–30.
93. Barnsley L, Lord S, Bogduk N. Comparative local anesthetic blocks in the diagnosis of cervical zygapophysial joints pain. *Pain*. 1993; **55**: 99–106.
94. Lord SM, Barnsley L, Bogduk N. The utility of comparative local anesthetic blocks versus placebo-controlled blocks for the diagnosis of cervical zygapophysial joint pain. *Clinical Journal of Pain*. 1995; **11**: 208–13.
95. International Spine Intervention Society. Sacroiliac joint blocks. In: Bogduk N (ed.). *Practice guidelines for spinal diagnostic and treatment procedures*. San Francisco: International Spinal Intervention Society, 2004: 66–85.
96. Schwarzer AC, Aprill CN, Bogduk N. The sacroiliac joint in chronic low back pain. *Spine*. 1995; **20**: 31–7.
*97. Maigne JY, Aivaliklis A, Pfefer F. Results of sacroiliac joint double block and value of sacroiliac pain provocation tests in 54 patients with low-back pain. *Spine*. 1996; **21**: 1889–92.
98. Dreyfuss P, Michaelsen M, Pauza K *et al*. The value of history and physical examination in diagnosing sacroiliac joint pain. *Spine*. 1996; **21**: 2594–602.
99. International Spine Intervention Society. Lumbar medial branch blocks. In: Bogduk N (ed.). *Practice guidelines for spinal diagnostic and treatment procedures*. San Francisco: International Spinal Intervention Society, 2004: 47–65.
*100. Dreyfuss P, Schwarzer AC, Lau P, Bogduk N. Specificity of lumbar medial branch and L5 dorsal ramus blocks: a computed tomographic study. *Spine*. 1997; **22**: 895–902.
*101. Kaplan M, Dreyfuss P, Halbrook B, Bogduk N. The ability of lumbar medial branch blocks to anesthetize the zygapophysial joint. *Spine*. 1998; **23**: 1847–52.
102. Schwarzer AC, Aprill CN, Derby R *et al*. The false-positive rate of uncontrolled diagnostic blocks of the lumbar zygapophysial joints. *Pain*. 1994; **58**: 195–200.
103. Manchikanti L, Pampati V, Fellows B, Bakhit CE. Prevalence of lumbar facet joint pain in chronic low back pain. *Pain Physician*. 1999; **2**: 59–64.
104. Manchikanti L, Pampati V, Fellows B, Bakhit CE. The diagnostic validity and therapeutic value of lumbar facet joint nerve blocks with or without adjuvant agents. *Current Review of Pain*. 2000; **4**: 337–44.
105. Barnsley L, Lord S, Wallis B, Bogduk N. False-positive rates of cervical zygapophysial joint blocks. *Clinical Journal of Pain*. 1993; **9**: 124–30.
*106. Bogduk N. Diagnostic nerve blocks in chronic pain. *Best Practice and Research Clinical Anaesthesiology*. 2002; **16**: 565–78.
*107. Derby R, Lee SH, Kim BJ *et al*. Pressure-controlled lumbar discography in volunteers without low back symptoms. *Pain Medicine*. 2005; **6**: 213–21.
108. International Spinal Intervention Society. Lumbar disc stimulation. In: Bogduk N (ed.). *Practice guidelines for spinal diagnostic and treatment procedures*. San Francisco: International Spinal Intervention Society, 2004: 20–46.
109. Carragee EJ, Tanner CM, Yang B *et al*. False-positive findings on lumbar discography: reliability of subjective concordance assessment during provocative disc injection. *Spine*. 1999; **24**: 2542–7.
110. Carragee EJ, Tanner CM, Khurana S *et al*. The rates of false-positive lumbar discography in select patients without low back symptoms. *Spine*. 2000; **25**: 1373–81.
111. Schellhas KP, Smith MD, Gundry CR, Pollei SR. Cervical discogenic pain: prospective correlation of magnetic resonance imaging and discography in asymptomatic subjects and pain sufferers. *Spine*. 1996; **21**: 300–12.
112. International Spine Intervention Society. Cervical disc stimulation. In: Bogduk N (ed.). *Practice guidelines for spinal diagnostic and treatment procedures*. San Francisco: International Spinal Intervention Society, 2004: 95–111.
*113. Grubb SA, Kelly CK. Cervical discography: clinical implications from 12 years of experience. *Spine*. 2000; **25**: 1382–9.

*114. Bogduk N, Aprill C. On the nature of neck pain, discography and cervical zygapophysial joint pain. *Pain*. 1993; **54**: 213–7.

115. Merskey H, Bogduk N (eds). *Classification of chronic pain. descriptions of chronic pain syndromes and definitions of pain terms*, 2nd edn. Seattle: IASP Press, 1994.

116. Yousem DM, Atlas SW, Grossman RI *et al*. MR imaging of Tolosa–Hunt syndrome. *American Journal of Neuroradiology*. 1989; **10**: 1181–4.

117. Goto Y, Hosokawa S, Goto I *et al*. Abnormality in the cavernous sinus in three patients with Tolosa–Hunt syndrome: MRI and CT findings. *Journal of Neurology, Neurosurgery, and Psychiatry*. 1990; **53**: 231–4.

118. Rowed DW, Kassel EE, Lewis AJ. Transorbital intracavernous needle biopsy in painful ophthalmoplegia. *Journal of Neurosurgery*. 1985; **62**: 776–80.

119. Tobias S, Lee JH, Tomford JW. Rare actinobacilis infection of the cavernous sinus causing painful ophthalmoplegia: case report. *Neurosurgery*. 2002; **51**: 807–09.

120. Deyo RA, Diehl AK. Cancer as a cause of back pain: frequency, clinical presentation and diagnostic strategies. *Journal of General Internal Medicine*. 1988; **3**: 230–8.

*121. Joines JD, McNuff RA, Carey TS *et al*. Finding cancer in primary care outpatients with low back pain. A comparison of diagnostic strategies. *Journal of General Internal Medicine*. 2001; **16**: 14–23.

122. El-Farhan N, Busuttil A. Sudden unexpected deaths from ruptured abdominal aortic aneurysms. *Journal of Clinical Forensic Medicine*. 1997; **4**: 111–6.

123. Bachulis BL, Long WB, Hynes GD, Johnson MC. Clinical indications for cervical spine radiographs in the traumatized patient. *American Journal of Surgery*. 1987; **153**: 473–7.

124. Kreipke DL, Gillespie KR, McCarthy MC *et al*. Reliability of indications for cervical spine films in trauma patients. *Journal of Trauma*. 1989; **29**: 1438–9.

125. Hoffman JR, Schriger DL, Mower W *et al*. Low-risk criteria for cervical-spine radiography in blunt trauma: a prospective study. *Annals of Emergency Medicine*. 1992; **21**: 1454–60.

126. Johnson MJ, Lucas GL. Value of cervical spine radiographs as a screening tool. *Clinical Orthopaedics and Related Research*. 1997; **340**: 102–08.

127. Deyo RA, Diehl AK. Lumbar spine films in primary care: current use and effects of selective ordering criteria. *Journal of General Internal Medicine*. 1986; **1**: 20–5.

128. Nice DA, Riddle DL, Lamb RL *et al*. Intertester reliability of judgements of the presence of trigger points in patients with low back pain. *Archives of Physical Medicine and Rehabilitation*. 1992; **73**: 893–8.

129. Njoo KH, Van der Does E. The occurrence and inter-rater reliability of myofascial trigger points in the quadratus lumborum and gluteus medius: a prospective study in non-specific low back pain patients and controls in general practice. *Pain*. 1994; **58**: 317–23.

*130. Schwarzer AC, Aprill CN, Derby R *et al*. The prevalence and clinical features of internal disc disruption in patients with chronic low back pain. *Spine*. 1995; **20**: 1878–83.

131. Schwarzer AC, Aprill CN, Derby R *et al*. Clinical features of patients with pain stemming from the lumbar zygapophysial joints. Is the lumbar facet syndrome a clinical entity? *Spine*. 1994; **19**: 1132–7.

*132. Bogduk N. A narrative review of intra-articular corticosteroid injections for low back pain. *Pain Medicine*. 2005; **6**: 287–96.

133. Laslett M, McDonald B, Aprill CN *et al*. Clinical predictors of screening lumbar zygapophyseal joint blocks: development of clinical prediction rules. *Spine Journal*. 2006; **6**: 370–9.

134. Schwarzer AC, Wang S, Bogduk N *et al*. Prevalence and clinical features of lumbar zygapophysial joint pain: a study in an Australian population with chronic low back pain. *Annals of the Rheumatic Diseases*. 1995; **54**: 100–06.

135. Osti OL, Fraser RD. MRI and discography of annular tears and intervertebral disc degeneration: a prospective clinical comparison. *Journal of Bone and Joint Surgery*. 1992; **74B**: 431–5.

136. Horton WC, Daftari TK. Which disc as visualized by magnetic resonance imaging is actually a source of pain? A correlation between magnetic resonance imaging and discography. *Spine*. 1992; **17**: S164–71.

137. Simmons JW, Emery SF, McMillin JN *et al*. Awake discography: a comparison study with magnetic resonance imaging. *Spine*. 1991; **16**: S216–21.

*138. Aprill C, Bogduk N. High intensity zone: a diagnostic sign of painful lumbar disc on magnetic resonance imaging. *British Journal of Radiology*. 1992; **65**: 361–9.

139. Schellhas KP, Pollei SR, Gundry CR, Heithoff KB. Lumbar disc high-intensity zone: correlation of magnetic resonance imaging and discography. *Spine*. 1996; **21**: 79–86.

*140. Ito M, Incorvaia KM, Yu SF *et al*. Predictive signs of discogenic lumbar pain on magnetic resonance imaging with discography correlation. *Spine*. 1998; **23**: 1252–8.

141. Saifuddin A, Braithwaite I, White J *et al*. The value of lumbar spine magnetic resonance imaging in the demonstration of anular tears. *Spine*. 1998; **23**: 453–7.

142. Bogduk N. Point of view. *Spine*. 1998; **23**: 1259–60.

143. Dvorak J, Hayek J, Zehnder R. CT-functional diagnostics of the rotatory instability of the upper cervical spine. Part 2. An evaluation on healthy adults and patients with suspected instability. *Spine*. 1987; **12**: 726–31.

144. Johansson BH. Whiplash injuries can be visible by functional magnetic resonance imaging. *Pain Research and Management*. 2006; **11**: 197–9.

145. Barnsley L, Lord SM, Wallis BJ, Bogduk N. The prevalence of chronic cervical zygapophysial joint pain after whiplash. *Spine*. 1995; **20**: 20–6.

*146. Lord S, Barnsley L, Wallis BJ, Bogduk N. Chronic cervical zygapohysial joint pain after whiplash: a placebo-controlled prevalence study. *Spine*. 1996; **21**: 1737–45.

147. Speldewinde GC, Bashford GM, Davidson IR. Diagnostic cervical zygapophysial joint blocks for chronic cervical pain. *Medical Journal of Australia*. 2001; **174**: 174–6.
148. Gibson T, Bogduk N, Macpherson J, McIntosh A. Crash characteristics of whiplash associated chronic neck pain. *Journal of Musculoskeletal Pain*. 2000; **8**: 87–95.
*149. Cooper G, Bailey B, Bogduk N. Cervical zygapophysial joint pain maps. *Pain Medicine*. 2007; **8**: 344–53.
150. Dwyer A, Aprill C, Bogduk N. Cervical zygapophysial joint pain patterns. I: A study in normal volunteers. *Spine*. 1990; **15**: 453–7.
151. Joseph B, Kumar B. Gallie's fusion for atlantoaxial arthrosis with occipital neuralgia. *Spine*. 1994; **19**: 454–5.
152. Ghanayem AJ, Leventhal M, Bohlman HH. Osteoarthrosis of the atlanto-axial joints – long-term follow-up after treatment with arthrodesis. *Journal of Bone and Joint Surgery*. 1996; **78**: 1300–07.
*153. Dreyfuss P, Halbrook B, Pauza K *et al*. Efficacy and validity of radiofrequency neurotomy for chronic lumbar zygapophysial joint pain. *Spine*. 2000; **25**: 1270–7.
*154. Schofferman J, Kine G. Effectiveness of repeated radiofrequency neurotomy for lumbar facet pain. *Spine*. 2004; **29**: 2471–3.
*155. Lord SM, Barnsley L, Wallis BJ *et al*. Percutaneous radiofrequency neurotomy for chronic cervical zygapophysial-joint pain. *New England Journal of Medicine*. 1996; **335**: 1721–6.
156. Lord SM, McDonald GJ, Bogduk N. Percutaneous radiofrequency neurotomy of the cervical medial branches: a validated treatment for cervical zygapophyseal joint pain. *Neurosurgery Quarterly*. 1998; **8**: 288–308.
157. McDonald GJ, Lord SM, Bogduk N. Long term follow-up of patients treated with cervical radiofrequency neurotomy for chronic neck pain. *Neurosurgery*. 1999; **45**: 61–8.
158. Govind J, King W, Bailey B, Bogduk N. Radiofrequency neurotomy for the treatment of third occipital headache. *Journal of Neurology, Neurosurgery, and Psychiatry*. 2003; **74**: 88–93.

13

Psychological effects of chronic pain: an overview

LANCE M McCRACKEN

KEY LEARNING POINTS

- Particular effects of chronic pain are as varied and complex as the people who suffer them.
- The language of "cause" and "effects" in chronic pain can be considered loosely, and for analytic purposes, without losing sight of the whole person, in context, with their own personal history.
- Among the most well-documented effects that come with chronic pain is emotional distress or mood disturbance, including three to six times the rates of anxiety and depressive disorders compared to the general population.
- Half or more of pain sufferers in the community report disturbed sleep, decreased lifting and exercise, and regular use of medication.
- Considering some effects of chronic pain as possible processes of suffering and disability is potentially useful.

INTRODUCTION

Any healthcare provider who has seen even a small sample of chronic pain sufferers will know the profound behavioral, cognitive, emotional, financial, physical, and social effects that can occur. Providing extensive literature citations to substantiate these effects appears almost unnecessary, as these effects are practically incontestable. However, even if most clinicians readily associate chronic pain with experiences of significant suffering and life disruption, this does not occur for every person with chronic pain, and universal effects of chronic pain can be difficult to describe. The particular effects are as varied and complex as the people who suffer them. Indeed, this variability requires examination.

There are many different models by which to understand the experience of chronic pain, such as those that are biological, psychological, social, or a blend of these. Each model comes with its own assumptions regarding cause and effect. Some of these assumptions resemble everyday thinking and speaking, or are highly influenced by them, and some are not (a point that is discussed below under Psychological domains of chronic pain assessment). These assumptions are also imbedded in the measures we use, the treatments we deliver, and what we call a "good outcome." With this in mind, the purpose of this chapter is to briefly present a practical description of the psychological effects of chronic pain, a description that is intended to be technically useful, for clinical applications, treatment development, and research. The focus of the chapter is intended to be broad, on situations inside and outside of healthcare contexts, and not only on specialty care, as can sometimes be the case. Examples of possible measures to employ in key assessment domains are presented. Recent advances in understanding both effects and processes of chronic pain are described to indicate directions for further research.

DEVELOPMENTS IN PSYCHOLOGICAL MODELS OF CHRONIC PAIN OVER TIME

There is a 40-year history of development in the behavioral and cognitive approaches to chronic pain, beginning with the operant approach,[1] including the cognitive-behavioral approaches,[2] up to the present day. As this history continues, any description of the psychological effects of chronic pain will be a snapshot in time and in a process of change. It is fortunate for this purpose, however, that interest in the contributory causes of chronic pain has been more changeable over time than interest in the effects of chronic pain, which has tended to yield greater consensus. In other words, psychologists and other professionals have considered an ever wider range of variables in the search for where suffering, disability, and life disruption come from, as opposed to what they are made of or how significant they are. If there is doubt about these trends, notice our changing interest in conversion disorders, pain behavior, reinforcement, social support, and responses from significant others, depression, neuroticism, locus of control, self-efficacy, coping, catastrophizing, stages of change, attention and hypervigilance, fear and avoidance, attachment style, and, more recently, acceptance and mindfulness, among others.

Greater attention to the influences on the experience of chronic pain is perhaps appropriate, as it is the processes by which patients suffer that should dictate how to help. In any case, the distinction between the causes and effects of chronic pain is probably best considered flexibly. The variables we define as causes and effects ought to serve practical purposes and not be regarded as absolutes. The lines we draw between initiating causes, maintaining or exacerbating causes, and effects, obviously do not exist in nature as such, but are analytic tools only. While we sometimes can take our variables too seriously, as if they are real or true entities, and not simply ways of speaking and writing, their truth or falsity will, perhaps, most usefully depend on how well they serve the purpose of the analysis at hand. It is, arguably, the whole person acting within a context of complex historical and situational events, both inside and outside their body, that is of primary clinical interest. With these caveats in mind, it is the effects of chronic pain that are the primary focus of this chapter.

PSYCHOLOGICAL DOMAINS OF CHRONIC PAIN ASSESSMENT

Every day clinicians come directly into contact with the many ways pain leads to changes in what the individual pain sufferer thinks, what they feel in their body and in their emotions, and, perhaps most importantly, what they do or do not do, including how they speak about their experiences, and what they do to seek relief. Standard self-report inventories administered along with these clinical encounters help to quantify some of these experiences. In turn, empirical analyses of large clinical databases, using factor analysis, show some consistency in the factors underlying the information collected for clinical purposes. These analyses reliably demonstrate that emotional distress, disability, and pain description are key domains.[3, 4, 5, 6] These domains are validated further by their inclusion in attempts to produce an integrated psychosocial assessment model for chronic pain,[7] in attempts to standardize a comprehensive assessment procedure from both the physician and patient perspective,[8] in attempts to develop comprehensive assessment instruments for young people with chronic pain,[9] and in recommendations for outcome domains in clinical trials for chronic pain.[10]

PSYCHOLOGICAL EFFECTS FROM PATIENTS SEEKING TREATMENT FOR CHRONIC PAIN

It may come as no surprise that among the most well-documented effects that come with chronic pain is emotional distress or mood disturbance. In their very useful review paper, Banks and Kerns[11] reported that depression is disproportionately prevalent in sufferers of chronic pain compared to other chronic medical conditions, that depression is most likely to be a result and not cause of chronic pain, and that 30.0–54.0 percent of patients seeking treatment for chronic pain suffer with a diagnosable depressive disorder. There is also evidence that patients with chronic pain have high prevalence rates of anxiety disorders, including panic disorder and generalized anxiety disorder, and substance use disorders, although the prevalence figures appear varied across studies.[12] Rates of current anxiety disorders may range from 16.5 to 28.8 percent and current substance use disorders from 15 to 28 percent.[12] In comparison with the clinical data, a recent nationally representative sample of the USA estimated that for chronic pain sufferers the prevalence of depression was 20.2 percent and for anxiety disorders it was 35.1 percent,[13] suggesting a much higher rate of depression in clinical samples, but a similar rate of anxiety disorders.

Naturally, chronic pain can present occasions when patients feel misunderstood or mistreated, feel threatened by poor health, experience interference with normal daily functioning, take medications that can produce side effects, and experience depression and anxiety, as noted above. As a result of these circumstances they also experience anger,[14, 15] and health anxiety.[16] Along with these emotions they experience a host of other distressing problems, such as loss of role functioning and personal identity,[17] impaired neuropsychological functioning,[18, 19] sexual dysfunction,[20] and sleep disturbance.[21, 22] In some cases they spend a disproportionate amount of their time seeking health care,[23] which will clearly take time away from other important concerns.

SURVEYS OF PAIN IN THE COMMUNITY

There have been a number of recent market research studies of chronic pain. These employ telephone surveys administered to people in the community prescreened for chronic pain. The largest of these was the *Survey of Chronic Pain in Europe* funded by Mundipharma International.[24] This study included interviews with 4839 individuals with chronic pain, about 300 per country, from 15 European countries and Israel. The purpose of the study was to estimate the prevalence of chronic pain, explore underlying features and correlations with demographic issues, to examine impact on quality of life and daily functioning, and understand individual attitudes. Overall they estimated that 19 percent of all those screened (N = 46,394) had chronic pain for at least six months, including the last month, at least twice a week, and rated at least five out of ten on a numerical rating scale of pain severity. The median duration of pain was seven years.

Selected findings from the more than 36 tables and figures presented by Breivik *et al.*[24] are shown in **Figure 13.1**. For example, of those with chronic pain surveyed, 40 percent reported they were less able to walk, 56 percent less able to sleep, and 21 percent were diagnosed with depression. Most respondents were seeking treatment for pain (69 percent) and taking prescription medications (52 percent). A few additional findings not included in **Figure 13.1** were that 32 percent of respondents considered themselves no longer able to work outside the home and around 50 percent considered themselves less able to do lifting or exercising. Mean time lost from work in the previous six months was 7.8 days. In terms of healthcare use, 58 percent of respondents had seen two or more doctors related to their pain, and 30 percent felt that their doctor did not know how to control their pain. Only 2 percent were currently treated by a pain management specialist and the same percentage reported having sought therapy or counseling.

There are a series of additional studies conducted over the past several years, typically in the USA, that similarly highlight the experience of chronic pain, its impact on daily living, and some of the frustrations of the treatment experience. One of these, reported in April 2004, was conducted for the American Chronic Pain Association, sponsored by Endo Pharmaceuticals, and conducted by Roper Public Affairs and Media.[25] It was a survey of 800 adults with chronic pain sampled from a process of random digit dialling. For the purpose of this study, chronic pain was defined as pain that occurs constantly or flares up frequently at least once per month, and not caused by cancer. Most of those surveyed (72 percent) had their pain for more than three years. The impacts on daily living were remarkably similar to those from the European survey: interference with daily routines (61 percent), household chores (67 percent), or sleep (78 percent); adverse effects on relationship with partner (28 percent), decreased productivity at work (51 percent), depression (46 percent), or feeling unable to cope (35 percent). Concerns about side effects of medications were common (56 percent), and nearly half of respondents reported that their pain was not under control (47 percent).

The findings from the surveys described here have been essentially duplicated many times using similar telephone survey-based approaches (see, for example, Ref. 26). Limitations of this method are important to take into account. The results obtained from these methods clearly represent the personal views of the respondents. These include complex judgments and are likely shaped by the survey methods used. They are, however, a unique perspective on pain sufferers outside a clinical situation.

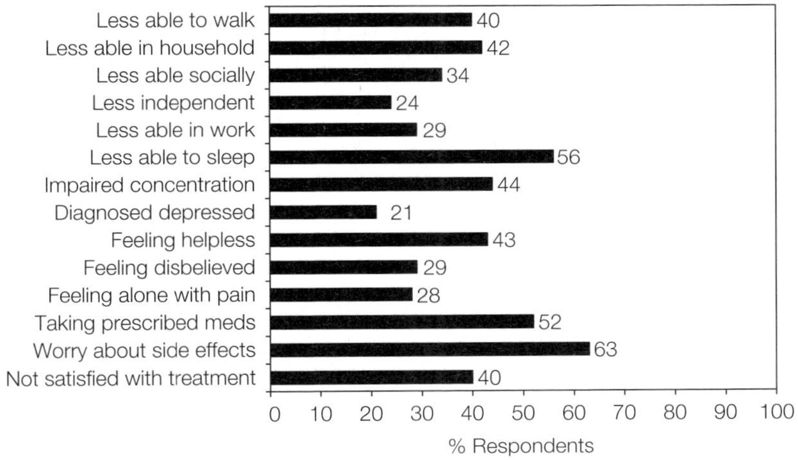

Figure 13.1 Selected results from Breivik *et al.*'s 2006 survey of individuals with chronic pain covering 15 European countries and Israel (n = 4839).[24]

ASSESSMENT METHODS FOR DISABILITY AND DAILY FUNCTIONING

There are a number of books on pain assessment that include the assessment of psychological effects of pain (see, for example, Ref. 27). The purpose here will be to give a brief summary of assessment methods, bearing in mind the discussion of psychological effects to this point. Although there are a number of direct observation, performance,[28, 29] daily diary,[30] or interview-based measures of psychological effects, the focus here will be on self-report methods, as these are the most practical to use in most settings. The recommendations presented are based on direct experience using each of the instruments discussed in both clinical and research applications.

Table 13.1 includes a set of recommended instruments. They are separated into single domain measures, such as those that focus only on one aspect of emotional functioning or global disability, and multidomain measures, which typically quantify pain, mood, and social or physical functioning. There are some variables that may be noticeably absent here, such as pain-coping strategies, beliefs or other cognitive variables, or measures of personality or trait-like variables, such as neuroticism, for example. While these are clearly important, depending on one's approach to chronic pain management, these are technically not considered effects of pain *per se*, but are, rather, potential processes of pain adjustment, or even personal qualities that precede the pain. Some of these processes are discussed below under Processes in chronic pain-related disability and suffering. Finally, this list highlights measures that are generally applicable to a range of chronic pain samples. Instruments focused on particular types of pain, such as the way the Oswestry Disability Questionnaire[43] is designed for low back pain, for example, were not included.

Table 13.1 Suggested instruments for assessment psychological effects of chronic pain.

Instrument	Domains assessed	No. items	References
Single domain measures			
Beck Depression Inventory	Depression	21	Beck *et al.*[31]
Center for Epidemiological Studies-Depression Scale	Depression	20	Radloff[32]
Pain Anxiety Symptoms Scale	Pain-related anxiety and avoidance	40 or 20 (short form)	McCracken *et al.*[33] McCracken and Dhingra[34]
Pain Disability Index	Disability	7	Pollard[35]
Roland–Morris Disability Questionnaire	Physical disability	24 or 11 (abbreviated)	Roland and Morris[36] Stroud *et al.*[37]
Multiple domain measures			
Brief Pain Inventory	Pain Interference with daily activity, mood, sleep, enjoyment of life	40 or 15 (short form)	Cleeland[38] Mendoza *et al.*[39]
Medical Outcomes Study Short Form 36-item	Physical functioning Role limitations (physical) Social functioning Bodily pain General mental health Role limitations (emotional) Vitality General health perception	36	Ware *et al.*[40]
Multidimensional Pain Inventory	Pain severity Interference Life control Affective distress Support Spouse responses Daily activities	52 or 61 (later version)	Kerns *et al.*[41]
Sickness Impact Profile	"Other" disability Physical disability Psychosocial disability	136	Bergner *et al.*[42]

For measuring overall functioning the Sickness Impact Profile (SIP) is comprehensive and well validated.[42] It has the advantage of providing scores for 12 separate aspects of daily functioning that can be combined into three domain scores. It is not a pain-specific measure as it is designed to assess overall functioning in relation to health in general. Its prime disadvantage is its length at 136 items, and scoring is extremely laborious if done by hand, as each item must be weighted by a different coefficient. Most will know that the Roland scale was derived from the SIP, is 20 items in length, and was developed to assess patients with low back pain.[36] The Roland scale has since been demonstrated as valid for chronic pain sufferers with pain in a variety of sites in their body, not just their back.[44] The Roland scale assesses physical disability only. It is, however, available in 20- and 11-item lengths,[37] and in 12 languages.[45]

Among the other comprehensive, multiple domain instruments that will help quantify effects of pain, the Multidimensional Pain Inventory (MPI), developed by Kerns and colleagues,[41] is probably the best known pain-specific measure. Its advantages include its demonstrated utility in a range of pain conditions, its development from a cognitive-behavioral framework, and the available patient subtyping or classification scheme that has been developed with it.[46] The MPI allows for a classification of patients as either dysfunctional, interpersonally distressed, or adaptive copers. Numerous studies have substantiated that this classification scheme is psychologically meaningful.[47]

Although the Brief Pain Inventory (BPI) was originally developed in the area of cancer pain assessment,[38] it has been validated for use with other pain, such as osteoarthritis,[39] and general nonmalignant chronic pain.[48] It is short and easy to use for repeat administrations in clinic settings. The Medical Outcomes Study Short Form instrument (SF-36) is another option for multidomain assessment in a relatively short format.[40] It has the advantages of being very brief and well-recognized, having comparative data available from many samples, and availability in multiple languages. There is an augmented version particularly for pain management contexts called the Treatment Outcomes in Pain Survey.[49] Finally, the Pain Disability Index is a very brief, seven-item, measure of disability in a combination of family/home, recreation, social, occupational, sexual, self-care, and life support activities.[35] It requires that patients rate their disability in each domain on a 0–10 scale, from no disability to total disability. Its advantages are its brief format and its inclusion of key aspects of functioning. A concern is that as it does not focus on particular behavior patterns or particular situations, but rather relies on global ratings, it may be more a measure of the patient's subjective sense or perception of disability, rather than a summary of particular tasks they are able or unable to do.

ASSESSMENT METHODS FOR EMOTIONAL DISTRESS

For assessment of emotional distress in chronic pain, depression is a key target. The Beck Depression Inventory (BDI) has long been a standard and is a very good measure. It is very useful clinically, as its content is comprehensive, and in research where it appears sensitive to psychological differences.[31] As each of the 21 items of the BDI potentially includes four statements to read, it may be too long for some applications. The BDI has been well studied in chronic pain samples.[50, 51] Concerns about the somatic item content of the BDI can be confusing. There is sometimes an assumption that these will contaminate or inflate judgments about the degree of depression present in an individual or sample.[50] It seems likely, however, that these can be managed with an examination of endorsed item content in clinical contexts, testing of effects of content in research contexts, and a flexible use of standard cut-off scores. Results from extensive factor analysis of the BDI in patients with chronic pain suggest a robust factor structure that differs from nonchronic pain samples and again suggests the need for careful examination of the item content that contributes to high scores.[51] A distinct advantage of the BDI in clinical assessment is the inclusion of an item assessing suicidal ideation. The Center for Epidemiological Studies-Depression Scale (CES-D)[32] is another measure of depression that is well established and is perhaps somewhat shorter to administer than the BDI. We have also used a less well-known measure called the British Columbia Major Depression Inventory.[52] It includes 20 items, requires an examination of separate symptom types for scoring and interpretation, rather than a straight interpretation of the total score, and includes assessment of both symptom severity and impact of symptoms.

For years, the standard assessment method for anxiety in relation to chronic pain included use of instruments such as the Spielberger State-Trait Anxiety Inventory (STAI).[53] We questioned the utility of the STAI in a study demonstrating that instruments assessing more pain-specific fear and anxiety responses appear more useful, and are stronger predictors than general measures, like the STAI, of patient functioning.[54] General measures of anxiety tend to be highly correlated with measure of depression and, thus, do not provide additional information in most clinical assessments. They also do not take into account the source of the distress and, thus, are not as helpful in the design or selection of treatment methods as they could be. As an alternative for measuring pain-related fear and avoidance, clinicians or researchers might use the Pain Anxiety Symptoms Scale (PASS).[33, 34] The distinction between the PASS and other measures related to fear of pain, such as the Fear Avoidance Beliefs Questionnaire (FABQ)[55] and the Tampa Scale for Kinesiophobia (TSK),[56] is that the latter scales appear to almost exclusively focus on beliefs, while the PASS focuses on a range of cognitive and physiological anxiety responses in addition to avoidance. Again, beliefs may be considered more as contributors to the experience of pain-related suffering and disability, rather than effects of it.

PROCESSES IN CHRONIC PAIN-RELATED DISABILITY AND SUFFERING

As mentioned above under Assessment methods for disability and daily functioning, there are many psychological responses to pain that are considered important for patient functioning. In recent clinical studies these include catastrophizing,[57, 58] coping,[59] self-efficacy,[60, 61] and stages of change,[62] among others.[63] Discussing all of these is well beyond the scope of the present chapter. However, there are a small number of other processes that have been the focus of work for our group, first in Chicago, and now in Bath. These are both effects of chronic pain, in the sense that they are changes in quality of behavior patterns resulting from the experience of chronic pain, and processes of suffering and disability, as they appear to lead to higher levels of emotional distress and greater restrictions in patient functioning. These processes include experiential avoidance, values-failures, and disturbances of awareness.[64]

When pain occurs, the pain sufferer naturally will try to avoid it. When chronic pain leads to painful emotions, memories, and other unwanted experiences (e.g. feelings and thoughts that come with facing unwelcome changes in life or from challenging social situations), the pain sufferer will naturally attempt to avoid these as well. This is normal human behavior. This process, called "experiential avoidance," is proposed as the source of much of human behavior disturbance and suffering.[65] The problem with experiential avoidance is that attempting to avoid private experiences, including psychological experiences that come from one's personal history, is often not possible, often brings the person, paradoxically, in contact with the material they are attempting to avoid, and can be extremely restricting of a person's functioning. If one is unwilling to feel painful or unwanted feelings, one will be unable to do any activity that brings one in contact with those feelings. Numerous studies demonstrate the disutility of avoidance in relation to chronic pain.[66, 67, 68] Our work has focused on a process that is intended to undermine experiential avoidance, namely, acceptance of chronic pain, and we have shown that acceptance is consistently correlated with higher patient emotional, physical, social, and work-related functioning.[47, 69, 70]

A second type of change in the quality of the pain sufferer's behavior that occurs with chronic pain is that it is increasingly influenced by pain and not by other concerns. Rest, medication consumption, seeking help, refusing invitations, seeking treatment, complaining, withdrawing socially, and using assistive devices can be behavior patterns that serve only as attempts to limit contact with pain, and do not serve purposes the pain sufferer would otherwise rate as most important and meaningful in their life. In essence, dealing with pain can move an individual, unwittingly, away from what they care about most. Part of this process can be referred to as a values failure or a failure of values-based action.[71] We have found that patients with chronic pain rate their success at living according to their values in areas of family, intimate relations, friends, work, health, and growth or learning, as significantly lower than the level of importance with which they hold their values in these domains.[72] We have also found that the losses that come with the failures of values to guide action contribute to significant anxiety, depression, and disability in patients with chronic pain. Additional analyses in this same study demonstrated that both acceptance of pain and values-based action contribute uniquely to patient functioning.[72]

A third behavioral dimension within the chronic pain experience that can demonstrate significant changes is the quality of contact the pain suffer has with the environment, or their level of awareness. For the purposes of discussing this process, the environment needs to be considered broadly as made up of experience available to the senses inside and outside the body and experience in the content of thought. When a person has chronic pain, their awareness of their social and physical situation can be disrupted by a number of experiences, including their sensations of pain[73] and experience of emotions, changes in the way they observe or try to block out these experiences, and by preoccupation or entanglement with the content of their own thinking in ways that limit their awareness of the actual situation around them.[74] When people suffer, they seem particularly prone to dwell on the past or to become distressingly preoccupied with the future – this seems to be particularly true for those with chronic pain. Processes of getting caught up with psychological influences of pain and related thoughts, experiencing the distress of reliving experiences from the past or from events in the future that likely will never come to pass, and having behavior disorganized from a loss of contact with what is occurring at that particular moment, each appear to contribute to the suffering and behavior-restricting effects of chronic pain. In a sense, data from studies of catastrophizing and pain document the impact of these cognitive processes.[57] Counteractive processes for some of these are included in what is referred to as "mindfulness." Mindfulness is full, accurate, moment-to-moment, present-focused, and nonreactive awareness.[75] Mindfulness methods of treatment have long been advocated as a way to undermine the otherwise natural effects of distressing experiences on emotions and behavior.[76] Uncontrolled treatment outcome studies of mindfulness support the role of awareness and disturbances of awareness in chronic pain.[76] An additional preliminary investigation of mindfulness demonstrated that it significantly predicts pain-related anxiety, depression, and physical and psychosocial disability, independent of patient age, gender, education, duration of pain, pain severity, and acceptance of pain.[77]

CONCLUSIONS

In some ways, the behavior of the individual pain sufferer, interacting with and in a broader psychological context, is an indivisible whole. To separate out parts of the individual's experience and behavior in context, some as causes and some as effects, changes the nature of what is being examined, so that it is not the same thing anymore. We can, however, look at individual parts, name them, and examine them in relation to one another, as an analytic tool, as an aid for understanding. We do this to understand how, in some cases, people with chronic pain come to suffer as much as they do, and how their participation in life can become so remarkably restricted. Along the way, the fact remains: these are simply ways of speaking designed, at best, to serve purposes of science and clinical service. In the end, the focus perhaps ought to return to the whole person, and their behavior, in context.

On the level of human experience, chronic pain brings loss, threats, uncertainty, restraint, apparent mistreatment, and failure into the lives of those who suffer with it. In turn, it brings depression, fear, anxiety, frustration, anger, and shame. It also brings all of the behavior patterns these experiences and emotions, and the sufferer's personal history, will naturally occasion. The behavior patterns include avoidance, withdrawal, complaints, passivity, and the persistent, sometimes urgent, search for relief. These effects generally are seen both in patients studied in clinical contexts and chronic pain sufferers contacted in the community to varying degrees.

It might be argued that some of the effects of chronic pain are more important than others in the sense that they represent core processes of suffering and disability. For example, experiential avoidance, failures of values-based action, and loss of accurate awareness of the present situation, seem to be key aspects of suffering both across behavior disorders generally[71] and in chronic pain,[64] and appear fully addressable with current treatment methods. The evolution of the behavioral and cognitive therapies for chronic pain seems to be including these in a process of integration in two directions, both with the history of successes from the operant behavioral and cognitive-behavioral approaches of the past and with developments in the broader field of clinical psychology.

Chronic pain is not always what it appears. It was mentioned at the start of this chapter that some of our assumptions about chronic pain resemble "everyday thinking and speaking." It could be argued that "everyday thinking and speaking" gets people into the suffering and disability of chronic pain and may not be the best means for getting them out of it. Chronic pain is possibly not best understood as a symptom or condition of the body that results in effects on the person and their functioning. It is in the whole experience of the person. When it becomes a problem it is always a fundamentally physical, emotional, cognitive, social, and behavioral process of the individual based in their situation and history. Particularly in cases where these processes represent profound areas of disturbance, recent research advocates for the utility of a contextual process-oriented model of chronic pain rather than an "effects" model that may be implied by the title of this chapter.

REFERENCES

1. Fordyce WE. *Behavioral methods for chronic pain and illness.* St Louis, MO: Mosby, 1976.
2. Turk DC, Meichenbaum D, Genest M. *Pain and behavioral medicine: a cognitive-behavioral perspective.* New York: Guilford Press, 1983.
3. Williams RC. Toward a set of reliable and valid measures for chronic pain assessment and outcome research. *Pain.* 1988; **35**: 239–51.
4. Tait RC, Chibnall JT, Duckro PN, Deshields TL. Stable factors in chronic pain. *Clinical Journal of Pain.* 1989; **5**: 323–8.
5. Mikail SF, DuBreuil S, D'Eon JL. A comparative analysis of measures used in the assessment of chronic pain patients. *Psychological Assessment.* 1993; **5**: 117–20.
6. DeGagne TA, Mikail SF, D'Eon JL. Confirmatory factor analysis of a 4-factor model of chronic pain evaluation. *Pain.* 1995; **60**: 195–202.
7. Strong J, Ashton R, Stewart A. Chronic low back pain: Toward an integrated psychosocial assessment model. *Journal of Consulting and Clinical Psychology.* 1994; **62**: 1058–63.
8. Rucker KS, Metzler HM, Kregel J. Standardization of chronic pain assessment: a multiperspective approach. *Clinical Journal of Pain.* 1996; **12**: 94–110.
9. Eccleston C, Jordan A, McCracken LM *et al.* The Bath Adolescent Pain Questionnaire (BAPQ): development and preliminary psychometric evaluation of an instrument to assess the impact of chronic pain on adolescents. *Pain.* 2005; **118**: 263–70.
10. * Turk DC, Dworkin RH, Allen RR *et al.* Core outcome domains for chronic pain clinical trials: IMMPACT recommendations. *Pain.* 2003; **106**: 337–45.
11. Banks SM, Kerns RD. Explaining high rates of depression in chronic pain: a diathesis-stress framework. *Psychological Bulletin.* 1996; **119**: 95–110.
12. * Dersh J, Polatin PB, Gatchel RJ. Chronic pain and psychopathology: research findings and theoretical considerations. *Psychosomatic Medicine.* 2002; **64**: 773–86.
13. McWilliams LA, Cox BJ, Enns MW. Mood and anxiety disorders associated with chronic pain: an examination in

a nationally representative sample. *Pain.* 2003; **106**: 127–33.

14. Okifuji A, Turk DC, Curran SL. Anger in chronic pain: investigations of anger targets and intensity. *Journal of Psychosomatic Research.* 1999; **47**: 1–12.
15. Lombardo ER, Tan G, Jensen MP, Anderson KO. Anger management style and associations with self-efficacy and pain in male veterans. *Journal of Pain.* 2005; **6**: 765–70.
16. Rode S, Salkovskis P, Dowd H, Magdi H. Health anxiety levels in chronic pain clinic attenders. *Journal of Psychosomatic Research.* 2006; **60**: 155–61.
17. Harris S, Morley S, Barton SB. Role loss and emotional adjustment in chronic pain. *Pain.* 2003; **105**: 363–70.
18. Sjøgren P, Christrup LL, Peterson M, Højsted J. Neuropsychological assessment of chronic non-malignant pain patients treated in a multidisciplinary pain centre. *European Journal of Pain.* 2005; **9**: 453–62.
19. Weiner DK, Rudy TE, Morrow L *et al.* The relationship between pain, neuropsychological performance, and physical function in community-dwelling older adults with chronic low back pain. *Pain Medicine.* 2006; **7**: 60–70.
20. Kwan KSH, Roberts LJ, Swalm DM. Sexual dysfunction and chronic pain: the role of psychological variables and impact on quality of life. *European Journal of Pain.* 2005; **9**: 643–52.
21. McCracken LM, Iverson GL. Disrupted sleep patterns and daily functioning in chronic pain. *Pain Research and Therapy.* 2002; **7**: 75–9.
22. Smith MT, Perlis ML, Smith MS *et al.* Sleep quality and presleep arousal in chronic pain. *Journal of Behavioral Medicine.* 2000; **23**: 1–13.
23. Blyth FM, March LM, Brnabic AJM, Cousins MJ. Chronic pain and frequent use of health care. *Pain.* 2004; **111**: 51–8.
24. * Breivik H, Collett B, Ventafridda V *et al.* Survey of chronic pain in Europe: prevalence, impact on daily life, and treatment. *European Journal of Pain.* 2006; **10**: 287–333.
25. Roper Public Affairs and Media. Americans living with pain survey: executive summary and results. Survey conducted on behalf of the American Chronic Pain Association. Last updated April 2004, cited February 2008. Available from: http://theacpa.org/documents/final pain survey results report.pdf.
26. David Michaelson & Company, LLC. Voices of chronic pain: a national study conducted for the American Pain Foundation. Last updated May 2006, cited February 2008. Available from: www.painfoundation.org/Voices/VoicesSurveyFactSheet.pdf.
27. Turk DC, Melzack R. *Handbook of pain assessment*, 2nd edn. New York: Guilford Press, 2001.
28. Lee CE, Simmonds MJ, Novy DM, Jones S. Self-reports and clinician-measured physical function among patients with low back pain: a comparison. *Archives of Physical Medicine and Rehabilitation.* 2001; **82**: 227–31.
29. Wittink H, Rogers W, Sukiennik A, Carr DB. Physical functioning: self-report and performance measures are related but distinct. *Spine.* 2003; **228**: 2407–13.
30. Peters ML, Sorbi MJ, Kruise DA *et al.* Electronic diary assessment of pain, disability, and psychological adaptation in patients differing in duration of pain. *Pain.* 2000; **84**: 181–92.
31. Beck AT, Ward CH, Mendelson M *et al.* An inventory for measuring depression. *Archives of General Psychiatry.* 1961; **4**: 561–71.
32. Radloff LS. The CES-D scale: a self-report depression scale for research in general populations. *Applied Psychological Measurement.* 1977; **1**: 385–401.
33. McCracken LM, Zayfert C, Gross RT. The Pain Anxiety Symptoms Scale: development and validation of a scale to measure fear of pain. *Pain.* 1992; **50**: 67–73.
34. McCracken LM, Dhingra L. A short version of the Pain Anxiety Symptoms Scale (PASS-20): preliminary development and validity. *Pain Research and Management.* 2002; **7**: 45–50.
35. Pollard CA. Preliminary validity study of the Pain Disability Index. *Perceptual and Motor Skills.* 1984; **59**: 974.
36. Roland M, Morris R. A study of the natural history of low back pain. Part 1: development of a reliable and sensitive measure of disability in low back pain. *Spine.* 1983; **8**: 141–4.
37. Stroud MW, McKnight PE, Jensen MP. Assessment of self-reported physical activity in patients with chronic pain: development of an abbreviated Roland-Morris Disability Scale. *Journal of Pain.* 2004; **5**: 257–63.
38. Cleeland S. Measurement of pain by subjective report. Issues in pain measurement. In: Chapman CR, Loeser JD (eds). *Advances in Pain Research and Therapy, 12.* New York: Raven Press, 1991: 391–403.
39. Mendoza T, Mayne T, Rublee D, Cleeland C. Reliability and validity of a modified Brief Pain Inventory short form in patients with osteoarthritis. *European Journal of Pain.* 2006; **10**: 353–61.
40. Ware JE, Sherbourne CD. The MOS 36-Item Short-Form Health Survey (SF-36) I. Conceptual framework and item selection. *Medical Care.* 1992; **30**: 473–83.
41. Kerns RD, Turk DC, Rudy TE. The West Haven-Yale Multidimensional Pain Inventory (WHYMPI). *Pain.* 1985; **23**: 345–56.
42. Bergner M, Bobbitt RA, Carter WB, Gilson BS. The Sickness Impact Profile: development and final revision of a health status measure. *Medical Care.* 1981; **19**: 787–805.
43. Fairbank JC, Couper J, Davies JB, O'Brien JP. The Oswestry Low Back Disability Questionnaire. *Physiotherapy.* 1980; **66**: 271–3.
44. Jensen MP, Strom SE, Turner JA, Romano JM. Validity of the Sickness Impact Profile Roland scale as a measure of dysfunction in chronic pain. *Pain.* 1992; **50**: 157–62.
45. Roland M, Fairbank J. The Roland-Morris Disability Questionnaire and the Oswestry Disability Questionnaire. *Spine.* 2000; **25**: 3115–24.
46. Turk DC, Rudy TE. Towards a comprehensive assessment of chronic pain patients. *Behaviour Research and Therapy.* 1987; **25**: 237–49.

47. McCracken LM, Spertus IL, Janeck AS *et al.* Behavioral dimensions of adjustment in person with chronic pain: pain-related anxiety and acceptance. *Pain.* 1999; **80**: 283–9.
48. Tan G, Jensen MP, Thornby JI, Shanti BF. Validation of the Brief Pain Inventory for chronic nonmalignant pain. *Journal of Pain.* 2004; **5**: 133–7.
49. Rogers WH, Wittink HM, Ashburn MA *et al.* Using the "TOPS," an outcomes instrument for multidisciplinary outpatient pain treatment. *Pain Medicine.* 2000; **1**: 55–67.
50. Geisser ME, Roth RS, Robinson ME. Assessing depression among persons with chronic pain using the Center for Epidemiological Studies-Depression Scale and the Beck Depression Inventory: a comparative analysis. *Clinical Journal of Pain.* 1997; **13**: 163–70.
51. Morley S, Williams ACdeC, Black S. A confirmatory factor analysis of the Beck Depression Inventory in chronic pain. *Pain.* 2002; **99**: 289–98.
52. Iverson GL, Remick R. Diagnostic accuracy of the British Columbia Major Depression Inventory. *Psychological Reports.* 2004; **95**: 1241–7.
53. Spielberger CD, Gorsuch RL, Lushene PR *et al. Manual for the State-Trait Anxiety Inventory.* Palo Alto, CA: Consulting Psychologists Press, 1983.
54. McCracken LM, Gross RT, Aikens J, Carnrike CLM. The assessment of anxiety and fear in persons with chronic pain: a comparison of instruments. *Behaviour Research and Therapy.* 1996; **34**: 927–33.
55. Waddell G, Newton M, Henderson I *et al.* A Fear-Avoidance Beliefs Questionnaire (FABQ) and the role of fear-avoidance beliefs in chronic low back pain and disability. *Pain.* 1993; **52**: 157–68.
56. Kori SH, Miller RP, Todd DD. Kinesiophobia: a new view of chronic pain behavior. *Pain Management.* 1990; **3**: 35–43.
* 57. Sullivan MJL, Thorn B, Haythornthwaite JA *et al.* Theoretical perspectives on the relation between catastrophizing and pain. *Clinical Journal of Pain.* 2001; **17**: 52–64.
58. Sullivan MJL, Lynch ME, Clark AJ. Dimensions of catastrophic thinking associated with pain experience and disability in patients with neuropathic pain conditions. *Pain.* 2005; **113**: 310–15.
59. Romano JM, Jensen MP, Turner JA. The chronic pain coping inventory-42: reliability and validity. *Pain.* 2003; **104**: 65–73.
60. Asghari A, Nicholas MK. Pain self-efficacy beliefs and pain behavior: a prospective study. *Pain.* 2001; **94**: 85–100.
61. Nicholas MK, Asghari A. Investigating acceptance in adjustment to chronic pain: is acceptance broader than we thought? *Pain.* 2006; **124**: 269–79.
62. Kerns RD, Wagner J, Rosenberg R *et al.* Identification of subgroups of persons with chronic pain based on profiles on the pain stages of change questionnaire. *Pain.* 2005; **116**: 302–10.
63. Keefe FJ, Rumble ME, Scipio CD *et al.* Psychological aspects of persistent pain: current state of the science. *Journal of Pain.* 2004; **5**: 195–211.
64. McCracken LM. *Contextual cognitive-behavioral therapy for chronic pain.* Seattle, WA: IASP Press, 2005.
* 65. Hayes SC, Wilson KG, Gifford EV *et al.* Emotional avoidance and behavioral disorders: a functional dimensional approach to diagnosis and treatment. *Journal of Consulting and Clinical Psychology.* 1996; **64**: 1152–68.
66. Fordyce WE, Shelton JL, Dundore DE. The modification of avoidance learning pain behaviors. *Journal of Behavioral Medicine.* 1982; **5**: 405–14.
* 67. Vlaeyen JWS, Linton SJ. Fear-avoidance and its consequences in chronic musculoskeletal pain: a state of the art. *Pain.* 2000; **85**: 317–32.
68. McCracken LM, Samuel VM. The role of avoidance, pacing, and other activity patterns in chronic pain. *Pain.* 2007; **130**: 199–25.
69. McCracken LM. Learning to live with the pain: acceptance of pain predicts adjustment in persons with chronic pain. *Pain.* 1998; **74**: 21–7.
70. McCracken LM, Eccleston C. A prospective study of acceptance of pain and patient functioning with chronic pain. *Pain.* 2005; **118**: 164–9.
71. Hayes SC, Strosahl KD, Wilson KG. *Acceptance and commitment therapy: an experiential approach to behavior change.* New York: Guilford Press, 1999.
72. McCracken L-M, Yang SY. The role of values in a contextual cognitive-behavioral approach to chronic pain. *Pain.* 2006; **123**: 137–45.
73. Eccleston C, Crombez G. Pain demands attention: a cognitive-affective model of the interruptive function of pain. *Psychological Bulletin.* 1999; **125**: 356–66.
74. McCracken LM. A contextual analysis of attention to chronic pain: what the patient does with their pain might be more important than their awareness or vigilance alone. *Journal of Pain.* 2007; **8**: 230–6.
75. Kabat-Zinn J. *Full catastrophe living: using the wisdom of your body and mind to fact stress, pain, and illness.* New York: Dell Publishing, 1990.
76. Kabat-Zinn J, Lipworth L, Burney R. The clinical use of mindfulness meditation for self-regulation of chronic pain. *Journal of Behavioral Medicine.* 1985; **8**: 163–90.
* 77. McCracken LM, Gauntlett-Gilbert J, Vowles K. The role of mindfulness in a contextual cognitive-behavioral analysis of chronic pain-related suffering and disability. *Pain.* 2007; **131**: 63–9.

14

Outcome measurement in chronic pain

TIM JOHNSON

KEY LEARNING POINTS

- Chronic pain is complex and can be assessed in many ways.
- Most individual treatments for chronic pain have low efficacy.
- Nonspecific treatment effects (including placebo) are substantial and may exceed the specific effects of treatment.
- It is difficult to measure the effect of some of the most valuable components of therapy (information, advice, reassurance, and encouragement).
- Treatments are very diverse and are often combined resulting in changes in several measures in different directions.
- Clinical trials are usually designed to maximize apparent drug efficacy and thereby overestimate treatment effects in clinical practice.
- Outcome measures such as number needed to treat (NNT) are population-, condition-, and treatment-specific, so comparisons between studies need to be made carefully.

INTRODUCTION

This chapter is intended to help the reader to understand how to assess all of the consequences, good and bad, of treating pain. Chapters on individual chronic pain conditions will include measures that have been used to measure the effect of the appropriate treatments. Specific pain measuring tools are also described elsewhere in this book (Chapter 3, Selecting and applying pain measures and Chapter 2, Practical methods for pain intensity measurements in the *Practice and Procedures* volume of this series). These and many other sources of data describe which pain measures are available. We will discuss who benefits from outcome measurement and the application of measures in a variety of different situations. It is necessary to know when measures can be applied and to have an understanding of how they may be used (and unfortunately abused) in research and clinical practice. It is impossible to specify all the possibilities for measuring outcome in chronic pain, but a wide range will be considered by the use of pertinent examples from the literature. These are included only to illustrate aspects of the process of outcome measurement rather than to demonstrate the superiority, or otherwise, of specific treatments. We will start by considering the reasons for measuring outcome.

WHY IS IT NECESSARY TO MEASURE OUTCOMES?

To determine the outcome of pain conditions

Our knowledge of the natural history of pain syndromes comes from longitudinal studies in which patients' symptoms and levels of function are documented over time together with risk factors that might affect them. It is important that the measures used are stable and reliable.

For example, patients with back pain who are female, have had long or frequent previous episodes of pain, who exercise less, and who have had a poor initial response to treatment are more likely to be disabled by their pain five years later.[1] Studies such as this illustrate the large number of factors that must be controlled in research involving chronic pain. The stakeholders of outcome measurement are summarized in **Table 14.1**.

As a guide to treatment

Very many treatments have been used in patients with chronic pain. Published studies describe techniques varying from the drug treatment of phantom limb pain with anticonvulsants,[2][II] to heating vertebral disks to treat back pain,[3][II] and from the physical exercise of yoga[4][II] to spiritual healing.[5][II] It is hardly surprising that interpretation of the results of these individual treatments is difficult for the clinician, even without the added complications of several sequential or concurrent treatments, some of which may be unknown to the treating clinician. Patients naturally demand the best, but many factors are involved in determining what is best. For example, whether the simplicity, safety, and availability of transcutaneous electrical nerve stimulation (TENS) outweighs the precise stimulation localization, but inevitable risk of complications with spinal cord stimulation (SCS) cannot be reduced to yes or no. A great deal will depend on the patient and their attitudes to risk and benefit.

The collection and analysis of large sets of data have now enabled the construction of algorithms to guide clinicians through sequences of treatment, for example when treating neuropathic pain,[6][I] and we will see how material is being made accessible for patients in order to help them with these decisions (www.nice.org.uk).

To determine specific treatments

Procedures for treating chronic pain sometimes involve either major surgery or the selective destruction of tissues with significant risks of complications. Preliminary evidence that these invasive procedures will be beneficial is therefore helpful. For example, the use of local anesthetic nerve blocks is able to identify patients who may respond to subsequent heat lesions of the nerves supplying the cervical facet joints;[7][II]; indeed, in this study, preliminary nerve blocks were used first to identify patients who were eligible for a later trial of the effects of the heat lesions. Similarly, patients who respond to provocative discography (where dye is injected into an intervertebral disk in order to provoke their pain symptoms) have been offered spinal fusion surgery in order to immobilize the affected segment, although the positive predictive value of this particular test in one study appears to be low at 50 to 60 percent.[8] The toss of a coin is almost as good.

To justify the safety of therapy

Some treatments may have inevitable risks. For example, the use of large doses of methadone in patients who have had problems with other opioid analgesics might be questioned in terms of safety or effectiveness. A detailed study has demonstrated that the technique can be used safely and that there are substantial benefits in terms of pain control, return to work, and global quality of life with a relatively low rate of drug diversion, side effects, or complications.[9] Again the very wide range of outcome measures that must accompany the assessment of pain is demonstrated. It is very important to note also that outcome is specific to the study and not the technique or drug – methadone can still be lethal if its use is not properly supervised.

To determine the benefit of therapy

As well as safety issues, pain clinics will be under increasing financial scrutiny and charged with justifying

Table 14.1 Stakeholders of outcome measurement.

Stakeholder	Interest
Patients	Document or validate symptoms and treatment effects
Clinic/hospital	Justify the funding of expensive treatments (cost benefit)
	Compete for business (effectiveness, cost–utility)
Pharmaceutical company	Demonstrate efficacy and cost–benefit
Government healthcare, e.g. NICE	Information on comparative treatment cost-effectiveness, cost–utility and cost–benefit to justify expenditure
Government, disability payments	To establish medical evidence to justify payments to claimant
Legal system	Document actual or likely outcome of pain condition or treatment

NICE, National Institute for Clinical Excellence.

their existence and improving quality.[10] Okifuji and Turk[11] give a stern warning:

> Make no mistake about it: the survival of pain medicine will not be possible without our knowledge of the effects of what we do...

These effects can be further defined as outlined below.[11]

EFFICACY

Efficacy can be defined as the benefit of treatment in a defined population under controlled conditions. This describes most clinical trials where a single treatment is investigated in order to determine its effect on the pain condition of willing and able subjects (volunteer patients). Patients with other pains or pathologies or who may have difficulty participating in data collection are excluded, so results will indicate only whether the treatment can be effective, for example, by reducing pain or the disability associated with pain. Studies are usually comparative with a placebo arm to determine the benefit over and above any nonspecific treatment effect.

EFFECTIVENESS

Effectiveness can be defined as the benefit of treatment when average clinicians deliver treatment under average conditions. This will be the case in most pain clinics which have to serve a geographical population and in which other medical diagnoses, infirmity, and communication difficulties will exist across the whole age range.

Example

Two studies of the effect of the anticonvulsant gabapentin as an analgesic illustrate the difference between efficacy and effectiveness. Rice and Maton[12] found that the number needed to treat (see below under Number needed to treat) for postherpetic neuralgia (PHN) was 5.34,[12, 13] [II] whereas Serpell reported a figure of 14.3 in a more diverse population of patients with mixed neuropathic pain.[14][II] Although efficacy is demonstrated for the drug, its effectiveness in the latter population appears to be low.

Table 14.2 illustrates some differences between efficacy and effectiveness.

UTILITY

Analgesia is unlikely to be useful if its use is limited by side effects or by poor compliance. For example, if a patient is prescribed amitriptyline, but objects to having a dry mouth or taking an antidepressant medication,[15] the utility of the otherwise efficacious treatment is reduced.

EFFICIENCY

Efficiency can be defined as the resources required producing the benefits of treatment:

Cost-effectiveness – the financial cost of achieving a specific clinical target, such as return to work or reduction in pain score by 30 percent. Turk[16] cautions against simple comparisons between different modalities of treatment because of the "broad differences in the pain syndromes and inclusion criteria used, the drug dosages, comparability of treatments, the definition of 'chronic' used, the outcome criteria selected to determine success, and societal differences between studies." It is necessary to have detailed knowledge and understanding of each study that is compared – simple reference to published abstracts is insufficient.

Cost-utility – the financial cost of improving patients' lives – usually more patient-focused outcomes, which are less objective and often cover a broad range of measures. Results from the SF36 questionnaire, may be converted to an abstract measure such the Quality Adjusted Life Year (QALY). One QALY can be demonstrated to cost about $60–70,000 for

Table 14.2 A summary of the differences between clinical trials and clinical practice.

	Clinical trial	Clinical practice
Demonstrates drug	Efficacy	Effectiveness
Purpose	To demonstrate that the drug works	To improve patient's condition
Population	Strictly defined, homogeneous	Mixed, variable, ill-defined
Confounding diagnoses	Absent	Frequent
Motivation	High	Often low
Compliance	Good, assured, low dropout rate	Often poor, failure to attend appointments
Outcome measures	Comprehensive	Often vague or nonexistent
Duration	Short, often concluded after enough time for initial improvement	Indefinite

interdisciplinary management of chronic spinal pain[17] or $15,000 for acupuncture for chronic neck pain[18] (up to $100,000 per QALY is usually considered to be justified). These measures are useful in order to help refine pharmacoeconomic models of managing pain.[19]

Cost benefit – the ratio of healthcare expenditure to financial benefit (i.e. the sum of treatment cost savings, reduced disability benefits, and wages earned) considered in purely monetary terms.

Example

By modelling a cohort of patients with diabetic and postherpetic pain, cost-utility was calculated using a measure of utility (which designates a pain-free outcome with no side effects as having utility equal to 1.0; pain free with minor side effects as 0.95, and persistent pain as 0.55) and allowing for the cost of monitoring laboratory tests and the differential rates of complications, such as myocardial infarction with amitriptyline.[20] Gabapentin fared badly against amitriptyline and tramadol, largely because of its high cost and lack of superior effectiveness.

WHY IS OUTCOME MEASUREMENT DIFFICULT?

The complexity of chronic pain

The definition of pain as chronic gives us a clue that it may not change much over time, indeed attempts to cure the problem are often disappointing. In addition, Chapman and Dunbar[21] note that:

> Pain is not an isolated symptom. Severe pain creates fatigue, impairs concentration, compromises mood, degrades sleep and diminishes overall activity level. The goal of intervention for chronic pain must include alleviating the functional impairment that pain produces as well as its discomfort. Evaluating treatment outcome requires:
>
> 1. quantification of both pain intensity and pain-related impairment; and
> 2. review of how the relationship between these variables changes as a function of treatment.
>
> Simply tracking pain intensity level as an indicator of pain relief is insufficient and can lead to misinterpretation of the effects of an intervention.

Important material losses and perceptions of loss that shape patients' views can only be discovered and understood by detailed questioning and exploration of individual narratives.[22] The losses are unlikely to be standardized between patients and therefore are difficult to group or categorize. We must nevertheless be careful to try to capture these important features rather than simply measure that which is easily measurable.

The biopsychosocial model of pain allows us to categorize outcomes into the following groups:

- **Biomedical** – e.g. pain, either spontaneous or evoked by touch or pressure (allodynia) or activity. This will almost always be included, but many patients find dysesthesia (e.g. numbness or tingling) to be as disruptive and in these, analgesic treatments will be ineffective. Physical functioning (e.g. time to walk 50 m), weight gain due to inactivity, medication use or dose reduction, and number of physician visits will also be of interest in some studies. McCracken and Eccleston[23] have noted that acceptance of chronic pain predicts physical function and this is yet another dimension to be taken into account.
- **Psychological** – there are many measures of depression and cognitions, such as pain beliefs, negative thoughts, or catastrophization (see also Chapter 10, The psychological assessment of pain in patients with chronic pain and Chapter 13, Psychological effects of chronic pain: an overview, as well as Ref. 24). It is well established that depression affects the measurement of pain.[25]
- **Social** – e.g. effects on relationships, family, leisure, and working. The relationship between psychological and social factors is reviewed by Stroud *et al.*[26]

Chronological issues

The enduring nature of chronic pain means that the duration of treatment effects can only be assessed in long-term studies. Twelve months is often considered to be a prolonged study but, for example, in a study of chronic neck and shoulder pain with delayed recurrence after treatment, follow up for 18–24 months was recommended.[27]

The pattern of pain may be very irregular with intermittent attacks, sometimes separated by many months. In conditions such as migraine[28] and trigeminal neuralgia,[29] recommendations have been made for reporting of the results of either medical or surgical treatments to take this periodicity into account. Frequency and duration of attacks will be as important as intensity of pain in determining the outcome of treatments.

Challenging populations

There are relatively few studies of treatment of chronic pain in children, but assessment methodology has been reviewed.[30] Adolescents present particular challenges and a suitable compact measure has been developed.[31]

The elderly are often excluded from studies of chronic pain and so treatments cannot be based on sound evidence. Weiner[32] sets an agenda for the improvement of analgesia in the elderly to include the improvement of measurement of outcome of studies. Unfortunately, the elderly with impaired mental function do even worse.[33]

Cultural and ethnic issues are starting to be taken into account in measurements of outcome[34] and these may address some of the disparities in treatment allocation to different racial groups.[35]

WHICH MEASURES?

A consensus

The Initiative on Methods, Measurement and Pain Assessment in Clinical Trials (IMMPACT)[36] has produced guidelines on choice of measures of efficacy and effectiveness in analgesic studies. The core domains and measures are summarized in **Table 14.3**. While these core domains and specific measures are recommended for use in clinical trials, their use in many different types of settings and patient populations is clearly applicable. Although McQuay[46] encouraged comment on these recommendations cautioning against acceptance of prescriptive measures selected on the basis of opinion rather than firm evidence, this author's review (October 2006) of articles citing the recommendations suggests that his challenge has not been taken up and thus the recommendations stand.

Other measures in clinical practice

Because of the diversity of chronic pain, a range of additional measures is also used depending on the clinical objectives. Rehabilitation approaches are likely to set specific objectives for function or social engagement and analyze healthcare resource use, such as clinic visits. Independent observation of activity can be captured by accelerometers that record patient movement and provide data for analysis for example in studies of migraine.[47] Covert video evidence may be obtained during legal proceedings, particularly when the extent of disability is in doubt. Clearly function rather than pain is assessed by this method, however, conclusions may be inferred from the consistency between reported and observed behaviors as to the reliability of the pain report.

Practical considerations for measurement

Compromises often have to be made between feasibility, patient acceptance, and methodological quality.[11] Brief measures have been developed and validated for specific conditions, e.g. back pain,[48] in order to reduce the respondent burden.

SENSITIVITY

It is unethical to recruit patients to studies that are not sensitive to the parameter being tested. The patients' time and effort is wasted and they may have to endure suboptimal treatment unnecessarily. Studies that draw negative conclusions because they are insensitive rather than because the treatment is ineffective mislead clinicians and can distort literature summaries, such as meta-analysis.[49]

Multiple design details can influence the sensitivity of a study. The "floor effect" occurs when the initial pain level is low so that it is difficult for a study to detect a decrease. Studies should therefore be on "properly painful conditions" (equivalent to 30 mm on a 100-mm visual analog scale (VAS)).[50] Assessment during standardized provocative movement rather than at rest may result in greater

Table 14.3 Measures of efficacy and effectiveness in analgesic studies.

Domain[37]	Example of suitable measures[38]
Pain	11-point (0–10) numerical rating scale of pain intensity Use of rescue analgesics Categorical rating of pain intensity (none, mild, moderate, severe) in circumstances in which numerical ratings may be problematic
Physical functioning	Multidimensional Pain Inventory (MPI)[39] – (interference scale) Brief Pain Inventory (BPI)[40, 41] (interference items)
Emotional functioning	Beck Depression Inventory (BDI)[42] and/or Profile of Mood States (POMS)[43]
Participant rating of global improvement and satisfaction with treatment	Patient Global Impression of Change (PGIC)[44]
Symptoms and adverse events	Passive capture of spontaneously reported adverse events and symptoms and use of open-ended prompts
Participant disposal	Detailed information regarding participant recruitment and progress through the trial, including all information specified in the CONSORT guidelines[45]

study sensitivity. Additionally, pain scores can be calibrated to take into account patient's previous experience of pain using individual responder analyses[51] – this may increase sensitivity of trials in diverse populations. In clinical trials aiming to demonstrate a difference in level of pain, concurrent treatments will be discouraged in order to maximize sensitivity (whereas in clinical practice, any measure that reduces symptoms will be encouraged).

Other strategies for maximizing study sensitivity include:

- eliminating placebo responders from the study by using a placebo run-in period in all groups;
- excluding patients who may have incentive not to improve (e.g. seeking or receiving disability compensation); and
- studying only severe and clearly defined cases.

This is particularly important where diagnosis is contentious, such as with complex regional pain syndrome or fibromyalgia.

It is important that investigators delivering treatment are trained to be effective, particularly when psychosocial interventions are delivered[52] and that patients are fully trained in completing the tests before and during the study.[53] There are subtle interpersonal effects at the point of assessment – if the experimenter has elevated professional status or is of the opposite sex to the subject, pain scores will be lower and pain threshold higher.[54] All these factors should, ideally be standardized in any study of efficacy.

Sensitive studies will be more powerful in detecting a genuine difference between two treatments. Wide patient variability accounts for lack of power in many analgesic studies and when the difference between the control and experimental event rate is small – studies may detect only statistically rather than clinically significant differences.[55]

Patient management often changes in subtle ways around a clinical study. Improvements in measures that can be attributed only to the fact that a study is being conducted are referred to as the Hawthorne effect.[56]

ABBREVIATED MEASURES

Simple brief measures are attractive and have in some cases been validated. A four-grade (none/mild/moderate/severe) scale compares favorably with a VAS in adult migraneurs and is easier to administer,[57] and the cut points (equivalent on a numerical scale) of this type of scale are generally reproducible.[58] Many factors will influence the level of rating:

> The action of arriving at a rating is better conceptualised as an attempt to construct meaning, influenced by and with reference to a range of internal and external factors and private meanings, rather than as a task of matching a distance or number to a discrete internal stimulus.[59]

Simple measures may therefore approach the validity and utility of more detailed and intensive measures of chronic pain[60] or acute pain,[61] particularly when large populations are studied.

DATA COLLECTION

Prompt recording of data (contemporaneous) is important for accuracy because delayed recall increasingly introduces interference from the condition at the time of recall.[62] Electronic recordings using hand-held or internet-based devices or via automated telephone systems have replaced many paper systems and are reliable in adults[63] and children.[64]

PUBLISHED GUIDELINES

In general, parallel group studies should conform to CONSORT guidelines;[45] however, as we have seen, there are many considerations relating to chronic pain. Surgical treatments avoid most problems of compliance and specific checklists for studies have been advocated for trigeminal neuralgia.[29] Progress with measures for complex, multicomponent treatments, such as pain management programmes, has also been reviewed and there are many difficulties remaining.[65] It is no surprise, therefore, that it is exceptionally difficult to compare surgical and nonsurgical treatments.[66]

"N of 1" studies

The heterogeneous nature of chronic pain populations (e.g. genetic or psychological differences) may result in only a proportion of patients being able to respond to a particular treatment, the effect of which will be underestimated if the whole population is included in a simple parallel design study. One solution to this problem is the "n of 1" design in which treatments are sequentially assessed in individuals and then the results are pooled for responders and nonresponders. This methodology has been used to explore combinations of antidepressants in fibromyalgia[67] – experience suggests that patients also benefit from this individualized approach to treatment and it has even been recommended that nonsteroidal anti-inflammatory drugs (NSAID) be withheld until the safer paracetamol has been shown to be ineffective by using 'n of 1' or Individualized Medication Effectiveness Tests (IMET).[68, 69, 70]

SOME CHALLENGES WITH CHRONIC PAIN STUDIES

Control group (or lack of)

Analyzing the progress of a single treatment group without comparison with a similar untreated group is usually of little help. Differences may arise in the course of randomization; for example, when patients local to a study center and participating in a study of inpatient versus outpatient may differentially opt into a particular group.[71]

Studies of the outcome of intrathecal (i.t.) opioids revealed improvement in the study groups; however, control groups were either nonexistent or consisted of treatment failures or treatment refusers, or a group of new referrals whose pain was less severe.[72][III] Although the intention of these studies was not necessarily to prove superiority of these treatments over no treatment, the data from them could be misused to come to this unsafe conclusion.

In two similar studies comparing surgical and conservative management of back pain,[73][II], [74][II] there was no difference demonstrated. It is therefore difficult to conclude which is the best treatment for an individual patient. Noninferiority was concluded in a study of surgery versus SCS for chronic back pain,[75][II] and in another of surgery versus intradiscal electrothermal therapy.[3] Unfortunately, without control groups, these studies cannot exclude it being better to offer no treatment at all!

Blinding

Comparative studies depend on effective blinding. Powerful placebo effects are influenced by patients' perception of the placebo treatment.[76] Ineffective blinding is known to exaggerate the difference between active and control treatments and is probably common.[77] Testing blindness and treatment credibility has been recommended[65] and in some studies active placebos, such as lorazepam[78] (sedative but not analgesic) have been used.

Concurrent treatments

Studying the effects of two treatments together is important because combinations are often found to be useful in clinical practice with synergism of effect and reduced side effects. Traditionally, different combinations of two drugs can be assessed and the results represented graphically as an isobologram[79] – an example is given in **Figure 14.1**, although other more sophisticated methods are available.[79] For example, Gilron *et al.*[78] found that gabapentin and morphine together were synergistic in effect (although side effects were not reduced) – the results would be represented as points below the diagonal line on an isobologram. Comparisons are more difficult when drug and psychological treatments are combined and lessons on this can be learnt from the psychiatry literature.[80] Since treatment combinations may interact to produce improvements or adverse events in different measurement domains, multidimensional outcomes are especially valuable.

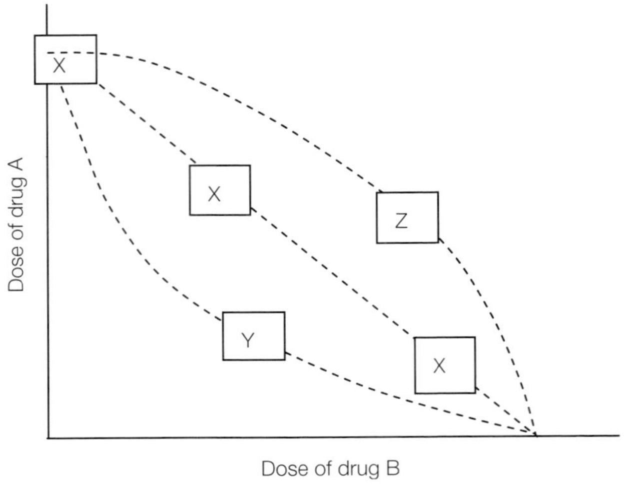

Figure 14.1 Isobologram. The points represent drug doses that result in a fixed clinical outcome (e.g. 30 percent pain reduction). Assuming that the effect of two drugs is simply additive, a series of trials of different combinations achieving the same clinical result will fall along the dotted line (X). Different drugs could alternatively: work synergistically to produce greater effect (e.g. point Y below the line); or interfere with (antagonize) each others' actions, such that a higher dose of each is required for the same effect (points for equivalent effect would be above the line, e.g. Z).

DATA ANALYSIS AND PRESENTATION

Pain measures

PAIN INTENSITY DIFFERENCE VERSUS PAIN RELIEF

Pain intensity scales may be categorical (e.g. none, mild, moderate, or severe), numerical rating (e.g. 11-point integer, 0–10), or numerical derived from a VAS. Pain relief scales are usually categorical (e.g. none, slight, moderate, good, or complete). Categorical data can often be converted directly to integers and analyzed as numerical data,[81] differences are calculated by subtraction. Pain relief (PAR) may be more meaningful to patients; however, they need to refer back to the initial pain and, particularly with chronic pain, this may increasingly be influenced by subsequent events.[62]

Large differences in pain intensity always imply significant change, whereas complete pain relief may be of less significance if the initial pain was only "mild."

When a series of measurements is made, the sum of the differences in pain intensity (SPID) or the area under the pain relief curve may be calculated as outcome data. As well as pain, patients often cite decreased medication use, increased function, and improved sleep, as worthy end points of therapy.[82]

WHAT END POINT?

There now seems to be reasonable consensus from a variety of sources that a change in pain intensity of 30–60 percent, or two to four points on an 11-point scale, represents a clinically useful reduction in chronic pain.[50, 83, 84, 85, 86] Percentage pain reduction correlates better with patient global impression of change than does pain intensity difference, particularly when the initial pain report is high. Patients may view an 80 percent reduction in both pain and disability as desirable, but will consider 25 and 35 percent, respectively, to be worthwhile.[87] Levels of depression and disability appear to modify expectations of outcome of treatment.[88] The minimum clinically important change (MCIC) has been reported for back pain and associated disability; smaller improvements are more valuable in chronic pain states than in acute ones.[89] Meanwhile, satisfaction with care may be rated as more important than satisfaction with improvement in pain score.[90]

Outcome success may be specifically defined for individual conditions using a number of measures grouped together, for example the ACR-20 (American College of Rheumatology) responder index for rheumatoid arthritis,[91] which includes pain and tenderness within a validated battery of measures to assess overall whether the treatment is effective. Similarly, a composite score has been defined for low back pain that attempts to amalgamate a number of measures into one index.[92]

A target end point may be used to direct therapy in clinical practice (e.g. 4 out of 10 on an 11-point VAS scale using i.t. hydromorphone for chronic benign pain[93]).

In summarizing group data, the proportion or percentage of patients achieving a specified level of analgesia (usually 30 or 50 percent) is used in preference to an averaged reduction in pain scores because it is more useful to know that 25 percent of patients in a study achieved 50 percent pain relief (definitely a helpful level of analgesia) than that there was a 20 percent reduction in pain scores across the whole study population (unlikely to be considered helpful).

Number needed to treat

Conceived as a basic tool of evidence-based medicine,[94, 95] it has been refined for chronic pain studies and found to be suitable as a common currency of treatment effect[81] for both medication and intervention[96] studies. It is calculated as the inverse of the absolute risk reduction between groups and is most usefully expressed with confidence intervals.[97] **Figure 14.2** illustrates a simple example.

NNT is unique to each treatment and may differ according to:

- drug dose;
- pain condition being treated;
- comparator (control group);
- conditions (environment) of the trial;
- duration of trial;
- patient population:
  - age;
  - sex;
  - baseline pain level.
- therapeutic outcome (e.g. 30 or 50 percent pain relief).

Given the variability between individual studies, it is not surprising that an analysis of NNTs for a wide variety of medications in several pain conditions has failed to confirm a pattern of efficacy between the various classes of medication that are available.[98]

NNTs are now widely used to define the effectiveness of treatments by health professionals[99] and patients (www.besttreatments.co.uk). Although the NNT is useful for comparing treatments, care must be exercised with its use because it can only be applied in similar circumstances to those patients and circumstances from which it was derived.

- NNT is context specific. The NNT for gabapentin from a brief clinical trial in adults with trigeminal neuralgia would certainly not apply to long-term therapy of octogenarians with PHN.

	Placebo group	Anticonvulsant group
□ = Less than 30% relief ■ = 30% relief or more	■ □ □ □	■ ■ □ □
Response rate (effectiveness)	25%	50%
Relative efficacy	1 (by definition)	2
Absolute risk reduction	0 (by definition)	25%
Number needed to treat		4.0

Figure 14.2 NNT: an example of a simple clinical trial. Eight patients with identical chronic pains receive treatment with medication, of whom four receive placebo and four receive an anticonvulsant. Thirty percent pain relief is considered to be a success. One of the placebo group and two of the anticonvulsant group gets 30 percent relief. It can be seen that for every four patients treated, one (one-quarter) will respond with anticonvulsant that would not have responded with placebo. Thus the NNT is 4 – and the anticonvulsant can be considered to be a moderately effective treatment for chronic pain. Obviously larger trials are required for statistical significance!

- NNT depends on the outcome measure used. The NNT for gabapentin (2400 mg per day) as a treatment of PHN in one study was 3.88 for 30 percent relief and 5.04 for 50 percent relief (the values are different again if a lower daily dose is used). Graphs illustrating how the proportion of responders changes according to the level of analgesia achieved have recently been advocated in order to understand this further.[100]

Graphical representation of outcomes

Displaying the results of several comparative studies of two treatments in the same pain condition is possible using the L'Abbé plot. This is illustrated in **Figure 14.3**.

THE FUTURE OF CHRONIC PAIN OUTCOME MEASUREMENT

Chronic pain must be addressed as a complex biopsychosocial condition.

Currently, it is more likely than not that the specific effect of any individual treatment will fail to control symptoms to an acceptable degree. This failure contrasts with the current popularity of our established pain clinics. The interpersonal aspects of treatment are therefore clearly important so that interest and advice from a physiotherapist, for example, is perhaps as valuable as physiotherapy treatment itself.[102, 103] Interdisciplinary input generally has a very significant impact so it is important that its effect can be measured in order that it can be further encouraged in the future.[17]

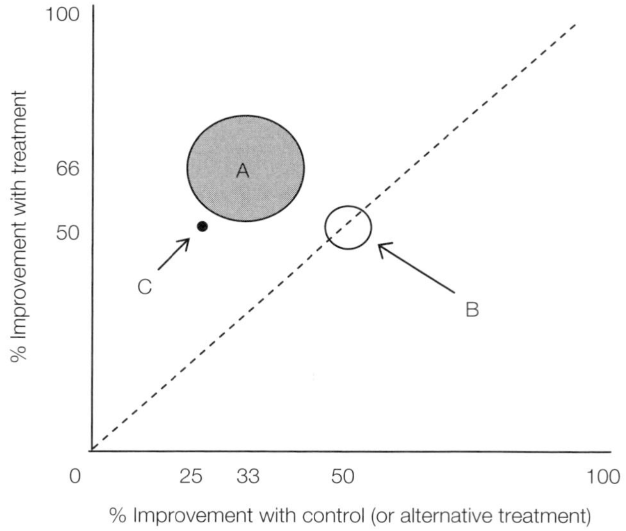

Figure 14.3 A range of studies presented on a L'Abbé plot.[101] Study A is positioned well above the diagonal line of equal effectiveness and as it includes many patients, it is represented by a larger circle. (The NNT is 3 (1/0.66–0.33)). Study B has fewer patients and indicates no advantage of treatment over control (the NNT will be very large or infinite if there is no difference between the treatments (1/0)). Study C is indicated by a small dot (NNT = 4).

REFERENCES

1. Enthoven P, Skargren E, Carstensen J, Oberg B. Predictive factors for 1-year and 5-year outcome for disability in a working population of patients with low back pain treated in primary care. *Pain*. 2006; **122**: 137–44.
2. Bone M, Critchley P, Buggy DJ. Gabapentin in postamputation phantom limb pain: a randomized, double-blind, placebo-controlled, cross-over study. *Regional Anesthesia and Pain Medicine*. 2002; **27**: 481–6.
3. Andersson GB, Mekhail NA, Block JE. Treatment of intractable discogenic low back pain. A systematic review of spinal fusion and intradiscal electrothermal therapy (IDET). *Pain Physician*. 2006; **9**: 237–48.
4. Williams KA, Petronis J, Smith D *et al.* Effect of Iyengar yoga therapy for chronic low back pain. *Pain*. 2005; **115**: 107–17.
5. Abbot NC, Harkness EF, Stevinson C *et al.* Spiritual healing as a therapy for chronic pain: a randomized, clinical trial. *Pain*. 2001; **91**: 79–89.

* 6. Finnerup NB, Otto M, McQuay HJ *et al.* Algorithm for neuropathic pain treatment: an evidence based proposal. *Pain*. 2005; **118**: 289–305.

7. Lord SM, Barnsley L, Wallis BJ *et al.* Percutaneous radiofrequency neurotomy for chronic cervical zygapophyseal-joint pain. *New England Journal of Medicine*. 1996; **335**: 1721–6.
8. Carragee EJ, Lincoln T, Parmar VS, Alamin T. A gold standard evaluation of the "discogenic pain" diagnosis as determined by provocative discography. *Spine*. 2006; **31**: 2115–23.
9. Rhodin A, Gronbladh L, Nilsson LH, Gordh T. Methadone treatment of chronic non-malignant pain and opioid dependence – A long-term follow-up. *European Journal of Pain*. 2006; **10**: 271–8.
10. Gordon DB, Dahl JL. Quality improvement challenges in pain management. *Pain*. 2004; **107**: 1–4.

* 11. Okifuji A, Turk DC. Assessment of treatment outcomes in clinical practice: A survival guide. In: Turk DC, Melzack R (eds). *Handbook of pain assessment*, 2nd edn. New York: Guilford, 2001: 639–58.

12. Rice ASC, Maton S. Gabapentin in postherpetic neuralgia: a randomised, double blind, placebo controlled study. *Pain*. 2001; **94**: 215–24.
13. Rice ASC, Maton S. Response to comment on Rice ASC, Maton S, the Postherpetic Neuralgia Study Group (UK), Gabapentin in postherpetic neuralgia: a randomized, double blind, placebo-controlled study (*Pain* 2001; 94: 215–24). *Pain*. 2002; **96**: 411–12.

14. Serpell MG. Gabapentin in neuropathic pain syndromes: a randomised, double-blind, placebo-controlled trial. *Pain.* 2002; **99**: 557–66.
15. Richeimer SH, Bajwa ZH, Kahraman SS *et al.* Utilization patterns of tricyclic antidepressants in a multidisciplinary pain clinic: a survey. *Clinical Journal of Pain.* 1997; **13**: 324–9.
* 16. Turk DC. Clinical effectiveness and cost-effectiveness of treatments for patients with chronic pain. *Clinical Journal of Pain.* 2002; **18**: 355–65.
17. Hatten AL, Gatchel RJ, Polatin PB, Stowell AW. A cost-utility analysis of chronic spinal pain treatment outcomes: converting SF-36 data into quality-adjusted life years. *Clinical Journal of Pain.* 2006; **22**: 700–11.
18. Willich SN, Reinhold T, Selim D *et al.* Cost-effectiveness of acupuncture treatment in patients with chronic neck pain. *Pain.* 2006; **125**: 107–13.
19. Thompson D. Toward a pharmacoeconomic model of neuropathic pain. *Clinical Journal of Pain.* 2002; **18**: 366–72.
20. Cepeda MS, Farrar JT. Economic evaluation of oral treatments for neuropathic pain. *Journal of Pain.* 2006; **7**: 119–28.
21. Chapman CR, Dunbar PJ. Measurement in pain therapy: is pain relief really the endpoint? *Current Opinion in Anaesthesiology.* 1998; **11**: 533–7.
22. Walker J, Sofaer B, Holloway I. The experience of chronic back pain: Accounts of loss in those seeking help from pain clinics. *European Journal of Pain.* 2006; **10**: 199–207.
23. McCracken LM, Eccleston C. A prospective study of acceptance of pain and patient functioning with chronic pain. *Pain.* 2005; **118**: 164–9.
24. Sletten C. Outcome measurement in chronic pain. In: Jensen T, Wilson P, Rice A (eds). *Chronic pain.* In: Rice A, Warfield C, Justins D, Eccleston C (eds). *Clinical Pain Management.* London: Arnold, 2003: 145–53.
* 25. Dworkin RHP, Katz JP, Gitlin MJMD. Placebo response in clinical trials of depression and its implications for research on chronic neuropathic pain. *Neurology.* 2005; **65**: S7–19.
26. Stroud MW, Thorn BE, Jensen MP, Boothby JL. The relation between pain beliefs, negative thoughts, and psychosocial functioning in chronic pain patients. *Pain.* 2000; **84**: 347–52.
27. Luime JJ, Koes BW, Miedem HS *et al.* High incidence and recurrence of shoulder and neck pain in nursing home employees was demonstrated during a 2-year follow-up. *Journal of Clinical Epidemiology.* 2005; **58**: 407–13.
28. Lipton RB, Bigal ME, Stewart WF. Clinical trials of acute treatments for migraine including multiple attack studies of pain, disability, and health-related quality of life. *Neurology.* 2005; **65**: S50–8.
29. Zakrzewska JM, Lopez BC. Quality of reporting in evaluations of surgical treatment of trigeminal neuralgia: recommendations for future reports. *Neurosurgery.* 2003; **53**: 110–22.
30. von Baeyer CL, Spagrud LJ. Systematic review of observational (behavioral) measures of pain for children and adolescents aged 3 to 18 years. *Pain.* 2007; **127**: 140–50.
31. Eccleston C, Jordan A, McCracken LM *et al.* The Bath Adolescent Pain Questionnaire (BAPQ): development and preliminary psychometric evaluation of an instrument to assess the impact of chronic pain on adolescents. *Pain.* 2005; **118**: 263–70.
32. Weiner DK. Improving pain management for older adults: an urgent agenda for the educator, investigator, and practitioner. *Pain.* 2002; **97**: 1–4.
33. Stolee P, Hillier LM, Esbaugh J *et al.* Instruments for the assessment of pain in older persons with cognitive impairment. *Journal of the American Geriatrics Society.* 2005; **53**: 319–26.
34. Edwards C, Keefe F. New directions in research on pain and ethnicity: a comment on Riley, Wade, Myers, Sheffield, Pappas, and Price (2002). *Pain.* 2002; **100**: 211–12.
35. Rollman GB. The need for ecological validity in studies of pain and ethnicity. *Pain.* 2005; **113**: 3–4.
* 36. IMMPACT. The initiative on methods, measurement and pain assessment in clinical trials. Cited January 2008. Available from: www.immpact.org.
37. Turk DC, Dworkin RH, Allen RR *et al.* Core outcome domains for chronic pain clinical trials: IMMPACT recommendations. *Pain.* 2003; **106**: 337–45.
* 38. Dworkin RH, Turk DC, Farrar JT *et al.* Core outcome measures for chronic pain clinical trials: IMMPACT recommendations. *Pain.* 2005; **113**: 9–19.
39. Kerns RD, Turk DC, Rudy TE. The West Haven-Yale multidimensional pain inventory (WHYMPI). *Pain.* 1985; **23**: 345–56.
40. Cleeland CS, Ryan KM. Pain assessment: global use of the Brief Pain Inventory. *Annals of the Academy of Medicine, Singapore.* 1994; **23**: 129–38.
41. Cleeland CS, Nakamura Y, Mendoza TR *et al.* Dimensions of the impact of cancer pain in a four country sample: new information from multidimensional scaling. *Pain.* 1996; **67**: 267–73.
42. Beck AT, Ward CH, Mendelson M *et al.* An inventory for measuring depression. *Archives of General Psychiatry.* 1961; **4**: 561–71.
43. McNair DM, Lorr M, Droppleman LF. *Profile of mood states.* San Diego, CA: Educational and Industrial Testing Service, 1971.
44. Guy W. *ECDEU assessment manual for psychopharmacology.* DHEW Publication No. ADM 76-338. Washington DC: US Government Printing Office, 1976.
* 45. Moher D, Schulz KF, Altman D, for the CG. The CONSORT statement: revised recommendations for improving the quality of reports of parallel-group randomized trials. *Journal of the American Medical Association.* 2001; **285**: 1987–91.
46. McQuay H. Consensus on outcome measures for chronic pain trials. *Pain.* 2005; **113**: 1–2.

47. Tulen JHM, Stronks DL, Bussmann JBJ *et al.* Towards an objective quantitative assessment of daily functioning in migraine: a feasibility study. *Pain.* 2000; **86**: 139–49.
48. Ferrer M, Pellise F, Escudero O *et al.* Validation of a minimum outcome core set in the evaluation of patients with back pain. *Spine.* 2006; **31**: 1372–9.
49. Kalso E, Smith L, McQuay HJ, Andrew Moore R. No pain, no gain: clinical excellence and scientific rigour – lessons learned from IA morphine. *Pain.* 2002; **98**: 269–75.
* 50. Farrar JT, Young J, James P *et al.* Clinical importance of changes in chronic pain intensity measured on an 11-point numerical pain rating scale. *Pain.* 2001; **94**: 149–58.
51. Dionne RA, Bartoshuk L, Mogil J, Witter J. Individual responder analyses for pain: does one pain scale fit all? *Trends in Pharmacological Sciences.* 2005; **26**: 125–30.
52. Macfarlane GJ, Jones GT, Hannaford PC. Managing low back pain presenting to primary care: Where do we go from here? *Pain.* 2006; **122**: 219–22.
53. Rosier EM, Iadarola MJ, Coghill RC. Reproducibility of pain measurement and pain perception. *Pain.* 2002; **98**: 205–16.
54. Kallai I, Barke A, Voss U. The effects of experimenter characteristics on pain reports in women and men. *Pain.* 2004; **112**: 142–7.
* 55. Moore RA, Gavaghan D, Tramer MR *et al.* Size is everything – large amounts of information are needed to overcome random effects in estimating direction and magnitude of treatment effects. *Pain.* 1998; **78**: 209–16.
56. Gillespie R. *Manufacturing knowledge: a history of the Hawthorne experiments.* Cambridge: Cambridge University Press, 1991.
57. Lines CR, Vandormael K, Malbecq W. A comparison of visual analog scale and categorical ratings of headache pain in a randomized controlled clinical trial with migraine patients. *Pain.* 2001; **93**: 185–90.
58. Anderson KO. Role of cutpoints: why grade pain intensity? *Pain.* 2005; **113**: 5–6.
* 59. Williams ACdC, Davies HTO, Chadury Y. Simple pain rating scales hide complex idiosyncratic meanings. *Pain.* 2000; **85**: 457–63.
60. Jensen MP, Turner JA, Romano JM, Fisher LD. Comparative reliability and validity of chronic pain intensity measures. *Pain.* 1999; **83**: 157–62.
61. Collins SL, Edwards J, Moore RA *et al.* Seeking a simple measure of analgesia for mega-trials: is a single global assessment good enough? *Pain.* 2001; **91**: 189–94.
62. Haas M, Nyiendo J, Aickin M. One-year trend in pain and disability relief recall in acute and chronic ambulatory low back pain patients. *Pain.* 2002; **95**: 83–91.
63. Cook AJ, Roberts DA, Henderson MD *et al.* Electronic pain questionnaires: A randomized, crossover comparison with paper questionnaires for chronic pain assessment. *Pain.* 2004; **110**: 310–17.
64. Palermo TM, Valenzuela D, Stork PP. A randomized trial of electronic versus paper pain diaries in children: impact on compliance, accuracy, and acceptability. *Pain.* 2004; **107**: 213–19.
* 65. Morley S, Williams ACdC. RCTs of psychological treatments for chronic pain: Progress and challenges. *Pain.* 2006; **121**: 171–2.
66. Polomano RC, Marcotte PJ, Farrar JT. Spinal fusion or exercise and cognitive intervention? In search of the answers. *Pain.* 2006; **122**: 4–5.
67. Zucker DR, Ruthazer R, Schmid CH *et al.* Lessons learned combining n-of-1 trials to assess fibromyalgia therapies. *Journal of Rheumatology.* 2006; **33**: 2069–77.
68. Nikles CJ, Yelland M, Glasziou PP, Del Mar C. Do individualized medication effectiveness tests (n-of-1 trials) change clinical decisions about which drugs to use for osteoarthritis and chronic pain? *American Journal of Therapeutics.* 2005; **12**: 92–7.
69. Nikles CJ, Yelland M, Del Mar C, Wilkinson D. The role of paracetamol in chronic pain: an evidence-based approach. *American Journal of Therapeutics.* 2005; **12**: 80–91.
70. Wegman AC, van der Windt DA, de Haan M *et al.* Switching from NSAIDs to paracetamol: a series of n of 1 trials for individual patients with osteoarthritis. *Annals of the Rheumatic Diseases.* 2003; **62**: 1156–61.
71. Williams ACdC, Nicholas MK, Richardson PH *et al.* Generalizing from a controlled trial: the effects of patient preference versus randomization on the outcome of inpatient versus outpatient chronic pain management. *Pain.* 1999; **83**: 57–65.
72. Thimineur MA, Kravitz E, Vodapally MS. Intrathecal opioid treatment for chronic non-malignant pain: a 3-year prospective study. *Pain.* 2004; **109**: 242–9.
73. Brox JI, Reikeras O, Nygaard O *et al.* Lumbar instrumented fusion compared with cognitive intervention and exercises in patients with chronic back pain after previous surgery for disc herniation: A prospective randomized controlled study. *Pain.* 2006; **122**: 145–55.
74. Fairbank J, Frost H, Wilson-MacDonald J *et al.* Randomised controlled trial to compare surgical stabilisation of the lumbar spine with an intensive rehabilitation programme for patients with chronic low back pain: the MRC spine stabilisation trial. *British Medical Journal.* 2005; **330**: 1233.
75. North RB, Kidd DH, Farrokhi F, Piantadosi SA. Spinal cord stimulation versus repeated lumbosacral spine surgery for chronic pain: a randomized, controlled trial. *Neurosurgery.* 2005; **56**: 98–107.
76. Vase L, Riley III JL, Price DD. A comparison of placebo effects in clinical analgesic trials versus studies of placebo analgesia. *Pain.* 2002; **99**: 443–52.
77. Turner JA, Jensen MP, Warms CA, Cardenas DD. Blinding effectiveness and association of pretreatment expectations with pain improvement in a double-blind randomized controlled trial. *Pain.* 2002; **99**: 91–9.
78. Gilron I, Bailey JM, Tu D *et al.* Morphine, gabapentin, or their combination for neuropathic pain. *New England Journal of Medicine.* 2005; **352**: 1324–34.
79. Black DR, Sang CN. Advances and limitations in the evaluation of analgesic combination therapy. *Neurology.* 2005; **65**: S3–6.

80. Haythornthwaite JAP. Clinical trials studying pharmacotherapy and psychological treatments alone and together. *Neurology.* 2005; **65**: S20–31.
* 81. McQuay HJ, Moore RA. *An evidence-based resource for pain relief.* Oxford: Oxford University Press, 1998.
* 82. Casarett D, Karlawish J, Sankar P *et al.* Designing pain research from the patient's perspective: what trial end points are important to patients with chronic pain? *Pain Medicine.* 2001; **2**: 309–16.
83. Rowbotham MC. What is a 'clinically meaningful' reduction in pain? *Pain.* 2001; **94**: 131–2.
84. ten Klooster PM, Drossaers-Bakker KW, Taal E, van de Laar MAFJ. Patient-perceived satisfactory improvement (PPSI): Interpreting meaningful change in pain from the patient's perspective. *Pain.* 2006; **121**: 151–7.
85. Forouzanfar T, Weber WEJ, Kemler M, van Kleef M. What is a meaningful pain reduction in patients with complex regional pain syndrome type 1? *Clinical Journal of Pain.* 2003; **19**: 281–5.
86. Robinson ME, Brown JL, George SZ *et al.* Multidimensional success criteria and expectations for treatment of chronic pain: the patient perspective. *Pain Medicine.* 2005; **6**: 336–45.
87. Yelland MJ, Schluter PJ. Research: Defining worthwhile and desired responses to treatment of chronic low back pain. *Pain Medicine.* 2006; **7**: 38–45.
* 88. Petrie KJ, Frampton T, Large RG *et al.* What do patients expect from their first visit to a pain clinic? *Clinical Journal of Pain.* 2005; **21**: 297–301.
89. Ostelo RW, de Vet HC. Clinically important outcomes in low back pain. Best Practice and Research. *Clinical Rheumatology.* 2005; **19**: 593–607.
90. Hirsh AT, Atchison JW, Berger JJ *et al.* Patient satisfaction with treatment for chronic pain: predictors and relationship to compliance. *Clinical Journal of Pain.* 2005; **21**: 302–10.
91. Felson DT, Anderson JJ, Boers M *et al.* American College of Rheumatology. Preliminary definition of improvement in rheumatoid arthritis. *Arthritis and Rheumatism.* 1995; **38**: 727–35.
92. Mannion AF, Elfering A, Staerkle R *et al.* Outcome assessment in low back pain: how low can you go? *European Spine Journal.* 2005; **14**: 1014–26.
93. Du Pen S, Du Pen A, Hillyer J. Intrathecal hydromorphone for intractable nonmalignant pain: a retrospective study. *Pain Medicine.* 2006; **7**: 10–15.
94. Cook RJ, Sackett DL. The number needed to treat: a clinically useful measure of treatment effect. *British Medical Journal.* 1995; **310**: 452–4.
95. McQuay HJ, Moore RA. Using numerical results from systematic reviews in clinical practice. *Annals of Internal Medicine.* 1997; **126**: 712–20.
96. Tramer MR, Glynn CJ. Magnesium bier's block for treatment of chronic limb pain: a randomised, double-blind, cross-over study. *Pain.* 2002; **99**: 235–41.
97. Altman DG. Confidence intervals for the number needed to treat. *British Medical Journal.* 1998; **317**: 1309–12.
98. Sindrup SH, Jensen TS. Efficacy of pharmacological treatments of neuropathic pain: an update and effect related to mechanism of drug action. *Pain.* 1999; **83**: 389–400.
* 99. Bandolier. Number needed to treat (NNT) (electronic version). Cited October 2006. Available from: www.jr2.ox.ac.uk/bandolier/band59/NNT1.html.
100. Farrar JT, Dworkin RH, Max MB. Use of the cumulative proportion of responders analysis graph to present pain data over a range of cut-off points: making clinical trial data more understandable. *Journal of Pain and Symptom Management.* 2006; **31**: 369–77.
101. L'Abbé KA, Detsky AS, O'Rourke K. Meta-analysis in clinical research. *Annals of Internal Medicine.* 1987; **107**: 224–33.
102. Rivero-Arias O, Gray A, Frost H *et al.* Cost-utility analysis of physiotherapy treatment compared with physiotherapy advice in low back pain. *Spine.* 2006; **31**: 1381–7.
103. Frost H, Lamb SE, Doll HA *et al.* Randomised controlled trial of physiotherapy compared with advice for low back pain. *British Medical Journal.* 2004; **329**: 708.

PART II

MANAGEMENT – THERAPIES

15

The use of NSAIDs and paracetamol (acetaminophen) in chronic pain

JOHN HUGHES AND K RIAZ KHAN

KEY LEARNING POINTS

- Nonsteroidal anti-inflammatory drugs (NSAIDs) are widely used by prescription and as over the counter medicines but their side effects may be life-threatening.
- Theoretically, the newer cyclooxygenase (COX)-2 antagonists have potential benefits but should be used with great caution in patients with concurrent cardiac disease.
- Clinically, NSAIDs with the lowest risk should be tried first, at the lowest recommended dose and only after having first assessed the efficacy of paracetamol (acetaminophen).
- There is good evidence for NSAID benefit in acute and chronic inflammatory pain but minimal evidence in neuropathic pain.
- Paracetamol is well tolerated and safe at recommended doses and is a first line agent in mild to moderate pain of osteoarthritis.
- Combinations of paracetamol with other agents offer little real benefit and have increased risk of side effects. They may be of benefit in short-term use.
- Elderly patients are at greater risk for NSAID side effects.
- Topical NSAIDs have been shown to be more effective than placebo in musculoskeletal pain for short-term pain relief with fewer side effects.

INTRODUCTION

The use of nonsteroidal anti-inflammatory drugs (NSAIDs) and paracetamol in chronic pain is discussed together because of their common convention of usage. The combined opioid paracetamol agents will also be considered.

NSAIDS

NSAIDs have been used for over 100 years. They possess anti-inflammatory, anti-pyretic and analgesic properties and inhibit thrombocyte aggregation. NSAIDs act by inhibiting cyclooxygenase (COX), a family of enzymes with at least two members involved in prostaglandin metabolism. See Chapter 4, Clinical pharmacology: traditional NSAIDs and selective COX-2 inhibitors in the *Acute Pain* volume of this series for full information on the pharmacology of both nonselective and selective NSAIDs. They have been the mainstay for treating chronic inflammatory conditions.[1] There is, however, a lack of evidence for their relative efficacy in chronic and neuropathic pain.

This generic group of drugs is one of the most commonly prescribed in clinical practice. It is estimated that over 100 million people take NSAIDs regularly worldwide.[2] Over 18 million prescriptions for NSAIDs were dispensed in England during 2005[3] (a reduction from 20 million in 1999[4]). In 1994 over $900 million was spent on over the counter analgesics in the US, $100 million was for aspirin approximating to 20,000 tons of aspirin consumed each year and averaging 225 tablets per head of population.[5]

NSAIDs have well-recognized side effects which creates a separate burden for health system budgets. The estimates for UK expenditure in 1999 for acute hospital admissions and coprescribing was £251 million.[6]

Assessing the real risks and benefits of NSAIDs is complicated by the fact that many agents are available without prescription. A Swedish survey from the general population aged over 18 years obtained 12,000 replies (79 percent response rate). It suggested that 7 percent of men and 12 percent of women used prescription analgesics with 20 and 30 percent using nonprescription analgesics respectively. Only 2 percent of men and 4 percent of women reported using both prescription and nonprescription medications together. Nonprescription analgesic use was higher in the under 44-year age group and prescription analgesic use increased with age.[7] A more recent survey by Porteous *et al.*[8] on a smaller sample in Scotland demonstrated similar results. This also confirmed that analgesics are the most common over the counter medication and that there is a problem with inappropriate use such as using multiple analgesics or ignoring contraindications. It is reasonable to assume that a large proportion of the nonprescription analgesics contain NSAIDs. A Canadian study[9][I] assessing the management of elderly patients (who were trained to present standard clinical scenarios in a blinded fashion to clinicians) suggested unnecessary prescribing and poor complication management of NSAIDs. If these results are generalizable, then current prescribing habits contribute to avoidable complications. A significant proportion of prescriptions are for elderly patients who are at greater risk of side effects but these drugs are safe and efficacious if used with caution in the elderly.[10] In another Canadian survey,[11] it was found that unnecessary NSAID prescriptions were written in more than one-third of physician visits. They were prescribed for elderly patients with relative contraindications and were started mostly at or near full adult dose.

Indications and contraindications

Generally, NSAIDs are prescribed for pain associated with the inflammatory arthritides (e.g. rheumatoid arthritis), osteoarthritis, musculoskeletal disorders, dysmenorrhea, and mild to moderate pain. The indications are licensed specifically for each agent and are found in the general pharmacopoeia for each country. The absolute and relative contraindications are also specified in the license for each agent but again some general principles apply. These include a history of hypersensitivity to aspirin or other NSAIDs, first trimester of pregnancy due to risk of miscarriage,[12] and those with coagulation disturbances. Caution should be used when prescribing for the elderly, lactating mothers, and those with renal, hepatic, or cardiac impairment.[13] The other common caution is for patients with a history of gastrointestinal ulceration or bleeding. For a comprehensive list, please refer to Chapter 4, Clinical pharmacology: traditional NSAIDs and selective COX-2 inhibitors in the *Acute Pain* volume of this series.

Administration and dosage

Several reviews[14][I], [15][I] suggest that current studies comparing analgesia and safety between different NSAIDs may be misleading if they only examine single doses, do not span the dose–response range, or use equianalgesic dosing. The ceiling effect for analgesia with NSAIDs is frequently not reached because toxicity prevents further dose escalation. There is individual variation with these agents and systematic drug rotation and dose titration allows the minimum effective dose to be reached whilst minimizing the risk of side effects. Patients who do not respond to one agent may well respond to another, even of the same class. This response variability is also seen in the side-effect profile of NSAIDs. When rotating NSAIDs, it is often suggested to try a representative from each group. This approach is pragmatic rather than scientific as an individual may respond to one member of a group but not another.[16] The formulation and dosing schedules for each agent vary. Use of the smallest effective dose should be the aim in every case. In some instances slow release preparations may be equally or more effective than intermittent standard release preparations with better side-effect profile and tolerance.[17] Analgesic benefits are usually seen soon after taking the first dose but it may take up to a week for full effect. The anti-inflammatory effects may take longer to be apparent.

The usual routes of administration are oral or rectal. Topical formulations are also popular. In a systematic review and meta-analysis of NSAID use for chronic musculoskeletal pain, Mason *et al.*[18] found that the number needed to treat (NNT) was 4.6 (95 percent CI 3.8 to 5.9) for one patient to experience improvement at two weeks with topical NSAIDs, compared with placebo. Patients treated with topical NSAIDs for knee osteoarthritis derived the same degree of pain relief as those treated for general musculoskeletal conditions.

Side effects and their management

Overall, NSAIDs have a good safety record but, due to the enormous quantities prescribed, they account for a large proportion of serious adverse drug events. In 1985, from all reported adverse drug reactions, NSAIDs accounted for 25 percent in men and 30 percent in women. The elderly account for approximately 40 percent of NSAID prescriptions and are at greater risk of side effects.[19] In a recent retrospective study conducted by Gallelli *et al.*,[20] NSAIDs were found to be responsible for 55.2 percent of the episodes of adverse drug reactions overall. Diclofenac and aspirin were the drugs most frequently involved, while the skin was the system most susceptible to NSAID-induced adverse drug reactions (43 percent). Withdrawal of NSAID therapy resulted in resolution of side effects in 86 percent of episodes. NSAID side effects may present with a life-threatening event. As well as the elderly, those at higher risk include patients who are hypovolemic, immunocompromised or taking corticosteroids and those who have gastroduodenal disease, cardiovascular disease, concomitant anticoagulant and diuretic use, renal impairment, a past history of NSAID intolerance, and asthma.[21, 22][III]

NSAIDS AND CARDIOVASCULAR RISK

There has been considerable interest in the development of COX-2 inhibitors in the hope that they may be associated with an improved side-effect profile. This was initially with the aim of reducing the gastrointestinal side effects and to avoid the antiplatelet effect of traditional NSAIDs. Studies suggest that this is the case.[23][II], [24][II], [25]

Since the launch of NSAIDs in the late 1990s, it has become apparent that there is also an associated increased cardiovascular risk. This led to the withdrawal of rofecoxib and a significant review of the literature.[26, 27, 28] There is now reliable evidence confirming increased risk of cardiovascular complications with both selective and nonselective NSAIDs taken long term. The evidence points to a potential COX-2 inhibitor class effect on cardiovascular events.

The evidence against celecoxib comes from the National Cancer Institute's Colorectal Adenoma Prevention with Celecoxib (APC) trial which showed a two- to three-fold increase in adverse cardiovascular events, such as myocardial infarction and stroke, with celecoxib compared to placebo after a mean duration treatment of 33 months.[29] These results were not replicated in two other trials that compared celecoxib 400 mg daily with placebo.[30, 31] Evidence against rofecoxib emerged in the Adenomatous Polyp Prevention on Vioxx (APPROVe) trial. For serious adverse cardiovascular events, a relative risk of approximately two was seen for rofecoxib compared to placebo over a three-year period.[32] This led to the withdrawal of rofecoxib in 2004 by the manufacturer. In contrast, two long-term placebo-controlled trials in patients with early Alzheimer's disease did not show a significant difference in cardiovascular events between rofecoxib 25 mg once daily and placebo.[31] In April 2005, the European Medicines Agency withdrew another COX-2 inhibitor, valdecoxib, following frequent reports of skin reactions, such as toxic epidermal necrolysis, in the USA. This warning was in addition to the associated cardiovascular risks.[33] There is also evidence as to the increased risk of cardiac events with nonselective NSAIDs in general.[22][III] A population-based nested case–control analysis to determine the comparative risk of myocardial infarction in patients taking COX-2 and conventional NSAIDs in primary care between 2000 and 2004 in the UK suggested an increased risk of myocardial infarction associated with current use of rofecoxib, diclofenac, and ibuprofen, despite adjustment for many potential confounders. No evidence was found to support a reduction in risk of myocardial infarction associated with current use of naproxen. In a meta-analysis,[34, 35] selective COX-2 inhibitors were associated with a moderate increase in the risk of vascular events, as are high-dose regimens of ibuprofen and diclofenac, but high-dose naproxen is not. In the Multinational Etoricoxib and Diclofenac Arthritis Long-term (MEDAL) program designed to provide a precise estimate of thrombotic cardiovascular events with the COX-2 selective inhibitor etoricoxib versus the traditional NSAID diclofenac, the results show that patients with arthritis treated with etoricoxib and those given diclofenac have nearly identical rates of thrombotic cardiovascular events.[36] In a matched case–control study of the relationship between recent use of NSAIDs and hospitalization with congestive heart failure (CHF), NSAIDs were responsible for approximately 19 percent of hospital admissions with CHF.[37] These concerns may warrant a reconsideration of the cardiovascular safety of all NSAIDs.[38] Currently, there continues to be debate as to the role of the COX-2 antagonists and how they should be prescribed.[26, 27, 39, 40][I] There is also debate as to the risk of cardiac events with NSAIDs in general.[22][III] In June 2005, after reviewing evidence for all COX-2 inhibitors available in the European Union, the European Medical Agency suggested the following measures:[41] (1) all COX-2 inhibitors are contraindicated in patients with established ischemic heart disease, stroke, and peripheral arterial disease; (2) physicians should exercise caution when prescribing COX-2 inhibitors to patients with cardiovascular risk factors; (3) the lowest effective dose should be used for the shortest possible duration of treatment; (4) the balance of cardiovascular and gastrointestinal risks should be carefully considered for patients who do not have heart disease but are taking low-dose aspirin (75–100 mg daily), as evidence indicates that any gastrointestinal safety advantage for COX-2 inhibitors is substantially reduced when given with aspirin; and (5) though hypersensitivity reactions are rare, serious, and sometimes fatal, skin reactions might occur with all COX-2 inhibitors. The majority of these reactions occur in the first month of use, and prescribers are warned that patients with a history of drug allergies may be at greater risk.

Gastrointestinal complications

Gastrointestinal (GI) side effects of NSAIDs range from mild dyspepsia to severe and even fatal perforated and bleeding ulcers. According to US national statistics, these drugs cause around 16,500 deaths each year and in the UK approximately 2500 people die annually from their GI side effects.[42] Patients taking long-term NSAIDs have a point prevalence for gastric or duodenal ulcers of up to 20 percent.[43] In the TARGET trial, estimates from the US suggest serious GI hemorrhage and perforation occur in 0.25 to 1.58 percent of users per year and result in at least 7000 deaths per annum in the USA and 1000 deaths every year in the UK.[44] Precise figures are not available as patients often have associated risk factors such as smoking, alcohol, and concomitant drug use.[2] The risk of fatal adverse reactions to NSAIDs may be higher; in the US NSAIDs carry a warning label stating a 2–4 percent risk of serious gastrointestinal reactions.[19] Many patients who take these agents will terminate therapy due to abdominal pain, irrespective of proven GI complications. Further evidence of this is seen in the drop-out rate of many trials and in clinical practice.[45] Up to 31 percent of the cost of managing arthritis patients is accounted for through the management of GI side effects. In a nested case–control study[46] conducted between August 2000 and July 2004 involving 367 general practices in the UK to determine the risk of adverse upper GI events in patients taking different COX-2 inhibitors compared with nonselective NSAIDs, the incidence of adverse upper GI events was 1.36 per 1000 person years (95 percent CI 1.34 to 1.39). Increased risks of adverse GI events were associated with current use of COX-2 inhibitors and with conventional NSAIDs. No consistent evidence was found of enhanced safety for GI events with any of the new COX-2 inhibitors compared with nonselective NSAIDs. The use of ulcer healing drugs reduced the increased risk of adverse GI outcomes with all groups of NSAIDs, but for diclofenac the increased risk remained significant. A cohort study[47] [III] examined 52,000 patients over 50 years old who had been prescribed one or more NSAID prescriptions over a two-year period against 74,000 controls. Follow-up was for three years looking at hospital admissions for gastrointestinal complaints. The risk was assessed as 0.2 percent per annum and remained the same with long-term use. A meta-analysis[48][I] of GI complications of NSAIDs showed ibuprofen to have the lowest risk and used it as the comparator. The authors commented that ibuprofen is generally used in a low-dose regimen (up to 1600 mg a day) and demonstrated a dose–response curve. Higher daily doses of ibuprofen increase the relative risk towards that of the other NSAIDs. There is also a risk of lower GI events with NSAIDs, which may account for up to 40 percent of the GI side effects.[49] They include bleeding, ulceration, stricture formation, and diverticulitis. A more recent systematic review highlights the elderly and those with a past history of GI side effects to be at higher risk; this reduces to baseline on withdrawal of the NSAID and confirms a dose–response effect with regard to gastric irritation.[50][I] In a randomized controlled trial,[51] GI toxicity with celecoxib versus NSAIDs for osteoarthritis and rheumatoid arthritis (the CLASS study), celecoxib was associated with a lower incidence of ulcer and ulcer-related complications combined, as well as other clinically important side effects compared with NSAIDs at standard dosages. The decrease in upper GI toxicity was strongest in those not taking aspirin concomitantly. In the TARGET trial,[44] two NSAIDs, naproxen and ibuprofen, were compared to a COX-2 inhibitor, lumiracoxib, to assess GI and cardiovascular safety. The latter showed a three- to four-fold decrease in ulcer related complications compared to NSAIDs, without an increase in the rate of serious cardiovascular events.

Prospective GI outcome studies show that COX-2 inhibitors significantly decrease the rate of endoscopic ulcers and clinical GI events as compared to nonselective NSAIDs. The NNT to avert one clinical event in one year is ~40 to 100. Their cost-effectiveness is higher in high risk patients (31 percent). An alternative to COX-2 agents is the concomitant use of gastroprotective agents with nonselective NSAIDs.[52][I] Commonly used groups include: H2 antagonists (e.g. ranitidine), prostaglandin analogs (e.g. misoprostol) or proton pump inhibitors (e.g. omeprazole). A systematic review examined the effect of adding a proton pump inhibitor (PPI) or using a COX-2 antagonist versus NSAID alone. With a PPI the absolute risk reduction was 9 percent and the NNT 11; with COX-2 antagonist, the figures were 37 percent and 27 for the NNT.[53][I]

Respiratory complications

NSAIDs may aggravate asthma and reversible airway disease.[54] Up to 10–20 percent of the general asthmatic population has hypersensitivity to aspirin and there is as much as 98 percent cross-reactivity with NSAIDs in those patients, but only 7 percent with paracetamol.[55] This may cause severe exacerbation of asthma and naso-ocular reactions. Approximately half of this group is steroid dependent.[56] This risk is highlighted in publications such as the British National Formulary.[57] Other respiratory risk factors include nasal polyps and rhinitis.[58] The NSAIDs are therefore relatively contraindicated in this group of patients. It is now clear that the specific COX-2 inhibitors do not cross-react with aspirin and are safe in patients with aspirin-sensitive airways and chronic obstructive pulmonary disease (COPD). The safety of COX-2 inhibitors in asthma and COPD does not imply that other hypersensitivity reactions do not occur.[59]

Renal complications

Normal individuals with healthy kidneys and no risk factors are at minimal risk of renal impairment from NSAID use as their renal perfusion is less dependent on prostaglandin mechanisms.[60] COX-1 is expressed constitutively in the kidney but constitutive COX-2 expression has also been reported to be extensively present in normal kidneys.[61]

NSAIDs are, however, the most common cause of drug-induced renal failure in clinical practice, but the overall proportion of patients on renal replacement therapy due to analgesic nephropathy fell from 5 percent in the 1970s to 0.6 percent in 1998.[62] Inhibition of intrarenal prostaglandin production from COX-1 inhibition has been hypothesized to cause a critical reduction in renal blood flow and glomerular filtration rate, especially in patients with concomitant renal impairment, cardiac failure, sepsis, or hypovolemia. It was originally hypothesized that the renal effects of nonselective NSAIDs were linked to COX-1 inhibition, hence COX-2 inhibitors were safe, but reports of renal damage following widespread use of selective COX-2 inhibitors has indicated important roles for COX-2 metabolites in both physiologic and pathophysiologic modulation of renal and cardiovascular function. The elderly and those undergoing surgery are also at higher risk. Most NSAIDs at full doses have the potential to cause acute renal failure within 24–48 hours of initiating treatment, but this is usually reversible.[63]

Other complications include sodium and water retention, elevated potassium causing hypertension, and edema, particularly in the elderly. Other drugs, which reduce renal blood flow when used with NSAIDs, increase the risk of renal failure (e.g. diuretics, angiotensin converting enzyme inhibitors, or angiotensin receptor antagonists and ciclosporine).[62] Sulindac and nabumetone may pose less risk than other NSAIDs.[64][III]

Nephrotoxic effects may occur but are less frequent. These may not relate to prostaglandin synthesis and the risk factors are not clear. Resolution occurs following withdrawal of the drug but may not be complete.[63] In a Medline search of clinical trials to determine the relative nephrotoxic potential of COX-2 inhibitors versus traditional NSAIDs, it was found that COX-2 inhibitors may not offer distinct advantages over nonselective NSAIDs with respect to kidney function.[65] In a population-based study to compare the association of both selective and nonselective COX-2 inhibitors with acute renal failure (ARF), investigators found that the relative risk (RR) of ARF within the first 30 days of therapy initiation was comparable for rofecoxib (RR 2.31, 95 percent CI 1.73–3.08) and naproxen (RR 2.42, 95 percent CI 1.52–3.85). The risk was comparable with other nonselective non-naproxen NSAIDs (RR 2.30, 95 percent CI 1.6–3.32), but lower with another COX-2 inhibitor, celecoxib (RR 1.52, 95 percent CI 1.14–2.09).[66]

Liver

NSAIDs tend to be plasma protein bound with low volumes of distribution and hepatically metabolized. Mild elevations in liver enzymes are common, with the elderly being at greatest risk. NSAIDs have been implicated in reports of liver injury, though the precise risk is unknown. In a systematic review of the published literature of population-based epidemiological studies reporting the incidence or comparative risk of NSAIDs for liver injury resulting in clinically significant events, defined as hospitalization or death, Rubenstein and Laine[67] concluded that there is the possibility of a small increase in the risk of clinically relevant hepatotoxicity with NSAID use. Hepatotoxicity is an uncommon, but potentially lethal complication, which usually occurs within 12 weeks of starting therapy. It can occur with any NSAIDs, but appears to be more common with diclofenac and particularly sulindac. Female patients aged >50 years, with autoimmune disease, and those on other potentially hepatotoxic drugs, appear to be particularly susceptible. Liver function test abnormalities generally settle within four to six weeks of stopping the causative drug. However, some patients may develop acute liver failure. Lumiracoxib, a COX-2 inhibitor, has been reported to cause elevated liver enzymes and there have been case reports of severe hepatic reactions including liver failure and death.[68] In November 2007 lumiracoxib was withdrawn from the UK.

Platelets

Apart from aspirin, all NSAIDs inhibit COX competitively, and the effects on platelet aggregation depend on the pharmacokinetic profiles of the agents. Aspirin irreversibly inhibits COX and prostaglandin synthesis for the seven- to ten-day life span of the platelet. The non-aspirin NSAIDs reversibly block COX. It is safe to proceed with central neuraxial block in patients taking these drugs, a view endorsed by the American Society of Regional Anesthesia. COX-2 is not expressed in platelets and therefore COX-2 inhibitors do not affect platelet function. They are safe when used alone, but can potentiate the effect of warfarin by increasing the prothrombin time.[69] The concurrent use of other medications affecting clotting mechanisms, such as oral anticoagulants, unfractionated heparin, and low molecular weight heparin, may increase the risk of bleeding complications.

Other side effects

Agranulocytosis and aplastic anemia are rare complications.[70] Hypersensitivity reactions are common with all NSAIDs. Rarely, more serious reactions occur such as Stevens–Johnson syndrome and toxic epidermal necrolysis.[71] NSAIDs run second, after antibiotics, mainly of the β-lactam group in causing skin reactions.[72]

Other rarely reported complications include alveolitis, pulmonary eosinophilia, pancreatitis, eye changes, and aseptic meningitis.[57, 73]

NSAIDs given during pregnancy have the potential to cause adverse maternal and fetal effects. Maternal effects include miscarriage, prolongation of pregnancy, and labor, whereas constriction of the ductus arteriosus, renal dysfunction, and hemostatic abnormalities can occur in the fetus and neonate. As weak acids, NSAIDs are excreted in small amounts into human breast milk with little risk for adverse effects in the suckling infant. In a population-based cohort study it was found that the risk of miscarriage was higher if NSAIDs or aspirin were taken around the time of ovulation or conception and for longer than one week. COX-2 inhibitors are classified as pregnancy category C due to increased peri-implantation and post-implantation losses and reduced fetal survival in rats and rabbits. It has been suggested that a delicate balance of the concentration of various types of prostanoids is essential for maintaining normal blood pressure during pregnancy.[12] NSAID use that suppresses the production of prostaglandins may have an adverse effect on placental perfusion and circulation. Without a healthy placenta, the risk of fetal demise can increase greatly.[74]

PHARMACEUTICAL AND PHARMACOLOGICAL ISSUES

Many preparations have been developed in an attempt to circumvent the side effects of NSAIDs. A systematic review comparing routes of administration suggests that the oral route should be used when patients can swallow. The intramuscular and rectal routes are associated with a higher adverse effects rate including pain on injection, rectal irritation, and diarrhea.[9][I]

A large *in vitro* analysis of COX-1 and COX-2 selectivity for NSAIDs has been performed for a wide range of agents.[75] This demonstrates the relative specificities for COX-1 against COX-2, but also demonstrates the level of COX-1 inhibition when COX-2 is inhibited by 80 percent. The postulate is that this is the level of COX-2 inhibition required for a therapeutic benefit. It is suggested that the agents with greatest COX-1 selectivity correlate with those that have higher GI side effects.

The NSAIDs are often grouped by chemical structure. This does not really aid drug choice and lack of efficacy of one member of a class does not exclude other members of the same class from being effective.[76]

EVIDENCE OF EFFECTIVENESS

The evidence is summarized in **Table 15.1**.

MUSCULOSKELETAL PAIN

Analgesics are commonly prescribed for musculoskeletal pain in the general population.[7] Many of the prescription and nonprescription agents commonly used are likely to contain NSAIDs. There is some good evidence for the beneficial role of NSAIDs in chronic low back pain compared to placebo, but it becomes limited when compared to paracetamol. When considering chronic low back pain there was insufficient evidence to perform subgroup analysis, suggesting that further research is required.[78][I] A more recent review of drugs used to treat low back pain again suggests further research is required.[77][I] A series of N-of-1 trials that examined the efficacy of NSAIDs for chronic musculoskeletal pain demonstrated the difficulties encountered with research in this area. There was no benefit for NSAIDs but there was a high incidence of side effects and high drop-out rates resulting in small numbers completing the trial.[86]

ARTHRITIC PAIN

Rheumatoid arthritis patients are frequently prescribed NSAIDs. A double-blind placebo-controlled trial comparing naproxen, celecoxib, and placebo demonstrated that the active agents were significantly more efficacious than placebo. There were fewer treatment failures in the active groups (approximately 25 percent) compared to placebo (45 percent). Adverse events were common in all groups, but few led to withdrawal from the study.[80][II] A further double-blind randomized trial comparing celecoxib with diclofenac over 24 weeks in rheumatoid arthritis came to a similar conclusion.[81][II] However, it should be noted that whilst NSAIDs are useful in treating rheumatoid arthritis, others agents are often more effective.[87][III]

In a survey assessing global preferences (effectiveness and side effects), which examined paracetamol and NSAIDs in patients with osteoarthritis (OA), rheumatoid arthritis, and fibromyalgia, 60 percent had a general preference for NSAIDs. The authors point out that this is a perception of effectiveness, which may differ from actual

Table 15.1 Review of evidence of effectiveness.

Condition	Comment	Agents	Outcome	Reference
Low back pain	Acute and chronic	NSAIDs systematic review	Limited evidence supports NSAIDs	[77][I]
		NSAIDs versus placebo	Statistical improvement for NSAID	[78][I]
	Acute	NSAIDs versus paracetamol	No difference	
Chronic back pain	Subgroup assessment	NSAIDs versus placebo	Unable to assess	
		NSAIDs versus paracetamol	Limited evidence of NSAID advantage	
		Paracetamol/codeine versus tramadol	Similar efficacy with combination being better tolerated	[79][II]
Rheumatoid arthritis	Response to treatment	NSAIDs, COX-2 antagonists and placebo	Significant improvement compared with placebo; no difference between active agents	[80][II], [81][II]
		Steroids versus NSAIDs	Steroids show advantage in low dose, short-term use	[82][I]
Rheumatic disease	Survey of patient preference for benefit and side-effects	NSAIDs and paracetamol	Preference for NSAIDs 60%, paracetamol 14%, and no preference 25%	[83][IV]
Osteoarthritis	Long-term comparison	Naproxen versus paracetamol	Similar efficacy with high drop-out rate suggesting neither is satisfactory	[45]
		Ibuprofen versus paracetamol	Similar effects both better than placebo	[84][II]
	Systematic review of relative efficacy	NSAIDs	Relative efficacy data not yet available	[13][I], [14][I]
Neuropathic	Review	NSAIDs	Probably no role to play	[85][II]

effectiveness. The results may be biased due to the beliefs and perceptions of both patients and physicians.[83][IV]

In OA, the NSAIDs are commonly used. A two-year double-blind comparison of naproxen and paracetamol, using a model of OA of the knee, showed little difference between treatments for those completing the trial, the withdrawal rates were high (65 percent). The reasons for withdrawal were not significantly different between groups, although GI reactions were higher in the naproxen group.[45][II] The Cochrane collaboration has reviewed the use of NSAIDs in OA of the knee.[13][I] The reviewers conclude that despite a large number of publications, few are randomized control trials and many have substantial design faults. The authors were unable to demonstrate a difference in efficacy between agents or for withdrawal rates, and suggested that prescribing be based on relative safety, patient acceptability, and cost. Similar comments were made in a review which used OA of the hip as the model.[14][I]

Pain can follow hip arthroplasty, as can heterotopic bone formation in the soft tissues surrounding the joint. A systematic review confirms that perioperative NSAIDs reduce the risk of heterotopic bone formation. The significance of this along with the short-term side effects is less clear and the long-term effect on pain and clinical outcome has not been fully elucidated.[88][I], [89][I] There is also concern about the effect of NSAIDs and bone healing. Currently, there is insufficient evidence to make clear comments other than that further research is required.[90]

Neuropathic pain often proves difficult to manage and the evidence suggests that NSAIDs are probably ineffective in this condition.[78][I]

Chronic pain in the elderly poses a major challenge for management. The population is aging and the elderly have a significantly higher incidence of chronic pain. Estimates from the USA suggest 70 million older people are prescribed regular analgesics and that the majority are NSAIDs. It is suggested that all NSAIDs should be used with caution and that high doses and long-term usage be avoided.[91] It has also been suggested that NSAID toxicity is a problem in this population and ibuprofen should be the NSAID of first choice.[92][V] There is a large individual variation with regard to the minimal effective and toxic doses. Dose titration is extremely valuable in this group and it is suggested that side effects are regularly monitored with long-term use.

PARACETAMOL AND ITS COMMON COMBINATIONS

Paracetamol has been available worldwide over the counter for over 40 years.[93] Today, it is an ingredient of a large number of prescription and nonprescription formulations and is one of the most commonly used drugs. In 2005, over 14 million prescriptions for paracetamol were filled in England.[3]

Mechanism of action and metabolism

Paracetamol is an effective analgesic with antipyretic but not anti-inflammatory activity.[45][II] The mechanism of its analgesic action is not fully understood, but has a central effect inhibiting COX.[94] At therapeutic dosages, it does not inhibit COX in peripheral tissues, which explains its lack of anti-inflammatory activity.[95] Recent research has shown the presence of a new COX enzyme, COX-3, found in the brain and spinal cord, which is selectively inhibited by paracetamol, and is distinct from the two already known COX enzymes COX-1 and COX-2. There are suggestions of selective inhibition of the enzyme COX-3 in the brain and spinal cord by paracetamol, which explains its effectiveness in relieving pain and reducing fever without having unwanted GI side effects.[96] Other reports suggest a selective COX-2 inhibition[97] (see Chapter 4, Clinical pharmacology: traditional NSAIDs and selective COX-2 inhibitors in the *Acute Pain* volume of this series for a full description of its pharmacology).

Administration and dosage

The proper use of paracetamol is crucial to optimizing its effectiveness and achieving pain relief. Patients may conclude that paracetamol is ineffective after taking only one or two tablets a day for short periods of time and subsequently terminate treatment. This is an inadequate trial period for chronic pain conditions, which require up to 4 g/day in divided doses for at least a week.[95] The oral route is preferable with suspensions and dispersible preparations being available. Rectal and parenteral preparations are also available (in some countries). Paracetamol is available in combination with several opioids such as codeine, dihydrocodeine, dextropropoxyphene, and tramadol, as well as other compounds such as caffeine and NSAIDs. The rationale behind such combinations is the theoretical enhancement of efficacy by combining two analgesics with different modes of action. Extended release paracetamol preparations are also available.

PARACETAMOL – WEAK OPIOID COMBINATIONS VERSUS PARACETAMOL ALONE

Studies have been performed which suggest that combinations provide improved analgesia compared to paracetamol alone but there is also an increase in side effects. A systematic review[98][I] assessing the efficacy and safety of paracetamol–codeine combinations versus paracetamol alone concluded that most trials were of good to very good quality. Only the single-dose studies could be combined for analysis of analgesic efficacy and pooled efficacy results indicated that paracetamol–codeine combinations added a 5 percent increase in analgesia using the sum pain intensity difference measure. This effect was small but statistically significant and comparable to the difference in analgesic effect between codeine and placebo. The cumulative incidence of side effects with each treatment was comparable in the single-dose trials. In the multidose studies a significantly higher proportion of side effects occurred with paracetamol–codeine preparations suggesting that for occasional pain relief paracetamol–codeine combination might be appropriate but repeated use increases the occurrence of side effects. More recent work reinforces this view that further studies are required looking at this as well as other paracetamol combinations.[99, 100] In a multicenter 91-day randomized placebo-controlled trial of tramadol 37.5 mg/paracetamol 325 mg versus placebo for treatment of chronic low back ache, patients reported better visual analog scale (VAS) scores, quality of life, and physical functioning with tramadol and paracetamol combination compared to placebo.[101] It has also been shown to deliver better efficacy than either agent alone and improved tolerability than the equianalgesic alternatives of conventional dose tramadol alone or paracetamol plus codeine in combination.[100]

There are many preparations available that combine paracetamol with other analgesics. In a large, double-blind, randomized, parallel group, placebo-controlled trial, Diener *et al.*[102] investigated efficacy, safety, and tolerability of two tablets of the fixed combination of 250 mg acetylsalicylic acid (ASA) + 200 mg paracetamol + 50 mg caffeine in comparison with two tablets of 250 mg ASA + 200 mg paracetamol, two tablets of 500 mg ASA, two tablets of 500 mg paracetamol, two tablets of 50 mg caffeine, and placebo in patients with episodic tension-type headache or migraine attacks. The fixed combination of ASA, paracetamol, and caffeine was statistically significantly superior to the other combinations.[102] Many over the counter remedies contain paracetamol with a wide variety of other agents and these have not been addressed in this chapter.

Side effects and their management

Paracetamol is generally well tolerated. Skin rashes and other allergic reactions occur occasionally, but generalized anaphylactic-type reactions are very rare.[103, 104] The rash is usually erythematous or urticarial, but may be more serious and accompanied by a drug fever and mucosal lesions.

In a few isolated cases, the use of paracetamol has been associated with neutropenia, pancytopenia, and leucopenia. The most serious adverse effect of acute over dosage of paracetamol is a dose-dependent, potentially fatal hepatic necrosis. Renal tubular necrosis and hypoglycemic coma may also occur.[105] There is some newer evidence suggesting a link between paracetamol and asthma or COPD.[106]

GASTRIC

Paracetamol causes little or no gastrointestinal irritation and is not associated with ulcer formation.[107]

RENAL

The effect of paracetamol on renal function is minimal because it does not influence renal prostaglandin synthesis. There is negligible evidence for the development of classical analgesic nephropathy (papillary necrosis, chronic interstitial nephritis) when used alone and it has not been conclusively associated with any evidence of end-stage renal disease.

Renal toxicity has been documented with paracetamol only in overdose and is thought to be secondary to acute hepatic failure.[95] In a 1996 position paper, the National Kidney Foundation (UK) recommended paracetamol as the non-narcotic analgesic of choice "for episodic use in patients with underlying renal disease." Both experimental and epidemiological data have found an association between combinations of aspirin, paracetamol, caffeine and/or codeine, and increased renal toxicity.[108][V]

HEPATIC

Paracetamol has been associated with liver toxicity in association with massive overdose or chronic unintentional overdose in patients with a history of chronic alcohol abuse, malnutrition, and prolonged starvation and it is one of the most common causes of acute liver failure in the USA.[109][III] Patients consuming more than three units of alcohol per day should consult with their physician before taking any analgesic.[95, 109][III]

There is no evidence that preexisting chronic liver disease increases the risk of hepatotoxicity after administration of paracetamol in therapeutic doses for short periods of time (up to five days). Cytochrome P-450 enzyme levels are not increased and excretion of various conjugates (including cysteine and mercapturic acid conjugates) remains unchanged in the presence of liver disease.[109, 79, 110, 111, 112] The elimination half-life of paracetamol is statistically prolonged, but clinically unimportant.

COPROXAMOL

Coproxamol (dextropropoxyphene in combination with paracetamol) was implicated in 300–400 deaths from overdose in the UK every year. It was implicated in almost one-fifth of drug-related suicides and was second only to tricyclic antidepressants as an agent of fatal overdose. After considering all the available data, the Committee on Safety of Medicines (CSM) in the UK advised that coproxamol should be withdrawn from the market on the grounds that the benefits of coproxamol did not outweigh the risks.[113]

PHARMACEUTICAL AND PHARMACOLOGICAL ISSUES

Paracetamol is rapidly absorbed with peak plasma concentrations occurring within one hour. If taken with food, peak concentrations may be delayed until four hours after ingestion. Paracetamol may be administered orally, intravenously, and rectally. Rectal absorption may be variable. The optimum dose is 1 g with a daily maximum of 4 g. There is, however, no correlation between plasma levels and dose.[114]

Paracetamol is metabolized and eliminated via three pathways.

1. Approximately 90 percent is conjugated with sulfate or glucuronide. Although the sulfate is less important in adults, it has been proposed as a more active pathway in children, which could account for their greater tolerance to higher doses.
2. Between 5 and 10 percent is metabolized by a cytochrome P-450 mixed function oxidase system. The intermediate metabolite of this pathway, *N*-acetyl-*p*-benzoquinoneimine (NAPQI) is detoxified by the addition of sulfhydryl groups. NAPQI has a half-life ($t_{1/2}$) that is three times longer than that of paracetamol (36 hours versus 12 hours, respectively). This is responsible for the hepatic injury associated with paracetamol toxicity. Normally, glutathione acts as the sulfhydryl group. In nutritionally depleted patients or in the presence of overdose, there may be insufficient glutathione to protect the liver. Renal injury is thought to occur via the same mechanism.
3. Less than 5 percent is eliminated unchanged in the urine. The volume of distribution of paracetamol is 0.75 to 1.0 L/kg, with protein binding of 35–50 percent.[115]

EVIDENCE OF EFFECTIVENESS

Osteoarthritis

Paracetamol is as effective as NSAIDs for the management of mild-to-moderate OA pain. There is evidence to suggest it should be first line management at up to 4 g a day.[116] A randomized, double-blind trial in OA of the hip or knee demonstrated that 4 g paracetamol daily was more effective than placebo and as effective as commonly used NSAIDs for the relief of joint pain and improvement of function.[84][II] Additionally, the majority of patients with OA were elderly and were at increased risk of NSAID-related GI and renal side effects. A prospective, double-blind control study over two years for the treatment of OA concluded that the efficacy of paracetamol and naproxen were similar.[62][II] In a double-blind study, slow release paracetamol (1300 mg three times daily) has been shown to be effective in managing moderately severe chronic OA of the hip and knee.[117][II]

Although paracetamol and NSAIDs are both effective for the relief of mild-to-moderate pain, NSAIDs may be necessary for treating pain resulting from inflammatory conditions. When treating pain associated with a largely noninflammatory condition such as OA, then paracetamol may be a more appropriate therapeutic option due to its lack of GI and renal adverse events compared to those seen with NSAIDs.[118]

Chronic back pain

A double-blind, multiple-dose, randomized, cross-over study comparing a fixed-dose capsule preparation of paracetamol/codeine with tramadol in patients with refractory chronic back pain found both were efficacious but the paracetamol combination was better tolerated.[119][II] An outpatient-based placebo-controlled study demonstrated superiority of tramadol/paracetamol over a three-month period.[101][II] However, there remains the need for further investigation into these combination preparations.[99]

Headache

Three double-blind, randomized, placebo-controlled trials concluded that the nonprescription combination of paracetamol, aspirin, and caffeine was highly effective for the treatment of migraine headache. It also alleviated the nausea, photophobia, and functional disability associated with migraine attacks, with an excellent safety profile and tolerability.[120][II] A more recent double-blind, randomized, placebo-controlled study looking at headache demonstrated the combination of acetylsalicylic acid, paracetamol, and caffeine to be superior.[121][II]

There are no good data to either support or refute a role for paracetamol in the management of neuropathic pain.

CONCLUSION

- Paracetamol is well tolerated and safe, except in overdose.
- Paracetamol is a first line agent in mild-to-moderate pain of OA.
- Combinations of paracetamol with other agents offer little real benefit and have increased risk of side effects. They may be of benefit in short-term use.
- There is good evidence for NSAIDs benefit in acute and chronic inflammatory pain but minimal evidence in neuropathic pain.
- NSAIDs are widely used by prescription and as over the counter medicines. The side effects of NSAIDs are potentially life-threatening but this must be examined in the context of the enormous scale of usage of this class of drugs.
- The newer COX-2 antagonists have potential benefits but should be used with caution because of the risks in patients with concurrent cardiac disease.
- Clinically, agents with lower risk should be tried first and at the lowest recommended dose before titration, having first assessed the efficacy of paracetamol. Trialing several agents and drug rotation may be beneficial with some patients.
- Elderly patients are at greater risk for side effects than the young.
- Further high quality systematic review or new research has to be carried out to evaluate:
  - relative efficacies between agents;
  - long-term effects in terms of risk and benefit;
  - the effects of common combinations in chronic pain;
  - what role, if any, there is in neuropathic pain for these agents.

REFERENCES

1. Talley JJ. Selective inhibitors of cyclooxygenase-2(COX-2). *Progress in Medicinal Chemistry.* 1999; **36**: 201–34.
2. Berd CB, Rowbotham MC. COX-2 Inhibitors: a status report. *Technical Corner, IASP Newsletter.* 1998.
3. The Information Centre. Prescription cost analysis: England 2005. Last updated April 2006, cited February 2008. Available from: www.ic.nhs.uk/pubs/prescostanalysis2005.
4. Anonymous. NSAIDs and aspirin as an analgesic. In: Summary of prescription items dispensed according to British National Formulary classification. UK Prescription Cost Analysis Data. England: Crown copyright, SDIE, Department of Health, 1999.
5. * Latham J, Davis BD. The socioeconomic impact of chronic pain. *Disability and Rehabilitation.* 1994; **16**: 39–44.
6. Moore RA, Phillips CJ. Cost of NSAID adverse effects to the UK National Health Service. *Journal of Medical Economics.* 1999; **2**: 45–55.
7. Antonov KIM, Isacson DGL. Prescription and nonprescription analgesic use in Sweden. *Annals of Pharmacotherapy.* 1998; **32**: 485–9.
8. Porteous T, Bond C, Hannaford P, Sinclair H. How and why are non-prescription analgesics used in Scotland? *Family Practice.* 2005; **22**: 78–85.

* 9. Tramer MR, Williams JE, Carroll D *et al.* Comparing analgesic efficacy of non-steroidal anti-inflammatory drugs given by different routes in acute and chronic pain: A qualitative systematic review. *Acta Anaesthesiologica Scandinavica.* 1998; **42**: 71–9.
10. Sager DS, Bennett RM. Individualizing the risk/benefit ratio of NSAIDs in older patients. *Geriatrics.* 1992; **47**: 24–31.
11. Tamblyn R, Berkson L, Dauphinee WD *et al.* Unnecessary prescribing of NSAIDs and the management of NSAID-related gastropathy in medical practice. *Annals of Internal Medicine.* 1997; **127**: 429–38.
12. Nielsen GL, Sørensen HT, Larsen H, Pedersen L. Risk of adverse birth outcome and miscarriage in pregnant users of non-steroidal anti-inflammatory drugs: population based observational study and case-control study. *British Medical Journal.* 2001; **322**: 266–70.
13. Jones SF, Power I. Postoperative NSAIDs and COX-2 inhibitors: cardiovascular risks and benefits. *British Journal of Anaesthesia.* 2005; **95**: 281–4.
* 14. Watson MC, Brookes ST, Kirwan JR, Faulkner A. Non-aspirin, non-steroidal anti-inflammatory drugs for osteoarthritis of the knee (Cochrane Review). *Cochrane Database of Systematic Reviews.* 2000; **CD000142**.
* 15. Towheed T, Shea B, Wells G, Hochberg M. Analgesia and non-aspirin, non-steroidal anti-inflammatory drugs for osteoarthritis of the hip (Cochrane Review). *Cochrane Database of Systematic Reviews.* 2000; **CD000517**.
16. Poole Arcangelo V, Peterson AM (eds). *Pharmacotherapeutics for advanced practice: a practical approach*, 2nd edn. Philadelphia: Lippincott, Williams and Wilkins, 2005: 519–56.
17. National Library for Health Evidence Based Medicine Q&A service. Is there any evidence for modified release NSAIDs compared to standard preparations, used for musculoskeletal pain relief; London: NLH. Last updated: April 8, 2005; cited January 2008. Available from: www.clinicalanswers.nhs.uk/index.cfm?question=394.
18. Mason L, Moore A, Edwards JE *et al.* Topical NSAIDs for chronic musculoskeletal pain: systematic review and meta-analysis. *BMC Musculoskeletal Disorders.* 2004; **5**: 28.
19. Shimp LA. Safety issues in the pharmacologic management of chronic pain in the elderly. *Pharmacotherapy.* 1998; **18**: 1313–22.
20. Gallelli L, Colosimo M, Pirritano D *et al.* Retrospective evaluation of adverse drug reactions induced by nonsteroidal anti-inflammatory drugs. *Clinical Drug Investigation.* 2007; **27**: 115–22.
21. Medicines and Healthcare products Regulatory Agency. Cardiovascular Safety of Non-Steroidal Anti-inflammatory Drugs: Overview of key data. Last updated August 2, 2005; cited January 2008. Available from: www.mhra.gov.uk/home/idcplg?IdcService=SS_GET_PAGE&useSecondary=true&ssDocName=CON1004301&ssTargetNodeId=221.
* 22. Hernandez-Diaz S, Varas-Lorenzo C, Garcia Rodriguez LA. Non-steroidal antiinflammatory drugs and the risk of acute myocardial infarction. *Basic and Clinical Pharmacology and Toxicology.* 2006; **98**: 266–74.
23. Bombardier C, Laine L, Reicin A *et al.* Comparison of upper gastrointestinal toxicity of rofecoxib and naproxen in patients with rheumatoid arthritis. *New England Journal of Medicine.* 2000; **343**: 1520–8.
24. Silverstein FE, Faich G, Goldstein JL *et al.* Gastrointestinal toxicity with celecoxib vs. nonsteroidal anti-inflammatory drugs for osteoarthritis and rheumatoid arthritis: The CLASS Study: a randomized controlled trial. *Journal of the American Medical Association.* 2000; **284**: 1247–55.
25. Laine L. Gastrointestinal effects of NSAIDs and coxibs. *Journal of Pain and Symptom Management.* 2003; **25**: S32–40.
26. Nielsen OH, Ainsworth M, Csillag C, Rask-Madsen J. Systematic review: coxibs, non-steroidal anti-inflammatory drugs or no cyclooxygenase inhibitors in gastroenterological high-risk patients? *Alimentary Pharmacology and Therapeutics.* 2006; **23**: 27–33.
27. Savage R. Cyclo-oxygenase-2 inhibitors: when should they be used in the elderly? *Drugs and Aging.* 2005; **22**: 185–200.
28. Sanghi S, MacLaughlin EJ, Jewell CW *et al.* Cyclooxygenase-2 inhibitors: a painful lesson. *Cardiovascular and Hematological Disorders Drug Targets.* 2006; **6**: 85–100.
29. Scott D. Solomon *et al.* Cardiovascular risk associated with Celecoxib in a clinical trial for colorectal adenoma prevention. *New England Journal of Medicine.* 2005; **352**: 1071–80.
30. Arber N, Eagle CJ, Spicak J *et al.* Celecoxib for the prevention of colorectal adenomatous polyps. *New England Journal of Medicine.* 2006; **355**: 885–95.
31. ADAPT Research Group. Cardiovascular and cerebrovascular events in the randomized, controlled Alzheimer's Disease Anti-Inflammatory Prevention Trial (ADAPT). *PLoS Clinical Trials.* 2006 Nov 17; **1**: e33.
32. Lagakos SW. Time-to-event analyses for long-term treatments–the APPROVe trial. *New England Journal of Medicine.* 2006; **355**: 113–7.
33. Joint Formulary Committee. *British National Formulary*, 54th edn. London: British Medical Association and Royal Pharmaceutical Society of Great Britain, 2007.
34. Kearney PM, Baigent C, Godwin J *et al.* Do selective cyclo-oxygenase-2 inhibitors and traditional non-steroidal anti-inflammatory drugs increase the risk of atherothrombosis? Meta-analysis of randomised trials. *British Medical Journal.* 2006; **332**: 1302–08.
35. Graham DJ, Campen D, Hui R *et al.* Risk of acute myocardial infarction and sudden cardiac death in patients treated with cyclo-oxygenase 2 selective and non-selective non-steroidal anti-inflammatory drugs: nested case-control study. *Lancet.* 2005; **365**: 475–81.
36. Cannon CP, Curtis SP, FitzGerald GA *et al.* Cardiovascular outcomes with etoricoxib and diclofenac in patients with osteoarthritis and rheumatoid arthritis in the Multinational Etoricoxib and Diclofenac Arthritis

Long-term (MEDAL) programme: a randomised comparison. *Lancet.* 2006; **368**: 1771–81.
37. Page J, Henry D. Consumption of NSAIDs and the development of congestive heart failure in elderly patients: an underrecognized public health problem. *Archives of Internal Medicine.* 2000; **160**: 777–84.
38. Hippisley-Cox J, Coupland C. Risk of myocardial infarction in patients taking cyclo-oxygenase-2 inhibitors or conventional non-steroidal anti-inflammatory drugs: population based nested case-control analysis. *British Medical Journal.* 2005; **330**: 1366.
39. Meagher EA. Balancing gastroprotection and cardioprotection with selective cyclo-oxygenase-2 inhibitors: clinical implications. *Drug Safety.* 2003; **26**: 913–24.
* 40. Hur C, Chan AT, Tramontano AC, Gazelle GS. Coxibs versus combination NSAID and PPI therapy for chronic pain: an exploration of the risks, benefits, and costs. *Annals of Pharmacotherapy.* 2006; **40**: 1052–63.
41. European Medicines Agency. European Medicines Agency concludes action on COX-2 inhibitors. Last updated: June 27, 2005; cited February 2008. Available from: www.emea.europa.eu/pdfs/human/press/pr/6275705N.pdf
42. Langford RM. Pain management today – what have we learned? *Clinical Rheumatology.* 2006; **25**: S2–S8.
43. Hawkey CJ. The gastroenterologist's caseload: Contribution of the rheumatologist. *Seminars in Arthritis and Rheumatology.* 1997; **26**: 11–15.
44. Schnitzer TJ, Burmester GR, Mysler E *et al.* Comparison of lumiracoxib with naproxen and ibuprofen in the Therapeutic Arthritis Research and Gastrointestinal Event Trial (TARGET), reduction in ulcer complications: randomised controlled trial. *Lancet.* 2004; **364**: 665–74.
* 45. Williams HJ, Ward JR, Egger MJ *et al.* Comparison of naproxen and acetaminophen in a two-year study of treatment of osteoarthritis of the knee. *Arthritis and Rheumatism.* 1993; **36**: 1196–206.
46. Hippisley-Cox J, Coupland C, Logan R. Risk of adverse gastrointestinal outcomes in patients taking cyclo-oxygenase-2 inhibitors or conventional non-steroidal anti-inflammatory drugs: population based nested case-control analysis. *British Medical Journal.* 2005; **331**: 1310–6.
47. MacDonald TM, Morant SV, Robinson GC *et al.* Association of upper gastrointestinal toxicity of non-steroidal anti-inflammatory drugs with continued exposure: cohort study. *British Medical Journal.* 1997; **315**: 1333–7.
48. Henry D, Lim LLY, Rodriguez LAG *et al.* Variability in risk of gastrointestinal complications with individual non-steroidal anti-inflammatory drugs: results of a collaborative meta-analysis. *British Medical Journal.* 1996; **312**: 1563–6.
49. Laine L, Connors LG, Reicin A *et al.* Serious lower gastrointestinal clinical events with nonselective NSAID or coxib use. *Gastroenterology.* 2003; **124**: 288–92.
50. Hernandez-Diaz S, Rodriguez LA. Association between nonsteroidal anti-inflammatory drugs and upper gastrointestinal tract bleeding/perforation: an overview of epidemiologic studies published in the 1990s. *Archives of Internal Medicine.* 2000; **160**: 2093–9.
51. Silverstein FE, Faich G, Goldstein JL *et al.* Gastrointestinal toxicity with celecoxib vs nonsteroidal anti-inflammatory drugs for osteoarthritis and rheumatoid arthritis: the CLASS study: A randomized controlled trial. Celecoxib Long-term Arthritis Safety Study. *Journal of American Medical Association.* 2000; **284**: 1247–55.
* 52. Rostom A, Dube C, Wells G *et al.* Prevention of NSAID-induced gastroduodenal ulcers. *Cochrane Database of Systematic Reviews.* 2002; **CD002296**.
53. Spiegel BM, Farid M, Dulai GS *et al.* Comparing rates of dyspepsia with Coxibs vs NSAID+PPI: a meta-analysis. *American Journal of Medicine.* 2006; **119**: 448.e27–36.
54. Sturtevant J. NSAID-induced bronchospasm – a common and serious problem. A report from MEDSAFE, the New Zealand Medicines and Medical Devices Safety Authority. *New Zealand Dental Journal.* 1999; **95**: 84.
55. Jenkins C, Costello J, Hodge L. Systematic review of prevalence of aspirin induced asthma and its implications for clinical practice. *British Medical Journal.* 2004; **328**: 434. Review.
56. Szczeklik A, Nizankowska E, Duplaga M. Natural history of aspirin-induced asthma. AIANE Investigators. European Network on Aspirin-Induced Asthma. *European Respiratory Journal.* 2000; **16**: 432–6.
57. British National Formulary (BNF). *Non-steroidal anti-inflammatory drugs.* London: British Medical Association and Royal Pharmaceutical Society of Great Britain, 2007: 10.1.1.
58. Nuki G. Pain control and the use of non-steroidal analgesic anti-inflammatory drugs. *British Medical Bulletin.* 1990; **46**: 262–78.
59. Crofford LJ. COX-2: Where are we in 2003? – Specific cyclooxygenase-2 inhibitors and aspirin-exacerbated respiratory disease. *Arthritis Research and Therapy.* 2003; **5**: 25–7.
60. Murray MD, Brater DC. Effects of NSAIDs on the kidney. *Progress in Drug Research.* 1997; **49**: 155–71.
61. Harris RC. An update on cyclooxygenase-2 expression and metabolites in the kidney. *Current Opinion in Nephrology and Hypertension.* 2008; **17**: 64–9.
62. Stuart R, Rodger C. Analgesic-induced renal damage. *Prescribers' Journal.* 2000; **40**: 151–64.
63. Pugliese F, Cinotti GA. Nonsteroidal anti-inflammatory drugs (NSAID's) and the kidney. *Nephrology Dialysis Transplantation.* 1997; **12**: 386–8.
64. Cangiano JL, Figuerao J, Palmer R. Renal hemodynamic effects of nabumetone, sulindac and placebo in patients with osteoarthritis. *Clinical Therapeutics.* 1999; **21**: 503–12.
65. Sandhu GK, Heyneman CA. Nephrotoxic potential of selective cyclooxygenase-2 inhibitors. *Annals of Pharmacotherapy.* 2004; **38**: 700–4. Review.
66. Schneider V, Levesque LE, Zhang B *et al.* Association of selective and conventional nonsteroidal anti-inflammatory

drugs with acute renal failure: a population-based, nested case- control analysis. *American Journal of Epidemiology*. 2006; **164**: 881–9.

67. Rubenstein JH, Laine L. Systematic review: the hepatotoxicity of non-steroidal anti-inflammatory drugs. *Alimentary Pharmacology and Therapeutics*. 2004; **20**: 373–80.
68. MHRA. Drug safety Update vol 1 issue 4. Last updated November 2007; cited February 2008. Available from: www.mhra.gov.uk/home/idcplg?IdcService=SS_GET_PAGE&useSecondary =true&ssDocName=CON2032916&ssTargetNodeId=1100.
69. Horlocker TT, Wedel DJ, Benzon H *et al*. Regional anesthesia in the anticoagulated patient: defining the risks. (The second ASRA Consensus Conference on Neuraxial Anesthesia and Anticoagulation). *Regional Anesthesia and Pain Medicine*. 2003; **28**: 172–97.
70. Galati G, Tafazoli S, Sabzevari O *et al*. Idiosyncratic NSAID drug induced oxidative stress. *Chemico-Biological Interactions*. 2002; **142**: 25–41.
71. Roujeau JC. Clinical aspects of skin reactions to NSAIDs. *Scandinavian Journal of Rheumatology. Supplement*. 1987; **65**: 131–4. Review.
72. Sánchez-Borges M, Capriles-Hulett A, Caballero-Fonseca F. Risk of skin reactions when using ibuprofen-based medicines. *Expert Opinion on Drug Safety*. 2005; **4**: 837–48. Review.
* 73. Tramer MR, Moore RA, Reynolds DJM, McQuay HJ. Quantitative estimation of rare adverse events which follow a biological progression: a new model applied to chronic NSAID use. *Pain*. 2000; **85**: 169–82.
74. Li DK, Liu L, Odouli R. Exposure to non-steroidal anti-inflammatory drugs during pregnancy and risk of miscarriage: population based cohort study. *British Medical Journal*. 2003; **327**: 368.
75. Warner TD, Giuliano F, Vojnovic I *et al*. Nonsteroid drug selectivities for cyclo-oxygenase-1 rather than cyclo-oxygenase-2 are associated with human gastrointestinal toxicity: A full in vitro analysis. *Pharmacology*. 1999; **96**: 7563–8.
76. Flynn BL. Rheumatoid arthritis and osteoarthritis: current and future therapies. *American Pharmacy*. 1994; **34**: 31–7.
* 77. Schnitzer TJ, Ferraro A, Hunsche E, Kong SX. A comprehensive review of clinical trials on the efficacy and safety of drugs for the treatment of low back pain. *Journal of Pain and Symptom Management*. 2004; **28**: 72–95.
78. van Tulder MW, Scholten RJ, Koes BW, Deyo RA. Non-steroidal anti-inflammatory drugs for low back pain. *Cochrane Database of Systematic Reviews*. 2000; **CD000396**.
79. Benson GD. Hepatotoxicity following the therapeutic use of antipyretic analgesics. *American Journal of Medicine*. 1983; **75**: 85–93.
80. Simon LS, Weaver AL, Graham DY *et al*. Anti-inflammatory and upper gastrointestinal effects of celecoxib in rheumatoid arthritis. *Journal of the American Medical Association*. 1999; **282**: 1921–8.
81. Emery P, Zeidler H, Kvien TK *et al*. Celecoxib versus diclofenac in long-term management of rheumatoid arthritis: randomised double-blind comparison. *Lancet*. 1999; **354**: 2106–11.
82. Gotzsche PC, Johansen HK. Short-term low-dose corticosteroids vs placebo and nonsteroidal antiinflammatory drugs in rheumatoid arthritis. *Cochrane Database of Systematic Reviews*. 2000; **CD000189**.
* 83. Wolfe F, Zhao S, Lane N. Preference for nonsteroidal antiinflammatory drugs over acetaminophen by rheumatic disease patients. A survey of 1,799 patients with osteoarthritis, rheumatoid arthritis, and fibromyalgia. *Arthritis and Rheumatism*. 2000; **43**: 378–85.
84. Bradley JD, Brandt KD, Katz BP *et al*. Treatment of knee osteoarthritis: relationship of clinical features of joint inflammation to the response to a nonsteroidal antiinflamatory drug or pure analgesic. *Journal of Rheumatology*. 1992; **19**: 1950–4.
85. Kingery WS. A critical review of controlled clinical trials for peripheral neuropathic pain and complex regional pain syndromes. *Pain*. 1997; **73**: 123–9.
86. Sheather-Reid RB, Cohen ML. Efficacy of analgesics in chronic pain: A series of N-of-1 studies. *Journal of Pain and Symptom Management*. 1998; **15**: 244–52.
87. Page J, Henry D. Consumption of NSAIDs and the development of congestive heart failure in elderly patients. An underrecoggnized public health problem. *Archives of Internal Medicine*. 2000; **160**: 777–84.
88. Neal B, Rodgers A, Dunn L, Fransen M. Non-steroidal anti-inflammatory drugs for preventing heterotopic bone formation after hip arthroplasty. *Cochrane Database of Systematic Reviews*. 2000; **CD001160**.
89. Fransen M, Neal B. Non-steroidal anti-inflammatory drugs for preventing heterotopic bone formation after hip arthroplasty. *Cochrane Database of Systematic Reviews*. 2004; **CD001160**.
90. Gerstenfeld LC, Einhorn TA. COX inhibitors and their effects on bone healing. *Expert Opinion on Drug Safety*. 2004; **3**: 131–6.
91. Ferrell BR, Ferrell BA. Management of chronic pain in the Elderly: Pharmacology of opioids and other analgesic drugs. In: Ferrell BR, Ferrell BA (eds). *Pain in the elderly*. Seattle, WA: IASP Press, 1996: 21–34.
92. Fick DM, Cooper JW, Wade WE *et al*. Updating the Beers criteria for potentially inappropriate medication use in older adults: results of a US consensus panel of experts. *Archives of Internal Medicine*. 2003; **163**: 2716–24.
93. D'Arcy PF. Paracetamol. *Adverse Drug Reactions and Toxicological Reviews*. 1997; **16**: 9–14.
94. Remy C, Marret E, Bonnet F. State of the art of paracetamol in acute pain therapy. *Current Opinion in Anaesthesiology*. 2006; **19**: 562–5.
95. Schnitzer TJ. Non-NSAID Pharmacologic treatment options for the management of chronic pain. *American Journal of Medicine*. 1998; **105**: 45S–52.
96. Chandrasekharan NV, Dai H, Roos KL *et al*. COX-3, a cyclooxygenase-1 variant inhibited by acetaminophen and

other analgesic/antipyretic drugs: cloning, structure, and expression. *Proceedings of the National Academy of Sciences of the United States of America.* 2002; **99**: 13926–31.

97. Hinz B, Cheremina O, Brune K. Acetaminophen (paracetamol) is a selective cyclooxygenase-2 inhibitor in man. *The FASEB journal: official publication of the Federation of American Societies for Experimental Biology.* 2008; **22**: 383–90.

* 98. de Craen AJ, Di Giulio G, Lampe-Schoenmaeckers JE *et al.* Analgesic efficacy and safety of paracetamol-codeine combinations versus paracetamol alone: a systemic review. *British Medical Journal.* 1996; **313**: 321–5.

99. Anonymous 2004. Weak opiate analgesics: modest practical merits. *Prescribe International.* 2004; **13**: 22–5.

100. Langford RM. Pain management today – what have we learned? *Clinical Rheumatology.* 2006; **25**: S2–8.

101. Peloso PM, Fortin L, Beaulieu A *et al.* Analgesic efficacy and safety of tramadol/ acetaminophen combination tablets (Ultracet) in treatment of chronic low back pain: a multicenter, outpatient, randomized, double blind, placebo controlled trial. *Journal of Rheumatology.* 2004; **31**: 2454–63.

102. Diener HC, Pfaffenrath V, Pageler L *et al.* The fixed combination of acetylsalicylic acid, paracetamol and caffeine is more effective than single substances and dual combination for the treatment of headache: a multicentre, randomized, double-blind, single-dose, placebo-controlled parallel group study. *Cephalalgia.* 2005; **25**: 776–87.

103. Jenkins C. Recommending analgesics for people with asthma. *American Journal of Therapeutics.* 2000; **7**: 55–61. Review.

104. Jenkins C, Costello J, Hodge L. Systematic review of prevalence of aspirin induced asthma and its implications for clinical practice. *British Medical Journal.* 2004; **328**: 434.

105. Insel PA. Analgesic-antipyretics and antiinflammatory agents; drugs employed in the treatment of rheumatoid arthritis and gout. In: Goodman LS, Gilman AG (eds). *The pharmacological basis of therapeutics*, 8th edn. New York: McGraw-Hill Inc, 1990.

106. McKeever TM, Lewis SA, Smit HA *et al.* The association of acetaminophen, aspirin, and ibuprofen with respiratory disease and lung function. *American Journal of Respiratory and Critical Care Medicine.* 2005; **171**: 966–71.

107. Vickers FN. Mucosal effects of aspirin and acetaminophen: report of a controlled gastroscopic study. *Gastrointestinal Endoscopy.* 1967; **14**: 94–9.

*108. Henrich WL, Agodoa LE, Barrett B *et al.* Analgesics and the kidney: summary and recommendations to the scientific advisory board of the National Kidney Foundation. *American Journal of Kidney Diseases.* 1996; **27**: 162–5.

109. Larson AM, Polson J, Fontana RJ *et al.* Acetaminophen-induced acute liver failure: results of a United States multicenter, prospective study. *Hepatology.* 2005; **42**: 1364–72.

110. Forrest JA, Adriaenssens P, Finlayson ND, Prescott LF. Paracetamol metabolism in chronic liver disease. *European Journal of Clinical Pharmacology.* 1979; **15**: 427–31.

111. Andreasen PB, Hutters L. Paracetamol (acetaminophen) clearance in patients with cirrhosis of the liver. *Acta Medica Scandinavica.* 1979; **624**: 99–105.

112. Farrell GC, Cooksley WGE, Powell LW. Drug metabolism in liver disease: activity of hepatic microzomal metabolizing enzymes. *Clinical Pharmacology and Therapeutics.* 1979; **26**: 483–92.

113. Hawton K, Simkin S, Deeks J. Co-proxamol and suicide: a study of national mortality statistics and local non-fatal self poisonings. *British Medical Journal.* 2003; **326**: 1006–08.

114. Bannwarth B, Pehourcq F. [Pharmacologic basis for using paracetamol: pharmacokinetic and pharmacodynamic issues]. *Drugs.* 2003; **63**: 5–13.

115. James B, Mowry R, Furbee B, Chyka PA. Poisoning. In: Chernow B (ed.). *The pharmacological approach to the critically ill patient*, 3rd edn. Philadelphia: Lippincott, Williams & Wilkins, 1994.

116. Bertin P, Keddad K, Jolivet-Landreau I. Acetaminophen as symptomatic treatment of pain from osteoarthritis. *Joint, Bone, Spine.* 2004; **71**: 266–74.

117. Altman RD, Zinsenheim JR, Temple AR, Schweinle JE. Three-month efficacy and safety of acetaminophen extended-release for osteoarthritis pain of the hip or knee: a randomized, double-blind, placebo-controlled study. *Osteoarthritis Cartilage.* 2007; **15**: 454–61.

118. Nikles CJ, Yelland M, Del Mar C, Wilkinson D. The role of paracetamol in chronic pain: an evidence-based approach. *American Journal of Therapeutics.* 2005; **12**: 80–91.

119. Muller FO, Odendaal CL, Muller FR *et al.* Comparison of the efficacy and tolerability of a paracetamol/codeine fixed-dose combination with tramadol in patients with refractory chronic back pain. *Arzneimittel-Forschung.* 1998; **48**: 675–9.

120. Lipton RB, Stewart WF, Ryan Jr RE *et al.* Efficacy and safety of acetaminophen, aspirin, and caffeine in alleviating migraine headache pain: three double-blind, randomized, placebo-controlled trials. *Archives of Neurology.* 1998; **55**: 210–7.

121. Diener HC, Pfaffenrath V, Pageler L *et al.* The fixed combination of acetylsalicylic acid, paracetamol and caffeine is more effective than single substances and dual combination for the treatment of headache: a multicentre, randomized, double-blind, single-dose, placebo-controlled parallel group study. *Cephalalgia.* 2005; **25**: 776–87.

16

Opioids and chronic noncancer pain

C ROGER GOUCKE AND ERIC J VISSER

KEY LEARNING POINTS

- The mean decrease in pain intensity for opioids in chronic noncancer pain (CNCP) is approximately 30 percent.
- Between 50 and 80 percent of patients developed at least one opioid-related adverse event.
- Only 30 percent of patients in randomized controlled trials (RCTs) remained on "long-term" opioid therapy.
- The average opioid dose escalation rate (ODER) for all opioids in CNCP was approximately 0.5 percent per day.
- The ODER was lower in the elderly, in neuropathic pain, and with buprenorphine analgesia.
- The optimum ceiling dose (if any) for opioids in CNCP is not known, but an equivalent of 100 mg of oral morphine per day seems a reasonable trigger for reevaluation.
- Up to 30 percent of patients may require opioid rotation (OR) at some stage during long-term opioid therapy for CNCP.

INTRODUCTION

There is increasing evidence that in some patients, opioids can relieve chronic noncancer pain (CNCP). However, the evidence is limited to relatively short-term studies which demonstrate a high drop-out rate because of opioid-related side effects or lack of efficacy. Patients who develop problems with opioid therapy, particularly those with dependency/addictive behavior traits, are time-consuming and frustrating to manage, their manipulative behavior stressing even the most tolerant staff. The long-term effects of opioids are not well quantified, but include suppression of both the immune system and the hypothalamic–pituitary axis and it is likely that their widespread use in society almost certainly leads to a greater availability for illicit use and abuse. For these reasons, proscriptive legal frameworks continue to discourage opioid prescribing. Despite this, the prescription of opioids in western countries is escalating.[1, 2]

Unfortunately, there is only limited evidence in the literature to guide clinicians in the appropriate use of opioids for the treatment of CNCP; however, consensus guidelines on the topic have been promulgated by authoritative bodies such as The Pain Society.[3]

To guide everyday clinical practice, the pain physician might ask the following questions when considering the use of opioids for the treatment of CNCP.

- What is the evidence that opioids are effective in the treatment of CNCP?
- What outcome measures do I use: pain relief, improved function, or quality of life?
- Is "opioid responsiveness" different for nociceptive or neuropathic pain (central or peripheral)?

- Are there differences between various long-acting opioids or between short- and long-acting preparations?
- Is there a place for "as-needed" opioid analgesia versus regular "by the clock" administration?
- Is there a place for multimodal analgesia including fixed-dose combinations (e.g. codeine–acetaminophen (paracetamol), combined opioid–opioid analgesia (COOA), or antineuropathic–opioid combinations?
- Are there significant differences between the routes of opioid administration?
- How do I select a patient? Does intravenous opioid (sensitivity) testing (IVOT) play a role?
- What are the causes and consequences of opioid dose escalation? Is their a maximum ceiling dose?
- How do I treat breakthrough pain?
- What about side effects?
- What about addiction, dependency, withdrawal, and diversion?
- What are some practical tips (such as the opioid contract)?
- Is there a place for opioid rotation in CNCP?

EVIDENCE FOR EFFICACY

There is evidence that opioids are effective in the treatment of certain pain states. They are widely used in the perioperative period for the management of acute pain where dose titration to effect to accommodate interindividual requirements is the norm.[4, 5] The use of opioids in the management of cancer pain also appears relatively straightforward, however opioid-resistant cancer pain is now a well-recognized problem.[6, 7, 8] The major reason for the variable reports of opioid efficacy in different pain states is that pain has a multifactorial etiology and presentation. Attempting to treat acute, cancer, or chronic pain with only one modality of treatment is likely to get poor and variable results. When the cause of the pain is not clear as in many chronic pain states, the failure rate of single modality opioid therapy will be even worse.

Patients with chronic pain present with a complex paradigm. Many, if not all, have significant biological pain generators, but this may not be the predominant factor determining their pain behavior. Consequently, treatment with opioids, which may only reduce part of the pain process, may be inappropriate at best and detrimental at worst. Many countries and societies have developed guidelines[9, 10, 11, 12] in an attempt to improve the success of opioid prescribing for this group of patients. A recent epidemiological study from Denmark reporting on 228 opioid users with pain found significant negative features in terms of quality of life, when compared with 1678 nonopioid users with pain. They strongly recommend caution when long-term opioid use for pain is being considered.[13]

What is the evidence that opioids are effective in the treatment of CNCP?

There have been a number of systematic reviews and meta-analyses of randomized controlled trials (RCTs).[14] [I], [15][I], [16][I] These reviews have included many of the same studies and identified similar problems with the current literature on opioids for CNCP. They do, however, attempt to answer some of the questions we have posed. A summary of the data from these meta-analyses and systematic reviews is listed below (note: approximate values are listed).

- No RCTs have tested opioids for the treatment of CNCP in doses greater than 300 mg morphine (equivalent) per day (or methadone 80 mg per day), for more than 16 weeks.
- It was difficult to determine the effects of opioids on functional or quality of life outcomes.
- There was a significant placebo effect.
- The mean decrease in pain intensity was 30 percent (15–30 percent for placebo).
- The mean decrease in visual analog scale (VAS) pain score was 15/100.
- Between 5 and 10 percent of patients withdrew due to lack of opioid efficacy (20 percent for placebo).
- Between 50 and 80 percent of patients developed at least one opioid-adverse effect (30–60 percent for placebo).
- Between 20 and 30 percent of patients withdrew due to opioid-adverse effects (5–15 percent for placebo).
- Only 30 percent of RCT patients remained on long-term opioid therapy for the management of chronic pain.

Is opioid responsiveness different for nociceptive or neuropathic pain (central or peripheral)?

Kalso *et al.*[14][I] provide some help here. They reviewed 15 randomized placebo controlled trials. Four looked at intravenous opioid testing and included 120 patients, the other 11 compared oral opioids with placebo in 1025 patients. The opioids tested were described as World Health Organization (WHO) step 3 analgesics, including fentanyl, hydromorphone, methadone, morphine, oxycodone, and oxymorphone and a wide variety of nociceptive and neuropathic pain disorders were treated.

Trials lasted between four days and eight weeks and mean daily opioid doses varied between 30 and 120 mg of morphine, 20–45 mg of oxycodone, and 15 mg of methadone. The maximum daily dose reached in some patients was morphine 300 mg, oxycodone 120 mg, and methadone 80 mg. Trial designs were generally of good quality; however, functional and quality of life outcomes were frequently not evaluated.

The mean reduction in pain intensity with opioids was approximately 30 percent for both nociceptive and neuropathic pain. Five of the studies that assessed function reported no change in a range of measures with one[17][II] reporting significant improvement in pain-related disability and two[18][II], [19][II] reporting disability scores lower during treatment with oxycodone over placebo.

In summary, the review by Kalso *et al.*[14] suggests that short-term, moderate-dose opioid therapy can produce a modest reduction in both nociceptive and neuropathic pain and may reduce pain-related disability.

Eisenberg *et al.*[15] specifically addressed the efficacy of opioids in neuropathic pain in a systematic review and meta-analysis of RCTs.[15][II] These reviewers analyzed 22 articles with neuropathic pain as an inclusion criteria using opioid agonists (partial agonists and agonist–antagonists being excluded) via the oral, rectal, transdermal, intravenous, intramuscular, or subcutaneous routes. Trials were classified as either short term (less than 24 hours; $n = 14$) or intermediate term (8–56 days; $n = 8$) with regards to the duration of opioid therapy. In the short-term group, morphine, fentanyl, alfentanil, pethidine (meperidine), or codeine were used and most trials were placebo controlled. The short-term studies provided equivocal evidence of opioid efficacy and no conclusions could be made.

In the intermediate group, morphine, oxycodone, methadone, and levorphanol were included; placebo was used in seven of the eight trials. Doses ranged from morphine 20–300 mg per day, oxycodone 20–120 mg per day, methadone 10–80 mg per day, and levorphanol with mean doses of 2.7–8.9 mg per day. The mean pain intensity was reduced by 14/100 VAS points (95 percent CI −18 to −10) in opioid-treated patients; however, the authors had difficulties commenting on functional or quality of life outcomes because the wide range of measures used prevented comparison.

Are there differences between various long-acting opioids or between short- and long-acting preparations?

Chou *et al.*, in a systematic review of 16 RCTs with 1427 patients, together with eight observational studies describing 1190 patients, address this issue.[20][I] Unfortunately, there was significant heterogeneity in the design, duration, and quality of these studies and difficulties in establishing the equivalent potency of the various opioid preparations. For the purposes of this review, a long-acting opioid was defined as a drug requiring administration no more than twice per day. Opioids studied included fentanyl, morphine, oxycodone, levorphanol, methadone, codeine, and dihydrocodeine.

COMPARISON OF LONG-ACTING OPIOIDS

Only two RCTs directly compared long-acting opioids in a head-to-head fashion. One trial included in the review – although criticized for its methodology – looked at patients with miscellaneous pain etiologies, comparing transdermal fentanyl and twice daily long-acting morphine.[21][II] This trial only met some of the systematic review's inclusion criteria (it was nonblinded and many patients had been on one of the drugs prior to the study) and the reviewers concluded that the study really measured the efficacy of fentanyl in those patients who had failed oral morphine therapy. There was also criticism of the finding that constipation was less prevalent in patients receiving fentanyl.

The second RCT, including patients with pain due to osteoarthritis, looked at morphine 30 mg once daily (either in the morning or evening) versus morphine 15 mg, twice a day There was no difference in analgesia or function, but the evening dose of morphine provided a better sleep score.[22][II]

The remaining 14 RCTs compared various long-acting opioids to other types of analgesia or placebo controls. Unfortunately, the data from these studies were too heterogeneous to allow for a comparison of long-acting opioids using this paradigm. However, data from open-label studies or comparative nonrandomized trials demonstrated some differences between various long-acting opioids.

Transdermal buprenorphine may cause less constipation than transdermal fentanyl or oral slow-release morphine, based on comparative data from open-label studies and postmarketing surveillance. The incidence of central nervous system (CNS) adverse effects, such as somnolence, hallucinations, or vertigo, may also be lower with transdermal buprenorphine.[23, 24, 25] In a retrospective, comparative data analysis of 631 patients with CNCP, the rate of dose escalation and number of dose changes was significantly lower with transdermal buprenorphine compared with fentanyl.[26]

In an open-label, randomized, parallel group trial, there was no difference in the analgesic efficacy of transdermal fentanyl 25 µg/hour or morphine SR (sustained release) 30 mg/day, however there was significantly less constipation with fentanyl.[27][III] In a review of pooled data from open-label, uncontrolled, and randomized controlled trials in 1220 patients with chronic pain, there was significantly less constipation and somnolence with transdermal fentanyl compared with controlled-release morphine.[28][III]

In conclusion, there are insufficient data from RCTs to determine if there are differences between long-acting opioids in terms of analgesic efficacy or adverse effects. However, transdermal buprenorphine or fentanyl may produce less somnolence and constipation compared with oral slow-release morphine, based largely on data from open-label, comparative studies. Transdermal buprenorphine may also produce less rapid dose escalation (see below under Buprenorphine).

COMPARISON OF SHORT-ACTING AND LONG-ACTING OPIOIDS

Most patients with CNCP are treated with long-acting (controlled-release) opioids rather than short-acting preparations, in the belief that steady plasma levels are associated with better pain control and fewer adverse effects, including withdrawal or dependency. Indeed, most consensus guidelines recommend the use of long-acting opioids for the treatment of CNCP.[9, 11]

However, the systematic review by Chou *et al.*[20][I] (568 patients in seven RCTs) found there was insufficient evidence to determine if either long- or short-acting opioids were superior in the treatment of CNCP. Again there were problems with heterogeneity and the quality of the trials. However, in a subanalysis of three RCTs, there was fair evidence that short- and long-acting preparations of oxycodone were equally effective. In addition, two RCTs found that the total daily opioid dose was lower using short-acting morphine or codeine compared with long-acting forms.

In conclusion, there are insufficient data to determine if there is a difference between short- and long-acting opioids in the treatment of CNCP, in terms of efficacy or safety. However, subanalysis of the data suggests that short-acting opioids may be just as effective as long-acting preparations and result in reduced daily opioid doses.

What about evidence for the use of individual opioids?

METHADONE

There is only limited literature on the use of methadone in chronic noncancer pain.[29] Morley *et al.*[30][II] studied 19 patients with neuropathic pain in a high quality (high Jadad score[31]) RCT that ran for 20 days. They demonstrated a statistically significant analgesic effect for methadone 10 mg twice a day over placebo.

The major analgesic effect of methadone is due to high affinity, stereospecific (R-enantiomer) binding at the mu-opioid receptor. The D-enantiomer of methadone also demonstrates *in vivo N*-methyl-D-aspartic acid (NMDA) receptor antagonism and this ketamine-like effect may be of advantage in the treatment of pathological pain states.[32]

Methadone is well absorbed from the gastrointestinal tract with an oral bioavailability of between 60 and 95 percent, reaching a peak plasma concentration at four hours.[33] Methadone undergoes oxidative biotransformation in the liver by cytochrome P450 3A4. Only 15 percent of a dose of methadone is excreted unchanged in the urine and its major metabolite (ethylidine-dimethyl-diphenylpyrrolidine (EDDP)) is metabolically inactive, thus making major dose adjustments unnecessary in patients with renal impairment.[34]

Single-dose studies with methadone show an analgesic effect of four to six hours. However, with multiple dosing, the main determinant of the duration of action is the slow terminal elimination phase. Plasma methadone concentrations decline in a biexponential manner after parenteral administration. The initial elimination phase lasts two to three hours, however the terminal half-life is extremely wide ranging (10–150 hours) compared with other opioids, such as morphine (two to four hours). This is largely due to significant interindividual variability (50-fold) in the activity of cytochrome P450 3A4 combined with methadone's relatively low hepatic clearance rate. However, variability in cytochrome P450 3A4 activity (and therefore methadone half-life) may also be due to drug interactions at that site. Methadone clearance is increased by concurrent use of phenytoin and decreased by use of amitriptyline and fluvoxamine.[35] The clearance of methadone is reduced with age and increased in females. All of these factors may lead to variable accumulation of methadone between individuals with long-term dosing, risking either overdose and or a lack of analgesia. As a result, extreme care must be taken when loading patients with methadone for chronic pain management.

Initial reports suggested that morphine and methadone were equipotent (dose conversion ratio of 1:1) and this is true to some extent for limited, low-dose administration of methadone, such as in acute pain management. However, recent guidelines recommend graded dose conversion ratios ranging from 2.5:1 to 14.3:1 (median 7.75:1) when changing from oral morphine to methadone,[36] with the ratio increasing as the dose of morphine increases (e.g.1000 mg of oral morphine per day at 14:1 is approximately 70 mg methadone per day; 200 mg morphine per day at 4:1 is approximately 50 mg methadone per day). It is therefore uncommon for any patient to need more than 100 mg of methadone per day, even when converting from very high doses of oral morphine. This variable conversion ratio is unique to methadone and reflects saturation of cytochrome P450's enzymatic capacity with higher doses (methadone will not be metabolized and will therefore accumulate). Increased analgesia and sedation with higher-dose methadone may also be due to pharmacodynamic effects such as NMDA receptor antagonism (ketamine-like effects) and 5-hydroxytryptamine reuptake inhibition (serotoneregic effects).

When commencing methadone in opioid-naive patients, small (2.5–5 mg) 8–12 hourly doses have been suggested. Ideally, dose changes should not be made more frequently than every five days (in case they are one of those patients with a very long half-life, e.g. 60–100 hours), and careful monitoring must be made until a stable effective dose has been established.[37] When using higher doses of methadone, such as during opioid conversion, hospital monitoring may be required.

Opioid toxicity is a potentially serious problem and may be particularly so in the chronic noncancer pain population. Deaths have been reported in the addiction literature when patients who were previously on a stable dose of methadone ceased their drug for a short period of time and then developed severe respiratory depression on restarting the same dose (apparently due to a rapid loss of tolerance).[38] Deaths in the addiction/forensic literature often report concomitant high levels of benzodiazepines and occasionally alcohol in postmortem blood and liver samples. It is important that patients with chronic noncancer pain are warned of these risks if opioids are to be used.[39, 40]

If methadone is ceased for more than two days, we would recommend a conservative restarting dose at 30 percent of the previous dose.

OXYCODONE

There are three RCTs evaluating the efficacy of oxycodone – all in neuropathic pain states. Watson *et al.*[19][II] looked at 36 patients with painful diabetic neuropathy and evaluated pain relief, safety, and health-related quality of life (QOL) as measured with the SF36. Maximum doses of controlled-release oxycodone were 40 mg twice a day compared to an active placebo (benztropine). The oxycodone group showed significantly lower pain scores (mean daily VAS pain scores 21.8/100 versus 48.6/100) and improved SF36 scores. The number needed to treat (NNT) for at least 50 percent pain relief was 2.6. In a larger multicentre study of 159 patients also with diabetic neuropathy, Gimbel *et al.*[41][II] found similar efficacy for controlled-release oxycodone. In a randomized, double-blind, placebo-controlled study that lasted six weeks, they demonstrated a statistically significant reduction in average daily pain intensity for days 28 to 42 of 4.1 in the oxycodone group versus 5.3 in the placebo group ($p = 0.002$). There were typical opioid-related side effects; however, the clinical significance of this small benefit is difficult to quantify.

In a previous study, Watson and Babul[18][II] also reported on the efficacy of controlled-release oxycodone in patients with postherpetic neuralgia. Using a double-blind crossover design allowing a maximum dose of oxycodone of 30 mg twice a day (mean dose of 45 mg at end of the study), 50 patients were enrolled with 38 completing the two four-week components. With regard to pain relief, there was a significant difference in VAS scores in the oxycodone group versus the placebo group (ongoing pain 34/100 (± 26) versus 55/100 (± 27), $p = 0.0001$; paroxysmal pain 22/100 $\pm$ 24 versus 42/100 $\pm$ 32, $p = 0.0001$; allodynia 1.6/100 $\pm$ 1 versus 2/100 $\pm$ 1.1, $p = 0.0155$). Disability was measured using a categorical scale (none, mild, moderate, or severe) at patient interview, and was less in the oxycodone group 0.3 versus 0.7 in the placebo arm.

MORPHINE

Moulin *et al.*[42][II] studied the use of oral morphine (in a sustained-release preparation) versus benztropine (an active placebo which has many of the side-effects of morphine – sedation, light-headedness, nausea, dry mouth, constipation, and urinary hesitancy) in a double-blind randomized crossover trial over nine weeks. Patients had stable noncancer pain of at least six months' duration. Average pain intensity of the previous week was classified as at least moderate on a categorical scale and at least 5 on a 0–10 VAS. The pain was of a myofascial, musculoskeletal, or rheumatic nature and had failed to respond to nonsteroidal anti-inflammatory drugs (NSAID) and at least one tricyclic antidepressant (TCA). Patients went through a treatment cycle that increased the dose of drug weekly for three weeks, followed by maintenance and evaluation for six weeks, then reducing the dose of drug in reverse order to the titration for two weeks. The cycle was then repeated with the other drug.

The doses of morphine were 15, 30, and 60 mg twice daily and the maintenance dose was the highest tolerated during the evaluation phase. Matching placebos ensured the study remained blinded. Paracetamol (acetaminophen) 500 mg was available as rescue medication. The patients' psychological status, quality of life, and pain intensity were assessed using standard methods.

One hundred and three patients were found suitable for the study, but only 43 patients completed the study; their mean daily dose of morphine was 83.5 mg and of benztropine was 1.5 mg. Patients showed a significant reduction in pain intensity (VAS) compared with placebo when the morphine was administered first ($p = 0.01$). Morphine (regardless of whether it was given as the first or second drug) also significantly reduced the sum of differences in pain intensity from baseline. Further analysis confirmed that the analgesic response was independent of the side effects. Morphine was not associated with any improvement in psychological state or level of function. Moulin concludes that morphine may confer analgesic benefit, but is unlikely to confer any improvement in psychological state.

Caldwell *et al.*[22][II] compared two different controlled-release oral morphine preparations (30 mg) with placebo in a randomized double-blind trial on patients with moderate to severe osteoarthritis who had failed to respond to nonsteroidal medication and paracetamol. The study was initially a four-week trial, but allowed an open label extension. One hundred and eighty-one patients completed the study. Both morphine groups demonstrated a 17–20 percent reduction in pain from baseline score compared to the placebo group. Statistically significant changes in physical function could not be demonstrated.

FENTANYL

Langford *et al.*,[43][II] in a multicountry randomized, placebo-controlled study running over six weeks, screened 553 subjects before enrolling 416 of them. Ninety-three patients completed the placebo arm and 106 completed the active transdermal fentanyl (TDF) arm. Outcome assessments for the patients, who had osteoarthritis of their hip or knee and were awaiting joint replacement surgery, were undertaken with pain being measured by VAS and function with the Western Ontario and McMaster Universities Osteoarthritis Index (WOMAC). By using their primary outcome measure (area under the curve for VAS scores), they demonstrated a significant difference between the TDF group (20/100) and the placebo group (14.6/100); however, at the conclusion of the study at six weeks there was little difference between the groups. There was a high dropout rate in both groups, those dropping out of the TDF group because of treatment related side effects such as nausea, vomiting, and somnolence, while dropouts from the placebo group were for lack of effect (leaving, of course, a high proportion of placebo responders in the study, demonstrating the difficulty in the design of such studies). The overall WOMAC index was significantly better in the TDF group; however, stiffness and physical function scores only showed nonsignificant trends in favor of the TDF group.

BUPRENORPHINE

Although there is significant confusion in the literature, buprenorphine is most commonly classified as a (partial) mu agonist/kappa antagonist. However, this is based largely on animal data and may not necessarily apply to the human clinical paradigm. There is some consensus that in lower doses commonly used in clinical pain management, buprenorphine acts more like a full mu agonist. The partial agonist effect only occurs at very high doses as used in the treatment of opioid addiction.[44]

The use of buprenorphine in the treatment of CNCP has increased significantly over recent years, mainly as a transdermal system in doses of 5–70 μg/hour. Transdermal buprenorphine is effective in the treatment of CNCP, based largely on open-label surveillance data[45, 46] and a limited number of randomized, placebo-controlled trials.[47][II]

Because of the confusion regarding the partial agonist/antagonist effects of buprenorphine, strategies for dealing with breakthrough pain are not clear. However, sublingual buprenorphine, tramadol, or possibly full opioid agonists in clinically appropriate doses may be effective. In an open-label study of patients treated with transdermal buprenorphine for cancer pain, standard doses of intravenous morphine were effective for the management of breakthrough pain.[48]

The rate of dose escalation is significantly less with buprenorphine compared with other opioids, possibly reflecting reduced opioid tolerance or hyperalgesia.[26] Although there is still liability for abuse, the development of dependence or addiction may also be less.[49][II]

Buprenorphine can be used safely without dose adjustment in patients with renal impairment, including those on hemodialysis,[50, 51] and is associated with less sedation, constipation, or pruritis compared with full opioid agonists.[25] The incidence of respiratory depression is also significantly less with buprenorphine due to partial agonist ceiling effects (which occurs at a lower dose than analgesia ceiling effects), although reversal with naloxone may be more difficult.[52]

TRAMADOL

Tramadol is a unique opioid analgesic combining mu, noradrenergic, and serotonergic receptor agonist effects. Tramadol is effective in the treatment of moderately severe chronic pain, particularly neuropathic pain such as postherpetic neuralgia and painful diabetic neuropathy.[53] [I] Tramadol also provides modest improvement in chronic low back pain and pain associated with fibromyalgia[54] or osteoarthritis.[55][I] Tramadol may produce less constipation, respiratory depression, dependence, abuse, and diversion compared with standard opioids.[56, 57] There are some concerns with regards to provoking fits in patients who have a reduced seizure threshold or the development of serotonergic syndrome, particularly when higher doses of tramadol are combined with tricyclic antidepressants or selective serotonin reuptake inhibitors (SSRI).[58, 59]

Is there a place for as-needed opioid dosing versus regular by-the-clock administration in the treatment of CNCP?

Although most patients are prescribed regular, by-the-clock opioids for CNCP, in practice it is not unusual for patients to skip doses when their pain is not as severe, effectively giving themselves (and their receptors) a short opioid holiday. In one review, up to 90 percent of patients with CNCP intermittently stopped or missed opioid doses with only 15 percent developing withdrawal symptoms.[60] In an RCT by the same authors, only 30 percent of patients with CNCP developed (usually mild) withdrawal symptoms following placebo interruption of their long-term opioid therapy for 60 hours.[61][II]

Given that not all CNCP is continuous or of the same intensity over time, it may be reasonable for patients to skip doses, at least within a 24-hour period, without substantial risk of developing withdrawal symptoms. In theory, these short opioid holidays may allow opioid receptors time to recover from being constantly bombarded by agonists (perhaps developing less tolerance or hyperalgesia). However, no trials have been performed to determine if as-needed opioid dosing is as effective or has any advantages (such as dose reduction or fewer side effects) over regular opioid dosing in the treatment of CNCP. When prescribing methadone to patients with CNCP, they should be cautioned about reducing their restart dose if they miss more than two days of methadone (see above under Methadone).

Is there a place for multimodal analgesia including fixed-dose combinations (e.g. codeine–paracetamol or combined opioid–opioid analgesia?

Multimodal analgesia is defined as the use of two or more analgesic drugs or techniques to improve analgesic efficacy and/or reduce adverse effects. This concept has been trialled extensively and found to be beneficial in acute pain management, but data for the treatment of CNCP are limited. Multimodal analgesia may take the form of either flexible or fixed-dose opioid, paracetamol, or NSAID combinations, or the use of adjuvant agents, such as ketamine or gabapentin.

OPIOIDS COMBINED WITH PARACETAMOL OR NSAID

Meta-analyses demonstrate that combining opioids, including tramadol, with paracetamol or NSAID significantly improves acute postoperative pain relief, usually with significant opioid-sparing and a reduction in related side effects.[62, 63][I], [64][I] However, in cancer pain, there was no clinical benefit in adding NSAID or paracetamol to opioids.[65][I]

Unfortunately, there are only limited data on the use of opioids combined with either paracetamol, NSAID, or COX-2-selective inhibitors (usually in fixed-dose combinations) in the treatment of CNCP. Except for Chou *et al.*,[20][I] none of the recent systematic reviews provided data on these combination analgesics.

Hydrocodone 7.5 mg plus ibuprofen 200 mg was of equal efficacy to codeine 60 mg plus paracetamol 600 mg[66][III] or oxycodone 5 mg plus paracetamol 325 mg in the treatment of chronic pain.[67][III]

TRAMADOL/PARACETAMOL COMBINATIONS

The unique opioid analgesic tramadol (37.5 mg), combined with paracetamol (325 mg) is highly effective in the treatment of chronic pain,[54] including osteoarthritis, low back pain,[68][III], [69][II], [70][II] and fibromyalgia,[71][II] using modest total daily doses of approximately 150 mg of tramadol and 1200 mg paracetamol with minimal side effects.

COMPARING COMBINATION ANALGESICS WITH LONG-ACTING OPIOIDS

Only five RCTs have directly compared opioid–paracetamol combinations with long-acting opioids and a systematic review of three of these trials was inconclusive.[20][I] In one trial, short-acting oxycodone/paracetamol was just as effective as long-acting oxycodone; however, side effects were greater with the combination therapy.[72][II] Two RCTs found that oxycodone 5 mg/paracetamol 325 mg or hydrocodone 7.5 mg/paracetamol 325 mg combinations were as effective as transdermal buprenorphine (5–20 μg/hour) in chronic low back pain.[73]

Although specific data are lacking, it seems logical to use multimodal analgesia with paracetamol, NSAIDs, or COX-2-specific inhibitors in patients on long-term opioids for chronic pain, if the risks associated with use of adjuvant agents (e.g. NSAIDs and gastrointestinal, renal, or cardiovascular effects) are acceptable. At the very least, multimodal analgesia may provide a degree of opioid-sparing, perhaps reducing dose escalation (due to tolerance or hyperalgesia), or side effects. The use of paracetamol or NSAIDs/COX-2 inhibitors may also be useful in the treatment of breakthrough pain or during opioid rotation.

Based on limited data, fixed-dose combinations of short-acting opioids (including tramadol) and paracetamol may be as effective as long-acting opioids in the treatment of mild-to-moderate CNCP.

Gabapentin and opioids

Based on evidence from a meta-analysis and systematic review in acute postoperative pain, gabapentin improves analgesia and reduces opioid consumption and related side effects.[74][I], [75][I] A combination of gabapentin and morphine was considerably more effective than either drug alone in attenuating cold pressor hyperalgesia in healthy volunteers, suggesting a possible benefit in patients with pain that is poorly opioid-responsive.[76][II] Based on these data, the addition of gabapentin to long-term opioid therapy may improve analgesic efficacy and reduce side effects, and may be a useful adjunct in opioid rotation or where neuropathic pain is present; however, further research is required.

Ketamine and opioids

There is level I evidence from studies of acute postoperative pain that ketamine is opioid-sparing, without significantly reducing pain scores or the incidence of opioid-adverse events.[77] However, ketamine is useful in the treatment of opioid nonresponsive (opioid tolerance or hyperalgesia) acute or cancer pain (as burst therapy), or in neuropathic, or visceral pain. The role of ketamine in pain management is as an antihyperalgesic, anti-allodynic, and tolerance-protective agent, rather than as an analgesic *per se*.[78]

Practically speaking, a short-term parenteral ketamine infusion may be useful in the treatment of severe breakthrough or incident pain (such as surgery), in patients on long-term opioid therapy. The use of regular sublingual or oral ketamine lozenges reduces opioid requirements and improves analgesia in selected patients with severe CNCP, although this practice has yet to be validated (personal data).

COMBINED OPIOID–OPIOID ANALGESIA: A FUTURE OPTION?

There are fascinating experimental data suggesting that combinations of opioid agonists or agonist–antagonists may improve analgesia and reduce adverse effects, including the development of tolerance, dependence, and withdrawal. Highly experimental bivalent opioids (a mu-opioid agonist and a delta antagonist tethered together with a spacer molecule of critical length), have proved effective in animal models. The administration of tramadol, morphine, or remifentanil to patients on long-term buprenorphine or methadone, reduced (opioid-induced) hyperalgesia on cold pressor testing.[79]

Limited clinical data suggest that COOA may be of added benefit, compared with single opioid therapy. RCTs have shown that the addition of tramadol (by coinfusion) to morphine PCA (patient-controlled analgesia) for postoperative pain control, significantly improved analgesia with morphine sparing,[80][I], [81][II] although no benefit was found when alfentanil was added to morphine PCA following cesarian section.[82][II]

The addition of low-dose (transdermal) fentanyl or methadone to morphine maintenance therapy for poorly controlled cancer pain, significantly improved pain scores and reduced morphine dose escalation, without increasing side effects.[83][III]

A combination of subanalgesic doses of oxycodone and morphine produced better analgesia (with a 40 percent reduction in opioid requirements) and less nausea compared with morphine alone, in patients with chronic pain due to osteoarthritis.[84][III] In a similar trial, combined oxycodone and ultralow-dose naltrexone was more effective than oxycodone alone.[85][II]

Although the mechanisms for COOA are likely to be complex and multifactorial, a synergistic analgesic effect has been demonstrated in isobolographic studies combining oxycodone or methadone with morphine in rodents.[86, 87] Mechanisms may include the differential effects of various opioids on mu, kappa, or delta receptors or their subtypes or the prevention of aberrant G-protein coupling.

Methadone (and other endogenous opioid ligands), but not morphine, promotes mu opioid receptor endocytosis, which in turn reduces NMDA receptor activity and the development of opioid tolerance, dependence, and withdrawal. The addition of low-dose methadone to morphine may have specific beneficial effects by inducing this protective endocytosis mechanism.[87] It is interesting to note that most animal and human studies of COOA have used morphine as the baseline opioid, adding in low-dose oxycodone, methadone, fentanyl, tramadol, or antagonists such as naltrexone.

Conceptually, COOA is a form of partial opioid rotation with similar indications, particularly the management of reduced analgesic efficacy. However, further clinical trials are required to determine if COOA is truly beneficial in pain management.

PATIENT SELECTION

Intravenous opioid testing

Selection of patients for long-term opioid therapy in the treatment of CNCP is a complex process. The first requirement is evidence that the patient's pain is actually opioid responsive, which is usually determined by a trial of oral medication over a period of weeks. In some centers, IVOT is used to determine opioid responsiveness, thus guiding the selection of patients for long-term opioid therapy. However, evidence for this approach is limited and none of the major consensus guidelines for the use of opioids in CNCP suggest using IVOT for patient selection. Some centers also use blood opioid level monitoring following IVOT or oral loading to assess opioid responsiveness; data for this approach are even more limited.

In the current literature, there were 15 RCTs of IVOT, which were largely designed to test short-term opioid responsiveness in patients with neuropathic pain.[15][I] Only two RCTs correlated short-term responsiveness with long-term opioid efficacy in the treatment of CNCP.[14][I], [88][II]

Most trials were of a (within-patient) cross-over design and some used an active control such as diazepam, ketamine, or lidocaine. Test opioids included morphine, fentanyl, alfentanil, buprenorphine, pethidine, or remifentanil, either as fixed-dose infusions or titrated to maximal analgesic effect (or side effects). Doses approximated 20-mg morphine (over 40–60 minutes) or 800 µg fentanyl (over five hours); PCA morphine or remifentanil[88][II] titration have also been used. Trial end points were usually a 50 percent reduction in pain (or at least 3/10 VAS points) or the development of intolerable side effects.

A meta-analysis of six RCTs using IVOT in patients with neuropathic pain found a significant reduction in mean-weighted VAS pain scores (30–60 percent reduction in pain) when doses were increased to maximum tolerable limits; however, side effects were common and often limited further dose escalation.[14][I], [15][I] Three RCTs found no correlation between opioid dose and analgesic response.[15][I] Overall, the outcomes of IVOT for opioid responsiveness in neuropathic pain were equivocal and contradictory.[89][I]

Only two RCTs correlated IVOT with long-term opioid therapy outcomes, approaching the paradigm of using IVOT to select patients for opioid analgesia in CNCP. Dellemijn *et al.* found a positive correlation between fentanyl IVOT response and analgesia with transdermal fentanyl in chronic neuropathic pain.[90][II]

Attal *et al.* found that 46 percent of patients with central pain responded to morphine IVOT, correlating with a beneficial effect with oral morphine one month later. However, only 20 percent of patients continued to use oral morphine for analgesia at one year.[91][II]

IVOT is probably most effective in predicting poor responders to opioid therapy. In other words, patients who fail to respond to IVOT are unlikely to benefit from long-term opioid therapy. However, a positive response to IVOT does not necessarily predict a successful outcome.[14] [I]

Further research is required to determine if IVOT is useful in selecting patients for long-term opioid therapy in CNCP. Studies should be randomized, within-patient, crossover trials with clearly defined opioid response end points, valid dose titration regimes, and most importantly, follow up of long-term opioid treatment outcomes.

The biopsychosocial approach to a diagnosis

It is essential that all reasonable attempts are made to establish a cause for the patient's pain behavior, including nociceptive, neuropathic, and psychological contributions. Pain behavior itself can obviously be modified by many other factors involving social and environmental influences. A demonstration of pathology commensurate with the degree of pain behavior is desirable. However, patients often have pathology which is difficult to interpret, e.g. degenerative changes on spinal radiographs. In some cases, the treating physician can be confident that these changes are relevant to the patient's pain behavior, but in others they can be the least important contributor.

Certain conditions result in neuropathic pain, which is usually a clinical diagnosis and may not be reflected in investigations, such as radiographs or nerve conduction studies. Examples include postherpetic neuralgia, trigeminal neuralgia, postlaminectomy syndrome, and painful peripheral small fiber neuropathies.

Investigations, such as the effects of local anesthetic blocks, must be taken into account along with other clinically relevant information to determine whether a nociceptive stimulus is the main cause of the patient's pain behavior.

There is increasing support for the use of opioids within a biopsychosocial perspective where opioids are used as one component of a pain management plan.[92] However, opioids are not appropriate for patients whose main problem is loneliness, fear, anxiety, hypervigilance, or activity intolerance.

Patients for whom opioids are being considered should be psychologically stable, although it is recognized that this is difficult to define. It is not uncommon for patients to develop psychological problems, including depression and anxiety states, as a result of their chronic pain, and therein lies a dilemma for the physician. Will treating the pain reverse some of the psychological abnormalities? Or are the psychological abnormalities a significant contributor to the overall pain behavior? Studies would suggest the former in most cases.[93]

It is important, however, to avoid treating distress with opioids. Some patients' lives degenerate into chaos for reasons unrelated to their pain syndrome. Opioids may appear to help with their distress, but may make little impact on their pain behavior or level of function. Of course, it is not always easy to differentiate distress related to sociodomestic disintegration from that related to severe pain. In this situation, it is vital to limit initial opioid therapy to a clearly defined and limited trial period with the provision of informed consent and a plan to cease therapy if required. Otherwise, in our experience, well-intentioned but uncontrolled prescribing usually results in escalating doses with a negative overall outcome.

For certain groups of patients, a formal psychological/psychiatric assessment is useful before prescribing opioids. This may include patients with poorly defined pathology, younger patients, those with high levels of distress, and those with previous or ongoing substance abuse. Such a formal assessment may lead to information related to personality disorders, identification of treatment-resistant depression, past history of sexual, physical or emotional abuse, and may be essential in designing alternative or complementary management plans. Specific treatment aimed at reducing anxiety, improving coping mechanisms and, where appropriate, cognitive behavioral therapy may potentiate the beneficial effects of opioid therapy. Screening tools to predict development of addictive behavior are being developed and might prove useful to the prescribing clinician.[94, 95] Consideration should be given to managing these more complex patients in a multidisciplinary pain center.

Having reached an appropriate diagnosis and identified significant psychological issues, it is important to determine that patients have had a thorough trial of previous conservative therapy before consideration is given to adding in the medium- to long-term use of opioids.[9] This may mean combined and continued intervention with:

- active exercise programs;
- attention to improving coping mechanisms;
- a formalized multidisciplinary pain management program;
- attention to psychosocial stresses;

- the use of appropriate invasive physical treatments;
- drug therapy, which should include trials of:
  - nonopioid analgesics;
  - tricyclic antidepressants;
  - anticonvulsant and membrane-stabilizing medications (e.g. sodium valproate, gabapentin, pregabalin, carbamazepine).

Opioids should be seen as a means to an end, not the end point of treatment. The analgesia obtained should ideally allow an increased participation in these therapies. As detailed already, the current evidence for opioid efficacy is limited to relatively low-dose and short-term use, consequently an expectation of a finite window to encourage involvement and compliance with these other therapies rather than an expectation of using opioids in the long term should be encouraged.

ADVERSE EFFECTS OF OPIOID THERAPY AND THEIR MANAGEMENT

Common adverse effects

Opioid-related adverse effects are common, particularly in the initial weeks of treatment for CNCP, and may lead to cessation of therapy in one out of every 12 patients.[14] [I] In a systematic review of RCTs by Moore and McQuay, the most common opioid-related adverse events were dry mouth (25 percent), nausea (21 percent), and constipation (15 percent). Dizziness (14 percent), drowsiness and somnolence (14 percent), pruritis (13 percent), and vomiting (10 percent) were also common; however, there was also a high incidence of these symptoms in the placebo group.[96][I]

In systematic reviews by Kalso *et al.*[14][I] and Eisenberg *et al.*,[15][I] the numbers needed to harm (NNH) for opioids in the treatment of CNCP were in the following ranges: nausea, 3.6–5.0; constipation, 3.4–4.6; drowsiness, 5.3; vomiting, 6.2–8.1; dizziness, 6.7–8.2; and itchiness, 13.

During RCTs lasting up to 16 weeks, 50 percent of patients treated with opioids experienced at least one adverse event (NNH 4.2, 3.1–6.4) with 22.0 percent having to withdraw from the trials as a result (NNH 12, 8.0–27).[14][I], [96][I]

Constipation as a regular side effect of opioid use requires prophylactic treatment. For some patients, regular intake of fruits and other high-fiber foods is sufficient, but most require a regular laxative. It is advisable to commence with bowel stimulants, for example senna-containing compounds, and graduate to osmotic agents (sorbitol), if required. There is limited evidence that transdermal fentanyl or buprenorphine may be less constipating than oral opioids.[28]

Adverse interaction between opioids and other sedatives, especially alcohol and benzodiazepines, is well recognized.

Cognitive dysfunction without overt sedation is more common early in treatment with opioids, but studies[97] suggest that regular use of opioids is much less likely to result in impairment of psychomotor or cognitive processes than in healthy volunteers. The cognitive dysfunction effects of pain alone are unknown. Haythornwaite *et al.*[98] measured cognitive function in patients with chronic pain, comparing those on long-term opioids with those having usual care, and concluded that long-acting opioid medications do not impair cognitive functioning in patients with CNCP.

With regard to driving, there is no evidence that regular use of opioids results in a significantly higher rate of accidents. In fact, Budd *et al.*[99] examined body fluids from fatally injured drivers in Los Angeles and identified opioids in only one in 594 samples. They surmised that opioid users "either don't drive or don't crash if they do drive." Two recent studies tend to support the lack of change in cognitive function and driving skills from prescribed opioids.[100, 101] However, we would recommend that patients be cautioned when commencing opioid use, and also after dosage escalations. They should not drive until they have been on a stable dose for one to two weeks. Motor vehicle insurance companies may insist that clients declare information regarding prescribed opioids in order to honor their policy.

Opioid-induced immunosuppression has had an increasing focus recently; however, its clinical relevance is yet to be quantified.[102]

Several investigators have reported suppression of the hypothalamo–pituitary axis following intrathecal and oral opioid administration.[103, 104, 105] The major clinical effect appears to be on libido and erectile dysfunction. From a population-based perspective, there may be implications for the development of early osteoporosis from the increasing number of males receiving oral opioids for CNCP. This risk remains unevaluated.

The potential for methadone to prolong the QTc and put the patient at risk of a malignant arrhythmia (torsades de pointes) has been recognized for a number of years; however, the significance of this feature is uncertain.[106] Initially, it was reported that only doses of methadone over 150 mg were likely to prolong the QTc; however, it is now recognized at lower doses. It is possible to screen patients at risk for prolonged QTc (advanced age, female gender, hypokalemia, bradycardia, congenital prolongation of the QT interval, use of other drugs known to prolong the QT interval, use of medicines that inhibit methadone metabolism, e.g. fluconazole and fluvoxamine) and perhaps offer alternative opioid therapy.[107]

There is agreement internationally that intramuscular opioids should play no part in the treatment of CNCP. In particular, intramuscular pethidine should be avoided. It has a short half-life, a possible increased risk of dependence due to its psychomimetic effects, and the potential for excitatory CNS effects from accumulated norpethidine concentrations following repeated dosage.

Opioid dose escalation

Apart from opioid-related side effects, the major problem with long-term opioid therapy is progressive dose escalation. Many societies are concerned with limiting opioid dose escalation in individuals and in the community, often through legislation, usually to control the adverse social effects of opioids, including addiction and criminality.

The major causes of opioid dose escalation are:

- decreased opioid analgesic efficacy:
  - opioid-induced neuroadaptation:
    - opioid tolerance (OT);
    - opioid-induced hyperalgesia (OIH).
  - increased pain:
    - development of chronic pain (e.g. central sensitization, neuropathic pain);
    - breakthrough pain (intercurrent illness or disease progression).
- increased opioid demand due to maladaptive behaviors:
  - opioid reward-center effects;
  - addiction;
  - opioid diversion (pseudoescalation);
  - associative tolerance (or hyperalgesia):
    - conditioned response: opioid nocebo effect.
- effects of opioid dependence and withdrawal:
  - neuroadaptation and behavioral factors;
  - motivation to continue or increase opioid dose is avoidance of withdrawal symptoms.

In patients with CNCP, the most frequent cause of opioid dose escalation is inadequate analgesia due to disease progression or the development of chronic pain, OT, or OIH. Maladaptive opioid-use behaviors, such as addiction, are far less common, occurring in fewer than 10 percent (3.2–18.9 percent) of patients treated for CNCP[108] and withdrawal symptoms are also infrequent.[60]

When considering opioid dose escalation in the treatment of chronic pain, the major issues are how frequently the problem occurs (prevalence), the rate of escalation and the final or ceiling dose, as well as causes, modifying factors, and treatments.

Most patients treated with opioids for chronic or cancer pain do not exhibit significant dose escalation, in contrast to those treated for addiction in which escalation seems to be more problematic.[109, 110] Only 10–30 percent of patients on long-term (nine months to five years) opioids for CNCP required significant dose escalation because of inadequate analgesia.[23, 26, 91, 111, 112][II], [19, 22, 109, 113] Fewer patients required dose escalation with transdermal buprenorphine compared with other opioids.[26]

The rate of dose escalation may be a significant factor in managing long-term opioid therapy for CNCP. The opioid escalation index (OEI), defined as the mean increase in dose compared with the starting dose (as a percentage or in milligrams), is used to measure dose escalation in cancer pain research.[114]

A crude estimate of the opioid dose escalation rate (ODER) for all opioids in the treatment of CNCP is 0.5 percent per day.[26, 115, 116, 117]

In a retrospective chart review of 288 patients with CNCP commenced on an oral morphine equivalent dose of 50 mg per day, the average ODER was 1.8 percent (0.88 mg of oral morphine) per day over 15 months.[115] The average ODER with transdermal fentanyl was 0.25–0.42 percent (0.42–1.32 mg oral morphine equivalent) per day (over 12–18 months); however, with transdermal buprenorphine, the ODER was only 0.10 percent, approximately half the rate of fentanyl and 1/15th that of oral morphine.[26, 116] The ODER for morphine, fentanyl, or buprenorphine in the treatment of cancer pain was approximately twice that seen in CNCP.[26, 118]

In older patients, the ODER was approximately half the rate of younger patients. The ODER was higher in the treatment of nociceptive pain compared with neuropathic pain, except in the elderly where there was no difference.[115]

In summary, the ODER was higher when treating cancer pain compared with CNCP. In contrast, the ODER was lower in the elderly, in neuropathic pain or using transdermal buprenorphine.

OPIOID CEILING: WHAT DOSE (IF ANY) IS TOO HIGH?

An issue of concern when considering opioid escalation is the maximum or "ceiling dose" deemed acceptable. Whilst the concept of monitoring the ODER may be a useful clinical tool, the actual dose prescribed and rate of change will depend not only on opioid pharmacology, but also on patient, physician, social, and legal factors.

Clearly, in CNCP, the dose of opioid cannot be escalated continually. What dose of opioid (if any) is too high and why? Concerns with high-dose opioid therapy include the development of OT and OIH, side effects, dependency (withdrawal), addiction, and diversion. In the treatment of cancer pain, there is less concern about opioid escalation; however, processes such as OIH may be an underrecognized cause of treatment failure in this context. Unfortunately, no trials have explored possible links between opioid dose and the development of OT or OIH.

The concept of an opioid ceiling dose in the treatment of CNCP was first discussed by Ballantyne and Mao in 2003,[119] who noted that RCTs had never tested doses greater than the equivalent of 180 mg of morphine per day for more than 16 weeks. However, data from a limited number of open label studies documented considerably higher ceiling doses, in a range equivalent to 300–900 mg of morphine per day. As with the ODER, the ceiling dose is higher in cancer pain and lower in the elderly and with buprenorphine.

Although authorities and consensus guidelines call for the use of stable and modest doses of opioids in the treatment of CNCP, there is no research data or expert consensus on what is considered an appropriate ceiling dose or whether dose limitation is actually of some benefit.

Generally speaking, in our clinics, we set an initial arbitrary ceiling dose equivalent to 100 mg oral morphine per day; when this limit is reached, we reassess the patient together with the treatment goals and expectations before further increasing the dose. We would seldom escalate the opioid dose beyond 200–300 mg of oral morphine equivalent per day in the treatment of CNCP without good reason.

The issue of an opioid ceiling dose is unresolved and potentially controversial, and further research is required to see if such restrictions actually impact on analgesic efficacy or side effects. At the very least, setting an initial ceiling dose of 100–200 mg morphine equivalent per day acts as a safety valve, at which time the patient's opioid therapy can be reassessed.

OPIOID TOLERANCE AND OPIOID-INDUCED HYPERALGESIA

OT is a state of reduced opioid potency, reflecting down-regulation or desensitization of opioid-dependent, anti-nociceptive systems in the CNS. In contrast, OIH is a neuroadaptive state where opioid administration is associated with an increased response to painful stimuli (hyperalgesia), due to up-regulation or increased sensitization of pronociceptive systems. These changes are reflected in a rightwards shift of the opioid dose–response curve in OT, in contrast to a downwards shift in OIH. Tolerance to opioid side effects, such as respiratory depression and nausea, may develop at different rates to analgesic tolerance. Differentiation of OT and OIH requires quantitative sensory testing and is difficult in the clinical setting.[120][I]

Both OT and OIH result in dose escalation in order to maintain analgesia and most likely share similar neurobiological mechanisms; however, technically and experimentally, they are different neuroadaptive states (see **Table 16.1**). Mechanisms include those associated with the development of central sensitization, such as opioid receptor changes, increased NMDA receptor-channel effects, changes in the neurochemistry and genetics of higher-order nociceptors (e.g. dorsal horn), the production of pronociceptive substances such as dynorphin or nitric oxide, modulation of descending inhibitory and excitatory pathways, and the effects of pronociceptive opioid metabolites (e.g. M3G).

Behavioral conditioning may produce an association between a painful stimulus and the effects of opioid therapy (e.g. euphoria, dysphoria) administered at the same time, resulting in an opioid nocebo effect which is expressed as apparent tolerance. Opioid responsiveness may also be modified by environmental cues. For example, an addict may exhibit a marked reduction in OT while in hospital, where opioid use is no longer associated with the cues of drug-seeking in the community. Reduced opioid efficacy due to behavioral conditioning or nocebo effects is known as associative tolerance (hyperalgesia).[119, 120][I]

There may also be neuropsychological mechanisms for the development of apparent OT/OIH. For example, opioid-induced suppression of the hypothalamo–pituitary axis may lower testosterone, which causes mood disturbance and, in turn, worsening pain behavior.

OT/OIH may develop within hours of starting opioid therapy, as demonstrated by increased postoperative pain and hyperalgesia following remifentanil-based anesthesia.[121] A recent clinical experiment using cold pressor testing found that OT/OIH developed within one month of commencing oral morphine for chronic low back pain.[122] It has long been recognized that former heroin addicts on long-term methadone maintenance therapy exhibit lower thresholds to cold pressor testing and are cross-tolerant to high doses of morphine.[123] Some authorities suggest that the presence of pain in some way reduces the development of OT/OIH in clinical pain, compared with addiction or animal models.[124] The rate of opioid dose escalation (possibly reflecting reduced OT

Table 16.1 The major features of opioid-induced hyperalgesia and opioid tolerance.

Opioid induced hyperalgesia	Opioid tolerance
Increased pain sensitivity (hyperalgesia)	Decreased analgesic potency
Up-regulation of pronociceptive systems	Down-regulation of antinociceptive systems
Downwards shift of dose–analgesia curve	Rightwards shift of dose–analgesia curve
Decreased relative analgesic potency	No change in relative analgesic potency
Hyperalgesia on QST	No hyperalgesia on QST
OIH persists following withdrawal	OT does not persist following withdrawal
Responds to NMDA antagonist	Responds to NMDA antagonist
Responds to opioid rotation	Responds to opioid rotation
Responds to opioid dose decrease?	Responds to opioid dose increase
Possible biological benefit	No obvious biological benefit

NMDA, *N*-methyl-D-aspartic acid; OIH, opioid-induced hyperalgesia; OT, opioid tolerance; QST, quantitative sensation testing.

and OIH) is lower in the elderly and in the treatment of neuropathic pain.

Although seemingly maladaptive in the clinical context, OIH may be of some evolutionary benefit. The production of endogenous opioids after an injury initially promotes analgesia, allowing the organism to escape from danger. However, the development of (endogenous) opioid-induced and injury-related hyperalgesia a few days later helps keep the damaged body part still to allow for healing and conditions the organism to avoid the circumstances of the injury in the future. Most animal models of OIH demonstrate a biphasic response (initially analgesia followed by hyperalgesia) which supports this concept. Animals that developed OIH remained vulnerable to OIH after withdrawal and with reexposure to further opioids – a form of OIH memory. There is no evolutionary reason why OT is adaptive, so it is likely that OIH is the primary neuroadaptive state.[125]

Cold pressor testing is the most sensitive method of determining OIH and OT; a comparative experimental trial found no difference between opioid-treated chronic pain patients and normal controls in responses to mechanical stimuli (mechanical allodynia) or heat hyperalgesia. However, numerous clinical and experimental studies have validated cold pressor testing for detecting OT/OIH in patients on long-term opioid therapy.[123, 126]

Clinically speaking, all patients on chronic opioid therapy will have some degree of OIH contributing to their clinical pain. A paradox arises where a patient may actually benefit from opioid dose reduction to improve analgesia. Unfortunately, there are no studies of opioid reduction in the treatment of (presumed) OIH and no way to clearly establish which patients may benefit. Nevertheless, in some patients (particularly those on "high doses"), a slow, steady reduction in opioid dose (approximately 10 percent per month) can lead to a significant reduction over time, often with improved analgesia and without precipitating withdrawal. However, it requires a clear explanation for the patient to understand the seemingly counterintuitive prospect of reducing their opioids to improve their pain, without precipitating withdrawal!

Buprenorphine or tramadol may be associated with the development of less OT/OIH. More established treatments for presumed OT/OIH include opioid rotation (see below under Opioid rotation in chronic noncancer pain) or the use of NMDA receptor antagonists, such as ketamine. The use of multimodal analgesia, particularly gabapentin or pregabalin or combined opioid –opioid analgesia may be useful in the prevention or treatment of OIH/OT, based on preliminary experimental data. It is interesting to speculate whether as-needed opioid dosing rather than by-the-clock administration could be associated with less OT/OIH, by reducing the constant stimulation of opioid receptors by the agonist.

Opioid rotation in chronic noncancer pain

Opioid rotation (OR) or switching is a therapeutic technique where the type of opioid or route of administration is changed in order to reduce adverse effects and/or improve analgesic efficacy, in other words to open up a therapeutic window.

The concept of OR is based largely on research and clinical experience in the treatment of cancer pain; however, the technique may also be of benefit in CNCP[127] or acute pain management.[128] However, according to a Cochrane review, OR is still not practiced commonly if there are problems with opioid therapy in CNCP.[129][I] In a prospective review of patients commencing opioids for CNCP, the rates of OR at six months were 10.6 percent (controlled-release oxycodone), 19 percent (transdermal fentanyl), and 26.0 percent (controlled-release morphine sulfate), respectively.[130]

The rationale for OR is based on the variability of opioids in their effects, both between and within patients, a concept known as "incomplete cross-tolerance."[131] Such variability in opioid effects is due to the following factors.

PHARMACODYNAMIC FACTORS

There are significant intra- and interopioid receptor differences, including at least seven subtypes of mu-receptors, based on pharmacogenomic evidence.[132] Opioids (and their metabolites) may have variable effects on particular opioid receptors (e.g. the partial agonist effect of buprenorphine on the mu-receptor or increased kappa affinity for oxycodone) or nonopioid receptors (NMDA effects of methadone, tramadol effects on neuroamide receptors). Based on limited animal data and case reports in cancer pain, OR from a phenanthrene-type opioid such as morphine, to a piperidine such as fentanyl, may lead to significant improvement of OIH.[133]

PHARMACOKINETIC FACTORS

Patients exhibit variable cytochrome P450 activity (e.g. reduced CYP2D6 expression and efficacy of codeine) affecting opioid metabolism, or altered renal function, leading to variable opioid half-lives.

OPIOID METABOLITES

Metabolites, such as morphine-6-glucuronide (M6G), may be active, thus contributing to analgesia or adverse effects, particularly at high doses or with impaired renal function. Fentanyl, oxycodone, and methadone have minimally active metabolites and may therefore be of some advantage in OR. In particular, fentanyl or buprenorphine are the opioids of choice in patients with renal failure.[50]

ROUTES OF ADMINISTRATION

The oral route may be lost due to bowel obstruction or difficultly swallowing, usually in cancer pain. Oral morphine is associated with a significant increase in M6G-related adverse effects due to first-pass metabolism, explaining symptomatic improvement with rotation from oral to subcutaneous morphine in cancer pain.[134] In CNCP, there is a trend to rotate from oral opioids, such as morphine, to transdermal preparations which may have fewer side effects.[28] Intrathecal administration allows a 10- to 100-fold reduction in the opioid dose and therefore fewer side effects. Unfortunately, intrathecal opioids are associated with a different profile of side effects.

OTHER FACTORS

OR may be required to manage practical or pharmaceutical problems, such as the loss of an oral route of administration or problems with concentrating opioids for infusion (e.g. morphine to hydromorphone). When rotating between different long-acting opioids, there was an improvement in analgesia and side effects in 59 percent of patients; when rotating from a short- to a long-acting opioid, analgesia improved in 73 percent of patients; however, the dose increased in the same percentage of patients.[127] COOA, which is conceptually partial OR, may improve analgesic efficacy and reduce adverse effects compared with single-opioid therapy; however, further research is required.

There are significant differences in the literature with regard to equipotent doses of opioids, primarily because much of the early work was undertaken on single-dose studies. Pereira *et al.*[135] critically address some of these issues. In chronic opioid dosing, perhaps because of incomplete receptor cross-tolerance and differing pharmacokinetics between opioids, precise dose equivalents are difficult to define. We suggest that the manufacturers' recommendation be reviewed and then the new opioid dose be reduced by at least 50 percent during OR.

The appropriate dose ratio when rotating from morphine to methadone or methadone to morphine, is particularly complex and caution is advised. There is some evidence that when rotating from low-dose morphine, the dose conversion to methadone is higher than when the morphine dose is high.[34, 36, 136, 137, 138]

By changing to a different opioid at a lower equivalent dose, side effects may be reduced, with similar or improved analgesic efficacy.[139] A Cochrane review concluded that OR was helpful to improve analgesic efficacy or reduce adverse effects, but the evidence was "largely anecdotal, based on case reports and observational studies."[129][I] A systematic review of OR for cancer pain came to essentially the same conclusions.[140][I]

In a review of OR in CNCP, the main reason for change was ineffective analgesia;[127] however, in cancer pain, OR was usually required to treat intolerable side effects. The majority of patients derived significant benefit from OR, particularly a reduction in myoclonus, confusion, and unrelieved pain, at about half the equipotent dose of the original opioid.[141]

In a retrospective review of 67 patients with CNCP, OR from morphine to hydromorphone, buprenorphine, or fentanyl was associated with a significant decrease in average pain scores (3/10 VAS points ($p<0.001$)).[142]

The key points of OR may be remembered as a set of 30/70 rules listed below.

- Thirty percent of patients treated with opioids for cancer or CNCP require OR at some stage.
- Seventy percent require OR to treat adverse effects, most commonly in cancer pain.
- Thirty percent require OR because of inadequate analgesia.
- Seventy percent of patients derive a significant therapeutic benefit from OR with:
  - 70–100 percent improvement in confusion or myoclonus;
  - 70 percent improvement in unrelieved pain;
  - 50 percent improvement in nausea;
  - 30 percent improvement in hallucinations.
- The most commonly performed ORs are from morphine to either hydromorphone, methadone, or transdermal fentanyl.
- Because of incomplete cross-tolerance, the equipotent dose of the new drug should be reduced by 50 percent during OR.
- OR rotation to methadone, although beneficial, may require a greater dose reduction (60–90 percent), particularly when converting from high-dose oral opioids, such as morphine (due to methadone's variable half-life and effects on nonopioid receptors, such as NMDA). Extreme care should be taken.
- Watch the patient closely during OR for features of over- or under-dosing, including withdrawal symptoms.
- The use of multimodal analgesia, including ketamine or possibly gabapentin/pregablin during OR may be beneficial, although this has yet to be proven in clinical trials.
- The act of rotation is probably more important than the properties of the new opioid.
- In summary, "if things aren't going great, remember to opioid rotate."

Breakthrough (or flare-up) pain

Breakthrough pain (BTP), a term derived from cancer pain management, is defined as a transient exacerbation of pain that breaks through an existing, effective analgesic regimen.[143]

Incident pain (IP) is a frequent, predictable pain exacerbation brought on by certain activities, such as weight-bearing in chronic low back pain or after surgery; this may occur on a background of continuous pain or the patient may be pain free between episodes.[3]

Episodic pain (EP) is defined as a spontaneous episode of recurrent, severe pain where the patient is pain free between episodes. Examples include pain exacerbations with sickle cell disease or rheumatoid arthritis.[3]

In CNCP, the term "flare-up pain" is sometimes used to describe these exacerbations. Flare-up pain may be due to an exacerbation of the underlying chronic pain disorder, the effects of intercurrent disease or procedures such as surgery.

Approximately 70 percent of patients treated with opioids for CNCP experience BTP, most commonly due to an exacerbation of their underlying chronic pain disorder. The median number of BTP episodes is two per day, lasting an average of 60 minutes. Most BTP is rated as severe and is related to physical activity (with an exacerbation of chronic low back pain being the most common presentation). In the hospice-care setting, BTP is more frequent (five episodes per day), severe, and often unpredictable, than in patients with noncancer pain.[144, 145, 146]

The underlying cause of the pain should be identified and treated where possible. Most cognitive behavioral pain management programs will teach patients how to manage flares of pain, by using pacing for prevention and then other nonpharmacological activities rather than using opioids or other medications.

Multimodal analgesia should be optimized, including the use of NSAIDs, COX-2 inhibitors, or antineuropathic agents. Tramadol may be a useful first-line analgesic for moderately-severe flare-up pain as it produces less respiratory depression, constipation, and dependency, and is highly effective in neuropathic pain.

Temporary use of short-acting opioids (approximately 1/5th the baseline daily opioid dose) as rescue analgesics to treat severe flare-up pain is effective and acceptable under controlled conditions, based on data from cancer pain management.[147]

Where there is severe, acute flare-up pain (e.g. postoperatively), intravenous opioid titration may be required to gain rapid control; intravenous morphine in a dose 1/5th that of the daily oral dose is safe and effective.[147] Intravenous morphine is also effective for the treatment of BTP in patients maintained on transdermal buprenorphine.[48][III]

Flare-up pain refractory to opioid analgesia may respond to intravenous ketamine, either as a bolus dose, or continuous infusion or as burst therapy, based on cancer pain studies[78] and intranasal ketamine has also been used effectively.[148][II]

One of the major issues in treating flare-up pain is whether to continue with rapidly acting rescue analgesia, including opioids, or to increase baseline opioid therapy. From a practical point of view, the frequency, duration, and predictability of the flare-up episodes determines the most effective approach. If flare-up pain requires the regular use of four (or more) doses of short-acting opioid per day without significant benefit, then opioid dose escalation or rotation should be considered. Conversion from short- to long-acting opioids is effective in reducing the frequency, duration, and intensity of BTP.[145]

CONSENT

Patients prescribed opioids for the treatment of CNCP should be fully informed of the potential consequences of this therapy.

Verbal consent may be sufficient for some patients, or a consent form can be presented in the form of a contract. Fishman *et al.*[149] and Gitlin[150] recently reviewed the possible contents of a consent form, and observed that the contract is an attempt to improve care through the use of an educational vehicle and to facilitate a course of treatment that has been mutually endorsed. It also provides a mechanism for obtaining informed consent.

Most importantly, the consent form should clearly define the goals of therapy. These goals may need adjustment as treatment progresses; however, the importance of unambiguous end points cannot be overstated, particularly if problems with prescribing develop. An information leaflet can be usefully incorporated into a consent form.

Informed consent should include the following:

- aims should be set for less pain rather than no pain;
- realistic functional goals should be set;
- there should be discussion regarding the likelihood of dependence and the risk of addictive behavior, i.e. that all patients will become dependent and are likely to experience withdrawal symptoms if opioids are suddenly ceased;
- there is lack of data on the long-term outcome of the effects of medically prescribed opioids;
- the potential for cognitive impairment should be discussed, including:
  - driving motor vehicles while commencing opioid therapy;
  - temporary worsening around the time of dose escalation;
  - the likelihood of increased sedation if benzodiazepines and/or alcohol are used;
- patients should be alerted to the possibility (for women) of physical dependence of children born to them if they continue to take opioids in late pregnancy;
- indications should be identified for the cessation of treatment with opioids and an indication of unacceptable behavior (included here could be practice rules about repeat prescriptions and amount of notice required);

- patients must accept responsibility for:
  - ensuring that their supply of medication does not run out after hours;
  - the security of their medication;
  - keeping review appointments;
  - using only one doctor (or their nominee in case of leave) to supply this medication.
- side effects and their management should be discussed, e.g. constipation, nausea, sedation, dry mouth, urinary hesitancy, possible hormonal effects;
- if methadone is the drug to be prescribed, emphasis on the risks of cessation and restarting, and unapproved dose escalations must be made.

In selected patients, it may be appropriate to discuss the definitions of the following terms and to include them in the information/consent form in order to increase compliance and ensure a more thorough understanding of consent.

Tolerance refers to decreasing pain control with the same dose of opioid over a given time period. Tolerance to side effects, such as sedation and nausea, appears earlier than it does to analgesia. It usually occurs in the first six months of dosing. Tolerance does not imply addiction.

Physical dependence refers to a constellation of physiological signs and symptoms seen on abrupt withdrawal of an opioid. The severity of symptoms varies between patients. They include coryza, tremor, sweating, abdominal cramps, arthralgia, myalgia, vomiting, and diarrhea. Patients can be reassured regarding this phenomenon. It is the same for opioids as it is for many other medications, e.g. antihypertensives, antiepileptics, or insulin.

Addiction is a psychosocial disorder characterized by the compulsive use of a substance and preoccupation with obtaining it. This is despite evidence that continued use results in physical, emotional, social, or economic harm.

MONITORING

One physician should institute and monitor the treatment. Goals and expectations (physician and patient) should be identified and the end points clearly stated. Goals may include restoration of function, improvement in the activities of daily living, return to work, psychological stability, improved family and social interactions, decreased use of healthcare resources, including use of other analgesics. Once identified, these goals could be incorporated into an individualized consent form.[10]

We recommend conservative starting doses, particularly in the elderly, and usually commence with the equivalent of sustained-release morphine (10–20 mg twice a day) and then assess weekly.

At each review it is essential to assess analgesic effect, level of function (goal achievement), side effects, and any aberrant behavior. The goals of therapy should be reinforced along with encouragement and appropriate adjuvant treatment.

The analgesic effect from the opioid should allow a significant reduction, if not cessation, of other analgesics.

Depending on the response, the dose could be increased or decreased. The prescriber should be aware of the occasional difficulty in determining the appropriate dose when rapid tolerance appears to be occurring. It is our practice to rigorously review the patient if reasonably good analgesia has not been achieved with the use of 100 mg morphine equivalents per day.

In general, round-the-clock medication is the accepted regimen. However, as already discussed, patients with fluctuating pain conditions (chronic recurrent or non-continuous) may be more appropriately treated using a variable dosing regimen with shorter-acting drugs, such as oxycodone or morphine elixir.

There is controversy regarding the expectation that patients will improve in function. Is it adequate for patients to achieve analgesia only? Is it adequate for patients to state that they feel better only? To some extent this is defined by the patient's clinical situation and, often, his or her age. Ideally, patients should demonstrate an improvement of function. Perception of improved analgesia and reduction of other analgesics should be the minimum requirement. Assessment with reports from significant others may be useful at this stage.

Most patients who experience minimal or no analgesic effect or significant adverse effects will cease the opioid themselves.

Patients should at first be reviewed fairly frequently (e.g. weekly) by the prescribing physician. The time interval between reviews can then be increased to monthly. At each review, analgesic efficacy, side effects, evidence of aberrant behavior, and any improvement in the level of function should be assessed. In many countries, the responsible regulatory authorities must be notified.

Over time, a degree of opioid tolerance may develop insidiously. The question then arises as to what is the maximum dose? While function is improved by the opioids and side effects are tolerated, some would argue that there is no need to restrict the dose.[151] However, as previously discussed, the development of tolerance and/or opioid-induced hyperalgesia should be born in mind, especially when there appears to be rapid dose escalation or when doses reach 200–300 morphine equivalents a day.

Evidence of aberrant behavior has been well characterized by Portenoy[152] and should be assessed at each visit. Aberrant behavior is variable in its importance and relevance. **Table 16.2** indicates factors which Portenoy considered to be less indicative of the development of addictive behavior. They indicate a need to assess the dose of drug, the psychological factors of relevance, the patient's expectations, or the type of medication.

Table 16.3 suggests behaviors which are more indicative of addictive behavior and should result in a serious reassessment of the appropriateness of opioid

Table 16.2 Less predictive features of aberrant drug-related behavior.

Behavior
Aggressive complaining about the need for more drug
Drug hoarding during periods of reduced symptoms
Requesting specific drugs
Openly acquiring similar drugs from other medical sources
Unsanctioned dose escalation
Unapproved use of the drug to treat other symptoms

Table 16.3 More predictive features of aberrant drug-related behavior.

Behavior
Selling prescription drugs
Prescription forgery
Stealing or borrowing drugs from others
Injecting oral formulations
Obtaining prescription drugs from nonmedical sources
Concurrent abuse of alcohol or illicit drugs
Multiple nonsanctioned dose escalations
Multiple episodes of prescription loss
Repeatedly seeking prescriptions from other physicians or emergency departments without informing the prescriber or after warnings to desist
Evidence of deterioration in function, at work, in the family, or socially, that appear to be drug related
Repeated resistance to therapy changes despite clear evidence of adverse physical or psychological effects from the drug

prescription. In many cases, it will be necessary to reduce and then cease the opioid. In other cases, a more regulated supply, such as daily or weekly prescriptions, may be appropriate. An initial written consent form, indicating those factors for which supply will be weaned and ceased, will make this easier.

SUMMARY

There is growing evidence that a small group of patients with CNCP pain may benefit from the use of opioids. We have tabulated a summary of the evidence to date (**Table 16.4**).

The challenge facing the medical profession rests with identifying responsive patients and alleviating suffering without significantly increasing illicit use, addiction, or medication-induced suffering.

Having mechanisms in place for monitoring patients using opioids with clear end points together with mutually acceptable rules to which all parties adhere, are essential. Best practice may mean a firm yet caring "No" where appropriate, rather than inappropriate prescribing of opioids.[153] It is more appropriate to initiate nonopioid treatment options for loneliness, fear, depression, anxiety hypervigilance, or activity intolerance. **Table 16.5** summarizes the questions we believe a treating doctor should ask himself/herself before prescribing opioids for a patient with CNCP.

We have provided a framework which is practical, is based on the evidence to date, and is combined with current clinical practice. Further research is required to identify the long-term outcomes and the cost–benefit ratios.

Table 16.4 A summary of data for opioid analgesia for chronic noncancer pain.

	For placebo (%)
The mean decrease in pain intensity with opioids was 30%[a]	15–30
5–10% of patients withdrew due to lack of opioid efficacy[a]	20
50–80% of patients developed at least one opioid-adverse effect[a]	30–60
20–30% of patients withdrew due to opioid-adverse effects[a]	5–15
Only 30% of patients remained on long-term opioid therapy	
Only 10–30% of patients on long-term opioid for analgesia required significant dose escalation because of inadequate analgesia	
The average ODER for all opioids in CNCP was approximately 0.5% per day	
The ODER was higher in cancer pain	
The ODER was lower in the elderly, in neuropathic pain and with buprenorphine analgesia	
The optimum ceiling dose (if any) for opioids in CNCP is not known, but an equivalent of 100 mg of oral morphine per day seems a reasonable trigger for reevaluation	
30% of patients required OR at some stage during long-term opioid therapy for chronic pain:	
30% required OR for failing analgesic efficacy	
70% required OR for side effects	
70% of patients "improved" after OR	

Approximate values only.
[a]Data from meta-analyses and systematic reviews of RCTs which lasted less than 16 weeks.
CNCP, chronic noncancer pain; ODER, opioid dose escalation rate; OR, opioid rotation.

Table 16.5 Questions to ask before prescribing opioids for chronic noncancer pain.

	Question
1	Has the patient tried opioids for this condition before?
2	Is the diagnosis established? (If not, are further investigations required?)
3	Does the patient have neuropathic (nerve damage) pain? If so, have nonopioids, membrane stabilizers, anticonvulsants, and antidepressants been tried?
4	Has the patient had a reasonable trial of nonpharmacological treatment, including assessment and treatment of psychosocial factors contributing to pain behavior?
5	Is the patient well known to me and psychologically stable?
6	Does the patient have a history of previous drug, alcohol, or substance abuse?
7	Does the patient understand the implications of long-term opioid therapy – is written consent necessary?
8	Do I have back-up resources (i.e. multidisciplinary support) when required?

REFERENCES

1. Caudill-Slosberg MA, Schwartz LM, Woloshin S. Office visits and analgesic prescriptions for musculoskeletal pain in US: 1980 vs. 2000. *Pain.* 2004; **109**: 514–9.
2. Australian Institute of Health and Welfare. *Statistics on drug use in Australia 2002.* Canberra: Australian Institute of Health and Welfare, 2003.
3. Anonymous. Recommendations for the appropriate use of opioids for persisitent non-cancer pain. 2004. Accessed 13 November 2006, www.britishpainsociety.org/opioids_doc_2004.pdf.
4. Macintyre PE, Jarvis DA. Age is the best predictor of postoperative morphine requirements. *Pain.* 1996; **64**: 357–64.
5. Australian and New Zealand College of Anaesthetists. *Acute pain management: scientific evidence.* Melbourne: Australian and New Zealand College of Anaesthetists, 2005.
6. Ballantyne JC. Chronic pain following treatment for cancer: the role of opioids. *Oncologist.* 2003; **8**: 567–75.
7. Breivik H. Opioids in cancer and chronic non-cancer pain therapy-indications and controversies. *Acta Anaesthesiologica Scandinavica.* 2001; **45**: 1059–66.
8. Mercadante S, Portenoy RK. Opioid poorly-responsive cancer pain. Part 1: clinical considerations. *Journal of Pain and Symptom Management.* 2001; **21**: 144–50.
9. Graziotti PJ, Goucke CR. The use of oral opioids in patients with chronic non-cancer pain. Management strategies. *Medical Journal of Australia.* 1997; **167**: 30–4.
10. Kalso E, Allan L, Dellemijn PL *et al.* Recommendations for using opioids in chronic non-cancer pain. *European Journal of Pain.* 2003; **7**: 381–6.
11. Anonymous. Recommendations for the appropriate use of opioids for persisitent non-cancer pain. 2004. Accessed 13 November 2006. Available from: www.britishpainsociety.org/opioids_doc_2004.pdf
* 12. Trescot AM, Boswell MV, Atluri SL *et al.* Opioid guidelines in the management of chronic non-cancer pain. *Pain Physician.* 2006; **9**: 1–39.
13. Eriksen J, Sjogren P, Bruera E *et al.* Critical issues on opioids in chronic non-cancer pain: an epidemiological study. *Pain.* 2006; **125**: 172–9.
* 14. Kalso E, Edwards JE, Moore RA, McQuay HJ. Opioids in chronic non-cancer pain: systematic review of efficacy and safety. *Pain.* 2004; **112**: 372–80.
* 15. Eisenberg E, McNicol ED, Carr DB. Efficacy and safety of opioid agonists in the treatment of neuropathic pain of nonmalignant origin: systematic review and meta-analysis of randomized controlled trials. *Journal of the American Medical Association* 2005; **293**: 3043–52.
* 16. Furlan AD, Sandoval JA, Mailis-Gagnon A, Tunks E. Opioids for chronic noncancer pain: a meta-analysis of effectiveness and side effects. *Canadian Medical Association Journal.* 2006; **174**: 1589–94.
17. Maier C, Hildebrandt J, Klinger R *et al.* Morphine responsiveness, efficacy and tolerability in patients with chronic non-tumor associated pain – results of a double-blind placebo-controlled trial (MONTAS). *Pain.* 2002; **97**: 223–33.
18. Watson CP, Babul N. Efficacy of oxycodone in neuropathic pain: a randomized trial in postherpetic neuralgia. *Neurology.* 1998; **50**: 1837–41.
* 19. Watson CP, Moulin D, Watt-Watson J *et al.* Controlled-release oxycodone relieves neuropathic pain: a randomized controlled trial in painful diabetic neuropathy. *Pain.* 2003; **105**: 71–8.
* 20. Chou R, Clark E, Helfand M. Comparative efficacy and safety of long-acting oral opioids for chronic non-cancer pain: a systematic review. *Journal of Pain and Symptom Management.* 2003; **26**: 1026–48.
21. Allan L, Hays H, Jensen NH *et al.* Randomised crossover trial of transdermal fentanyl and sustained release oral morphine for treating chronic non-cancer pain. *British Medical Journal* 2001; **322**: 1154–8.
22. Caldwell JR, Rapoport RJ, Davis JC *et al.* Efficacy and safety of a once-daily morphine formulation in chronic, moderate-to-severe osteoarthritis pain: results from a randomized, placebo-controlled, double-blind trial and an

open-label extension trial. *Journal of Pain and Symptom Management.* 2002; **23**: 278–91.
23. Griessinger N, Sittl R, Likar R. Transdermal buprenorphine in clinical practice – a post-marketing surveillance study in 13,179 patients. *Current Medical Research and Opinion.* 2005; **21**: 1147–56.
24. Radbruch L, Sabatowski R, Petzke F *et al.* Transdermal fentanyl for the management of cancer pain: a survey of 1005 patients. *Palliative Medicine.* 2001; **15**: 309–21.
25. Shipton E. Safety and tolerability of buprenorphine. In: Budd KRR (ed.). *Basic pharmacology of buprenorphine.* Stuttgart: Georg Thieme Verlag, 2005: 102–15.
* 26. Sittl R, Nuijten M, Nautrup BP. Changes in the prescribed daily doses of transdermal fentanyl and transdermal buprenorphine during treatment of patients with cancer and noncancer pain in Germany: results of a retrospective cohort study. *Clinical Therapy.* 2005; **27**: 1022–31.
27. Allan L, Richarz U, Simpson K, Slappendel R. Transdermal fentanyl versus sustained release oral morphine in strong-opioid naive patients with chronic low back pain. *Spine.* 2005; **30**: 2484–90.
* 28. Clark AJ, Ahmedzai SH, Allan LG *et al.* Efficacy and safety of transdermal fentanyl and sustained-release oral morphine in patients with cancer and chronic non-cancer pain. *Current Medical Research and Opinion.* 2004; **20**: 1419–28.
* 29. Sandoval JA, Furlan AD, Mailis-Gagnon A. Oral methadone for chronic noncancer pain: a systematic literature review of reasons for administration, prescription patterns, effectiveness, and side effects. *Clinical Journal of Pain.* 2005; **21**: 503–12.
30. Morley JS, Bridson J, Nash TP *et al.* Low-dose methadone has an analgesic effect in neuropathic pain: a double-blind randomized controlled crossover trial. *Palliative Medicine.* 2003; **17**: 576–87.
* 31. Jadad AR, Moore RA, Carroll D *et al.* Assessing the quality of reports of randomized clinical trials: is blinding necessary? *Controlled Clinical Trials.* 1996; **17**: 1–12.
32. Gorman AL, Elliott KJ, Inturrisi CE. The d- and l-isomers of methadone bind to the non-competitive site on the N-methyl-D-aspartate (NMDA) receptor in rat forebrain and spinal cord. *Neuroscience Letters.* 1997; **223**: 5–8.
33. Fainsinger R, Schoeller T, Bruera E. Methadone in the management of cancer pain: a review. *Pain.* 1993; **52**: 137–47.
34. Fredheim OM, Borchgrevink PC, Klepstad P *et al.* Long term methadone for chronic pain: A pilot study of pharmacokinetic aspects. *European Journal of Pain.* 2007; **11**: 599–604.
35. Gourlay G (ed.). *Different opioids – same actions.* In: Kalso EMH, Weisenfeld-Hallin Z (eds). Progress in pain research and management 14. Seattle, WA: IASP Press, 1991.
36. Ripamonti C, Groff L, Brunelli C *et al.* Switching from morphine to oral methadone in treating cancer pain: what is the equianalgesic dose ratio? *Journal of Clinical Oncology.* 1998; **16**: 3216–21.
37. Toombs JD, Kral LA. Methadone treatment for pain states. *American Family Physician.* 2005; **71**: 1353–8.
38. Cooper GA, Seymour A, Cassidy MT, Oliver JS. A study of methadone in fatalities in the Strathclyde Region, 1991–1996. *Medicine, Science, and the Law.* 1999; **39**: 233–42.
39. Caplehorn JR, Drummer OH. Fatal methadone toxicity: signs and circumstances, and the role of benzodiazepines. *Australian and New Zealand Journal of Public Health.* 2002; **26**: 358–62; discussion 62–3.
40. Milroy CM, Forrest AR. Methadone deaths: a toxicological analysis. *Journal of Clinical Pathology.* 2000; **53**: 277–81.
41. Gimbel JS, Richards P, Portenoy RK. Controlled-release oxycodone for pain in diabetic neuropathy: a randomized controlled trial. *Neurology.* 2003; **60**: 927–34.
42. Moulin DE, Iezzi A, Amireh R *et al.* Randomised trial of oral morphine for chronic non-cancer pain. *Lancet.* 1996; **347**: 143–7.
43. Langford R, McKenna F, Ratcliffe S *et al.* Transdermal fentanyl for improvement of pain and functioning in osteoarthritis: a randomized, placebo-controlled trial. *Arthritis and Rheumatism.* 2006; **54**: 1829–37.
44. Cowan A FE, Strassburger W, Rafa RB. Basic pharmacology of buprenorphine. In: Budd KRR (ed.). *Buprenorphine – the unique opioid analgesic. Pharmacology and clinical application.* Stuttgart: Georg Thieme Verlag, 2005: 3–21.
45. Likar R, Kayser H, Sittl R. Long-term management of chronic pain with transdermal buprenorphine: a multicenter, open-label, follow-up study in patients from three short-term clinical trials. *Clinical Therapy.* 2006; **28**: 943–52.
46. Sittl R. Transdermal buprenorphine in the treatment of chronic pain. *Expert Review of Neurotherapeutics.* 2005; **5**: 315–23.
47. Sorge J, Sittl R. Transdermal buprenorphine in the treatment of chronic pain: results of a phase III, multicenter, randomized, double-blind, placebo-controlled study. *Clinical Therapy.* 2004; **26**: 1808–20.
48. Mercadante S, Villari P, Ferrera P *et al.* Safety and effectiveness of intravenous morphine for episodic breakthrough pain in patients receiving transdermal buprenorphine. *Journal of Pain and Symptom Management.* 2006; **32**: 175–9.
49. Jasinski DR, Pevnick JS, Griffith JD. Human pharmacology and abuse potential of the analgesic buprenorphine: a potential agent for treating narcotic addiction. *Archives of General Psychiatry.* 1978; **35**: 501–16.
50. Murphy EJ. Acute pain management pharmacology for the patient with concurrent renal or hepatic disease. *Anaesthesia and Intensive Care.* 2005; **33**: 311–22.
51. Filitz J, Griessinger N, Sittl R *et al.* Effects of intermittent hemodialysis on buprenorphine and norbuprenorphine plasma concentrations in chronic pain patients treated with transdermal buprenorphine. *European Journal of Pain.* 2006; **10**: 743–8.

52. Dahan A. Opioid-induced respiratory effects: new data on buprenorphine. *Palliative Medicine*. 2006; **20** (Suppl. 1): s3–8.

* 53. Finnerup NB, Otto M, McQuay HJ *et al.* Algorithm for neuropathic pain treatment: an evidence based proposal. *Pain*. 2005; **118**: 289–305.

54. Schug SA. Combination analgesia in 2005 – a rational approach: focus on paracetamol-tramadol. *Clinical Rheumatology*. 2006; **25** (Suppl. 7): 16–21.

55. Cepeda MS, Camargo F, Zea C, Valencia L. Tramadol for osteoarthritis. *Cochrane Database of Systematic Reviews*. 2006; **CD005522**.

56. Preston KL, Jasinski DR, Testa M. Abuse potential and pharmacological comparison of tramadol and morphine. *Drug and Alcohol Dependence*. 1991; **27**: 7–17.

57. Adams EH, Breiner S, Cicero TJ *et al.* A comparison of the abuse liability of tramadol, NSAIDs, and hydrocodone in patients with chronic pain. *Journal of Pain and Symptom Management*. 2006; **31**: 465–76.

58. Labate A, Newton MR, Vernon GM, Berkovic SF. Tramadol and new-onset seizures. *Medical Journal of Australia*. 2005; **182**: 42–3.

59. Kitson R, Carr B. Tramadol and severe serotonin syndrome. *Anaesthesia*. 2005; **60**: 934–5.

* 60. Cowan DT, Wilson-Barnett J, Griffiths P, Allan LG. A survey of chronic noncancer pain patients prescribed opioid analgesics. *Pain Medicine*. 2003; **4**: 340–51.

61. Cowan DT, Wilson-Barnett J, Griffiths P *et al.* A randomized, double-blind, placebo-controlled, cross-over pilot study to assess the effects of long-term opioid drug consumption and subsequent abstinence in chronic noncancer pain patients receiving controlled-release morphine. *Pain Medicine*. 2005; **6**: 113–21.

62. *Oxford league table of analgesic efficacy*. Accessed November 26, 2006. Available from: www.jr2.ox.ac.uk/bandolier/booth/painpag/Acutrev/Analgesics/Leagtab.html

63. Elia N, Lysakowski C, Tramer MR. Does multimodal analgesia with acetaminophen, nonsteroidal antiinflammatory drugs, or selective cyclooxygenase-2 inhibitors and patient-controlled analgesia morphine offer advantages over morphine alone? Meta-analyses of randomized trials. *Anesthesiology*. 2005; **103**: 1296–304.

64. Romsing J, Moiniche S, Mathiesen O, Dahl JB. Reduction of opioid-related adverse events using opioid-sparing analgesia with COX-2 inhibitors lacks documentation: a systematic review. *Acta Anaesthesiologica Scandinavica*. 2005; **49**: 133–42.

65. McNicol E, Strassels SA, Goudas L *et al.* NSAIDS or paracetamol, alone or combined with opioids, for cancer pain. *Cochrane Database of Systematic Reviews*. 2005: **CD005180**.

66. Palangio M, Damask MJ, Morris E *et al.* Combination hydrocodone and ibuprofen versus combination codeine and acetaminophen for the treatment of chronic pain. *Clinical Therapy*. 2000; **22**: 879–92.

67. Palangio M, Morris E, Doyle Jr RT *et al.* Combination hydrocodone and ibuprofen versus combination oxycodone and acetaminophen in the treatment of moderate or severe acute low back pain. *Clinical Therapy*. 2002; **24**: 87–99.

68. Mullican WS, Lacy JR. Tramadol/acetaminophen combination tablets and codeine/acetaminophen combination capsules for the management of chronic pain: a comparative trial. *Clinical Therapy*. 2001; **23**: 1429–45.

69. Ruoff GE, Rosenthal N, Jordan D *et al.* Tramadol/acetaminophen combination tablets for the treatment of chronic lower back pain: a multicenter, randomized, double-blind, placebo-controlled outpatient study. *Clinical Therapy*. 2003; **25**: 1123–41.

70. Peloso PM, Fortin L, Beaulieu A *et al.* Analgesic efficacy and safety of tramadol/acetaminophen combination tablets (Ultracet) in treatment of chronic low back pain: a multicenter, outpatient, randomized, double blind, placebo controlled trial. *Journal of Rheumatology*. 2004; **31**: 2454–63.

71. Bennett RM, Kamin M, Karim R, Rosenthal N. Tramadol and acetaminophen combination tablets in the treatment of fibromyalgia pain: a double-blind, randomized, placebo-controlled study. *American Journal of Medicine*. 2003; **114**: 537–45.

72. Caldwell JR, Hale ME, Boyd RE *et al.* Treatment of osteoarthritis pain with controlled release oxycodone or fixed combination oxycodone plus acetaminophen added to nonsteroidal antiinflammatory drugs: a double blind, randomized, multicenter, placebo controlled trial. *Journal of Rheumatology*. 1999; **26**: 862–9.

73. Johnson RE, Fudala PJ, Payne R. Buprenorphine: considerations for pain management. *Journal of Pain and Symptom Management*. 2005; **29**: 297–326.

* 74. Hurley RW, Cohen SP, Williams KA *et al.* The analgesic effects of perioperative gabapentin on postoperative pain: a meta-analysis. *Regional Anesthesia and Pain Medicine*. 2006; **31**: 237–47.

75. Ho KY, Gan TJ, Habib AS. Gabapentin and postoperative pain – a systematic review of randomized controlled trials. *Pain*. 2006; **126**: 91–101.

76. Eckhardt K, Ammon S, Hofmann U *et al.* Gabapentin enhances the analgesic effect of morphine in healthy volunteers. *Anesthesia and Analgesia*. 2000; **91**: 185–91.

77. Subramaniam K, Subramaniam B, Steinbrook RA. Ketamine as adjuvant analgesic to opioids: a quantitative and qualitative systematic review. *Anesthesia and Analgesia*. 2004; **99**: 482–95.

* 78. Visser E, Schug SA. The role of ketamine in pain management. *Biomedicine and Pharmacotherapy*. 2006; **60**: 341–8.

79. Somogyi A, White J. *Opioid-induced hyperalgesia: implications for pain management in the opioid-dependent subject. 11th World Congress on Pain*. Sydney. Seattle: IASP Press, 2005.

80. Kocabas S, Karaman S, Uysallar E, Firat V. The use of tramadol and morphine for pain relief after abdominal

hysterectomy. *Clinical and Experimental Obstetrics and Gynecology.* 2005; **32**: 45–8.

81. Webb AR, Leong S, Myles PS, Burn SJ. The addition of a tramadol infusion to morphine patient-controlled analgesia after abdominal surgery: a double-blinded, placebo-controlled randomized trial. *Anesthesia and Analgesia.* 2002; **95**: 1713–8.
82. Ngan Kee WD, Khaw KS, Wong EL. Randomised double-blind comparison of morphine vs. a morphine-alfentanil combination for patient-controlled analgesia. *Anaesthesia.* 1999; **54**: 629–33.
83. Mercadante S, Villari P, Ferrera P, Casuccio A. Addition of a second opioid may improve opioid response in cancer pain: preliminary data. *Supportive Care in Cancer.* 2004; **12**: 762–6.
84. Smith MT, de la Iglesia FA. Co-administration of oxycodone and morphine and analgesic synergy re-examined. *British Journal of Clinical Pharmacology.* 2005; **59**: 486–7; author reply 7–8.
85. Chindalore VL, Craven RA, Yu KP *et al.* Adding ultralow-dose naltrexone to oxycodone enhances and prolongs analgesia: a randomized, controlled trial of Oxytrex. *Journal of Pain.* 2005; **6**: 392–9.
86. Ross FB, Wallis SC, Smith MT. Co-administration of sub-antinociceptive doses of oxycodone and morphine produces marked antinociceptive synergy with reduced CNS side-effects in rats. *Pain.* 2000; **84**: 421–8.
87. He L, Whistler JL. An opiate cocktail that reduces morphine tolerance and dependence. *Current Biology.* 2005; **15**: 1028–33.
* 88. Gustorff B. Intravenous opioid testing in patients with chronic non-cancer pain. *European Journal of Pain.* 2005; **9**: 123–5.
89. Eisenberg E, McNicol E, Carr DB. Opioids for neuropathic pain. *Cochrane Database of Systematic Reviews.* 2006; **CD006146**.
* 90. Dellemijn PL, van Duijn H, Vanneste JA. Prolonged treatment with transdermal fentanyl in neuropathic pain. *Journal of Pain and Symptom Management.* 1998; **16**: 220–9.
91. Attal N, Guirimand F, Brasseur L *et al.* Effects of IV morphine in central pain: a randomized placebo-controlled study. *Neurology.* 2002; **58**: 554–63.
* 92. Nicholas MK, Molloy AR, Brooker C. Using opioids with persisting noncancer pain: a biopsychosocial perspective. *Clinical Journal of Pain.* 2006; **22**: 137–46.
* 93. Waddell G, Pilowsky I, Bond MR. Clinical assessment and interpretation of abnormal illness behaviour in low back pain. *Pain.* 1989; **39**: 41–53.
94. Wu SM, Compton P, Bolus R *et al.* The addiction behaviors checklist: validation of a new clinician-based measure of inappropriate opioid use in chronic pain. *Journal of Pain and Symptom Management.* 2006; **32**: 342–51.
95. Akbik H, Butler SF, Budman SH *et al.* Validation and clinical application of the Screener and Opioid Assessment for Patients with Pain (SOAPP). *Journal of Pain and Symptom Management.* 2006; **32**: 287–93.
96. Moore RA, McQuay HJ. Prevalence of opioid adverse events in chronic non-malignant pain: systematic review of randomised trials of oral opioids. *Arthritis Research and Therapy.* 2005; **7**: R1046–51.
97. Vainio A, Ollila J, Matikainen E *et al.* Driving ability in cancer patients receiving long-term morphine analgesia. *Lancet.* 1995; **346**: 667–70.
98. Haythornthwaite JA, Menefee LA, Quatrano-Piacentini AL, Pappagallo M. Outcome of chronic opioid therapy for non-cancer pain. *Journal of Pain and Symptom Management.* 1998; **15**: 185–94.
99. Budd RD, Muto JJ, Wong JK. Drugs of abuse found in fatally injured drivers in Los Angeles County. *Drug and Alcohol Dependence.* 1989; **23**: 153–8.
100. Gaertner J, Radbruch L, Giesecke T *et al.* Assessing cognition and psychomotor function under long-term treatment with controlled release oxycodone in non-cancer pain patients. *Acta Anaesthesiologica Scandinavica.* 2006; **50**: 664–72.
101. Menefee LA, Frank ED, Crerand C *et al.* The effects of transdermal fentanyl on driving, cognitive performance, and balance in patients with chronic nonmalignant pain conditions. *Pain Medicine.* 2004; **5**: 42–9.
102. Wei G, Moss J, Yuan CS. Opioid-induced immunosuppression: is it centrally mediated or peripherally mediated? *Biochemical Pharmacology.* 2003; **65**: 1761–6.
103. Roberts LJ, Finch PM, Pullan PT *et al.* Sex hormone suppression by intrathecal opioids: a prospective study. *Clinical Journal of Pain.* 2002; **18**: 144–8.
104. Abs R, Verhelst J, Maeyaert J *et al.* Endocrine consequences of long-term intrathecal administration of opioids. *Journal of Clinical Endocrinology and Metabolism.* 2000; **85**: 2215–22.
105. Daniell HW. Hypogonadism in men consuming sustained-action oral opioids. *Journal of Pain.* 2002; **3**: 377–84.
106. Fredheim OM, Borchgrevink PC, Hegrenaes L *et al.* Opioid switching from morphine to methadone causes a minor but not clinically significant increase in QTc time: A prospective 9-month follow-up study. *Journal of Pain and Symptom Management.* 2006; **32**: 180–5.
107. Medsafe. Cardiac vigilance recommended for methadone. 2005; Accessed November 29, 2006. Available from: www.medsafe.govt.nz/profs/puarticles/methadone.htm.
108. Fishbain DA, Rosomoff HL, Rosomoff RS. Drug abuse, dependence, and addiction in chronic pain patients. *Clinical Journal of Pain.* 1992; **8**: 77–85.
109. Cowan DT, Allan LG, Libretto SE, Griffiths P. Opioid drugs: a comparative survey of therapeutic and "street" use. *Pain Medicine.* 2001; **2**: 193–203.
110. Collett BJ. Chronic opioid therapy for non-cancer pain. *British Journal of Anaesthesia.* 2001; **87**: 133–43.
111. Maier C, Schaub C, Willweber-Strumpf A, Zenz M. [Long-term efficiency of opioid medication in patients with chronic non-cancer-associated pain. Results of a survey 5 years after onset of medical treatment]. *Schmerz.* 2005; **19**: 410–7.

112. Zenz M, Strumpf M, Tryba M. Long-term oral opioid therapy in patients with chronic nonmalignant pain. *Journal of Pain and Symptom Management*. 1992; **7**: 69–77.

*113. Jensen MK, Thomsen AB, Hojsted J. 10-year follow-up of chronic non-malignant pain patients: opioid use, health related quality of life and health care utilization. *European Journal of Pain*. 2006; **10**: 423–33.

114. Mercadante S, Dardanoni G, Salvaggio L *et al*. Monitoring of opioid therapy in advanced cancer pain patients. *Journal of Pain and Symptom Management*. 1997; **13**: 204–12.

*115. Buntin-Mushock C, Phillip L, Moriyama K, Palmer PP. Age-dependent opioid escalation in chronic pain patients. *Anesthesia and Analgesia*. 2005; **100**: 1740–5.

*116. Milligan K, Lanteri-Minet M, Borchert K *et al*. Evaluation of long-term efficacy and safety of transdermal fentanyl in the treatment of chronic noncancer pain. *Journal of Pain*. 2001; **2**: 197–204.

117. Mystakidou K, Parpa E, Tsilika E *et al*. Long-term management of noncancer pain with transdermal therapeutic system-fentanyl. *Journal of Pain*. 2003; **4**: 298–306.

118. Sloan P, Melzack R. Long-term patterns of morphine dosage and pain intensity among cancer patients. *Hospice Journal*. 1999; **14**: 35–47.

*119. Ballantyne JC, Mao J. Opioid therapy for chronic pain. *New England Journal of Medicine*. 2003; **349**: 1943–53.

*120. Angst MS, Clark JD. Opioid-induced hyperalgesia: a qualitative systematic review. *Anesthesiology*. 2006; **104**: 570–87.

121. Guignard B, Bossard AE, Coste C *et al*. Acute opioid tolerance: intraoperative remifentanil increases postoperative pain and morphine requirement. *Anesthesiology*. 2000; **93**: 409–17.

122. Chu LF, Clark DJ, Angst MS. Opioid tolerance and hyperalgesia in chronic pain patients after one month of oral morphine therapy: a preliminary prospective study. *Journal of Pain*. 2006; **7**: 43–8.

*123. Athanasos P, Smith CS, White JM *et al*. Methadone maintenance patients are cross-tolerant to the antinociceptive effects of very high plasma morphine concentrations. *Pain*. 2006; **120**: 267–75.

124. South SM, Smith MT. Analgesic tolerance to opioids. *Pain Clinical Updates*. 2001; IX: 5 (accessed at wwwiasp-painorg/PCU01-5html).

125. Simonnet G, Rivat C. Opioid-induced hyperalgesia: abnormal or normal pain? *Neuroreport*. 2003; **14**: 1–7.

126. Doverty M, White JM, Somogyi AA *et al*. Hyperalgesic responses in methadone maintenance patients. *Pain*. 2001; **90**: 91–6.

*127. Thomsen AB, Becker N, Eriksen J. Opioid rotation in chronic non-malignant pain patients. A retrospective study. *Acta Anaesthesiologica Scandinavica*. 1999; **43**: 918–23.

128. Woodhouse A, Ward ME, Mather LE. Intra-subject variability in post-operative patient-controlled analgesia (PCA): is the patient equally satisfied with morphine, pethidine and fentanyl? *Pain*. 1999; **80**: 545–53.

*129. Quigley C. Opioid switching to improve pain relief and drug tolerability. *Cochrane Database of Systematic Reviews*. 2004; **CD004847**.

130. Berger A, Hoffman DL, Goodman S *et al*. Therapy switching in patients receiving long-acting opioids. *Annals of Pharmacotherapy*. 2004; **38**: 389–95.

*131. Kalso E, Vainio A. Morphine and oxycodone hydrochloride in the management of cancer pain. *Clinical Pharmacology and Therapeutics*. 1990; **47**: 639–46.

132. Pasternak GW. Incomplete cross tolerance and multiple mu opioid peptide receptors. *Trends in Pharmacological Sciences*. 2001; **22**: 67–70.

133. Yaksh TL, Harty GJ. Pharmacology of the allodynia in rats evoked by high dose intrathecal morphine. *Journal of Pharmacology and Experimental Therapeutics*. 1988; **244**: 501–07.

134. Enting RH, Oldenmenger WH, van der Rijt CC *et al*. A prospective study evaluating the response of patients with unrelieved cancer pain to parenteral opioids. *Cancer*. 2002; **94**: 3049–56.

135. Pereira J, Lawlor P, Vigano A *et al*. Equianalgesic dose ratios for opioids a critical review and proposals for long-term dosing. *Journal of Pain and Symptom Management*. 2001; **22**: 672–87.

136. Auret K, Goucke CR, Ilett KF *et al*. Pharmacokinetics and pharmacodynamics of methadone enantiomers in hospice patients with cancer pain. *Therapeutic Drug Monitoring*. 2006; **28**: 359–66.

137. Ayonrinde OT, Bridge DT. The rediscovery of methadone for cancer pain management. *Medical Journal of Australia*. 2000; **173**: 536–40.

138. Fredheim OM, Kaasa S, Dale O *et al*. Opioid switching from oral slow release morphine to oral methadone may improve pain control in chronic non-malignant pain: a nine-month follow-up study. *Palliative Medicine*. 2006; **20**: 35–41.

139. Portenoy R. Clinical strategies for the management of cancer pain poorly responsive to systemic opioid therapy. In: Giamberardino M (ed.). *An updated review*. Refresher Course Syllabus of the 10th World Congress on Pain. Seattle: IASP Press, 2002: 19–27.

140. Mercadante S, Bruera E. Opioid switching: a systematic and critical review. *Cancer Treatment Reviews*. 2006; **32**: 304–15.

141. de Stoutz ND, Bruera E, Suarez-Almazor M. Opioid rotation for toxicity reduction in terminal cancer patients. *Journal of Pain and Symptom Management*. 1995; **10**: 378–84.

142. Grilo RM, Bertin P, Scotto di Fazano C *et al*. Opioid rotation in the treatment of joint pain. A review of 67 cases. *Joint, Bone, Spine*. 2002; **69**: 491–4.

143. McQuay HJ, Jadad AR. Incident pain. *Cancer Surveys*. 1994; **21**: 17–24.

144. Portenoy RK, Bennett DS, Rauck R *et al*. Prevalence and characteristics of breakthrough pain in opioid-treated

patients with chronic noncancer pain. *Journal of Pain.* 2006; **7**: 583–91.

145. Svendsen KB, Andersen S, Arnason S *et al.* Breakthrough pain in malignant and non-malignant diseases: a review of prevalence, characteristics and mechanisms. *European Journal of Pain.* 2005; **9**: 195–206.

146. Zeppetella G, O'Doherty CA, Collins S. Prevalence and characteristics of breakthrough pain in patients with non-malignant terminal disease admitted to a hospice. *Palliative Medicine.* 2001; **15**: 243–6.

*147. Mercadante S, Villari P, Ferrera P *et al.* Safety and effectiveness of intravenous morphine for episodic (breakthrough) pain using a fixed ratio with the oral daily morphine dose. *Journal of Pain and Symptom Management.* 2004; **27**: 352–9.

148. Carr DB, Goudas LC, Denman WT *et al.* Safety and efficacy of intranasal ketamine for the treatment of breakthrough pain in patients with chronic pain: a randomized, double-blind, placebo-controlled, crossover study. *Pain.* 2004; **108**: 17–27.

149. Fishman SM, Bandman TB, Edwards A, Borsook D. The opioid contract in the management of chronic pain. *Journal of Pain and Symptom Management.* 1999; **18**: 27–37.

150. Gitlin MC. Contracts for opioid administration for the management of chronic pain: a reappraisal. *Journal of Pain and Symptom Management.* 1999; **18**: 6–8.

151. Horning MR. Chronic opioids: a reassessment. *Alaska Medicine.* 1997; **39**: 103–10, 20.

152. Portenoy RK. Opioid therapy for chronic nonmalignant pain: a review of the critical issues. *Journal of Pain and Symptom Management.* 1996; **11**: 203–17.

153. Bendtsen P, Hensing G, Ebeling C, Schedin A. What are the qualities of dilemmas experienced when prescribing opioids in general practice? *Pain.* 1999; **82**: 89–96.

17

Topical analgesics for neuropathic pain

CHARLES E ARGOFF AND K RIAZ KHAN

KEY LEARNING POINTS

- Topical analgesics work locally without producing significant systemic drug concentrations.
- Their mode of action involves reduction in peripheral sensitization, but central sensitization may also be affected.
- They have a better side-effect profile compared to similar agents given systemically due to less absorption.
- The most commonly prescribed agents are preparations of capsaicin, lidocaine alone or as a mixture with other agents, and nonsteroidal anti-inflammatory agents formulated as cream, paste, gel, patch, or spray.
- Evidence from clinical trials suggests that there is a role for the use of certain topical analgesics in the management of neuropathic pain.
- New topical analgesics are currently being developed for both neuropathic as well as other painful conditions.

INTRODUCTION

The term "topical analgesic" has been used to describe analgesic preparations that are applied locally and directly to painful areas and whose site of action is local to the site of analgesic application. The term also suggests the primary site of action of an analgesic and should not be confused with the term "transdermal analgesic," which in contrast requires systemic absorption to be effective. In some instances, analgesics have been loosely considered as "topical agents" even when formal pharmacological studies to demonstrate a lack of systemic activity or drug concentration have not been completed.

Topical analgesics are different from systemic analgesics in that they exert their analgesic activity locally over the skin, the underlying tissues, and the nerves that innervate them without significant systemic absorption as compared to systemic analgesics. They achieve high local tissue concentrations relative to systemic levels. The mechanism of action of a specific topical analgesic depends upon the specific medication being used for topical application. Topical analgesics are being studied in an ever increasing number of painful clinical conditions and will be discussed in this chapter. The potential for topical analgesics in affecting not only the peripheral processing of pain, but also in painful states considered to be central is also discussed.

The experience of pain cannot occur without the activation of relevant brain areas as has been clearly established over the past few decades. Yet even though the role of the central nervous system, and especially the brain, in the pain experience is underscored by this fact, an increasing number of chronic pain syndromes with a central pathology have been shown to respond to specific topical analgesics even though they are believed to exert their principle analgesic activity peripherally. Furthermore, while there exist certain painful conditions, such as central poststroke pain and spinal cord injury pain, in which the mechanisms of the pain almost exclusively lie within the brain and/or central nervous system, in many other commonly encountered pain syndromes, including postherpetic neuralgia (PHN), chronic low back pain, and osteoarthritis, the pain-inducing mechanisms ultimately likely result from a combination of both peripheral, as well as central nervous system mechanisms. Since nociception is not equivalent to pain and since interfering with nociception can potentially result in the experience of less pain, topical analgesics by their effects on peripheral processing of pain transmission may actually lead to a reduction of central pain mechanisms and thus pain. In other words, if pain is not pain until such pain-producing information reaches the brain, clearly if less such information arrives from the periphery for central processing, it is likely that fewer central mechanisms will be activated and thus less pain experienced. This article will review the use of topical analgesics in the treatment of a variety of painful conditions and provide an update to previously published similar reviews.[1][III], [2][III]

The effectiveness of any analgesic agent may be diminished by its adverse effect profile, toxicity, and drug–drug interactions. For most topical analgesics, the risk and severity of significant adverse effects, as well as of drug–drug interactions are less than for the identical agents given systemically.[3][III] Localized reactions such as rash or unpleasant skin sensations have been described, but are not commonly experienced.[4][III] Additionally, since a topical analgesic does not result in a significant systemic concentration of the analgesic (in contrast to the use of oral analgesics or a transdermal preparation, such as the fentanyl patch), it does not produce significant systemic accumulation of the specific analgesic. Few currently commercially available US Food and Drug Administration (FDA)-approved topical analgesics exist, although several are in various stages of clinical development and others may be available in other countries. Of the FDA-approved topical analgesics, the 5 percent lidocaine patch has been the most extensively studied. Using this preparation to illustrate some of the principles noted above, results of formal analysis of the tolerability and safety of daily 24-hour/day use of four lidocaine 5 percent patches have demonstrated that there were no significant systemic side effects experienced and measured plasma lidocaine levels remained below those associated with interference with cardiac activity. Comparable safety and tolerability was established in this report regardless of whether or not the subject used the patch for 12 or 24 hours daily.[5] In an unrelated study, patients with a history of chronic low back pain were treated safely with four lidocaine 5 percent patches every 24 hours for extended periods.[6][III] No significant dermal reactions or other side effects were experienced in either of these reports. [5][III], [6][III]

Beyond the potential experience of dermal sensitivity, other adverse effects may be associated with the use of specific topical analgesic. Upon application of topical capsaicin, as an example, severe burning of the skin at the site of application has been reported to occur in the overwhelming majority of treated patients, though the incidence of burning may decrease with repeated use. This adverse effect may in fact lead to a reduced effectiveness of this type of topical analgesic because of reduced patient compliance and, as a result, may potentially hinder a patient's ability to benefit from it.[7][III]

The fact that drug–drug interactions may be minimized when using topical analgesics may be of enormous importance for a patient who may use systemic medications concurrently for additional medical conditions. Consider for example, a 72-year-old patient who suffers from hypertension and diabetes. This person now requires analgesic treatment for his PHN and osteoarthritis (OA). He is using a number of medications for his diabetes and hypertension. Assuming that acceptable pain relief is experienced, the use of a topical analgesic in this setting may offer several advantages over a systemic agent due to the lack of drug–drug interactions.[8][III] The use of a topical analgesic in place of or in addition to a systemic analgesic may have an additional advantage in that the use of a topical analgesic does not often, if ever, require dose titration – this property also makes these agents relatively simple medications to use.

We need to keep in mind that in reality, not all "topical" analgesics are prescribed as commercially available agents. Thus, when prescribing a topical analgesic, one must distinguish between those which are FDA- or other similar agency-approved commercially available agents with consistent manufacturing standards and quality control, from those that may be manufactured on an individualized basis by a specialized compounding pharmacy. Without a doubt, many of the "topical" analgesics currently in use are not commercially available products and for many years healthcare providers have ordered other so-called topical agents from compounding pharmacies. Often the agents prescribed and thus made are combinations of medications put into a single product. This chapter will only review the use of those topical agents which are commercially available or for which there is clear evidence that they were manufactured in an unswerving and dependable manner. For many compounding pharmacies, no matter the good intentions of the prescriber or pharmacy, there is no proof of such quality control or consistency from one batch to another. Even so, the reader might appreciate that compounded, noncommercially available agents are prescribed as topical agents quite often. For example, in a recent survey of members of the American Society of Regional Anesthesia and Pain Medicine, 27 percent of the survey responders indicated that they prescribed such an agent and 47 percent of the responders reported that they felt that their patient responded positively to the prescribed agent(s).[9] [V] Overall, there appears to be increasing interest in the commercial development of new topical analgesics. Nonsteroidal anti-inflammatory drugs (NSAIDs), capsaicin, and local anesthetics are established topical agents in many countries already. Other agents with potential for topical use are antidepressants, glutamate receptor antagonists, alpha-adrenergic receptor agonists, adenosine, cannabinoids, cholinergic receptor agonists, GABA agonists, prostanoids, bradykinin, ATP, biogenic amines, and nerve growth factor.[10][V] The combination of different topical therapies may by synergistic and, as an example, the antinociceptive effects of topical morphine have been shown to be enhanced by a topical cannabinoid in a recent study in rats, in which the radiant tail-flick test was utilized.[11]

MECHANISMS OF ACTION OF TOPICAL AGENTS

Obviously, the mechanism of action of each topical analgesic depends upon the specific analgesic. This section deals with some of the possible mechanisms of action.

Capsaicin

Capsaicin-containing topical analgesics appear to achieve their action through their agonist activity at the transient receptor potential of vanilloid receptor 1 (TRPV1) on A-delta and C-fibers.[12][V], [13][V] This results in the release of substance P, as well as calcitonin gene-related peptide (CGRP). Therapeutic responses to capsaicin are generally achieved only with repeated topical application. It has been suggested that reduced peripheral, as well as central excitability with resulting less pain through reduced afferent input, is the outcome of the depletion of substance P in C fibers.[7][III], [12][V], [13][V] Histopathological examination results of human nerve biopsies, as well as of animal experiments, have suggested that application of capsaicin may lead to nerve fiber degeneration in the skin underneath the site of application. This neurodegenerative effect of capsaicin has been hypothesized to be one of its mechanisms of pain relief.[14][III]

NSAIDs

In contrast to capsaicin, the mechanism of action of an NSAID is probably related to the inhibition of prostaglandin synthesis and associated anti-inflammatory effect; however, because the anti-inflammatory effect is not always proportional to the amount of pain relief experienced, additional mechanisms of action might also be important to consider.[15]

Local anesthetic agents

While other mechanisms of action are being investigated, such as the role of reduced peripheral nociception on the dampening of central pain mechanisms, the analgesic action of local anesthetic agents based upon currently available evidence appears to be related to the ability of these agents to suppress the activity of peripheral sodium channels within the sensory afferents and subsequent pain transmission. They also cause a reduction in paroxysmal ectopic activity in these nerve fibers. Reduced expression of mRNA for specific sodium channel subtypes following local anesthetic use has also been reported.[1][III], [4][III]

Other agents

The current development of tricyclic antidepressants as topical analgesics is just being evaluated and is quite novel. The tricyclic antidepressants as a group are known to have multiple mechanisms of action and of these, the potential clinical benefit of their ability to block sodium channels when topically applied is being actively investigated at this time.[16, 17][III] In fact, in the United States, there is currently one commercially available topical antidepressant, Zonalon® (doxepin) cream. While it is indicated for use by the FDA for the short-term treatment of adult patients with pruritus associated with atopic dermatitis or lichen simplex chronicus, there are sporadic anecdotal reports of use of this agent in an "off-label" manner as a topical analgesic.[18] Other topical agents including topical opioids, glutamate receptor antagonists, and cannabinoids have stimulated great interest among basic and clinical scientists in their potential as topical analgesics. Several of the more recent studies of some of these agents are discussed below under Other uses of topical analgesics.

SIDE EFFECTS

Local anesthetics

Systemic adverse reactions following appropriate use of local anesthetic patches are unlikely due to the small dose absorbed. Allergic and anaphylactoid reactions associated with lidocaine can occur rarely. Erythema and pruritus at patch site are more common.[3][III], [4][III], [5][III], [6][III]

NSAIDs

Unfortunately, despite low systemic concentrations, the risks of side effects are not eliminated by topical NSAIDs.[19] The most common side effects are skin reactions such as urticaria, pruritus, irritation, and contact dermatitis. These occur in approximately 2 per cent of patients and tend to be self-limiting.[20] Because their incidence was similar in treatment and placebo groups, they may be related to the composition of the vehicle rather than the NSAID component. Published evidence suggests that topical NSAIDs are associated with fewer systemic side effects compared to oral therapy, although the risk is likely to increase if excessive quantities of topical NSAIDs are used. Hypersensitivity, dyspepsia, asthma, and renal toxicity have all been reported.[20, 21, 22]

Capsaicin

Burning, itching, and stinging at the site of application are common and are most commonly responsible for premature cessation of treatment. Other side effects are rare.[7][III]

CLINICAL USES

The clinical uses of topical agents will be summarized below under Neuropathic pain, Soft tissue injuries and osteorthritis, and Low back and myofascial pain.

Neuropathic pain

Clinical trial data provide varying levels of evidence for the use of certain topical analgesics in the treatment of neuropathic pain and various published reviews of the treatment of neuropathic pain have emphasized the role of these agents.[23][III], [24][I], [25][III]

LOCAL ANESTHETICS

Several local anesthetic-containing analgesics which may be considered topical agents are currently commercially available. Knowing which topical analgesic to use clearly depends upon the clinical setting in which the medication is being used. A mechanism of action of the lidocaine 5 percent patch as a topical agent, which is unrelated to the active medication, is that the patch itself may help to reduce the allodynia seen especially with neuropathic pain states, such as PHN, through the patch's ability to protect the skin.[1][III] The lidocaine 5 percent patch is FDA-approved for the treatment of PHN. Completed clinical trials of PHN patients which led to its FDA approval collectively demonstrated that use of the lidocaine 5 percent patch compared to placebo patches resulted in statistically significant pain reduction and was in addition safe and well tolerated.[26][II], [27][II] Following the FDA approval of this drug for PHN, a completed open label study was designed to examine the effect, if any, of the lidocaine 5 percent patch on various quality of life measures. A total of 332 patients with PHN were studied and a validated pain assessment tool, the Brief Pain Inventory (BPI), utilized. Up to three lidocaine 5 percent patches, 12 hours each day, were utilized by enrolled patients and the BPI was completed daily over four weeks. Of the 332 patients, 204 (67 percent) reported reduced pain intensity with repeated lidocaine 5 percent patch application by the end of the first week of the study. Pain intensity reduction was noted by the second week of patch use in over 40 percent of the remaining patients. At the conclusion of the study, approximately 70 percent of patients experienced notable improvement.[28][III]

Patients with neuropathic pain states other than PHN have been studied in various manners with the lidocaine 5 percent patch. A randomized, double-blind, placebo-controlled trial completed in Europe studied the efficacy of the lidocaine 5 percent patch in the treatment of "focal" neuropathic pain syndromes, such as mononeuropathies, intercostal neuralgia, and ilioinguinal neuralgia. Results of this trial suggested that when the lidocaine 5 percent patch is added to other pharmacotherapeutic regimens, the 5 percent lidocaine patch can reduce ongoing pain, as well as allodynia, as quickly as in the first eight hours of use, but also over a period of seven days.[29][II] An earlier reported smaller open-label study of 16 patients with various chronic neuropathic pain conditions (postthoracotomy pain, complex regional pain syndrome, postamputation pain, painful diabetic neuropathy, meralgia paresthetica, postmastectomy pain, neuroma pain), had suggested that the lidocaine 5 percent patch was able to provide pain relief without significant side effects in 81 percent of these patients.[30][III] Of note is that, according to the study's authors, patients enrolled in this study prior to the use of the lidocaine 5 percent patch, had experienced suboptimal outcomes with numerous other agents, including those typically used in the treatment of neuropathic pain. Several other non-controlled studies, each enrolling patients with painful diabetic neuropathy who were then treated with the lidocaine 5 percent patch have been completed. Patients in these studies were advised that they could use as many as four lidocaine 5 percent patches for as long as 18 hours per day. As a group, these studies have reported pain relief for the majority of patients with an acceptable adverse effect profile with this agent (data on file, Endo Pharmaceuticals, Chadds Ford, PA, USA).[31][III], [32, 33][III] In a three-week single center, open-label study of the lidocaine 5 percent patch in patients with painful idiopathic sensory polyneuropathy, significant improvements in both pain and quality of life measures were noted over the treatment period.[34][III]

Changes in the quality of the pain of patients with PHN treated with the lidocaine 5 percent patch compared to placebo were examined in a separate study. In this multicenter, randomized, vehicle-controlled study, 150 PHN patients were treated with either active or placebo lidocaine 5 percent patches (up to three lidocaine 5 percent or vehicle patches for 12 hours each day). The use of the lidocaine 5 percent patch, but not the vehicle patch, was found to reduce the intensity of certain, but not all neuropathic pain qualities utilizing the Neuropathic Pain Scale (NPS). The results demonstrated that some of the qualities of neuropathic pain (deep, sharp, and burning) which were reduced had previously been assumed not to be related to peripheral, but to central nervous system mechanisms. While the precise meaning of these findings remains unclear, the authors of this study proposed that their results suggested that peripheral mechanisms of neuropathic pain might also indeed play a role in the development of these neuropathic pain qualities.[35][II]

EMLA® cream is another local anesthetic preparation (the eutectic mixture of 2.5 percent lidocaine and 2.5 percent prilocaine). It is indicated as a topical anesthetic for use on normal intact skin for analgesia, but it is not FDA-approved for any specific neuropathic pain disorder. Nevertheless, several studies of the use of EMLA cream in the treatment of PHN have been completed. In a randomized, controlled study of PHN patients, treatment with EMLA resulted in similar efficacy as did treatment with placebo.[36][III]. Two uncontrolled studies have had more encouraging results suggesting that use of EMLA cream might relieve the pain associated with PHN.[37][III], [38][III] Although use of the lidocaine 5 percent patch is associated with an analgesic effect without creating anesthetic skin, the use of EMLA cream may create both analgesia and anesthesia when applied topically. In certain clinical settings, e.g. venepuncture, lumbar puncture, intramuscular injections, and circumcision, this property of EMLA may actually be desirable. In other clinical situations it might not be.[4][III]

CAPSAICIN

There has been great interest in using capsaicin in a number of neuropathic pain disorders, such as diabetic polyneuropathy, PHN, and postmastectomy pain, but currently available strengths of capsaicin (0.025 and 0.075 percent) have yielded disappointing results with the treatment being poorly tolerated, regimens poorly adhered to, and not enough pain relief experienced.[39][III] In contrast, examining the results of a capsaicin preparation currently in clinical development, notable analgesia has been reported by patients with painful HIV neuropathy receiving a 7.5 percent topical capsaicin cream. The patients, to be able to tolerate this medication, required concurrent treatment with epidural anesthesia.[40][V] At the 2004 Annual Scientific Meeting of the American Academy of Neurology, two open-label studies, one in patients with PHN and one in patients with painful HIV-associated distal symmetrical polyneuropathy, reported notable pain relief for the majority of patients following the single application of a high-concentration (8 percent) trans-capsaicin patch. The duration of pain relief lasted as long as 48 weeks (PHN).[41][III], [42][III] A review of the published randomized trials involving the use of topical capsaicin in the treatment of either neuropathic or musculoskeletal pain syndromes, concluded that "although topically applied capsaicin has moderate to poor efficacy in the treatment of chronic musculoskeletal or neuropathic pain, it may be useful as an adjunct or sole therapy for a small number of patients who are unresponsive to, or intolerant of, other treatments".[43][I]

A novel study comparing the analgesic effect of a topical preparation containing either 3.3 percent doxepin alone or 3.3 percent doxepin combined with 0.075 percent capsaicin to placebo in patients with various chronic neuropathic pain problems demonstrated that each treatment resulted in equal degrees of analgesia and each was superior to placebo.[44][II]

OTHER AGENTS

As suggested above under Mechanisms of action of topical agents, there has been interest in the use of topical tricyclic antidepressants in the treatment of neuropathic pain. Two recently published studies by a similar group of investigators have yielded some information regarding the development of such. In each of these studies, the preparation tested was a combination of amitriptyline 2 percent/ketamine 1 percent. The results of one of these studies, a double-blind, randomized, placebo-controlled study of 92 patients with neuropathic pain (diabetic polyneuropathy/PHN/postsurgical/posttraumatic), there was no difference in pain relief among the four treatment groups (placebo, amitriptyline 2 percent alone, ketamine 1 percent alone, or a combination of amitriptyline 2 percent/ketamine 1 percent).[45][II] Of interest is that a similar group of investigators studied 28 patients with neuropathic pain for 6–12 months in an open-label study of the combination topical analgesic amitryptyline 2 percent/ketamine 1 percent and concluded that on average patients experienced 34 percent pain reduction.[46][III] In yet another open-label study by similar investigators, assessing the potential benefit of a combination of topical amitriptyline and ketamine for neuropathic pain has yielded encouraging results, but no controlled study has yet been published.[47][III] Additional noncontrolled studies, one in patients with PHN and one in patients with complex regional pain syndrome type 1, have suggested that topical ketamine may be an effective topical analgesic; however, serum ketamine levels were not measured in either study.[48][III] A recent report has suggested that the topical application of geranium oil may be helpful in providing temporary relief from PHN.[49][V]

Case example

A 65-year-old female with painful diabetic peripheral neuropathy and hypertension chiefly affecting both lower extremities presents to your office for evaluation and treatment. She is utilizing several medications and complains of numbness in both lower extremities as well as severe, burning pain, with a visual analog scale score of

6/10. The pain is continuous and worst at night. She has achieved 30 percent pain relief taking both duloxetine and pregabalin at maximally tolerated doses. Should this person be treated with a topical analgesic as well, even in an "off-label" manner? If so, which and what evidence do we use in making this decision? In our opinion, this patient would be an appropriate candidate for a trial of a topical analgesic – although there is no such agent specifically FDA-approved for this indication.

Soft tissue injuries and osteorthritis

Soft tissue injuries and osteoarthritis are each commonly experienced musculoskeletal pain states. The use of topical analgesics for these heterogeneous conditions is actively being studied. We are well acquainted with the various systemic analgesics and various injection therapies which have been utilized in this setting, used perhaps not without the risk of significant side effects (especially with long-term and repeated use). The successful development of topical analgesics for these conditions is of great potential value to a patient. A number of studies in this area have been completed, primarily outside the United States.

NSAIDS

In a French 14-day randomized, placebo-controlled study of 163 patients with an ankle sprain, the use of a topical ketoprofen patch (100 mg) was superior to placebo in reducing pain after one week of treatment.[50][II] A similar group of investigators studied a similar ketoprofen preparation in patients with tendonitis. The results of this randomized, double-blind, placebo-controlled study were also positive and the treatment was in general, except for skin irritation, well tolerated.[51][II] Ketoprofen gel has been studied as adjunctive therapy to physical therapy in a child with Sever disease, a common cause of heel pain in athletic children.[52][V] In a randomized controlled study of a diclofenac patch in 120 individuals experiencing acute pain following a "blunt" injury, use of the patch was well tolerated, as well as significantly better than placebo in reducing the pain associated with this injury.[53][III] In one open-label study of patients generally described as suffering "soft tissue pain," the investigators concluded that topical flurbiprofen was associated with greater pain reduction than oral diclofenac with fewer adverse effects reported.[54][III] In two additional studies performed separately by different investigators, one an open-label study and the other a multicenter, randomized, controlled two-week study of pain associated with acute sports injuries, a diclofenac patch was found to be effective in providing pain relief and well tolerated. On average, patients experienced 60 percent pain relief in the open label study.[55][II], [56][III] In another controlled study, the use of topical ibuprofen cream in the management of acute ankle sprains has been examined. Ibuprofen cream was found, in this study, to be superior to placebo in reducing pain.[57][II] In a controlled study of the use of ketoprofen gel in the management of acute soft tissue pain, the gel was found to be more effective than placebo in providing pain relief.[58][II] The potential efficacy of a topical formulation of ibuprofen 5 percent gel was examined in a placebo-controlled study in patients with painful soft tissue injuries. Patients received either the ibuprofen 5 percent gel ($n = 40$) or placebo gel ($n = 41$) for a maximum of seven days. Pain intensity levels, as well as limitations of physical activity, were assessed daily using visual analog and other scales. There was a significant difference ($p < 0.001$) in pain reduction, as well as improvement in physical activities, for those patients who received the active gel compared to placebo recipients.[59][II] In a second study performed by the same investigators involving similar types of patients, similar outcomes were noted.[60][II]

There has also been interest in studying the use of topical analgesics in the treatment of osteoarthritis. A diclofenac patch has been studied in a randomized, double-blind controlled study assessing the potential benefits of such an agent in patients with osteoarthritis of the knee. This study has demonstrated that this patch may be safe and effective for this condition.[61][II] A separate randomized controlled study comparing the efficacy and side effects of a topical diclofenac solution to oral diclofenac in the treatment of osteoarthritis of the knee concluded that use of this topical diclofenac solution in patients with osteoarthritis of the knee produced symptom relief which was equivalent to oral diclofenac with significantly reduced incidence of diclofenac-related gastrointestinal complaints.[62][II] In a study of patients with pain in the temporomandibular joint, a group of patients received diclofenac solution applied topically several times daily and a second group received oral diclofenac. Although there was no significant difference seen from an analgesic viewpoint, there were significantly fewer gastrointestinal side effects experienced by the patients receiving the diclofenac topical solution.[63][II] A placebo-controlled trial has demonstrated the efficacy of topical diclofenac gel 1.16 percent for patients with osteoarthritis of the knee.[64][II] Another randomized controlled study has demonstrated the benefit of application of a topical diclofenac solution compared to placebo after six weeks of treatment for patients with painful osteoarthritis of the knee.[65][II] A meta-analysis examining the use of topical NSAIDs in the treatment of osteoarthritis concluded that there was evidence that topical NSAIDs are superior to placebo during the first two weeks of treatment, but not afterwards. In addition, this meta-analysis also concluded that available evidence suggested that topical NSAIDs were inferior to oral NSAIDs during the first week of treatment.[66][I] A separate meta-analysis examining the evidence for the use of topical NSAIDs for chronic musculoskeletal pain concluded that topical NSAIDs are effective and safe in treating chronic musculoskeletal conditions for two weeks. The investigators suggested that larger and longer trials must be completed to fully understand the practical role of topical NSAIDs in clinical settings.[67][I] Yet another meta-analysis of the use of topical NSAIDs for osteoarthritis suggested that of the four studies which had been completed in which a topical NSAID was compared to placebo or vehicle lasting four weeks or more for patients with osteoarthritis of the knee, pain relief did occur for a longer duration than placebo, but not all preparations had uniform results.[68][I] Commonly, topical salicylates are used by patients in non-prescription preparations. A meta-analysis examining the potential benefit of topical salicylates in acute and chronic pain concluded that based on the few studies that could be reviewed, topically applied rubefacients containing salicylates might be helpful in the treatment of acute pain, but that available trials of musculoskeletal and arthritic pain resulted in moderate to poor efficacy. Adverse events were rare in studies of acute pain and poorly reported in those of chronic pain. The authors emphasized that efficacy estimates for rubefacients were at present unreliable since there is a lack of appropriate clinical trials.[69][I]

A randomized controlled study completed in Germany examined the effect of topical eltenac, another NSAID, compared to placebo in 237 patients with osteoarthritis of the knee. It demonstrated efficacy and safety of the use of topical eltenac in the treatment of osteoarthritis of the knee compared to placebo.[70][II] In a separate study, topical eltenac gel was compared to oral diclofenac and placebo in patients with osteoarthritis of the knee. While both therapies were found to be superior to placebo with respect to analgesia, as reported in the meta-analysis above, the incidence of gastrointestinal side effects was notably lower in the group treated with topical eltenac gel compared to those treated with oral diclofenac.[71][II] Three additional studies have demonstrated that topical diclofenac may be effective in reducing the pain associated with various types of degenerative joint disease. [72][II], [73][II], [74]

OTHER TOPICAL AGENTS

Other agents have also been studied in these conditions. There was no benefit of 0.025 percent capsaicin cream over vehicle (not active) cream in a randomized, double-blind study of 30 patients with pain in the temporomandibular joint.[75][II] A randomized controlled study of a topical cream containing glucosamine sulfate, chondroitin sulfate, and camphor for osteoarthritis of the knee showed a significant reduction of pain in the treatment group after eight weeks compared to the placebo group.[76][II] To date, no randomized controlled trial results have been published regarding the use of a topical local anesthetic agent in the treatment of an acute soft tissue injury or in the treatment of osteoarthritis; however, two anecdotal reports of the use of the lidocaine 5 percent patch for an acute sports injury are of novel interest. A professional basketball player with a ligamentous strain in his left fifth toe was advised by the team doctor to use the lidocaine 5 percent patch for pain relief with a good outcome and a professional football player with chronic acromioclavicular joint pain due to a dislocation was anecdotally reported to experience pain relief with use of the lidocaine 5 percent patch as well. The basis for using such an agent in this setting may be the awareness that local anesthetics do in fact have anti-inflammatory properties.

A recently published case series has reported the potential benefit of "topical" morphine in the management of chronic osteoarthritis-related pain; however, the report did emphasize that morphine or its metabolites were identifiable in the urine of treated patients, hence calling into question just how truly "topical" this preparation was.[77][V]

Case example

Consider an 84-year-old female with osteoarthritis of both knees, who cannot tolerate any NSAID due to esophageal reflux, has had no response to short-acting opioids, injection therapy, and/or physical therapy and is not a candidate for knee replacement – she might be an excellent candidate for the use of a topical analgesic.

Low back and myofascial pain

Few published studies of any topical analgesic in chronic low back or myofascial pain exist. In a double-blind, placebo-controlled study comparing topical capsaicin to placebo in 154 patients with chronic low back, 60.8 percent of capsaicin-treated patients compared with 42.1 percent of placebo patients experienced 30 percent pain relief after three weeks of treatment ($p<0.02$). Fifteen of the capsaicin-treated and nine of the placebo-treated patients experienced adverse effects, none of which were believed to be harmful.[78][II]

Other studies, even if they have been presented in abstract form only, nevertheless are interesting and novel and will be reviewed briefly. For example, an open-label study of 120 patients with acute (<6 weeks), subacute (<3 months), short-term chronic (3–12 months), or long-term chronic (>12 months) low back pain was completed at eight sites in the United States. During the six-week study period, participants applied four lidocaine 5 percent patches to areas of maximal low back pain every 24 hours. Initial analysis of the first two weeks of data was presented at the Tenth World Congress on Pain.[6] Initial evaluation suggests that the majority of patients experienced moderate or greater degree of pain relief. Significant positive changes in quality of life indicators on this scale have been noted, as well as demonstrated, by the use of the NPS in this study. A more complete analysis of these data, as well as additional studies, are expected soon.[6][III] In an open-label study of patients with chronic myofascial pain presented at the 2002 Scientific Meeting of the American Pain Society, 16 patients with chronic myofascial pain were treated with the lidocaine 5 percent patch. After 28 days of treatment, statistically significant improvements were noted for average pain, general activity level, ability to walk, ability to work, relationships, sleep and overall enjoyment of life in approximately 50 percent of the patients studied.[79][V]

OTHER USES OF TOPICAL ANALGESICS

Based upon the results of a number of small studies, mostly case reports, topical analgesics of various types including opioids may be very helpful in reducing the pain associated with pressure ulcers or dressing changes.[80][I], [81][II], [82][II], [83][III], [84][II], [85] Patients undergoing any surgical procedure might benefit from the use of a topical analgesic to treat postoperative pain and reduce the need for systemic analgesics. Controlled studies have demonstrated the benefit of EMLA cream in the reduction of pain associated with circumcision and venepuncture, as well as for the pain associated with breast cancer surgery.[4][III], [86][II] Newly approved by the FDA for "local dermal analgesia" for superficial venous access and dermatological procedures is the lidocaine/tetracaine topical patch (Synera™). Several studies have suggested that either ketamine or morphine may be used topically for mucositis-associated pain following chemotherapy or radiation therapy in patients with head and neck carcinomas.[87][II], [88][V] There is also a recent report of two children with epidermolysis bullosa who were treated successfully with topical opioids.[89][V] A rather interesting recent report suggests that the analgesic effect of menthol, an ingredient common to many over-the-counter analgesic preparations, may exert part of its analgesic effect through the activation of kappa opioid receptors.[90] Burn pain has been reported to be treated effectively with a topical loperamide preparation.[91][V] Two randomized controlled studies – one involving postoperative pain (diclofenac patch) and one involving wound pain treatment (capsicum plaster topically applied at acupuncture sites) – have also been published recently.[92][II], [93][II]

In a single case report, a patient with a condition known as "central neuropathic itch" has been treated apparently successfully with the lidocaine 5 percent patch.[94][V] Several studies recently presented at professional association meetings are also worthy of mention. At the 2004 Joint Meeting of the American Pain Society/Canadian Pain Society, two new studies of new topical analgesic preparations were reported. The results of an enriched enrollment study in which an open-label initial study led to the randomization of responders in a placebo-controlled study of the use of either a 4 percent amitriptyline/2 percent ketamine cream, 2 percent amitriptyline/1 percent ketamine cream or placebo for patients with PHN demonstrated that after three weeks of treatment the average daily pain intensity was lowest in patients receiving the higher concentration combination cream compared to the lower concentration combination or placebo ($p = 0.026$ high concentration cream versus placebo). Plasma levels of either drug were detected in fewer than 10 percent of those patients receiving active treatment.[95][II] An open-label study of the use of a 0.25 percent capsaicin topical agent in a lidocaine-containing vehicle in 25 patients with painful diabetic polyneuropathy and seven patients with PHN demonstrated pain relief in the majority of patients who were studied.[96][III]

CONCLUSIONS

The use of topical analgesics may be considered for a variety of painful conditions. Although few FDA- or other similar agency-approved agents are currently available, studies involving the "off-label" use of several agents suggest a potential role for new topical therapies in the management of a variety of painful disorders. Because the use of a topical analgesic is generally associated with a better side effect profile than oral, transdermal, parenteral, or spinally administered analgesics, the successful development and availability of topical analgesics may be of particular importance. Additional controlled studies including comparative trials with "conventional" analgesics are undoubtedly required to further explore the role of topical analgesics in the management of acute and chronic pain.

REFERENCES

1. Argoff CE. New analgesics for neuropathic pain: the lidocaine patch. *Clinical Journal of Pain.* 2000; **16** (Suppl.): S62–5.
2. Argoff CE. Topical treatments for pain. *Current Pain and Headache Reports.* 2004; **8**: 261–7.
3. Argoff CE. Targeted topical peripheral analgesics in the management of pain. *Current Pain and Headache Reports.* 2002; **7**: 34–38.
4. * Galer BS. Topical medications. In: Loeser JD (ed.). *Bonica's management of pain.* Philadelphia: Lippincott-Williams & Wilkins, 2001: 1736–41.
5. Gammaitoni AR, Alvarez NA. 24-hour application of the lidocaine patch 5% for 3 consecutive days is safe and well tolerated in healthy adult men and women. Paper presented at the 54th Annual American Academy of Neurology Meeting, Denver, CO, April 13–20, 2002 (abstract P06.20).
6. Argoff C, Nicholson B, Moskowitz M *et al.* Effectiveness of lidocaine patch 5% (Lidoderm®) in the treatment of low back pain. Paper presented at the 10th World Congress on Pain, San Diego, CA, August 17–22, 2002.

7. Watson CPN. Topical capsaicin as an adjuvant analgesic. *Journal of Pain and Symptom Management*. 1994; **9**: 425–33.
8. Gammaitoni AR, Davis MW. Pharmacokinetics and tolerability of lidocaine 5% patch with extended dosing. *Annals of Pharmacotherapy*. 2002; **36**: 236–40.
9. Ness TJ, Jones L, Smith H. Use of compounded topical analgesics – results of an internet survey. *Regional Anesthesia and Pain Medicine*. 2002; **27**: 309–12.
* 10. Sawynok J. Topical and peripherally acting analgesics. *Pharmacological Reviews*. 2003; **55**: 1–20.
11. Yesilyurt O, Dogrul A, Gul H *et al*. Topical cannabinoid enhances topical morphine antinociception. *Pain*. 2003; **105**: 303–08.
12. Robbins W. Clinical applications of capsaicinoids. *Clinical Journal of Pain*. 2000; **16** (Suppl.): S86–89.
13. Bley KR. Recent developments in transient receptor potential vanilloid receptor 1 agonist based therapy. *Expert Opinion on Investigational Drugs*. 2004; **13**: 1445–56.
14. Rowbotham MC. Topical analgesic agents. In: Fields HL, Liebeskind JC (eds). *Pharmacologic approaches to the treatment of chronic pain: new concepts and critical issues*. Seattle: IASP Press, 1994: 211–27.
15. Cashman JN. The mechanism of action of NSAIDs in analgesia. *Drugs*. 1996; **52**: 13–23.(Suppl. 5)
* 16. Sawynok J, Esser MJ, Reid AR. Antidepressants as analgesics: an overview of central and peripheral mechanisms of action. *Journal of Psychiatry and Neuroscience*. 2001; **26**: 21–9.
17. Gerner P, Kao G, Srinivasa V *et al*. Topical amitriptyline in health volunteers. *Regional Anesthesia and Pain Medicine*. 2003; **28**: 289–93.
18. *Physicians desk reference*, 55th edn. Montvale, NJ: Medical Economics, 2002.
19. Skinner DV. *Cambridge textbook of accident and emergency medicine*. Cambridge: Cambridge University Press, 1997: 187.
20. Vaile JH, Davis P. Topical NSAIDs for musculoskeletal conditions. *Drugs*. 1998; **56**: 783–99.
21. Watson M. Management of patients with osteoarthritis. *Pharmaceutical Journal*. 1997; **259**: 296–7.
22. O'Callaghan CA. Acute renal failure associated with NSAIDS. *British Medical Journal (Clinical research ed.)*. 1994; **308**: 857–8.
23. Sawynok J. Topical analgesics in neuropathic pain. *Current Pharmaceutical Design*. 2005; **11**: 2995–3004.
24. Attal N, Crucci G, Haanpaa M *et al*. EFNS guidelines on pharmacological treatment of neuropathic pain. *European Journal of Neurology*. 2006; **13**: 1153–69.
25. Rowbotham MC. Pharmacologic management of complex regional pain syndrome. *Clinical Journal of Pain*. 2006; **22**: 425–9.
26. Rowbotham MC, Davies PS, Verkempinck C *et al*. Lidocaine patch: double-blind controlled study of a new treatment method for post-herpetic neuralgia. *Pain*. 1996; **65**: 39–44.
27. Galer BS, Rowbotham MC, Perander J *et al*. Topical lidocaine patch relieves post-herpetic neuralgia more effectively than vehicle patch: results of an enriched enrollment study. *Pain*. 1999; **80**: 533–8.
28. Katz NP, Davis MW, Dworkin RH. Topical lidocaine patch produces a significant improvement in mean pain scores and pain relief in treated PHN patients: results of a multicenter open-label trial. *Journal of Pain*. 2001; **2**: 9–18.
29. Meier T, Wasner G, Faust M *et al*. Efficacy of lidocaine patch 5% in the treatment of focal peripheral neuropathic pain syndromes: a randomized, double-blind, placebo-controlled study. *Pain*. 2003; **106**: 151–8.
30. Devers A, Galer BS. Topical lidocaine patch relieves a variety of neuropathic pain conditions: an open-label study. *Clinical Journal of Pain*. 2000; **16**: 205–08.
31. Hart-Gouleau S, Gammaitoni A, Galer BS *et al*. Open-label study of the effectiveness and safety of the lidocaine patch 5% (Lidoderm®) in patients with painful diabetic neuropathy. Paper presented at the 10th World Congress on Pain, San Diego, CA, August 17–22, 2002.
32. Galer BS, Jensen MP. Development and preliminary validation of a pain measure specific to neuropathic pain: the Neuropathic Pain Scale. *Neurology*. 1997; **48**: 332–8.
33. Barbano RL, Herrmann DN, Hart-Gouleau S *et al*. Effectiveness, tolerability and impact on quality of life of lidocaine patch 5% in diabetic polyneuropathy. *Archives of Neurology*. 2004; **61**: 914–18.
34. Herrmann DN, Barbano RL, Hart-Gouleau S *et al*. An open-label study of the lidocaine patch 5% in painful polyneuropathy. *Pain Medicine*. 2005; **6**: 379–84.
35. Galer BS, Jensen MP, Ma T *et al*. The lidocaine patch 5% effectively treats all neuropathic pain qualities: results of a randomized, double-blind, vehicle-controlled, 3-week efficacy study with use of the Neuropathic Pain Scale. *Clinical Journal of Pain*. 2002; **18**: 297–301.
36. Lycka BA, Watson CP, Nevin K *et al*. EMLA® cream for the treatment of pain caused by post-herpetic neuralgia: a double-blind, placebo-controlled study. Proceedings of the Annual Meeting of the American Pain Society, 1996, A111 (abstract).
37. Attal N, Brasseur L, Chauvin M *et al*. Effects of single and repeated applications of a eutectic mixture of local anesthetics (EMLA®) cream on spontaneous and evoked pain in post-herpetic neuralgia. *Pain*. 1999; **81**: 203–09.
38. Litman SJ, Vitkun SA, Poppers PJ. Use of EMLA® cream in the treatment of post-herpetic neuralgia. *Journal of Clinical Anesthesia*. 1996; **8**: 54–7.
39. Rains C, Bryson HM. Topical capsaicin: a review of its pharmacological properties and therapeutic potential in post-herpetic neuralgia, diabetic neuropathy, and osteoarthritis. *Drugs and Aging*. 1995; **7**: 317–28.
40. Robbins WR, Staats PS, Levine J *et al*. Treatment of intractable pain with topical large-dose capsaicin: preliminary report. *Anesthesia and Analgesia*. 1998; **86**: 579–83.

41. Backonja M, Malan P, Brady S *et al.* One-hour high concentration trans-capsaicin applications provide durable pain relief in initial and repeat treatment of post herpetic neuralgia. Paper presented at the Annual Scientific Meeting of the American Academy of Neurology, San Francisco, CA, 2004.
42. Simpson D, Brown S, Sampson J *et al.* A single application of high-concentration trans-capsaicin leads to 12 weeks of pain relief in HIV-associated distal symmetrical polyneuropathy: results of an open label trial. Paper presented at the Annual Scientific Meeting of the American Academy of Neurology, San Francisco, CA, 2004.
43. Mason L, Moore RA, Derry S *et al.* Systematic review of topical capsaicin for the treatment of chronic pain. *BMJ (Clinical research ed.).* 2004; **328**: 991–6.
44. McCleane G. Topical application of doxepin hydrochloride, capsaicin and a combination of both produces analgesia in chronic neuropathic pain: a randomized, double-blind, placebo-controlled study. *British Journal of Clinical Pharmacology.* 2000; **49**: 574–9.
45. Lynch ME, Clark AJ, Sawynok J *et al.* Topical 2% amitriptyline and 1% ketamine in neuropathic pain syndromes: a randomized, double-blind, placebo-controlled trial. *Anesthesiology.* 2005; **103**: 140–6.
46. Lynch ME, Clark AJ, Sawynok J *et al.* Topical amitriptyline and ketamine in neuropathic pain syndromes: an open-label study. *Journal of Pain.* 2005; **6**: 644–9.
47. Lynch ME, Clark AJ, Sawynok J. A pilot study examining topical amitriptyline, ketamine, and a combination of both in the treatment of neuropathic pain. *Clinical Journal of Pain.* 2003; **19**: 323–8.
* 48. Quan D, Wellish M, Gilden DH. Topical ketamine treatment of postherpetic neuralgia. *Neurology.* 2003; **60**: 1391–2.
49. Greenway FL, Frome BM, Engels TM *et al.* Temporary relief of postherpetic neuralgia pain with topical geranium oil. *American Journal of Medicine.* 2003; **115**: 586–7.
50. Mazieres B, Rouanet S, Velicy J *et al.* Topical ketoprofen patch (100 mg) for the treatment of ankle sprain: a randomized, double-blind, placebo-controlled study. *American Journal of Sports Medicine.* 2005; **33**: 515–23.
51. Mazieres B, Rouanet S, Guillon Y *et al.* Topical ketoprofen patch in the treatment of tendonitis: a randomized, double blind, placebo controlled study. *Journal of Rheumatology.* 2005; **32**: 1563–70.
52. White RL. Ketoprofen gel as an adjunct to physical therapy management of a child with Sever disease. *Physical Therapy.* 2006; **86**: 424–33.
53. Predel HG, Koll R, Pabst H *et al.* Diclofenac patch for topical treatment of acute impact injuries: a randomized, double blind, placebo controlled, multicenter study. *British Journal of Sports Medicine.* 2004; **38**: 318–23.
54. Marten M. Efficacy and tolerability of a topical NSAID patch (local action transcutaneous flurbiprofen) and oral diclofenac in the treatment of soft-tissue rheumatism. *Clinical Rheumatology.* 1997; **16**: 25–31.
* 55. Galer BS, Rowbotham MC, Perander J *et al.* Topical diclofenac patch significantly reduces pain associated with minor sports injuries: results of a randomized, double-blind, placebo-controlled, multicenter study. *Journal of Pain and Symptom Management.* 2000; **19**: 287–94.
56. Jenoure P, Segesser B, Luhti U *et al.* A trial with diclofenac HEP plaster as topical treatment in minor sports injuries. *Drugs under Experimental and Clinical Research.* 1993; **19**: 125–31.
57. Campbell J, Dunn T. Evaluation of topical ibuprofen cream in the treatment of acute ankle sprains. *Journal of Accidental and Emergency Medicine.* 1994; **11**: 178–82.
58. Airaksinen O, Venalainen J, Pietilainen T. Ketoprofen 2.5% gel versus placebo gel in the treatment of acute soft tissue injuries. *International Journal of Clinical Pharmacology, Therapy, and Toxicology.* 1993; **31**: 561–3.
59. Machen J, Whitefield M. Efficacy of a proprietary ibuprofen gel in soft tissue injuries: a randomized, double-blind, placebo-controlled study. *International Journal of Clinical Practice.* 2002; **56**: 102–06.
60. Whitefield M, O'Kane CJ, Anderson S. Comparative efficacy of a proprietary topical ibuprofen gel and oral ibuprofen in acute soft tissue injuries: a randomized, double-blind study. *Journal of Clinical Pharmacy and Therapeutics.* 2002; **27**: 409–17.
61. Bruhlmann P, Michel BA. Topical diclofenac patch in patients with knee osteoarthritis: A randomized, double-blind, controlled clinical trial. *Clinical and Experimental Rheumatology.* 2003; **21**: 193–8.
62. Tugwell PS, Wells GA, Shainhouse JZ. Equivalence study of a topical diclofenac solution (pennsaid) compared with oral diclofenac in symptomatic treatment of osteoarthritis of the knee: a randomized, controlled trial. *Journal of Rheumatology.* 2004; **31**: 2002–12.
63. Di Rienzo BL, Di Rienzo BA, D'Emilia E *et al.* Topical versus systemic diclofenac in the treatment of temporo-mandibular joint dysfunction symptoms. *Acta Otorhinolaryngologica Italica.* 2004; **24**: 279–83.
64. Niethard FU, Gold MS, Solomon GS *et al.* Efficacy of topical diclofenac diethylamine gel in osteoarthritis of the knee. *Journal of Rheumatology.* 2005; **32**: 2384–92.
65. Baer PA, Thomas LM, Shainhouse Z. Treatment of osteoarthritis of the knee with a topical diclofenac solution: A randomized, controlled, 6 week trial (ISRCTN53366886). *BMC Musculoskeletal Disorders.* 2005; **6**: 44.
66. Lin J, Zhang W, Jones A *et al.* Efficacy of topical non-steroidal anti-inflammatory drugs in the treatment of osteoarthritis: meta-analysis of randomized controlled trials. *British Medical Journal (Clinical research ed.).* 2004; **329**: 324–8.
67. Mason L, Moore RA, Edwards JE *et al.* Topical NSAIDS for chronic musculoskeletal pain: a systematic review and meta-analysis. *BMC Musculoskeletal Disorders.* 2004; **5**: 28.
68. Biswal S, Medhi B, Pandhi P. Longterm efficacy of topical nonsteroidal anti-inflammatory drugs in knee osteoarthritis: metaanalysis of randomized placebo

controlled clinical trials. *Journal of Rheumatology.* 2006; **33**: 1841–4.
69. Mason L, Moore RA, Edwards JE *et al.* Systematic review of topical rubefacients containing salicylates for the treatment of acute and chronic pain. *British Medical Journal (Clinical research ed.).* 2004; **328**: 995.
70. Ottillinger B, Gomor B, Michel BA *et al.* Efficacy and safety of eltenac gel in the treatment of knee osteoarthritis. *Osteoarthritis Cartilage.* 2001; **9**: 273–80.
71. Sandelin J, Harilainen A, Crone H *et al.* Local NSAID gel (eltenac) in the treatment of osteoarthritis of the knee. A double-blind study comparing eltenac with oral diclofenac and placebo gel. *Scandinavian Journal of Rheumatology.* 1997; **26**: 287–92.
72. Dreiser RL, Tisne-Camus M. DHEP plasters as a topical treatment of knee osteoarthritis: a double-blind placebo-controlled study. *Drugs under Experimental and Clinical Research.* 1993; **19**: 107–15.
73. Galeazzi M, Marcolongo R. A placebo-controlled study of the efficacy and tolerability of a nonsteroidal anti-inflammatory drug, DHEP plaster in inflammatory peri- and extra-articular rheumatological diseases. *Drugs under Experimental and Clinical Research.* 1993; **19**: 107–15.
74. Gallachia G, Marcolongo R. Pharmacokinetics of diclofenac hydroxyethylpyrrolidine (DHEP) plasters in patients with monolateral knee joint effusion. *Drugs under Experimental and Clinical Research.* 1993; **19**: 95–7.
75. Winocur E, Gavish A, Halachmi M *et al.* Topical application of capsaicin for the treatment of localized pain in the temporomandibular joint area. *Journal of Orofacial Pain.* 2000; **14**: 31–6.
76. Cohen M, Wolfe R, Mai T *et al.* A randomized, double blind placebo-controlled trial of a topical crème containing glucosamine sulfate, chondroitin sulfate and camphor for osteoarthritis of the knee. *Journal of Rheumatology.* 2003; **30**: 523–8.
77. Wilken M, Ineck JR, Rule AM. Chronic arthritis pain management with topical morphine: case series. *Journal of Pain and Palliative Care Pharmacotherapy.* 2005; **19**: 39–44.
78. Keitel W, Frerick H, Kuhn U *et al.* Capsicum pain plaster in chronic non-specific low back pain. *Arzneimittelforschung.* 2001; **51**: 896–903.
79. Lipman AG, Dalpiaz AS, London SP. Topical lidocaine patch therapy for myofascial pain. Paper presented at the Annual Scientific Meeting of the American Pain Society, Baltimore, MD, March 14–17, 2002, abstract 782.
80. Briggs M, Nelson EA. Topical agents or dressings for pain in venous leg ulcers. *Cochrane Database of Systematic Reviews.* 2003; **CD001177**.
81. Flock P. Pilot study to determine the effectiveness of diamorphine gel to control pressure ulcer pain. *Journal of Pain and Symptom Management.* 2003; **25**: 547–54.
82. Zeppetella G, Ribeiro PJ. Analgesic efficacy of morphine applied topically to painful ulcers. *Journal of Pain and Symptom Management.* 2003; **25**: 555–8.
83. Gallagher RE, Arndt DR, Hunt KL. Analgesic effects of topical methadone: a report of four cases. *Clinical Journal of Pain.* 2005; **21**: 190–2.
84. Vernassiere C, Cornet C, Trechot P *et al.* Study to determine the efficacy of topical morphine on painful chronic skin ulcers. *Journal of Wound Care.* 2005; **14**: 289–93.
85. Ashfield T. The use of topical opioids to relieve pressure ulcer pain. *Nursing Standard.* 2005; **19**: 90–2.
86. Fassoulaki A, Sarantopoulos C, Melemeni A *et al.* EMLA reduces acute and chronic pain after breast surgery for cancer. *Regional Anesthesia and Pain Medicine.* 2000; **25**: 350–5.
87. Cerchietti LC, Navigante AH, Bonomi MR *et al.* Effect of topical morphine for mucositis-associated pain following concomitant chemoradiotherapy for head and neck carcinoma. *Cancer.* 2002; **95**: 2230–6.
88. Slatkin NE, Rhiner M. Topical ketamine in the treatment of mucositis pain. *Pain Medicine.* 2003; **4**: 298–303.
89. Watterson G, Howard R, Goldman A. Peripheral opiates in inflammatory pain. *Archives of Disease in Childhood.* 2004; **89**: 679–81.
90. Galeotti N, DeCesare Mannelli L, Mazzanti G *et al.* Menthol: a natural analgesic compound. *Neuroscience Letters.* 2002; **322**: 145–8.
91. Ray SB. Loperamide: a potential topical analgesic for the treatment of burn pain. *Journal of Burn Care and Research.* 2006; **27**: 121–2.
92. Alessandri F, Lijoi D, Mistrangelo E *et al.* Topical diclofenac patch for postoperative wound pain in laparoscopic gynecologic surgery: a randomized study. *Journal of Minimally Invasive Gynecology.* 2006; **13**: 195–200.
93. Kim KS, Nam YM. The analgesic effects of capsicum plaster at the Zusanli point after abdominal hysterectomy. *Anesthesia and Analgesia.* 2006; **103**: 709–13.
94. Sandroni P. Central neuropathic itch: A new treatment option? *Neurology.* 2002; **59**: 778–9.
95. Lockhart E. Topical combination of amitriptyline and ketamine for post herpetic neuralgia. *Journal of Pain.* 2004; **5** (Suppl. 1): 82.
96. Bernstein J, Phillips S, Group T. A new topical medication for the adjunctive relief of painful diabetic neuropathy and post herpetic neuralgia. *Journal of Pain.* 2004; **5** (Suppl. 1) 82.

18

Chronic pain and depression

W MICHAEL HOOTEN

KEY LEARNING POINTS

- Chronic pain and depression are epidemiologically linked.
- Individuals with chronic pain and depressive symptoms have altered responses to pain stimuli and opioids.
- Functional neuroimaging techniques demonstrate differences in brain activity among adults with chronic pain and depression.
- Antidepressants have proven efficacy for treatment of chronic pain of diverse etiologies.
- Serotonin syndrome, serotonin withdrawal syndrome, and suicide are associated with use of antidepressants.

INTRODUCTION

Clinicians have long recognized the close association between depression and chronic pain. Findings from epidemiologic and experimental pain studies now provide empirical evidence to support this longstanding clinical observation. Knowledge of the epidemiologic associations and pathophysiological processes that interrelate chronic pain and depression provide a broad framework for understanding the clinical use of antidepressants in the treatment of chronic pain. Advancements in the understanding of drug mechanisms and awareness of adverse effects unique to antidepressant medications could further enhance clinical outcomes and improve patient safety.

EPIDEMIOLOGY

Epidemiologic studies have demonstrated an indirect association between depressive symptoms and chronic pain.[1] More recently, investigators have identified a direct relationship between the severity of depressive symptoms and the propensity to develop chronic pain. In a population-based study that involved a random sample of 2184 participants, 1131 respondents completed a mailed survey.[2] Depressive symptoms were measured using the Center for Epidemiological Studies-Depression (CES-D) scale and the severity of neck and back pain was measured using the Chronic Pain Questionnaire (CPQ). The primary outcome was the time to onset of an episode of disabling neck or low back pain, as assessed at 6- and 12-month follow up. Compared to subjects with CES-D scores in the lowest quartile, study participants in the second (hazard rate ratio (HRR) 2.46, 95 percent CI, 1.07–5.67), third (HRR 2.35, 95 percent CI, 1.01–5.45), and fourth (HRR 3.97, 95 percent CI, 1.81–8.72) quartiles were at greater risk for developing disabling neck or back pain, after adjusting for baseline general health, pain, age, education, and the occurrence of injuries during the study period. Furthermore, for every single point increase on the CES-D, the rate of developing disabling pain rose by 4 percent.[2]

These findings have been replicated in a second population-based study where the temporal relationship between major depression and chronic back pain was investigated over a two-year period.[3] This particular study involved 9909 individuals who participated in a national health survey conducted in Canada. At baseline, the presence of major depression was determined by way of a validated structured interview utilizing Diagnostic and Statistical Manual of Mental Disorders IV (DSM-IV)[4] criteria for major depression. Participants were also assessed for the presence of chronic back pain. Pain-free individuals diagnosed with major depression at study inclusion were more likely to develop chronic back pain (odds ratio (OR) 2.9, 95 percent CI, 1.2–7.0) at two-year follow up. Furthermore, each additional DSM-IV depressive symptom identified at study intake increased the rate of developing chronic back pain by 20 percent.[3] While these epidemiological studies demonstrate a temporal association between the severity of depressive symptoms and the development of chronic spinal pain, the relationship between chronic pain and the development of depression requires further consideration.

Currie and Wang[5] used similar methodologies in a separate study to investigate the association between chronic pain and development of depression. The occurrence of major depression and chronic back pain were assessed in a population-based sample of 10,600 individuals. Chronic back pain was found to be the strongest predictor of major depression (OR 6.17, 95 percent CI, 5.2–7.6) compared to other established risk factors for depression, including chronic medical illness, age, gender, and marital status.[5]

EXPERIMENTAL PAIN STUDIES AND DEPRESSION

Consistent with epidemiologic studies which have identified a direct association between chronic pain and depression, experimental studies have demonstrated that patients with depression have altered pain thresholds and tolerances.[6] In a recent study, 30 patients diagnosed with major depressive disorder, using DSM-IV criteria, were matched with 30 nondepressed control subjects.[7] Pain thresholds and tolerances were assessed bilaterally in response to experimentally induced thermal, electrical, and ischemic pain. Compared to controls, the depressed group was hypoalgesic to heat and electrical pain, but hyperalgesic to ischemic muscle pain. Similar findings have been reported for a group of patients diagnosed with adjustment disorder, depressed subtype.[8]

These differences in pain thresholds and tolerances suggest patients with depression may experience a differential analgesic response to opioid medications compared to patients without depression. In a randomized, cross-over, double-blind, placebo-controlled study, 60 patients with chronic low back pain were stratified into three groups based on the severity of depressive, anxiety, and neurotic symptoms.[9] Subjects in each of the three groups were administered 4–6 mg of morphine intravenously and pain severity was assessed over three hours. The total analgesic response was significantly greater in the low psychopathology group compared to the high psychopathology group. Additionally, the analgesic placebo response was significantly greater in the high psychopathology group compared to the low group. While the mechanisms mediating the association between chronic pain, depression, and analgesia remain to be fully elucidated, alterations in emotional processing could be important contributing factors.[10, 11, 12]

FUNCTIONAL IMAGING, PAIN, AND DEPRESSION

Advances in neuroimaging techniques, including functional magnetic resonance imaging and positron emission tomography, have revealed brain regions involved in the experience of acute pain. In a seminal study, investigators using functional imaging techniques demonstrated release of endogenous opioids and interaction of these opioids with mu-opioid receptors in response to experimentally induced acute pain.[13] Activation of the endogenous opioid system was associated with reductions in the sensory and affective intensity of the acute pain experience. In a meta-analysis, six brain structures were found to be consistently activated by acute pain stimuli including the primary and secondary somatosensory cortices, insular cortex, anterior cigulate cortex, prefrontal cortex, and the thalamus.[14] In general, the primary and secondary somatosensory cortices have been implicated in the sensory-discriminative processes of pain, whereas the thalamus, insula, anterior cigulate, and prefrontal cortices have been associated with the affective-motivational dimension of pain. Sensory-discriminative processes involve recognition of the quality and intensity of pain stimuli, including spatial and temporal characteristics. The affective-motivational dimension of pain refers to the negative emotions associated with pain experiences, including the innate sense of unpleasantness. Other brain structures, including the amygdala and periaqueductal gray matter, can be activated to a lesser extent by acute pain stimuli.[15] Furthermore, significant interindividual variation exists in the level to which various brain structures can be activated by acute pain stimuli. Variations in these observed effects can be explained, in part, by interindividual differences in peripheral neurotransmission. For example, polymorphisms of catechol-O-methyl transferase have been shown to alter activation of the endogenous opioid system.[16] Other factors which could account for variations in the activation of brain structures include gender and interindividual differences in how anticipation alters the response to nociceptive stimuli.[17, 18]

Activation of brain structures by acute pain stimuli is different among individuals with chronic pain. In general, the primary and secondary somatosensory, anterior cingulate, insula, and thalamus are activated significantly less compared to normal subjects. In the aforementioned meta-analysis, the average incidence of activation of these brain regions in normal controls was 82 percent compared to 42 percent for individuals with chronic pain.[14] Alternatively, among adults with chronic pain, the incidence of prefrontal cortex activation was 81 percent compared to 55 percent in normal subjects.[14] The observation that activity in brain structures associated with the affective-motivational dimension of pain are accentuated in patients with chronic pain is consistent with clinical observations that these patients experience more pain-related emotions and affective distress. This postulate is also consistent with neuroimaging findings from patients with comorbid depression and chronic pain. In a cohort of patients with fibromyalgia, which represented a homogenous group of patients with chronic pain, symptoms of depression were not correlated with the magnitude of experimentally induced pain.[19] Furthermore, no correlation was found between the severity of pain or depressive symptoms and activation of brain structures implicated in processing the sensory-discriminative dimensions of pain. However, a significant correlation was found between measures of depression and activation of brain structures responsible for processing the affective-motivational qualities of pain, including the prefrontal cortices. Whereas these findings require further study and replication by other investigators, they provide the impetus for the assertion that chronic pain, with or without comorbid depressive symptoms, is associated with dysregulation in an entire network of brain regions subserving both the sensory and affective components of pain.[15] Findings from functional neuroimaging studies could also provide the basis for further understanding the analgesic mechanisms of antidepressant medications.

TRICYCLIC ANTIDEPRESSANTS

Tricyclic antidepressants (TCA) were the first class of drugs widely used for the treatment of depression. These compounds were also the first class of antidepressants used to treat pain.

Structure and mechanism of action

Tricyclic antidepressants have a central three-ring structure with a single side chain. Tertiary amine tricyclics, including amitriptyline and imipramine, have two methyl groups at the end of the side chain while secondary amines, such as desipramine and nortriptyline, have one methyl group. Tetracyclic antidepressants, such as maprotiline and mianserin, are a related group of drugs that are not as widely used as the tricyclic compounds.

The analgesic effects of TCAs are mediated in part by activation of the descending inhibitory pathways that project from supraspinal centers and terminate in the dorsal horn of the spinal cord.[20] The principal mechanism of action appears to be related to blockade of serotonin and norepinephrine transport by the side chain and not the central three-ring structure. Tertiary tricyclics are more potent in blocking serotonin transport, whereas the secondary amines have greater affinity for blocking norepinephrine transport.[21] As a result of reuptake inhibition, serotonin levels rise. Inhibitory presynapic autoreceptors are desensitized while postsynapic receptors are up-regulated. The overall effect of these pre- and postsynaptic changes enhances the transmission of serotonin. Reuptake inhibition of norepinephrine enhances transmission by desensitizing inhibitory presynaptic autoreceptors in a process mediated by α_2-adrenergic receptors. Other proposed mechanisms of action include blockade of voltage-gated sodium channels,[22] inhibition of *N*-methyl-D-asparate receptors[23] and interaction with opioid receptors.[24] Major secondary effects include blockade of muscarinic, histamine (H_1), and α_1-receptors, which are responsible for many adverse side effects (**Table 18.1**).

Pharmacology and adverse effects

Absorption of tricyclics occur in the small intestine where, following first-pass metabolism, peak levels are achieved in two to eight hours. The principal method of clearance is hepatic metabolism via demethylation of the side chain and hydroxylation of the central ring structure. Tertiary amines are demethylated to the secondary amines which are conjugated to inactive forms. Several cytochrome P450 enzymes are responsible for the metabolism of TCAs including the 1A2, 3A4, 2C19, and 2D6 pathways.[25] Drugs or other substances that either inhibit or induce these enzymatic pathways can alter serum TCA levels.

In general, undesirable effects related to TCA use stem from blockade of various receptor systems (**Table 18.1**). Secondary amines are associated with fewer side effects compared to tertiary amines. Anticholinergic effects can

Table 18.1 Profile of antidepressant dosages, reuptake activity, and receptor affinities.

	Dose range	Serotonin reuptake	Norepinephrine reuptake	Adrenergic blockade	Histaminergic blockade	Cholinergic blockade	Sodium channel
Tricyclics							
Amitriptyline	25–200	++	++	++	++	+++	++
Imipramine	25–200	++	++	++	++	++	++
Nortriptyline	30–150	+	++	+	+	+	+
Desipramine	50–200	+	+++	+	–	+	+
Selective serotonin reuptake inhibitors							
Fluoxetine	20–60	++	–	–	–	–	+
Paroxetine	20–60	+++	+	–	+	+	–
Citalopram	20–60	+++	–	–	–	–	–
Serotonin–norepinephrine reuptake inhibitors							
Duloxetine	60–120	+++	+++	–	–	–	–
Venlafaxine[a]	75–225	++	++	–	–	–	–
Milnacipran	100–200	+	++	–	–	–	–

[a]Norepinephrine reuptake is dose dependent.

lead to urinary retention, constipation, tachycardia, blurred vision, and delirium. Antihistaminergic effects include sedation, increased appetite, and weight gain. Orthostatic hypotension results from blockade of α_1-receptors and could contribute to the increased risk of fall-related hip fractures among patients receiving TCAs.[26, 27, 28] Tricyclics also have type 1 antiarrhythmic properties in that cardiac conduction is prolonged by inhibition of sodium channels. These antiarrhythmic effects could, in part, account for the increased risk of sudden cardiac death and myocardial infarction in patients treated with TCAs.[29, 30] The use of TCAs in combination with methadone, which increases the QTc interval, has been associated with an increased risk of death related to accidental overdose.[31, 32] Tricyclics also increase the risk of seizure by inhibiting chloride channels.

EVIDENCE-BASED OUTCOMES FOR TRICYCLIC ANTIDEPRESSANTS

Tricyclic antidepressants are predominantly used in the treatment of neuropathic pain, but these drugs have shown efficacy in the treatment of chronic low back pain and fibromyalgia.

Neuropathic pain

Multiple randomized, placebo-controlled trials have demonstrated the efficacy of tricyclics for treatment of neuropathic pain syndromes. These pain syndromes can be generally categorized as painful polyneuropathy,[33, 34, 35, 36, 37, 38, 39, 40, 41, 42] including diabetic peripheral neuropathy, postherpetic neuralgia,[43, 44, 45, 46, 47][I] and centrally mediated pain.[48, 49][II] The outcomes of these trials have been summarized in several systematic reviews.[50, 51, 52, 53, 54] [I] The number needed to treat (NNT) in order to achieve greater than 50 percent pain relief among individuals with neuropathic pain has been shown to be 3.1 (95 percent CI, 2.7–3.7).[52]

One previous trial of postamputation limb pain found no difference between placebo and amitriptyline; however, the mean pain intensity on the numerical rating scale at study inclusion ranged from 3.0 to 3.9.[55] [II] A separate trial of postamputation pain, where the mean pain score on the visual analog scale at study inclusion ranged from 44 to 49, found significant reductions in pain following use of amitriptyline compared to placebo.[56][II]

Two trials of HIV-related neuropathy[57, 58][II] and one trial of spinal cord injury[59][II] found no difference between the tricyclics and placebo. Low medication dosages could, in part, explain the negative outcomes of these particular trials which has led some investigators to advocate for the use of plasma drug monitoring.[60]

Low back pain

Tricyclic and heterocyclic antidepressants have beneficial effects on pain intensity among patients with chronic low back pain. Specific medications used in randomized placebo-controlled trials include nortriptyline,[61, 62][II] maprotiline,[63][II] doxepin,[64][II] desipramine,[65][II] imipramine,[66, 67][II] and amitriptyline.[68][II] In these trials, the dose of nortriptyline ranged from a mean of 84 to 100 mg/day and the dose of imipramine ranged from

75 to 150 mg/day. In general, the favorable effects of improved pain intensity occurred independent of depression status, but functional status was not consistently improved.[69, 70, 71]

Fibromyalgia

Amitriptyline is the most widely used tricyclic antidepressant for treatment of fibromyalgia.[72][I] Numerous randomized placebo-controlled trials have documented the clinical benefits of amitriptyline for fibromyalgia-related symptoms including pain, fatigue, sleep, and quality-of-life.[73, 74, 75, 76, 77, 78, 79, 80, 81][II] In these trials, the dose of amitriptyline ranged from 25 to 50 mg/day. In general, the symptomatic improvements occurred independent of changes in depressive symptoms.[82, 83]

SEROTONIN-NOREPINEPHRINE REUPTAKE INHIBITORS

The selectivity for serotonin and norepinephrine reuptake distinguishes these drugs from the tricyclic group. Duloxetine, venlafaxine, and milnacipran are three widely available medications in this particular drug class.

Structure and mechanism of action

The chemical structures of duloxetine, venlafaxine, and milnacipran are individually distinct. These drugs selectively inhibit the reuptake of serotonin and norepinephrine and are referred to as serotonin-norepinephrine reuptake inhibitors (SNRI). Similar to tricyclics, the analgesic effects of SNRIs are most likely mediated by increases in serotonin and norepinephrine levels, which in turn facilitate activation of the descending inhibitory pathways. Venlafaxine has greater affinity for the serotonin transporter, but noradrenergic reuptake activity increases in a dose-dependent fashion.[84]

Pharmacology and adverse effects

Venlafaxine is metabolized by the liver to an equipotent metabolite, *O*-desmethylvenlafaxine. The half-life of venlafaxine is four hours, but the active metabolite has a half-life of ten hours. Duloxetine is hepatically metabolized and 70 percent renally excreted. The dose should be reduced in patients with impaired renal function and is contraindicated for use by patients with alcohol use disorders. Milnacipran does not significantly inhibit or induce P450 isoenzymes, thereby reducing the potential for adverse drug–drug interactions.[85]

In general, the adverse effects associated with SNRIs include nausea, vomiting, diarrhea, constipation, insomnia, somnolence, dizziness, dry mouth, hyperhydrosis, reduced appetite, and sexual dysfunction. The SNRIs do not promote weight gain. One of the most common side effects of venlafaxine and duloxetine is nausea. This effect is generally abated with continued use by down-regulation of central and peripheral serotonin receptors. An adverse effect associated with venlafaxine is blood pressure elevation that returns to baseline in approximately 50 percent of patients with continued medication use.

EVIDENCE-BASED OUTCOMES FOR SEROTONIN-NOREPINEPHRINE REUPTAKE INHIBITORS

Neuropathic pain

Among the three SNRIs, duloxetine is the most widely studied drug for neuropathic pain. In three randomized placebo-controlled trials, duloxetine improved pain intensity and functioning of patients with diabetic peripheral neuropathy.[86, 87, 88][II] Two doses of duloxetine, 60 mg daily and 60 mg twice daily, were used in these three trials. Metabolic parameters of diabetic control were not adversely affected. Venlafaxine extended-release, at a dose of 150–225 mg daily, was found to improve pain intensity among a cohort of patients with diabetic peripheral neuropathy; however, subjects randomized to receive 75 mg daily failed to respond.[89] The NNT in order to achieve 50 percent reduction in pain intensity was 4.5. In a separate randomized placebo-controlled trial, venlafaxine provided moderate pain relief for patients with polyneuropathy where the number needed to treat was 5.2.[42] In less commonly studied neuropathic pain syndromes, venlafaxine reduced pain in a small group of patients with cancer treatment-related neuropathic pain.[90]

Fibromyalgia

Of the three SNRIs, duloxetine has the most randomized trial data to support its use in the treatment of fibromyalgia. Among fibromyalgia patients with or without major depressive disorder, duloxetine improved pain and functioning independent of depression.[91, 92][II] The clinical improvements were evident in patients randomized to receive either duloxetine 60 mg/day or 60 mg twice daily. Using a similar study design, fibromyalgia patients with and without depression were randomized to receive milnacipran once (mean dose, 174 mg) or twice (mean dose, 191 mg) daily.[93][II] At study completion, both treatment groups experienced significant improvements in pain and global well-being, but patients in the higher-dose group experienced improvements in physical functioning. The less favorable outcomes of the once-daily dosage group could have been due in part to the short half-life of the drug. Randomized trial data are not available for venlafaxine in the treatment of fibromyalgia, but two prospective open-label trials found significant improvements in both pain and physical functioning.[94, 95][III]

Generalized painful symptoms of depression

Several randomized controlled trials of duloxetine for depression reported significant improvements in a variety of pain symptoms, including back pain, shoulder pain, and headache.[96, 97, 98][II] The findings from these and other similar trials have been summarized and subjected to further pooled analyses.[99, 100, 101][I] Painful physical symptoms among patients with depression was the primary outcome measure for a randomized placebo-controlled trial of duloxetine.[102] In this particular study, subjects who received duloxetine 60 mg daily experienced significant improvements in pain and activity-related pain interference. These clinical improvements occurred independent of changes in depressive symptoms.

SELECTIVE SEROTONIN REUPTAKE INHIBITORS

Numerous selective serotonin reuptake inhibitors (SSRIs) are available including fluoxetine, paroxetine, sertraline, citalopram, escitalopram, and fluvoxamine. The ensuing material will be limited to those medications with proven efficacy for treatment of pain.

Structure and mechanism of action

Fluoxetine, paroxetine, and citalopram inhibit serotonin reuptake but differences in structure and activity exist. Compared to fluoxetine, paroxetine and citalopram are more potent serotonin reuptake inhibitors, whereas paroxetine is a weak inhibitor of norepinephrine reuptake (**Table 18.1**).[103] The antinociceptive mechanisms of SSRIs are poorly understood. In general, SSRIs block serotonergic reuptake which desensitizes feedback receptors leading to accumulation of serotonin in the synaptic cleft. Apart from serotonergic mechanisms, animal studies suggest the analgesic effects of SSRIs are also mediated by opioid and cholinergic pathways,[104, 105] inhibition of sodium channels,[106] and activation of the descending inhibitory pathways.[103]

Pharmacology and adverse effects including suicide

Fluoxetine, paroxetine, and citalopram are hepatically metabolized by the cytochrome P450 system. The half-life of fluoxetine is 84 hours and the principal metabolite is equipotent with an extended half-life of seven days. The half-life of paroxetine (21 hours) and citalopram (36 hours) are prolonged in geriatric patients and the dose of paroxetine should be reduced in patients with renal dysfunction. Fluoxetine and paroxetine are both substrates and inhibitors of the 2D6 enzyme. The inhibition of 2D6 by fluoxetine and paroxetine could elevate serum levels of other analgesic medications, including tricyclic antidepressants and tramadol.[107] The metabolism of citalopram is more balanced in that the drug is metabolized by three different cytochrome enzymes including 2D6, 2C19, and 3A4.

Side effects associated with use of these medications are related to enhanced serotonergic transmission. Frequently encountered side effects include nausea, vomiting, tremor, anxiety, agitation, sweating, sleep disturbance, diarrhea, and sexual dysfunction. Paroxetine has affinity for muscarinic receptors which account for mild anticholinergic effects, predominantly dry mouth, constipation, and blurred vision. Long-term use of paroxetine has been associated with weight gain.[108]

One of the most important controversies related to use of SSRIs is the potential increased risk of suicide, particularly among adolescents with depression.[109, 110, 111] However, further research is needed to firmly establish the overall risks and benefits of antidepressant therapy on both attempted and completed suicide.[112, 113, 114] Knowledge of the potential association between SSRIs and suicide is particularly important for pain medicine specialists given the high incidence of depression among patients with chronic pain. In the context of this ongoing controversy, physicians who prescribe antidepressant medications should be vigilant in accounting for the potential risk of this uncommon, but devastating, adverse event.

EVIDENCE-BASED OUTCOMES FOR SELECTIVE SEROTONIN REUPTAKE INHIBITORS

Neuropathic pain

Serotonin reuptake inhibitors are not commonly used to treat neuropathic pain. Four randomized trials have compared fluoxetine, paroxetine, and citalopram to placebo. In three trials, fluoxetine 20 and 40 mg, paroxetine 40 mg, and citalopram 40 mg was more effective compared to placebo in the treatment of diabetic neuropathy.[38, 115, 116][II] In a small randomized comparative trial involving antidepressant naive patients diagnosed with postherpetic neuralgia, fluoxetine 60 mg was found to be less effective compared to desipramine and amitriptyline at dosages of 150 mg.[117][II] The NNT in order to achieve 50 percent pain relief among patients with neuropathic pain treated with SSRIs is 6.8 (95 percent CI, 3.4–441).[52][I]

Fibromyalgia

Trials of fluoxetine for treatment of fibromyalgia have yielded contradictory results. In two randomized placebo-controlled trials, fluoxetine was superior to placebo in the treatment of fibromyalgia-related symptoms.[118, 119][II] The dose of fluoxetine in one trial was 20 mg, whereas a flexible-dose schedule ranging from 10 to 80 mg was employed in the second trial. In a third placebo-controlled trial, the clinical outcomes of subjects randomized to receive fluoxetine 20 mg were similar to placebo.[120] Citalopram at doses of 20–40 mg/day was no more effective than placebo in two randomized placebo-controlled trials.[121, 122][II]

Low back pain

Limited evidence exists to support the use of SSRIs in the treatment of low back pain. In two placebo-controlled trials, improvement in pain was similar between subjects randomized to paroxetine 20–30 mg/day compared to placebo.[63, 123][II]

MISCELLANEOUS ANTIDEPRESSANTS

Bupropion

Bupropion is a monocyclic compound with an aminoketone side chain. Whereas the structure is similar to sympathominetics, bupropion has no stimulant abuse potential. Bupropion effects dopaminergic and noradrenergic activity with negligible effects on serotonergic activity. The half-life of the parent compound is 21 hours, but the half-life of two active metabolites is in excess of 40 hours.

Common adverse side effects include insomnia, agitation, headache, nausea, and dry mouth. Due to minimal effects on histaminergic, α-adrenergic, cholinergic, or serotonergic activity, bupropion is relatively free of many side effects commonly encountered with use of other antidepressants including sedation, weight gain, and sexual dysfunction.[124] However, bupropion is associated with a small increase risk of seizure.

The efficacy of bupropion in treatment of neuropathic pain has been demonstrated in a single cross-over trial. In this study, 41 subjects with neuropathic pain of multiple etiologies were randomized to receive either bupropion sustained release 150–300 mg daily or placebo.[125][II] Subjects in the bupropion group experienced significant improvement in pain intensity compared to the placebo. In a separate study of 44 patients with low back pain, outcomes of subjects randomized to receive bupropion sustained release 150–300 mg daily were no different compared to placebo.[126][II]

ANTIDEPRESSANT DISCONTINUATION SYNDROME

The antidepressant discontinuation syndrome is predominately characterized by the acute onset of dizziness, headache, nausea, fatigue, vomiting, ataxia, and paresthesias following abrupt discontinuation of antidepressants with serotonergic activity.[127] This clinical syndrome can occur with the use of SSRIs, SNRIs, and tricyclic antidepressants. Whereas the syndrome generally occurs following abrupt discontinuation of antidepressants, clinical symptoms can emerge following dose reductions. Diagnostic criteria have been proposed as outlined in **Table 18.2**.[128, 129] The physiologic mechanisms which mediate the clinical manifestations of this syndrome are presumably related to the rapid decline in serotonin availability, but alterations in noradrenergic and cholinergic activity could also account for some associated symptoms.[130]

The half-life of the antidepressant is also an important contributing factor in that drugs with a short half-life are more likely to result in discontinuation symptoms. Fluoxetine has a long half-life and is rarely associated with antidepressant discontinuation syndrome.[131] Comparatively, discontinuation symptoms are more likely to occur following abrupt discontinuation of paroxetine and duloxetine, each of which has a relatively short half-life.[131, 132] A recent consensus panel recommended slowly tapering antidepressants with serotonergic activity over a three- to

Table 18.2 Diagnostic criteria for antidepressant discontinuation syndrome.

Criterion	Description
A	Discontinuation or reduction in serotonergic antidepressant after ≥one month exposure
B	Two (or more) symptoms within one to seven days of criterion A Dizziness Vertigo Light-headedness Headache Visual disturbances Paresthesia Tremor Fatigue Insomnia Anxiety Nausea or vomiting Diarrhea
C	Symptoms in criterion B cause clinically significant distress or impairment in social, occupational, or other important areas of functioning
D	The symptoms are not due to a general medical condition or other concomitant psychiatric disorder.

Adapted with permission from Selective serotonin reuptake inhibitor discontinuation syndrome: proposed diagnostic criteria – Reprinted from *JPN* May 2000; 25(3), Pages 255–61 by permission of the publisher. © 2000 Canadian Medical Association.

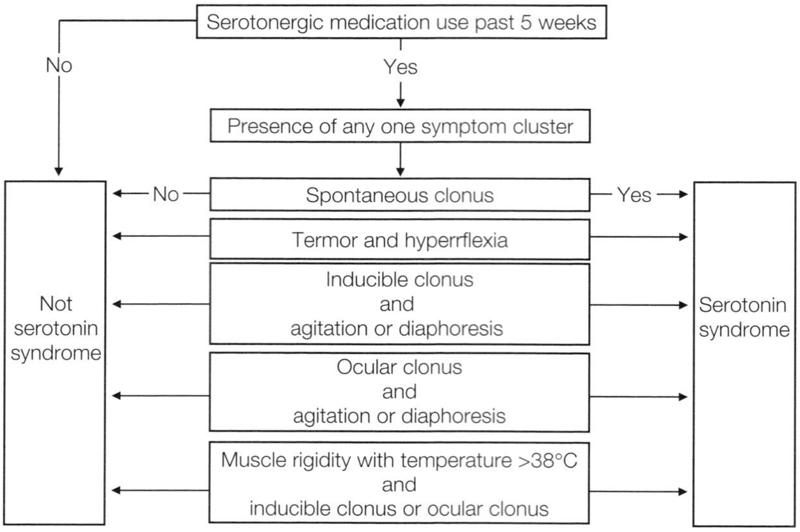

Figure 18.1 Diagnostic algorithm for serotonin syndrome.

four-week period in order to prevent or attenuate discontinuation symptoms.[133] The exception to this recommendation was fluoxetine which does not require tapering.

SEROTONIN SYNDROME

Serotonin syndrome refers to a spectrum of symptoms stemming from excessive serotonergic stimulation of the central nervous system. The syndrome has been most commonly associated with SSRIs and drug combinations involving these medications.[134] Serotonin syndrome has also been associated with drug combinations involving venlafaxine, duloxetine, oxycodone, and tramadol.[135, 136, 137] The clinical triad of autonomic and neuromuscular hyperactivity with associated alterations in mental status characterize the clinical presentation of many patients.[129, 138] Mild or early symptoms include tremor, hyperreflexia, tachycardia, mydriasis, and akathisia. As the syndrome progresses, neurologic findings include delirium, hypertension, diaphoresis, and inducible clonus. In the latter, life-threatening stages, core body temperature can be $>41^{\circ}$C and patients have profound muscle rigidity. Laboratory findings include metabolic acidosis and abnormalities consistent with rhabdomyolysis, renal failure, and coagulopathy. Treatment is primarily supportive following identification and removal of the offending agent or drug combination. The majority of cases resolve within one to two days.

No single symptom, physical finding, or laboratory test is pathognomonic for serotonin syndrome. However, a clinically oriented diagnostic algorithm has been developed with a reported sensitivity and specificity of 85 and 97 percent, respectively (**Figure 18.1**).[139] Increased physician awareness coupled with use of objective diagnostic criteria could lead to early recognition and successful management of this potentially life-threatening adverse drug effect.

CONCLUSIONS

Epidemiologic and experimental pain studies provide empirical data which provide the framework to define further the physiologic substrates and mechanisms that link chronic pain and depression. Randomized, placebo-controlled studies demonstrate the efficacy of antidepressants in the treatment of neuropathic pain, fibromyalgia, and, to a lesser extent, low back pain and painful symptoms related to depression. However, further clinical trials are needed to investigate the interplay between the antinociceptive and antidepressant effects of these medications. While antidepressants are generally well tolerated, an understanding of the unique and devastating adverse effects, including the potential risk of suicide and serotonin syndrome, are vital to the safe use of these medications.

ACKNOWLEDGMENTS

This chapter is adapted and expanded from Sindrup SH. Antidepressants and chronic pain. In: Jensen TS, Wilson PR and Rice ASC (eds). *Clinical Pain Management: Chronic Pain*. London: Hodder Arnold, 2002: 403–16.

REFERENCES

1. Ohayon MM, Schatzberg AF. Using chronic pain to predict depressive morbidity in the general population. *Archives of General Psychiatry.* 2003; **60**: 39–47.
2. Carroll LJ, Cassidy JD, Cote P. Depression as a risk factor for onset of an episode of troublesome neck and low back pain. *Pain.* 2004; **107**: 134–9.

3. Currie SR, Wang JL. More data on major depression as an antecedent risk factor for first onset of chronic back pain. *Psychological Medicine*. 2005; **35**: 1275–82.
4. American Psychiatric Association. *Diagnostic and statistical manual of mental disorders*, 4th edn. Arlington: American Psychiatric Association, 2000.
5. Currie SR, Wang JL. Chronic back pain and major depression in the general Canadian population. *Pain*. 2004; **107**: 54–60.
6. Dickens C, McGowan L, Dale S. Impact of depression on experimental pain perception: A systematic review of the literature with meta-analysis. *Psychosomatic Medicine*. 2003; **65**: 369–75.
7. Bar KJ, Brehm S, Boettger MK *et al*. Pain perception in major depression depends on pain modality. *Pain*. 2005; **117**: 97–103.
8. Bar KJ, Brehm S, Boettger MK *et al*. Decreased sensitivity to experimental pain in adjustment disorder. *European Journal of Pain*. 2006; **10**: 467–71.
9. Wasan AD, Davar G, Jamison R. The association between negative affect and opioid analgesia in patients with discogenic low back pain. *Pain*. 2005; **117**: 450–61.
10. Klossika I, Flor H, Kamping S *et al*. Emotional modulation of pain: a clinical perspective. *Pain*. 2006; **124**: 264–8.
11. Meredith PJ, Strong J, Feeney JA. The relationship of adult attachment to emotion, catastrophizing, control, threshold and tolerance, in experimentally-induced pain. *Pain*. 2006; **120**: 44–52.
12. Meredith P, Strong J, Feeney JA. Adult attachment, anxiety, and pain self-efficacy as predictors of pain intensity and disability. *Pain*. 2006; **123**: 146–54.
13. Zubieta JK, Smith YR, Bueller JA *et al*. Regional mu opioid receptor regulation of sensory and affective dimensions of pain. *Science*. 2001; **293**: 311–5.

* 14. Apkarian AV, Bushnell MC, Treede RD, Zubieta JK. Human brain mechanisms of pain perception and regulation in health and disease. *European Journal of Pain*. 2005; **9**: 463–84.

* 15. Tracey I, Mantyh PW. The cerebral signature for pain perception and its modulation. *Neuron*. 2007; **55**: 377–91.

16. Zubieta JK, Heitzeg MM, Smith YR *et al*. COMT val158met genotype affects mu-opioid neurotransmitter responses to a pain stressor. *Science*. 2003; **299**: 1240–3.
17. Fairhurst M, Wiech K, Dunckley P, Tracey I. Anticipatory brainstem activity predicts neural processing of pain in humans. *Pain*. 2007; **128**: 101–10.
18. Zubieta JK, Smith YR, Bueller JA *et al*. Mu-opioid receptor-mediated antinociceptive responses differ in men and women. *Journal of Neuroscience*. 2002; **22**: 5100–7.
19. Giesecke T, Gracely RH, Williams DA *et al*. The relationship between depression, clinical pain, and experimental pain in a chronic pain cohort. *Arthritis and Rheumatism*. 2005; **52**: 1577–84.
20. Millan MJ. Descending control of pain. *Progress in Neurobiology*. 2002; **66**: 355–474.
21. Tatsumi M, Groshan K, Blakely RD, Richelson E. Pharmacological profile of antidepressants and related compounds at human monoamine transporters. *European Journal of Pharmacology*. 1997; **340**: 249–58.
22. Amir R, Argoff CE, Bennett GJ, Cummins TR. The role of sodium channels in chronic inflammatory and neuropathic pain. *Journal of Pain*. 2006; **7**: S1–29.
23. Li YF, Zhang YZ, Liu YQ *et al*. Inhibition of *N*-methyl-D-aspartate receptor function appears to be one of the common actions for antidepressants. *Journal of Psychopharmacology*. 2006; **20**: 629–35.
24. Zarrindast MR, Vousooghi N, Sahebgharani M. Imipramine-induced antinociception in the formalin test – Receptor mechanisms involved and effect of swim stress. *Pharmacology*. 2003; **68**: 154–61.
25. Nemeroff CB, DeVane CL, Pollock BG. Newer antidepressants and the cytochrome P450 system. *American Journal of Psychiatry*. 1996; **153**: 311–20.
26. Hubbard R, Farrington P, Smith C *et al*. Exposure to tricyclic and selective serotonin reuptake inhibitor antidepressants and the risk of hip fracture. *American Journal of Epidemiology*. 2003; **158**: 77–84.
27. Liu B, Anderson G, Mittmann N *et al*. Use of selective serotonin-reuptake inhibitors or tricyclic antidepressants and risk of hip fractures in elderly people. *Lancet*. 1998; **351**: 1303–7.
28. Ray WA, Griffin MR, Malcolm E. Cyclic antidepressants and the risk of hip fracture. *Archives of Internal Medicine*. 1991; **151**: 754–6.
29. Tata LJ, West J, Smith C *et al*. General population based study of the impact of tricyclic and selective serotonin reuptake inhibitor antidepressants on the risk of acute myocardial infarction. *Heart*. 2005; **91**: 465–71.
30. Ray WA, Meredith S, Thapa PB *et al*. Cyclic antidepressants and the risk of sudden cardiac death. *Clinical Pharmacology and Therapeutics*. 2004; **75**: 234–41.
31. Chan GM, Stajic M, Marker EK *et al*. Testing positive for methadone and either a tricyclic antidepressant or a benzodiazepine is associated with an accidental overdose death: Analysis of medical examiner data. *Academic Emergency Medicine*. 2006; **13**: 543–7.
32. Krantz MJ, Lowery CM, Martell BA *et al*. Effects of methadone on QT-interval dispersion. *Pharmacotherapy*. 2005; **25**: 1523–9.
33. Sindrup SH, Ejlertsen B, Froland A *et al*. Imipramine treatment in diabetic neuropathy: relief of subjective symptoms without changes in peripheral and autonomic nerve function. *European Journal of Clinical Pharmacology*. 1989; **37**: 151–3.
34. Sindrup SH, Gram LF, Skjold T *et al*. Clomipramine vs desipramine vs placebo in the treatment of diabetic neuropathy symptoms. A double-blind cross-over study. *British Journal of Clinical Pharmacology*. 1990; **30**: 683–91.
35. Sindrup SH, Tuxen C, Gram LF *et al*. Lack of effect of mianserin on the symptoms of diabetic neuropathy. *European Journal of Clinical Pharmacology*. 1992; **43**: 251–5.

36. Max MB, Culnane M, Schafer SC *et al.* Amitriptyline relieves diabetic neuropathy pain in patients with normal or depressed mood. *Neurology.* 1987; **37**: 589–96.
37. Max MB, Kishore-Kumar R, Schafer SC *et al.* Efficacy of desipramine in painful diabetic neuropathy: a placebo-controlled trial. *Pain.* 1991; **45**: 3–9.
38. Max MB, Lynch SA, Muir J *et al.* Effects of desipramine, amitriptyline, and fluoxetine on pain in diabetic neuropathy. *New England Journal of Medicine.* 1992; **326**: 1250–6.
39. Gomez-Perez FJ, Rull JA, Dies H *et al.* Nortriptyline and fluphenazine in the symptomatic treatment of diabetic neuropathy. A double-blind cross-over study. *Pain.* 1985; **23**: 395–400.
40. Kvinesdal B, Molin J, Froland A, Gram LF. Imipramine treatment of painful diabetic neuropathy. *Journal of the American Medical Association.* 1984; **251**: 1727–30.
41. Vrethem M, Boivie J, Arnqvist H *et al.* A comparison of amitriptyline and maprotiline in the treatment of painful polyneuropathy in diabetics and nondiabetics. *Clinical Journal of Pain.* 1997; **13**: 313–23.
42. Sindrup SH, Bach FW, Madsen C *et al.* Venlafaxine versus imipramine in painful polyneuropathy – a randomized, controlled trial. *Neurology.* 2003; **60**: 1284–9.
43. Graff-Radford SB, Shaw LR, Naliboff BN. Amitriptyline and fluphenazine in the treatment of postherpetic neuralgia. *Clinical Journal of Pain.* 2000; **16**: 188–92.
44. Kishore-Kumar R, Max MB, Schafer SC *et al.* Desipramine relieves postherpetic neuralgia. *Clinical Pharmacology and Therapeutics.* 1990; **47**: 305–12.
45. Max MB, Schafer SC, Culnane M *et al.* Amitriptyline, but not lorazepam, relieves postherpetic neuralgia. *Neurology.* 1988; **38**: 1427–32.
46. Watson CP, Evans RJ, Reed K *et al.* Amitriptyline versus placebo in postherpetic neuralgia. *Neurology.* 1982; **32**: 671–3.
47. Raja SN, Haythornthwaite JA, Pappagallo M *et al.* Opioids versus antidepressants in postherpetic neuralgia: a randomized, placebo-controlled trial. *Neurology.* 2002; **59**: 1015–21.
48. Panerai AE, Monza G, Movilia P *et al.* A randomized, within-patient, cross-over, placebo-controlled trial on the efficacy and tolerability of the tricyclic antidepressants chlorimipramine and nortriptyline in central pain. *Acta Neurologica Scandinavica.* 1990; **82**: 34–8.
49. Leijon G, Boivie J. Central post-stroke pain – a controlled trial of amitriptyline and carbamazepine. *Pain.* 1989; **36**: 27–36.
* 50. Sindrup SH, Jensen TS. Efficacy of pharmacological treatments of neuropathic pain: an update and effect related to mechanism of drug action. *Pain.* 1999; **83**: 389–400.
* 51. Sindrup SH, Otto M, Finnerup NB, Jensen TS. Antidepressants in the treatment of neuropathic pain. *Basic and Clinical Pharmacology and Toxicology.* 2005; **96**: 399–409.
* 52. Finnerup NB, Otto M, McQuay HJ *et al.* Algorithm for neuropathic pain treatment: An evidence based proposal. *Pain.* 2005; **118**: 289–305.
53. Lynch ME. Antidepressants as analgesics: a review of randomized controlled trials. *Journal of Psychiatry and Neuroscience.* 2001; **26**: 30–6.
54. Saarto T, Wiffen PJ. Antidepressants for neuropathic pain. *Cochrane Database of Systematic Reviews.* 2005; **CD005454**.
55. Robinson LR, Czerniecki JM, Ehde DM *et al.* Trial of amitriptyline for relief of pain in amputees: Results of a ramdomized controlled study. *Archives of Physical Medicine and Rehabilitation.* 2004; **85**: 1–6.
56. Wilder-Smith CH, Hill LT, Laurent S. Postamputation pain and sensory changes in treatment-naive patients – characteristics and responses to treatment with tramadol, amitriptyline, and placebo. *Anesthesiology.* 2005; **103**: 619–28.
57. Kieburtz K, Simpson D, Yiannoutsos C *et al.* A randomized trial of amitriptyline and mexiletine for painful neuropathy in HIV infection. *Neurology.* 1998; **51**: 1682–8.
58. Shlay JC, Chaloner K, Max MB *et al.* Acupuncture and amitriptyline for pain due to HIV-related peripheral neuropathy – a randomized controlled trial. *Journal of the American Medical Association.* 1998; **280**: 1590–5.
59. Cardenas DD, Warms CA, Turner JA *et al.* Efficacy of amitriptyline for relief of pain in spinal cord injury: results of a randomized controlled trial. *Pain.* 2002; **96**: 365–73.
60. Rasmussen PV, Jensen TS, Sindrup SH, Bach FW. TDM-based imipramine treatment in neuropathic pain. *Therapeutic Drug Monitoring.* 2004; **26**: 352–60.
61. Atkinson JH, Slater MA, Williams RA *et al.* A placebo-controlled randomized clinical trial of nortriptyline for chronic low back pain. *Pain.* 1998; **76**: 287–96.
62. Khoromi S, Cui L, Nackers L, Max MB. Morphine, nortriptyline and their combination vs. placebo in patients with chronic lumbar root pain. *Pain.* 2007; **130**: 66–75.
63. Atkinson JH, Slater MA, Wahlgren DR *et al.* Effects of noradrenergic and serotonergic antidepressants on chronic low back pain intensity. *Pain.* 1999; **83**: 137–45.
64. Hameroff SR, Weiss JL, Lerman JC *et al.* Doxepin's effects on chronic pain and depression: a controlled study. *Journal of Clinical Psychiatry.* 1984; **45**: 47–53.
65. Ward N, Bokan JA, Phillips M *et al.* Antidepressants in concomitant chronic back pain and depression: doxepin and desipramine compared. *Journal of Clinical Psychiatry.* 1984; **45**: 54–9.
66. Alcoff J, Jones E, Rust P, Newman R. Controlled trial of imipramine for chronic low back pain. *Journal of Family Practice.* 1982; **14**: 841–6.
67. Jenkins DG, Ebbutt AF, Evans CD. Tofranil in the treatment of low back pain. *Journal of International Medical Research.* 1976; **4**: 28–40.
68. Pheasant H, Bursk A, Goldfarb J *et al.* Amitriptyline and chronic low-back pain. A randomized double-blind crossover study. *Spine.* 1983; **8**: 552–7.

* 69. Salerno SM, Browning R, Jackson JL. The effect of antidepressant treatment on chronic back pain – a meta-analysis. *Archives of Internal Medicine*. 2002; **162**: 19–24.
* 70. Schnitzer TJ, Ferraro A, Hunsche E, Kong SX. A comprehensive review of clinical trials on the efficacy and safety of drugs for the treatment of low back pain. *Journal of Pain and Symptom Management*. 2004; **28**: 72–95.
* 71. Staiger TO, Gaster B, Sullivan MD, Deyo RA. Systematic review of antidepressants in the treatment of chronic low back pain. *Spine*. 2003; **28**: 2540–5.
* 72. Goldenberg DL, Burckhardt C, Crofford L. Management of fibromyalgia syndrome. *Journal of the American Medical Association*. 2004; **292**: 2388–95.
73. Carette S, Bell MJ, Reynolds WJ *et al*. Comparison of amitriptyline, cyclobenzaprine, and placebo in the treatment of fibromyalgia. A randomized, double-blind clinical trial. *Arthritis and Rheumatism*. 1994; **37**: 32–40.
74. Carette S, Oakson G, Guimont C, Steriade M. Sleep electroencephalography and the clinical response to amitriptyline in patients with fibromyalgia. *Arthritis and Rheumatism*. 1995; **38**: 1211–7.
75. Goldenberg DL, Felson DT, Dinerman H. A randomized, controlled trial of amitriptyline and naproxen in the treatment of patients with fibromyalgia. *Arthritis and Rheumatism*. 1986; **29**: 1371–7.
76. Goldenberg D, Mayskiy M, Mossey C *et al*. A randomized, double-blind crossover trial of fluoxetine and amitriptyline in the treatment of fibromyalgia. *Arthritis and Rheumatism*. 1996; **39**: 1852–9.
77. Scudds RA, McCain GA, Rollman GB, Harth M. Improvements in pain responsiveness in patients with fibrositis after successful treatment with amitriptyline. *Journal of Rheumatology Supplement*. 1989; **19**: 98–103.
78. Jaeschke R, Adachi J, Guyatt G *et al*. Clinical usefulness of amitriptyline in fibromyalgia: the results of 23 N-of-1 randomized controlled trials. *Journal of Rheumatology*. 1991; **18**: 447–51.
79. Ginsberg F, Mancaux A, Joos E *et al*. A randomized placebo-controlled trial of sustained-release amitriptyline in primary fibromyalgia. *Journal of Musculoskeletal Pain*. 1996; **4**: 37–47.
80. Hannonen P, Malminiemi K, Yli-Kerttula U *et al*. A randomized, double-blind, placebo-controlled study of moclobemide and amitriptyline in the treatment of fibromyalgia in females without psychiatric disorder. *British Journal of Rheumatology*. 1998; **37**: 1279–86.
81. Kempenaers C, Simenon G, Vander Elst M *et al*. Effect of an antidiencephalon immune serum on pain and sleep in primary fibromyalgia. *Neuropsychobiology*. 1994; **30**: 66–72.
82. Arnold LM. Biology and therapy of fibromyalgia – new therapies in fibromyalgia. *Arthritis Research and Therapy*. 2006; **8**: 212.
83. O'Malley PG, Balden E, Tomkins G *et al*. Treatment of fibromyalgia with antidepressants – a meta-analysis. *Journal of General Internal Medicine*. 2000; **15**: 659–66.
84. Bymaster FP, Dreshfield-Ahmad LJ, Threlkeld PG *et al*. Comparative affinity of duloxetine and venlafaxine for serotonin and norepinephrine transporters in vitro and in vivo, human serotonin receptor subtypes, and other neuronal receptors. *Neuropsychopharmacology*. 2001; **25**: 871–80.
85. Puozzo C, Lens S, Reh C *et al*. Lack of interaction of milnacipran with the cytochrome p450 isoenzymes frequently involved in the metabolism of antidepressants. *Clinical Pharmacokinetics*. 2005; **44**: 977–88.
86. Goldstein DJ, Lu YL, Detke MJ *et al*. Duloxetine vs. placebo in patients with painful diabetic neuropathy. *Pain*. 2005; **116**: 109–18.
87. Raskin J, Pritchett YL, Wang FJ *et al*. A double-blind, randomized multicenter trial comparing duloxetine with placebo in the management of diabetic peripheral neuropathic pain. *Pain Medicine*. 2005; **6**: 346–56.
88. Wernicke JF, Pritchett YL, D'Souza DN *et al*. A randomized controlled trial of duloxetine in diabetic peripheral neuropathic pain. *Neurology*. 2006; **67**: 1411–20.
89. Rowbotham MC, Goli V, Kunz NR, Lei D. Venlafaxine extended release in the treatment of painful diabetic neuropathy: a double-blind, placebo-controlled study. *Pain*. 2004; **110**: 697–706.
90. Tasmuth T, Hartel B, Kalso E. Venlafaxine in neuropathic pain following treatment of breast cancer. *European Journal of Pain*. 2002; **6**: 17–24.
91. Arnold LM, Lu YL, Crofford LJ *et al*. A double-blind, multicenter trial comparing duloxetine with placebo in the treatment of fibromyalgia patients with or without major depressive disorder. *Arthritis and Rheumatism*. 2004; **50**: 2974–84.
92. Arnold LM, Rosen A, Pritchett YL *et al*. A randomized, double-blind, placebo-controlled trial of duloxetine in the treatment of women with fibromyalgia with or without major depressive disorder. *Pain*. 2005; **119**: 5–15.
93. Gendreau RM, Thorn MD, Gendreau JF *et al*. Efficacy of milnacipran in patients with fibromyalgia. *Journal of Rheumatology*. 2005; **32**: 1975–85.
94. Sayar K, Aksu G, Ak I, Tosun M. Venlafaxine treatment of fibromyalgia. *Annals of Pharmacotherapy*. 2003; **37**: 1561–5.
95. Dwight MM, Arnold LM, O'Brien H *et al*. An open clinical trial of venlafaxine treatment of fibromyalgia. *Psychosomatics*. 1998; **39**: 14–7.
96. Detke MJ, Lu YL, Goldstein DJ *et al*. Duloxetine, 60 mg once daily, for major depressive disorder: A randomized double-blind placebo-controlled trial. *Journal of Clinical Psychiatry*. 2002; **63**: 308–15.
97. Detke MJ, Lu YL, Goldstein DJ *et al*. Duloxetine 60 mg once daily dosing versus placebo in the acute treatment of major depression. *Journal of Psychiatric Research*. 2002; **36**: 383–90.
98. Goldstein DJ, Mallinckrodt C, Lu YL, Demitrack MA. Duloxetine in the treatment of major depressive disorder: A double-blind clinical trial. *Journal of Clinical Psychiatry*. 2002; **63**: 225–31.

99. Goldstein DJ, Lu YL, Detke MJ *et al.* Effects of duloxetine on painful physical symptoms associated with depression. *Psychosomatics.* 2004; **45**: 17–28.

100. Fava M, Mallinckrodt CH, Detke MJ *et al.* The effect of duloxetine on painful physical symptoms in depressed patients: Do improvements in these symptoms result in higher remission rates? *Journal of Clinical Psychiatry.* 2004; **65**: 521–30.

*101. Garcia-Cebrian A, Gandhi P, Demyttenaere K, Peveler R. The association of depression and painful physical symptoms – a review of the European literature. *European Psychiatry.* 2006; **21**: 379–88.

102. Brannan SK, Mallinckrodt CH, Brown EB *et al.* Duloxetine 60 mg once-daily in the treatment of painful physical symptoms in patients with major depressive disorder. *Journal of Psychiatric Research.* 2005; **39**: 43–53.

103. Gilmor ML, Owens MJ, Nemeroff CB. Inhibition of norepinephrine uptake in patients with major depression treated with paroxetine. *American Journal of Psychiatry.* 2002; **159**: 1702–10.

104. Anjaneyulu M, Chopra K. Possible involvement of cholinergic and opioid receptor mechanisms in fluoxetine mediated antinociception response in streptozotocin-induced diabetic mice. *European Journal of Pharmacology.* 2006; **538**: 80–4.

105. Singh VP, Jain NK, Kulkarni SK. On the antinociceptive effect of fluoxetine, a selective serotonin reuptake inhibitor. *Brain Research.* 2001; **915**: 218–26.

106. Lenkey N, Karoly R, Kiss JP *et al.* The mechanism of activity-dependent sodium channel inhibition by the antidepressants fluoxetine and desipramine. *Molecular Pharmacology.* 2006; **70**: 2052–63.

107. Garcia-Quetglas E, Azanza JR, Sadaba B *et al.* Pharmacokinetics of tramadol enantiomers and their respective phase I metabolites in relation to CYP2D6 phenotype. *Pharmacological Research.* 2007; **55**: 122–30.

108. Dannon PN, Iancu I, Cohen A *et al.* Three year naturalistic outcome study of panic disorder patients treated with paroxetine. *BMC Psychiatry.* 2004; **4**: 16.

*109. Dubicka B, Hadley S, Roberts C. Suicidal behaviour in youths with depression treated with new-generation antidepressants – meta-analysis. *British Journal of Psychiatry.* 2006; **189**: 393–8.

*110. Gunnell D, Saperia J, Ashby D. Selective serotonin reuptake inhibitors (SSR1s) and suicide in adults: meta-analysis of drug company data from placebo controlled, randomised controlled trials submitted to the MHRA's safety review. *British Medical Journal.* 2005; **330**: 385–388A.

*111. Jick H, Kaye JA, Jick SS. Antidepressants and the risk of suicidal behaviors. *Journal of the American Medical Association.* 2004; **292**: 338–43.

112. Moller HJ. Evidence for beneficial effects of antidepressants on suicidality in depressive patients – A systematic review. *European Archives of Psychiatry and Clinical Neuroscience.* 2006; **256**: 329–43.

*113. Moller HJ. Is there evidence for negative effects of antidepressants on suicidality in depressive patients? A systematic review. *European Archives of Psychiatry and Clinical Neuroscience.* 2006; **256**: 476–96.

114. Tiihonen J, Lonnqvist J, Wahlbeck K *et al.* Antidepressants and the risk of suicide, attempted suicide, and overall mortality in a nationwide cohort. *Archives of General Psychiatry.* 2006; **63**: 1358–67.

115. Sindrup SH, Bjerre U, Dejgaard A *et al.* The selective serotonin reuptake inhibitor citalopram relieves the symptoms of diabetic neuropathy. *Clinical Pharmacology and Therapeutics.* 1992; **52**: 547–52.

116. Sindrup SH, Gram LF, Brosen K *et al.* The selective serotonin reuptake inhibitor paroxetine is effective in the treatment of diabetic neuropathy symptoms. *Pain.* 1990; **42**: 135–44.

117. Rowbotham MC, Reisner LA, Davies PS, Fields HL. Treatment response in antidepressant-naive postherpetic neuralgia patients: double-blind, randomized trial. *Journal of Pain.* 2005; **6**: 741–6.

118. Goldenberg D, Mayskiy M, Mossey C *et al.* A randomized, double-blind crossover trial of fluoxetine and amitriptyline in the treatment of fibromyalgia. *Arthritis and Rheumatism.* 1996; **39**: 1852–9.

119. Arnold LM, Hess EV, Hudson JI *et al.* A randomized, placebo-controlled, double-blind, flexible-dose study of fluoxetine in the treatment of women with fibromyalgia. *American Journal of Medicine.* 2002; **112**: 191–7.

120. Wolfe F, Cathey MA, Hawley DJ. A double-blind placebo controlled trial of fluoxetine in fibromyalgia. *Scandinavian Journal of Rheumatology.* 1994; **23**: 255–9.

121. Anderberg UM, Marteinsdottir I, von Knorring L. Citalopram in patients with fibromyalgia – a randomized, double blind, placebo-controlled study. *European Journal of Pain.* 2000; **4**: 27–35.

122. Norregaard J, Volkmann H, Danneskioldsamsoe B. A randomized controlled trial of citalopram in the treatment of fibromyalgia. *Pain.* 1995; **61**: 445–9.

123. Dickens C, Jayson M, Sutton C, Creed F. The relationship between pain and depression in a trial using paroxetine in sufferers of chronic low back pain. *Psychosomatics.* 2000; **41**: 490–9.

124. Clayton AH, Montejo AL. Major depressive disorder, antidepressants, and sexual dysfunction. *Journal of Clinical Psychiatry.* 2006; **67**: 33–7.

125. Semenchuk MR, Sherman S, Davis B. Double-blind, randomized trial of bupropion SR for the treatment of neuropathic pain. *Neurology.* 2001; **57**: 1583–8.

126. Katz J, Pennella-Vaughan J, Hetzel RD *et al.* A randomized, placebo-controlled trial of bupropion sustained release in chronic low back pain. *Journal of Pain.* 2005; **6**: 656–61.

127. Fava M. Prospective studies of adverse events related to antidepressant discontinuation. *Journal of Clinical Psychiatry.* 2006; **67**: 14–21.

*128. Black K, Shea C, Dursun S, Kutcher S. Selective serotonin reuptake inhibitor discontinuation syndrome: proposed diagnostic criteria. *Journal of Psychiatry and Neuroscience.* 2000; **25**: 255–61.

129. Sternbach H. The serotonin syndrome. *American Journal of Psychiatry*. 1991; **148**: 705–13.
130. Blier P, Tremblay P. Physiologic mechanisms underlying the antidepressant discontinuation syndrome. *Journal of Clinical Psychiatry*. 2006; **67**: 8–13.
131. Rosenbaum JF, Fava M, Hoog SL *et al*. Selective serotonin reuptake inhibitor discontinuation syndrome: A randomized clinical trial. *Biological Psychiatry*. 1998; **44**: 77–87.
132. Perahia DG, Kajdasz DK, Desaiah D, Haddad PM. Symptoms following abrupt discontinuation of duloxetine treatment in patients with major depressive disorder. *Journal of Affective Disorders*. 2005; **89**: 207–12.
*133. Schatzberg AF, Blier P, Delgado PL *et al*. Antidepressant discontinuation syndrome: Consensus panel recommendations for clinical management and additional research. *Journal of Clinical Psychiatry*. 2006; **67**: 27–30.
134. Nieuwstraten C, Labiris NR, Holbrook A. Systematic overview of drug interactions with antidepressant medications. *Canadian Journal of Psychiatry– Revue Canadienne De Psychiatrie*. 2006; **51**: 300–16.
135. Houlihan DJ. Serotonin syndrome resulting from coadministration of tramadol, venlafaxine, and mirtazapine. *Annals of Pharmacotherapy*. 2004; **38**: 411–3.
136. Karunatilake H, Buckley NA. Serotonin syndrome induced by fluvoxamine and oxycodone. *Annals of Pharmacotherapy*. 2006; **40**: 155–7.
137. Keegan MT, Brown DR, Rabinstein AA. Serotonin syndrome from the interaction of cyclobenzaprine with other serotoninergic drugs. *Anesthesia and Analgesia*. 2006; **103**: 1466–8.
*138. Boyer EW, Shannon M. The serotonin syndrome. *New England Journal of Medicine*. 2005; **352**: 1112–20.
*139. Dunkley EJC, Isbister GK, Sibbritt D *et al*. The Hunter Serotonin Toxicity Criteria: simple and accurate diagnostic decision rules for serotonin toxicity. *QJM – an International Journal of Medicine*. 2003; **96**: 635–42.

19

Antiepileptic and antiarrhythmic agents

TURO J NURMIKKO

KEY LEARNING POINTS

ANTIEPILEPTIC DRUGS: ANTICONVULSANTS

- Antiepileptic drugs (AEDs) are moderately effective in the management of neuropathic pain with the number needed to treat (NNT) ranging from 1.9 to 7.1.
- AEDs may also have efficacy in conditions not considered neuropathic (fibromyalgia, orofacial myalgia).
- Gabapentin and pregabalin are of equal efficacy and should be considered as first line therapy for neuropathic pain.
- Carbamazepine and oxcarbazepine are of equal efficacy and may be considered first line therapy for trigeminal neuralgia.
- Gabapentin, pregabalin, and lamotrigine have a role in the management of central neuropathic pain.
- Safety issues vary from one AED to another, are complex, and require the full attention of the prescribing clinician.

ANTIARRHYTHMICS

- Several isoforms of sodium channels have been identified but no selective channel blockers are available.
- Systemic lidocaine occasionally affords prolonged pain relief.
- Oral congeners of lidocaine have limited usefulness.

INTRODUCTION

The two families of drugs are discussed together because as membrane stabilizing agents they are capable of inhibiting ion channels, thereby reducing excessive firing. In recent years, however, evidence has accumulated that other mechanisms, some known (such as release of excitatory neurotransmitters by inhibition of the α2δ receptors) and some unknown, are decisive in mediating many of the effects of antiepileptic drugs (AEDs). The clinical applications of the two families of drugs have subsequently separated somewhat, with AEDs finding a new role in non-neuropathic pain.

ANTIEPILEPTIC DRUGS

Carbamazepine and oxcarbazepine

Carbamazepine and oxcarbazepine, the 10-keto analog of carbamazepine, have relatively similar pharmacological profiles. Both have been shown to block tetrodotoxin-resistant Na^+ channels in brain tissue.[1] Neuronal hyperexcitability, linked to accumulation of sodium channels in injured peripheral axons and cell bodies, is reduced by carbamazepine, as is similar excitability in dorsal horn neurons[2, 3] and possibly elsewhere in the central nervous system (CNS) where sodium channel may be up-regulated.[4] The selectivity of Na^+ channel blockade remains to be determined, but interaction with a low activation state of $Na_V1.8$ channels may be one of the key mechanisms of carbamazepine.[5] In addition, both carbamazepine and oxcarbazepine appear to antagonize the A_1 adenosine receptor, increase dopaminergic transmission, and potentiate voltage-gated potassium channels, all potentially useful properties in chronic pain.[1] Both drugs inhibit L-type voltage-gated calcium channels and presynaptic glutamate release, although it is uncertain whether this happens in sufficient concentrations in clinical conditions.[1] Oxcarbazepine and its metabolites are also thought to modulate other calcium channels.[6] Both carbamazepine and oxcarbazepine have been shown to possess some antihyperalgesic effects in experimental models of inflammatory pain, probably mediated by indirect activation of adrenergic α_2 receptors.[7]

CARBAMAZEPINE

Almost all clinical trials were conducted in the 1960s and 1970s. A Cochrane review on all publications up to November 2004 identified 11 studies on chronic pain, seven on trigeminal neuralgia, two on diabetic neuropathy, one on postherpetic neuralgia (PHN) and one on poststroke pain.[8][I] No new clinical trials evaluating the efficacy of carbamazepine have since been published.

Evidence for the efficacy of carbamazepine in trigeminal neuralgia remains solid, and while the original trials were small and used rather superficial methods, vast clinical experience since has established the position of this drug as first line treatment in trigeminal neuralgia. The bulk of the evidence comes from four randomized controlled studies totaling 147 patients, showing that carbamazepine is more effective than placebo in reducing the intensity and frequency of pain attacks. The number needed to treat (NNT) for pain relief for carbamazepine was calculated as 1.9 (95 percent CI 1.4–2.8).[8][I] In a comparator trial, pimozide appeared more effective than carbamazepine but is no longer in use, while in another small study tocainade showed equal efficacy but it has since been withdrawn because of serious side effects.[9][I] Tizanidine, in turn, was less effective than carbamazepine.[10][III] Comparison with oxcarbazepine suggests similar efficacy in trigeminal neuralgia, which will be discussed below under Oxcarbazepine.[11][II], [12][II]

For diabetic neuropathy, two small controlled trials with carbamazepine have been published. In a cross-over placebo-controlled trial, patients on carbamazepine 200–600 mg/day improved in 28/30 cases versus 19/30 on placebo; there was no pain increase in any of the patients on carbamazepine, while 11/30 on placebo reported worse pain.[13][III] Similarly, Gomez-Perez *et al.*[14][III] reported no difference in efficacy between carbamazepine (200 mg/day) and a combination of nortriptyline (10 mg) and fluphenazine (0.5 mg). International guidelines on the treatment of diabetic neuropathy do not contain a robust recommendation for the use of carbamazepine due to concerns regarding study methodology.[9][I], [15][I], [16][I]

A drug combination of carbamazepine (up to 1000 mg/day) and clomipramine (up to 75 mg/day) was more effective than transcutaneous electrical nerve stimulation (TENS) in PHN.[17][III] A placebo-controlled cross-over comparator study of 15 patients with central poststroke pain showed carbamazepine (800 mg/day) to have a pain ameliorating effect of similar magnitude to that of amitriptyline (75 mg/day) (OR 3.3, 95 percent CI 0.8–13.8).[18][III], [19][I] There were 10/15 patients on amitriptyline who improved versus 5/9 on carbamazepine. The latter caused more frequent side effects, prompting the investigators to recommend amitriptyline over carbamazepine in this indication.[18][III]

OXCARBAZEPINE

Despite being a structural analog of carbamazepine, oxcarbazepine has some unique characteristics that distinguish it from the former.[6] It is metabolized via a P450-independent pathway and there are fewer clinically meaningful drug–drug interactions. Its active metabolite, a monohydroxy-derivative, has a better safety and tolerability profile than that of 10,11 carbamazepine epoxide, the main metabolite of carbamazepine.[6] It has a linear pharmacokinetic profile, and titration and dose adjustments are relatively simple.[12] Oxcarbazepine and its metabolites are almost completely excreted in urine and therefore patients with renal impairment require dose reduction. Oxcarbazepine seems to be associated with hyponatremia more frequently than carbamazepine.[6]

Evidence of clinical efficacy of oxcarbazepine in chronic pain is derived from controlled trials in diabetic neuropathy and trigeminal neuralgia. In three pivotal large studies, totaling 634 patients, oxcarbazepine only inconsistently provided better pain relief than placebo.[20][II], [21][II], [22][II]

In a double-blind placebo-controlled parallel group trial of 16 weeks duration involving 146 patients with painful diabetic polyneuropathy of more than six months but less than five years duration, oxcarbazepine appeared effective. There was an adjusted treatment difference in average daily pain score (0 to 100) of 11.2 (CI 95 percent –19.8, –2.6), $p = 0.01$. The NNTs for reduction of pain ≥ 50 percent and ≥ 30 percent was reported to be 6.0 for both. Compared to placebo, oxcarbazepine was more effective in improving sleep, mood, and other quality of life measures.[20][II]

One hundred and forty-one patients with painful diabetic neuropathy (DPN) were recruited into another similar study but using a target dose of 1200 mg/day.[21][II] No difference was shown between oxcarbazepine and placebo in any of the outcome measures. In a third dose ranging study in which 347 patients with painful DPN participated, the results were mixed.[22][II] No significant difference was seen between groups receiving 600, 1200, and 1800 mg/day. When a further analysis was carried out based only on those who completed the study, a significant difference in pain relief was found in favor of the 1200 and 1800 mg group over placebo. Impact of withdrawals (43 percent of the group) on the outcome was clear in those receiving 1800 mg/day but this was negligible in the placebo group. This translates to a clinical usefulness of the drug only to those who can tolerate high doses. Numbers needed to harm (NNH) was low, 6.2, for the 1200 mg/day group but high, 2.1, for the 1800 mg/day group. The NNTs were reported at 7.9 and 8.3.[22][II]

The message from these three studies remains unclear. The lack of efficacy in two of three studies suggests that oxcarbazepine is not a drug of first choice in painful DPN. However, in certain situations, for example if there is evidence that sodium channel blockers have helped but the effect is lost, or poor tolerability prevents their use, oxcarbazepine may be worth considering. Recommendations in guidelines are mixed[9][I], [16][I] (see **Table 19.1**).

In trigeminal neuralgia, open-label studies suggest a rapid onset of effect for oxcarbazepine. Three double-blind, cross-over comparator studies with carbamazepine have been completed, although only one has been published as an original communication.[23][III] In a study of 48 patients with newly diagnosed trigeminal neuralgia, oxcarbazepine and carbamazepine, individually titrated to optimal dose, reduced intensity of attacks, and in both groups 50 percent of patients became pain free.[23][III] A meta-analysis of this study and two other double-blind, randomized controlled studies evaluating a further 84 patients with refractory trigeminal neuralgia, has been published in review papers.[11][II], [12][II] The daily doses in the latter two studies ranged from 1050 to 1200 mg for oxcarbazepine and from 700 to 900 mg for carbamazepine. The results showed comparable efficacy between oxcarbazepine and carbamazepine in reducing attacks and improving sleep and activities in daily living.[11][II], [12][II]

Safety

Carbamazepine and oxcarbazepine have similar dose-dependent adverse effect profiles (see **Table 19.2**). Gastrointestinal (nausea) and central (dizziness, vertigo, somnolence, fatigue, headache) side effects are common, but apparently less common and less severe with oxcarbazepine.[6] Allergic rash is relatively common and includes Stevens–Johnson syndrome and toxic epidermal necrolysis. There is approximately 25 percent allergic cross-reactivity between carbamazepine and oxcarbazepine.[6, 12] Mild hyponatremia is common, while clinically significant hyponatremia (<125 mmol/L) prompted discontinuation of the drug in 1 percent of those started on oxcarbazepine.[24][II] High doses of both drugs can induce liver enzymes. NNH for all combined adverse effects with carbamazepine is estimated at 3.7 (95 percent CI 2.4, 7.8).[19][I] A 12-month open-label follow-up of 594 patients on oxcarbazepine showed reasonably good tolerability with 20 percent withdrawing; serious side effects were rare and mostly dermatological.[24][II]

General comment on oxcarbazepine and carbamazepine

Both of these drugs may be considered as first line treatment in trigeminal neuralgia and in similar cranial neuralgias.[9][I], [15][I], [16][I] There are no controlled studies for efficacy in conditions with predominant shooting or explosive pain that could be speculated to have an Na^+ channel-mediated mechanism.

Table 19.1 Commonly used antiepileptic drugs featuring in guidelines for the management of neuropathic pain by three Task Forces.

Drug	Dworkin *et al.*[16]	Attal *et al.*[9]	Moulin *et al.*[15]	Comment
Gabapentin	1st line	1st line	1st line	
Pregabalin	1st line	1st line	1st line	
Lamotrigine	2nd or 3rd line	2nd line	4th line	No distinction made between central and peripheral NP
Valproate	2nd or 3rd line	2nd line	4th line	
Topiramate	2nd or 3rd line	Not effective	4th line	
Carbamazepine	2nd or 3rd line	No recommendation	No recommendation	Attal *et al.* question methodology
Oxcarbazepine	2nd or 3rd line	Not effective	No recommendation	
Specific indications				
Carbamazepine for TGN	1st line	1st line	1st line	
Oxcarbazepine for TGN	NR	1st line	No recommendation	

NP, neuropathic pain; TEN, trigeminal neuralgia.

Table 19.2 Indications, doses and side effects of antiepileptic drugs effective in the management of chronic pain (headache not included).

Drug	Indication	Titration phase (weeks)[a]	Initial dose (mg/day)[b]	Maintenance dose (mg/day)[b]	Common adverse effects
Gabapentin	PHN	2–4	300	1200–3600	Dizziness, somnolence, weight gain, peripheral edema, memory disturbances, blurred vision, dry mouth, constipation
	DPN	2–4	300	900–3600	
	Other peripheral NP	2–4	300–400	1200–2400	
	Spinal cord injury	4–8	300	1800–3600	
	Fibromyalgia	2–4	300	1200–2400	
	CMM	3–6	300	2400–3600	
Pregabalin	PHN	1	150	150–600	Same as gabapentin
	DPN	1–3	75–300	300–600	
	Spinal cord injury	1–2	150	(150) 300–600	
	Fibromyalgia	1	150–300	450	
Carbamazepine	Trigeminal neuralgia	<1	300–600	300–1200	Dizziness, somnolence, fatigue, nausea, rash, hyponatraemia, headache. *Caveat* Drug interactions
	Diabetic neuropathy		300–600	200–600	
Oxcarbazepine	Trigeminal neuralgia	4	150–300	1200–1800	Same as carbamazepine
	Diabetic neuropathy	4	300–600	900–1800	
Lamotrigine	Central pain	8	25	200–400	Rash, dizziness, somnolence, nausea, headache
Lacosamide	DPN	6	100	400	Dizziness, anxiety, nausea

[a]Refers to the minimum period of time needed to reach a clinically useful dose, as reported in clinical trials. In clinical practice, a slower titration pattern using lower initial dose is recommended;
[b]From clinical trials. Maximum tolerated dose escalation or maintenance dose may be less.
CMM, chronic masticatory myalgia; DPN, diabetic neuropathy; NP, neuropathic pain; PHN, postherpetic neuralgia.
Dose recommendations have been extrapolated from several clinical trials and case series. In the elderly, slower titration and lower doses are needed.

Gabapentin and pregabalin

Gabapentin and pregabalin have very similar pharmacological profiles. Both exert their effects through to the $\alpha 2\delta$ type 1 subunits of voltage-dependent calcium channels, which experimental studies show are up-regulated in dorsal root ganglia and central terminals of neurones.[25, 26, 27, 28] This pharmacological effect results in moderate decrease in calcium influx and release of neurotransmitters (glutamate, noradrenaline, and substance P), leading to a subtle reduction in postsynaptic neuronal hyperexcitability.[28, 29] Pregabalin differs from gabapentin because of its linear pharmacokinetics after oral administration, with low inter-subject variability.[28, 29] This makes dose escalation a more straightforward exercise than with gabapentin. Pregabalin is administered twice and gabapentin three times a day. Neither has major interaction with other drugs, neither is metabolized, and both are excreted almost exclusively through the kidneys.[29]

GABAPENTIN

A Cochrane review consisting of publications up to November 2004 identified 13 randomized controlled trials (RCTs) in chronic neuropathic pain with sufficient data to include in the analysis of efficacy of gabapentin.[30][I] There were two studies on PHN, six on DPN, and one each for mixed neuropathic pain, cancer-related neuropathic pain, phantom limb pain, Guillain–Barré syndrome, and spinal cord injury. The overall NNT calculated from seven studies with binary data available was 4.3 (95 percent CI 3.5, 5.7) and NNH for minor harm (side effects not requiring withdrawal) 3.7 (95 percent CI 2.4, 5.4).[30][I]

In PHN, two large trials of eight weeks duration, with 334 and 229 participants and gabapentin titrated to a maximum tolerated dose up to 3600 mg/day, showed gabapentin to be superior to placebo.[31][II] Judged on the Patient Global Impression of Change Scale, 43 percent of patients on gabapentin and 12 percent on placebo improved. In another, dose-ranging study, Rice and Maton[32][II] used enriched enrollment with previous gabapentin nonresponders excluded. Both doses, 1800 and 2400 mg/day, reduced daily pain scores more than placebo (35, 34, and 16 percent, respectively, $p<0.01$). NNT for ≥ 50 percent pain relief from these two studies was 3.9 (95 percent CI 3.0, 5.7). Both studies showed improvement in several secondary efficacy measures including sleep, mood, fatigue, and some aspects of quality of life.

The conclusion to be drawn from four placebo-controlled studies, with daily doses ranging from 900 to 3600 mg and involving 269 patients in total, is that with adequate dosing, gabapentin is also effective in painful diabetic neuropathy.[9][I], [16][I] The decisive study was that of Backonja and coworkers[33][II] who demonstrated in 165 patients an adjusted treatment difference between gabapentin and placebo of –1.2 (95 percent CI –1.9, –0.6). Patients were titrated up to 3600 mg of gabapentin or maximum tolerated dose; 14/84 on gabapentin and 16/81 on placebo withdrew. Using a similar study protocol, Simpson[34][II] reported 65 percent of patients on the active drug to be much or moderately improved as opposed to 26 percent on placebo, giving an NNT of 1.5 (95 percent CI 2.2, 4.3) Two other studies used lower doses with variable results.[35][III], [36][III] The combined NNT (50 percent) for effectiveness of gabapentin in diabetic neuropathy from all the four studies was 2.9 (95 percent CI 2.2, 4.3); 68 percent of patients receiving gabapentin experienced improvement as opposed to 18 percent receiving placebo.[30][I]

Two small studies have compared gabapentin with amitriptyline in diabetic neuropathy; neither showed convincing evidence of superiority of one over the other.[37][III], [38][III]

In a double-blind parallel group eight-week study of 305 patients with mixed neuropathic pain up-titrated to 2400 mg/day according to their response, gabapentin was narrowly better than placebo in reducing daily pain by a mean of 1.5 (on a 0–10 scale) compared to 1.0 achieved on placebo.[39][II] The treatment difference of 0.5 is among the lowest reported in neuropathic pain and no effect was seen on allodynia, hyperalgesia, or shooting/burning pain.[39][II] Two small studies suggest a rapid onset effect in hospitalized patients with Guillain–Barré syndrome and neuropathic cancer pain.[40][III], [41][III]

Since the Cochrane review, several studies have appeared that have explored the potential of wider use of gabapentin. In a unique placebo-controlled double-blind, four-period, cross-over comparative study, 57 patients with either PHN ($n = 22$) or painful diabetic polyneuropathy ($n = 35$) were randomized to either gabapentin, morphine, combination of the two, or active placebo (lorazepam).[42][II] Each treatment arm lasted five weeks and drugs were up-titrated to maximum tolerated dose. The gabapentin–morphine combination (mean maximum tolerated doses: gabapentin 1705 ± 83 mg, morphine 34.4 ± 2.6 mg) was more effective in controlling pain than was morphine alone (mean maximum tolerated dose 45.3 ± 3.9 mg) or gabapentin alone (mean maximum tolerated dose 2207 ± 89 mg), and all treatments were significantly better than placebo. During the combination phase, patients reported more constipation than during gabapentin alone, and more dry mouth than during morphine alone.[42][II]

No significant difference was seen from gabapentin in several small studies of complex regional pain syndrome type I (58 patients),[43][III], HIV neuropathy, [44][III], and chemotherapy-induced pain,[45][III] whereas there was a marginal improvement after six weeks of therapy in phantom limb pain.[46][III]

Gabapentin was reported to be astonishingly effective in a double-blind, placebo-controlled cross-over trial of 20 patients with tetraplegia due to spinal cord injury.[47][III] A highly significant ($p = 0.000$) treatment difference in favor of gabapentin of –4.3 was reported at the end of each eight weeks arm. Gabapentin was titrated to maximum tolerated dose, and in this group of relatively young patients (mean age 39) the mean was 2850 ± 750 mg. Several types of the pain reported on the Neuropathic Pain Scale improved, as did sleep and disability.

Other pain conditions

Single studies have been published in musculoskeletal pain and headache (for the latter, see Chapter 34, Headache). Fifty patients with orofacial pain due to myalgia of the masticatory muscles benefited from high-dose gabapentin (mean 3400 mg/day) reporting an improvement in pain and tenderness which continued after dosing had peaked.[48][II] Pain was reduced by 52 percent in the gabapentin group versus 19 percent in the placebo group.

Another controlled trial was conducted to assess the efficacy of gabapentin in fibromyalgia.[49][II] Seventy-five patients were randomized to a flexible dose of gabapentin 1200–2400 mg/day, or placebo. Pain severity measured on the 11-point Brief Pain Inventory Likert subscale was greater in those on gabapentin versus those on placebo, with an adjusted treatment difference after 12 weeks of treatment (95 percent CI –1.75, –0.71). Improvement was seen in scales measuring sleep disturbance, impact of fibromyalgia, and mood, but there was no reduction in the number of tender spots. The results are similar to those obtained in a clinical trial of pregabalin in this condition.[50][II]

A bewildering number of open label studies exploring the clinical usefulness of gabapentin in numerous conditions have been published. They are too numerous to be reviewed here. Sadly, despite recognition that gabapentin is prescribed in conditions with a poor prognosis for recovery, long-term, prospective, open label studies are few and far between.

PREGABALIN

The first RCT on the effect of pregabalin in chronic pain was published in 2003, and in the following four years results from 11 such trials were published. Eight reports dealt with diabetic polyneuropathy and/or PHN, two with central pain, and one fibromyalgia. In addition, reports on the usefulness of pregabalin as a perioperative adjunct medication to reduce postoperative pain have started to emerge. In 7 out of 11 chronic pain studies an enriched enrollment method was used, in the sense that the patients who previously had not responded to a moderate dose of gabapentin (1200 mg/day) were excluded. Two studies specifically stated that all patients with previous exposure to gabapentin were included (gabapentin had to be withdrawn seven days before the trial).[51][II], [52][II]

Postherpetic neuralgia

Three fixed dose parallel-group studies with a similar design show superiority of pregabalin to placebo.[53][II], [54][II], [55][II] The duration of the trial ranged from 8 to 13 weeks, including a one-week titration phase. Stable previous medications (including opioids, antiepileptic, and antidepressant drugs) were permitted and the primary outcome measure was change in pain at the end of the study, with sleep, mood, and quality of life as secondary outcome measures. Allodynia was not systematically assessed. In the first study, the dose was forced titrated to 600 mg/day (with one third remaining on 300 mg/day due to low creatinine clearance). Reduction in mean pain scores rated at baseline and at end point over seven days (primary efficacy measure) was significantly greater in the pregabalin than placebo group ($p<0.001$; mean treatment difference −1.69 (95 percent CI −2.33, −1.05). Of the secondary outcome measures, sleep and mood improved but quality of life did not (apart from general health perception and, inevitably, bodily pain).[53][II] In the second multicenter trial of eight weeks duration, 238 patients were randomized either to receive pregabalin 150 mg day, 300 mg/day, or placebo. Pregabalin was well tolerated at these lower doses. The reduction in daily pain was significantly greater than placebo in both the 150 mg/day group (mean difference −1.20 (95 percent CI 11.81, −0.58)) and 300 mg/day group (mean difference −1.57 (95 percent CI −2.20, −0.95). Sleep and mood but not quality of life also improved significantly.[54][II]

In the third study, 370 patients with PHN were randomized to receive either placebo or three doses of pregabalin: 150, 300, and 600 mg/day, in a 13-week trial (including a one-week titration phase).[55][II] Pregabalin showed an increase in effect with increasing dosage. Weekly mean pain scores rated on an 11-point scale improved steadily in all groups and were greatest in the 600 mg/day group. Sleep improved in all active drug groups more than in the placebo group. Patients in the 150 and 600 mg/day group, but not 300 mg/day, reported global improvement more than those receiving placebo.

Painful peripheral diabetic neuropathy

Five randomized, placebo-controlled, parallel group trials on painful DPN involving 1463 patients in total were reported between 2004 and 2007. In four of them, multiple doses were used ranging from 75 to 600 mg/day. No concomitant neuropathic pain medications were permitted. In one study a group with flexible dosing of 150–600 mg/day was included. The titration period varied from one to three weeks. The shortest maintenance period was four weeks, the longest 11 weeks.[56][II], [57][II] In another study both patients with DPN and PHN were included, with similar results reported between groups and presented as a single group.[51][II]

Of the tested doses, 600 mg/day reduced pain in all four studies. The mean treatment difference (from placebo) on the visual analog scale (VAS) scale of 0–10 ranged from −1.45 (−2.1, −0.9) to −0.97 (−1.6, −0.3). NNT for 50 percent pain relief ranged from 3.3 to 6.3. Superior efficacy of a lower dose of 300 mg/day over placebo was found in two of three studies.[56][II], [58][II] At this dose, treatment differences to placebo ranged from −1.5 (−2.2, −0.9) to −0.1 (−0.7, 0.5) and NNT 50 percent from 2.8 to 23. In the two studies that included a group assigned to a fixed dose regimen of 150 mg/day, no benefit was shown over placebo in regard to pain, sleep, or global impression of change.[59][II], [57][II] Freynhagen *et al.*[51][II] showed that only 11 percent of patients in the flexible dosing group remained at 150 mg/day; also, in that group the average dose was 372 mg/day and therefore those on the lowest dose will not have dictated the favorable response. The conclusion will have to be that for an adequate clinical response in diabetic neuropathy one needs to aim at a daily dose of 300 mg or higher.

Central pain

Two randomized, placebo-controlled, flexible dose (150–600 mg) trials show that pregabalin has an analgesic effect in central pain.[60][II], [52][II] In 137 patients with incomplete and complete lesions and central pain, the treatment difference between pregabalin (at an average dose of 460 mg/day) and placebo was 1.79 (95 percent CI 0.9, 2.7).[60][II] The effect was seen for the first week and did not seem to diminish over the duration of the study (12 weeks). NNT 30 percent was 3.9 and NNT 50 percent 7.1.[60][II] In a study based on a similar design, 40 patients with supraspinal or intraspinal lesions, a similar large treatment difference was found: end point pain relief at four weeks was 2.1 (0.57–3.80) on a 0–10 scale.[52][II] While NNT 50 percent was reported to be 4.0 (95 percent CI: 2.0, 328) and NNT 30 percent 3.3 (95 percent CI: 1.9, 14.3), it is important to acknowledge the presence of large confidence intervals due to the small number of patients enrolled. Both studies showed significant improvement in sleep, anxiety, and some aspects of quality of life. Interestingly, in these studies pregabalin seemed better tolerated than in other studies, possibly reflecting the flexible dosing pattern the investigators had adopted, and the lower age of participants.

Fibromyalgia

A single dose ranging multicenter controlled trial involving 530 patients with fibromyalgia showed that pregabalin as monotherapy at a dose of 450 mg/day improved pain, sleep, and fatigue, whereas lower doses (300 or 150 mg/day) did not.[50][II] In the 450 mg/day group, tender spots also became less sensitive although the significance was borderline. However, at the last eight week visit, those who were still in the trial failed to demonstrate significant improvement over placebo, irrespective of the dose they received. Because the study was not designed to last longer than eight weeks it is not known if this effect is explained by a loss of analgesic effect of pregabalin over time in this patient population, or some other mechanism. Side effects were very similar to those in other studies.[50][II]

General comments on pregabalin and gabapentin

Systematic reviews and meta-analysis have confirmed the efficacy of both drugs in neuropathic pain, including central pain.[9][I], [15][I], [16][I], [30][I] Emerging evidence suggests an effect superior to placebo in some non-neuropathic pain conditions.[48, 49, 50] There is little difference to be found between the two drugs, either in indications, contraindications, efficacy, tolerability, or drug interactions (**Tables 19.2** and **19.3**). The arguably more straightforward pharmacokinetics of pregabalin offers some benefits but with a patient who will need individual titration anyway, this may not be decisive. The relative safety and lack of interactions are properties that justify choosing either pregabalin or gabapentin as a first-line treatment in neuropathic pain, with good potential to be used in combination therapy if needed (**Table 19.1**).

Safety

The pharmacological similarity of pregabalin and gabapentin is confirmed in the frequency of adverse events reported across most clinical trials. Withdrawals range from one-third to one-fifth. The most commonly reported side effects include dizziness, somnolence, peripheral edema, weight gain, vertigo, asthenia, blurred vision, dry mouth, and constipation (see **Table 19.2**). NNH is reported at 2.5 (95 percent CI 2.0, 3.2).[19][I] Cognitive problems are highlighted ranging from memory disturbance to confusion. Balance problems are frequent, and the tendency to injury reported in some studies.[56, 59] Dose reduction, albeit leading to reduced efficacy, should be considered, especially in the elderly with PHN. NNTs of 5.3–6.3 for 150 mg/day and 5.3–5.3 for 300 mg/day of pregabalin suggest that there still may be a reasonable response,[54][II], [55][II] and consideration should only be given to higher doses when tolerability is good.[9][I]

TOPIRAMATE

Topiramate is a broad-spectrum AED with multiple pharmacological actions, making it a potentially effective antinociceptive agent. It inhibits voltage-gated sodium and calcium type L-channels, inhibits neurotransmission at the AMPA/kainite receptor, enhances GABA-mediated inhibition and activates potassium conductance.[61] It is a weak carbonic anhydrase inhibitor which explains its propensity to cause paresthesias. Its use is shown to lead to weight loss in approximately 25–75 percent of those taking it for long periods, and it may therefore correct some weight-related metabolic abnormalities.[61, 62] Over the years it has shown most potential in headache prophylaxis, which is discussed elsewhere in Chapter 34, Headache.

Neuropathic pain

Four moderate size and large RCTs have been conducted in diabetic neuropathy. Three of these were identical in design and published as one paper in 2004.[62][II] In total, 1259 patients were randomized to 100, 200 and 400 mg of topiramate or placebo; the duration of each trial arm was 18–22 weeks with the titration phase lasting eight weeks. No dose provided any benefit over placebo either for pain relief, sleep, mood, or quality of life. The fourth placebo-controlled trial of 323 patients differed in its approach in details of pain assessment and rating, but otherwise employed the same study design as the three other studies. A high dose of 400 mg/day of topiramate was shown to reduce pain more than placebo.[63][II] However, at that dose the drop-out rates were very high, nearly 48 percent in the topiramate group (some 25 percent withdrew due to side effects) and 27 percent in the placebo group, much higher than in the three large negative trials. The NNT 30 percent was 6.3. Poor tolerability, the requirement of a long titration phase, and limited efficacy make this drug a poor contender in painful DPN and should only be considered after adequate trials of other drugs with a more promising profile.[15][I] A small study with 27 patients suffering from chronic radicular pain also narrowly failed to show benefit and the authors did not recommend its use in this indication except in exceptional cases.[64][II]

Other pain conditions

Muehlbacher *et al.*[65][II] carried out a double-blind study on the effect of topiramate 300 mg/day in chronic low back patients with moderate levels of pain and disability. Up-titration was conducted over five weeks to a daily dose of 300 mg of topiramate or placebo, which was maintained for a further five weeks. There were 48 assessable patients in each group. Topiramate was modestly superior to placebo as measured using the Pain Rating Scale from McGill Pain Questionnaire, Oswestry Disability Index, and SF-36. As an interesting observation, anger reduction was also greater in the topiramate group. Topiramate was used as an add-on medication and the authors did not declare whether there were dose changes in the ongoing medication and did not discuss what other treatments the patients were receiving (e.g. physiotherapy).[65][II] Given the almost complete lack of pharmacotherapy available for patients with chronic low back pain who have failed to benefit from conventional analgesics, these results are encouraging enough to warrant larger, decisive studies.

Safety

Of all AED used for chronic pain, topiramate probably has the poorest adverse effect record. CNS effects are common and include dizziness, impaired concentration, confusion, fatigue, and speech disturbances. Kidney stone formation

Table 19.3 Efficacy of antiepileptic drugs based on randomized controlled trials.

Condition	Gabapentin	Pregabalin	Carbamazepine	Oxcarbazepine	Lamotrigine	Topiramate	Lacosamide	Valproate/ divalproex
Peripheral neuropathic pain								
DPN	Effective [I] NNT 2.9	Effective [I] NNT 3.9	Effective [I] NNT 2.3	Conflicting evidence [I]	Not effective [I]	Conflicting evidence [II]	Effective [II]	Conflicting [II]
PHN	Effective [I] NNT 4.9	Effective [I] NNT 4.4					Not effective [II]	Effective [III] NNT 2.1
CRPS	Not effective [II]							
Guillain–Barré Syndrome	Effective [II]							
Radiculopathy						Not effective [II]		
Cancer-related NP	Effective [II]							
Mixed NP	Effective [II] NNT 14							
Trigeminal neuralgia			Effective [I] NNT 1.8	Effective [I]	Effective [III]			
Central pain								
Spinal cord injury	Effective [II]	Effective [II] NNT 7.1			In subgroup effective [III]			
CPSP			Possibly effective [III]		Effective [II]			
Phantom limb pain	Effective [III]							
Other								
								Effective [II]
SUNCT	Possibly effective [V]				Possibly effective [V]			
Fibromyalgia	Effective [II]	Effective [II] NNT 6.3						
Masticatory myalgia	Effective [II] NNT 3.4							
Low back pain						Effective [III]		

occurs in approximately 2 percent on topiramate, reflecting changes in urine pH as a result of inhibition of carbonic anhydrase.[66, 67] Paresthesias in hands and feet and around the mouth occur commonly, in approximately 50 percent.[65, 67] A significant percentage on topiramate will experience some weight loss with a mean loss of up to 4–6 percent of body weight in those on 200–300 mg/day.[65, 67] Dose effects are dose dependent and a lesser problem, especially if a slow up-titration is used to reach a low maintenance level, such as the 100 mg/day commonly used in migraine prophylaxis.[68][I] NNHs for separate adverse effects were calculated by Chronicle and Mulleners[68][I] to be 2.4 (95 percent CI 21, 27) for tremor and paresthesia, 11.1 (95 percent CI 8.3, 16.6) for weight loss, and 1.6 (95 percent CI 11.2, 32.4) for memory impairment.

Comment

While topiramate appears to be effective in migraine prophylaxis (see Chapter 34, Headache), its role in neuropathic pain appears very limited. Preliminary evidence suggests some efficacy in chronic low back pain but its true value in this refractory condition remains to be determined.

LAMOTRIGINE

Lamotrigine blocks activation of voltage-sensitive sodium channels and inhibits presynaptic release of glutamate.[61] Early studies suggested efficacy in diabetic neuropathy[69][II] and human immunodeficiency virus (HIV)-related painful sensory neuropathy[70][II] but subsequent large RCTs have yielded less promising results.

A Cochrane review up to August 2006[71][I] consisted of seven studies; two on central pain (one in central poststroke pain[72][II] and one in spinal cord injury pain,[73][II], two in HIV-associated neuropathy,[70][II], [74][II] and one each in trigeminal neuralgia[75][II] diabetic neuropathy,[69][II] and nonspecific neuropathic pain.[76][II] The Cochrane reviewers concurred with the interpretation of the authors of the original reports in five cases and disagreed in two.[69][II], [75][I] In central poststroke pain, 30 patients randomized to lamotrigine 200 mg/day or placebo for eight weeks with ten crossed over to the active arm of the trial after a two-week washout reported a reduction in median pain score of approximately 30 percent in comparison with placebo.[72][II] In another cross-over study by the Danish group, 30 patients with spinal cord injury pain were randomized to lamotrigine 400 mg/day or placebo; each arm lasted for nine weeks with a two-week washout.[73][II] No group-wise differences were found in any efficacy parameter; however subgroup analysis showed modest improvement in those with incomplete lesions and presence of allodynia. In HIV-related polyneuropathy, a subgroup of those on antiretroviral therapies (88 patients out of the original 205 randomized) reported marginally greater pain relief on lamotrigine (400 mg/day) than placebo. Those not on antiretrovirals experienced no benefit, possibly reflecting the role of treatment-induced neuropathy.[74][II] In a small cross-over study involving 14 patients with refractory trigeminal neuralgia, lamotrigine 400 mg/day was more effective than placebo based on the Composite Efficacy Index, which combined the intensity and frequency of paroxysms. In global evaluation, 7/13 on lamotrigine and 1/14 on placebo reported an improvement.[75][II] In nonspecific neuropathic pain, lamotrigine 200 mg/day was no better than placebo.[76][II] Evidence from several case series suggests efficacy in SUNCT but controlled trials are lacking.[77][I]

In two replicate randomized placebo-controlled trials of a total of 720 patients with painful diabetic neuropathy, lamotrigine at doses of 200 or 300 mg/day was ineffective, with the higher dose of 400 mg/day showing efficacy in one study only.[78][II] Another study evaluated the efficacy of lamotrigine up to 400 mg/day in 213 patients with common painful neuropathies and found no difference compared to placebo.[79][II] Only three patients had central pain, with no separate analysis for this subgroup.

Safety

Side effects associated with lamotrigine are dose dependent and similar to side effects reported with other CNS drugs: dizziness, somnolence, fatigue, nausea, and headache. In the three large trials quoted above[78, 79] the withdrawal percentages due to adverse effects in those on 400 mg/day of lamotrigine ranged from 17 to 24. Interestingly, cognitive disturbances were relatively rare. The main concern with lamotrigine is its potential for severe rash (including Stevens–Johnson syndrome and toxic epidermal necrolysis) which are best avoided by very slow up-titration.[80] The risk of any rash is about 5 percent.[80, 81] The drug should be discontinued at the appearance of a rash, however mild. It has been suggested that after discontinuation, lamotrigine may be reintroduced using a very slow dose escalation regimen.[82] When fever, lymphadenopathia, and other systemic involvement are associated with rash, the patient may have anticonvulsant hypersensitivity syndrome which will require prompt and aggressive treatment. The risk for this very serious condition is calculated at 2.5 per 10,000 new users.[80]

Comment

Converging evidence suggests that the effect of lamotrigine in neuropathic pain of peripheral origin has limited efficacy. The question of its efficacy in trigeminal neuralgia, SUNCT, and central pain, all conditions in which pathophysiological mechanisms appear different from peripheral neuropathic pains, remains open. Sodium channel blockade in these conditions may be advantageous,[4] and because there is a paucity of sodium channel blockers available to the clinician, lamotrigine may still be considered in refractory cases not responding to first line therapy.[9][I], [16][I]

SODIUM VALPROATE AND DIVALPROEX

Sodium valproate and divalproex (a combination of sodium valproate and valproic acid in a molar ratio of 1:1) were reported to be effective in painful diabetic neuropathy in two small studies from a single center.[83][II], [84][II] Valproate at a dose of 1200 or 1000 mg/day was compared with placebo for one and three months, respectively. Significant improvement was claimed with a combined NNT for moderate or better pain relief of 1.5 (95 percent CI 1.2, 2.2).[9][I] However, one must raise concerns regarding methodology, especially as the nature of randomization, blinding, and statistical analyses used in these studies were inadequately described. Moreover, in another small placebo-controlled cross-over study of 37 patients with polyneuropathy, mostly diabetic, valproate showed no benefit.[85][II] Unusually, a placebo response was minimal or lacking in all these trials.[83][II], [85][II] All were probably underpowered to detect a genuine difference. A further small controlled study conducted in 42 patients with PHN randomized to valproic acid (1000 mg/day) or placebo was positive in favor of the former, with an NNT of 2.1 (95 percent CI 1.4, 4.2) but no corroborative studies have been published.[86][II] While inconsistent results from these small studies prevent firm conclusions, some guidelines do recommend sodium valproate as second, third, or fourth line option for the management of neuropathic pain of peripheral origin.[9][I], [15][I], [16][I]

Safety

Common side effects reported in the above studies and long-term randomized follow-up studies in patients with epilepsy include tremor, dizziness, drowsiness, weight gain, nausea, and hair loss.[81][II], [83][II], [84][II], [85][III] NNHs for nausea was calculated by a Cochrane review to be 7.0 (95 percent CI 5.1, 7.0).[68][I] The same for tremor was 12.5 (9.0, 20.9) and dizziness 16.3 (95 percent CI 9.5, 57.9).[68][I] The two most notorious yet rare problems associated with valproate are its known potential hepatotoxic and teratogenic effects.[67]

LACOSAMIDE

A single randomized placebo-controlled trial of 119 patients with diabetic neuropathy showed superiority of lacosamide, a third generation novel AED, over placebo.[87][II] Adverse effects were mostly mild or moderate with CNS-related effects (dizziness, nausea, and anxiety) more common with lacosamide. Despite borderline efficacy, its relative tolerability associated with probably a novel mode of action, justifies larger trials.

OTHER ANTIEPILEPTIC DRUGS

Several small case series are reported in which most of the second and third generation antiepileptic drugs have been used in various chronic pain conditions, usually neuropathic pain and/or headache. The results are mostly disappointing and the few that claim efficacy are far from convincing. Some clearly negative results from large trials involving antiepileptic drugs remain unpublished. The clinician should therefore resist the temptation to try just another drug from this class when others have failed; many old and new AEDs require good understanding of their pharmacological properties and attention to detail if they are to be used safely.

ANTIARRHYTHMICS

Local anesthetic drugs administered systemically do not seem to alter the threshold for pain perception in healthy subjects.[88, 89] However, once various pathophysiological mechanisms have activated and hyperalgesia has developed, systemic lidocaine and mexiletine are effective in interrupting abnormal discharges and associated neuropathic sensory symptoms.[89, 90, 91] The sites of action are multiple, with inhibition of ectopic activity shown at the neuroma, dorsal root ganglia, dorsal horn, rostroventromedial medulla, and the periaqueductal gray.[91, 92, 93, 94, 95] All local anesthetic-like drugs are nonspecific blockers of Na^+ channels making them better suited for topical than systemic therapy. Following injury, time-dependent changes in the expression and function of sodium channels occur throughout the nervous system and are likely to play a significant role in the generation of neuropathic pain and possibly in other forms of chronic pain.[91] Many sodium channel isoforms have been identified, and at present $Na_v1.3$, $Na_v1.7$, $Na_v1.8$, and $Na_v1.9$ have attracted most interest. However, by 2007, no specific antagonist was available for clinical use.

In a systematic review, published in 2005, systemic lidocaine and its oral analogs, mexiletine and tocainide – the latter no longer in use – were shown to be consistently better than placebo in alleviating neuropathic pain.[96][I] In 11 trials with sufficient data available, doses of intravenous lidocaine ranged from 1 to 5 mg/kg and duration of infusion from 30 to 120 minutes (in one study a bolus injection only was given).[97][II] For the meta-analysis there were data from a total of 187 patients who received lidocaine and 186 who received saline.[96][I] Lidocaine was superior to placebo in reducing ongoing pain levels with a weighted mean difference calculated (using VAS of 0–100) at –11 (95 percent CI: –15, –7), and NNT 30 percent about 4. The effect was present at the end of the infusion and frequently continued for hours and in one study three days following the infusion. In a subsequent small trial of 15 patients with painful diabetic neuropathy randomized to receive 5 and 7.5 mg/kg, the effect was present at 14 days.[98][II] Another well-controlled dose ranging study confirmed the postinfusion effect of lidocaine but only when a dose of 5 mg/kg was used.[99][II]

In a meta-analysis of 184 patients on mexiletine and 193 on placebo, the weighted mean difference was 11 (95 percent CI 16, –6) in favor of mexiletine.[96][I] Comparison of mexiletine and lidocaine with other neuropathic analgesics showed no difference in five small studies.[96][I] Although the adverse effect profile in these studies was not particularly exceptional, the situation appears different in the clinic. Because of the small effect size, mexiletine does not seriously feature as a candidate in neuropathic pain.[9][I] Topical lidocaine is discussed elsewhere in this book (see Chapter 17, Topical analgesics for neuropathic pain).

REFERENCES

1. Ambrosio AF, Soares-da-Silva P, Carvalho CM, Carvalho AP. Mechanisms of action of carbamazepine and its derivates, oxcarbazepine, BIA 2-093, and BIA 2-024. *Neurochemical Research*. 2002; **17**: 121–30.
2. Waxman SG, Dib-Hajj S, Cummins TR, Black JA. Sodium channels and pain. *Proceedings of the National Academy of Sciences of the United States of America*. 1999; **96**: 7635–9.
3. Chapman V, Suzuki R, Chamarette HLC *et al.* Effects of systemic carbamazepine and gabapentin on spinal neuronal responses in spinal nerve ligated rats. *Pain*. 1998; **75**: 261–72.
4. Max MB, Hagen NA. Do changes in brain sodium channels cause pain? *Neurology*. 2000; **54**: 544–5.
5. Cardenas CA, Cardenas CG, de Armendi AJ, Scroggs RS. Carbamazepine interacts with a slow style inactivation state of Nav 1.8-like sodium channels. *Neuroscience Letters*. 2006; **408**: 129–34.
6. Schmidt D, Elger CE. What is the evidence that oxcarbazepine and carbamazepine are distinctly different antiepileptic drugs? *Epilepsy Behaviour*. 2004; **5**: 627–35.
7. Vuckovic SM, Tomic M, Stepanovic-Petrovic RM *et al.* The effects of α2-adrenoceptor agents on anti-hyperalgesic effects of carbamazepine and oxcarbazepine in a rat model of inflammatory pain. *Pain*. 2006; **125**: 10–19.
8. * Wiffen PJ, McQuay HJ, Moore RA. Carbamazepine for acute and chronic pain. *Cochrane Database of Systematic Reviews*. 2005; **CD005451**.
9. * Attal N, Cruccu G, Haanpää M *et al.* EFNS guidelines on pharmacological treatment of neuropathic pain. *European Journal of Neurology*. 2006; **13**: 1153–69.
10. Vilming ST, Lyberg T, Lataste X. Tizanidine in the management of trigeminal neuralgia. *Cephalalgia*. 1986; **6**: 181–2.
11. Beydoun A. Clinical use of tricyclic anticonvulsants in painful neuropathies and bipolar disorders. *Epilepsy Behavior*. 2002; **3**: S18–22.
12. Carrazana E, Mikoshiba I. Rationale and evidence for the use of oxcarbazepine in neuropathic pain. *Journal of Pain and Symptom Management*. 2003; **5S**: S31–5.
13. Rull J, Quibrera R, Gonzales-Millan H, Lozano Castenado O. Symptomatic treatment of peripheral diabetic neuropathy with carbamazepine; double-blind, cross-over study. *Diabetologia*. 1969; **5**: 215–20.
14. Gomez-Perez F, Choza R, Rios JM *et al.* Nortriptyline-Fluphenazine vs. Carbamazepine in the symptomatic management of diabetic neuropathy. *Archives of Medical Research*. 1996; **27**: 525–9.
15. * Moulin DE, Clark AJ, Gilron I *et al.* Pharmacologic management of chronic neuropathic pain – Consensus statement and guidelines from the Canadian Pain Society. *Pain Research and Management*. 2007; **12**: 13–21.
16. * Dworkin RH, O'Connor AB, Backonja M *et al.* Pharmacologic management of neuropathic pain: evidence-based recommendations. *Pain*. 2007; **132**: 237–51.
17. Gerson GR, Jones RB, Luscombe DK. Studies on the concomitant use of carbamazepine and clomipramine for the relief of post-herpetic neuralgia. *Postgraduate Medical Journal*. 1977; **53**: 104–09.
18. Leijon G, Boivie J. Central post-stroke pain – a controlled trial of amitriptyline and carbamazepine. *Pain*. 1989; **36**: 27–36.
19. * Wiffen PJ, McQuay HJ, Moore RA. Anticonvulsant drugs for acute and chronic pain. *Cochrane Database of Systematic Reviews*. 2005; **CD001133**.
20. Dogra S, Beydoun S, Maxzzola J *et al.* Oxcarbazepine in painful diabetic neuropathy: a randomized, placebo-controlled trial. *European Journal of Pain*. 2005; **9**: 543–54.
21. Grosskopf J, Mazzola J, Wan Y, Hopwood MA. A randomized, placebo-controlled study of oxcarbazepine in painful diabetic neuropathy. *Acta Neurologica Scandinavica*. 2006; **114**: 177–80.
22. Beydoun A, Shaibani A, Hopwood M, Wan Y. Oxcarbazepine in painful diabetic neuropathy: results of a dose-ranging study. *Acta Neurologica Scandinavica*. 2006; **113**: 395–404.
23. Liebel JT, Menger N, Langohr H. Oxcarbazepine in der Behandlung der Trigeminusneuralgie. *Nervenheilkunde*. 2001; **20**: 461–5.
24. Beydoun S, Alarcon F, Mangat S, Wan Y. Long-term safety and tolerability of oxcarbazepine in painful diabetic neuropathy. *Acta Neurologica Scandinavica*. 2007; **115**: 284–8.
25. Li C-Y, Zhang X-L, Matthews EA *et al.* Calcium channel α2δ subunit mediates spinal hyperexcitability in pain modulation. *Pain*. 2006; **125**: 20–34.
26. Melrose H, Kinloch RA, Cox PJ *et al.* [3 H] pregabalin binding is increased in ipsilateral dorsal horn following chronic constriction injury. *Neuroscience Letters*. 2007; **417**: 187–92.
27. Field MJ, Cox PJ, Stott E. Identification of the α-2-δ subunit of voltage dependent calcium channels as a molecular target for pain mediating the analgesic actions of pregabalin. *Proceedings of the National Academy of*

Sciences of the United States of America. 2006; **46**: 17537–42.
28. Dooley DJ, Taylor CP, Donevan S, Feltner D. Ca2+ channel α2δ ligands: novel modulators of neurotransmission. *Trends in Pharmacological Sciences Sci.* 2007; **28**: 75–82. doi:10.1016/j.tips.2006.12.006.
29. Sills GJ. The mechanisms of action of gabapentin and pregabalin. *Current Opinion in Pharmacology.* 2006; **6**: 108–13.
* 30. Wiffen PJ, McQuay HJ, Edwards JE, Moore RA. Gabapentin for acute and chronic pain. *Cochrane Database of Systematic Reviews*. 2005; **CD005452**.
* 31. Rowbotham MC, Harden N, Stacey B *et al.* Gabapentin for the treatment of postherpetic neuralgia. *Journal of the American Medical Association*. 1998; **280**: 1837–42.
* 32. Rice AS, Maton S. Postherpetic Neuralgia Study Group. Gabapentin in postherpetic neuralgia: a randomised, double blind, placebo controlled study. *Pain*. 2001; **94**: 215–24.
* 33. Backonja M, Beydoun A, Edwards KR *et al.* Gabapentin for the symptomatic treatment of painful neuropathy in patients with Diabetes mellitus. *Journal of the American Medical Association*. 1998; **280**: 1831–6.
34. Simpson DA. Gabapentin and venlafaxine for the treatment of painful diabetic neuropathy. *Journal of Clinical Neuromuscular Disease*. 2001; **3**: 53–62.
35. Perez HE, Sanches GE. Gabapentin therapy for diabetic neuropathic pain [letter]. *American Journal of Medicine*. 2000; **108**: 689.
36. Gorson KC, Schott C, Herman R *et al.* Gabapentin in the treatment of painful diabetic neuropathy: a placebo controlled, double blind, cross over trial. *Journal of Neurology, Neurosurgery, and Psychiatry.* 1999; **66**: 251–2.
37. Dallocchio C, Buffa C, Mazarello P *et al.* Gabapentin vs. amitriptyline in painful diabetic neuropathy: an open-label pilot study. *Journal of Pain and Symptom Management*. 2000; **20**: 280–5.
38. Morello CM, Leckband SG, Stoner CP *et al.* Randomized double-blind study comparing the efficacy of gabapentin with amitriptyline on diabetic peripheral neuropathy pain. *Archives of Internal Medicine*. 1999; **159**: 1931–7.
39. Serpell MG. Neuropathic Pain Study Group. Gabapentin in neuropathic pain syndromes: a randomised, double-blind, placebo-controlled trial. *Pain*. 2002; **99**: 557–66.
40. Pandey CK, Bose N, Garg G *et al.* Gabapentin for the treatment of Guillain-Barre syndrome: a double-blind, placebo controlled, crossover study. *Anesthesia and Analgesia*. 2002; **95**: 1719–23.
41. Caraceni A, Zecca E, Bonezzi C *et al.* Gabapentin for neuropathic cancer pain: a randomised controlled trial from the Gabapentin Cancer Pain Study Group. *Journal of Clinical Oncology.* 2004; **22**: 2909–17.
* 42. Gilron I, Bailey JM, Tu D *et al.* Morphine, gabapentin, or their combination for neuropathic pain. *New England Journal of Medicine*. 2005; **352**: 1324–34.
43. Hahn K, Arendt G, Braun JS *et al.* A placebo-controlled trial of gabapentin for painful HIV-associated sensory neuropathies. *Journal of Neurology.* 2004; **251**: 1260–6.
44. van de Vusse AC, Stomp-van den Berg SG, Kessels AH, Weber EJ. Randomized controlled trial of gabapentin in complex regional pain syndrome type 1. *BMC Neurology.* 2004; **4**: 13.
45. Rao RD, Michalak JC, Sloan JA *et al.* Efficacy of gabapentin in the management of chemotherapy induced peripheral neuropathy: a phase 3 randomized, double-blind, placebo-controlled, crossover trial (N00C3). *Cancer.* 2007; **110**: 2110–18.
46. Bone M, Critchley P, Buggy DJ. Gabapentin in postamputation phantom limb pain: a randomised double-blind, placebo-controlled, cross-over study. *Regional Anesthesia and Pain Medicine*. 2002; **27**: 481–6.
47. Levendoğlu F, Öğün Ö, Özerbil Ö *et al.* Gabapentin is the first line drug for the treatment of neuropathic pain in spinal cord injury. *Spine*. 2004; **29**: 743–51.
48. Kimos P, Biggs C, Mah J *et al.* Analgesic action of gabapentin on chronic pain in the masticatory muscles: a randomised controlled trial. *Pain*. 2007; **127**: 151–60.
49. Arnold LM, Goldenberg DL, Stanford SB *et al.* Gabapentin in the treatment of fibromyalgia. *Arthritis and Rheumatism*. 2007; **56**: 1336–44.
50. Crofford LJ, Rowbotham MC, Mease PJ *et al.* Pregabalin for the treatment of fibromyalgia syndrome. Results of a randomised, double-blind, placebo-controlled trial. *Arthritis and Rheumatism*. 2005; **52**: 1264–73.
51. Freynhagen R, Strojek K, Griesing T *et al.* Efficacy of pregabalin in neuropathic pain evaluated in a 12 week, randomised, double-blind, multicentre, placebo-controlled trial of flexible- and fixed-dose regimens. *Pain*. 2005; **115**: 254–63.
52. Vranken JH, Dijkgraaf MGW, Kruis M *et al.* Pregabalin in patients with central neuropathic pain: a randomized, double-blind, placebo-controlled trial of a flexible-dose regimen. *Pain*. 2008; **136**: 150–7.
* 53. Dworkin RH, Corbin AE, Young Jr JP *et al.* Pregabalin for the treatment of postherpetic neuralgia. *Neurology.* 2003; **60**: 1274–83.
* 54. Sabatowski R, Galvez R, Cherry DA *et al.* Pregabalin reduces pain and improves sleep and mood disturbances in patients with postherpetic neuralgia: results of a randomised, placebo-controlled trial. *Pain*. 2004; **109**: 26–35.
* 55. Van Seventer R, Feister HA, Young JP *et al.* Efficacy and tolerability of twice-daily pregabalin for treating pain and related sleep interference in postherpetic neuralgia: a 13-week, randomized trial. *Current Medical Research and Opinion*. 2006; **2**: 375–84.
* 56. Lesser H, Sharma U, LaMoreaux L, Poole RM. Pregabalin relieves symptoms of painful diabetic neuropathy. *A randomized controlled trial. Neurology.* 2004; **63**: 2104–10.
57. Tölle T, Freynhafe R, Varsavel V *et al.* A randomized, double-blind, placebo-controlled study evaluating twice

daily dosing of pregabalin for relief of neuropathic pain associated with diabetic peripheral neuropathy. *European Journal of Pain.* 2007; **12**: 203–13.

* 58. Rosenstock J, Tuchman M, LaMoreaux L, Sharma U. Pregabalin for the treatment of painful diabetic peripheral neuropathy: a double-blind, placebo-controlled trial. *Pain.* 2004; **110**: 628–38.

59. Richter RW, Portenoy R, Sharma U *et al.* Relief of painful diabetic peripheral neuropathy with pregabalin: a randomized, placebo-controlled trial. *Journal of Pain.* 2005; **6**: 253–60.

* 60. Siddall PJ, Cousins MJ, Otte A *et al.* Pregabalin in central neuropathic pain associated with spinal cord injury: a placebo-controlled trial. *Neurology.* 2006; **67**: 1792–800.

61. Stefan H, Feuerstein TJ. Novel anticonvulsant drugs. *Pharmacology Therapeutics.* 2007; **113**: 165–83.

* 62. Thienel U, Neto W, Schwabe SK *et al.* The Topiramate Diabetic Neuropathic Pain Study Group. Topiramate in painful diabetic polyneuropathy: findings from three double-blind placebo-controlled trials. *Acta Neurologica Scandinavica.* 2004; **110**: 221–31.

63. Raskin P, Donofrio PD, Rosenthal NR *et al.* Topiramate vs placebo in painful diabetic neuropathy: analgesic and metabolic effects. *Neurology.* 2004; **63**: 865–73.

64. Khoromi S, Patsalides A, Parada S *et al.* Topiramate in chronic lumbar radicular pain. *Journal of Pain.* 2005; **6**: 829–36.

65. Muehlbacher M, Nickel MK, Kettler C *et al.* Topiramate in treatment of patients with chronic low back pain. A randomized, double-blind, placebo-controlled study. *Clinical Journal of Pain.* 2006; **22**: 526–31.

66. Guay DRP. Oxcarbazepine, topiramate, zonisamide, and levetiracetam: potential use in neuropathic pain. *American Journal of Geriatric Pharmacotherapy.* 2003; **1**: 18–37.

67. Walia KS, Khan EA, Ko DH *et al.* Side effects of antiepileptics – a review. *Pain Practice.* 2004; **4**: 194–203.

* 68. Chronicle EP, Mulleners WM. Anticonvulsant drugs for migraine prophylaxis. *Cochrane Database of Systematic Reviews.* 2004; **CD003226**.

69. Eisenberg E, Lurie Y, Braker C *et al.* Lamotrigine reduces painful diabetic neuropathy. *Neurology.* 2001; **57**: 505–09.

70. Simpson DM, Olney R, McArthur JC *et al.* A placebo-controlled trial of lamotrigine for painful HIV-associated neuropathy. *Neurology.* 2000; **54**: 2115–19.

71. Wiffen PJ, Rees J. Lamotrigine for acute and chronic pain. *Cochrane Database of Systematic Reviews.* 2007; **CD006044**.

72. Vestergaard K, Andersen G, Gottrup H *et al.* Lamotrigine for central poststroke pain. A randomized controlled trial. *Neurology.* 2001; **56**: 184–90.

73. Finnerup NB, Sindrup SH, Bach FW *et al.* Lamotrigine in spinal cord injury pain: a randomized controlled trial. *Pain.* 2002; **96**: 375–83.

74. Simpson DM, McArthur JC, Olney R *et al.* Lamotrigine for HIV-associated painful sensory neuropathies. A placebo-controlled trial. *Neurology.* 2003; **60**: 1508–14.

75. Zakrzewska JM, Chaudury Z, Nurmikko TJ *et al.* Lamotrigine (Lamictal) in refractory trigeminal neuralgia: results from a double-blind placebo-controlled crossover trial. *Pain.* 1997; **73**: 223–30.

76. McCleane G. 200 mg daily of lamotrigine has no analgesic effect in neuropathic pain: a randomised, double-blind, placebo-controlled trial. *Pain.* 1999; **83**: 105–07.

* 77. May A, Leone M, Áfra J *et al.* EFNS guidelines on the treatment of cluster headache and other trigeminal-autonomic cephalalgias. *European Journal of Neurology.* 2006; **13**: 1066–77.

* 78. Vinik AI, Tuchman M, Safirstein B *et al.* Lamotrigine for treatment of pain associated with diabetic neuropathy: results of two randomized, double-blind, placebo-controlled studies. *Pain.* 2007; **128**: 169–79.

79. Silver M, Blum D, Grainger J *et al.* Double-blind, placebo-controlled trial of lamotrigine in combination with other medication for neuropathic pain. *Journal of Pain and Symptom Management.* 2007; **34**: 446–54.

80. Mockenhaupt M, Messenheimer J, Tennis P, Sclingmann J. Risk of Stevens-Johnson syndrome and toxic epidermal necrolysis in new users of antiepileptics. *Neurology.* 2005; **64**: 1134–8.

81. Marson AG, Al-Karushi AM, Alwaidh M *et al.* The SANAD study of effectiveness of valproate, lamotrigine, or topiramate for generalised and unclassifiable epilepsy: an unblinded randomised controlled trial. *Lancet.* 2007; **369**: 1016–26.

82. Besag FMC, NG GYT, Pool F. Successful re-introduction of lamotrigine after initial rash. *Seizure.* 2000; **9**: 282–6.

83. Kochar DK, Jain A, Agrawal RP *et al.* Sodium valproate in the management of painful diabetes in type 2 diabetes – a randomized placebo controlled study. *Acta Neurologica Scandinavica.* 2002; **106**: 248–52.

84. Kochar DK, Raat N, Agrawal RP *et al.* Sodium valproate for painful diabetic neuropathy: a randomized double-blind placebo-controlled study. *Quarterly Journal of Medicine.* 2004; **97**: 33–8.

85. Otto M, Bach FW, Jensen TS, Sindrup SH. Valproic acid has no effect on pain in polyneuropathy: a randomized, controlled trial. *Neurology.* 2004; **62**: 285–8.

86. Kochar DK, Garg P, Bumb RA *et al.* Divalproex sodium in the management of post-herpetic neuralgia: a randomized double-blind placebo-controlled study. *Quarterly Journal of Medicine.* 2005; **98**: 29–34.

87. Rauck RL, Shaibani A, Biton V *et al.* Lacosamide in painful diabetic neuropathy. A Phase 2 double-blind placebo-controlled study. *Clinical Journal of Pain.* 2007; **23**: 150–8.

88. Nielsen JC, Arendt-Nielsen L, Bjerring P, Carlsson P. Analgesic efficacy of low doses of intravenous lidocaine on experimental laser-induced pain: a placebo controlled study. *Regional Anesthesia.* 1991; **16**: 28–33.

89. Koppert W, Zeck S, Sittl R *et al.* Low-dose lidocaine suppresses experimentally induced hyperalgesia in humans. *Anesthesiology.* 1998; **89**: 1345–53.

90. Chabal C, Russell LC, Burchiel K. The effect of intravenous lidocaine, tocainide, and mexiletine on spontaneously

active fibers originating in the rat sciatic neuroma. *Pain.* 1989; **38**: 333–8.

91. Devor M, Wall PD, Catalan N. Systemic lidocaine silences ectopic neuroma and DRG discharge without blocking nerve conduction. *Pain.* 1992; **48**: 261–8.
92. Amir R, Argoff CE, Bennett GJ *et al.* The role of sodium channels in chronic inflammatory and neuropathic pain. *Journal of Pain.* 2006; **7**: S1–29.
93. Pertovaara A, Wei H, Hamalainen MM. Lidocaine in the rostroventromedial medulla and the periaqueductal gray attenuates allodynia in neuropathic rats. *Neuroscience Letters.* 1996; **218**: 127–30.
94. Chapman V, Ng J, Dickenson AH. A novel spinal action of mexiletine in spinal somatosensory transmission of nerve injured rats. *Pain.* 1998; **77**: 289–96.
95. Waxman SG, Dib-Hajj S, Cummins TR, Black JA. Sodium channels and pain. *Proceedings of the National Academy of Sciences of the United States of America.* 1999; **96**: 7635–9.
* 96. Challapalli V, Tremont-Lukats IW, McNicol ED *et al.* Systemic administration of local anesthetic agents to relieve neuropathic pain. *Cochrane Database of Systematic Reviews.* 2005; **CD003345**.
97. Marchettini P, Lacerenza M, Marangoni C *et al.* Lidocaine test in neuralgia. *Pain.* 1992; **48**: 377–42.
98. Viola V, Newnham HH, Simpson RW. Treatment of intractable painful diabetic neuropathy with intravenous lignocaine. *Journal of Diabetes and its Complications.* 2006; **20**: 34–9.
99. Tremont-Lukats IW, Hutson PR, Backonja M-M. A randomised, double-masked, placebo-controlled trial of extended IV lidocaine infusion for relief of ongoing neuropathic pain. *Clinical Journal of Pain.* 2006; **22**: 266–71.

20

Neurostimulation techniques

MARC A HUNTOON

KEY LEARNING POINTS

- Although spinal stimulation has been in existence for 40 years, the lack of suitable controls (patient, electrical, paresthesia, sensation) has hampered the performance of randomized trials.
- The mechanism of action of neurological stimulation appears to include gate control systems at the spinal level, as well as changes in neurotransmitter modulation of neural function.
- Technological advances in stimulation leads and battery power sources have made virtually any neurological site a potential target for neuromodulation.
- Spinal stimulation for the multiple operated back and radicular pain has been buoyed by a recent key randomized trial comparing stimulation to reoperation. Likewise, spinal stimulation for intractable angina pectoris is best supported by published trials.
- Due to the difficulty with sham controls, and resulting evidential problems, interventional pain physicians should develop best practice approaches to safety to limit adverse events from implantation of these devices.

INTRODUCTION

Spinal cord stimulation (SCS) is a treatment that was first described in the late1960s by Shealy *et al.*,[1] but has undergone significant technological improvement, and is being applied to an increasingly larger scope of potential neural targets. SCS is currently used in failed back surgery syndrome with predominately neuropathic extremity pain, an emerging capability to better target low back pain,[2][III] some ischemic cardiac and peripheral vascular conditions, complex regional pain syndromes, some peripheral polyneuropathies and mononeuropathies, advanced postherpetic neuralgia, phantom pain syndromes, and several other neuropathic pain states. Recent advances in the technology and extensive research have broadened the clinical indications to include other syndromes that are not neuropathic/ischemic pain states in the conventional sense, e.g. visceral pain. Peripheral nerve stimulation utilization has also increased substantially, with indications including sacral stimulation for urge incontinence and interstitial cystitis, occipital stimulation for occipital head pain, supraorbital and infraorbital nerve stimulation (postherpetic neuralgia), and other peripheral upper and lower extremity nerves. In some cases, where discrete nerve targets are not easily identifiable, the use of peripheral field stimulation has become popular. Peripheral field stimulation has been utilized for ilioinguinal neuralgia and other abdominal regions, intercostal neuralgia and trunk pain syndromes, and many other conditions. The use of deep brain stimulation has reemerged for a variety of syndromes, as well as motor cortex stimulation for chronic facial pain and some deafferentation syndromes. One of the main problems plaguing stimulation therapies to date has been the lack of randomized controlled trials. Deyo and colleagues[3] discussed the problem of difficulty in blinding participants in a research trial when physical treatments are being used. They surveyed participants after attempting to produce sham transcutaneous electrical nerve stimulation (TENS) to evaluate efficacy of blinding. The authors noted that their efforts were only partially effective, in spite of attempts to replicate controllable aspects of the sights and sounds of real TENS.[3] Motor cortex stimulation may offer some advantage for the ability to perform randomized controlled trials in this respect, as this physical treatment does not have a perceived paresthesia.

MECHANISM OF ACTION

The gate control theory[4] was originally thought to be the major mechanism of pain relief afforded by spinal cord dorsal column stimulation. Thus, large afferent fibers were thought to functionally close the gate to small diameter myelinated and unmyelinated fiber pain input. The gate control theory is probably inadequate to explain the mechanism of action of spinal stimulation as a sole theory. Experimental evidence suggests that altered neurochemical transmitter pools, conduction block of ascending pain transmission, activation of descending pain inhibiting neural tracts, supraspinal gating activity, and potentially other mechanisms are operative as well (**Figure 20.1**).[5]

Neurotransmitter effects

In rat models of neuropathic pain, the intrathecal administration of the gamma aminobutyric acid b (GABA-b) agonist baclofen will change spinal stimulation nonresponding rats to responders. Likewise, a GABA-b antagonist will reverse the effect.[6] Purinergic mechanisms appear to be operative in SCS induced analgesia and adenosine-A receptor agonists potentiate the effect of spinal stimulation in nonresponder rats. Interestingly, it appears that adenosine is synergistic with baclofen in these mononeuropathic animals.[7] These animal studies led to pilot data in humans that further suggest that these neurotransmitter systems and others (e.g. α-adrenergic activation) are important in SCS function. Intrathecal clonidine has been extensively studied for safety, and its use in cancer neuropathic pain states via the epidural route is Food and Drug Administration (FDA) approved. In addition, current consensus guidelines suggest that it is an effective agent when used as an intrathecal adjunct for

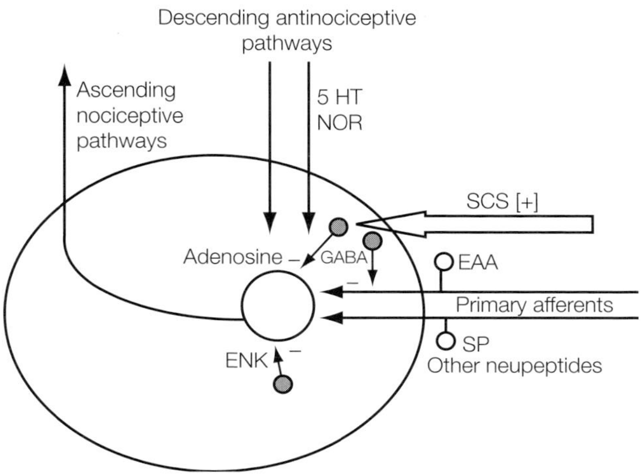

Figure 20.1 Noxious afferent pain pathways utilize excitatory amino acids (EAA) and peptides, e.g. substance P (SP), to signal local interneurons and centrally projecting pathways. Spinal cord stimulation may modulate pain projection by promoting the available balance of inhibitory neurotransmitters, including gamma aminobutyric acid-b (GABA-b), adenosine, and others. Additional mechanisms of stimulation analgesia might include conduction blockade of spinothalamic central projections, and/or descending modulation of tracts utilizing noradrenaline (NE) and 5-hydroxytryptamine (5-HT). Redrawn with permission from Meyerson BA, Linderoth B. Mechanisms of spinal cord stimulation in neuropathic pain. *Neurological Research.* 2000; **22**: 285–92.

a variety of neuropathic pain states. Schechtmann and colleagues[8] studied the addition of clonidine at small (1–20 μg) subeffective doses in nerve-injured animals in which SCS failed to suppress tactile hypersensitivity. The combination of clonidine and SCS in these animals was synergistic and effectively decreased the hypersensitivity. In a nerve ligation model of neuropathic pain, depolarization-induced acetylcholine release was enhanced by clonidine only in nerve-injured animals, but not in the control animals. This implies that clonidine-induced acetylcholine release is important in analgesia, but first requires depolarization.[9] Animal data led to a human study that examined the role of baclofen or adenosine phosphate as an adjunct to spinal stimulation. Forty-eight patients with peripheral neuropathic pain unresponsive to spinal stimulation were recruited, of whom 28 responded to drug bolus. Seven patients ultimately had both intrathecal pumps and spinal stimulators implanted, of whom five patients kept both systems. These patients had a decrease in pain on visual analog scale (VAS) from 82 to 33.[10] In an ischemia-induced sciatic nerve injury model, both gabapentin and pregabalin were able to suppress tactile allodynia when both the drug and SCS were utilized in subtherapeutic doses.[11] Importantly, these animal and human studies may lead to randomized trials whereby adjuvant pharmacotherapy is coincidentally applied to patients being treated with spinal stimulation.[5]

Supraspinal mechanisms

Saadè *et al.*[12] examined a potential role for a supraspinal gating mechanism by transecting the spinal cord dorsal columns, both above and below the level of stimulation electrode placement in rats. When the dorsal columns were transected above the electrode, the effects on phasic and tonic pain were abolished. When the spinal dorsal columns were transected below the level of stimulation, there was preservation of stimulation-induced analgesia.

Descending modulation

Stiller and colleagues[13] examined the role of spinal stimulation on neurotransmitter release in the periaqueductal gray (PAG) area in freely moving rats. Ongoing stimulation resulted in a decrease of PAG release of GABA. As GABA is an inhibitory neurotransmitter in the PAG, this effect may facilitate descending nociceptive inhibitory pathways.

Ascending tract conduction block

Spinal stimulation may produce a conduction blockade of ascending (e.g. spinothalamic) tract input. Studies indicate that lesioning of the fasciculus gracilus at T10 via midline myelotomy will abolish visceral pelvic pain from cancer.[14] Furthermore, visceral nociceptive activity may preferentially utilize fasciculus gracilus dorsal column pathways that project to the ventral posterolateral thalamus instead of the spinothalamic tracts.[15] Case series of spinal stimulation for patients with visceral pelvic pain have shown some efficacy.[16]

TECHNICAL CONSIDERATIONS

Modern stimulation electrodes are either "paddle"-type laminectomy electrodes or cylindrical percutaneously placed electrodes. The spacing between each contact varies from 1 to 10 mm, depending on the application. Spinal stimulation requires depolarization of a target neuron (making the neuron positively charged) which is done by activating a negatively charged electrode (cathode). Positively charged electrodes hyperpolarize the neuron, limiting propagation of action potentials. Therefore, the cathode is the stimulus site for active neuronal targeting and the resultant electrical field is conformed or limited by the anodal effects.[17] As most electrodes are placed epidurally, the conductivity of various substances in the anatomical vicinity are important in determining the extent of electrical field propagation. Within the spinal cord itself, longitudinally arrayed white matter tracts are most conductive, while fat within the epidural space is not very conductive. Vertebral bone is least conductive of all, and cerebrospinal fluid is most conductive (see **Table 20.1**). The conductivity of cerebrospinal fluid can become important in those cases where accidental dural puncture has occurred, as stimulation occurs at significantly lower amplitudes, and may propagate paresthesias to larger areas. The goals of SCS are to stimulate midline sensory fibers electrically without stimulating the more lateral nerve roots, which may cause abdominal cramping or other irritating sensations. Depending on the anatomical location in the spine, the distance between the electrode(s) and the spinal cord can vary significantly. The thickness of the area between the electrode and the cord (the δCSF) is maximal in the mid-thoracic spine, and this has implications for the occurrence of some variable postural effects of stimulation for patients. Thus, in some patients, simply flexing or extending the torso can create stimulation that is either imperceptible or painful (see **Figure 20.1**).[18] Oakley and Prager[17] describe the concepts of "perception threshold" (the point at which the patient first detects the paresthesia), and "discomfort threshold" (the point at which the paresthesia is uncomfortable). The area between these thresholds is then called the "usage range." Power consumption increases with increasing δCSF, which has implications for recharging frequency and pulse generator longevity.

Computer models

Holsheimer *et al.*[19] have performed computer modelling of electrode designs and suggested that optimal lead configuration is a transverse tripole with a central cathode with longer lateral anodes separated by 2.5–3 mm. A narrow bipole or tripole is optimal for dorsal column stimulation (**Figures 20.2** and **20.3**), as this keeps the stimulation over the posterior spinal cord better with anodal effects forcing the stimulus to penetrate more over the physiological midline. Many of the leads with large intercontact distances lead to dorsal root stimulation first, as the anode is not close enough to the cathode to exert

Table 20.1 Conductivity of intraspinal elements.

Tissue	Conductivity
Gray matter	0.23
White matter	
Longitudinal	0.6
Transverse	0.08
Cerebrospinal fluid	1.7
Epidural fat	0.04
Dura mater	0.03
Vertebral bone	0.02
Electrode insulation	0.002

Reprinted with permission from Oakley JC, Prager JP. Spinal cord stimulation. Mechanisms of action. *Spine*. 2002; **27**: 2574–83.

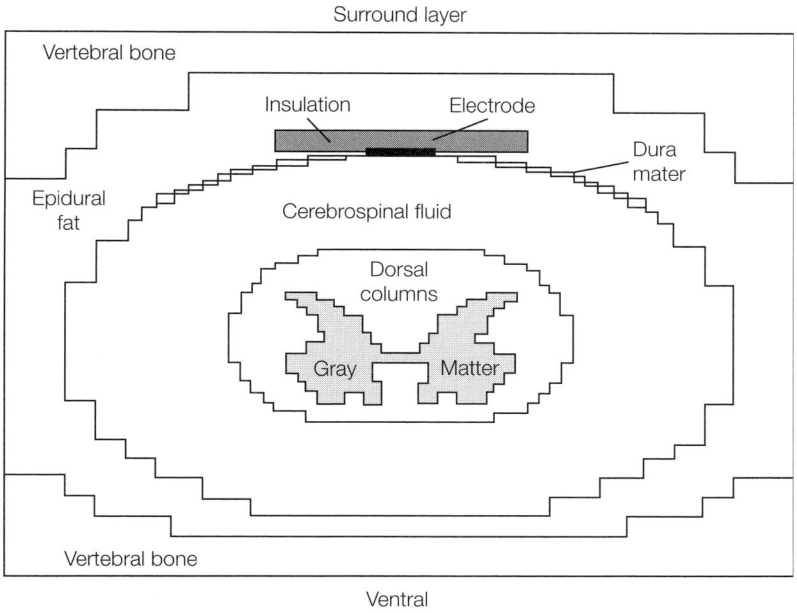

Figure 20.2 Computer model of the low thoracic region demonstrating an electrode in the dorsal epidural space. Spinal stimulation requires that the electrode conducts the distance through the layer of cerebrospinal fluid to reach the dorsal spinal cord. Redrawn with permission from Aló KM, Holsheimer J. New trends in neuromodulation for the management of neuropathic pain. *Neurosurgery.* 2002; **50**: 690–703.

any significant shaping of the vertical or horizontal extent of the electrical field. The threshold for dorsal column to dorsal root stimulation will increase, the greater the distance between the lead and the spinal cord. The highest threshold occurs at T4-T7 (**Figure 20.4**).[19] Optimization of the usage range (avoiding nerve root stimulation) often requires anodal guarding, which will establish field boundaries around the primary stimulating cathode, and produce more penetration of the dorsal spinal cord in a longitudinal guarded cathode. A transversely oriented guarded cathode (which may require using adjacent parallel leads) with a central cathode and flanking anodes as envisioned by Holsheimer *et al.*[19] allows for greater paresthesia steering to better cover the "sweet spot."

PROGRAMMING

The concept of multiple electrodes placed in parallel has become popular with many authors (**Figure 20.5**),[20] although others have suggested that a single electrode at the physiologic midline is not inferior to dual lead configurations for initial paresthesia coverage of the axial low back.[2] Newer electrodes may have independently variable voltages that allow the voltage ratio to be blended between the midline cathode and lateral anodes to better treat complex pain presentations.[18] Barolat and colleagues[21] carried out initial mapping of where various cathodal stimulations would produce paresthesias. In general, the areas of stimulation are several levels above the target dermatome, e.g. a foot paresthesia requires targeting the extremely low thoracic spine.

Initial targets for lead placement for the treatment of extremity pain are approximately a C3/4 location for stimulation of upper extremities, and T9/10 for lower extremity stimulation paresthesia coverage. Narrow contact spacing of bipoles or tripoles produces optimized coverage of painful areas, and maximal paresthesia coverage of the painful area has been a long-standing fundamental concept of spinal stimulation.[18]

SCS for spinal pain syndromes

The multiple operated back, often termed "failed back surgery syndrome" (FBSS) or postlaminectomy syndrome is currently the most common indication for spinal stimulation.[22] The care of the multiple operated back pain patients is difficult, and requires a multimodal approach that includes physical modalities, cognitive-behavioral therapies, procedural and pharmacologic therapies. Patients with ongoing postsurgical pain have complex pain patterns that often include both back and leg pains of various types (nociceptive, mixed, and neuropathic pains). Causes vary, but include cauda equina syndrome, arachnoiditis, epidural scarring or fibrosis, chronic radicular pain, and many others. Choosing the correct diagnosis is extremely important, as is the proper therapy for each diagnosis. Many patients simply want resolution and will repeatedly opt for more surgery in spite of little evidence of efficacy. An algorithmic approach within an established spinal care network can be useful. Several retrospective and prospective long-term studies have established SCS as a viable choice for these patients.[23] [III], [24][II] There are few randomized trials for FBSS. However, a recent trial by North and colleagues of a series of 50 patients randomized to either SCS or reoperation is important. Patients were all thought to be operative candidates by a staff surgeon, due to recurrent or persistent pain in a radicular pattern. Patients were allowed

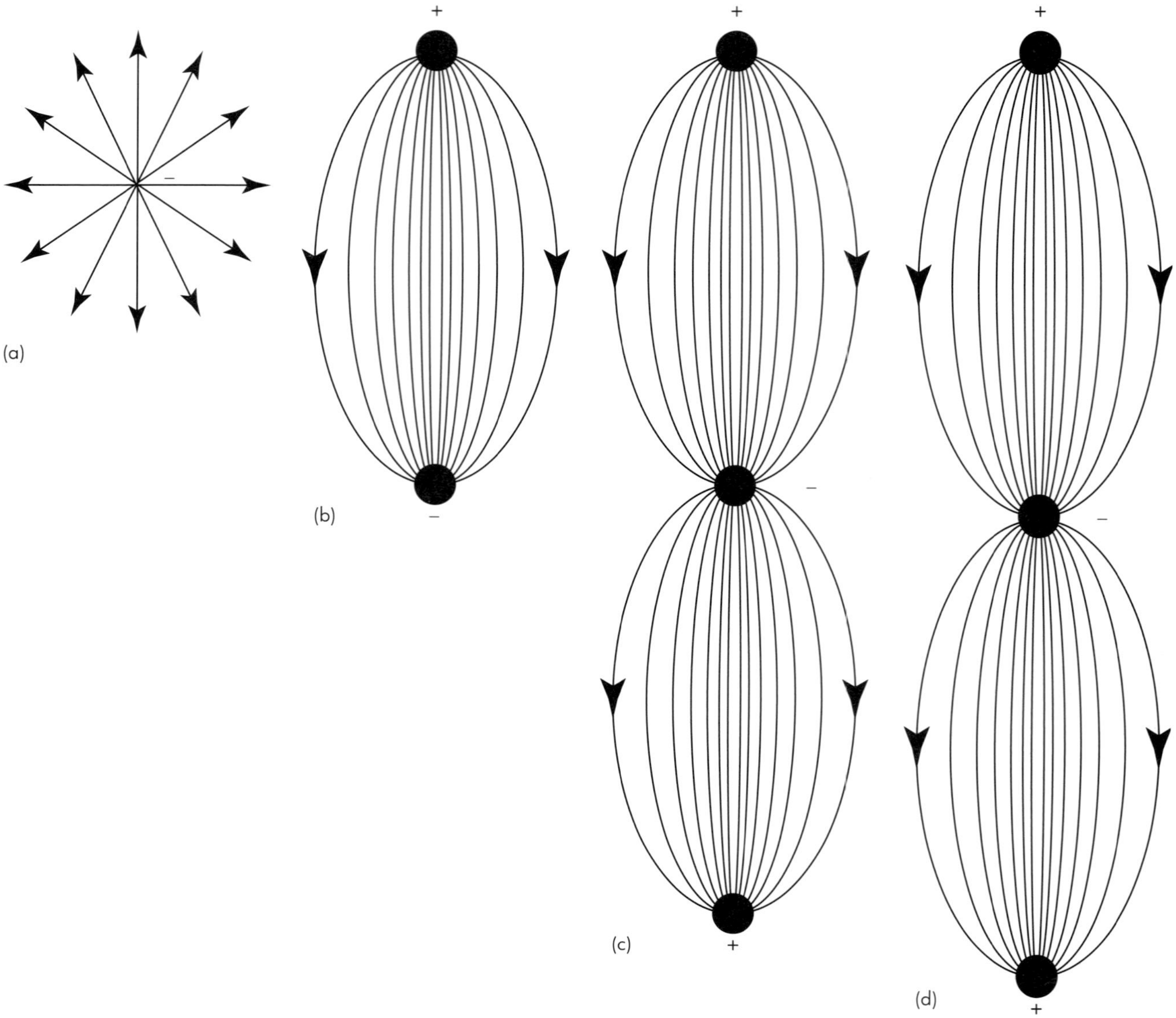

Figure 20.3 Stimulation may be (a) unipolar, (b) bipolar, (c) tripolar, or (d) narrow tripolar. The computer model predicts narrow tripolar stimulation as optimal. Redrawn with permission from Aló KM, Holsheimer J. New trends in neuromodulation for the management of neuropathic pain. *Neurosurgery.* 2002; **50**: 690–703.

to crossover to the other group as warranted. In the SCS group, 9 of 19 patients were successful versus only 3 of 26 in the reoperation group. Patients randomized to reoperation were much more likely to crossover to SCS (14/26) from which an additional 6/14 patients were successful.[24][II]

Although extremity neuropathic pain has long been thought to be the best indication for SCS, it is only recently that low back pain coverage for these patients has been achievable. The problem in years past has been that the approximate areas of stimulation required for low back coverage are from about L2 to L5. Stimulation of these areas is prone to also stimulate the anterior thighs, a less common area of pain for many patients (**Figure 20.6**). As the stimulation amplitude is increased, the abdomen will also be stimulated.[25] The sensory homunculus for the low back is quite small compared to the extremities (**Figure 20.7**), and low back fibers are not uniformly situated within the dorsal columns. Thus, the problem is one of penetrating the stimulus deeply enough into the spinal cord without activating the more prevalent fibers that are not desirably stimulated. Wide pulse widths may help to some extent with this problem.[25] Both Barolat *et al.*[26][III] and North *et al.*[2][II] have recently published trials demonstrating efficacy in low back pain patients.

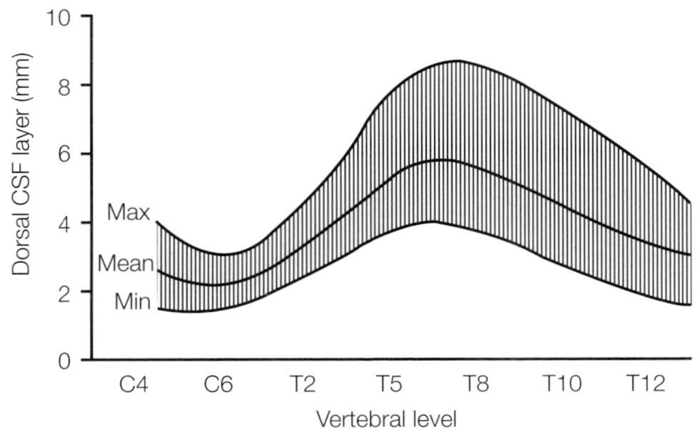

Figure 20.4 The distance from the spinal cord surface to the epidural electrode (d-CSF) is highest in the mid-thoracic spinal cord. High d-CSF decreases the usage range between stimulation threshold and uncomfortable dorsal root stimulation. Redrawn with permission from Aló KM, Holsheimer J. New trends in neuromodulation for the management of neuropathic pain. *Neurosurgery*. 2002; **50**: 690–703.

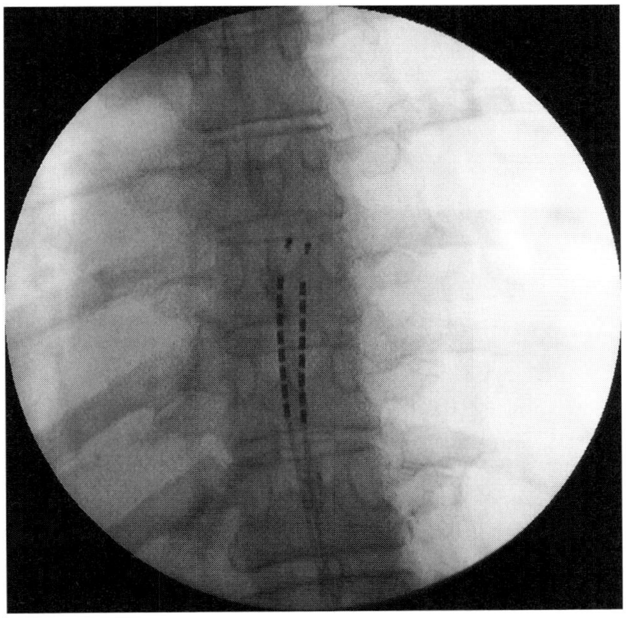

Figure 20.5 A dual-octapolar contact lead array spanning the eighth and ninth vertebral bodies in an anteroposterior projection. Note the cephalad aspect of the rightward lead is beginning to move too far lateral and might produce thoracic root stimulation.

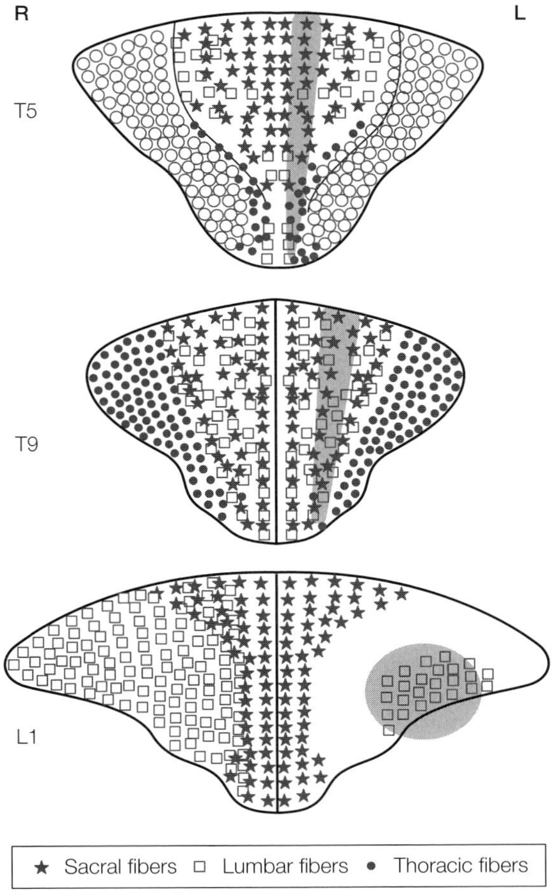

Figure 20.6 Low back stimulation coverage is often difficult and requires stimulation at thoracic levels where the lumbar roots from, e.g. L2, have moved centrally nearer the physiologic midline. At lower thoracic and upper lumbar levels, excessive stimulation paresthesias will be noted by patients in the anterior thighs and abdomen, because of the more lateral location of the representative L2 fibers. L2 fibers depicted in squares. Redrawn with permission from Oakley JC. Spinal cord stimulation in axial low back pain: Solving the dilemma. *Pain Medicine*. 2006; **7**: S58–63.

SCS in ischemic syndromes

The pain of intractable cardiac ischemia and ischemic peripheral vascular disease is often difficult to control despite attempts at revascularization, multimodal pharmacologic therapy, and other techniques. Ischemic disease results in increased morbidity, frequent hospitalizations, emergency room visits, and overall poor quality of life. Many patients are not candidates for revascularization procedures, such as bypass procedures, and it is unclear which of many newer therapies constitute "best practice."

SCS has emerged as one potentially beneficial therapy with previous prospective trials, retrospective case series and meta-analysis suggesting benefit of stimulation for several ischemic conditions. Unfortunately, little class I evidence for the technique exists because of the difficulty in performing randomized controlled trials for spinal and peripheral stimulation techniques in general.[3] Patients must be able to feel somatotopically correct stimulation paresthesia to verify appropriate coverage for all stimulation techniques.

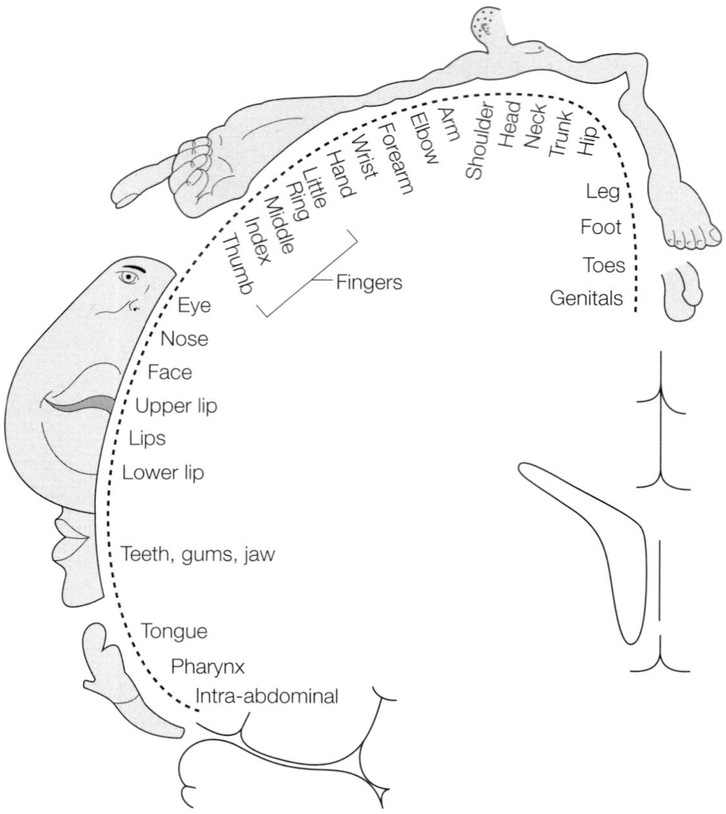

Figure 20.7 The sensory homunculus has a small representation of low back neuronal targets relative to the larger fields devoted to the feet and toes. Redrawn with permission from Oakley JC. Spinal cord stimulation in axial low back pain: Solving the dilemma. *Pain Medicine.* 2006; **7**: S58–63.

SCS in refractory angina pectoris

SCS was first applied two decades ago for the treatment of angina pectoris.[27] Since that time, several authors have noted significant improvement in a variety of clinical indices of ischemia. Spinal stimulation has enjoyed great popularity, particularly in Europe, but some resistance as well.[28] Reasons for this ongoing controversy are varied, but may include cardiologists' unfamiliarity with the technology, an incomplete mechanistic understanding of SCS, and the required utilization of noncardiac practitioners for ongoing therapy. Therefore, spinal stimulation has competed with other therapies, such as (1) percutaneous laser revascularization, (2) enhanced external counter pulsation (EECP), and (3) gene therapies. A recent comparison study of SCS and percutaneous myocardial laser revascularization is typical of the literature, with no difference demonstrated for the primary outcome measure (exercise treadmill time) between the groups. Several shortcomings are apparent with this type of comparative study, however, as the trial did not even mention the lead type, contact spacing, or programming sequences for what the authors admitted was their group's initial use of stimulation techniques. Furthermore, because the stimulation technology used is always changing, the implants were the older, nonrechargeable units.[29]

Despite these detractors, there is ample evidence of the efficacy of spinal stimulation for angina pectoris, as well as a potentially large number of patients who may qualify for this therapy. Many of these patients are not candidates for coronary bypass grafts or coronary stenting procedures. Some are at maximal medical therapy with optimized beta-blocker therapy, nitrates, vasodilators, and other pharmacologic agents. Many patients have nonatherosclerotic coronary disease, such as syndrome X, which is attributable to incomplete endothelial relaxation caused by dysfunctional adenosine receptors or other causes.[30] Pathologically, cardiac ischemia represents an imbalance of myocardial oxygen supply and demand. Numerous basic science and clinical studies have attempted to explain the mechanism of SCS beneficial effects, potentially attributable to redistribution of myocardial blood flow.

MECHANISM OF ACTION

The cardiac plexus in man was described in detail by Mizeres.[31] Cardiac fibers emanating from both vagal and sympathetic trucks form ganglionated plexus that exist in several areas including the pulmonary trunk, right and left pulmonary arteries, aortic arch, and atrial plexus. Intrinsic cardiac plexus neurons most important for SCS effects are likely found in the fat pads of the atria. Gagliardi and colleagues[32] identified these spontaneously firing cardiac neurons in the epicardial fat around the pulmonary veins and right atrium. Occlusion of the aorta and increased arterial pressure induced increased neuronal firing. Foreman and colleagues[33] placed spinal stimulation electrodes at T1, T2 in a canine study. During 90 percent motor threshold stimulation at 50 Hz and 0.2 millisecond trials with left anterior descending coronary ligatures placed to induce left heart ischemia, the previously increased cardiac intrinsic neuronal activity was decreased by SCS. Later, Armour *et al.*[34] demonstrated that SCS induced persistently decreased cardiac neuronal firing for approximately 20 minutes even after the cessation of stimulation. This after-effect suggests more than just a transient coronary vasodilatation during SCS. The question of whether spinal stimulation acts via coronary blood flow increase is not clear at present.

Chauhan and colleagues[35] had studied a cohort of coronary atherosclerotic disease (CAD) patients, syndrome X patients, and cardiac transplant patients with TENS. Both syndrome X and CAD patients had increased coronary flow velocity by Doppler study.

In contrast however, Norssel's group[36] studied patients with a pacing-induced ischemic episode with no consistent effect on coronary blood flow velocity. Norepinephrine spillover through the heart, a viable measure of increased coronary flow, was unchanged in their study. However, total body norepinephrine spillover did decrease.

Clinical effects

Multiple studies have demonstrated consistent clinical improvement from the application of SCS. Early work by Mannheimer *et al.*[37][III] involved a study of 20 patients with refractory, treatment-resistant angina pectoris. Atrial pacing-induced tachycardia and myocardial oxygen consumption were compared with or without spinal stimulation. During SCS, patients tolerated higher levels of pacing, prolonged time of pacing-induced chest pain, and reduced oxygen consumption. Hautvast and his group prospectively compared chronic angina patients with or without SCS.[38][III] Both duration of exercise and time period to angina increased during SCS. Nitrate consumption and angina attack frequency decreased during the study. Pain relief and quality of life were improved. Later, the same group assessed myocardial blood flow by positron emission tomography (PET) and were not able to demonstrate a change in blood flow despite substantial decreases in angina attacks, improved exercise and decreased S-T segment depression. It appeared that SCS worked by homogenization of cardiac blood flow at the expense of reserve flow.[39]

Technical considerations

Thoracic epidural needle placement is usually at approximately T4/5, but can be entered at lower levels as needed. Targeting the C7-T2 areas is optimal for most patients producing paresthesiae in the anterior chest and into the left or right arms as needed. Midline to slightly left of midline positioning is optimal (**Figure 20.8**). Lead migration and other technical problems are seemingly less than with other approaches, perhaps due to a less vigorous patient population and less effect by extremity and trunk movement. Early use of widely spaced (10-mm intercontact distance) bipoles and single leads has changed to tighter contact distances and dual eight-contact leads in many cases to better cover the pain topography.

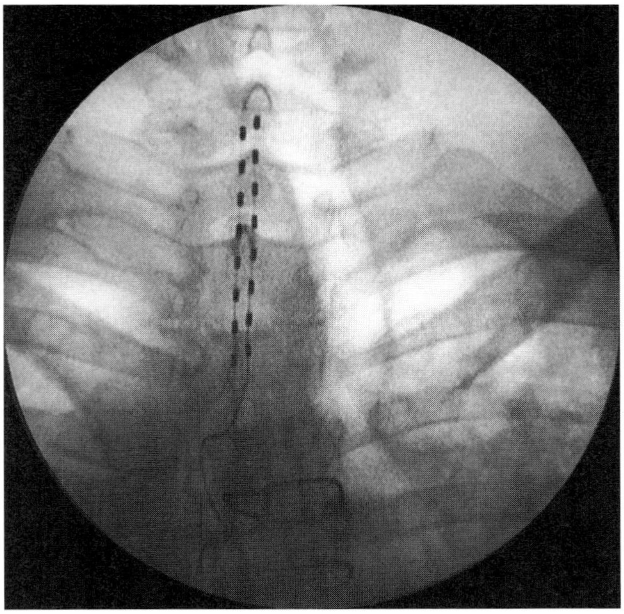

Figure 20.8 Two eight-contact electrodes placed for angina pain. The electrodes are central to slightly leftward and span from C7 to T3. Note the sternal wires from previous coronary bypass surgery in inferior aspect of film.

Peripheral vascular disease and SCS

Patients with critical limb ischemia from peripheral vascular disease (PVD) are at risk of significant ongoing morbidity and mortality. Limb salvage is important as a primary outcome for this group, as well as ulcer formation/healing and control of ischemic rest pain and claudication. Cook *et al.*[40] was the first to utilize SCS for PVD. Patients in that study had improvement in ulcer healing and pain symptoms. Multiple trials have shown some efficacy of SCS for PVD.[41, 42, 43, 44, 45, 46][II], [III]

BASIC SCIENCE

Both reduction of sympathetic efferent activity (decreased peripheral vasoconstriction) and antidromic dorsal afferent activation triggering release of calcitonin gene-related peptide (CGRP) and nitric oxide are important mechanistically. For example, Croom and colleagues[47] were able to block the cutaneous vasodilatation caused by

SCS at 90 percent motor threshold by dorsal rhizotomy at L3-L5, but not by rhizotomy at T10-12 or T12-L2. However, Tanaka and colleagues[48] did not see inhibition of SCS-induced rat hindpaw dilatation by hexamethonium ganglionic blockade at any level (30, 60, or 90 percent motor threshold) of stimulation. The use of a CGRP antagonist did reverse the beneficial effects of SCS in this animal model. Thus, it appears that both sympathetic and neurohumeral-induced vasodilatation may be important for SCS effects, but the exact stimulation parameters necessary and timing of each mechanistic contribution is not yet clear (**Figure 20.9**).

Complications are an ongoing and significant problem in caring for this group of vasculopathic patients.[49] Multiple complications of SCS were recorded in the large retrospective trial of Horsch *et al.*, including 30 lead dislocations, 12 broken leads, seven device-related infections, three patients with breakdown of tissue over the generator site, and two cerebrospinal fistulas in a cohort of 177 patients. These complications of SCS systems confound interpretation of outcomes for these patients with significant disease-related morbidities.[50] A total of 60 patients in another trial had implantation technical problems.[51]

Those patients who have baseline intermediate level $\text{Tc}p\text{O}_2$ values between 10 and 30 mmHg, reflecting availability of some vascular reserve, appear to be the best candidates. SCS trials should demonstrate an increase by >10 mmHg of the $\text{Tc}p\text{O}_2$ to warrant implantation.[52][III]

SCS for visceral pain syndromes

Nociceptive pain has long been regarded as difficult to treat with spinal stimulation, but visceral pain may involve several mechanisms, including inflammatory pain, mixed autonomic neuropathic pain, ischemia, and other causes. Visceral pain is often poorly localized and thus specific diagnoses are often difficult. Conditions treated can vary from cancer-related organ involvement, mesenteric ischemia syndromes, interstitial cystitis, urge incontinence, chronic pancreatitis, and many others.

The recent development of animal models of visceral pain has seen exciting findings with potential therapeutic implications. Animals with irritant-induced inflammatory colonic hypersensitivity will have measurable muscular abdominal contractions in response to pressure distention of the rectum. Rats that received irritant versus saline enemas had evidence of colonic hypersensitivity. Spinal stimulation attenuated these visceromotor abdominal contractions, providing speculation that SCS may be useful in certain inflammatory bowel conditions for pain control.[53] In a similar animal model, Al-Chaer and colleagues[15] noted that dorsal column pathways are important in signalling of the ventroposterolateral (VPL) thalamus projections in visceral pain, and dorsal column lesioning decreased the VPL response to colorectal distention. This and other studies, plus the fact that midline myelotomy (lesioning the fasciculus gracilus) helped patients with pelvic cancer-related pain, imply that spinal stimulation may have a role in many visceral pain syndromes.[14]

Human study to date on SCS for visceral pain is minimal. Khan *et al.* reported a case series of nine patients with chronic pancreatitis and other conditions which were improved with thoracic SCS.[54][V] Kapural and colleagues[16] recently described a small series of patients with chronic visceral pelvic pain who were helped with SCS.[16][V] The use of selective stimulation of sacral roots for interstitial cystitis[55] and the description of retrograde percutaneous approaches to the sacral roots[56] has improved the technical access to stimulation. Visceral pain appears to be a promising area of future applications for stimulation techniques.

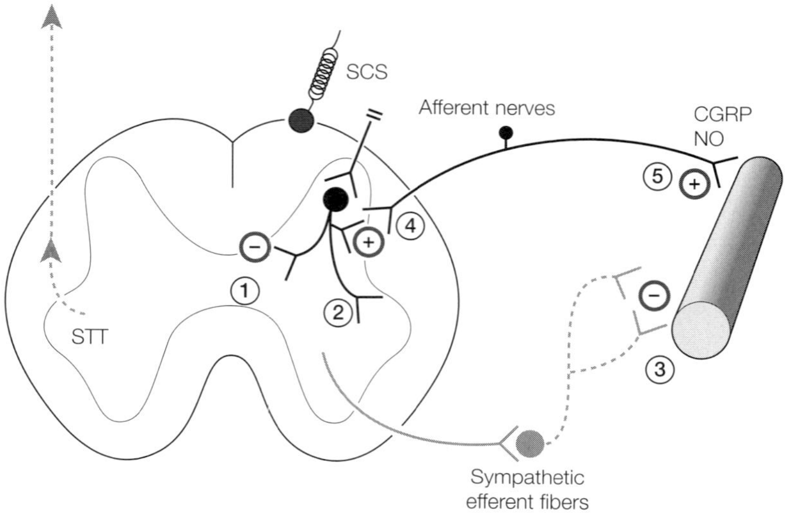

Figure 20.9 Spinal stimulation activates interneurons that may lead to: (1) decreased spinothalamic tract activity; (2) a decrease in sympathetic preganglionic firing; (3) reduction in postganglionic norepinephrine release at the vessels; (4) antidromic activation of dorsal root afferent fibers; and (5) peripheral release of vasodilator transmitters nitric oxide (NO) and calcitonin gene-related peptide (CGRP). Redrawn with permission from Linderoth B, Foreman RD. Mechanisms of spinal cord stimulation in painful syndromes: Role of animal models. *Pain Medicine.* 2006; **7**: S14–26.

SCS in complex regional pain syndrome

Complex regional pain syndrome (CRPS) occurs in association either with medical diseases such as post-myocardial infarction, systemic lupus erythematosus (SLE), post-cerebrovascular accident (CVA), in association with diabetes mellitus (DM) or as a posttraumatic limb pain syndrome with autonomic abnormalities. Complex regional pain syndrome is often arbitrarily diagnosed based on a constellation of signs and symptoms and the diagnostic criteria can easily be misapplied to multiple conditions. Objective evidence of CRPS requires three-phase bone scans, quantitative sudomotor axon reflex testing, or other specific tests to increase diagnostic accuracy, but some of these tests (quantitative sudomotor axon reflex test (QSART)) are only available at specialized centers (see Chapter 27, Complex regional pain syndromes for additional information). Recent evidence suggests that CRPS may be due to minimal distal nerve injury. Axonal densities were diminished at test sites in 17/18 patients by an average of 29 percent. These small fiber axonal changes would not be easily detected in most patients.[57] The IASP criteria for CRPS include: (1) the presence of a noxious inciting event or immobilization; (2) pain, allodynia, or hyperalgesia that is disproportional to the inciting event; (3) edema, skin blood flow abnormalities, or sudomotor abnormalities in the painful region at some time; (4) exclusion by other conditions that could account for the pain and dysfunction in some way.[58] The criteria do not help significantly in cases where patients have, for example, vasomotor changes and edema, but do not have sudomotor, motor changes, or a clear inciting noxious event. These diagnostic challenges make the study of CRPS difficult because of the likely presence of patients within one or another arm of a trial with differing pathological presentations. Nonetheless, previous prospective trials of SCS for CRPS have been positive. Harke and colleagues[59][III] implanted SCS systems in 29 patients with a previous provocative analgesic response to sympathetic blockade. Deep pain and allodynia were permanently reduced. Pain medication use was reduced as well ($p < 0.01$). Eight of ten patients who had been disabled with lower extremity CRPS resumed walking without crutches. Long-term functional status and quality of life were improved.

One randomized controlled study compared 36 patients who received physical therapy plus SCS and 18 patients who received physical therapy alone. Test stimulation of SCS yielded 24 patients with a positive response. Intention-to-treat analysis between the two groups demonstrated a 2.4-cm reduction in pain intensity at six months in the SCS and physical therapy (PT) group compared to PT alone ($p < 0.001$). Global perceived effect was much higher in the SCS group, 39 versus 6 percent ($p = 0.01$). No clinically significant outcomes related to functional improvement were seen.[60][II] Unfortunately, unlike the Harke study where patients demonstrated a positive response to sympathetic blockade, 22/24 patients in this study had previously undergone surgical, chemical, or radiofrequency sympathectomy. Measures of laser Doppler flow and skin microcirculation were measured while the SCS was either switched on or off. The study failed to demonstrate any SCS effects on microcirculation in patients with CRPS and low sympathetic tone. The authors suggested that their results were consistent with the theory that SCS causes an inhibition of sympathetically induced vasoconstriction, and thus the pain relief of SCS did not depend on vasodilatation.[61] Kemler and colleagues[62] recently published a five-year follow up to their previous randomized prospective study. Thirty-one of the original 36 patients in the SCS group were available, as were 13 patients in the control group. Twenty-two of the 31 SCS group patients were actually implanted with the device (intention to treat). The analysis demonstrated a diminution of the SCS effect over time, such that by three years the results favoring SCS were no longer statistically significant.[62][II] The five-year follow-up conclusions, as well as those from the original study, are potentially flawed because of the nearly universal inclusion of patients with sympathectomies, the use of outdated equipment and techniques, as well as the limited information on the specific physical therapies employed.

SCS for other neuropathic pain states

Postherpetic neuralgia (PHN) is a syndrome of persistent (> six months after acute zoster) pain and dysesthesia in the dermatomal topography of the original zoster outbreak. There is a definite predilection for the dormant varicella zoster virus to reoccur in the aged and immunocompromised patients (e.g. lymphoma patients). The pain of PHN is variously described as constant, aching, sharp, or shooting. Patients often have severe allodynia, dysesthesia, or hypoesthesia, and may not be able to tolerate even their own clothing touching the area involved. Pharmacologic therapies have been the mainstays of treatment, although various sympathetic and somatic blocks, epidural and intrathecal corticosteroid injections, TENS, and topical treatments are advocated by some. Pharmaceutical agents generally are utilized, such as ion channel modulating anticonvulsant class agents, nonselective reuptake inhibition by tricyclic antidepressants and newer agents, opioids, topical local anesthetics, or intravenous lidocaine infusions. SCS is usually considered after other less invasive therapies have failed. What is often not considered though, are the side effects of these pharmacologic agents, particularly the opioids, anticonvulsants, and antidepressants, or combinations thereof, in a predominately geriatric age group. The fall risk and cognitive impairment from many of these agents is not insignificant, particularly at higher dosages.

Harke and colleagues[63][III] studied 28 patients prospectively over a median period of 29 months. In addition, they implanted SCS in four patients with acute herpes zoster pain. As PHN often slowly resolves over time, the results of many therapies may appear more successful than is actually the case. To prevent undue emphasis on the results from SCS, the authors employed quarterly SCS inactivation tests to note any spontaneous resolution of pain with the SCS turned off. The results of this study were a median decrease in the visual analog pain scores from 9 to 1 ($p<0.001$). Long-term pain relief was noted by 82 percent of patients with PHN, and 8 of 29 were able to cease therapies. In the acute herpes zoster pain group, resolution occurred by 2.5 months on average.

PAINFUL DIABETIC PERIPHERAL NEUROPATHY

Like PHN, painful diabetic peripheral neuropathy (PDPN) is prevalent in society and treated with nearly identical pharmacologic agents. These drug therapies are often ineffective, and SCS has been attempted in previous trials for that reason. PDPN may be related to ischemia of the small vasa nervorum, metabolic impairments, or other causes. In a study of ten PDPN patients who were unresponsive to conventional treatments, eight of ten had positive responses to SCS trials and received implants. A control group received sham placebo screening. Mean duration of neuropathy was five years. Improvement was noted in both background and peak neuropathic pain, and exercise tolerance. These results were statistically significant in comparison to the sham group. The authors recommended SCS for drug-refractory patients.[64][III] In another study, eight male patients with long-term treatment of PDPN were followed over a three-year or greater period. Although some patients developed diabetes-related cardiovascular complications over time, the four long-term survivors continued to have significant reduction in pain over a range of 7–8.5 years.[65][III]

Peripheral nerve and peripheral nerve field stimulation

INTRODUCTION

Recently, stimulation technologies have been utilized to target more superficial areas of the body to treat predominately neuropathic pain sites not easily targeted by spinal cord stimulation. Currently, TENS, PENS (percutaneous electrical nerve stimulation), and peripheral field stimulation for abdominal, trunk, chest wall, face, and neck targets, as well as occipital nerve, trigeminal end branches, and upper and lower extremity peripheral nerve stimulation techniques, have been described in the literature. Although many of these techniques are similar, their mechanisms of action are as yet unclear.

INDICATIONS

Occipital neuralgia treatment was originally described by Picaza *et al.*,[66] but was popularized by Weiner and Reed utilizing modern electrodes and pulse generator technologies.[67, 68]

Small case series have substantiated successful treatment of intractable occipital neuralgia.[69][V] Many patients with occipital headaches may not have occipital neuralgia *per se*, but may also respond to peripheral stimulation in treating occipital headaches, cervicalgia, and other headache syndromes. Weiner and Aló (unpublished reports) have noted approximately a 75 percent improvement in some 150 patients over the last several years.[70] Success in treatment of occipital neuralgia has given rise to other peripheral nerve targets including both the supraorbital and infraorbital nerves, and others (**Figure 20.10**). Johnson and Burchiel[71] studied ten patients with pain after trigeminal PHN or post-traumatic V1 or V2 trigeminal branch neuropathic pain. These patients received quadripolar electrodes over the supraorbital or infraorbital nerves. Peripheral nerve stimulation was noted to provide at least 50 percent relief in 70 percent of the patients with long-term satisfaction and 70 percent decline in medication use. The authors suggested that prospective trials are indicated to study these outcomes further.[71][V]

Peripheral nerve field stimulation is a relatively new concept, wherein spinal stimulation cylindrical leads are introduced percutaneously into the subcutaneous tissues in the area of pain to stimulate small afferents which may not be as amenable to single peripheral nerve stimulation placement by open technique.

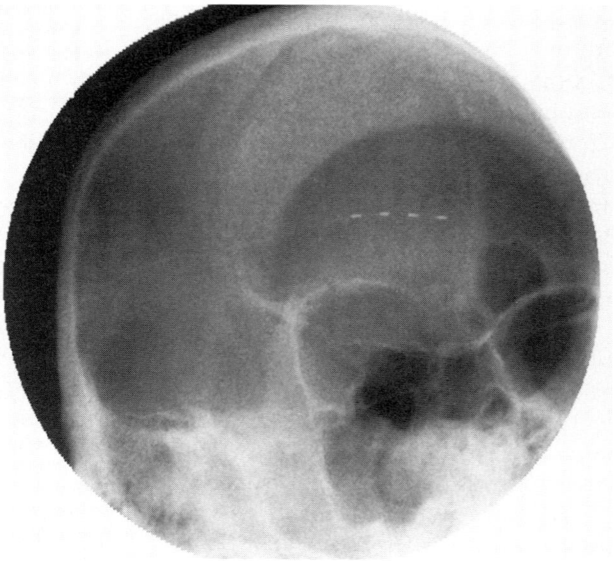

Figure 20.10 A four-contact subcutaneous electrode is *in situ* for peripheral nerve stimulation in a patient with supraorbital nerve (V1) distribution postherpetic neuralgia pain.

Paicius and colleagues[72][V] treated patients with subcutaneous electrodes placed for inguinal neuralgia, post-liver transplant abdominal wall pain, and chronic pancreatitis. All three patients noted substantial pain relief and reduction or elimination of opioid use. Peripheral nerve field stimulation may have similar mechanism to PENS. Hamza and colleagues[73] had previously shown benefit of PENS for diabetic neuropathic pain in 50 patients who were randomly assigned to receive PENS or sham PENS. Pain scores were decreased, and activity scores increased with active PENS.

Mechanistically, it is thought that PENS may cause central release of opioid peptides, induce neuromodulation, cause vasodilatation at peripheral sites, and improve wound healing. It is possible that peripheral field stimulation works through comparative means or perhaps other unknown mechanisms. Another recent case series[74] [V] of an additional three patients with regional chest wall and trunk targets were successfully treated with peripheral nerve field stimulation systems.

INTRACRANIAL STIMULATION

Stimulation of central neuronal targets has been performed for several decades with variable results. Deep brain stimulation and motor cortex stimulation have emerged as the most commonly employed and successful uses of this rapidly evolving field. While deep brain stimulation is quite commonly utilized for movement disorders and Parkinson's disease, it is useful in some painful disorders as well. As many of these painful neurological conditions are highly resistant to multiple therapies, cranial stimulation may be preferable to long-term opioids or many ablative neurosurgical techniques.

Motor cortex stimulation

Motor cortex stimulation is a technique of delivering a subthreshold stimulus to the contralateral motor cortex. This stimulation is, therefore, not perceived by the patient subsequent to initial intraoperative testing, and as the brain tissue is not broached, has less risk of hemorrhage than does deep brain stimulation. Motor cortex stimulation does not require stereotactic frame application, and leads are placed over the dura, either through a burr hole, or more commonly via a frontoparietal craniotomy. Early localization of the motor cortex utilized somatosensory evoked potential (SEP) wave reversal (N20/P20), but both electrophysiologic and magnetic resonance navigation is utilized in more modern centers to locate the position of the central sulcus. Electromyographic and visual monitoring of the muscles within the area of pain (e.g. facial muscles) is important to accuracy of electrode placement. One center commonly places two contiguous vertically oriented quadripolar electrodes, which are sutured to the dura. Various programs of stimulation may be required to achieve optimum results. Central pain after thalamic or lateral medullary stroke, or various facial neuropathic pain syndromes, such as trigeminal nerve injuries or postherpetic facial pain, are common indications. In addition, other neuropathic pain conditions, such as phantom pain and spinal cord injury pain, are potential applications for this technique. Initially, it was thought that stimulation of the sensory cortex might be analgesic for some of these pain conditions, but Tsubokawa and colleagues found that stimulation of the precentral gyrus was more effective in producing analgesia in their first publication of motor cortex stimulation for thalamic and post-stroke pain.[75][V] Prophylactic antiseizure drugs, such as phenytoin intravenously, are given,[76] as seizure is a known complication of motor cortex stimulation. However, most seizures resolve quickly after stimulation is turned off. A recent prospective trial of motor cortex stimulation was published involving 31 patients over a four-year period.[77][III] The primary outcome of excellent ($>$70 percent) or good pain relief (40–69 percent) occurred in 52 percent of the patients. In the first month after implantation, the level of pain relief was highly predictive of ultimate long-term relief (regression analysis, $r = 0.744$: $p < 0.0001$).

Deep brain stimulation

Contrary to the more recent introduction of motor cortex stimulation, deep brain stimulation has been utilized for decades, but its early use was not associated with universal acceptance due to the lack of randomized trials and often poor outcomes. Deep brain stimulation requires a stereotactic frame application and utilization of x, y, z coordinates to target specific brain sites. In general, the targets for nociceptive pain syndromes are usually the more medial areas (periaquaductal or periventricular gray (PAG/PVG)). Targets for neuropathic pain states tend to be deeper thalamic areas, often the VPL nucleus for bodily pain, or the ventroposteriomedial (VPM) nucleus for facial pain syndromes. Early trials for various neuropathic, nociceptive, or mixed pain syndromes were disappointing, with the Medtronic 3380 model trial showing 17.8 percent of 169 internalized (system implanted) patients with ongoing $>$50 percent pain relief at 24 months versus 13.5 percent of 37 internalized patients in the 3387 trial.[78][III] A more recent trial of 21 patients, although retrospective in nature, demonstrated better efficacy. Thirteen patients had electrodes implanted in the ventrocaudalis (VC) thalamic nucleus, or both the VC and PAG/PVG ($n = 8$). Those patients with 50 percent or greater analgesia were implanted, yielding 13/21 patients. One patient had a prolonged insertional effect from the placement, and did not require lead activation. The authors suggested that if an insertional or microlesion effect occurred during placement, the leads should be buried until pain recurrence and then a new trial of stimulation could be initiated. Eight of the 13 patients discontinued stimulation within the first year and only five had ongoing relief, four of whom had VC stimulation.[79][V] Overall, the lack of suitable prospective controlled studies continues to hamper the utilization of this therapy.

Complications of neurostimulation

As with any implanted device, the potential for adverse occurrences is always present. Most of the complications of stimulation devices are related to movement of the electrodes relative to the target of stimulation. Other complications of stimulation systems include infection, hardware failure, lead fracture or disconnection, hematoma, spinal fluid leak and resulting spinal headache, discomfort over the pulse generator site, and many other rarer complications.[80][V] In a large retrospective trial encompassing 22 years of implanting spinal stimulators, the authors noted a 21.5 percent incidence of displaced electrodes.[80] Overall, most lead migrations were easily revised with prompt resumption of effective stimulation. Infection occurred in the same series at a rate of 3.4 percent. Infections sometimes responded to antibiotics, but often required explantation of the device. Significant and recurrent lead migrations are usually treated with replacement of percutaneous systems with "paddle type electrodes" that are surgically placed via laminectomy. Of perhaps more concern to implanters is the late development of failure of analgesia, despite continued optimal paresthesia coverage. This has been called "tolerance" by some investigators,[80] but is not thought to be a pharmacologic stimulation dose requirement change, but rather a change in either central neural processing or other unknown process.[81][V] In spite of the apparent frequency of complications approaching 43 percent in one review,[82][V] there are to date no major spinal cord injuries, deaths, or other major catastrophic reports associated with these devices.

CONCLUSIONS

Neuromodulation technological advances and new applications continue to outpace the evidence to support their use. There is great enthusiasm for these techniques within the interventional pain physician community and the evidence from the available trials, and the reports of thousands of patients suggest that many painful syndromes can indeed be ameliorated by neuromodulation implants. There is a significant need to answer critics of stimulation therapies with greater creativity in designing randomized sham controlled studies which may answer questions of efficacy. The future of neuromodulation appears to be exciting, and likely will flourish if these studies are published.

REFERENCES

1. Shealy CN, Mortimer JT, Reswick JB. Electrical inhibition of pain by stimulation of the dorsal columns: preliminary clinical report. *Anesthesia and Analgesia.* 1967; **46**: 489–91.
2. North RB, Kidd DH, Olin J *et al.* Spinal cord stimulation for axial low back pain: a prospective, controlled trial comparing dual with single percutaneous electrodes. *Spine.* 2005; **30**: 1412–8.
3. Deyo RA, Walsh NE, Schoenfeld LS, Ramamurthy S. Can trials of physical treatments be blinded? The example of transcutaneous nerve stimulation for chronic pain. *American Journal of Physical Medicine and Rehabilitation.* 1990; **69**: 6–10.
4. Melzack R, Wall PD. Pain mechanisms, a new theory. *Science.* 1965; **150**: 971–9.
5. * Linderoth B, Foreman RD. Mechanisms of spinal cord stimulation in painful syndromes: Role of animal models. *Pain Medicine.* 2006; **7**: S14–26.
6. Cui JG, Linderoth B, Meyerson BS. Effects of spinal cord stimulation on touch-evoked allodynia involve GABAergic mechanisms. An experimental study in the mononeuropathic rat. *Pain.* 1996; **66**: 287–95.
7. Meyerson BA, Cui JG, Yakhnitsa V *et al.* Modulation of spinal pain mechanisms by spinal cord stimulation and the potential role of adjuvant pharmacotherapy. *Stereotactic and Functional Neurosurgery.* 1997; **68**: 129–40.
8. Schechtmann G, Wallin J, Meyerson BA, Linderoth B. Intrathecal clonidine potentiates suppression of tactile hypersensitivity by spinal cord stimulation in a model of neuropathy. *Anesthesia and Analgesia.* 2004; **99**: 135–9.
9. Obata H, Li X, Eisenach JC. Alpha-2-Adrenoceptor activation by clonidine enhances stimulation-evoked acetylcholine release from spinal cord tissue after nerve ligation in rats. *Anesthesiology.* 2005; **102**: 657–62.
10. Lind G, Meyerson BA, Winter J, Linderoth B. Intrathecal baclofen as adjuvant therapy to enhance the effect of spinal cord stimulation in neuropathic pain: a pilot study. *European Journal of Pain.* 2004; **8**: 377–83.
11. Wallin J, Cui JG, Yakhnitsa V *et al.* Gabapentin and pregabalin suppress tactile allodynia and potentiate spinal cord stimulation in a model of neuropathy. *European Journal of Pain.* 2002; **6**: 261–72.
12. Saadè NE, Tabet MS, Banna NR *et al.* Inhibition of nociceptive evoked activity in spinal neurons through a dorsal column–brainstem–spinal loop. *Brain Research.* 1985; **339**: 115–58.
13. Stiller C-O, Linderoth B, O'Connor W *et al.* Repeated spinal stimulation decreases the extracellular level of GABA in the periaquaductal grey matter of freely moving rats. *Brain Research.* 1995; **699**: 231–41.
14. Hirshberg RM, Al-Chaer ED, Lawand NB *et al.* Is there a pathway in the posterior funiculus that signals visceral pain. *Pain.* 1996; **67**: 291–305.

15. Al-Chaer ED, Lawand NB, Westlund KN, Willis WD. Visceral nociceptive input into the ventral posterolateral nucleus of the thalamus – a new function for the dorsal column pathway. *Journal of Neurophysiology.* 1996; **76**: 2661–74.
16. Kapural L, Narouze SN, Janicki TI, Mekhail N. Spinal cord stimulation is an effective treatment for the chronic intractable visceral pelvic pain. *Pain Medicine.* 2006; **7**: 440–3.
17. Oakley JC, Prager JP. Spinal cord stimulation. *Spine.* 2002; **27**: 2574–83.
18. Aló KM, Holsheimer J. New trends in neuromodulation for the management of neuropathic pain. *Neurosurgery.* 2002; **50**: 690–703.
* 19. Holsheimer J, Struijk JJ, Wesselink WA. Analysis of spinal cord stimulation and design of epidural electrodes by computer modeling. *Neuromodulation.* 1998; **1**: 14–18.
20. Alo KM, Yland MJ, Kramer DL *et al.* Computer assisted and patient interactive programming of dual octrode spinal cord stimulation in the treatment of chronic pain. *Neuromodulation.* 1998; **1**: 30–45.
* 21. Barolat G, Massaro F, He J *et al.* Mapping of sensory responses to epidural stimulation of the intraspinal neural structures in man. *Journal of Neurosurgery.* 1993; **78**: 233–9.
22. Van Buyten J-P. Neurostimulation for chronic neuropathic back pain in failed back surgery syndrome. *Journal of Pain and Symptom Management.* 2006; **31**: S25–9.
23. Van Buyten J-P, Van Zundert P, Vueghs P, Vanduffel L. Efficacy of spinal cord stimulation: 10 years of experience in a pain centre in Belgium. *European Journal of Pain.* 2001; **5**: 299–307.
* 24. North RB, Kidd DH, Farrokhi F, Piantdosi SA. Spinal cord stimulation versus repeated lumbosacral spine surgery for chronic pain: a randomized, controlled trial. *Neurosurgery.* 2005; **56**: 98–106.
25. Oakley JC. Spinal cord stimulation in axial low back pain: Solving the dilemma. *Pain Medicine.* 2006; **7**: S58–63.
26. Barolat G, Oakley JC, Law JD *et al.* Epidural spinal cord stimulation with a multiple electrode paddle lead is effective in treating intractable low back pain. *Neuromodulation.* 2001; **4**: 59–66.
27. Murphy DF, Giles KE. Dorsal column stimulation for pain relief from intractable angina pectoris. *Pain.* 1987; **28**: 365–8.
28. Buchser E, Durrer A, Albrecht E. Spinal cord stimulation for the management of refractory angina pectoris. *Journal of Pain and Symptom Management.* 2006; **31**: S36–40.
29. McNab D, Khan SN, Sharples LD *et al.* An open label, single-centre, randomized trial of spinal cord stimulation vs. percutaneous myocardial laser revascularization in patients with refractory angina pectoris: The SPiRiT trial. *European Heart Journal.* 2006; **27**: 1048–53.
30. Panza JA. Myocardial ischemia and the pains of the heart. *New England Journal of Medicine.* 2002; **346**: 1934–5.
31. Mizeres NJ. The cardiac plexus in man. *American Journal of Anatomy.* 1963; **112**: 141–51.
32. Gagliardi M, Randall WC, Bieger D *et al.* Activity of in vivo canine cardiac plexus neurons. *American Journal of Physiology.* 1988; **255**: H789–800.
* 33. Foreman RD, Linderoth B, Ardell JL *et al.* Modulation of intrinsic cardiac neurons by spinal cord stimulation: implications for its therapeutic use in angina pectoris. *Cardiovascular Research.* 2000; **47**: 367–75.
34. Armour JA, Linderoth B, Arora RC *et al.* Long term modulation of the intrinsic cardiac nervous system by spinal cord neurons in normal and ischemic hearts. *Autonomic Neuroscience.* 2002; **95**: 71–9.
35. Chauhan A, Mullins PA, Thuraisingham SI *et al.* Effects of transcutaneous electrical nerve stimulation on coronary blood flow. *Circulation.* 1994; **89**: 694–702.
36. Norssel HA, Eliasson TA, Albertson PB *et al.* Effects of spinal cord stimulation on coronary blood flow velocity. *Coronary Artery Disease.* 1998; **9**: 273–8.
* 37. Mannheimer C, Eliasson T, Anderson B *et al.* Effects of spinal cord stimulation in angina pectoris induced by pacing and possible mechanisms of action. *British Medical Journal.* 1993; **307**: 477.
38. Hautvast RWM, DeJonste MJL, Staal MJ *et al.* Spinal cord stimulation in chronic intractable angina pectoris: A randomized controlled efficacy study. *American Heart Journal.* 1998; **136**: 1114–20.
39. Hautvast RWM, Blanksma PK, DeJonste MJL *et al.* Effect of spinal cord stimulation on myocardial blood flow assessed by positron emission tomography in patients with refractory angina pectoris. *American Journal of Cardiology.* 1996; **77**: 462–7.
40. Cook AW, Oygar A, Baggenstos P *et al.* Vascular disease of extremities: electrical stimulation of spinal cord and posterior roots. *New York State Journal of Medicine.* 1976; **76**: 366–8.
41. Suy R, Gybels J, VanDamme H *et al.* Spinal cord stimulation for ischemic rest pain. The Belgian randomized study. In: Horsd S, Claeys L (eds). *Spinal cord stimulation: An innovative method in the treatment of PVD.* Darmstadt: Steinhhof, 1994: 197–202.
42. Jivegard LL, Augustinsson LE, Holm J *et al.* Effects of spinal cord stimulatin (SCS) in patients with inoperable sever lower limb ischemia: a prospective randomized controlled study. *European Journal of Vascular and Endovascular Surgery.* 1995; **9**: 421–5.
43. Claey SLG, Horsch S. Transcutaneous oxygen pressure as predictive parameter for ulcer healing in end stage vascular patients treated with spinal cord stimulation. *International Angiology.* 1996; **15**: 344–9.
44. Klomp HM, Spincemaille GH, Steyerberg EW *et al.* Spinal cord stimulation in critical limb ischemia: a randomized trial ESES Study Group. *Lancet.* 1999; **353**: 1040–4.
45. Spincemaille GH, Klomp HM, Steyeberg EW, Habbema JD. Spinal cord stimulation in patients with critical limb ischemia: a preliminary evaluation of a multicenter trial. *Acta Chirurgica Austriaca.* 2000; **32**: 49–51.
* 46. Amann W, Berg P, Gersbach PA *et al.* Spinal cord stimulation in the treatment of non-reconstructible stable

critical leg ischemia: results of the European Peripheral Vascular disease outcome study (SCS-EPOS). *European Journal of Vascular and Endovascular Surgery.* 2003; **26**: 280–6.

47. Croom J, Foreman R, Chandler M *et al.* Cutaneous vasodilation during dorsal column stimulation is mediated by dorsal roots and CGRP. *American Journal of Physiology.* 1997; **272**: H950–7.
48. Tanaka S, Barron K, Chandler M *et al.* Low intensity spinal cord stimulation may induce cutaneous vasodilation via CGRP release. *Brain Research.* 2001; **896**: 183–7.
49. Tiede JM, Huntoon MA. Review of spinal cord stimulation in peripheral arterial disease. *Neuromodulation.* 2004; **7**: 168–75.
50. Horsch S, Claeys L. Epidural spinal cord stimulation in the treatment of severe peripheral arterial occlusive disease. *Annals of Vascular Surgery.* 1994; **8**: 468–74.
51. Spincemaille GH, Klomp HM, Steyerberg EW *et al.* ESES Study Group. Technical Data and Complications of spinal cord stimulation: data from a randomized trial on critical limb ischemia. *Stereotactic and Functional Neurosurgery.* 2000; **74**: 63–72.
52. Gersbach P, Hasdenir MG, Stevens RD *et al.* Discriminative microcirculation screening of patients with refractory limb ischemia for dorsal column stimulation. *European Journal of Vascular and Endovascular Surgery.* 1997; **13**: 464–71.

* 53. Greenwood-VanMeerveld B, Johnson AC, Foreman RD, Linderoth B. Spinal cord stimulation attenuates visceromotor reflexes in a rat model of post-inflammatory colonic hypersensitivity. *Autonomic Neuroscience.* 2005; **122**: 69–76.

54. Khan YN, Raza SS, Khan EA. Application of spinal cord stimulation for the treatment of abdominal visceral pain syndromes: case reports. *Neuromodulation.* 2005; **8**: 14–27.
55. Maher CF, Carey MP, Dwyer PL, Schlucter PI. Percutaneous sacral nerve root neuromodulation for intractable interstitial cystitis. *Journal of Urology.* 2001; **165**: 884–6.
56. Alo KM, Gohel R, Corey CL. Sacral nerve root stimulation for the treatment of urge incontinence and detrusor dysfunction utilizing a cephalocaudal intraspinal method of lead insertion: A case report. *Neuromodulation.* 2001; **4**: 53.
57. Oaklander AL, Rissmiller JG, Gelman LB *et al.* Evidence of focal small-fiber axonal degeneration in complex regional pain syndrome-1 (reflex sympathetic dystrophy). *Pain.* 2006; **120**: 235–43.
58. Merskey H, Bogduk N. *Classification of chronic pain: description of chronic pain syndromes and definition of pain terms*, 2nd edn. Seattle: IASP Press, 1994.
59. Harke H, Gretenkort P, Ladleif HU, Rahman S. Spinal cord stimulation in sympathetically maintained complex regional pain syndrome type I with severe disability. *A prospective clinical study. European Journal of Pain.* 2005; **9**: 363–73.
60. Kemler MA, Barendse GAM, VanKleef M *et al.* Spinal cord stimulation in patients with chronic reflex sympathetic dystrophy. *New England Journal of Medicine.* 2000; **343**: 618–24.
61. Kemler MA, Barendse GAM, van Kleef M, Egbrink MGA. Pain relief in complex regional pain syndrome due to spinal cord stimulation does not depend on vasodilation. *Anesthesiology.* 2000; **92**: 1653–60.
62. Kemler MA, de Vet HCW, Barendse GAM *et al.* Spinal cord stimulation for chronic reflex sympathetic dystrophy – 5 year follow up. *New England Journal of Medicine.* 2006; **354**: 2394–6.
63. Harke H, Gretenkort P, Ladleif HU *et al.* Spinal cord stimulation in postherpetic neuralgia and acute herpes zoster pain. *Anesthesia and Analgesia.* 2002; **94**: 694–700.
64. Tesfaye S, Watt J, Benbow SJ *et al.* Electrical spinal-cord stimulation for painful diabetic peripheral neuropathy. *Lancet.* 1996; **348**: 1698–701.
65. Daousi C, Benbow SJ, MacFarlane IA. Electrical spinal cord stimulation in the long term treatment of chronic painful diabetic neuropathy. *Diabetic Medicine.* 2004; **22**: 393–8.
66. Picaza JA, Hunter SE, Cannon BW. Pain suppression by peripheral nerve stimulation: Chronic effects of implanted devices. *Applied Neurophysiology.* 1977/8; **40**: 223–34.
67. Weiner RL, Reed KL. Peripheral neurostimulation for the control of intractable occipital neuralgia. *Neuromodulation.* 1999; **2**: 369–75.
68. Weiner RL. The future of peripheral nerve neurostimulation. *Neurological Research.* 2000; **22**: 299–304.
69. Slavin KV, Nersesyan H, Wess C. Peripheral neurostimulation for treatment of intractable occipital neuralgia. *Neurosurgery.* 2006; **58**: 112–9.
70. Weiner RL. Occipital neurostimulation (ONS) for treatment of intractable headache disorders. *Pain Medicine.* 2006; **7**: S137–9.
71. Johnson JD, Burchiel KJ. Peripheral stimulation for treatment of trigeminal post-herpetic neuralgia and trigeminal post-traumatic neuropathic pain: A pilot study. *Neurosurgery.* 2004; **55**: 135–42.
72. Paicius RM, Bernstein CA, Lempert-Cohen C. Peripheral nerve field stimulation. *Pain Physician.* 2006; **9**: 261–6.
73. Hamza MA, White PF, Craig WF *et al.* Percutaneous electrical nerve stimulation. *Diabetes Care.* 2000; **23**: 365–70.
74. Goroszeniuk T, Kothari S, Hamann W. Subcutaneous neuromodulating implant targeted at the site of pain. *Regional Anesthesia and Pain Medicine.* 2006; **31**: 168–71.
75. Tsubokawa T, Katayama Y, Yamamoto T *et al.* Chronic motor cortex stimulation for the treatment of central pain. *Acta Neurochirurgica. Supplement.* 1991; **52**: 137–9.
76. Osenbach R. Neurostimulation for the treatment of intractable facial pain. *Pain Medicine.* 2006; **7**: S126–36.
77. Nuti C, Peyron R, Garcia-Larrea L *et al.* Motor cortex stimulation for refractory neuropathic pain: Four year outcome and predictors of efficacy. *Pain.* 2005; **118**: 43–52.

78. Coffey RJ. Deep brain stimulation for chronic pain: results of two multicenter trials and a structured review. *Pain Medicine.* 2001; **2**: 183–92.
79. Hamani C, Schwalb JM, Rezai AR *et al.* Deep brain stimulation for chronic neuropathic pain: Long-term outcome and the incidence of insertional effect. *Pain.* 2006; **125**: 188–96.
80. Kumar K, Hunter G, Demeria D. Spinal cord stimulation in treatment of chronic benign pain: Challenges in treatment planning and present status, a 22 year experience. *Neurosurgery.* 2006; **58**: 481–96.
* 81. North RB, Kidd DH, Olin J *et al.* Spinal cord stimulation for chronic intractable pain: Experience over two decades. *Neurosurgery.* 1993; **32**: 384–94.
* 82. Taylor RS, Van Buyten JP, Buchser E. Spinal cord stimulation for chronic back and leg pain and failed back surgery syndrome: A systematic review and analysis of prognostic factors. *Spine.* 2005; **30**: 152–60.

21

Spinal administration

KATE GRADY AND JON RAPHAEL

KEY LEARNING POINTS

- Spinal administration refers to the delivery of drugs to the intrathecal or epidural space.
- The principle of spinal administration is to deliver drugs directly to the intrathecal or epidural space so that therapeutic concentrations can be achieved at the dorsal horn of the spinal cord, which cannot be achieved by systemic administration or only with extremely high systemic doses.
- Enhanced therapeutic effects can thereby be achieved, and as smaller doses are needed than for systemic administration there is sparing of side effects.
- The epidural route has in the past been used more commonly than the intrathecal route. The intrathecal route is physiologically preferable, offers improved pain control, and a better side-effect profile. Now that technically the intrathecal route can confidently be used, it is the technique of preference.
- Intrathecal drug delivery (ITDD) is widely used for the management of cancer pain, chronic nonmalignant pain (CNMP) and painful spasticity; there is a supportive evidence base.
- The drugs used are opioids, membrane stabilizers, alpha-2 adrenergic agonists, gamma aminobutyric acid (GABA) agonists and more recently ziconotide, an N-type calcium channel blocker.
- ITDD should be delivered in a multiprofessional, carefully planned, and well-resourced context; patient selection is important and previous and alternative treatments should be considered[1] (see also Chapter 31, Intrathecal drug delivery in the *Practice and Procedures* volume of this series).

PHYSIOLOGY OF SPINAL ADMINISTRATION

Analgesia

- In 1973, opioid receptors were discovered in the brain and spinal cord by Pert and Snyder.[2]
- In 1976, animal studies demonstrated powerful and selective analgesic effects of intrathecal opioids.[3]
- In 1979, Behar *et al.*[4] demonstrated that the epidural administration of a 2 mg dose of morphine produced profound analgesia.
- In 1979, Wang *et al.*[5] demonstrated the profound analgesic effect of intrathecal opioids.

It has been shown that the analgesic effect of opioids delivered to the epidural or intrathecal space is mainly due to the drug being taken up directly into the spinal cord and cerebrospinal fluid.[6] By delivering analgesic drugs directly to the spinal cord and cerebrospinal fluid, a selective concentration of the drug is allowed to act at an important site of pain transmission, the dorsal horn of the spinal cord.

Spinal administration can therefore be extremely effective in terms of analgesia and further, it can overcome unwanted motor, sensory, and autonomic effects from the systemic administration of what are inevitably larger doses of drugs (**Figure 21.1**).

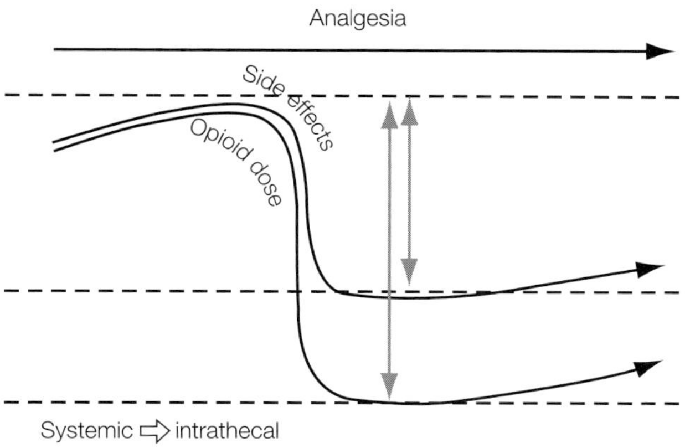

Figure 21.1 Greater analgesia with fewer side effects through spinal drug delivery.

The term selective spinal analgesia, originally used by Cousins *et al.*[7] in 1979, has come into common usage. The drugs most commonly used for spinal administration are opioids. Spinal administration can be the route of delivery of other drugs and can enable patients to be exposed to drugs that are unstable by nonspinal routes of administration. Other drugs which are delivered by spinal administration are local anesthetics, clonidine (an alpha-2 adrenergic agonist), and more recently ziconotide. Intrathecal baclofen is used to treat severe spasticity, which in turn has an impact on the pain of spasticity and the pain caused by deformities and disabilities of spasticity. There are reports of the use of other drugs, but there is no high quality evidence for these.

It is recognized that single shot spinal doses are only appropriate in the acute perioperative setting. The use of the techniques in the management of ongoing pain requires systems for the continuous delivery of drugs.

The blood–brain barrier

For systemic medications to reach tissues they must cross the endothelial lining of capillaries. These differ in different organs and relevant to this discussion is the lack of fenestrations of central nervous system endothelial cells acting as a barrier to drug passage (**Figure 21.2**). This is clearly a teleological protection mechanism from neurotoxins but hampers therapeutic drug delivery by the systemic route (**Figure 21.3**, indicator 3). It can be overcome by direct administration into the cerebrospinal fluid (indicator 2).

Central nervous system blood flow

The vast majority of central nervous system blood flow is to the more metabolically active brain when compared with the spinal cord (**Figure 21.4**).

As a result, systemic drugs that are distributed as a function of blood flow lead to a much greater delivery to the brain than spinal cord. Whilst both are important sites of analgesia, they have a differing spectrum of nonanalgesic (side) effects, with more derived from the brain. Again, direct spinal cerebrospinal fluid administration can overcome this.

Spasticity

In normality, muscle tone is maintained by constant activity from alpha neurones whose cell bodies are located in the anterior horn of the spinal cord. If the stretch receptors within muscle indicate lengthening of the muscle then the muscle contracts. The threshold at which the stretch receptor fires is controlled by gamma neurones. In pathophysiological states there is a failure of

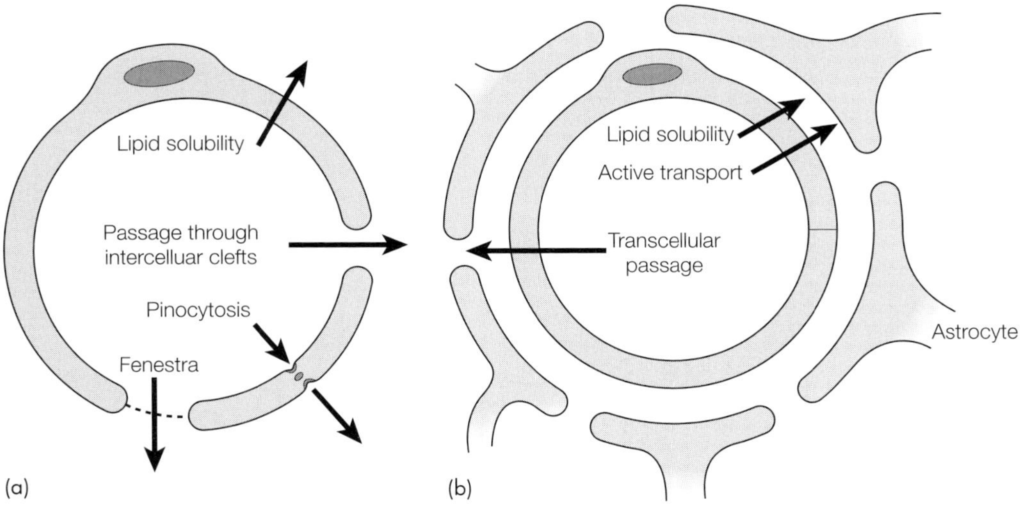

Figure 21.2 Differences between (a) normal and (b) brain capillaries.

GABA-mediated inhibition of alpha neurones and an imbalance between active and passive muscles results. Baclofen (a GABA-B agonist) corrects this.

PHARMACOLOGY OF SPINAL ADMINISTRATION

Opioids

It is perhaps fortuitous that the dorsal horn, the important site of pain transmission, is in the superficial layers of the spinal cord, enabling drugs reaching the cerebrospinal fluid to more readily exert their effects (**Figure 21.5**).

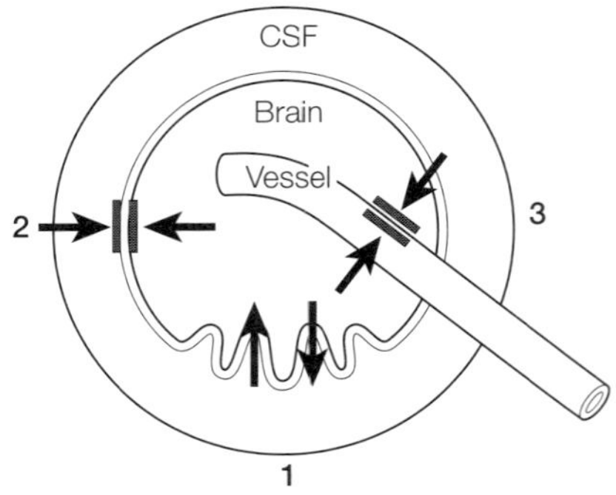

Figure 21.3 Blood/cerebrospinal fluid–brain barrier. 1, cerebrospinal fluid–brain barrier, chorioidal part; 2, cerebrospinal fluid–brain barrier, extrachoroidal part; 3, blood–brain barrier.

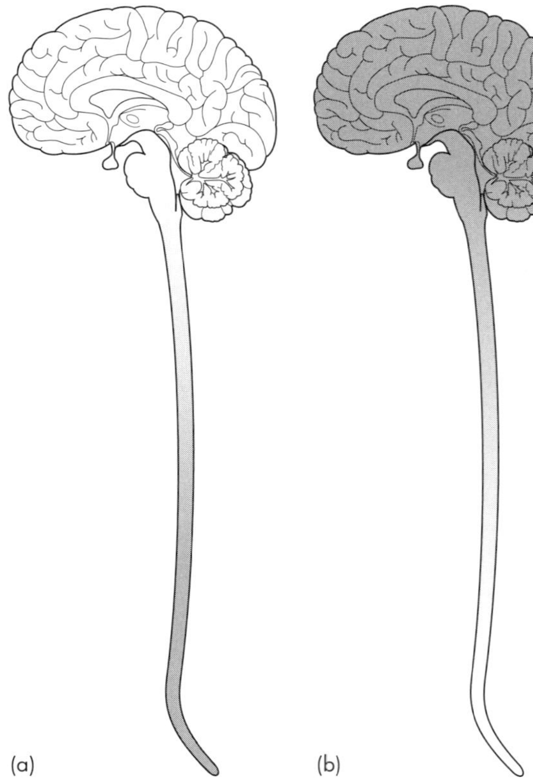

Figure 21.4 Central nervous system distribution of systemic and spinal analgesics: (a) spinal; (b) systemic.

Spinal opioids exert their analgesic effect at the spinal cord pre- and postsynaptically by reducing neurotransmitter release and by hyperpolarizing the membrane of dorsal horn neurons.[8]

SPINAL OPIOID PHARMACOKINETICS

Whilst spinal administration overcomes adverse effects secondary to distribution to the brain, there are other pharmacokinetic factors to consider; delivery of a spinally administered drug to respective receptor sites within the brain and spinal cord depends on a drug's lipophicity. A lipophilic drug remains localized reasonably near the site of intrathecal delivery whereas a hydrophilic drug spreads within the cerebrospinal fluid. The practical implications of this are that a lipophilic drug should be delivered by placing the catheter near to the spinal level of the pain.[9]

With hydrophilic drugs, a greater proportion spreads within the cerebrospinal fluid and can diffuse cranially and have a direct effect on the respiratory center. The relatively high concentration that can reach the respiratory center can cause respiratory depression. Close monitoring is necessary until drugs have equilibrated. Notwithstanding, in the longer term, the adverse effects of spinal administration are significantly less than systemic.[10][III]

Morphine is the opioid most commonly used in spinal delivery. It is considered to be the drug of choice because of its stability, increased receptor affinity, and the extensive experience of its use.[11][IV] It is recommended in current guidelines.[1] Morphine has been shown to be stable in intrathecal pumps for 90 days. The intrathecal dose of morphine is 0.1–20.0 mg per 24 hours.

Hydromorphone is approximately five times more potent than morphine. It can be used for patients who

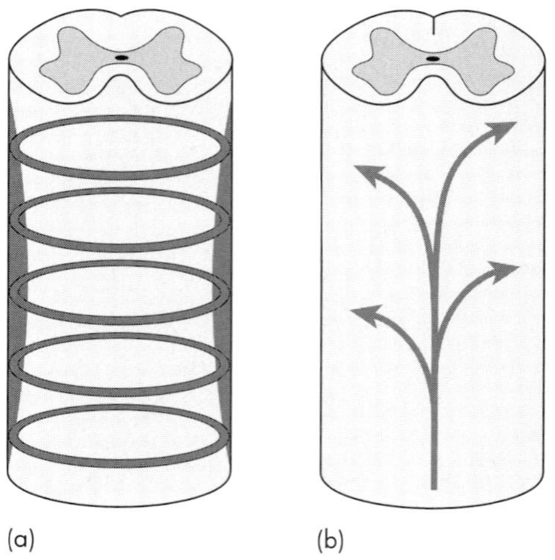

Figure 21.5 Distribution of analgesics in the spinal cord: (a) spinal; versus (b) systemic administration.

become unresponsive or develop intolerable side effects to intrathecal morphine. Its side-effect profile is equivalent to, or surpasses, that of morphine.

The intrathecal dose of hydromorphone is 0.2–12.0 mg per 24 hours.

Di-acetyl morphine (Diamorphine) is used in the UK. Its high solubility may reduce the likelihood of granulomata (see also Chapter 31, Intrathecal drug delivery in the *Practice and Procedures* volume of this series).

Di-acetyl morphine is highly soluble in saline, bupivacaine, and clonidine enabling high volume local anesthetic delivery. It rapidly breaks down into mono-acetyl morphine and morphine, but is equipotent with morphine.[12]

Spinal opioids which are used less commonly include buprenorphine (which is favored for having less effect on the bladder sphincter when urinary retention remains a problem), fentanyl, and sufentanil.

Membrane stabilizers

These drugs are in use as local anesthetics. They block sodium channels to inhibit action potentials in the dorsal horn and the intrathecal portion of the nerve and thereby inhibit nerve conduction. They have been found useful as systemic analgesics in neuropathic pain, but have a narrow therapeutic window with effects on cardiac conduction of concern.[13][III] Direct spinal delivery overcomes this. Intrathecally local anesthetics are used in the management of chronic nonmalignant pain and cancer pain.[14, 15, 16]

There is evidence that intrathecal bupivacaine acts synergistically with morphine, reducing the progression of intrathecal morphine dosage.[17] The intrathecal dose of bupivaciane is 4–30 mg per 24 hours.

Ropivaciane has been used; it is less toxic, more selective for sensory blockade, and offers better segmental spread but is less potent than bupivacaine.[18]

Local anesthetics are less selective than opioids and block motor and autonomic as well as sensory fiber transmission. Care is needed to locate the spinal catheter at the site of pain and to titrate the dose. Long-term use can be associated with tachyphylaxis.

Alpha-2 adrenergic agonists

The intrathecal application of alpha-2 agonists modulates pain transmission by depression of the release of substance P and calcitonin gene-related peptide (CGRP) from C fibers and enhancement of noradrenaline descending inhibition.[19] They may also suppress preganglionic sympathetic outflow and may have analgesic effects in sympathetically maintained pains.

There are studies of the greater efficacy of clonidine in the treatment of neuropathic pain when administered spinally as opposed to systemically.[20]

Intrathecal clonidine has been used in the management of cancer pain and neuropathic pain.[21, 22] The intrathecal dose of clonidine is 50–1000 μg per 24 hours.

GABA B agonists

Baclofen is used in the treatment of severe spasticity and its painful and disabling consequences. In pathophysiological states, in which there is an imbalance between active and passive muscles due to a failure of GABA-mediated inhibition, baclofen (a GABA-B agonist) corrects this. It is believed that the majority of GABA receptors lie in the dorsal horn and the expression of these receptors increases in pathological states; therefore, baclofen is more effective in pathological states.

Baclofen may have a primary analgesics effect; this is predominantly seen in central pain states.[23]

Voltage-gated calcium channel blockers

Ziconotide is an antagonist at N-type voltage-sensitive calcium channels (VSCCs) found at presynaptic terminals in the dorsal horn of the spinal cord. The blockade produced by ziconotide is more specific for nociceptive than somatosensory transmission. There is increased expression of N-type VSCCs in chronic pain states which may explain its greater specificity for chronic rather than acute pain states.

In contrast to opioids and local anesthetics, ziconotide is not associated with the development of tolerance.

Although experience with ziconotide is more limited, its other advantage is that it does not cause respiratory depression.

Drug admixtures are commonly used such as opioids and local anesthetics, clonidine and morphine, and/or bupivacaine. Those with ziconotide result in significantly reduced concentrations of this drug.

Potential drugs

N-METHYL-D-ASPARTIC ANTAGONISTS

Dorsal horn *N*-methyl-D-aspartic (NMDA) receptors have a core role in central sensitization and modulate alterations in synaptic plasticity, pivotal to the generation of persistent pain.

Racemic ketamine acts as a co-analgesic with opioid analgesic effects in neuropathic pain states. Clinically, there is limited efficacy data and a report of potential neurotoxicity.[24]

GABA A AGONISTS

These agents suppress afferent evoked excitation in the substantia gelatinosa by binding to the benzodiazepine

(BDZ) site of GABA-A receptor complex. There are several reports of efficacy. However, there are troublesome side effects of sedation and degradation of motor function.[25]

Safety remains of concern following two rabbit studies showing behavioral indices of neurotoxicity[26] and a number of human case reports showing the same. There is, however, no histological evidence and there has been a large cohort study of intrathecal midazolam in an obstetric population with less than 2 percent incidence of neurological dysfunction and no evidence of increased risk of neurotoxicity.[27]

For clinical use of drugs and side effects, see Chapter 31, Intrathecal drug delivery in the *Practice and Procedures* volume of this series.

EVIDENCE FOR SPINAL ADMINISTRATION

Cancer pain

There is a systematic review which demonstrates that cancer pain that has not been controlled by systemic drugs can be managed by intrathecal opioid therapy.[28][I] There are randomized controlled studies which demonstrate the intrathecal route to be superior to conventional routes in the management of cancer pain.[29][II]

Smith and coworkers[29][II], [30][III], [31][III] demonstrated in a multicenter randomized controlled trial that quality of life was improved (because of improved pain control) and drug toxicity was significantly less in patients undergoing intrathecal administration of drugs compared to those undergoing comprehensive medical management.

One study[30][III] also demonstrated that at six months, 53 percent of those undergoing intrathecal therapy were still alive compared to 32 percent of those undergoing comprehensive medical management. Survival was not a primary outcome measure, but the finding resulted from an intention to treat analysis; however, it does suggest that longevity might be increased in those underoing intrathecal delivery compared to those undergoing conventional medical management. This may be due to improved mobility and activity. There is also evidence, however, that systemic morphine inhibits the immune system and may therefore have an adverse effect on survival.[32][IV] This may explain the findings of difference in survival.

There are many case reports to support the efficacy of spinal drug delivery in the management of cancer pain. There is a randomized controlled trial which demonstrates the usefulness of intrathecal ziconotide in the treatment of cancer pain or acquired immunodeficiency syndrome (AIDS).[33][II]

Chronic nonmalignant pain

There is a single-blind, prospective placebo-controlled study, which looked at short-term efficacy, showing spinal morphine to be of benefit in the short term in patients with CNMP who have responded to systemic morphine but in whom side effects have become intolerable.[34][III]

There are many studies of good quality to support the long term use of intrathecal drug delivery in CNMP.[35][III], [36][III], [37][III], [38][III]

There are two randomized double blind placebo controlled trials supporting the use of intrathecal ziconotide in CNMP; however, the clinical significance was small, experience is extremely limited, and side effects were troublesome.[39][II], [40][II]

For CNMP in particular, patient characteristics have to be clearly considered in selection; a three year prospective study of intrathecal opioid treatment for CNMP in patients with extreme pain showed improvement but that overall severity of pain remained high.[41][III]

Trialing is mandatory (see Chapter 31, Intrathecal drug delivery in the *Practice and Procedures* volume of this series).

Spasticity

Baclofen is very efficacious in the treatment of spasticity in multiple sclerosis, cerebral plasy, and spinal cord injury.[42][III], [43][III], [44][III], [45][III], [46][III], [47][III]

The ongoing effect on function can be assessed by infusion trial.

Cost-effectiveness

For cancer pain, ITDD is more cost effective than systemic medication beyond 3–6 months and for 11–22 months for noncancer pain.[10, 48][III] Intrathecal baclofen has a favorable cost–benefit ratio in the management of spasticity in carefully selected patients.[49][III]

CLINICAL APPLICATION

The following is an empirical guide to the application of ITDD to the various categories of pain. It is not a substitute for thorough assessment of individual patients and their conditions nor an assessment of the availability of resources (see Chapter 31, Intrathecal drug delivery in the *Practice and Procedures* volume of this series).

Cancer pain

The greatest interest in ITDD has been in its application to advanced cancer pain. Particular consideration should be given to risk to benefit ratio. It is important to assess the effect of advancing disease on the safe conduct of the technique and carry out investigations, for example radiological scanning where there is suspected intracranial or vertebral disease. Ten to fifteen percent of cancer patient's pain will not be controlled by the use of systemic medication as per the World Health Organization (WHO) guidelines.[50, 51, 52] As above, this is for reasons of inadequacy or intolerable side effects of systemic analgesia.

Both nociceptive and neuropathic cancer pain can be managed by ITDD. It is likely that nociceptive pain, for example bone pain, will be most responsive to opioids and neuropathic, visceral and incident pain will be more responsive when local anesthetics ± clonidine are added to the infusate.

Other treatments should be considered, such as neuroablative or neurolytic techniques.

Chronic nonmalignant pain

ITDD can be considered as a potential treatment in the management of some nociceptive pain, particularly mechanical back pain, cases of mixed neuropathic and nociceptive pain, and cases of widespread pain, for example back and leg pain. In a retrospective study, Raphael *et al.*[53][III] found ITDD systems appeared to confer advantage over spinal cord stimulation in failed postsurgical spine pain and chronic mechanical back pain.

Other treatments such as cognitive behavioral therapy should not be excluded.

Spasticity

There is good evidence for the efficacy of intrathecal baclofen in the management of spasticity of various causes. Its effect on function and quality of life should be assessed by trial.

ACKNOWLEDGMENTS

The authors would like to thank H Mueller for preparing the figures.

REFERENCES

∗ 1. Intrathecal drug delivery for the management of pain and spasticity in adults; recommendations for best clinical practice. London: British Pain Society, April 2007.

∗ 2. Pert CB, Snyder SH. Opioid receptor: demonstration in nervous tissue. *Science*. 1973; **179**: 1011–14.

∗ 3. Yaksh TL, Rudy TA. Narcotic analgesia produced by a direct action on the spinal cord. *Science*. 1976; **192**: 1357–8.

4. Behar M, Magora F, Olshwang D, Davidson JT. Epidural morphine in treatment of pain. *Lancet*. 1979; **1**: 527–9.

5. Wang J, Nauss LA, Thomas JE. Pain relief by intrathecally applied morphine in man. *Anesthesiology*. 1979; **50**: 149–51.

6. Gourlay GK, Cherry DA, Cousins MJ. Cephalad migration of morphine in cerebrospinal fluid following lumbar epidural administration in patients with cancer pain. *Pain*. 1985; **23**: 317–26.

7. Cousins MJ, Mather LE, Glynn CJ *et al*. Selective spinal analgesia. *Lancet*. 1979; **1**: 1141–2.

8. Dickenson AH. Recent advances in the physiology and pharmacology of pain: plasticity and its implications for clinical analgesia. *Journal of Psychopharmacology*. 1991; **5**: 342–51.

9. Penn RD. Central nervous system drug infusion for pain. In: Tindall GT, Cooper PR, Barrow DL (eds). *The practice of neurosurgery*. Baltimore: Williams and Wilkins, 1996.

10. Mueller-Schwefe G, Hassenbusch SJ, Reig E. Cost-effectiveness of intrathecal therapy for pain. *Neuromodulation*. 1999; **2**: 77–87.

11. Paice JA, Penn RD, Shotts I. Intraspinal morphine for chronic pain: Retrospective multicentre study. *Journal of Pain and Symptom Management*. 1996; **11**: 71–80.

12. Raphael JH, Palfrey SM, Rayen A *et al*. Stability and analgesic efficacy of di-acetyl morphine(diamorphine) compared with morphine in implanted intrathecal pumps in vivo. *Neuromodulation*. 2004; **7**: 197–200.

13. Raphael JH, Southall JL, Treharne GJ, Kitas GD. Adverse effects of Intravenous lignocaine therapy in fibromyalgia syndrome. *Rheumatology (Oxford)*. 2003; **42**: 185–6.

14. Berde CB, Sethna NF, Conrad LS *et al*. Subarachnoid bupivavacaine analgesia for seven months for a patient with a spinal cord tumour. *Anaesthesiology*. 1990; **72**: 1094–6.

15. Dahm P, Nitescu P, Appelgrenb L, Curelaru I. Continuous intrathecal infusion of opioid and bupivacaine in the treatment of refractory pain due to post herpetic neuralgia; a case report. *Neuromodulation*. 1998; **1**: 85–9.

16. Krames ES, Lanning RM. Intrathecal infusional analgesia for non-malignant pain: analgesic efficiacy of intrathecal opioid with our without bupivacaine. *Journal of Pain and Symptom Management*. 1993; **8**: 539–48.

∗ 17. Van Dongen RTM, Crul BJP, Van Egmond J. Intrathecal coadministration of bupivacaine diminishes morphine dose progression during long-term intrathecal infusion in cancer patients. *Clinical Journal of Pain*. 1999; **15**: 166–72.

18. Markham A, Faulds D. Ropivacaine: a review of its pharmacology and therapeutic use in regional anesthesia. *Drugs*. 1996; **52**: 429–49.

∗ 19. Eisenach JC, De Kock M, Klimscha W. Alpha$_2$-adrenergic agonists for regional anesthesia: a clinical review of clonidine (1984–1995). *Anesthesiology*. 1996; **85**: 655–74.

20. Glynn CJ, Jamous MA, Teddy PJ. Cerebrospinal fluid kinetics of epidural clonidine in man. *Pain*. 1997; **49**: 361–7.

21. Eisenach JC, Du Pen S, Dubois M *et al*. The epidural clonidine study group. Epidural clonidine analgesia for intractable cancer pain. *Pain*. 1995; **61**: 391–9.

22. Eisenach JC. Three novel spinal analgesics: Clonidine, neostigmine, amitriptyline. *Regional Anesthesia.* 1996; **21**: 81–3.
23. van Hilten BJ, van de Beek W-JT, Hoff JI *et al.* Intrathecal baclofen for the treatment of dystonia in patients with reflex sympathetic dystrophy. *New England Journal of Medicine.* 2000; **343**: 625–30.
24. Hassenbusch SJ, Satterfield WC, Gradert TL *et al.* Preclinical toxicity study of intrathecal administration of the pain relievers dextrorphan, dextromethorphan, and memantine in the sheep model. *Neuromodulation.* 1999; **2**: 230–40.
25. Walker SM, Goudas LC, Cousins MJ, Carr DB. Combination spinal analgesic chemotherapy: a systematic review. *Anesthesia and Analgesia.* 2002; **95**: 674–715.
26. Malinovsky JM, Cozian A, Lepage JY *et al.* Ketamine and midazolam neurotoxicity in the rabbit. *Anesthesiology.* 1991; **75**: 91–7.
27. Tucker AP, Mezzatesta J, Nadeson R, Goodchild CS. Intrathecal midazolam II: Combination with intrathecal fentanyl for labor pain. *Anesthesia and Analgesia.* 2004; **98**: 1521–7.
28. Ballantyne JC, Carwood CM. Comparative efficacy of epidural, subarachnoid and intracerebroventricular opioids in patients with pain due to cancer. *Cochrane Database of Systematic Reviews.* 2005; **CD005178**.
29. Smith TJ, Staats PS, Deer T *et al.* Implantable drug delivery systems study group. Randomised clinical trial of an implantable drug delivery system compared with comprehensive medical management for refractory cancer pain; impact on pain, drug related toxicity and survival. *Journal of Clinical Oncology.* 2002; **20**: 4040–9.
30. Smith TJ, Coyne PJ, Staats PS *et al.* An implantable drug delivery syatem (IDSS) for refractory cancer pain provides sustained pain control, less drug related toxicity and possibly better survival compared with comprehensive medical management (CMM). *Annals of Oncology.* 2005; **16**: 825–33.
31. Smith TJ, Coyne PJ. Implantable drug delivery systems (IDSS) after failure of comprehensive medical management (CMM) can palliate symptoms in the refractory cancer pain patients. *Journal of Palliative Medicine.* 2005; **8**: 736–42.
32. Hamra JG, Yaksh TL. Equianalgesic doses of subcutaneous but not intrathecal morphine alter phenotypic expression of cell surface markers and mitogen induced proliferation in rat lymphocytes. *Anesthesiology.* 1996; **85**: 355–65.
33. Staats P, Yearwood T, Charapata SG *et al.* Intrathecal ziconotide in the treatment of refractory pain in patients with cancer or AIDS. *Journal of the American Medical Association.* 2004; **291**: 63–70.
34. Raphael JH, Gnanadurai TV, Southall JL *et al.* Placebo controlled single blind study of short term efficacy of spinal morphine in chronic non malignant pain. *Regional Anesthesia and Pain Medicine.* 2006; **31**: 47.
35. Anderson VC, Burchiel KJ. A prospective study of long term intrathecal morphine in the management of non malignant pain. *Neurosurgery.* 1999; **44**: 289–300.
36. Hassembusch SJ, Stanton-Hicks M, Covington EC *et al.* Long term intraspinal infusions of opioids in the treatment of neuropathic pain. *Journal of Pain and Symptom Management.* 1995; **10**: 527–43.
37. Tutak U, Doleys DM. Intrathecal infusion systems for treatment of chronic low back pain and leg pain of noncancer origin. *Southern Medical Journal.* 1996; **89**: 295–300.
38. Winkelmüller M, Winkelmüller W. Long term effects of continuous intrathecal opioid treatment in chronic pain of nonmalignant aetiology. *Journal of Neurosurgery.* 1996; **85**: 458–67.
39. Wallace MS, Charapata SG, Fisher R. Intrathecal ziconotide in the treatment of chronic nonmalignant pain: a randomised double blind controlled clinical trial. *Neuromodulation.* 2006; **9**: 75–86.
40. Rauch RL, Wallace MS, Leong M *et al.* A randomised, double blind, placebo controlled study of intrathecal ziconotide in adults with severe chronic pain. *Journal of Pain and Symptom Management.* 2006; **31**: 393–406.
41. Thimineur MA, Kravitz E, Vodapally MS. Intrathecal opioid treatment for chronic nonmalignant pain; a 3 year prospective study. *Pain.* 2004; **109**: 242–9.
42. Penn RD, Savoy SM, Corcos D *et al.* Intrathecal baclofen for severe spinal spasticity. *New England Journal of Medicine.* 1989; **320**: 1517–21.
43. Penn RD. Intrathecal baclofen for spasticity of spinal origin: seven years of experience. *Journal of Neurosurgery.* 1992; **77**: 236–40.
44. Ochs G, Struppler A, Myerson B *et al.* Intrathecal baclofen for long term treatment of spasticity: a multi centre study. *Journal of Neurology, Neurosurgery and Psychiatry.* 1989; **52**: 933–9.
45. Lazorthes Y, Sallerin-Caute B, Verdic JC. Chronic intrathecal baclofen administration for the control of severe spasticity. *Journal of Neurosurgery.* 1990; **72**: 393–402.
46. Loubser PG, Narayan RK, Sandin KJ *et al.* Intrathecal baclofen: long term effects on spasticity in spinal cord injury. *Paraplegia.* 1991; **29**: 48–64.
47. Coffey RJ, Cahill D, Steers W *et al.* Intrathecal baclofen for intractable spasticity of spinal origin. *Journal of Neurosurgery.* 1993; **78**: 226–32.
48. Southall J, Beddall C, Raphael JH. Cost utility analysis of intrathecal pump implant for chronic non malignant low back pain. *Neuromodulation.* 2006; **9**: 156–7.
49. Sampson FC, Hayward A, Evans G *et al.* Functional benefits and cost/benefit analysis of continuous baclofen for the management of severe spasticity. *Journal of Neurosurgery.* 2002; **96**: 1052–7.
* 50. Grond S, Zech D, Schug SA *et al.* Validation for the World Health Organisation guidelines for cancer pain relief in the

last days or hours of life. *Journal of Pain and Symptom Management.* 1991; **6**: 411–22.

* 51. Zech DFJ, Grond S, Lyon J *et al.* Validation of the World Health Organisation guidelines for cancer pain relief: a 10 year prospective study. *Pain.* 1995; **63**: 65–76.
* 52. Stjernsward J, Colleau SM, Ventafridda V. The World Health Organisation Cancer Pain and Palliative Care Program: past, present and future. *Journal of Pain and Symptom Management.* 1996; **12**: 65–72.

53. Raphael JH, Southall JL, Gnanadurai TV *et al.* Long term experience with implanted intrathecal systems for failed back syndrome and chronic mechanical back pain. *BMC Muskuloskeletal Disorders.* 2002; **3**: 17–25.

22

Cognitive-behavior therapy for chronic pain in adults

STEPHEN MORLEY AND CHRISTOPHER ECCLESTON

KEY LEARNING POINTS

- Cognitive-behavior therapy (CBT) is a complex treatment developed from principles of learning theory and empirical studies of cognition.
- Effective implementation of CBT should be based on an explicit treatment protocol, careful attention to multidisciplinary teamwork, and supervision.
- Chronic pain patients frequently experience comorbid symptoms of anxiety and depression. Patients' approach to pain is construed as one of inappropriate and ineffective problem solving.
- The aims of CBT are to increase physical and occupational activity and to decrease disability and emotional distress through behavioral strategies for managing activity and social interactions, and cognitive strategies to address the subjective and emotional experience of chronic pain.
- CBT is delivered via a collaborative engagement between the patient and the therapist or therapeutic team.
- CBT is an effective treatment for chronic pain as judged by evidence from meta-analyses of randomized controlled trials (RCT).

INTRODUCTION

This chapter introduces the principles of cognitive-behavior therapy, its therapeutic aims, and the evidence for its effectiveness. Finally, we discuss possible developments for treatment.

The most common psychological treatments in the fields of pain, physical health, and rehabilitation are cognitive-behavioral. Other psychological treatments are practiced, but are rarely researched or reported. The treatment of choice for the rehabilitation of patients presenting with persistent and unremitting chronic pain is cognitive-behavior therapy (CBT) for which the evidence of effectiveness has been reported.[1, 2, 3][I] Contemporary CBT has developed from several sources. The earliest was operant behavioral analysis, in which the focus of treatment is the manipulation of the contingencies and reinforcer value.[4] The second development was the respondent formulation of pain that identified the pain–tension cycle as a focus of treatment and led to the introduction of relaxation to break the pain–tension cycle. The third development introduced cognitive therapy, first with methods of distraction and imagery and later with methods of self-talk.[5] Both manipulations were aimed at changing the way in which individuals experienced pain. These elements have been combined in varying degrees with a generic cognitive-behavioral approach and additional elements drawn from cognitive therapy for depression, particularly identifying and challenging unhelpful thought content and processes, are also included. At present, most psychological treatments for pain are multicomponent and frequently delivered in a multidisciplinary format to groups of patients as a Pain Management Program (PMP).[1]

THE ADULT WITH CHRONIC PAIN

Adults with chronic pain present to healthcare settings primarily with the symptom of persistent or recurrent pain. The overall population reporting chronic pain is large (see Chapter 5, Epidemiology of chronic pain: classical to molecular approaches to understanding the epidemiology of pain). However, we are concerned here with those who report chronic pain but who are also highly distressed and disabled, and who repeatedly present for a wide range of treatments.

Chronic pain patients often complain of disability and enforced inactivity associated with poor sleep patterns and fatigue. Chronic pain and disability may lead to an impoverished social environment and loss of valued work, family, and social roles.[6] Particularly distressing can be an unwanted and countertherapeutic reliance upon social care and medical support systems. It is common, for example, for people to continue to seek and receive ineffective treatments over long periods of time.[7]

The constant demand to react and adapt to pain and its associated disabling consequences also results in emotional problems. Principal among them is the development of a pattern of pain-related fear that is itself distressing, but is also thought to be a factor in the maintenance of chronic disability.[8][IV] Typical targets of fear (or fear-provoking stimuli) for chronic pain patients are physical activity and movement, or even the thought of physical activity and movement. Movement is often associated with the catastrophic belief that increased pain and (re)injury will occur.[9] These fears may be specific to the patient group, e.g. the fear for chronic low back pain patients that a back-stressing movement, such as lifting, will lead to disk damage.

Chronic pain patients also report low mood and depression, anger, and frustration.[10, 11, 12, 13][IV] In general medical practice, there is a longstanding concern about the underdiagnosis of depression associated with illness or disability, a situation that is also relevant to chronic pain. There is a less well-recognized risk of overdiagnosis when almost all the widely used diagnostic criteria and self-report questionnaires include somatic symptoms, such as low energy, fatigue, sleep disturbance, and poor libido, which may also be attributable to pain.[14] The dominant psychological model is the diathesis and stress model: the diathesis, or vulnerability to depression, consists of previous depression or pre-pain experiences which may heighten the risk of becoming depressed; and the stress consists of pain and its negative impact on the individual's life.[10] There is an urgent need for better understanding of the significance of previous depression, and the process of acceptance and adaptation.[15, 16, 17] There may also be depressive content and cognitive processing specific to chronic pain which warrants more careful identification and targeted treatment. As in depression without chronic pain, it may be that the efficacy of antidepressants has been overestimated and cognitive-behavior treatment is appropriate for depression or depressed mood in the context of chronic pain. Severe depression in the context of chronic pain needs immediate attention because of the risk of suicide and because pain treatment cannot proceed until the patient is able to foresee some worthwhile future.[18, 19][I]

Prolonged pain, disability, and depression will affect everyday cognition. Patients commonly complain of cognitive problems, such as difficulties in concentration and focused attention.[20, 21] These effects are likely to reduce everyday problem-solving abilities and to affect confidence in attempting social re-entry. Chronic pain patients often present with a range of problems in addition to persistent pain. This complex presentation has often been referred to as a syndrome, as it is largely a collection of associated and interlocking problems.

There is often a danger in this summarizing of a complex clinical presentation that we might unintentionally imply that an underlying vulnerability of psychopathology is the common feature of chronic pain patients. There is no evidence, however, for the claim that all chronic pain patients share a common psychopathology. Instead, this syndrome of distress can usefully be understood as resulting from a normal response of people to a fundamentally abnormal situation: pain that does not subside. People persevere and sometimes perseverate in ineffective and frustrating attempts to escape from pain and distress.[22, 23, 24][IV]

AIMS OF TREATMENT

Aims or targets of treatment are constructed within healthcare systems largely in reflection of the value system of a specific culture. Wealthy medicalized cultures often have two sets of competing values clasped nervously together: first, the prolongation of life in complete mental and physical perfection, characterized by the total absence of illness or decay (see, for example, the World Health Organization's definition of health, "Health is not only the absence of infirmity and disease but also a state of physical, mental and social well-being"); second, the personal and social management of a natural progression of aging, characterized by the shift to nonphysical life goals and the investment in social and community services.

The pain clinic is an environment where there exists a clash on an almost daily basis of these two broad social values. Services for most people with chronic pain are often provided within acute medical settings by practitioners trained in methods of symptom control. However, chronic pain patients present with the syndrome of physical, psychological, and social problems outlined. Some studies have attempted to capture this clash of values in action. One example is of the physician focused on symptom control, while the patient seeks the solution to a wider range of problems. A second example is of the contrary situation in which the patient is focused on the need for the problem of pain to be fixed and the physician is attempting to introduce a broader behavioral context of the problem and its treatment. Cognitive-behavior therapy is often used with chronic pain patients for some, and occasionally all, of the following goals:

- improved physical fitness;
- reduced disability;
- (re)introduction into a work environment;
- increase in effective problem solving;
- increase in adaptive behavior;
- reduction in pain-related fear;
- reduction in pain-related depression.

At this point one might be forgiven for asking, "Is there anything CBT doesn't do?" The point is, of course, that CBT is an inclusive term for a range of techniques framed within a common philosophical approach and implemented as a complex, multicomponent treatment. This approach characterizes the average pain patient as suffering from the ineffective and repetitive application of normal psychological processes within the fundamentally abnormal context of intractable pain. CBT is not the right approach for all patients and the same package of CBT will not work for all patients. Ideally, any program of therapy should be tailored to patient need given the available skills and resources of the treatment environment. Of critical importance to the effectiveness of any program of CBT is a working consensus on: (1) the aims of treatment; (2) how to measure change; and (3) which active components of treatment are to be used and in what format.

PRINCIPLES OF CBT-BASED PAIN MANAGEMENT PROGRAMS

General requirements

The description of components listed below does not constitute a set of instructions for the uninitiated. It is a description of what is carried out by trained professionals with the relevant skills and knowledge.

QUALIFIED STAFF

The success of CBT is critically dependent upon the expertise and experience of the staff. Most programs include personnel with qualifications in medicine, psychology, nursing, and physical and occupational therapy. These staff should have received additional training in pain management. It is important to note that unlike pharmacological interventions, where the quality of the medicine is controlled in the manufacturing process, psychological treatments are essentially manufactured *de novo* each time they are delivered.[25] Programs should therefore use protocols that provide clear guidance to the sequence and structure of therapy sessions and provide a framework in which clinical skills are practiced. Regular supervision should occur to ensure adherence to the protocol, facilitate sustained clinical competence and development, and aid problem solving when the team need to deviate from the protocol for therapeutic purposes. Staff cohesion flourishes where they have good opportunities to work together, to discuss patient's needs and how they are best met, to train together, and where there is mutual respect and clarity of the roles of different disciplines. This is not to suggest that there is no substantial overlap between disciplines in some skills and knowledge, but in a team which functions well this contributes to a consistent message to patients and not to disputes about professional boundaries.

COLLABORATIVE AND CONSULTATIVE ENGAGEMENT

Eliciting and working with material of personal relevance to participants is of paramount importance. Staff should aim for an interactive collaborative and consultative engagement with patients to elicit patients' difficulties and struggles as the material for demonstrating applicability of pain management methods. This consultative style also maximizes involvement of patients in sharing solutions, with the benefits of easing the burden on the staff member, facilitating motivation, and increasing the credibility of solutions discussed.[26][V]

EMPATHIC DISCUSSION AND RECOGNITION OF LIMITATIONS

Life can be very hard for some patients and difficulties raised may be partly or entirely outside the remit of pain management or the influence of staff. Many housing and social welfare difficulties, and family disturbances, come in this category. Empathic discussion and recognition of limitations (and of possible other sources of support or help) is preferable to either negation of the problem or overambitious suggestions that pain management will solve it.

ACTIVE PRACTICING OF SKILLS

A major goal of CBT is to produce behavior change to enhance patients' behavioral repertoire and coping strategies. Behavior change requires practice: even work on very minor or small-scale goals under the supervision of staff will establish the methods of behavior change and ensure that the patient is trying what they have been taught. Attempts to cover all information of possible use to all members of the group tend to result in a didactic style and little opportunity for behavioral experiment. It is better to back up teaching with written information and to provide time and support for patients to attempt and practice desired changes. We make a distinction between active practicing of skills and behavioral experiments in that behavioral experiments are specific technical strategies employed in CBT to test patients' hypotheses and predictions about their behavior.[27] [V]

INTEGRATION AND SYNERGY

Program components should build on and facilitate one another, rather than being additive or complementary. For instance, education on how the spine works helps the patient to challenge unrealistic fears about possible damage from lifting; challenging those fears enables the patient to work both on back strength in exercise sessions and on practical lifting tasks related to work requirements.

Components of CBT

The following constitute the major – but not all – components provided by CBT-based chronic PMPs. The integrated and multidisciplinary delivery of PMPs means that components are not necessarily delivered by a single discipline and may characterize some of the work of all disciplines.

EDUCATION

In some programs, education about pain is restricted to specific information about pain management strategies, or about models of pain, most often drawing the distinctions between acute and chronic pain and explaining the integration of psychological and physical influences on the pain experience. More extensive implementations include comprehensive and integrated educational material that explicitly underpins changes in behavior and cognition practiced in other parts of the program. Ideally, general educational material should be enhanced by specific information that enables formulation of patients' problems to be made to guide specific interventions. This approach is most explicit in individualized programs such as that developed from the fear-avoidance model.[28, 29] Evidence from RCTs shows that education *per se* has a small but significant effect and CBT adds to this effect.[3] [I]

Programs frequently provide written supplements to educational sessions and workbooks for patients to review their learning and improve their understanding. Written information facilitates the communication of program aims and methods. The source of communication is also important. The most credible source of information about the body and pain is a medical doctor specialized in pain who is willing to answer questions on treatment and to acknowledge the uncertainties in our understanding of pain. Similarly, a pharmacist's professional knowledge of drug treatments, their side effects, and interactions is often highly valued by patients.

GOAL SETTING

Goal setting may encompass targeting particular areas for all patients, e.g. work or domestic duties, to individualized and iterative goal setting. Patients find it hard to set goals and aiming to restore pre-pain activities may not be appropriate. Goals, such as reducing work hours, may be the means to improve quality of life and should not be rejected. Obstacles, pain-related or otherwise, to goal attainment should be identified and consideration given to how other aspects of the program might address these. A good strategy is to teach the specification of interim and proximal goals, often as simple as sitting or walking tolerances, and the application of a steady incremental approach known as pacing, with the particular activity carried out in a time-contingent manner. Thus, a patient would be encouraged to plan to do a task for a specific period of time rather than engaging in it until the task is completed. For example, the task of doing the family ironing can be partitioned into periods of 10 or 15 minutes with intermittent rest rather than achieving it in an unrelenting period of an hour or more.

RELAXATION

This may be taught using a single technique, such as diaphragmatic breathing or progressive muscular relaxation, but patients may find one technique easier to use than another and may learn to use different techniques in different settings.[30, 31] [V] It is preferable to aim for a well-integrated and broadly applied set of techniques that facilitate goal attainment. Biofeedback is an effective technique for pain control and is more commonly used in the USA than elsewhere,[32] but it is not essential to the process of achieving relaxation. Practice of techniques while moving, exercising, and otherwise working on goals is necessary to improve generalization.

EXERCISE AND FITNESS TRAINING

Many programs include regular exercise and fitness training. This may range from written or verbal advice on posture, body mechanics, ergonomics, and recommended exercise routines through to specific exercises and techniques targeted at movement and exercise integrated with the patient's physical strength and deficits and with their personal goals. In the spirit of self-management, the use of hands-on techniques by therapists, which cannot be reproduced by patients in their own environments, is best kept to a minimum. The easily quantifiable nature of exercise (by repetitions, time, or resistance) makes recording of goal attainment simple, and contingency management (see below under Operant principles) can be applied by staff and by patients to enable them to recognize and reward successes and steady progress.

Behavioral change

The methods outlined above will have an impact on behavior and this section considers two methods that specifically target behavior change using explicit psychological principles. Behavioral change is achieved by a set of techniques requiring systematic application to the patients' own personal difficulties, which demand ingenuity in application. At a simple level, patients can be given information on changing habits using cues, practice techniques, and targeted reinforcement.

OPERANT PRINCIPLES

Historically, the application of operant-conditioning principles to chronic pain[4] focused on several aspects of behavior: verbal expression of pain – including paravocalizations, nonverbal behavior such as guarding and bracing, reduced general activity levels, and medication consumption.[33] Application of operant principles requires a functional analysis of the target behavior(s) to identify the antecedents (e.g. presence of others, type of social interaction, physical setting) where the behavior is most likely to occur or where the behavior appears to be inhibited.[34] Identification of the setting conditions and discriminative stimuli that appear to control the behavior is a critical component of the functional analysis. The second part of the analysis identifies current reinforcement contingencies. Two types of reinforcement maintain behavior: positive reinforcement, i.e. the contingent occurrence of an event (subjectively perceived as a pleasant event) that increases the behavior (in pain it may be the expression of concern by another) and negative reinforcement of a behavior, i.e. the removal of an event (subjectively often experienced as aversive), which similarly increases the behavior. Given that pain is inherently aversive it is easy to see that activities (or lack of activity) that reduce pain are readily negatively reinforced (i.e. the reduction of pain serves to increase the behavior that reduces pain). There are several strategies available to the therapist including the removal of the positive reinforcers (extinction), changing the antecedents, and gradually shaping new behavioral repertoires that are incompatible with pain behavior. Operant principles are often incorporated into CBT programs and used to help patients and partners change the way in which they interact.[35, 36][II]

BEHAVIORAL EXPERIMENTS: THE EXAMPLE OF EXPOSURE AND RESPONSE PREVENTION

Behavioral experiments are an integral part of mainstream cognitive therapy[27] and seen as a significant vehicle for producing cognitive and behavioral change. Behavioral experiments are developed to test individual's beliefs about the consequences (emotional, behavioral, and cognitive) of either engaging or not engaging in particular behaviors. Behavioral experiments can be used to help with many of the problems that are experienced by patients with chronic pain. The clearest example of the use of behavioral experimentation has emerged in the therapeutic application of the fear-avoidance model.[28, 29] [III] This model proposes that a proportion of chronic pain patients are inactive because they fear that movement will produce physical damage to their bodies, i.e. their behavior is negatively reinforced by the avoidance and reduction of anxiety. Treatment comprises analyses of the patient's avoidance behavior and the development of a hierarchy of feared situations. Patients' predictions about what will happen if they engage in the feared behavior are elicited and subsequently tested by helping them to complete the behavior while not escaping from the situation; this leads to disconfirmation of their predictions, fear reduction, and increased behavioral activity.

Cognitive therapy

ATTENTION MANAGEMENT

At its simplest, attention management consists of provision of advice on one or more methods, such as the use of distraction or imagery control techniques. More advanced forms require patients to practice a range of attention-centering techniques that provoke a dissociation of self from both pain and pain-related automatic negative thoughts, providing an internal observation or metacognitive perspective on harmful self-talk.[37] A free comprehensive manual is available at www.leeds.ac.uk/hsphr/psychiatry/staff/morley.htm.

COGNITIVE RESTRUCTURING

This includes a variety of methods aimed at changing both the content and process of thinking. Cognitive change requires access to emotionally significant material and written or verbal instruction alone is unlikely to have sufficient impact except in the most resourceful and least distressed patients. Therapists aim to elicit the appraisals, attributions, biased thinking patterns, and negative emotions from patients. These become the material on which the techniques are demonstrated and practiced. Instruction in a variety of coping skills may well expose patients to novel strategies, but teaching cognitive coping skills is best undertaken with reference to patients' existing skills, their range of skills, and the appropriateness with which they apply particular strategies to difficult situations. Beverly Thorn has written a comprehensive manual.[38, 39][V]

PROBLEM SOLVING

Problem solving is often implicit in programs rather than taught as a separate component. It involves identification of the problem, generation of a range of possible solutions, prioritizing among those solutions according to opportunities, resources, and risks, and then attempting them. Many patients appear to use a narrow range of strategies, such as forcing themselves to persist when they meet an obstacle, which succeeds in some situations but rarely in chronic pain. Experimenting with different ways of tackling problems is an important experience for changing habits and beliefs about "the right/best way to do things." Although specific problem-solving strategies are still being researched,[23, 24, 40][IV] creative attempts are needed by therapists to introduce patients to new methods of problem solving and to recognition that some problems are insoluble.[22]

Generalization and maintenance strategies

A thorough program will pay attention to generalizing treatment gains and developing maintenance strategies.[41] Although this component of CBT remains under-researched, strategies include scheduled reviews of homework with a therapist, and developing strategies for relapse prevention, e.g. *a priori* recognition of vulnerabilities and learning how to handle crises. Where possible, the involvement of family members and other important people in the patient's environment should be incorporated into the program. Communication skills, particularly where family members cannot attend the treatment, include assertion skills, discussion of pain behavior and its effects on other people, and listening skills. Particular areas for application of communication skills, which may be discussed during the program, include consultation with health professionals and negotiations with potential or actual employers.

For all of the components, adherence to program content and methods is important. One dimension of this is checking that patients are, in fact, doing as instructed, whether it is relaxing during relaxation sessions or monitoring thoughts when distressed. Staff adherence to the treatment protocol, irrespective of discipline, is important: inconsistency in therapy or in providing explanations undermines the efficacy of the technique and patents' confidence in staff. To help maintain consistency, protocols for each component of the program should be regularly reviewed in the light of local outcomes and published evidence.

THE EVIDENCE BASE

Despite the complexity of CBT and the heterogeneity of the client group, there are a large number of treatment evaluations reported and a respectable number of randomized controlled trials. Reviews of CBT for chronic pain in adults have reported strong evidence for the efficacy of CBT in restoring function and mood and in reducing pain and disability-related behavior. Evidence for CBT ranges from unimodal treatments, such as biofeedback to complex multicomponent packages and studies fall into the top three categories of Bandolier's criteria:

[I] At least one systematic review of multiple RCTs, for example, Refs 2, 3, 42, 43.

[II] At least one RCT of appropriate size and setting. There are approximately 50 RCTs. Early publications reported small samples ($n<20$ per arm), but more recent ones have used adequate statistical power.[44]

[III] Well designed, nonrandomized ... time series. There are many good pre-post studies and more recently researchers have used single case methods to evaluate new treatments.[45, 46, 47]

Perhaps the most detailed analysis of CBT for chronic pain is that published by Morley *et al.*[3] This work is currently being updated with additional refinements, but it is not sufficiently advanced to include the results in this chapter. We therefore report our earlier analysis in some depth to illustrate some of the complexities in evaluating CBT as a treatment for chronic pain. This will highlight some of the methodological problems in both conducting meta-analytic reviews and individual RCTs and report on some recent developments.

Critical evaluation of a meta-analysis of CBT

In preparing this study,[3] we made a number of *a priori* assumptions and exclusions. First, chronic pain was accepted as a label for a heterogeneous group of pain problems in which diagnosis, site of pain, or medical findings were not apparent major sources of variance in any of the targets of treatment. This probably reflects the assumptions made in many PMPs in clinical settings. Second, we excluded studies of psychological treatments of headache because the episodic nature of chronic headache is markedly different from nonheadache. Third, we also excluded trials reporting the effectiveness of psychological treatments for children with chronic pain, see Ref. 48[I]. The study was designed to answer two questions.

1. Absolute efficacy – is CBT an effective treatment for chronic pain, i.e. is it "better" than no treatment?
2. Relative efficacy – is CBT more effective than alternative active treatments?

To answer the first question, we compared active CBT with waiting list control groups, and to answer the second question we identified active non-CBT treatments as the contrast. We identified papers in the English language reporting 25 trials containing controlled comparisons of CBT and data suitable for analysis. Information from the trials was extracted and coded using criteria developed for the study including details of trial design, participants, the treatments, and outcome measures used, and statistical data on differences in outcomes. As an ideal, all trials would use the same outcome measures and have similar design features, e.g. identical treatment and control conditions, homogeneous diagnostic groups. While pharmacological treatments approximate this (comparison between active and placebo groups and a single "simple" outcome such as pain reduction), the situation is substantially different where complex interventions such as psychological treatments are concerned. Meta-analysts face a number of problems concerning the methods of how to aggregate and combine information.

OUTCOMES: EFFECT SIZES AND CLINICAL SIGNIFICANCE

The first problem concerned the type of data available for analysis. Many psychological measures are continuous rather than dichotomous. As a consequence, results are reported as mean differences between groups rather than as proportions of patients meeting a predetermined criterion of wellness. The metric used for continuous measures is the effect size (ES). The ES is computed by dividing the difference between the treatment and control group scores at the end of treatment by the pooled standard deviations of the samples. Adjustments are made for differing sample sizes and we also made a further adjustment to try to estimate the "true" difference between treatments by correcting the ES for the impact of the reliability of the measures used. This is important when the analysis includes ES values estimated from a range of measures which differ in reliability as the variation in reliability adds unwanted "noise" to the data.

MULTIPLE OUTCOMES IN TRIALS

The second problem concerned how to manage data from trials containing multiple different outcome measures. First, we identified different measurement domains (see **Table 22.1**) and conducted separate analyses on these domains. Outcomes were allocated to domains, although there were too few data in some of the domains to permit analysis. Second, where studies used more than one outcome measure in a given domain, one measure was selected using the criteria of widespread use and reliability.

MULTIPLE TRIAL ARMS

The third problem was how to manage multiarmed trials, i.e. trials that compared two or more treatments with a control. This presents two issues: (1) how to classify and combine treatment groups and (2) the choice of comparison (control) group for estimating ES values. We estimated treatment effects by including all treatment arms within a trial and acknowledged that the mean of the combined ES estimates in this comparison were not independent because those drawn from a single trial had a common control condition. Coding the details of treatments reported in the papers revealed wide variation between treatments described with a generic term, for example cognitive therapy, but there was marked variability between studies in the detail provided. We categorized the treatments into three primary classes: biofeedback and relaxation, behavior therapy, and cognitive-behavior therapy. We anticipated that further

Table 22.1 Outcome domains for cognitive-behavior therapy.

Domain name	Definition and example measures
Pain experience	Measures of subjective pain experience: McGill Pain Questionnaire, visual and numerical scales
Mood/affect	Primary measure of mood or affective state: Beck Depression Inventory
Cognitive – coping and appraisal	Reports of cognitive strategies – subsequently divided into negative strategies known to be associated with poor outcome, e.g. catastrophizing, and positive strategies, e.g. active coping strategies: Cognitive Strategies Questionnaire
Pain behavior	Overt behavioral acts associated with pain – there were two subcategories: pain behavior referring to behavior that signals the presence of pain, e.g. guarding, and activity level, e.g. distance walked: Pain Observation Scale
Social role performance	Assessments of the impact of pain on the ability of a person to function in various social roles: Sickness Impact Profile
Biological and physical fitness measures	Assessment of biological function: VO_{max}, joint flexibility
Use of healthcare services	Clinic visits and drug consumption
Miscellaneous	All other measures: pain drawings, repertory grids

analyses might be possible by estimating the mean ES values for treatments with common ingredients. Ultimately, these analyses were not possible as there were too few trials in some of the classes. We identified two classes of control group: (1) waiting list control (WLC), where no new treatment was prescribed, although some WLC patients obtained some treatment, e.g. continued medication; and (2) treatment control (TC), in which a participant was allocated to a new or defined treatment for the duration of the trial. The TC conditions comprised a heterogeneous collection of treatments, including access to regular treatment provided in a pain clinic, physiotherapy, occupational therapy, and the provision of a standard educational and advice package.

We conducted two analyses comparing active treatments with WLC and then comparing active treatments with TC. As the studies also used more than one potential control group, some studies contributed data to both comparisons. The results of the analyses are shown in **Figures 22.1** and **22.2**. **Figure 22.1** shows the ES values when active CBT was compared with waiting list controls. The average effect sizes are shown with their 95 percent confidence intervals. In no case does the lower confidence interval cross the x-axis where the ES = 0, providing evidence that receiving CBT is reliably more effective than merely waiting for treatment. Treatment gains cannot therefore be explained by the passage of time or the effects of repeated measurement.

Figure 22.2 shows the results when CBT is compared with other active treatments. In this figure, the range bars representing the 95 percent confidence intervals for the mean ES either embrace the horizontal dashed line, which represents no difference between treatments or, in the case of three comparisons, shows that CBT is superior. The overall conclusion is that as a class of treatment CBT is at least as good as other active treatments for chronic pain.

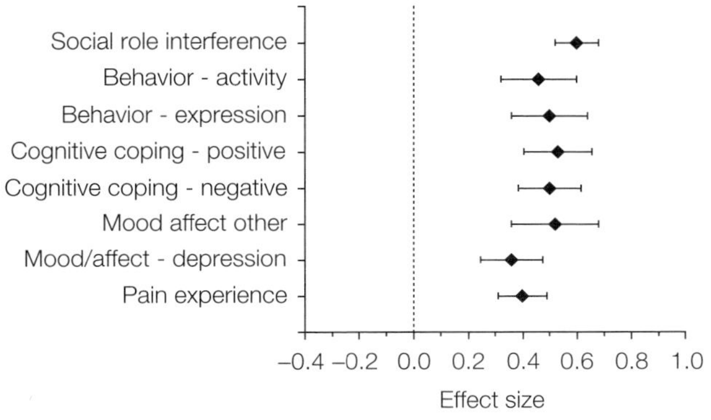

Figure 22.1 The mean effect size values and 95% confidence intervals for all the measurement domains when active cognitive therapy is compared with waiting list control. The vertical dotted line indicates an effect size = 0, i.e. no effect.

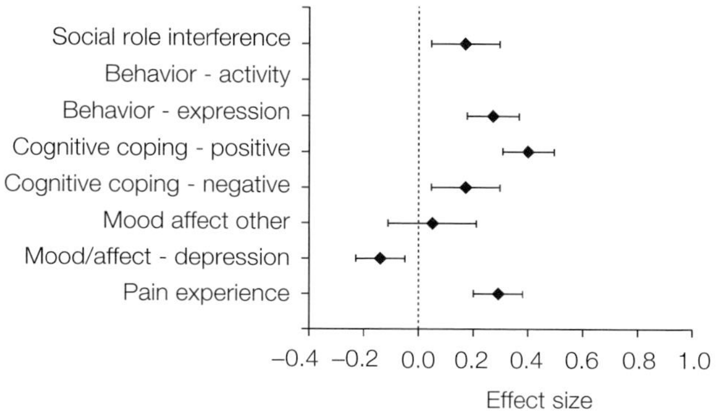

Figure 22.2 The mean effect size values and 95% confidence intervals for all the available measurement domains when active cognitive therapy is compared with active treatment control. The vertical dotted line indicates an effect size = 0, i.e. no effect.

CRITICAL OVERVIEW OF THE STUDY – ISSUES OF TRIAL QUALITY

While this work concluded that CBT is an effective treatment, improvement to the design and conduct of treatment trials can be made. For example, we concluded that most trials were statistically underpowered and that some trials were overcomplex with multiple treatment and control groups. The content and differentiation of control groups from treatment requires more consideration. Patients assigned to a waiting list in one trial may continue to receive existing treatments that may be equivalent to the treatment control in another trial. The distinction between the content of an active treatment and a control condition can be a fine one. Allocation to a control condition will have different psychological consequences from allocation to an active treatment, even if that treatment is based on predominantly non-psychological principles, e.g. physical therapy. There was variation in quality and quantity of treatment given. Some authors gave explicit accounts of the treatment procedures with reference to manualized interventions which were appropriately monitored, but this was not universally so. We also noted a paucity of information about the impact of CBT on economically important outcomes.

We have sought to quantify the quality of trials by developing a quality scale (QS) designed specifically for complex psychological treatments. Most published quality scales evaluate important biases (e.g. compromised randomization), but some of these are not applicable to psychological treatments. The extant quality scales pay scant attention to important aspects of treatment administration. Yates *et al.*[49] obtained consensus agreement on the desirable content of a QS from a set of experts. The final scale contained items measuring both methodological quality and the quality of treatment implementation. Studies were carried out to assess the scale's reliability and validate its use and these provided formal evidence of our conclusions about trial quality. Yates *et al.* also examined six more recently published trials and the analysis indicated that the quality of trials appears to be improving. Future meta-analysis of trials will be able to examine the influence of overall trial quality and of specific features, for example duration of treatment, on outcome. Furthermore, more advanced statistical analysis that can incorporate the complexities of trial design (multiple trial arms and multiple outcomes) will circumvent some of the compromises made in the original meta-analysis.

Finally, trialists are beginning to report outcomes as the proportion of patients showing clinical improvement on a given variable, rather than a mean difference score. The main method for this is the application of the reliable change index and clinically significant change criteria[50, 51, 52] to dichotomize continuous measures using the statistical and normative properties of the outcome measure. Although this approach is not free of problems, it enables researchers to express outcomes in terms that might be more widely understood.[25]

FUTURE OF CBT FOR CHRONIC PAIN

Clinical researchers are constantly striving to improve the effectiveness of treatments. A traditional strategy has been to try to identify characteristics that define patient responsiveness to treatment and to use these criteria in several ways: (1) to select patients; (2) to attempt to understand what it is about these characteristics that influence responsiveness to treatments; or (3) to develop customized treatments for specific subgroups of patients. On balance, this approach has yet to be successful. The major issues in developing customized treatments are discussed in a special section of the *Clinical Journal of Pain.*[53][V] Rather than pursue these arguments in detail, we suggest that future development in this field may occur in the following ways.

- Refining the theoretical understanding of chronic pain and the development of more specific treatments. The fear-avoidance model[9] is an example of a model-driven approach for which there is some evidence from replicated single case series[45, 47][III] and two small RCTs.[54, 55][II] A second example is the development of a new formulation of chronic pain. Whereas traditional CBT has focused directly on teaching coping strategies and restoring behavioral function, "third-wave CBT" based around the concept of acceptance approaches the problem from a different stance.[56] It is not possible to convey the details of this approach here, but the key issue is that it invites pain sufferers to consider how they can develop valued lives in the presence of persistent pain (see Chapter 13, Psychological effects of chronic pain: an overview). Initial studies, including uncontrolled case series and a small RCT,[57][II], [58, 59][IV] indicate the feasibility and promise of the approach.
- Identifying key cognitive and behavioral changes that mediate outcomes and the therapeutic actions that facilitate these changes. Despite a significant number of randomized controlled trials, there are relatively few studies that have examined processes of change. RCTs provide an opportunity to identify moderators and mediators of treatment and the statistical techniques to model these data are available. Burns and colleagues have tested these methods in single cohort studies[60, 61][IV] and Turner *et al.* have recently applied the method to data from a high quality RCT.[62][II]

CONCLUSIONS

Psychological therapy and, in particular, CBT therapy, for adults with chronic pain are effective treatments for helping patients to manage the deleterious effects of chronic pain. Multidisciplinary CBT has been established practice for over 30 years and the evidence base is now sufficiently robust to allow the research and development of critical aspects of treatment.

REFERENCES

* 1. Gatchel RJ, Okifuji A. Evidence-based scientific data documenting the treatment and cost-effectiveness of comprehensive pain programs for chronic nonmalignant pain. *Journal of Pain.* 2006; **7**: 779–93.
* 2. Hoffman BM, Papas RK, Chatkoff DK, Kerns RD. Meta-analysis of psychological interventions for chronic low back pain. *Health Psychology.* 2007; **26**: 1–9.
* 3. Morley S, Eccleston C, Williams A. Systematic review and meta-analysis of randomized controlled trials of cognitive behaviour therapy and behaviour therapy for chronic pain in adults, excluding headache. *Pain.* 1999; **80**: 1–13.
4. Fordyce WE. *Behavioral methods for chronic pain and illness.* St Louis: Mosby, 1976.
5. Turk DC, Meichenbaum D, Genest M. *Pain and behavioral medicine: a cognitive-behavioral perspective.* New York: Guilford Press, 1983.
6. Harris S, Morley S, Barton SB. Role loss and emotional adjustment in chronic pain. *Pain.* 2003; **105**: 363–70.
7. Sharpe M, Mayou R, Seagroatt V *et al.* Why do doctors find some patients difficult to help? *Quarterly Journal of Medicine.* 1994; **87**: 187–93.
8. Morley S, Eccleston C. The object of fear in pain. In: Asmundson GJ, Vlaeyen J, Crombez G (eds). *Understanding and treating fear of pain.* Oxford: Oxford University Press, 2004: 163–88.

* 9. Vlaeyen JW, Linton SJ. Fear-avoidance and its consequences in chronic musculoskeletal pain: a state of the art. *Pain.* 2000; **85**: 317–32.
* 10. Banks SM, Kerns RD. Explaining high rates of depression in chronic pain: A diathesis-stress framework. *Psychological Bulletin.* 1996; **119**: 95–110.
11. Fernandez E, Turk DC. The scope and significance of anger in the experience of chronic pain. *Pain.* 1995; **61**: 165–75.
12. Wade JB, Dougherty LM, Archer CR, Price DD. Assessing the stages of pain processing: a multivariate analytical approach. *Pain.* 1996; **68**: 157–67.
13. Wade JB, Price DD, Hamer RM *et al.* An emotional component analysis of chronic pain. *Pain.* 1990; **40**: 303–10.
14. Pincus T, Williams A. Models and measurements of depression in chronic pain. *Journal of Psychosomatic Research.* 1999; **47**: 211–9.
15. Pincus T, Morley S. Cognitive-processing bias in chronic pain: a review and integration. *Psychological Bulletin.* 2001; **127**: 599–617.
16. Conner TS, Tennen H, Zautra AJ *et al.* Coping with rheumatoid arthritis pain in daily life: within-person analyses reveal hidden vulnerability for the formerly depressed. *Pain.* 2006; **126**: 198–209.
17. Tennen H, Affleck G, Zautra A. Depression history and coping with chronic pain: a daily process analysis. *Health Psychology.* 2006; **25**: 370–9.
18. Edwards RR, Smith MT, Kudel I, Haythornthwaite J. Pain-related catastrophizing as a risk factor for suicidal ideation in chronic pain. *Pain.* 2006; **126**: 272–9.
* 19. Tang NK, Crane C. Suicidality in chronic pain: a review of the prevalence, risk factors and psychological links. *Psychological Medicine.* 2006; **36**: 575–86.
20. Grisart JM, Plaghki LH. Impaired selective attention in chronic pain patients. *European Journal of Pain.* 1999; **3**: 325–33.
21. Grisart JM, Van der Linden M. Conscious and automatic uses of memory in chronic pain patients. *Pain.* 2001; **94**: 305–13.
22. Aldrich S, Eccleston C, Crombez G. Worrying about chronic pain: vigilance to threat and misdirected problem solving. *Behaviour Research and Therapy.* 2000; **38**: 457–70.
23. De Vlieger P, Bussche EV, Eccleston C, Crombez G. Finding a solution to the problem of pain: conceptual formulation and the development of the Pain Solutions Questionnaire (PaSol). *Pain.* 2006; **123**: 285–93.
24. De Vlieger P, Crombez G, Eccleston C. Worrying about chronic pain. An examination of worry and problem solving in adults who identify as chronic pain sufferers. *Pain.* 2006; **120**: 138–44.
* 25. Morley S. Trial design in psychological treatments: What can we tell patients? In: Moore RA, McQuay HJ (eds). *Systematic reviews in and meta-analyses in pain: Lessons from the past leading to pathways for the future.* Seattle: IASP Press, 2008: 217–32.
* 26. Jensen MP. Enhancing motivation to change in pain treatment. In: Turk DC, Gatchel RJ (eds). *Psychological approaches to pain management: A practitioner's handbook*, 2nd edn. New York: Guilford, 2002: 71–93.
* 27. Bennet-Levy J, Butler G, Fennell M *et al.* (eds). *Oxford guide to behavioural experiments in cognitive therapy. Cognitive Behaviour Therapy: Science and Practice Series.* Oxford: Oxford University Press, 2004: 461.
28. Leeuw M, Vlaeyen J, de Jong J, Goossens ME. *Exposure in vivo bij chronische lage rugpijn (Exposure in vivo for chronic low back pain): A treatment manual.* Amsterdam: Boom, 2006: 64.
* 29. Vlaeyen J, de Jong J, Seiben J, Crombez G. Graded exposure in vivo for pain-related fear. In: Turk DC, Gatchel RJ (eds). *Psychological approaches to pain management: A practitioner's handbook*, 2nd edn. New York: Guilford Press, 2002: 210–33.
30. Bernstein D, Borkovec TD. *Progressive relaxation therapy: A manual for the helping professions.* Champaign, IL: Research Press, 1973.
31. Syrjala KL, Abrams JR. Hypnosis and imagery in the treatment of pain. In: Turk DC, Gatchel RJ (eds). *Psychological approaches to pain management: A practitioner's handbook*, 2nd edn. New York: Guilford Press, 2002: 187–209.
32. Arena JG, Blanchard EB. Biofeedback training for chronic pain disorders. In: Turk DC, Gatchel RJ (eds). *Psychological approaches to pain management: A practitioner's handbook*, 2nd edn. New York: Guilford Press, 2002: 138–58.
33. Sanders SH. Operant conditioning with chronic pain: Back to basics. In: Turk DC, Gatchel RJ (eds). *Psychological approaches to pain management: A practitioner's handbook*, 2nd edn. New York: Guilford Press, 2002: 128–37.
34. Sarafino EP. *Principles of behavior change: understanding behavior modification techniques.* New York: Wiley, 1996.
35. Romano JM, Turner JA, Friedman LS *et al.* Sequential analysis of chronic pain behaviors and spouse responses. *Journal of Consulting and Clinical Psychology.* 1992; **60**: 777–82.
36. Romano JM, Turner JA, Jensen MP *et al.* Chronic pain patient-spouse behavioral interactions predict patient disability. *Pain.* 1995; **63**: 353–60.
37. Morley S, Shapiro DA, Biggs J. Developing a treatment manual for attention management in chronic pain. *Cognitive Behaviour Therapy.* 2004; **33**: 1–11.
* 38. Thorn BE. *Cognitive therapy for chronic pain: A step-by-step guide.* New York: Guilford Press, 2004.
39. Thorn BE, Kuhajda MC. Group cognitive therapy for chronic pain. *Journal of Clinical Psychology.* 2006; **62**: 1355–66.
40. van den Hout JH, Vlaeyen JW, Heuts PH *et al.* Secondary prevention of work-related disability in nonspecific low back pain: does problem-solving therapy help? A randomized clinical trial. *Clinical Journal of Pain.* 2003; **19**: 87–96.
41. Turk DC, Rudy TE. Neglected topics in the treatment of chronic pain patients – relapse, noncompliance, and adherence enhancement. *Pain.* 1991; **44**: 5–28.

42. Guzman J, Esmail R, Karjalainen K *et al.* Multidisciplinary rehabilitation for chronic low back pain: systematic review. *British Medical Journal.* 2001; **322**: 1511–6.
43. Ostelo RW, van Tulder MW, Vlaeyen JW *et al.* Behavioural treatment for chronic low-back pain. *Cochrane Database of Systematic Reviews.* 2005; **CD002014**.
* 44. Turner JA, Mancl L, Aaron LA. Short- and long-term efficacy of brief cognitive-behavioral therapy for patients with chronic temporomandibular disorder pain: a randomized, controlled trial. *Pain.* 2006; **121**: 181–94.
45. Boersma K, Linton S, Overmeer T *et al.* Lowering fear-avoidance and enhancing function through exposure in vivo. A multiple baseline study across six patients with back pain. *Pain.* 2004; **108**: 8–16.
46. de Jong JR, Vlaeyen JW, Onghena P *et al.* Reduction of pain-related fear in complex regional pain syndrome type I: the application of graded exposure in vivo. *Pain.* 2005; **116**: 264–75.
47. Vlaeyen JW, de Jong J, Geilen M *et al.* Graded exposure in vivo in the treatment of pain-related fear: a replicated single-case experimental design in four patients with chronic low back pain. *Behaviour Research and Therapy.* 2001; **39**: 151–66.
48. Eccleston C, Morley S, Williams A *et al.* Systematic review of randomised controlled trials of psychological therapy for chronic pain in children and adolescents, with a subset meta-analysis of pain relief. *Pain.* 2002; **99**: 157–65.
49. Yates SL, Morley S, Eccleston C, Williams ACdeC. A scale for rating the quality of psychological trials for pain. *Pain.* 2005; **117**: 314–25.
50. Atkins DC, Bedics JD, McGlinchey JB, Beauchaine TP. Assessing clinical significance: does it matter which method we use? *Journal of Consulting and Clinical Psychology.* 2005; **73**: 982–9.
* 51. Jacobson NS, Roberts LJ, Berns SB, McGlinchey JB. Methods for defining and determining the clinical significance of treatment effects: description, application, and alternatives. *Journal of Consulting and Clinical Psychology.* 1999; **67**: 300–7.
52. Jacobson NS, Truax P. Clinical significance: a statistical approach to defining meaningful change in psychotherapy research. *Journal of Consulting and Clinical Psychology.* 1991; **59**: 12–9.
53. Vlaeyen JW, Morley S. Cognitive-behavioral treatments for chronic pain: what works for whom? *Clinical Journal of Pain.* 2005; **21**: 1–8.
54. Woods MP, Asmundson GJG. Evaluating the efficacy of graded in vivo exposure for the treatment of fear in patients with chronic back pain: A randomized controlled clinical trial. *Pain.* 2007 Aug 21 [Epub ahead of print] (in press).
55. Leeuw M, Goossens MEJB, Breukelen GJP *et al.* Exposure in vivo versus operant graded activity in chronic low back pain patients: results of a randomized controlled trial. *Pain* (in press).
56. McCracken LM. *Contextual cognitive-behavioral therapy for chronic pain.* Progress in Pain Research and Management 33. Seattle: IASP Press, 2005: 148.
57. Dahl J, Wilson KG, Nilsson A. Acceptance and commitment therapy and the treatment of persons at risk for long-term disability resulting from stress and pain symptoms: a preliminary randomized trial. *Behavior Therapy.* 2004; **35**: 785–801.
58. McCracken LM, Mackichan F, Eccleston C. Contextual cognitive-behavioral therapy for severely disabled chronic pain sufferers: Effectiveness and clinically significant change. *European Journal of Pain.* 2007; **11**: 314–22.
59. McCracken LM, Vowles KE, Eccleston C. Acceptance-based treatment for persons with complex, long standing chronic pain: a preliminary analysis of treatment outcome in comparison to a waiting phase. *Behaviour Research and Therapy.* 2005; **43**: 1335–46.
60. Burns JW, Glenn B, Bruehl S *et al.* Cognitive factors influence outcome following multidisciplinary chronic pain treatment: a replication and extension of a cross-lagged panel analysis. *Behaviour Research and Therapy.* 2003; **41**: 1163–82.
61. Burns JW, Kubilus A, Bruehl S *et al.* Do changes in cognitive factors influence outcome following multidisciplinary treatment for chronic pain? A cross-lagged panel analysis. *Journal of Consulting and Clinical Psychology.* 2003; **71**: 81–91.
* 62. Turner JA, Holtzman S, Mancl L. Mediators, moderators, and predictors of therapeutic change in cognitive-behavioral therapy for chronic pain. *Pain.* 2007; **127**: 276–86.

23

Evaluation of complementary and alternative therapies

MILES J BELGRADE AND CASSANDRA D SCHAMBER

KEY LEARNING POINTS

- Between a quarter to half of the population in developed countries are using complementary or alternative therapies at a cost of nearly $30 billion in the United States alone.
- Complementary and alternative medicine (CAM) spans many broad categories such as culturally based systems of medicine, other systems of medicine such as chiropractic and homeopathy, and individual practices such as massage and meditation.
- Acupuncture has ancient roots, but remains one of the most well-researched of practices.
- Originating in the late eighteenth century as the brainchild of mainly one man, Samuel Hahnemann, homeopathy is based on unique concepts of the energetic properties of matter and the paradoxical idea that potency increases as dilution increases. It is widely practiced in Europe, India, and Asia.
- Based on the premise that spinal misalignment contributes to disease, chiropractic has often been at odds with conventional medicine. It has nevertheless gained legitimacy with recognized licensing and widespread use.
- Botanical therapies may be the oldest alternative medical practice. It is part of many world systems of medicine. Efforts to classify herbs for their safety and efficacy are ongoing.
- Mindful CAM therapies include relaxation breathing, meditation, mindfulness-based stress reduction, self-hypnosis, guided imagery, autogenic training, and progressive muscle relaxation.
- Therapeutic touch, healing touch, Reiki, Qi Gong, and shamanic healing are all examples of energy healing therapies. These therapies are based on the construct that energy flow can be manipulated by practitioners and brought into balance to induce healing and pain relief.
- Helping patients choose CAM therapies should take into consideration the individual and the goals of therapy.
- Unproven herbs or supplements should be avoided in the pregnant patient.
- Active self-care therapies should be emphasized in the passive patient who needs physical rehabilitation.
- Integrating CAM with needed conventional care is critical for the patient with complex medical problems.

INTRODUCTION

The practices of acupuncture, chiropractic, homeopathy, herbal medicine, traditional Chinese medicine are often described as CAM therapies because they lie outside the dominant health system of a western industrialized society. Yet, in many cultures these techniques may be mainstream. Indeed, world health practices are so varied and culturally based that allopathic medicine is a subordinate and foreign alternative to the indigenous medicine of many societies. A chapter such as this one discussing CAM must be written from a regional point of view. This chapter is written from the perspective of a western industrialized society in which allopathic medicine dominates health care, where a biological model of health and disease dictates the approach to healing.

Mainstream medicine relies on pathophysiologic diagnoses derived from history and laboratory investigations, and treatment using pharmaceutical agents, surgery, physical rehabilitation, and radiation therapies. To a lesser extent, a restricted set of behavioral and psychological therapies are also parts of this tradition. The axiomatic foundations of this medicine are the scientific method and the biological sciences that evolve from it. Although many if not most therapies in this system are empirically derived, those therapies that are scientifically derived or validated are the most valued. Those disease states in which the pathophysiology is undetermined or vague tend to be poorly served by this system of medicine that depends so heavily on well-defined pathophysiologic causes of disease.

WHY DO PAIN PATIENTS SEEK CAM?

Pain management is an excellent example of where the biomedical model falls short. First, pain management is, by definition, an experience that is subjective[1] and cannot be measured directly. Second, the pathophysiologic processes that produce clinical pain problems are still incompletely understood. We can only infer what the pathology is in broad generalities – for example, inflammatory, neuropathic, or mechanical. Complex social and psychological factors play such an important role in chronic pain problems that attempts to treat chronic pain exclusively using scientific principles are doomed to fail under our current state of scientific knowledge. Pain has a motivational component, i.e. it is accompanied by a drive to eliminate it. The result is that patients continually seek alternative treatments to eliminate their pain.

All of these conditions lead patients to seek CAM for pain: incomplete pathophysiologic characterization, lack of scientifically derived treatments, inability of allopathic treatments to control the social and psychological components of complex chronic pain, high motivation for symptom elimination, and lack of physician enthusiasm for treatment. In fact, chronic pain may be the affliction physicians are most loath to treat. Many physicians shun the chronic pain patient because they feel powerless to help these individuals who often have unrealistic expectations and require large amounts of time during and after office hours. It is no wonder that these patients look elsewhere for help.

Astin[2] identified chronic pain as a predictor of CAM use. Other predictors included poorer health status, more education, anxiety, back problems, urinary tract problems, interest in spirituality and personal growth psychology, and having had a change in philosophy of life. Interestingly, dissatisfaction with conventional medicine did not predict the use of CAM. In fact, only about 4 percent of individuals report relying exclusively on CAM.[2, 3]

The discomfort of allopathic treatments is often a deterrent for patients. Surgical treatments carry inevitable discomfort and recovery periods of varying degrees. Pharmaceuticals' side effects frequently interfere with normal functioning. The public's perception of these agents as foreign substances can even result in avoidance of medicines that are usually well tolerated. These "costs" of allopathic treatment also fuel the flight to "natural" alternatives.

Patients seeking treatment for pain want physicians to listen to them and to believe them. These elements of the physician–patient relationship are as important as successful pain reduction.[4] Yet, time constraints and productivity expectations on physicians by disinterested third parties may reduce the listening time to ten minutes or less. The solo practitioner of a complementary or alternative therapy may offer 30 to 60 minutes of unhurried time to listen to their patients and satisfy that essential ingredient of success.

Prevalence

Several large surveys in the United States, Europe, and Australia have demonstrated the extent of CAM use by the public. According to the Centers for Disease Control and Prevention, in 2002 36 percent of US adults used some form of CAM therapy and if prayer was included, the number increased to 62 percent.[5] Use of these therapies was most prominent for back problems, upper respiratory infections, and neck problems. In 2001, Millar[6] reported that 17 percent of Canadians visited an alternative health care practitioner in 1998/1999. MacLennan *et al.*[7] reported that approximately 49 percent of Australians used CAM in 1993. In England in 1998 the prevalence of CAM use was 28 percent.[8] The prevalence in Denmark in 2003 was 20 percent.[9] A survey published in Germany in 2004 found a prevalence of CAM use of 70 percent for women and 54 percent for men.[10] The use of CAM is increasing at a rapid rate. In Italy the prevalence almost doubled from 1991 to 1999 to an estimated use of 15 percent.[11] Estimates of prevalence may vary widely depending on the study methods used. The choice of study population and the scope of what is considered complementary or alternative medicine will greatly impact prevalence estimates. For example, the use of prayer or local heat and ice are such common practices that it would be misleading to include these in survey data.

In the United States, the high rates of CAM use crosses socioeconomic, racial, and geographic boundaries; but those who used CAM in 2002 were more likely to be white, female, college-educated, with age less than 65, living in the western US, with a higher annual household income.[12] The types of therapies that patients use will depend on many factors besides patient preference, such as availability and cost. As reported in a 2002 survey by Tindle *et al.*,[12] the most common therapies were herbal medicine (18.6 percent) and relaxation techniques (14.2 percent), chiropractic care (7.4 percent), and yoga (5 percent), while acupuncture was used by 1 percent of the population. The number of visits to a CAM practitioner varies depending on the nature of the therapy. Thus, chiropractic, acupuncture, and massage therapy will require more visits to a practitioner in a given time period than herbal medicine or homeopathy.

Cost

A conservative estimate of out-of-pocket costs to consumers for CAM in the US is $27 billion. This compares with out-of-pocket expenses of $9.1 billion for hospitalizations and $29.3 billion for physician services.[3] Payment by insurers for CAM has become a greater issue as the popularity and demand has increased, virtually all health plans now cover chiropractic services and most health plans offer coverage for at least some of the other CAM therapies.[13] In Britain, Pal and Morris[14] surveyed 20 private medical insurers regarding payment for complementary treatment. Most of the responders indicated that they paid for chiropractic, osteopathy, homeopathy, and the Alexander technique – sometimes only with a consultant referral.

Physician attitudes

Acceptance of CAM by physicians is not uniform. Many physicians themselves are practitioners of one or more complementary therapies. Others are skeptical, misinformed, or oppositional. All physicians share a culture that respects logical thinking, responsibility, and evidence-based treatment. Physicians as a whole abhor magical thinking and pandering, particularly in regard to patients with serious illness. Many physicians have seen patients die with cancer who were led to alternative therapies by alternative practitioners who pandered to vulnerable patients. These practitioners often exploit patients fear of medical treatment and its side effects by promising "natural" cures.

For chronic conditions that are not life threatening, physicians tend to be more forgiving of complementary and alternative therapies and less rigid about their lack of scientific foundation. In a meta-analysis of 12 surveys of physician perceptions regarding complementary medicine, Ernst and co-authors[15] concluded that most of the surveys implied that physicians perceived complementary therapies as moderately useful and/or effective. Manipulative therapies (osteopathy or chiropractic), acupuncture, and homeopathy were deemed most useful or effective in the majority of these surveys. All but one of the 12 surveys was of physicians in general practice in the UK, Europe, New Zealand, and Israel.

Training of allopathic physicians in CAM therapies is becoming more common. Approximately 20 percent of Scotland's general practitioners have received basic training in integrating homeopathy with orthodox practice.[16] In the United States, a new residency program called the Integrative Family Medicine Program was introduced in 2003. It is a four-year combined family medicine residency and integrative medicine fellowship created in joint partnership between universities in six states. It was designed with the purpose of combining the training of family practice and CAM therapies.[17]

Medical schools in the US and Europe are responding to the new awareness of CAM's pervasiveness. Forty percent of European medical schools offer some form of CAM training.[18] A survey of family practice residency program directors and US medical school family medicine department chairs revealed that nearly 30 percent were currently teaching some form of complementary or alternative medicine.[19] Another 12 percent were either starting to teach or considering teaching such a course. Most of these courses were elective. According to another survey of CAM course directors from 53 medical schools in the US, course topics included acupuncture, herbs and botanicals, meditation and relaxation, spirituality/faith/prayer, chiropractic, homeopathy, and nutrition and diets.[20]

The US congress has shown its support of research into CAM by establishing the Office of Alternative Medicine (OAM) at the National Institutes of Health in 1992; and designating that office as the National Center for Complementary and Alternative Medicine with an annual budget of US$50 million.[21] This organization has started a number of large clinical trials that are expected to stimulate further research. In addition, the OAM has funded 13 research centers at institutions across the US that are carrying out a research agenda in various broad clinical areas. These areas include pain, HIV/AIDS, addiction, aging, cancer, women's health issues, general medical conditions, pediatric conditions, neurological disorders, cardiovascular diseases, chiropractic, and asthma, allergy and immunology.

Definitions

In 1993, Eisenberg *et al.*[22] utilized a working definition of alternative medical therapies as interventions neither taught widely in medical schools nor generally available in US hospitals. As we have seen, these alternative therapies are becoming more available in conventional medical settings and are being taught in medical schools.[18, 20] A broader definition of complementary and alternative medicine is those medical systems, practices, interventions, applications, theories, or claims that are currently not part of the dominant or conventional medical system in that society.[23] Under this definition, the list of practices that are considered complementary or alternative medicine will continually change as society changes and as those practices supported by research become incorporated into mainstream medicine. Eskinazi[24] proposed a refined definition of alternative medicine as a broad set of healthcare practices that are not readily integrated into the dominant healthcare model because they pose challenges to diverse societal beliefs and practices. The idea of a challenge to conventional practice is important. It highlights the difference between what is called "alternative" and what is called "complementary."

The terminology used to describe the broad scope of practices that are considered "complementary" or "alternative" to mainstream medical practice is diverse and often confusing. Alternative medicine, complementary medicine, holistic medicine, integrative therapies, natural medicine and traditional medicine are all terms that have been used nearly synonymously to represent an approach to health that is different from the biomedical system that is so entrenched in the western industrialized world. Each of the adjectives, alternative, holistic, complementary integrative, etc., have slightly different connotations which define a relationship with mainstream medicine. The term **alternative** implies "instead of" or "apart from" conventional medicine, whereas **complementary** connotes "in addition to" as a way of completing an approach to healing. **Integrative** medicine suggests multiple approaches that are applied "together" or "in concert" with one another. **Holistic** is an older term which was used to emphasize an "all-encompassing" approach to the person rather than the disease, illness, or symptom. Traditional medicines usually refer to a culturally based system such as traditional Chinese medicine, traditional Native American healing practices, and Ayurvedic medicine. In industrialized western societies, the term **traditional medicine** is sometimes used misleadingly to refer to the allopathic or biomedical model. Perhaps a more suitable term for those systems of healing that arise from one of the world's cultures is **world medicine**.

Even more problematic is the term **natural** as in natural healing, natural medicine, or naturopathy. The term generally implies techniques that rely only on botanicals and substances that are used in their natural form, i.e. are not modified by chemical or physical processes. The scope of what natural healing means has expanded to include techniques such as massage and acupuncture and other approaches that purport to promote the body's own power to heal itself by correcting mechanical or energy imbalances.[25]

Currently, the term **complementary and alternative medicine** (CAM) is the most commonly used term to describe the wide variety of complementary and alternative therapies offered in western culture.

Understanding the scope of CAM

The definition of CAM developed above is almost equivalent to defining it as everything except conventional medicine. This creates a challenge to categorize and classify countless therapies and systems of healing in a way that makes sense and provides an intellectual handle on a large and disparate field.

We can broadly separate all of CAM into three main classifications: world medicine systems, other comprehensive systems of medicine that are not culturally based, and individual therapies (**Figure 23.1**). Unlike individual therapies, a system of medicine provides treatment for a whole spectrum of symptoms, illnesses, or diseases. It is generally a complete system of medicine with its own philosophy or science of health and disease, and its own diagnostic approach. A world medicine system evolves from the belief system and cultural practices of a society. Examples of world medicine are traditional Chinese medicine and Ayurvedic medicine, which originates from India. Other systems of medicine, such as homeopathy, may evolve from a philosophical construct of health and disease, but is not part of a world cultural tradition.

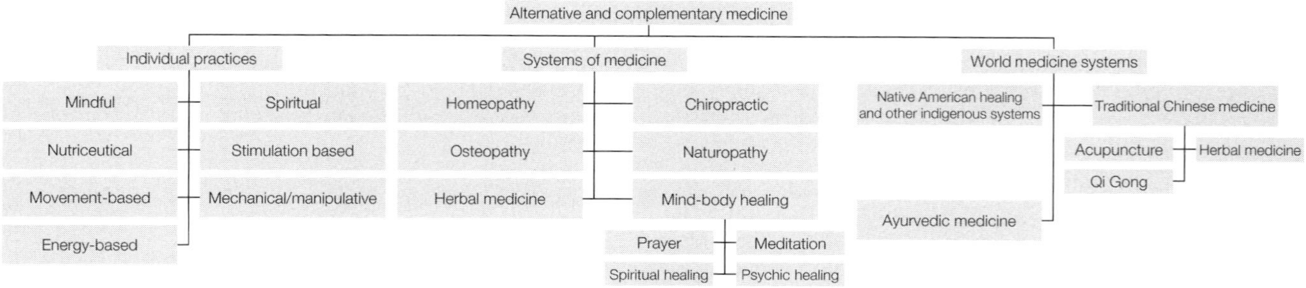

Figure 23.1 Organization of alternative and complementary therapies.

Individual therapies treat a narrower range of conditions with a specific type of intervention; but do not by themselves provide a model of health and illness. Hypnosis, massage, vitamin therapy, and relaxation techniques are examples of individual therapies.

To further classify individual therapies it is useful to think of them as falling into one or more of seven functional categories of treatment:

1. mindful;
2. spiritual;
3. energy-based;
4. stimulation-based;
5. movement-based;
6. mechanical or manipulative;
7. nutriceutical.

These are shown in **Table 23.1** with examples in each category. Mindful therapies utilize the mind to produce changes in physical and emotional status. Meditation, hypnosis, and yoga fall into this category. Spiritual therapies imply a letting go of the mind, giving up control to a higher power as with prayer. Energy-based techniques rely on a construct of a vital energy or energy field that exists in living systems. When the flow of energy is out of balance or obstructed, disease can occur. The goal of energy-based treatments is to restore the optimal energy balance to achieve health. Therapeutic touch and acupuncture use this concept as their foundation. Note that yoga can be considered as mindful, spiritual, energy-based, and movement-based. Acupuncture is a stimulation-based technique, but it is part of a world medicine system, traditional Chinese medicine, which uses the concept of a vital energy (Qi). Aromatherapy is also a stimulation-based approach to healing. It consists of inhaled essences of plants or topically applied essential oils. The absorption of micromolecules through the skin or respiratory mucosa is believed to produce favorable chemical changes; thus aromatherapy may also be a form of nutriceutical treatment. Vitamins, herbs, and diets are also examples of nutriceutical therapies which involve the absorption and assimilation of substances into the body to produce a change in state that is favorable to the living system.

Movement-based therapies include dance therapy, T'ai chi ch'uan, exercise, yoga, and other techniques that rely on movement and posture to promote health. Many of these movement-based therapies also rely on concepts of energy medicine as part of their foundation. Mechanical or manipulative therapies include chiropractic, osteopathic, cranio-sacral therapy, and massage. These approaches usually apply external forces to correct a mechanical problem of the spine, bones, muscle, or other soft tissues.

Organizing the universe of CAM into these seven functional categories helps the clinician plan a treatment strategy. When a patient is not having success achieving pain control, and has tried several therapies within one or two categories, suggesting choices from a different category makes sense. When faced with a vulnerable patient, certain types of treatment may pose challenges that are best avoided. The abuse victim may have difficulty with mindful and spiritual therapies that require a process of letting go. They also may not tolerate the vigorous physical contact inherent in some of the manipulative therapies. If they are seeking complementary treatment, the clinician should discuss these issues and may recommend less threatening types of treatment from the nutriceutical or movement-based groups.

In the following sections we will describe selected complementary and alternative treatments that span the three main groups (world medicine systems, other complete systems, and individual therapies) and most of the seven functional categories of alternative treatments. We will also describe CAM treatments most commonly used in pain clinics in the United States.

ACUPUNCTURE AND TRADITIONAL CHINESE MEDICINE

In our classification scheme, acupuncture is part of a world medicine system (traditional Chinese medicine) and is categorized as both a stimulation-based and an energy-based technique. Its origin dates to at least 600BC, preceding the availability of iron and steel for fashioning needles.[26] Acupuncture theory postulates a system of channels or meridians on the body named after organs or

Table 23.1 Categories of individual CAM therapies with examples.

Mindful	Spiritual	Energy based	Stimulation-based	Movement-based	Mechanical/manipulative	Nutriceutical
Hypnosis	Prayer	Massage	TENS	Exercise	Chiropractic	Vitamins
Imagery	Spiritual healing	Therapeutic touch	Acupuncture	Dance therapy	Osteopathy	Diet
Meditation	Psychic healing	Homeopathy	Massage	Alexander technique	Massage	Herbal medicine
Relaxation	Yoga	Acupuncture	Aromatherapy	Tai chi	Cranio-sacral therapy	Homeopathy
Biofeedback		Qi gong	Therapeutic touch	Qi gong	Rolfing	Aromatherapy
Yoga		Yoga	Music	Yoga		

TENS, trancutaneous electrical nerve stimulation.

bodily systems, and a vital energy called qi that flows through the channels. Acupuncture points lie along the channels. Good health and well-being occur when the flow of energy is balanced. Illness occurs when the energy flow is out of balance. It may be depleted from a channel or it may accumulate within a channel at a point of obstruction. By needling acupuncture points, the flow of qi can be restored to its proper balance.

Acupuncture technique and theory are embedded in traditional Chinese medicine, which in turn springs from Taoist philosophy. Taoism emphasizes the inextricable relationship between humans and the natural world drawing upon three fundamental concepts: yin and yang, the system of five phases or elements, and the vital energy qi.[27] Yin and yang conceptualize the dualistic nature of the universe and living systems in particular. Cold (yin) and heat (yang), internal (yin) and external (yang), deficiency (yin) and excess (yang) help characterize the balance of nature and the processes leading to disease. Another way to characterize the properties of matter or of processes that occur in the universe is with the system of five phases or five elements: wood, fire, earth, metal, and water. These are not elements in the same way we think of the more than 100 universal elements of modern science. The five elements of traditional Chinese medicine are metaphors describing different properties or behavior of things in nature. Unlike yin and yang and the five elements, which pertain to both living and nonliving things in the universe, the concept of qi defines living systems. It is created and replenished by breathing and eating. It flows through the 12 pairs of meridians throughout a 24-hour day, so it takes about two hours to traverse from one channel to the next.

The traditional acupuncturist will access information about the balance of qi in the various organs through a systematic diagnostic process that relies on history, and some unique physical assessments such as the appearance of the tongue and a complex analysis of the characteristics of the radial pulse. Pain indicates stagnation of qi in one or more of the channels or invasion of the channel by wind, heat, or cold. All of these concepts are crystallized in the world's first medical text entitled *Huang Ti Nei Ching* translated as *The Yellow Emperor's Classic of Internal Medicine*, which dates at least as early as 200BC.[27]

Brief history of acupuncture

During the fourth to the tenth centuries, acupuncture became ingrained in Chinese medicine and was officially recognized as an independent specialty of the Imperial Medical Academy of the Tang government in 618AD. During this same period, acupuncture, together with other branches of Chinese medicine, was introduced to other countries such as Japan.[28] During the eleventh to the early twentieth century, volumes of written material came out on acupuncture prescriptions. Acupuncture training programs became established in China, which allowed the growth of clinical experience with acupuncture and refinement in techniques. Complications of acupuncture were documented, lists of dangerous points appeared, and indications for acupuncture were identified.

As western medicine was introduced in China in the eighteenth century, acupuncture began to lose official favor. It was banned from the imperial court in 1822, but was still practiced widely and its use spread in Europe and other countries even as western medicine was making its way into China. In the 1940s, Mao Tse Tung revived the status of acupuncture practice as he found it a useful, inexpensive, and expedient alternative to western medicine, which was expensive and difficult to access during his quest for power against Chang Kai Shek. Chairman Mao encouraged the development of acupuncture and fostered simplification of acupuncture practice so that large numbers of nonphysicians (barefoot doctors) could use it in their communities together with herbal remedies.

In 1971, *New York Times* journalist James Reston wrote about his experience with acupuncture for postoperative pain while covering the American–Chinese ping-pong games. His report heralded a new beginning for acupuncture in the West. National magazines ran stories on acupuncture. Teams of medical investigators from the United States flocked to China to find out more about this mysterious and apparently wondrous treatment that was so different from pharmaceutical or surgical therapies familiar to the western mind. The initial frenzy of excitement settled down as some of the unrealistic expectations were not met; but acupuncture continued to be an important part of the CAM arena in the United States.

The National Institutes of Health (NIH) of the US sponsored a consensus conference in November 1997 to determine the status and role of acupuncture in American medicine.[29][I] The objectives of the conference were to form conclusions about the efficacy of acupuncture, its role in various conditions, its biological mechanisms, and what remaining issues must be addressed to incorporate acupuncture into today's healthcare system; and to identify directions for future research. The 12-member panel represented a wide spectrum of interests and expertise from public citizens to medical specialists to acupuncturists. They concluded the following.

- Acupuncture is widely practiced in the US.
- Sufficient evidence exists to support the use of acupuncture as primary therapy for adult postoperative and chemotherapy-induced nausea and vomiting, and postoperative dental pain.
- Sufficient evidence exists to support adjunctive use of acupuncture for various other conditions such as addiction, stroke rehabilitation, headache, menstrual cramps, tennis elbow, fibromyalgia, myofascial pain, osteoarthritis, low back pain, carpal tunnel syndrome, and asthma.

- Findings from basic research have begun to elucidate the mechanisms of acupuncture, including the release of opioids and other peptides in the central and peripheral nervous system and changes in neuroendocrine function.
- Issues of training, licensure, and reimbursement remain to be clarified.
- There is sufficient evidence of acupuncture's potential value to encourage further studies and to expand its use into conventional medicine.

These conclusions from an authoritative agency of the US government help to legitimize acupuncture practice and development.

A number of studies have recently been published evaluating efficacy of acupuncture. Manheimer *et al.*[30][I] published a meta-analysis of 33 randomized, controlled trials that compared acupuncture to sham, other active, or no treatment. They found evidence that acupuncture is more effective than sham or no treatment for patients with chronic low back pain. Evidence about acupuncture's effectiveness compared with other active treatments for acute low back pain was inconclusive. The quality of the included trials varied. According to a prospective, partially blinded, controlled, randomized clinical trial by Martin *et al.*,[31][II] acupuncture was found to significantly improve symptoms of fibromyalgia. Another randomized, double-blinded, controlled trial carried out by Assefi *et al.*[32][II] found no improvement over sham acupuncture. For knee osteoarthritis, a recent randomized, controlled, double-blinded trial carried out by Berman *et al.*[33][II] found that compared to sham acupuncture treatment or no treatment, acupuncture decreased pain by 40 percent and similarly improved function.

Acupuncture technique

Needles are generally made of stainless steel, but are sometimes gold or silver to achieve energizing or sedating effects. Twenty-eight- to 32-gauge solid needles are used. The length of the needle and depth of penetration depends on the thickness of the underlying soft tissue. Many acupuncture points overlie muscle and the depth of needle insertion is usually to the center of the muscle belly. Needles may be inserted perpendicularly, obliquely, or tangentially. The acupuncturist usually tries to elicit a special needling sensation called deqi, which refers to a deep, heavy, warm, spreading or aching sensation that is felt to be crucial to achieve a therapeutic effect.

Stimulation of the acupuncture points is a necessary part of treatment. Needles may be stimulated in a variety of ways: manually by thrusting up and down or twisting back and forth or by tapping or scraping the handle of the needle. Electrical current can be applied to pairs of needles at frequencies of 3–5 Hz or higher frequencies in the 100- or 1000-Hz range. The amplitude of stimulation is adjusted to patient tolerance (**Figure 23.2**). Needles and

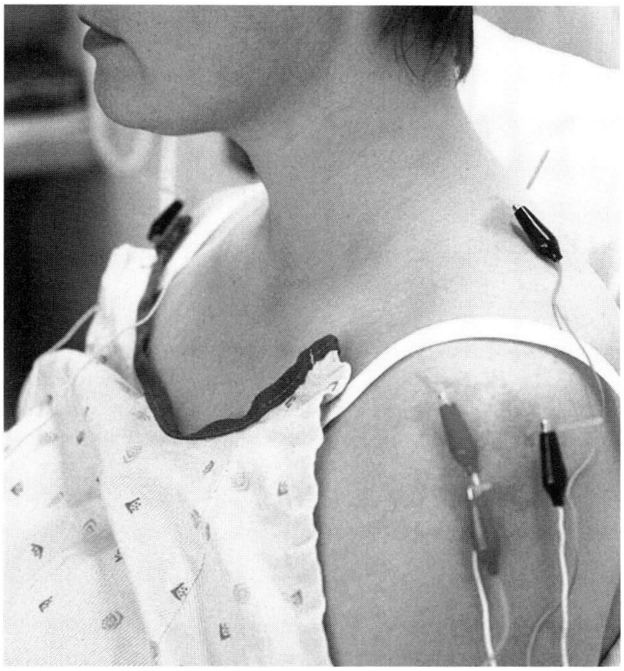

Figure 23.2 Electroacupuncture for rheumatoid arthritis affecting the shoulder.

acupuncture points may also be heated in various ways including the use of moxa, a plant that is burned near the acupuncture point or on the needle.

The duration of an acupuncture session is approximately 20–45 minutes. The frequency of sessions is variable depending on the clinical problem, its chronicity, and availability of resources. Typically, treatments are carried out once to three times per week. Sometimes treatments are offered daily or as infrequently as once or twice a month. A course of treatment consists of 10–20 sessions, but for intractable chronic conditions periodic maintenance therapy may be offered. Ultimately, the intervals between treatments and the duration of a course of acupuncture remain empiric.[34]

Points are chosen for acupuncture either through traditional Chinese diagnostic analysis or by a formula approach, which utilizes a limited number of basic rules for point selection.

- For localized symptoms, needle points in that same region on any meridian. For example, for shoulder pain, needle points on or near the shoulder.
- Tender points are considered acupuncture points and can often be chosen for therapy.
- Points on a meridian will influence symptoms or disorders along the entire meridian.
- Six important distal points on the upper and lower limbs have effects on specific regions of the head, neck, and trunk. For example, the point Hoku (large intestine – 4) in the first dorsal interosseous muscle between the thumb and first finger, affects the head and neck.

- There are subsets of points that have certain general effects such as sedation, tonification (energizing), and immune system regulation, or that influence certain tissues, such as muscle and tendons, bone and cartilage, etc.
- There is a somatotopic organization on the surface of the ear, so that points on the ear can be chosen to influence any other part of the body.

Acupuncture risks

Common side effects of acupuncture include syncope or near-syncope in approximately 1 percent of patients, bruising around the needle site in less than 1 percent of needle sticks, and persistent soreness from needling that outlasts the treatment by hours to days. Contact dermatitis has been reported and attributed to the nickel content in most stainless steel needles.[35] Acupuncture should be avoided during pregnancy or used with caution due to the apparent effect of uterine muscle contraction and cervical dilation that has been produced by stimulating certain points.[36, 37] Other risks of acupuncture can be divided into organ or tissue damage and infections. The lung is the organ most likely to be injured during acupuncture. Several reports of unilateral and bilateral pneumothorax have emerged.[35, 38, 39, 40] Cases of spinal cord and peripheral nerve injuries have been associated with acupuncture due to migration of a broken needle fragment or a purposefully retained needle.[41, 42, 43, 44] Boxall[45] reported 29 cases of serologically proven hepatitis B traced to an acupuncture clinic in Birmingham, UK. Four cases of hepatitis B were reported and traced to acupuncture treatment received at a chiropractic clinic in Florida in 1980.[46] In both clinics poor needle management was used: reusable needles, use of hollow syringe-type needles, and unsterilized needles.

The documentation of serious complications of acupuncture is an argument in favor of state regulation. This would help insure that practitioners meet certain standards of knowledge and practice that would limit public harm.

Scientific basis

Acupuncture, more than any other CAM therapy, has been studied scientifically. The discovery of opioid receptors and endorphins has led to a large number of investigations into the role these receptors and ligands play in experimental acupuncture analgesia. Few of these studies contradict the involvement of the endorphin system, and several lines of evidence demonstrate that the endogenous opioid system is part of acupuncture analgesia. Acupuncture analgesia can be reversed with opioid antagonists such as naloxone.[47, 48, 49, 50] Increased endogenous opioid production has been measured directly after acupuncture.[51, 52] Antiserum to opioid receptors has been shown to block acupuncture analgesia.

By 1982, biogenic amines had been implicated in acupuncture analgesia in numerous studies reviewed by Han and Terenius.[53] Ablating the descending inhibitory pathway for pain at the dorsal and medial raphe nuclei blunted acupuncture analgesia. Blocking serotonin receptors in rabbits and rats also diminished acupuncture analgesia. Administration of a serotonin precursor potentiates acupuncture analgesia. Measurements of serotonin and its byproducts showed increases in the lower brain stem during acupuncture analgesia.

Other neurochemical mediators have been implicated in experimental acupuncture analgesia including substance P, CGRP, CCK, and C-fos, but these investigations represent more preliminary individual findings.[35]

HOMEOPATHY

Homeopathy is classified as a comprehensive healing system that is not embedded in a world culture. The techniques of homeopathy are both nutriceutical and energy based.

Homeopathy originated primarily as the discovery of one man, Samuel Hahnemann. He was a German physician in the late eighteenth and early nineteenth centuries that rejected the conventional medical practices of his time such as bloodletting and the medicinal use of various toxic agents. Curious about the curative properties of cinchona bark for malaria, he experimented with it on himself and discovered that it produced a malaria-like illness in him. He concluded that such symptoms represented resistance to disease and that substances producing certain symptoms or effects in normal individuals would be effective in treating diseases that caused those same symptoms.[54] This led to the "doctrine of similars" or "like cures like." Hahnemann carried out innumerable "provings" on himself and others using hundreds of substances including botanical, animal, and mineral extracts. He developed the *Materia Medica*, a text of remedies that identified the substances and their associated effects. Many remedies were noxious and themselves toxic. Repeated dilutions would reduce the toxicity and apparently preserved and even increased the curative effect. This concept, called "potentization by dilution," is central to homeopathic practice and puzzling to the scientific mind. Typical dilutions of remedies are designated 2X, 6X, 12X, 30c, 200c, 1000c, 10,000c, and 50,000c. 2X refers to a dilution of $1{:}10^2$; 6X is a dilution of $1{:}10^6$ and so on. 30c is a $1{:}100^{30}$ dilution. Substances that are diluted beyond $1{:}10^{24}$ result in a liquid without a single molecule of the original substance since the number of dilutions exceeds Avogadro's number. Such dilutions are common in homeopathy and impart some confidence in the safety and tolerability of the remedy. How such a liquid can exert a healing property forms the basis of homeopathy theory.

Substances are believed to contain an essential energetic property that is not diluted out, but increases with successive dilutions. It is this energy or essence that strengthens the body's defenses against an illness. The preparation of remedies involves dilution and "succussion" or shaking the diluent vigorously to release or increase its energy. The potency of a remedy is determined both by the number of dilutions and the number of succussions.[55]

The homeopathic physician must take a different kind of history from the patient than an allopathic physician would. The homeopathic history is a detailed inquiry into the symptom complex and the environment and mind of the patient with respect to the symptoms. The purpose of this is to individualize the selection of remedies to match the symptoms. Classification of diseases and pathophysiology are not as important as the nature of the symptoms. Thus, diabetic neuropathy is not as relevant to a homeopathic assessment as burning, sensitive skin, interference with sleep, etc. This construct becomes useful to the allopathic practitioner, particularly when the pathophysiology of symptoms, such as chronic pain, may be obscure.

Homeopathy is widely practiced in Europe, India, and Asia. It has a growing popularity in the United States as a complementary and alternative therapy, but was systematically excluded and obstructed by the American Medical Association in the early 1900s.[56] Forty percent of general practitioners in the Netherlands practice homeopathy and 42 percent of general practitioners in Britain refer patients to homeopaths.[57]

Research

There have been many reports of the efficacy of homeopathic remedies, but few well-designed clinical trials. A randomized, double-blind, placebo-controlled trial of Arnica 30x for muscle soreness in 519 long distance runners found the remedy no more effective than placebo.[58][II] Ernst and Pittler[59][I] systematically reviewed the published controlled trials on Arnica montana and concluded that, on balance, the studies do not support the notion that arnica is more efficacious than placebo. A controversial study of the concept of biological effects of ultra-high dilutions was published in *Nature*.[60] In this study, human basophils were found to release histamine when exposed to homeopathic dilutions of IgE antiserum.

In a prospective, multicenter cohort study of 3981 patients in 103 primary care practices with additional specialization in homeopathy in Germany and Switzerland, Witt *et al.*[61][III] found that there were marked and sustained improvements in disease severity and quality of life during the two-year study period using homeopathic treatment. The most frequent diagnoses treated were allergic rhinitis in men, headache in women, and atopic dermatitis in children. Cucherat *et al.*[62][I] performed a meta-analysis evaluating homeopathy in 1998. Of 118 randomized controlled trials, only 16 trials met the inclusion criteria. The results showed that there is some evidence that homeopathic treatments are more effective than placebo; however, the strength of this evidence is low because of the low methodological quality of the trials. Studies of high methodological quality were more likely to be negative than the lower quality studies. Further high quality studies are needed to confirm these results. Another meta-analysis published in 1997 by Linde *et al.*,[63] [I] evaluating 89 double-blind and/or randomized placebo-controlled trials of homeopathic treatment, found that although the effects of homeopathy do not appear to be completely due to placebo, there is insufficient evidence that homeopathy is clearly efficacious for any single clinical condition.

Patients seek out homeopathic treatment for a large array of mostly chronic conditions. In the USA, one survey reported that patients tended to be highly educated, but uninformed about homeopathy. More than 70 percent reported getting some improvement in their primary symptom and nearly all were satisfied with the treatment regardless of the outcome.[64]

Risks

The extremely high dilutions of homeopathic remedies suggest the absence of risk. However, the use of toxic agents such as heavy metals, arsenic, bromide, etc., combined with improper handling, can result in adverse effects.[65] The reliability of the manufacturer is therefore an important safety factor. Avoiding remedies that use heavy metals, such as mercury or cadmium, may also be a warranted safety measure.

CHIROPRACTIC AND MANUAL THERAPIES

Chiropractic literally means "hand work" or "manual therapy." It can be classified as a comprehensive system of medicine or as an individual therapy in the mechanical–manipulative category. How one classifies chiropractic depends on how broadly one defines its scope. There is the school that sees chiropractic as a complete system of medicine applicable to a wide range of ailments from musculoskeletal pain to asthma and diabetes. On the other side, many chiropractors profess a narrower scope that primarily addresses neuromusculoskeletal symptoms.

History

The origination of chiropractic medicine is attributed to DD Palmer in the Midwestern United States in the late nineteenth century. The story goes that on September 18, 1895, Palmer cured a janitor in Iowa of deafness by manipulating a single cervical vertebra. Palmer developed a system of manual medicine techniques based on the folk medicine tradition of bonesetters and drawing on the philosophical constructs of mesmerism and vital energy, which he termed "innate intelligence." Illness was explained by a blockage of flow of vital energy, which in turn was caused by "subluxations" of the vertebrae. Chiropractic manipulation corrects those subluxations and restores the energy flow.

In the United States, there has been a longstanding battle between the institution of conventional medicine (embodied by the American Medical Association (AMA)) and chiropractic. The AMA was largely successful at suppressing the legitimization of chiropractic in the first quarter of the twentieth century. By the mid-1970s every state had come to recognize chiropractic as a legitimate healing art by providing for licensing. The federal government of the United States then covered chiropractic treatment through its healthcare programs for the poor, the elderly, and Worker's Compensation. Finally, in 1990, the United States Supreme Court upheld a lower court's ruling against the AMA and allied organizations for conspiring against chiropractors by prohibiting members from referring to a chiropractor.[66] More recently, the Agency for Health Care Policy and Research, a division of the Department of Health and Human Services of the US Government, approved of chiropractic for the management of acute low back pain in its 1994 guidelines for acute low back problems in adults.[67]

Scope of practice

Many chiropractors do not adhere to the vitalistic view of innate intelligence, preferring a more mechanical interpretation of what goes wrong in the spine to cause disease. All schools of chiropractic rely on a construct of the subluxation complex, which is the target of their treatment. Other differences that distinguish various practitioners lie in the scope of techniques used. Many chiropractors employ techniques of conventional physical therapy such as the application of heat, ice, ultrasound, or electrical stimulation to the soft tissues as supplementary treatment. Some chiropractors are also trained in and practice acupuncture and many provide counseling about nutrition, offering various nutriceuticals to augment their practice. Patients may seek out these eclectic practitioners as general CAM healthcare providers, but the central core of chiropractic treatment is still the therapeutic manual manipulation of the spine.

During its 100-year existence, numerous types of chiropractic adjustments have emerged. The goal of any adjustment is two-fold: to manipulate and to reposition. Palmer's original technique involved using the spinous and transverse processes of the spine as levers. A later technique relies on recoil or a rapid release after manipulating a vertebra. Osteopathic manipulation generally utilizes a long-lever technique in which movement of a limb helps to accomplish the adjustment. Cranio-sacral techniques use tiny forces and very low amplitude of movement. There may be between 100 and 200 different types of adjustments.[67]

Accompanying the spinal adjustment a patient will often experience a characteristic "crack" or "pop" at the moment the adjustment occurs. It is arguable what the mechanism of the sound or experience is – release of gas bubbles from synovial tissue or a ligamentous structure snapping into place? However, it does serve to emphasize that a change has taken place with expectant relief.

Value and efficacy

Survey data show a high degree of satisfaction of the public with chiropractic treatment. One study published in a general medical journal found that 66 percent of patients receiving chiropractic care for low back pain were "very satisfied" with their treatment, whereas only 22 percent of patients were as satisfied with treatment from family physicians.[68] Patients, especially pain patients, yearn for validation of their pain. Chiropractic provides such validation through a mechanistic view of pain that is devoid of psychological underpinnings. Furthermore, the practice of chiropractic is usually more responsive to the patient as customer with short waiting times and hands-on therapies.

In 2003, Assendelft *et al.*[69][I] performed a meta-analysis of 39 randomized controlled trials evaluating spinal manipulation in low back pain. They concluded that spinal manipulation was superior to sham therapy and to therapies that have been judged to be ineffective or harmful, but it had no advantage when compared with general practitioner care, analgesics, physical therapy, exercises, or back school. Results were similar for acute and chronic low back pain. A Cochrane review by Gross *et al.*[70][I] concluded that manipulation and/or gentle mobilization were not beneficial when performed alone, but they were beneficial when used with exercise. The review also concluded that neither was superior to the other and that there was insufficient evidence about their effects with radicular findings. The review acknowledged the methodological limitations of many of the underlying trials. Fernandez *et al.*[71][I] published a meta-analysis evaluating whether manual therapies have proven efficacy in reducing in tension-type headache. Only six studies met inclusion criteria and the authors found no rigorous evidence that manual therapies have a positive effect. At this time, evidence remains inadequate to draw firm conclusions about the efficacy of spinal manipulation for neck pain or tension-type headache.

Risks

Mild unpleasant reactions after spinal manipulative therapy are common but usually short-lived. According to a Norwegian study, 55 percent of patients had local discomfort, headache, tiredness, or radiating discomfort.[72] Most reactions resolved within 24 hours.

Serious adverse events associated with spinal manipulation include disk herniation and cauda equina syndrome with lumbar manipulation, and vertebrobasilar artery ischemic events with cervical manipulation. Estimates of the incidence of these complications range from 1 per 2 million to 1 per 400,000 manipulations.[73] Postulated causes include herniated nucleus pulposus, an underlying coagulation disorder, misdiagnosis, failure to recognize the onset and progression of neurological signs, improper technique, and manipulation of the cervical spine.[74] A population-based, case-control study found that in patients under the age of 45, those with vertebrobasilar dissection or occlusion were five times more likely than controls to have visited a chiropractor in the previous week and to have had three or more cervical chiropractic visits in the previous month.[75] No association was found for older individuals. The reason for this finding is unclear.

BOTANICAL THERAPIES

Botanical or herbal medicine is an important part of many broader systems of medicine, such as traditional Chinese medicine, Ayurvedic medicine, and other folk medicines. Of all the CAM practices, the use of botanicals is the oldest and most prevalent. Even allopathic pharmacological therapies can be considered as a highly evolved refinement of botanical medicine. Digitalis was originally isolated from the foxglove plant. Vinca alkaloids come from the Madagascar periwinkle (*Catharathus roseus*). Taxol is derived from the yew plant. Opioids are derived from the poppy. Many healthy individuals exploit plant products for their physiologic effects. For example, ginger and coffee are used worldwide as stimulants. In a strict sense, herbs are derived from soft-stemmed plants, but botanical therapies include an array of other products derived from fruits, berries, roots, bark, and other components of plants. The spectrum of "herbal therapies" often includes nonplant materials such as horn, bone, and cartilage. In the broadest sense, substances assimilated into the body for a therapeutic effect are called "nutriceuticals."

In 1998, approximately 32 percent of adults in the United States used some sort of herbal remedy with an estimated US$4 billion spent on these products.[76] By contrast, the prevalence of herbal product use was only 3 percent in 1991.[3] Awareness of this large market has driven the investment and promotion of herbal treatment, and acceptance by pharmacies and pharmaceutical companies.

Safety

Paradoxically, in spite of the widespread use of botanical remedies, the potential risks of this form of therapy are probably the least well defined of any CAM therapy. This is because botanical products are complex, having multiple potentially active or toxic ingredients with multiple physiologic effects. The array of botanicals is so vast as to make thorough analysis of all of them a slow process. Funding for such studies is inhibited unless there is a strong financial potential or strong evidence of public harm. A number of organizations exist that provide evidence-based consumer information to the public about botanical therapies. These include the World Health Organization (WHO) which publishes the *Guidelines for the Assessment of Herbal Medicines*,[77] the German Commission E, the European Scientific Cooperative of Phytotherapy (ESCOP), the American Herbal Products Association (AHPA), the American Botanical Council (ABC), and the Herb Research Foundation.

In Germany, phytomedicines are regulated as drugs. The German Commission E consists of a panel of medical, pharmaceutical, and research specialists, which makes determinations about the appropriate use and safety of herbal medicines. They also review applications by manufacturers for new botanical medicinal products.

In the United States, herbal remedies are under the jurisdiction of the Food and Drug Administration (FDA) which considers them as food supplements rather than as drugs. Thus, herbal products are not subject to the same scrutiny as drugs. Manufacturers must simply not make any claims for cure or treatment of a specific disease. They may only promote products as enhancing well-being or certain physiologic processes, such as the immune system or kidney function or energy level, etc. Products must be safe but efficacy is not required. The burden of proof of safety is on the FDA rather than on the manufacturer.[78]

In Minnesota, Fairview Health Services convened an Integrated Formulary and Drug Use Committee to establish policy and oversee the use of herbal and other alternative therapies. That committee is classifying alternative therapies and combinations of therapies into one of three categories: **Category I** agents have some data suggesting efficacy and appear to be safe in recommended doses. While not granted formulary status, they will be provided to hospitalized patients upon physician order and will be available to outpatients. **Category II** agents have insufficient information regarding efficacy but appear to be reasonably safe. They also include products that may be safe but for conditions not appropriate for self-treatment. A physician order for such a product will prompt the pharmacist to contact the prescribing physician and discuss the relative benefits and risks before making the product available to a patient. **Category III** agents are deemed unsafe. Such agents will not be provided to Fairview patients. **Tables 23.2** and **23.3**

Table 23.2 Category I herbs. Evidence suggests efficacy and safety.

Herb	Uses	Dose	Drug/disease interactions	Adverse effects
Chamomile	Antispasmodic, anti-inflammatory used for a variety of GI conditions	Consumed as tea	Anticoagulants: chamomile contains coumarin	Rare allergic reactions (cross allergenicity with ragweed, asters, mums)
Echinacae	Prevention and treatment of colds, flu and other infections	0.75–1.5 mL of hydroalcoholic extract 2–5 times/day; 1 g/day plant extract	Avoid in autoimmune disease, TB, multiple sclerosis, transplant patients, pregnancy/lactation	Rare allergic reactions
Feverfew	Migraine prophylaxis	250–500 µg parthenolide/day	Has antiplatelet activity. Avoid with anticoagulants. Not recommended in pregnancy/lactation	Nervousness and GI upset
Garlic	Hypercholesterolemia	600–900 mg powder/day or enteric coated	Has antiplatelet activity. Avoid with anticoagulants. Avoid with lactation	Heartburn, flatulence
Ginger	Antiemetic; motion sickness	1 g/day or 250 mg qid	May increase bleeding time; avoid with anticoagulants; insufficient safety information for pregnancy	None reported
Ginkgo	Dementia, peripheral vascular disease, sexual dysfunction, other vascular insufficiency problems	40 mg standardized extract tid	None known	None known
Grapeseed extract	Antioxidant	50–100 mg extract/day	None known	None known
Milk thistle	Hepatitis and cirrhosis of the liver	Silymarin 140 mg tid	None known	None known
Peppermint oil	Carminative, digestive aid, irritable bowel syndrome	0.2–0.4 mL bid	None known	Rectal burning
Pygeum	Benign prostatic hypertrophy	100 mg/day	None known	GI irritation
Saw palmetto	Benign prostatic hypertrophy	160 mg bid	Avoid during pregnancy/lactation	GI irritation
Slippery elm	Lozenge for throat	prn	None known	None known
St John's Wort	Depression and anxiety	300 mg standardized extract tid	Avoid concomitant serotonergic medication (antidepressants); contraindicated with MAOIs. Not recommended in pregnancy/lactation	Uncommon photosensitivity, fatigue, hypomania
Valerian	Insomnia	450 mg at bedtime	Other CNS depressants. Not recommended in pregnancy/lactation	None known

Table 23.3 Category III. Unsafe agents not recommended for use.

Herb	Purported use	Toxicity
Aloe (oral)	Cathartic	Safe when used topically; rarely recommended for oral use
Chapparal	Antioxidant, retard aging, skin and other disorders	Prepared from the leaves of the evergreen desert shrub known as creosote. Many case reports of fulminant hepatic failure and death
Comfrey	Demulcent, anti-inflammatory, GI disorders	Contains pyrrolizidine alkaloids that are hepatotoxic and carcinogenic in rats. Banned in Canada
Dong quai (angelica)	Stimulate menstrual flow, prevent cramping	Contraindicated in pregnancy. May contain a carcinogen
Germander		Hepatotoxicity
Licorice extracts		High doses can cause pseudoaldosteronism with hypertension, edema, hypokalemia
Life root		Hepatotoxicity
Ma huang (ephedra)	Used as a stimulant and appetite suppressant	Fatal cardiovascular events (stroke, myocardial infarction) and serious psychiatric adverse events in healthy individuals reported
Mistletoe		Hepatotoxicity
White willow	Herbal source of aspirin	Safer standardized sources available
Yohimbe	Impotence	CNS stimulation, blood pressure changes, tachycardia, nausea, vomiting, psychosis. Not recommended for self-treatment

summarize the committee's classification of category I and category III herbal products commonly available in the USA.

Application

Herbs are taken in many ways including capsules, aromatics, as a tea or infusion, as a decoction, or as a tincture. Steeping the herb in a covered pot with hot water makes an infusion. Decoctions require simmering of coarser leaves, stems, bark, and roots for about an hour in a covered or uncovered pot (depending on the volatile oil content). Tinctures are highly concentrated extracts that can be kept for long periods because they are prepared with alcohol.

MINDFUL CAM THERAPIES

Pain clinics in the United States frequently utilize mindful therapies (MT) for patients with pain because they have been found experientially to be beneficial. Frequently, nurses or psychologists receive training in one or more of these therapies and teach the patients to utilize them on a regular basis, for both prevention of pain and to manage pain flares. These therapies include relaxation breathing, meditation, mindfulness-based stress reduction (MBSR), self-hypnosis, guided imagery, autogenic training, and progressive muscle relaxation (PMR).[79]

Biofeedback is another MT frequently used for pain treatment. Biofeedback is a method that gives the patient conscious control over a physiologic function not normally under conscious control. This control is achieved by using computer technology to give the patient visual or auditory feedback over one or more physiologic functions including muscle tension, skin temperature, skin resistance, or brain wave activity. Surface electromyography (EMG), galvanic skin response monitors, and skin temperature monitors can be attached to the patient. Then, as the patient practices one of the mindful therapies, such as meditation, they will receive input from the computer about the changes they are making in their bodies. This input helps them understand their mind/body connection on a practical level.

Research

Astin[80][I] reviewed evidence from multiple randomized controlled trials and systematic reviews involving MT for a number of different pain states and his conclusion was that mindful therapies may be an appropriate adjunctive treatment for chronic low back pain, rheumatoid arthritis, osteoarthritis, tension headaches, postoperative pain, and pain during invasive medical procedures. Multiple MT were evaluated, including relaxation, meditation, imagery, and cognitive-behavioral therapy, biofeedback, and hypnosis. It was recommended that further research is needed, including comparisons of MT to credible shams and conventional medical therapies, comparisons of the different therapies with each other, and evaluations of which of the individual therapies are most effective for each of the individual pain diagnoses. Although it is difficult to create credible placebo conditions, it is important for future research to examine the relative contribution of nonspecific placebo factors in the efficacy of mindful therapies.

Findings regarding the efficacy of MT in fibromyalgia are equivocal. A recent Cochrane review of 13 controlled trials (the majority of which were of poor methodological quality), found limited evidence that MT are more effective than usual care controls and inconclusive evidence that these therapies are more effective than physical therapy or education/attention controls.[81][I]

ENERGY HEALING

Energy healing therapies are energy-based CAM modalities currently being used in over 50 hospitals across the US.[82] Therapeutic touch, healing touch, Reiki, Qi Gong, and shamanic healing are all examples of energy healing therapies. These therapies are based on the construct that energy flow can be manipulated by practitioners and brought into balance to induce healing and pain relief. To heal using energy healing, the practitioner acts as a conduit of the healing energy force and directs it to others or back to him or herself. The energy can be directed either with gentle hand placement on the body or at a distance from the body. The various energy healing therapies differ in the location of hand placement and also in the preparatory meditations the practitioners make prior to the treatment.

Research

Few studies involving the measurement of energy are noted in scientific literature.[82] The scientific explanation of the mechanism by which energy healing therapies works remains unknown. There have been a number of studies evaluating the efficacy of energy healing. A recent review of healing touch studies by Wardell and Weymouth[83][I] found that only 6 of 28 studies examined were of appropriate quality for inclusion. They concluded that although no generalizable results were found, a foundation exists for further research to test its benefits. In a meta-analytic review of therapeutic touch, Peters[84][I] found that only 9 of 36 studies met methodologic requirements for inclusion and the results supporting efficacy were mixed. A number of studies funded by the NIH are currently examining the efficacy of energy healing therapies, including Reiki, healing touch, Qi Gong, and shamanic healing.

No adverse effects of energy healing have been mentioned thus far in any scientific studies. Therapeutic touch founders have mentioned potential adverse effects including being so sated with energy that the patient experiences irritability, restlessness, anxiety, or increased pain.[82, 85] Dizziness, nausea, tension headache, and crying have been anecdotally reported.

CASE EXAMPLES

Case 1

A 29-year-old woman who suffers from migraine becomes pregnant. She is on prophylactic and abortive drugs for headache management. Her physician advises her to discontinue all of them if possible. What alternative therapies can be recommended? This case highlights the importance of CAM in the everyday practice of medicine. Herbal or nutriceutical treatments will most likely be avoided because of the uncertainty of these agents in pregnancy. Acupuncture may also carry at least a theoretical risk of premature labor. Self-management techniques such as biofeedback, yoga, and hypnosis can all be recommended. Osteopathic and chiropractic treatment can be beneficial, particularly if musculoskeletal factors trigger or influence headache. The herbal agent feverfew, which is commonly used in migraine, should be avoided during pregnancy.

Case 2

A 47-year-old man with a ten-year history of chronic low back pain due to several work-related injuries sees his chiropractor three times each week for an adjustment. He also sees a massage therapist once a week. His family assists him with many of his daily needs such as putting on his socks and tying his shoes. He is completely sedentary and has been disabled from work for the last six years. He relies on daily opioid analgesics, yet he says he is sick of taking drugs. He has become increasingly isolated from social activities. He has a friend whose back pain was cured with acupuncture and is asking for a referral. Neurological examination is normal. A musculoskeletal examination reveals decreased range of motion and muscle tenderness. X-rays and scans show mild to moderate lumbar degenerative changes.

This case challenges the physician to analyze the pain problem comprehensively using a biopsychosocial model, and then to diplomatically steer the patient away from his misguided path toward a healthier approach that will more likely make a sustainable difference in his life. Although acupuncture can be helpful in the management of low back pain, offering one more passive modality in this case would reinforce this patient's passive maladaptation. Instead, a closely supervised exercise and educational program is needed. Classes in a movement-based therapy like tai chi chuan or yoga would have a self-actualizing effect. A heated pool would provide a tolerable transition toward activity. Frequent counseling and supervision would lead the patient away from self-defeating behaviors. One could negotiate with this patient by offering acupuncture if he would discontinue the other treatments, which have only provided brief symptom relief, and participate in the more comprehensive program outlined above.

Case 3

A 63-year-old woman with metastatic breast cancer is not able to tolerate her opioid analgesics due to intractable nausea. She has had sequential trials of many different opioids and has not tolerated any of them; nor has she had success with antiemetics. Without opioids, bone pain is intolerable. She is growing increasingly hopeless and withdrawn, yet she will not take antidepressant medication for fear of side effects and because she insists that the pain and nausea are the cause of her depression.

The clinician must identify alternatives at this crucial moment. At the same time, this patient must remain connected to the primary physician or oncologist because of the progressive nature of the pain problem and the likely need for opioid and other aggressive analgesic measures. From the classification scheme of CAM therapies, one can rule out movement-based therapies and manipulative therapies, which would certainly aggravate bone pain. The goal for a complementary or alternative therapy may be to manage nausea rather than pain since some opioid is likely to be needed no matter what alternatives are applied. Acupuncture has been shown to improve nausea in several controlled trials in a variety of settings, including nausea due to cancer chemotherapy. It may be worthwhile to offer it for opioid-induced nausea. Acupressure can be applied more frequently at the same well-defined point on the volar aspect of the wrist (P-6) by a caregiver or by using a wristband with a pressure bead over the point. Other complementary options include hypnosis, guided imagery, healing touch, music therapy, and spiritual counseling, or careful application of herbal remedies or homeopathic remedies. Once nausea is reduced and pain is a little better with complementary tools, opioid titration may be more successful.

ACKNOWLEDGMENT

The authors wish to thank Richard Branson DC for his valuable information on chiropractic.

REFERENCES

1. International Association for the Study of Pain. Pain terms: A list with definitions and notes on usage. *Pain.* 1979; **6**: 249–52.
2. Astin JA. Why patients use alternative medicine: results of a national study. *Journal of the American Medical Association.* 1998; **279**: 1548–53.
3. Eisenberg DM, Davis RB, Ettner SL *et al.* Trends in alternative medicine use in the United States, 1990-1997: Results of a follow-up national survey. *Journal of the American Medical Association.* 1998; **280**: 1569–75.
4. Stewart MA. Effective physician–patient communication and health outcomes: a review. *Canadian Medical Association Journal.* 1995; **153**: 1064–5.
5. Barnes PM, Powell-Griner E, McFann K, Nahin RL. Complementary and alternative medicine use among adults. United States, 2002. *Advance Data.* 2004; **343**: 1–19.
6. Millar WJ. Patterns of use – alternative health care practitioners. *Health Reports.* 2001; **13**: 9–21.
7. MacLennan AH, Wilson DH, Taylor AW. Prevalence and cost of alternative medicine in Australia. *Lancet.* 1996; **347**: 569–73.
8. Thomas KJ, Nicholl JP, Coleman P. Use and expenditure on complementary medicine in England: a population based survey. *Complementary Therapies in Medicine.* 2001; **9**: 2–11.
9. Lonroth HL, Ekholm O. [Alternative therapies in Denmark – use, users and motives for the use]. *Ugeskrift for Laeger.* 2006; **168**: 682–6 (in Danish).
10. Hartel U, Volger E. [Use and acceptance of classical natural and alternative medicine in Germany – findings of a representative population-based survey]. *Forschende Komplementarmedizin und Klassische Naturheilkunde.* 2004; **11**: 327–34 (in German).
11. Menniti-Ippolito F, Gargiulo L, Bologna E *et al.* Use of unconventional medicine in Italy: a nation-wide survey. *European Journal of Clinical Pharmacology.* 2002; **58**: 61–4.
12. * Tindle HA, Davis RB, Phillips RS, Eisenberg DM. Trends in use of complementary and alternative medicine by US adults: 1997–2002. *Alternative Therapies in Health and Medicine.* 2005; **11**: 42–9.
13. Sipkoff M. Steadily, plans increase coverage of unorthodox medical therapies. *Managed Care.* 2005; **14**: 59–60.
14. Pal B, Morris J. Rheumatologists and complementary medicine. *Rheumatology in Practice.* 1996; **3**: 18–20.
15. Ernst E, Resch K-L, White AR. Complementary medicine. What physicians think of it: A meta-analysis. *Archives of Internal Medicine.* 1995; **155**: 2405–08.
16. Reilly D. Comments on complementary and alternative medicine in Europe. *Journal of Alternative and Complementary Medicine.* 2001; **7**: S23–31.
17. Maizes V, Silverman H, Lebensohn P *et al.* The integrative family medicine program: an innovation in residency education. *Academic Medicine.* 2006; **81**: 583–9.
18. Varga O, Marton S, Molnar P. Status of complementary and alternative medicine in European medical schools. *Forschende Komplementarmedizin.* 2006; **13**: 41–5.
19. Carlston M, Stuart MP, Jonas W. Alternative medicine instruction in medical schools and family practice residency programs. *Family Medicine.* 1997; **29**: 559–62.
20. Brokaw JJ, Tunnicliff G, Raess BU, Saxon DW. The teaching of complementary and alternative medicine in U.S. medical schools: a survey of course directors. *Academic Medicine.* 2002; **77**: 876–81.
21. Marwick C. Alterations are ahead at the OAM. *Journal of the American Medical Association.* 1998; **280**: 1553–4.
22. Eisenberg DM, Kessler RC, Foster C *et al.* Unconventional medicine in the United States. *New England Journal of Medicine.* 1993; **328**: 246–52.
23. Alternative medicine: Expanding medical horizons: A report to the National Institutes of Health on alternative

medical systems and practices in the United States. Washington DC: US Government Printing Office, 1994; (017-040-00537-7).

24. Eskinazi DP. Factors that shape alternative medicine. *Journal of the American Medical Association*. 1998; **280**: 1621–3.
25. Dunne R, Watkins J. Complementary medicine – some definitions. *Journal of the Royal Society of Health*. 1997; **117**: 287–91.
26. Gwei Djen L, Needham J. *Celestial lancets: A history and rationale of acupuncture and moxa*. New York: Cambridge University Press, 1980.
27. Veith I. *The Yellow Emperor's classic of internal medicine*. Berkeley: University of California Press, 1949.
28. Ma K-W. The roots and development of Chinese acupuncture: from pre-history to early 20th century. *Acupuncture in Medicine*. 1992: 1092–9.
29. * Acupuncture. NIH Consensus Statement Online. November 3–5, 1997, 15(5):1–34. Available from: http://consensus.nih.gov.
30. Manheimer E, White B, Berman B *et al*. Meta-analysis: Acupuncture for low back pain. *Annals of Internal Medicine*. 2005; **142**: 651–63.
31. Martin DP, Sletten CD, Williams BA, Berger IH. Improvement in fibromyalgia symptoms with acupuncture: Results of a randomized controlled trial. *Mayo Clinic Proceedings*. 2006; **81**: 749–57.
32. Assefi NP, Sherman KJ, Jacobsen C *et al*. A randomized clinical trial of acupuncture compared with sham acupuncture in fibromyalgia. *Annals of Internal Medicine*. 2005; **143**: 10–19.
33. Berman BM, Lao L, Langenberg P *et al*. Effectiveness of acupuncture as adjunctive therapy in osteoarthritis of the knee. *Annals of Internal Medicine*. 2004; **141**: 901–10.
34. Belgrade M. Two decades after Ping-Pong diplomacy: Is there a role for acupuncture in American pain medicine? *APS Journal*. 1994; **3**: 73–83.
35. Romaguera C, Grimalt F. Nickel dermatitis from acupuncture needles. *Contact Dermatitis*. 1979; **5**: 195.
36. Dunn PA, Rogers D, Halford K. Transcutaneous electrical nerve stimulation at acupuncture points in the induction of uterine contractions. *Obstetrics and Gynecology*. 1989; **73**: 286–90.
37. Yn YK, Lin JT, Robins J. Acupuncture for the induction of cervical dilation in preparation for first trimester abortions and its influence on HCG. *Journal of Reproductive Medicine*. 1985; **30**: 530–4.
38. Bodner G, Toplisky M, Greif J. Pneumothorax as a complication of acupuncture in the treatment of bronchial asthma. *Annals of Allergy*. 1983; **51**: 401–03.
39. Muzal DA, King T, Harvey J *et al*. Bilateral pneumothorax after acupuncture (letter). *New England Journal of Medicine*. 1980; **302**: 1365–6.
40. Ritter HD, Tarala R. Pneumothorax after acupuncture. *British Journal of Medicine*. 1978; **2**: 602–03.
41. Kondo A, Tsunemaro K, Ishikawa J *et al*. Injury to the spinal cord produced by acupuncture needle. *Surgical Neurology*. 1979; **11**: 155–6.
42. Murata K, Nishio A, Nishikawa M *et al*. Subarachnoid hemorrhage and spinal root injury caused by acupuncture needle. *Neurologia Medico-Chirurgica*. 1990; **30**: 956–9.
43. Siraishi S, Goto I, Kuroiwa Y *et al*. Spinal cord injury as a complication of acupuncture. *Neurology*. 1979; **29**: 1180–2.
44. Southworth SR, Hartwig RH. Foreign body in the median nerve: a complication of acupuncture. *Journal of Hand Surgery*. 1990; **15**: 111–12.
45. Boxall EH. Acupuncture hepatitis in the West Midlands, 1977. *Journal of Medical Virology*. 1979; **2**: 377–9.
46. Hepatitis B associated with acupuncture – Florida. *MMWR*. 1981; **30**: 1–3.
47. Mayer DJ, Price DD, Rafii A. Antagonism of acupuncture analgesia in man by the narcotic antagonist naloxone. *Brain Research*. 1977; **121**: 368–72.
48. Ha H, Tan E, Fukunaga H *et al*. Naloxone reversal of acupuncture analgesia in the monkey. *Experimental Neurology*. 1981; **73**: 298–303.
49. Pomeranz B, Cheng R. Suppression of noxious responses in single neurons of cat spinal cord by electroacupuncture and reversal by the opiate antagonist naloxone. *Experimental Neurology*. 1979; **64**: 327–49.
50. Tsunoda Y, Shakahira K, Nakano S *et al*. Antagonism of acupuncture analgesia by naloxone in unconscious man. *Bulletin of Tokyo Medical and Dental University*. 1980; **27**: 89–94.
51. Clement-Jones V, McLoughlin L, Tomlin S *et al*. Increased beta endorphin but not met-enkephalin levels in human cerebrospinal fluid after acupuncture for recurrent pain. *Lancet*. 1980; **2**: 946–9.
52. Pert A, Dionne R, Ng L *et al*. Alteration in rat central nervous system endorphins following transauricular electroacupuncture analgesia in the periaqueductal gray of the rabbit. *Brain Research*. 1984; **322**: 289–96.
53. Han JS, Terenius L. Neurochemical basis of acupuncture analgesia. *Annual Review of Pharmacology and Toxicology*. 1982; **22**: 193–220.
54. Fugh-Berman A. *Alternative medicine: what works*. Tucson, AZ: Odonian Press, 1996.
55. Vithoulkas G. *The science of homeopathy*. New York: Grove Press, 1980.
56. Coulter H. *Homeopathic science and modern medicine: the physics of healing with microdoses*. Berkeley: North Atlantic Books, 1980.
57. Vallance AK. Can biological activity be maintained at ultra-high dilution? An overview of homeopathy, evidence, and Bayesian philosophy. *Journal of Alternative and Complementary Medicine*. 1998; **4**: 49–76.
58. Vickers AJ, Fisher P, Smith C *et al*. Homeopathic Arnica 30x is ineffective for muscle soreness after long-distance running: a randomized, double-blind, placebo-controlled trial. *Clinical Journal of Pain*. 1998; **14**: 227–31.

59. Ernst E, Pittler MH. Efficacy of homeopathic arnica: a systematic review of placebo controlled-trials. *Archives of Surgery.* 1998; **133**: 1187–90.
60. Davenas E, Beauvais F, Amara J *et al.* Human basophil degranulation triggered by very dilute antiserum against IgE. *Nature.* 1988; **333**: 816–18.
61. Witt CM, Ludtke R, Baur R, Willich SN. Homeopathic medical practice: long-term results of a cohort study with 3981 patients. *BMC Public Health.* 2005; **5**: 115.
62. Cucherat M, Haugh MC, Gooch M, Boissel JP. Evidence of clinical efficacy of homeopathy. A meta-analysis of clinical trials. HMRAG. Homeopathic Medicines Research Advisory Group. *European Journal of Clinical Pharmacology.* 2000; **56**: 27–33.
63. Linde K, Clausius N, Ramirez G *et al.* Are the clinical effects of homeopathy placebo effects? A meta-analysis of placebo-controlled trials. *Lancet.* 1997; **350**: 834–43.
64. Goldstein MS, Glik D. Use of and satisfaction with homeopathy in a patient population. *Alternative Therapies in Health and Medicine.* 1998; **4**: 60–5.
65. Potier JP. Bromate intoxication due to the ingestion of a dose prescribed by a homeopathist (letter). *Nephrology, Dialysis, Transplantation.* 1998; **13**: 2978–9.
66. Kaptchuk TJ, Eisenberg DM. Chiropractic: origins, controversies, and contributions. *Archives of Internal Medicine.* 1998; **158**: 2215–24.
67. Bigos S, Bowyer O, Braen B *et al.* Clinical practice guideline No. 14: Acute low back problems in adults. Rockville, MD: US Dept of Health and Human Services, Agency for Health Care Policy and Research, 1994, publication 95-0842.
68. Cherkin DC, MacCormack FA. Patient evaluation of low back pain care from family physicians and chiropractors. *Western Journal of Medicine.* 1989; **150**: 351–5.
69. Assendelft WJ, Morton SC, Yu EI *et al.* Spinal manipulative therapy for low back pain. A meta-analysis of effectiveness relative to other therapies. *Annals of Internal Medicine.* 2003; **138**: 871–81.
70. Gross AR, Hoving JL, Haines TA *et al.* A Cochrane review of manipulation and mobilization for mechanical neck disorders. *Spine.* 2004; **29**: 1541–8.
71. Fernandez-de-Las-Penas C, Alonso-Blanco C, Cuadrado ML *et al.* Are manual therapies effective in reducing pain from tension-type headache?: A systematic review. *Clinical Journal of Pain.* 2006; **22**: 278–85.
72. Senstad O, Leboeuf-Yde C, Borchgrevink C. Frequency and characteristics of side effects of spinal manipulative therapy. *Spine.* 1997; **22**: 435–40.
73. Stevinson C, Ernst E. Risks associated with spinal manipulation. *American Journal of Medicine.* 2002; **112**: 566–71.
74. Powell PC, Hanigan WC, Olivero WC. A risk/benefit analysis of spinal manipulation therapy for relief of lumbar or cervical pain. *Neurosurgery.* 1993; **33**: 73–8.
75. Rothwell DM, Bondy SJ, Williams JI. Chiropractic manipulation and stroke; a population-based case-control study. *Stroke.* 2001; **32**: 1054–60.
76. Integrative Medicine Communications. *A physician's reference to botanical medicines.* The Integrative Medicine Consult (supp) 1999.
77. World Health Organization. *Guidelines for the assessment of herbal medicine.* Geneva: WHO, 1991.
78. Mitka M. FDA never promised an herb garden – but sellers and buyers eager to see one grow. *Journal of the American Medical Association.* 1998; **280**: 1554–6.
79. Barrows KA, Jacobs BP. Mind-body medicine, an introduction and review of the literature. *Medical Clinics of North America.* 2002; **86**: 11–31.
80. Astin JA. Mind-body therapies for the management of pain. *Clinical Journal of Pain.* 2004; **20**: 27–32.
81. Hadhazy VA, Ezzo J, Creamer P, Berman BM. Mind-body therapies for the treatment of fibromyalgia. A systematic review. *Journal of Rheumatology.* 2000; **27**: 2911–8.
82. DiNucci EM. Energy healing: a complementary treatment for orthopaedic and other conditions. *Orthopaedic Nursing.* 2005; **24**: 259–69.
83. Wardell D, Weymouth K. Review of studies of healing touch. *Journal of Nursing Scholarship.* 2004; **36**: 147–54.
84. Peters RM. The effectiveness of therapeutic touch: A meta-analytic review. *Nursing Science Quarterly.* 1999; **12**: 52–61.
85. Astin JA, Harkness E, Ernst E. The efficacy of distant healing: a systematic review of randomized trials. *Annals of Internal Medicine.* 2000; **132**: 903–10.

PART III

MANAGEMENT – CLINICAL SITUATIONS

24

Pain in neurological disease

PAUL R NANDI

KEY LEARNING POINTS

- Pain in neurologic disease is common and may be severe.
- The clinical features of pain in neurologic disease are seldom disease-specific.
- Pain presentations in neurologic disease are diverse, reflecting diverse mechanisms.
- Nociceptive, as well as neuropathic, pain commonly occurs.
- Individual patients may have more than one pain phenotype.
- For each pain phenotype, the physiological nature of the generation of pain has implications for treatment.

INTRODUCTION

There is a commonly held view among many physicians (including some neurologists) that pain in the context of neurologic disease is rare, but when it does occur it is neuropathic in nature and extremely resistant to treatment. This chapter will show that the reality is that pain in neurologic disease is very common, multifactorial, and protean in its manifestations.

Despite its diversity, most pain in neurologic disease falls into one of two major mechanistic categories, and some other pain forms a third category:

1. Neuropathic pain resulting directly from the effects of the disease on somatosensory neurons – peripheral or central (for example, burning limb pain in syringomyelia, postherpetic neuralgia (PHN)).
2. Nociceptive pain resulting directly or indirectly from the motor effects of the disease on the locomotor system; activating the familiar nociceptive system responding to tissue damage (for example, painful lower limb muscle spasm in multiple sclerosis, "frozen shoulder" poststroke).

A third category can also be considered:

3. Neuropathic pain resulting from the effects of the disease on peripheral nerves/roots, secondary to motor changes (for example, meralgia paresthetica in spastic paraplegia, radiculopathy in cervical dystonia).

These distinctions are of practical value, as the rational management of each is different. In many conditions where both motor and sensory pathways are damaged (e.g. multiple sclerosis), combinations of two or all three types of pain are seen. It follows that an assessment of the nature of pain in an individual with neurologic disease relies upon an assessment of the pathophysiologic effects of that disease in that individual. Definitive diagnosis of the primary condition *per se* will not usually clarify this.

The prevalence of chronic pain across the spectrum of neurologic disorders is unknown. However, the data available from two common disorders – multiple sclerosis and Parkinsonism – suggest that the scale of the problem of pain in those two diseases is almost certainly underestimated, which suggests that the problem is also likely to be underestimated in less common disorders.

A classification of neurologic diseases is presented in **Table 24.1**. For each category, one or two representative examples of painful disorders are given. However, it may be argued that traditional classifications such as this have limited utility in pain evaluation, in that there is usually no clear link between the pathologic nature of the disease and the presence (and type) of pain. It may be more useful to consider categories of painful disorders presenting to neurology clinics, as proposed by Cervero and Jensen (see **Table 24.2**). In some neurologic disorders, pain is a well-recognized and predominant symptom and may be a prerequisite to diagnosis. Several such disorders are deservedly allocated chapters of their own in this volume and will be discussed little, if at all, in this chapter. These are:

- trigeminal neuralgia (Chapter 35, Facial pain);
- peripheral neuropathy (Chapter 25, Peripheral neuropathies);
- postherpetic neuralgia (Chapter 32, Herpes zoster pain including shingles and postherpetic neuralgia);
- complex regional pain syndrome (Chapter 27, Complex regional pain syndromes).

Other topics that to some degree overlap with this chapter and are covered elsewhere are:

- management of painful spasticity (Chapter 33, Management of painful spasticity);
- postamputation pain (Chapter 31, Postamputation pain);
- central pain syndromes (Chapter 28, Central neuropathic pain: syndromes, pathophysiology, and treatments).

It is not possible to provide a comprehensive list of every neurologic disease that may give rise to pain in this chapter.

What follows may be considered an overview of the scope and nature of pain in neurologic disease, largely exemplified by two conditions which are common and which illustrate some important general points – multiple sclerosis and parkinsonism. Additional brief notes are included on Guillain–Barré syndrome and dystonia.

MULTIPLE SCLEROSIS

There are two reasons to choose multiple sclerosis (MS) as a representative model on which to base generalizations about pain in neurologic disease.

Table 24.1 A suggested classification of neurological diseases associated with pain.

Etiologic category	Example	Nature of pain (location of lesion)
Hereditary	DMD	Nociceptive (muscular)
	HMSN	Either nociceptive or neurogenic (sensorimotor neuropathy)
Metabolic	DM	Neurogenic (small-fiber neuropathy)
Infective – viral	Herpes zoster	Neurogenic (ganglioneuropathy)
Infective – bacterial	Syphilis (Tabes dorsalis)	Neurogenic (myelopathy)
Inflammatory	Guillain–Barré syndrome	Neurogenic (neuropathy)
Structural/degenerative	Intervertebral disk herniation	Neurogenic (compressive radiculopathy)
Developmental	Syringomyelia	Neurogenic (myelopathy)
Vascular	Cerebral infarct	Neurogenic (central)
Demyelination – central	MS	Neurogenic (central)+nociceptive (musculoskeletal)
Demyelination – peripheral	AIDP	Neurogenic
Movement disorders – hypokinetic	PD	Nociceptive+? neurogenic (musculoskeletal+? central)
Movement disorders – hyperkinetic	Primary dystonia	Nociceptive (musculoskeletal)
Trauma	Spinal cord transection	Neurogenic (myelopathy)
Iatrogenic	Radiation plexopathy	Neurogenic (plexus)
Neoplastic	Intracerebral glioma	Nociceptive (headache ↑ ICP)

AIDP, acute inflammatory demyelinating polyneuropathy; DM, diabetes mellitus; DMD, Duchenne muscular dystrophy; HMSN, hereditary motor and sensory neuropathy; ICP, intracranial pressure MS, multiple sclerosis; PD, Parkinson's disease.

NB Some overlap between etiologic categories occurs. Guillain–Barré syndrome/AIDP is given as an example; it may be classified either as inflammatory or peripheral demyelinating.

Table 24.2 Painful conditions presenting to neurology clinics.

Painful conditions	
Pain after nerve injury	Complex regional pain syndrome
	Painful entrapment disorders
	Pain after surgical intervention
Facial pain	Trigeminal neuralgia
	Atypical facial pain
Painful neuropathies	Painful diabetic neuropathy
	Other painful polyneuropathies
	Postherpetic neuralgia
	Postamputation pain
Central neuropathic pain	Spinal cord injury pain
	Syringomyelia
	Central poststroke pain
	Pain in multiple sclerosis
	Pain in Parkinson's disease
Others	Fibromyalgia
	Chronic low back pain
	Whiplash
	Pain in dementia

First, it is common and has a high profile in the eyes of the lay public as well as the medical establishment, with vigorous support groups funding research and disseminating information about the disease. One might therefore expect reasonably accurate epidemiologic data to be available. Despite this, the prevalence of chronic pain as a major problem for persons with MS is widely underestimated. Until recently, the disease was regarded as typically painless, and described as such[1] in authoritative texts of neurology and reviews. Even now, the myth persists; a contemporary textbook of neurology for medical generalists states that pain in MS is so rare that the diagnosis should be questioned in its presence.[2]

Second, the disease can give rise to a wide variety of pains, both neuropathic and nociceptive, encompassing most of the pain patterns observed across the entire spectrum of neurologic disorders.

The nature of the disease

MS is characteristically a disease of young adults. The etiology remains unknown but both genetic and environmental factors probably contribute; the histopathologic lesion is a central nervous system (CNS) perivenular inflammatory demyelination consistent with an autoimmune response directed at myelin antigens. These lesions can occur almost anywhere in the CNS, accounting for the great diversity of clinical presentation seen in this disease. The clinical course is notoriously variable, but is typically relapsing/remitting with a tendency to cumulative neurologic deficit as the disease progresses. Optic neuritis or peripheral paresthesiae are the most common presenting features. Rarely, pain is the first clinical manifestation of the disease.[3] Motor and/or cerebellar symptoms tend to present later and are associated with a poorer prognosis. Approximately one-third of patients do not develop permanent functional impairment and less than one-third will become severely disabled. Typical features of the severe advanced case include spastic paraparesis or tetraparesis, variable somatosensory deficits, cerebellar ataxia with scanning dysarthria, incontinence, disorders of mood, and cognitive impairment.

Epidemiology

In northern Europe and North America, the incidence rates and prevalence of MS are in the order of 4–8 and 60–100 per 100,000, respectively. It is therefore about ten times as common as syringomyelia or myasthenia gravis.

Although the epidemiology of pain in the disease is less certain, several surveys suggest that a majority of sufferers experience pain of at least moderate severity.[4, 5, 6, 7, 8, 9] Moreover, these studies show a striking concordance in the breakdown of the distribution and probable cause of the reported pain patterns. A recent publication indicates that pain in MS is a major problem in registered sufferers in the community and not just in hospital clinic attenders (who may be more severely affected).[10] The most familiar type of pain quoted in neurology textbooks – trigeminal neuralgia – is relatively rare.[4, 5, 6, 7, 8, 9, 11] By contrast, myelopathic pain involving the lower limbs is common, as is pain of nociceptive musculoskeletal origin. This last feature should come as no surprise, as the consequences of the disease on motor function might be expected to cause nociceptive pain directly from spastic muscles and their mechanical effects on neighboring structures. In general, pain in MS appears comparable in severity to that of rheumatoid and osteoarthritis, and its intensity correlates with reduced quality of life.[12]

Patterns of pain presentation in multiple sclerosis

A suggested approach to the analysis of pain in MS is outlined in **Box 24.1**. It is intended to encourage the clinician to consider the pathophysiologic basis of the pain before considering which treatment modalities are most appropriate.Pains of primary neurogenic origin are divided into paroxysmal and nonparoxysmal. Paroxysmal pains may be more likely to respond to anticonvulsant drugs, whereas ongoing central pains may be more likely to respond to other groups of drugs such as antidepressants and *N*-methyl-D-aspartic acid (NMDA) receptor antagonists, and in some cases opioids.

Box 24.1 Pain classification in multiple sclerosis

- Pains of primary neurogenic origin
  - Paroxysmal
    - Trigeminal neuralgia
    - Lhermitte's phenomenon
    - Seizures
- Painful spasms
- Visceral pain
  - Nonparoxysmal central pain
- Nociceptive musculoskeletal pain
  - Chronic back pain
  - Peripheral muscle spasticity/spasm
- Miscellaneous
  - "Mechanical" neuropathic
- Nonspecific exacerbating factors
  - Infection
  - Iatrogenic

PAINS OF PRIMARY NEUROGENIC ORIGIN

Paroxysmal

Trigeminal neuralgia occurs in multiple sclerosis approximately 300 times more often than in the general population. It is generally similar in its presentation to the idiopathic condition, but tends to occur at a younger age and is more likely to be bilateral (which is extremely rare in the idiopathic disorder). It is generally responsive to treatment along similar lines to idiopathic tic douloureux,[13] although microvascular decompression (in a small series) appeared less effective,[14] and there also appears to be relative refractoriness to neurolytic surgical procedures.[15] A 1994 study[7] suggests a prevalence in the order of 5 percent (rather higher than formerly believed). Unlike most pain syndromes in MS, trigeminal neuralgia may be a presenting symptom of the disease, and the underlying diagnosis should therefore be considered particularly in a young patient or one with bilateral symptoms. The clinical manifestations and treatment of trigeminal neuralgia are discussed at greater length in Chapter 35, Facial pain.

Lhermitte's phenomenon is a classical finding in MS. It consists of rapidly evolving paresthesiae or dysesthesiae, provoked by neck flexion, and typically spreading down the back and into the extremities. It is suggested that traction on the dorsal columns actively involved in the inflammatory process is the trigger. A recent study indicates that it may occur in over 41 percent of individuals with MS at some point in the course of their disease, and is significantly correlated with magnetic resonance imaging (MRI) signal change in the cervical cord.[16]

Epileptiform seizures are rare in MS, and in general are a rare cause of pain. However, a syndrome of spreading dysesthesiae and muscle spasm, either spontaneous or evoked by trivial stimuli such as light touch, active or passive movement, or a startling event, is recognized. The prevalence of this symptom complex varies in the limited literature describing it.[7, 17]

Nonparoxysmal central pain

This is probably the most common neurogenic pain manifestation in MS. It is typically burning and/or aching in quality[4, 5, 7, 11] and often anatomically extensive (e.g. from the waist down). Although it is impossible to exclude supraspinal mechanisms in the genesis of pains of this sort, it seems likely that demyelinating myelopathy is the primary cause in most cases. This may be inferred from the similarity of the pain to that described in many cases of traumatic spinal cord damage with no evidence of rostral neural injury.[18] This type of pain is much more common in the lower extremities than the upper. A characteristic complaint is of a sensation of constriction of the painful territory, like wearing a tight corset or an undersized boot. Allodynia undoubtedly occurs but is uncommon in the author's experience and most published material.

Nociceptive musculoskeletal pain

There is no doubt that many patients with MS suffer pains in this category – perhaps in the order of 20 percent – and that such pains are more troublesome than in the general population. It seems obvious that many patients with myelopathy and/or cerebral disease will be susceptible to pains of both true central and peripheral nociceptive nature, the latter consequent on spasticity and immobilization. In some cases, analysis of the separate pain components may be difficult on clinical grounds. Nevertheless, it seems desirable to try to separate central neurogenic and peripheral nociceptive components of pain because of the different implications for treatment.

Painful spasticity of muscles, particularly of the spinal muscles and muscles of the lower limbs, is a common problem in advanced MS.[13] The management of painful spasticity is covered elsewhere in this volume (Chapter 33, Management of painful spasticity).

Low back pain is common and probably the consequence of a combination of factors. Lumbar paraspinal muscle spasticity may result directly in muscular pain and also produce increased mechanical stress on nonmuscular components of the spine (such as ligaments, disks, and zygapophysial joints). Additionally, the immobilization and weakness that occurs with advancing disability may predispose to musculoskeletal spinal pain in the same way as is believed to occur in patients with chronic back pain without neurologic disease.

Miscellaneous

"Mechanical neuropathic"

On the basis of the above, one would expect lumbar radiculopathic pain to be more common in people with MS than in the general population. Analysis of pain patterns in the aforementioned prevalence studies identifies pain of this type. The author has seen a number of patients with meralgia paresthetica associated with flexor spasms of the thigh.

Nonspecific exacerbating factors

Infections in persons with MS may worsen spasticity and spasm.[14] Pressure sores may be painful although typically they are not.

Iatrogenic

This includes pain, for example, related to surgical procedures such as intrathecal pump implants.

ACUTE INFLAMMATORY POLYNEUROPATHY (GUILLAIN–BARRÉ SYNDROME)

Guillain–Barré syndrome (GBS) is an acute onset, predominantly motor polyneuropathy with an immunologic basis. There is often an antecedent history of infection or immunization but in many cases no such trigger can be identified. Despite the predominance of motor over sensory deficit, pain is common (approximately 50–70 percent of cases in a fairly recent review[19]) and may manifest itself in a wide variety of ways including both neurogenic and nocigenic presentations. A more recent prospective study suggests an even higher frequency (nearly 90 percent), with nearly 50 percent reporting pain "distressing" or worse.[20] Pain can be a prominent symptom even in otherwise mild cases.[21] The most commonly encountered pains were deep, aching back/leg pain and dysesthetic extremity pain. Although complete recovery has widely been considered to be the rule, more recent data suggest that many patients report aching and cramping pain years after the onset of symptoms, that the pain is correlated with persisting sensory, but not motor, deficits,[22] and gabapentin appears to be effective.[23, 24][II]

MOVEMENT DISORDERS

Many neurologic diseases may result in disordered movement. However, those conditions traditionally grouped together under the heading "movement disorders" comprise a collection of disorders in which disease or dysfunction of the extrapyramidal system is the principal feature.

In common with multiple sclerosis, it seems likely that pain is underestimated in these conditions, although there are fewer data available from the medical literature to support this assertion. The likelihood of nociceptive pain in patients with impaired/involuntary movement seems intuitively obvious, but there is evidence of neuropathic pain in some of these disorders as well, focusing attention on involvement of sensory, as well as motor tract pathology.

Movement disorders can be subdivided into two categories: **hypokinetic**, characterized by impaired volitional movement, of which parkinsonism is much the commonest (see **Box 24.1**), and **hyperkinetic**, characterized by involuntary movements of various types (see **Box 24.2**).

Box 24.2 Causes of parkinsonism

- Parkinson's disease
- "Parkinson plus" syndromes
  - Progressive supranuclear palsy
  - Multiple system atrophy
  - Spinocerebellar ataxias
  - Corticobasal degeneration
- Other
  - Drug-induced/toxic
  - Vascular
  - Infectious/transmissible (including Creutzfeldt–Jakob disease)

Notes on some terms relating to movement disorders

A number of descriptive terms are used to differentiate patterns of disordered muscle tone and movement, and may give rise to confusion among non-neurologists. Some of these terms, and their corresponding meanings, are listed below:

- Spasticity is the type of muscle hypertonia seen following a lesion of the corticospinal tract. Resistance to passive movement of an affected limb is maximal at its outset and reduced once movement is initiated ("clasp-knife" effect). Tendon reflexes are increased. The Babinski response is extensor. Clonus (rhythmic repetitive contractions) may occur.
- Rigidity is a uniform increase of muscle tone seen in extrapyramidal lesions, notably parkinsonism. Resistance to passive movement is evenly encountered throughout the range ("lead-pipe" rigidity). In cases where tremor is superimposed, rapid fluctuations in the degree of resistance may be felt ("cog-wheel" effect).
- Dyskinesia is a term used to cover the range of involuntary movements seen in extrapyramidal disturbance:
  - chorea: jerky, quasi-purposive movements, typically of the face/upper limbs;
  - athetosis: slower, more writhing movements;
  - hemiballismus: violent excursions of an entire limb;
  - dystonia: sustained, often repetitive, muscle contraction, typically giving rise to twisting movements and/or abnormal postures;
  - tremor: rhythmic rapid oscillations;
  - myoclonus: brief isolated jerks which may involve part of a muscle, an entire muscle, or several muscle groups.

PARKINSONISM

The distinction should be made between the broad clinical syndrome of bradykinesia, rigidity, and tremor (parkinsonism) – which may result from several causes – and the idiopathic condition, Parkinson's disease (PD). Causes of parkinsonism are listed in **Box 24.2**. The relevance of the distinction between these conditions from the pain management perspective is that some of these conditions may be associated with somatosensory deficit, increasing the likelihood of neuropathic pain (although this has been proposed in idiopathic PD as well).

The nature of the disease

In contrast to MS, PD is typically a disorder of the middle-aged and elderly. Some secondary causes of parkinsonism may present earlier. Pain in PD has been the subject of a recent review article.[25]

Parkinsonism provides a useful second model of a neurologic disorder in which chronic pain is both common and underestimated.[26, 27] The etiology very probably involves both genetic and environmental factors; various toxic environmental chemicals have been implicated in the disease, as well as familial clustering of cases consistent with autosomal dominant inheritance. Concerning the pathology, degeneration of dopaminergic neurons of the substantia nigra is the hallmark of the idiopathic disease. The prevalence in the USA is in the order of 0.4 percent overall, increasing to 1 percent in individuals over age 55.

Parkinsonian syndromes classically present with a triad of features:

1. bradykinesia – slowness of spontaneous movement;
2. rigidity;
3. tremor – typically at rest.

Of this triad of components, it is usually the first two which are associated with pain.

PD is now hardly ever seen in its unmodified form in advanced cases as treatment with L-dopa and other dopaminergic drugs is more or less universal in developed countries. While L-dopa therapy has dramatic therapeutic benefit early on, its continued use ultimately typically gives rise to a state of clinical fluctuation between bradykinesia/rigidity and dyskinesia ("on–off" phenomenon). In this state, the parkinsonian patient may exhibit pain associated with both hyperkinetic and hypokinetic disorder.

Although pain has long been recognized in PD, there were few data on which to base estimates of its prevalence until the important paper by Snider *et al.* in 1976.[28] On the basis of this study, the prevalence is probably in the order of 40–50 percent (similar to MS), although the authors quote a lower figure on the basis of excluding burning sensations and also muscular pains clearly resulting directly from increased tone. A later study by Goetz *et al.*[29] closely mirrors these findings; however, Snider *et al.* attribute much of the limb pain to central mechanisms, whereas Goetz's paper places more emphasis on nociceptive pain attributable to the effects of the disease on muscle tone, movement, and posture.

Although Snider *et al.* cite a lack of correlation between muscle hypertonia and pain as evidence of a central cause for the pain, it is usually worse on the side with most motor dysfunction, and the character of the pain suggests a musculotendinous origin. In advanced treated cases with an "on–off" pattern, pain may be a feature of both the "on" and the "off" phase. Sufferers typically complain of a constant aching, cramp-like discomfort of the muscles while "off," and "muscle-strain" pain while "on."

However, some pains cannot be explained on this basis and seem likely to be neuropathic in nature, such as the reports of oral/genital pain.[30, 31] A fairly recent study suggests that in approximately 8 percent of parkinsonian patients with pain, the pain is neuropathic.[27] A small proportion of patients with PD have sensory symptoms (including pain) which precede any clinically apparent motor effects of the disease. Burning pain is often, though not invariably, related to L-dopa therapy.

There is evidence that the prevalence of pain in multiple system atrophy, the most common cause of secondary parkinsonism, is similar to that of PD.[32]

Quinn *et al.*[33] have proposed a classification of pain in Parkinson's disease largely based on its relation to medication, although this sheds no light on putative pain mechanisms.

HYPERKINETIC DISORDERS

Hyperkinetic disorders are categorized in **Box 24.3**. Usually, pains in these conditions are considered to be nociceptive and muscular/arthralgic in origin. However, a recent paper on pain in spasmodic torticollis,[34] the most frequent form of cervical dystonia, questions this and suggests that central mechanisms may be an important cause. This suggestion is largely based on the observation

Box 24.3 Classification of hyperkinetic disorders

- Chorea/athetosis/hemiballism
- Dystonia
- Myoclonus
- Tics

that the correlation between markedly hypertonic muscles and pain in those muscles is weak, rather than on any positive evidence of central sensory disturbance.

Neuropathic pain may undoubtedly occur if sensory pathways are damaged, in which case clinical evidence of such damage should be apparent. Certainly, dyskinesia giving rise to abnormal mechanical stress on the axial skeleton may cause radicular pain. In a study of cervical dystonia, Jancovic *et al.*[35] reported evidence of secondary radiculopathy in 32 percent of their patients.

MANAGEMENT OF PAIN IN NEUROLOGIC DISEASE

General considerations

Effective treatment of pain in neurologic disease is seldom, if ever, disease specific. Burning central neuropathic pain is probably as likely to respond to a tricyclic antidepressant whether the disorder responsible is syringomyelia, multiple sclerosis, or spinal cord injury. Conversely, an antiepileptic drug that successfully treats trigeminal neuralgia in a patient with MS may be completely ineffective for lumbar back pain in the same patient. Rational management of pain in any patient with neurologic disease must start with an attempt to identify the nature of the likely pathophysiology giving rise to the pain (or pains).

The following fundamental questions may form a useful starting point:

- Is the pain nociceptive or neurogenic?
- If neurogenic, is it central or peripheral?
- If peripheral, is it directly due to the primary disease process or the result of motor dysfunction?
- If nociceptive, is there spasticity, rigidity, or dyskinesia?

Almost all treatment modalities advocated and practiced in the treatment of pain in neurologic disease are described and discussed at length in the relevant chapters on treatments elsewhere in this volume. They will therefore be considered relatively briefly here, with the focus of attention on their use in the context of neurologic disorders and neuropathic pain states. As in other chapters, they will be discussed under the following headings:

- Pharmacologic;
- Physical treatments;
- Invasive treatments;
- Surgical treatment;
- Psychologic treatment;
- Alternative medicine.

The evidence scores given for each treatment modality generally refer to efficacy in treating neuropathic pain.

Pharmacologic

The pharmacologic treatment of neuropathic pain, including topical as well as systemic administration, has been the subject of a recent publication by a Task Force of the European Federation of Neurological Societies.[36]

TOPICAL TREATMENTS

Nonsteroidal anti-inflammatory drugs, capsaicin, and local anesthetics may be useful in clinical situations where pain is evoked or exacerbated by superficial nociceptors (or in some cases non-nociceptive afferents). Topical treatments are discussed in depth in Chapter 17, Topical analgesics for neuropathic pain, and their use in postherpetic neuralgia in Chapter 32, Herpes zoster pain including shingles and postherpetic neuralgia.

OPIOIDS

Some controversy still exists concerning the value of potent opioids such as morphine in chronic nonmalignant pain generally, as well as whether these drugs are effective in neuropathic pain. These issues are discussed in depth in Chapter 16, Opioids and chronic noncancer pain, but it is perhaps appropriate to cite here one well-conducted study demonstrating efficacy of opioids in neuropathic pain,[37][II] and another publication[38] reporting little or no benefit.

A reasonable interpretation of the medical literature overall addressing this issue is that there are some individual patients with individual neuropathic pains that are opioid responsive and others which are not. Whether or not a given individual will prove responsive to this group of drugs is not reliably predictable on the basis of pathologic diagnosis. A suggested practical management approach is to offer patients a limited trial of opioid therapy if it seems justified by clinical need, only continuing treatment in the long term if the trial results in substantial symptomatic and functional benefit without unacceptable side effects.

In general, nociceptive pain in neurologic disease should respond to opioids in a manner similar to that in the patient without neurologic disease.

ANTIDEPRESSANTS

The use of antidepressants in neuropathic pain has been subject to recent systematic review.[39, 40][I] This can be briefly summarized by stating that there was clear benefit compared with placebo in a variety of conditions, including diabetic neuropathy, PHN, and central pain. The number needed to treat (NNT) for pooled data was between two and three. Amitriptyline, in particular, appears effective in central poststroke pain.[41][I] Selective serotonin-reuptake inhibitors (SSRIs) generally appeared less effective than tricyclic antidepressants (although they were associated with fewer side effects), suggesting that the noradrenergic action of some tricyclics may be important for their analgesic effect. In this review, the character of the pain was not predictive of response to these drugs, and favorable response was typically achieved in a few days.

Beneficial effects of antidepressants on pain have been demonstrated in a wide variety of pain syndromes, including rheumatoid arthritis, low back pain, tension headache, and cancer pain. It is clear that these drugs may be helpful for both neurogenic and nociceptive pains. It is reasonable to try them in patients with neurologic disease whose pain falls into either category or both categories. The evidence of benefit in MS is conflicting. Clifford and Trotter[11][V] report relief of pain by tricyclic antidepressants in more than 50 percent of their series of patients, whereas Moulin *et al.*[5][V] found this group of drugs relatively ineffective.

ANTICONVULSANTS

The use of anticonvulsants in chronic pain has also been subject to fairly recent systematic review.[42][I]

To summarize the findings, the majority of studies were of neuropathic pain states, with three examining diabetic neuropathy. Results were conflicting. Overall, NNT for both effectiveness and adverse effects were similar to the corresponding figures for the antidepressants. The relatively new adjunctive anticonvulsant gabapentin was not included in this review, but a number of subsequent publications report benefit in pains associated with multiple sclerosis,[43, 44, 45, 46][V] diabetic neuropathy, PHN, and other neuropathic pain states. Pregabalin is also clearly effective,[47] although good evidence of superiority over gabapentin is lacking. There is also growing evidence of benefit from lamotrigine in central pain.[41][I], [48][V] Adverse effects frequently limit the practical utility of antiepileptic drugs, with a recent study of patients with MS showing that carbamazepine was associated with worse adverse effects than either gabapentin or lamotrigine, in some cases mimicking disease relapse.[49]

SYSTEMIC SODIUM CHANNEL BLOCKERS

Although this group of drugs comprises the local anesthetics and related "membrane-stabilizing" cardiac antiarrhythmics, it should be appreciated that sodium channel inhibition is a property of many other groups of drugs, including many anticonvulsants, antidepressants, and "mainstream" analgesics such as pethidine (meperidine), and it is possible that at least some of the therapeutic effects of these drugs are mediated through sodium channel inhibition.

A systematic review has been undertaken of systemic local anesthetic-type drugs in chronic pain.[50][I] The findings can be summarized as follows: the most convincing evidence for benefit is seen in neuropathic pain of peripheral nerve injury or peripheral neuropathy, with no evidence of benefit in dysesthesia from spinal cord injury or painful neuropathy (including plexopathy) in malignant disease. However, one recent publication supports their use in MS.[51][V]

NEUROLEPTICS

At the time of writing, the author is unaware of any convincing evidence in support of the use of these drugs for any pain-related indication. In addition, the risk of producing persisting tardive dyskinesia should be borne in mind by anyone tempted to prescribe these drugs on the basis of anecdotal evidence.

BENZODIAZEPINES AND OTHER GABA-AMINOBUTYRIC ACID AGONISTS

Generally speaking, drugs of the benzodiazepine group have been viewed with caution in long-term pain management because of the increasingly recognized problems of tolerance and dependence. However, although under most circumstances they are not analgesic, they are anxiolytic and, to varying degrees, antispastic. This last property may be valuable in the treatment of pain associated with muscular hypertonia. Spasticity may be relieved by both benzodiazepines and baclofen. Dantrolene, which acts peripherally on striated muscle, is of dubious value as a sole antispastic agent but may act synergistically with baclofen.[14] Baclofen has an antinociceptive action distinct from its antispastic effect, but the clinical effect in most pain associated with neurologic disease is probably marginal when it is given systemically (see below under Spinal drug administration).

Tizanidine, a centrally acting α_2-agonist, has also been reported as beneficial in a variety of spastic disorders, including MS.[52][II]

NMDA RECEPTOR ANTAGONISTS

The availability of drugs for human use with established effects on the NMDA receptor is limited. It is postulated, but not proven, that gabapentin may exert some effect through this mechanism; drugs with an established action are ketamine, dextromethorphan, and amantadine, all of which have been shown to be effective in studies of neuropathic pain.[53, 54, 55] The practical utility of these drugs is limited by side effects which, so far, seem inextricably linked with the desired pharmacologic effect. In addition, ketamine has well-recognized abuse potential and uncertain long-term adverse effects.

CANNABINOIDS

The use of cannabinoids as specific analgesics in neuropathic pain remains controversial. A recent study of a cannabis-based preparation in the treatment of pain in MS indicated that it was effective and well tolerated.[56][II]

Physical treatments

Included in this category are the range of "hands-on" techniques of physiotherapy, osteopathy, and chiropractic and the treatment modalities of transcutaneous electrical nerve stimulation (TENS) and acupuncture which are often offered by physiotherapists but which are also extensively practiced by other healthcare professionals. There is also some overlap with the treatment modalities espoused by alternative and complementary medicine.

An increasingly recognized role of physiotherapists in pain management is their contribution to cognitive/behavioral programs which will not be discussed further here.

Evidence-based evaluation of physical treatments is inherently difficult, partly because of the problems of blinding of the recipient and providing a placebo that is both credible and physiologically inert, and partly because of the difficulty of standardizing many of these treatments.

Not surprisingly, most clinical studies of physical treatments have focused on musculoskeletal/inflammatory disorders and there is little information about outcome when these techniques are applied specifically to sufferers of neurologic disease. A number of studies have reported reduction of spasticity following topical cooling, but the effects have generally been too brief to suggest a practical role for such treatment.

The problems of evaluating the use of TENS in chronic pain generally are discussed in a systematic review by McQuay and Moore,[57][I] who conclude that there is no good evidence in support of its use and that more studies are needed. Only one of the 38 randomized controlled trials included in this study looked specifically at a neurologic disorder (postherpetic neuralgia) and this compared TENS with acupuncture, as did many of the studies in this paper. The difficulty of blinding (especially the recipient) seems insuperable at present, but some problems with much of the literature to date can be remedied – larger numbers of subjects, longer periods of use of the treatment, and longer follow up. Evidence-based evaluation of acupuncture presents similar problems. At the time of writing, the author is unaware of any specific unimodal physical therapy of proven value for treatment of pain in neurologic disease. Kidd *et al.*[58][V] draw attention to the value of rehabilitation in the global management of patients with MS, but it is unclear whether there is any specific effect on pain.

Invasive treatments

There is an inevitable overlap between these therapies and (systemic) pharmacologic treatments, which is perhaps most obvious in the use of implanted spinal drug delivery systems to increase the therapeutic effect, and/or reduce side effects, of a drug previously given systemically.

Invasive treatments can be classified as follows:

- reversible local/regional block with local anesthetic, with or without the use of additional corticosteroid;
- spinal injection/infusion of some drugs considered largely effective only by this route (e.g. benzodiazepines, clonidine) or more effective/better tolerated in selected cases (e.g. opioids, baclofen);
- neurolytic procedures;
- botulinum toxin injection;
- miscellaneous.

LOCAL ANESTHETIC BLOCK

The indications for local anesthetic nerve blocks have been categorized by Bonica into:

- diagnostic;
- prognostic;
- prophylactic;
- therapeutic.

The practical value of this classification is as relevant to pain in neurological disease as in any other clinical context. The indications for, and practical use of, peripheral nerve blocks is discussed in Chapter 23, Peripheral nerve blocks: practical aspects in the *Practice and Procedures* volume of this series. It now seems clear that serial local anesthetic blocks – with or without the addition of corticosteroid – may provide extended periods of relief of chronic pain, long outlasting the anticipated direct duration of action of the local anesthetic drug.[59][V] More studies are needed to establish the indications and general utility of this form of treatment for pain in various neurologic disorders. The role, if any, of steroids is not established.

SPINAL DRUG ADMINISTRATION

Intrathecal baclofen is clearly effective in reducing spasticity and would therefore be expected to reduce nociceptive pain directly attributable to spasticity.[14][V] However, there is also evidence that it might be effective in the treatment of central pain.[60, 61][V]

There is some evidence of benefit from spinally administered clonidine in neuropathic pain of multiple sclerosis/spinal cord injury[62] and cancer,[63][V] and a study indicating pain relief in relapsing MS from spinally administered corticosteroid (triamcinolone).[64][III]

Spinal opioid delivery is discussed in Chapter 21, Spinal administration.

NEUROLYTIC PROCEDURES

There is some evidence for benefit from procedures in this category in the treatment of pain in neurologic disease, especially characterized by disabling and painful spasticity. Favorable results using hyperbaric intrathecal phenol in such cases were reported nearly 50 years ago by Nathan,[65][V] and similar results have emerged from a study by the author and others in patients with advanced MS.[66][V]

Use of neurolytic procedures interrupting sensory pathways in an attempt to relieve pain may expose the patient to the risk of recurrent, resistant central pain consequent upon deafferentation, which may be extremely difficult to treat. By contrast, treatment of nociceptive, spasticity-contingent pain by selective motor neuronal/axonal lesioning should be free of this risk provided it is sufficiently selective.

Because of the invasive and potentially irreversible nature of these treatments, they have been largely restricted to patients with severe pain and disability; there are some data concerning their use in neurologic disease with severe spasticity.

BOTULINUM TOXIN

Botulinum toxin injection is now a well established treatment for disorders of muscular hypertonia; it is discussed in a separate chapter (Chapter 33, Management of painful spasticity) and will not be further considered here.

Surgical treatment

Most surgical interventions deemed appropriate for pain in neurologic disease involve interruption or augmentation of neural pathways and therefore lie within the province of the neurosurgeon. However, there are obvious special situations where other surgical specialists may contribute to relief of pain as well as other symptoms – tenotomy, plastic surgical treatment of pressure sores, etc. A recent large review of neurosurgical interventions in MS suggests that good outcomes can be achieved with appropriate selection criteria.[67][III] Neurosurgical procedures for treating chronic pain are discussed in Chapter 28, Central neuropathic pain: syndromes, pathophysiology, and treatments and Chapter 20, Neurostimulation techniques, and will not be considered further here.

Psychologic treatment

The application of psychology-based treatment to chronic pain is extensively covered in Chapter 13, Self-regulation skills training for adults, including relaxation; Chapter 14, Biofeedback; Chapter 15, Contextual cognitive-behavioral therapy; and Chapter 16, Graded exposure *in vivo* for pain-related fear in the *Practice and Procedures* volume of this series. In principle, the management approach is as appropriate to chronic pain sufferers with neurologic disease as to other groups, with perhaps two qualifications.

First, cognitive impairment is a feature of some neurologic disorders and may limit the feasibility of cognitive modification.

Second, physical disability in many painful neurologic diseases may be directly attributable to motor/sensory deficit or dysfunction, in contrast with, for example, the patient with musculoskeletal back pain without neurologic disease whose disability is pain contingent. This may limit the capacity for improving physical function with a cognitive–behavioral management approach.

Alternative medicine

The evidence for efficacy of complementary and alternative medicines in MS has been the subject of a recent review by Huntley,[68][III] in which the paucity of well-conducted studies is emphasized and no firm conclusions reached for any specific therapy. A review of acupuncture concluded that there was no good evidence for symptomatic benefit from this treatment in either MS or PD, but highlighted the difficulties of trial design.[69][III]

CONCLUSION

Pain in neurologic disease is frequently underestimated in its importance, both in terms of its seriousness to those afflicted and its prevalence. Pains may be neuropathic or nociceptive, and the two types of pain frequently coexist in individual cases. Pain phenotype in neurologic disease is hardly ever disease-specific, and attention should be focused on likely mechanisms of pain generation in an attempt to determine the likelihood of response to therapeutic interventions.

REFERENCES

1. Tourtellotte WW, Baumhefner WW. Comprehensive management of multiple sclerosis. In: Hallpike JF, Adams CWM, Tourtellotte WW (eds). *Multiple sclerosis.* Baltimore, MD: Williams & Wilkins, 1983: 513–78.
2. Rolak LA. Immune mediated diseases. In: Samuels MA, Feske S (eds). *Office practice of neurology.* New York: Churchill Livingstone, 1996: 350.
3. Marchettini P, Formaglio F, Lacerenza M. Pain as heralding symptom in multiple sclerosis. *Neurological Sciences.* 2006; **27**: s294–6.

4. Vermote R, Ketelaer P, Carton H. Pain in multiple sclerosis patients. *Clinical Neurology and Neurosurgery.* 1986; **88**: 87–93.
5. Moulin DE, Foley KM, Ebers GC. Pain syndromes in multiple sclerosis. *Neurology.* 1988; **38**: 1830–4.
* 6. Stenager E, Knudsen L, Jensen K. Acute and chronic pain syndromes in multiple sclerosis. *Acta Neurologica Scandinavica.* 1991; **84**: 197–200.
* 7. Österberg A, Boivie J, Holmgren H *et al.* The clinical characteristics and sensory abnormalities of patients with central pain caused by multiple sclerosis. In: Gebhart GF, Hammond DL, Jensen TS (eds). *Progress in pain research and management.* Seattle, WA: IASP Press, 1994: 789–96.
* 8. Osterberg A, Boivie J, Thuomas KA. Central pain in multiple sclerosis – prevalence and clinical characteristics. *European Journal of Pain.* 2005; **9**: 531–42.
9. Solaro C, Brichetto G, Amato MP *et al.* The prevalence of pain in multiple sclerosis: a multicenter cross-sectional study. *Neurology.* 2004; **63**: 919–21.
10. Hadjimichael O, Kerns RD, Rizzo MA *et al.* Persistent pain and uncomfortable sensations in persons with multiple sclerosis. *Pain.* 2007; **127**: 35–41.
11. Clifford DB, Trotter JL. Pain in multiple sclerosis. *Archives of Neurology.* 1984; **41**: 1270–2.
12. Kalia LV, O'Connor PW. Severity of chronic pain and its relationship to quality of life in multiple sclerosis. *Multiple Sclerosis.* 2005; **11**: 322–7.
13. Shibasaki H, Kuroiwa Y. Painful tonic seizure in multiple sclerosis. *Archives of Neurology.* 1974; **30**: 47–51.
14. Thompson AJ. Multiple sclerosis: symptomatic treatment. *Journal of Neurology.* 1996; **243**: 559–65.
15. Cheng JS, Sanchez-Mejia RO, Limbo M *et al.* Management of medically refractory trigeminal neuralgia in patients with multiple sclerosis. *Neurosurgical Focus.* 2005; **18**: e13.
16. Al-Araji AH, Oger J. Reappraisal of Lhermitte's sign in multiple sclerosis. *Multiple Sclerosis.* 2005; **11**: 398–402.
17. Resnick DK, Jannetta PJ, Lunsford LD, Bissonette DJ. Microvascular decompression for trigeminal neuralgia in patients with multiple sclerosis. *Surgical Neurology.* 1996; **46**: 358–61.
18. Beri A. Spinal cord damage: injury. In: Wall PD, Melzack R (eds). *Textbook of pain*, 4th edn. Edinburgh: Churchill Livingstone, 1999: 915–29.
* 19. Pentland B, Donald SM. Pain in the Guillain–Barré syndrome: a clinical review. *Pain.* 1994; **59**: 159–64.
20. Moulin DE, Hagen N, Feasby TE *et al.* Pain in Guillain–Barré syndrome. *Neurology.* 1997; **48**: 328–31.
21. Green DM, Ropper AH. Mild Guillain-Barre syndrome. *Archives of Neurology.* 2001; **58**: 1098–101.
22. Bernsen RA, Jager AE, Schmitz PI, van der Meche FG. Long term sensory deficit after Guillain-Barré syndrome. *Journal of Neurology.* 2001; **248**: 483–6.
23. Pandey CK, Bose N, Garg G *et al.* Gabapentin for the treatment of pain in Guillain-Barré syndrome: a double-blinded, placebo controlled crossover study. *Anaesthesia and Analgesia.* 2002; **95**: 1719–23.
24. Pandey CK, Raza M, Tripathi M *et al.* The comparative evaluation of gabapentin and carbamazepine for pain management in Guillain-Barré syndrome patients in the intensive care unit. *Anesthesia and Analgesia.* 2005; **101**: 220–5.
* 25. Drake DF, Harkins S, Outubuddin A. Pain in Parkinson's disease: pathology to treatment, medication to deep brain stimulation. *Neurorehabilitation.* 2005; **20**: 335–41.
26. Giuffrida R, Vingerhoets FJ, Bogousslavsky J, Ghika J. Pain in Parkinson's disease. *Revue Neurologique.* 2005; **161**: 407–18.
27. Etchipare F, Rozenberg S, Mirault T *et al.* Back problems in Parkinson's disease: an underestimated problem. *Joint, Bone, Spine.* 2006; **73**: 298–302.
28. Snider SR, Fahn S, Isgreen WP, Cote LJ. Primary sensory symptoms in Parkinsonism. *Neurology.* 1976; **26**: 423–9.
* 29. Goetz CG, Tanner CM, Levy M *et al.* Pain in Parkinson's disease. *Movement Disorders.* 1986; **1**: 45–9.
30. Schott GD. Pain in Parkinson's disease. *Pain.* 1985; **22**: 407–11.
31. Ford B, Louis ED, Greene P, Fahn S. Oral and genital pain syndromes in Parkinson's disease. *Movement Disorders.* 1996; **11**: 421–6.
32. Tison F, Wenning GK, Volonte MA *et al.* Pain in multiple system atrophy. *Journal of Neurology.* 1996; **243**: 153–6.
33. Quinn NP, Koller WC, Lang AE, Marsden CD. Painful Parkinson's disease. *Lancet.* 1986; **1**: 1366–9.
34. Kutvonen O, Dastidar P, Nurmikko T. Pain in spasmodic torticollis. *Pain.* 1997; **69**: 279–86.
35. Jankovic J, Leder S, Warner D, Schwartz K. Cervical dystonia: clinical findings and associated movement disorders. *Neurology.* 1991; **41**: 1088–91.
36. Attal N, Cruccu G, Haanpaa M *et al.* EFNS guidelines on pharmacological treatment of neuropathic pain. *European Journal of Neurology.* 2006; **13**: 1153–69.
37. Rowbotham M, Reisner-Keller L, Fields H. Both intravenous lidocaine and morphine reduce the pain of postherpetic neuralgia. *Neurology.* 1991; **41**: 1024–8.
38. Arner S, Meyerson BA. Lack of analgesic effect of opioids on neuropathic and idiopathic forms of pain. *Pain.* 1988; **33**: 11–23.
* 39. McQuay HJ, Tramer M, Nye BA *et al.* A systematic review of antidepressants in neuropathic pain. *Pain.* 1996; **68**: 217–27.
* 40. Saarto T, Wiffen PJ. Antidepressants for neuropathic pain. *Cochrane Database of Systematic Review.* 2005; **CD005454**.
* 41. Frese A, Husstedt IW, Ringelstein EB, Evers S. Pharmacologic treatment of central post-stroke pain. *Clinical Journal of Pain.* 2006; **22**: 252–60.
* 42. McQuay H, Carroll D, Jadad AR *et al.* Anticonvulsant drugs for management of pain: a systematic review. *British Medical Journal.* 1995; **311**: 1047–52.
43. Khan OA. Gabapentin relieves trigeminal neuralgia in multiple sclerosis patients. *Neurology.* 1998; **51**: 611–4.

44. Solaro C, Lunardi GL, Capello E *et al.* An open-label trial of gabapentin treatment of paroxysmal symptoms in multiple sclerosis patients. *Neurology.* 1998; **51**: 609–11.
45. Houtchens MK, Richert JR, Sami A, Rose JW. Open-label gabapentin treatment for pain in multiple sclerosis. *Multiple Sclerosis.* 1997; **3**: 250–3.
46. Samkoff LM, Daras M, Tuchman AJ, Koppel BS. Amelioration of refractory dysesthetic limb pain in multiple sclerosis by gabapentin. *Neurology.* 1997; **49**: 304–05.
47. Freynhagen R, Strojek K, Griesing T *et al.* Efficacy of pregabalin in neuropathic pain evaluated in a 12 week, randomised, double-blind, multicentre, placebo controlled trial of flexible- and fixed-dose regimens. *Pain.* 2005; **115**: 254–63.
48. Cianchetti C, Zuddas A, Randazzo AP *et al.* Lamotrigine adjunctive therapy in painful phenomena in MS: preliminary observations. *Neurology.* 1999; **53**: 433.
49. Solaro C, Brichetto G, Battaglia MA *et al.* Antiepileptic medications in multiple sclerosis: adverse effects in a three-year follow-up study. *Neurological Sciences.* 2005; **25**: 307–10.
* 50. Kalso E, Tramer MR, McQuay HJ, Moore RA. Systemic local anaesthetic-type drugs in chronic pain: a systematic review. *European Journal of Pain.* 1998; **2**: 3–14.
51. Sakurai M, Kanazawa I. Positive symptoms in multiple sclerosis: their treatment with sodium channel blockers, lidocaine and mexiletine. *Journal of the Neurological Sciences.* 1999; **162**: 162–8.
52. United Kingdom Tizanidine Trial Group. A double blind, placebo-controlled trial of tizanidine in the treatment of spasticity caused by multiple sclerosis. *Neurology.* 1994; **44**: S70–8.
53. Eide PK, Jorum E, Stubhaug A *et al.* Relief of post-herpetic neuralgia with the *N*-methyl-D-aspartic acid receptor antagonist ketamine: a double-blind, cross-over comparison with morphine and placebo. *Pain.* 1994; **58**: 347–54.
54. Nelson KA, Park KM, Robinovitz RN *et al.* High-dose oral dextromethorphan versus placebo in painful diabetic neuropathy and postherpetic neuralgia. *Neurology.* 1997; **48**: 1212–8.
55. Pud D, Eisenberg E, Spitzer A *et al.* The NMDA receptor antagonist amantadine reduces surgical neuropathic pain in cancer patients: a double-blind, randomized, placebo-controlled trial. *Pain.* 1998; **75**: 349–54.
56. Rog DJ, Nurmikko TJ, Friede T, Young CA. Randomized, controlled trial of cannabis-based medicine in central pain in multiple sclerosis. *Neurology.* 2005; **65**: 812–9.
* 57. McQuay HJ, Moore RA. Transcutaneous electrical nerve stimulation (TENS) in chronic pain. In: McQuay HJ, Moore RA (eds). *An evidence-based resource for pain relief.* Oxford: Oxford University Press, 1998: 207–11.
58. Kidd D, Howard RS, Losseff NA, Thompson AJ. The benefit of inpatient neurorehabilitation in multiple sclerosis. *Clinical Rehabilitation.* 1995; **9**: 198–203.
59. Arner S, Lindblom U, Meyerson BA, Molander C. Prolonged relief of neuralgia after regional anesthetic blocks: a call for further experimental and systematic clinic studies. *Pain.* 1990; **43**: 287–97.
60. Herman RM, Luzansky SCD, Ippolito R. Intrathecal baclofen suppresses central pain in patients with spinal lesions. *Clinical Journal of Pain.* 1992; **8**: 338–45.
61. Taira T, Tanikawa T, Kawamura H *et al.* Spinal intrathecal baclofen suppresses central pain after stroke. *Journal of Neurology, Neurosurgery, and Psychiatry.* 1994; **57**: 381–2.
62. Glynn CJ, Jamous MA, Teddy PJ *et al.* Role of spinal noradrenergic system in transmission of pain in patients with spinal cord injury. *Lancet.* 1986; **2**: 1249–50.
63. Eisenach JC, DuPen S, Dubois M *et al.* Epidural clonidine analgesia for intractable cancer pain. The Epidural Clonidine Study Group. *Pain.* 1995; **61**: 391–9.
64. Hellwig K, Lukas C, Brune N *et al.* Repeat intrathecal triamcinolone acetonide application reduces acute occurring painful dysesthesia in patients with relapsing remitting multiple sclerosis. *Scientific World Journal.* 2006; **6**: 460–5.
65. Nathan PW. Intrathecal phenol to relieve spasticity in paraplegia. *Lancet.* 1959; **2**: 1099–102.
66. Jarrett L, Nandi P, Thompson AJ. Managing severe lower limb spasticity in multiple sclerosis: does intrathecal phenol have a role? *Journal of Neurology, Neurosurgery and Psychiatry.* 2002; **73**: 705–9.
67. Patwardhan RV, Minaqar A, Kelley RE, Nanda A. Neurosurgical treatment of multiple sclerosis. *Neurological Research.* 2006; **28**: 320–5.
68. Huntley A. A review of the evidence for efficacy of complementary and alternative medicines in MS. *International MS Journal.* 2006; **13**: 5–12.
69. Rabinstein AA, Shulman LM. Acupuncture in clinical neurology. *Neurologist.* 2003; **9**: 137–48.

25

Peripheral neuropathies

RAVIKIRAN SHENOY, KATHERINE ROBERTS, AND PRAVEEN ANAND

KEY LEARNING POINTS

- Identify the diagnostic points in peripheral neuropathies.
- Learn the mechanisms which result in pain in peripheral neuropathies.
- Outline the methods of investigation.
- Diagnose various types of peripheral neuropathies based on etiology and clinical findings.
- Learn the principles of therapy.
- Discuss and compare the differences between various modalities of treatment.

INTRODUCTION

The peripheral nervous system (PNS) is defined anatomically as the part of the nervous system in which neurons or their processes are related to Schwann cells. It includes the cranial nerves (with exception of the optic nerve), spinal nerve roots, dorsal root ganglia, peripheral nerve trunks, and nerve terminals. Any disorder of motor, sensory, or autonomic nerve fibers within the PNS could be classified as a neuropathy. The pathological processes that affect peripheral nerves may involve different sites and components of the PNS.

Peripheral neuropathies are described in different ways, based on (1) the pattern of neurological signs and symptoms as sensory, motor, autonomic, or mixed; (2) the distribution of affected nerves, as symmetrical versus asymmetrical, and distal or proximal; (3) the fiber type involved, as large versus small fiber; (4) the nature and brunt of the pathological process as axonal versus demyelinating; and (5) the time-course, as acute, subacute, or chronic. For example, multiple spinal roots are involved acutely in the Guillain–Barré syndrome, and in most cases preferentially affect the myelin sheath. The condition is thus described as an acute demyelinating inflammatory polyradiculopathy. The classification of the neuropathy narrows down the diagnostic possibilities. To illustrate, an acute onset suggests an inflammatory, immunologic, toxic, or vascular etiology. A polyneuropathy evolving subacutely over weeks and months is indicative of toxic, nutritional, or systemic diseases, whereas evolution over many years is indicative of a hereditary or metabolic disease. The dysfunction of an individual peripheral nerve is termed a "mononeuropathy." The syndrome of peripheral neuropathy, however, has many causes. Therefore, it is essential to first attempt to find the cause (which is not always possible) so that the patient can be informed about prognosis and receive specific treatment. The diagnostic process can also help with choice of symptomatic treatment, as for pain, based on the understanding of pathophysiological mechanisms in different conditions.

DIAGNOSTIC POINTS IN PERIPHERAL NEUROPATHIES

1. Pathological process:
   a. axonal;
   b. demyelinating.
2. Fiber type:
   a. large fiber;
   b. small fiber;
   c. mixed.
3. Distribution of symptoms:
   a. symmetrical;
   b. asymmetrical.
4. Onset of symptoms:
   a. acute;
   b. subacute;
   c. chronic.

GENERAL CLINICAL DESCRIPTION OF NEUROPATHIC SYNDROMES

Polyneuropathies

Symptoms and signs are symmetrical and distal in most polyneuropathies.

MOTOR FUNCTION

The feet and legs are usually affected earlier and more severely than the upper limbs. Truncal and cranial regions are the last to be affected, and are only involved in severe cases. Most of the common metabolic, toxic, and nutritional neuropathies show this predominantly distal pattern. An exception is seen in acute inflammatory neuropathies, where cranial nerve, respiratory, and upper limb involvement can occur early in the course of the disease. Facial and other cranial nerve paralyses can occur with sarcoidosis, Lyme disease, Sjögren syndrome, neoplastic invasion of meninges and nerve root infiltrations, or in rare metabolic neuropathies (Refsum, Tangier, and Riley–Day). Predominant involvement of upper limbs is unusual, but may be seen in Sjögren syndrome, the chronic immune neuropathies, porphyric, lead, and amyloid polyneuropathy, and some inherited neuropathies.

TENDON REFLEXES

Deep tendon reflexes are diminished or lost in peripheral neuropathies as a rule. Reflexes may be diminished early in the course of neuropathy, but not absent. Reflexes may, however, be retained in small-fiber neuropathies.

SENSORY LOSS

Like motor function, sensation is affected symmetrically and in distal segments in polyneuropathies. As the neuropathy worsens, sensory loss may spread from distal to proximal parts. In most polyneuropathies, all sensory modalities are impaired (pain and temperature, indicating small-fiber involvement; joint position and vibration sense, suggesting large-fiber dysfunction). Occasionally, selective damage to large or small fibers predominates. In polyneuropathy affecting mainly small nerve fibers, patients often present with burning, painful dysesthesiae, alteration of pinprick and temperature sensation, and autonomic dysfunction. Motor function, balance, and tendon jerks may be preserved. Some cases of amyloid and early distal diabetic polyneuropathies fall into this group. Large-fiber neuropathy, in contrast, is characterized by loss of joint position and vibration sense, ataxia, areflexia, and variable but often severe loss of motor function. In sensory neuronopathies (primary involvement of dorsal root ganglion), there is usually no motor loss.

POSITIVE SYMPTOMS IN PERIPHERAL NEUROPATHIES

Dysesthesiae, paresthesiae, and pain

Paresthesiae tend to be specially marked in the feet and hands in polyneuropathies, and localized to the affected part in other neuropathies. Pins and needles, stabbing, pricking, tingling, electric, and band-like sensations are some of the terms used to describe these symptoms. Positive symptoms or numbness may be the only features in some neuropathies, with no objective sensory loss on clinical examination. Certain types of diabetic, nutritional, and alcohol-related neuropathies may present as burning feet, which may be hypersensitive to touch and pinprick.

Peripheral neuropathic pain may manifest as spontaneous pain (stimulus-independent pain), often in a numb region, or pain and hypersensitivity elicited by a stimulus (stimulus-evoked pain). Hyperalgesia is an increased response to a stimulus that is normally painful and is due to abnormal processing of nociceptor inputs. Allodynia is a pain elicited by a stimulus that does not normally provoke pain. Stimulus-evoked pain is common after peripheral nerve injury, and early small-fiber polyneuropathies. Many patients with neuropathic pain suffer from spontaneous and paroxysmal pain, with different mechanisms operating in the same subject.

MECHANISMS OF PAIN IN PERIPHERAL NEUROPATHY

Normally, impulses are generated at sensory nerve terminals or in cell bodies. In pathological states, impulses may arise from the damaged part of the axon and propagate toward both the central nervous system and the periphery. Such ectopic discharges may also arise from local patches of demyelination, neuromas, and soma in the dorsal root ganglia. The mechanisms underlying neuropathic pain have been reviewed elsewhere.[1, 2, 3] Persistent primary pain is attributed to activity in nociceptor C-fibers, which in turn leads to central changes. Similar activity in large myelinated A-fibers may produce paresthesiae, and they mediate secondary allodynia and hyperalgesia in the setting of central changes. The mechanism of ectopic discharges is attributed to changes in the expression and distribution of membrane ion channels, especially sodium channels. Two types of sodium channel are found in sensory neurons. The first are sensitive to a neurotoxin derived from the puffer fish – tetrodotoxin (TTX) – and are found in all sensory neurons. The second types are resistant to tetrodotoxin, and are found predominantly in nociceptor sensory neurons. The TTX-resistant channels have much slower activation and inactivation kinetics than TTX-sensitive channels and are implicated in pathological pain states. Channel proteins are synthesized in the cell body and transported by axoplasmic mechanisms to their peripheral targets, which include nodes of Ranvier and axon terminals. Accumulation of sodium channels at sites of ectopic impulse generation has been postulated to play a role in the ectopic discharges.[4] Changes in the distribution of two TTX-resistant channels – Na_v 1.8 (SNS/PN3) and Na_v 1.9 (NaN/SNS2), preferentially expressed in nociceptors – have been identified in sensory neurons.[5, 6, 7] Na_v 1.8 (SNS/PN3) has been shown to accumulate preferentially at the site of nerve injury and also in nerve fibers in skin from patients with mechanical allodynia and hyperalgesia,[5] and appears to be an attractive target for the development of novel sensory neuron-specific sodium channel blockers for mechanism-based analgesia. Changes in other ion channels have also been implicated in the pathogenesis of pain. Specific potassium channels have been found to be decreased in the rat dorsal root ganglion after axotomy.[8] Thus, changes in potassium and sodium channel expression following axonal injury have the potential to change the electrical excitability of dorsal root ganglion (DRG) neurons and lead to chronic pain states.[8] Other mechanisms contributing to pain include ephaptic transmission, nociceptor sensitization, adrenergic chemosensitivity of regenerating axons, and nerve trunk inflammation.

There are many sensory symptoms of peripheral nerve disorders, such as their spread beyond the territory of the injured nerve, which could not be explained solely in terms of alterations in peripheral functions. It is now well established that peripheral stimuli can lead to central changes in spinal cord, including wind up, disinhibition, and sensitization,[9, 10] and altered rostral processing.[1, 2, 3] These mechanisms need to be understood in molecular terms, and targeted in association with peripheral strategies.

ETIOLOGICAL CLASSIFICATION AND INVESTIGATION OF NEUROPATHIES

When dealing with a patient, a clinician is faced with two tasks:

1. establishing the existence and nature of a disorder of the peripheral nervous system;
2. providing specific and symptomatic treatment.

For the clinical differential diagnosis, it is convenient to group the neuropathy into types (see **Table 25.1**). The next step is to determine whether polyneuropathy is axonal or demyelinating. This requires the use of nerve conduction studies (NCS) and needle examination of muscles by electromyography (EMG). These help to determine:

- that the primary process is a disorder of the nerves;
- the distinction between a generalized polyneuropathic process, multifocal neuropathy (mononeuritis multiplex), or a mononeuropathy;
- the distinction between a primary demyelinating neuropathy and axonal neuropathy.

The limitation of NCS is that it is a measure of large-fiber function, and does not provide information about small-fiber function, particularly nociceptors.

Quantitative sensory and autonomic testing (QST) provides information about small myelinated and unmyelinated fiber function, as well as large-fiber function. These tests can be particularly useful in patients with hypoalgesia and hyperalgesia/allodynia in providing objective assessment of abnormalities and establishing a diagnosis of pure small-fiber neuropathy.[11] QST is also useful for epidemiological and therapeutic studies of peripheral neuropathy.[12]

Other useful tests include the following:

- **blood tests** – to identify metabolic, nutritional, or toxic states, to measure immunoglobulins and antineural antibodies that relate to immune-mediated neuropathies,[13] and to perform genetic screens in the diagnosis of inherited neuropathies;
- **cerebrospinal fluid examination** – increased protein levels and cellular responses indicate radicular or meningeal involvement;
- **nerve and muscle biopsy** – progress in clinical electrophysiology and molecular genetics has resulted in fewer indications for nerve biopsy in clinical practice.[14] Biopsy should be reserved for carefully selected cases.[15] The main indications include:
  - mononeuritis multiplex, in which the etiology is still undetermined after extensive laboratory investigations, and the diagnostic possibilities include vasculitis, amyloidosis, leprosy, and sarcoidosis;

Table 25.1 Etiological classification of neuropathies.

Classification			
Painful neuropathies			
Symmetrical	Metabolic	Diabetes mellitus	
		Hypoglycemic (usually with insulinoma)	
		Hypothyroidism	
	Nutritional/deficiency	Pellagra (niacin deficiency)	
		Beriberi (thiamine deficiency)	
		Multiple nutritional deficiencies	
	Toxic	Drugs	Alcohol (ethanol)
			Antiretroviral drugs
			Cytostatic drugs
			Isoniazid, hydralazine, etc.
		Metals	Thallium
			Arsenic
			Mercury
	Immune mediated	Acute or chronic inflammatory demyelinating neuropathies	
		Neuropathies associated with paraproteinemia and cryoglobulinemia	
		Acquired amyloidosis	
		Paraneoplastic neuropathies	
	Hereditary	Hereditary sensory and autonomic neuropathy (type I)	
		Fabry's disease	
	Idiopathic		
Asymmetrical	Mononeuritis/mononeuritis multiplex	Diabetic	
	Vasculitic neuropathies	Cranial neuropathy	
		Trunk and limb mononeuropathy	
		Diabetic amyotrophy	
		Systemic vasculitis of the vasa nervorum associated with:	Polyarteritis nodosa
			Churg–Strauss syndrome
			Rheumatoid arthritis
			Lupus erythematosus
			Systemic sclerosis
			Wegener's granulomatosis
		Isolated angiitis of peripheral nerves	
		Infectious/parainfectious neuropathies	HIV related
			Borreliosis
			Herpes zoster
	Physical injuries	Nerve entrapment – carpal tunnel and other nerve compression	
		Root compression (intervertebral disk herniation)	
		Neuroma: post-traumatic, postsurgical, postamputation	
	Plexus neuropathies	Idiopathic neuritis of brachial or lumbosacral plexus	
		Post-traumatic	
		Tumor infiltration	
	Radiation induced		
	Cranial neuralgias: trigeminal and glossopharyngeal neuralgia		

(*Continued over*)

Table 25.1 Etiological classification of neuropathies (continued).

Classification		
Painless neuropathies		
	Neuropathies with selective loss of pain sensation	Congenital insensitivity to pain with anhidrosis – HSAN type IV Congenital analgesia without anhidrosis – HSAN type V
	Neuropathies (predominantly painless)	Leprosy

– distal, symmetric, polyneuropathies of subacute or chronic evolution when all other diagnostic measures have been exhausted and the condition continues to progress;
– in establishing diagnosis in genetically determined pediatric disorders, such as metachromatic leukodystrophy, Krabbe's disease, giant axonal neuropathy, and infantile neuroaxonal dystrophy.

PREDOMINANTLY PAINFUL NEUROPATHIES

These neuropathies are characterized by dysesthesiae as a major symptom.

Metabolic neuropathies

DIABETIC NEUROPATHY

Diabetes mellitus is the most common cause of neuropathy in the western world,[16] affecting approximately 50 percent of diabetic patients over time.[17] It is usually seen in diabetics over 50 years of age and is uncommon in children. Diabetes can affect different components of the PNS. As a result, diabetic neuropathy is not a uniform disorder, but rather a group of distinct clinical syndromes, each reflecting the site and components of the PNS affected by the pathological process. Several clinical syndromes have been delineated.

ACUTE DIABETIC MONONEUROPATHY

This is presumably due to infarction of the nerve.

Cranial neuropathy

Acute ophthalmoplegia due to third-nerve involvement is the most common cranial neuropathy. The onset is usually abrupt, and pain is seen in up to 50 percent of patients (owing to involvement of trigeminal branches in the cavernous sinus or involvement of pain-sensitive nerve endings within the connective tissue of the affected nerve[17]). Pain is aching and is located behind or above the eye. Most patients are usually over 50 years old and the pupils are often spared.

Peripheral nerves

Acute involvement of most individual peripheral nerves has been described. The most commonly involved nerves are the median, ulnar, radial, femoral, lateral cutaneous nerve of the thigh, and common peroneal nerves. Onset is often sudden, presumably due to infarction of the nerve, and pain may be a prominent feature in such cases. Isolated peripheral nerve lesions tend to occur at the common sites for pressure palsies, and nerves in diabetic subjects are more susceptible to compression injury.[17]

ASYMMETRIC NEUROPATHY AND RADICULOPATHY

Lower limb asymmetric motor neuropathy (diabetic amyotrophy)

A painful, asymmetrical neuropathy is sometimes seen in older patients with mild or undetected diabetes, and occasionally in patients with long-standing diabetes. Pain often begins in the lower back or hip and spreads down the leg on one side. Pain tends to be more severe at night and has a deep, aching quality with superimposed sharp jabs. Pelvic girdle and thigh muscles are usually affected and show weakness and wasting. The knee jerk is lost on the affected side. Sensory involvement is minimal. Most patients do recover, although in some recovery may be incomplete. The syndrome may recur on the opposite side. Pathologically, the site of involvement is multiple and affects roots, spinal nerve, or lumbosacral plexus. Pathologic changes appear to be the result of ischemic injury from microscopic vasculitis affecting small epineural vessels.[18]

Thoracoabdominal radiculopathy

This is usually seen in older patients with long-standing diabetes and may be associated with marked weight loss. Most patients describe girdle-like pain around the trunk that may be unilateral or bilateral. Abdominal wall weakness, cutaneous hyperesthesiae, or superficial sensory loss over the involved area may be seen on examination. EMG changes can be detected in paraspinal and abdominal wall muscles, in adjacent myotomes, and, on this basis, the lesion is presumed to be very proximal – in the nerve roots. The pain is difficult to treat and recovery may be protracted, but the ultimate prognosis for recovery is good.

DISTAL SYMMETRIC SENSORIMOTOR POLYNEUROPATHY

This predominantly sensory form is the most common type of diabetic neuropathy. Symptoms are variable, but when the polyneuropathy becomes symptomatic the main complaints are persistent and often distressing numbness and tingling. This is often confined to the feet and lower legs and is worse at night. Pain may be a troublesome feature and is felt as aching and deep as if "arising in the bones." Lancinating pain and burning paresthesiae may also occur. In the early stages, signs are confined to the distal part of the legs and include decreased light touch, pain, and vibration sensation. As the neuropathy progresses, sensory loss may spread to proximal parts, hands, and the trunk. Ankle jerks are decreased or absent and weakness is usually mild. If there is more severe distal motor involvement, other causes of neuropathy need to be excluded.

SMALL-FIBER NEUROPATHY

Patients present with distal burning pain in the extremities and have cutaneous hyperesthesiae and autonomic dysfunction as a prominent feature. They have loss of pain and temperature sensation, but preservation of large-fiber modalities, including tendon reflexes. Small-fiber loss has been demonstrated in nerve biopsies.[19] Such patients are believed to have small-fiber neuropathy. Small-fiber involvement is an early consistent feature in diabetic polyneuropathy to varying degrees.[17]

ACUTE PAINFUL DIABETIC NEUROPATHY

Rarely, patients present with burning pain that is worse during the night and profound weight loss. This type of neuropathy can follow an episode of ketosis or establishment of tight glycemic control. There is very little sensory and motor loss and tendon reflexes are usually preserved. However, there is hyperalgesia and contact with clothing and bedclothes is unpleasant. With weight gain and adequate diabetic control, the neuropathic symptoms tend to improve.

TREATMENT-INDUCED NEUROPATHY

Occasionally, paresthesiae and pain may develop following the institution of insulin therapy, raising the suspicion of neuropathy. The symptoms, however, tend to improve slowly with glycemic control.

Nerve biopsies show loss of myelinated and unmyelinated nerve fibers, regenerating nerve sprouts, axonal atrophy, and segmental demyelination and remyelination of axons in the distal symmetrical type of diabetic polyneuropathy. However, there is no simple correlation between presence of pain and morphological changes in painful neuropathies associated with diabetes. Loss of both large and small myelinated fibers has been shown in diabetic autonomic neuropathy associated with painful or painless sensory neuropathy.[20] The neuropathology of diabetic neuropathy is reviewed in detail elsewhere.[17]

The pathogenesis of diabetic neuropathies, and mechanisms of pain, are still uncertain and are likely to be multifactorial. The mononeuropathies and asymmetrical neuropathies are thought to be ischemic in origin, secondary to disease of the vasa nervorum. In other forms of diabetic neuropathy, a metabolic basis has been favored. Recently, oxidative stress, as a consequence of hyperglycemia, has been proposed as an inciting event in diabetic polyneuropathy.[21] Whatever may be the pathophysiological mechanisms underlying diabetic neuropathy, it is generally accepted that tight glycemic control helps in prevention and amelioration of neuropathy, including pain symptoms.[22]

HYPOTHYROID NEUROPATHY

Apart from the high incidence of carpal tunnel syndrome, a sensorimotor polyneuropathy also occurs in hypothyroidism. Sensory symptoms dominate the clinical picture and include painful dysesthesiae and lancinating pains in hands and feet. Usually, there is glove and stocking sensory loss, and occasionally distal weakness and wasting may be seen. The neuropathy tends to improve with thyroxine replacement therapy.

Deficiency states

Neuropathy due to nutritional deficiency is uncommon in developed countries and is usually seen in the setting of alcoholism, malabsorption, various gastrointestinal procedures leading to weight loss, and prolonged stay in intensive care units.

VITAMIN B_1 DEFICIENCY

Deficiency of vitamin B_1 (thiamine) causes a neuropathy that begins with painful paresthesiae in the feet (burning feet). If the nutritional deficiency is not corrected, the sensory symptoms progress and spread proximally, and distal motor weakness may develop. Prognosis is generally good and, with thiamine supplementation, most patients show recovery unless severe axonal degeneration has occurred.

VITAMIN B_6 DEFICIENCY

Peripheral neuropathy due to vitamin B_6 (pyridoxine) deficiency is usually seen in patients receiving the antituberculous drug isoniazid and the antihypertensive drug hydralazine.[23] Symptoms consist of symmetrical tingling and pain, and are reversible after stopping medication. The neuropathy could be prevented by daily supplementation of 10–20 mg of B_6 per day during treatment with these drugs. Paradoxically, the prolonged administration of extremely high doses of pyridoxine may actually cause a disabling sensory neuropathy.[24]

NIACIN DEFICIENCY

Pellagra is a nutritional deficiency state characterized by dermatitis, diarrhea, and mental changes. Neuropathic symptoms often described in association with pellagra are believed to be due to a coexistent deficiency of pyridoxine or other B vitamins as neuropathic symptoms do not improve with niacin alone.[23]

Toxic neuropathies

ALCOHOL

It is considered that neuropathy associated with chronic alcoholism is due to vitamin B_1 deficiency.[23] Symptoms are nonspecific and the diagnosis needs to be established carefully by excluding other causes and by establishing history of alcohol excess and nutritional imbalance or deficiency.

ARSENICAL POLYNEUROPATHY

The neuropathy associated with arsenic ingestion presents in the context of a systemic illness. In the case of chronic poisoning, neuropathic symptoms develop slowly in the distal part of the extremities. The first symptoms are usually pain, which is aching or burning, and tingling or numbness beginning in the fingers and toes and then spreading proximally. Motor symptoms soon follow in similar distribution. Gastrointestinal symptoms may precede the polyneuropathy. Other associated symptoms include anemia, jaundice, hyperkeratosis of palms and soles, and later white transverse banding of the nails (Mees lines). Following a single, large dose of arsenic, a rapidly evolving neuropathy may appear after a period of one to three weeks. It may be preceded by severe gastrointestinal symptoms, renal and hepatic failure, and mental disturbances. The disease is accompanied by an excess of arsenic in urine, nails, and hair. Most cases recognized nowadays are following homicidal or suicidal attempts.[25] A high index of suspicion is usually necessary for diagnosis. The diagnosis could be established by demonstrating high levels of arsenic in the hair or nails. Recovery from neuropathy may be very slow and the prognosis for recovery is related to the duration and severity of symptoms and success in removing the source of exposure.

THALLIUM POISONING

Sporadic instances of thallium poisoning usually occur as a result of accidental or suicidal ingestion of thallium-containing rodenticides and rarely from overuse of depilatory agents. Rapidly progressing painful sensory neuropathy develops if the patient survives acute poisoning. Persistent pain with allodynia can be a dominant feature. Rapid loss of hair is a striking feature (within one to two weeks). Cranial nerves may also be affected. The early onset of painful paresthesiae, relative preservation of proximal reflexes, and rapid loss of hair help to differentiate this neuropathy from Guillain–Barré syndrome and other acute polyneuropathies.[25] Prognosis for the recovery depends on the severity of peripheral nervous system involvement.

MERCURY POISONING

Chronic poisoning with organic mercury affects the central nervous system, predominantly producing symptoms such as visual field defects, ataxia, and mental impairments. However, one of the earliest complaints in many patients is paresthesiae, which start distally and progress proximally and may involve the tongue. A painful neuropathy of children due to mercury exposure from interior latex paint, calomel (mercurous chloride), teething powders, and a mercuric fungicide used in washing diapers has been described.[26, 27]

CYTOSTATIC DRUGS

Peripheral neurotoxicity is the significant dose-limiting side effect of many chemotherapeutic drugs, including vinca alkaloids, cisplatin, and taxols. Some of these agents interfere with microtubule-based axonal transport and cause length-dependent axonal injury. Although distal paresthesiae are the initial manifestations with vinca alkaloids, there are very few sensory signs, and motor abnormalities dominate the clinical picture. It is important to be aware of these neuropathies, as there may be a unique opportunity to initiate preventive measures before the damage occurs. A neuroprotective effect of neurotrophins has been demonstrated in tissue culture and animal models.[28]

ANTIRETROVIRAL DRUGS

A severe dose-limiting axonal peripheral neuropathy may develop in subjects receiving treatment with the nucleoside analogs didanosine (ddI), zalcitabine (ddC), and stavudine (d4T) for human immunodeficiency infection. It is estimated that around 10 percent of subjects receiving ddC or d4T, and 1–2 percent of ddI recipients, may have to discontinue therapy because of development of neuropathy.[29] It usually develops within weeks of starting therapy, and severe pain may be the chief complaint. It is a painful and predominantly sensory distal polyneuropathy. The symptoms and signs tend to resolve gradually with the withdrawal of the therapy, although symptoms may continue to worsen for some time after stopping the drug.[30] It has been demonstrated that those who develop neuropathy on antiretrovirals have lower levels of acetyl carnitine in the serum than subjects who did not develop neuropathy.[31] The main function of acetyl carnitine is in mitochondrial β-oxidation of fatty acids for membrane energy balance. It is suggested that levacecarnine (acetyl-L-carnitine) and nerve growth factors, such as recombinant human nerve growth factor, may have a role in managing this condition.[29]

Autoimmune neuropathies

Pain, paresthesiae, and dysesthesiae may occur in a significant proportion of patients with acute inflammatory demyelinating polyradiculoneuropathy (Guillain–Barré syndrome) and chronic inflammatory demyelinating neuropathy, although motor abnormalities dominate the clinical picture.

Pain is a common symptom in vasculitic neuropathy, and the extent of sensory loss and motor dysfunction depends on the nerves affected. The clinical picture is usually that of mononeuritis multiplex. If the involvement is extensive, the deficit may be more or less symmetrical, simulating a polyneuropathy. The neuropathy may occur on the background of a systemic illness or occasionally may be the presenting feature. Included in this category are polyarteritis nodosa, Churg–Strauss syndrome, rheumatoid arthritis, lupus erythematosus, systemic sclerosis, and Wegener's granulomatosis.

A symmetric polyneuropathy or a mononeuritis multiplex may occur in essential mixed cryoglobulinemia. Painful dysesthesiae are the common manifestation of polyneuropathy. The topic of paraproteinemia and neuropathy has been reviewed recently.[32]

Primary amyloidosis presents with painful dysesthesiae and numbness. Small-fiber modalities (pain and temperature) and autonomic functions are predominantly affected. Symptoms are more prominent in lower limbs. Most of the patients are elderly and diagnosis is established through biopsy.

Hereditary neuropathies

Spontaneous burning, aching, or lancinating pain can be a feature of hereditary sensory and autonomic neuropathy (HSAN) type I. It is characterized by autosomal dominant inheritance, onset is in the second to fourth decades, and there is preferential affection of lower limbs. Progression is very slow and may be associated with foot ulceration and other complications. Loss of pain and temperature sensations are the main findings upon examination.

Painful burning sensations in the hands and lower legs, and tender legs in boys or young men, may be the presenting feature in Fabry's disease. The pains may be so severe that walking is often restricted. It is an X-linked disease and other manifestations include maculopapular rash on the body, red angiectases under the nail beds, and renal impairment. Fabry's disease and hereditary sensory and autonomic neuropathy are discussed in detail elsewhere.[33, 34]

Hereditary (or primary) erythromelalgia, an autosomal dominant painful neuropathy, characterized by reddening of the skin and a burning sensation in the extremities, has been shown to be due to a gain of function mutation in the *SCN9A* gene, which encodes the $Na_v1.7$ sodium channel.[35, 36] The mutation in the ion channel causes a lowering of the threshold for single and high frequency action potential firing, causing hyperexcitability of the neuron and the symptoms of erythromelalgia.

Human immunodeficiency virus-associated painful peripheral neuropathy

Human immunodeficiency virus (HIV) infection may be complicated by various forms of peripheral neuropathy. Distal symmetrical polyneuropathy is the most common type of neuropathy that occurs in patients with HIV infection and is a result of HIV infection itself.[37] It is a predominantly sensory neuropathy and burning feet is the most common symptom. The signs are those of distal axonal sensorimotor polyneuropathy. Similar neuropathy in HIV-positive subjects could result from antiretroviral drugs[29, 30] and vitamin B_{12} deficiency, and these need to be excluded before diagnosis could be established.

Painful mononeuropathy multiplex related to focal vasculitis or subacute cauda equina syndrome due to cytomegalovirus infection are other painful neuropathies that are associated with HIV infection. Neuropathies associated with HIV infection are discussed elsewhere.[38]

For further discussion of this topic, see Chapter 26, HIV and AIDS.

Nerve compression and entrapment neuropathies

This refers to isolated peripheral nerve injuries that occur at specific locations. A nerve is usually mechanically constricted in a fibrous or fibro-osseous tunnel or deformed by a fibrous band. Symptoms come on gradually (sensory more than motor, other than in elderly subjects) and tend to fluctuate with activity and rest. Median nerve compression at the wrist is the most frequent nerve entrapment syndrome. Dysesthesiae and pain in the fingers is made worse by excessive use of the hands.

Other sites of entrapment are the ulnar nerve in the cubital tunnel at the elbow and in Guyon's canal at the wrist, suprascapular nerve at the spinoglenoid notch, posterior interosseous nerve in the radial tunnel, lateral femoral cutaneous nerve of thigh (meralgia paresthetica) at the inguinal ligament, obturator nerve in the obturator canal, posterior tibial nerve in the tarsal tunnel, and interdigital plantar nerve (Morton metatarsalgia) in the plantar fascia between the heads of the third and fourth metatarsals.

It is important to exclude systemic processes while dealing with entrapment neuropathies that make nerves prone to compression. This includes conditions such as diabetes, hypothyroidism, pregnancy, and amyloid and hereditary liability to pressure palsies.

Diagnosis is usually easy and should be confirmed by electrophysiological studies. Most of these neuropathies are amenable to surgery designed to relieve compression.

Postherpetic neuralgia

Postherpetic neuralgia (PHN) follows herpes zoster infections, mainly in the elderly. It occurs in the affected area in about 50 percent of patients over 50 years old following healing of the skin lesions, and persists for more than 12 weeks. It presents as a continuous burning or intense paroxysmal pain, and may be associated with tactile allodynia. It can be severe, debilitating, and reduce quality of life. The time-course is variable. It may abate within months, but may also continue for years. Certain human leukocyte antigen (HLA) class I antigens, such as HLA-A33 and -B44, have been shown to be associated with the development of PHN in Japanese patients.[39] The results of randomized, controlled trials and meta-analyses suggest that treatment with acyclovir, famciclovir, and valaciclovir reduce the risk of developing PHN.[40, 41, 42] It is now accepted that corticosteroids do not prevent the development of PHN.[43] Topically applied capsaicin and lidocaine have both been shown to be effective in the treatment of the pain associated with PHN.[44, 45, 46, 47, 48] A live, attenuated varicella-voster vaccine (Zostavax) has been developed and approved by the US Food and Drug Administration (FDA). In a randomized, double-blind, placebo-controlled trial of 34,546 patients over the age of 60 years by the Shingles Prevention Study Group, use of the vaccine reduced incidence of herpes zoster by 51.3 percent ($p<0.001$) and PHN by 61.1 percent ($p<0.001$).[49] For further discussion of this topic, see Chapter 32, Herpes zoster pain, including shingles and postherpetic neuralgia.

Complex regional pain syndrome

Complex regional pain syndrome (CRPS) is divided into type I (without) and type II (with) nerve injury. These types occur as a consequence of major or minor trauma, and are often characterized by allodynia, hyperpathia, and autonomic signs. After partial nerve injury, there is expression of α-adrenoreceptors in the injured and uninjured axons, making them sensitive to norepinephrine.[50, 51] Also, the sympathetic axons which normally innervate blood vessels within the dorsal root ganglion sprout to form basket-like terminals around the cell bodies of sensory neurons.[52] It may be postulated that sympathetic stimulation can activate these neurons repetitively.[52] These types of pain can respond strikingly to sympatholytic procedures, such as sympathetic blocks (either at the sympathetic ganglia or intravenous guanethidine). Reflex sympathetic dystrophy and causalgia are now included in a more general term – complex regional pain syndrome. For further discussion of this topic, see Chapter 27, Complex regional pain syndromes.

Brachial plexus neuropathies

NEURALGIC AMYOTROPHY

This may develop suddenly in an otherwise healthy individual or follow an infection, surgical procedure, childbirth, or an injection of vaccine or antibiotic. It usually begins as a severe pain around the shoulder on one side, followed by rapid development of weakness and atrophy. The muscles of C5 and C6 myotome are commonly involved, and the affected muscles may be very weak to the extent of being totally paralyzed. The pain is made worse by movement involving the affected muscles. It can be distinguished from cervical radicular lesions by the fact that weakness is usually not so severe in radicular lesions. It is usually unilateral, but occasionally bilateral. Rarely, it may be restricted to one or two nerve territories, or can present as an isolated phrenic nerve palsy. Pain usually disappears within a few days or weeks, and most patients show good recovery.

TRAUMATIC LESIONS OF THE BRACHIAL PLEXUS

Brachial plexus injury leading to spinal cord avulsion produces a constant crushing and intermittent shooting pain, which is often intractable. Pain in patients with brachial plexus injury can be severe, disabling, and persist for years. Pain tends to be worse in patients who do not show recovery. Deafferentation pain is particularly difficult to treat. It is suggested that this pain might be alleviated after successful repair with intercostal nerve transfer, and coincides with or is preceded by the return of function.[53]

BRACHIAL PLEXUS NEUROPATHY FOLLOWING RADIATION THERAPY AND MALIGNANCY

This usually occurs as a complication of surgery and/or irradiation of the axilla for carcinoma of the breast. The upper plexus is commonly involved, and may be associated with painless lymphedema.

Brachial plexopathy following neoplastic infiltration tends to involve the lower plexus more than the upper and is often associated with severe pain and Horner syndrome.

Paraneoplastic neuropathies

These occur as remote effects of a carcinoma and can precede detection of malignancy by months to years. Of the various types, a predominantly distal, symmetrical sensory, or sensorimotor polyneuropathy is the most common. A purely sensory neuronopathy (Denny–Brown syndrome, dorsal root ganglionitis), in which pain can be a distressing symptom, is rarely observed. There are three major manifestations of neuronopathy: an ataxic syndrome, a hyperalgesic–ataxic syndrome, and an ataxic or hyperalgesic–ataxic syndrome with prominent gastrointestinal dysmotility.[54] In patients with the hyperalgesic type, painful paresthesiae, burning sensations, and shooting limb pains are the usual presenting symptoms. These may be associated with ataxia or abdominal complaints. There is usually very little motor loss, and the sensory loss may be either proximal or distal. This syndrome is typically associated with small-cell carcinoma of lung, but can occur with other malignancies. The prognosis is related to that of the underlying carcinoma. The paraneoplastic neuropathies have been reviewed.[54, 55]

Idiopathic neuropathies

After a careful diagnostic work up, a cause can be found in the majority of neuropathies. However, in a proportion of cases, no cause can be found, despite extensive investigations. Such cases constitute a heterogeneous group of disorders. Some of them have small-fiber sensory neuropathy and suffer from burning pain, restricted initially to the feet and toes but extending more proximally to involve legs and hands with time. Most patients present with slowly progressive symptoms. Foot ulceration is uncommon in these patients, even though small fibers are involved. Rarely, the presentation can be acute with generalized small-fiber dysfunction. Pathologically, widespread loss of small fibers from the epidermis has been demonstrated.[56] Some patients resemble those with erythromelalgia.

Predominantly painless neuropathies

Loss of pain sensation can be such a dominant feature in some neuropathies that it may lead to severe mutilations. HSAN type IV is a prototypic example. Tangier disease and leprosy, although predominantly painless, can be associated with pain.

CONGENITAL INSENSITIVITY TO PAIN

Many entities, such as sensory neuropathy, central lesions at the level of reticular formation or dorsal horn of the spinal cord, or a central indifference to, or asymbolia for, pain have been described under this rubric.[57] It is now thought that most cases with congenital indifference to pain may have had HSAN type IV or V.[34] Type IV cases are characterized by onset of symptoms in infancy or early childhood, recurrent episodes of unexplained fever, anhidrosis, absence of reaction to painful stimuli, self-mutilation, and mental retardation. Unlike other types of HSAN, sensory action potentials are normal in HSAN type IV.[58] Ultrastructural and morphometric studies of the peripheral nerves demonstrate a loss of the unmyelinated and small myelinated fibers.[59] Mutations of the *TrkA* gene have been shown in some families with HSAN type IV,[60, 61] and these defects are suggested to cause HSAN-IV. TrkA is the high-affinity receptor for nerve growth factor (NGF) which induces neurite outgrowth and promotes survival of embryonic small sensory and sympathetic neurons.

TANGIER DISEASE

Tangier disease, a disorder of lipoprotein transport, can be associated with neuropathy with marked loss of pain sensation. Neuropathy can be transient, can be relapsing and asymmetrical, or can be slowly progressing and symmetrical with onset in upper or lower limbs. It may simulate syringomyelia, especially when the onset is in the upper limbs. Studies have shown than Tangier disease is associated with lancinating pains.[62] Other features that may be associated are corneal opacities, enlarged tonsils, and hepatosplenomegaly. Biochemical abnormalities include hypocholesterolemia and normal or elevated triacylglycerol levels. Normal or elevated triacylglycerol levels help in distinguishing this condition from abetalipoproteinemia and hypobetalipoproteinemia. Nerve biopsy reveals loss of small myelinated and unmyelinated fibers.

LEPROSY

Leprosy, caused by infection with *Mycobacterium leprae*, is the most common treatable neuropathy in the world. It is characterized by hypopigmented skin lesions, thickened nerves, and loss of small-fiber modalities, especially pain sensations in the affected regions. Recent studies, however, have shown that neuropathic pain can be an important feature of leprosy.[63] Diagnosis can be established by clinical examination. Depending on the immunological status, the clinical manifestations vary. Loss of pain sensation can lead to painless burns and trophic ulcers. It has been demonstrated that NGF, which plays an important role in nociception, is reduced in skin and nerve fibers from patients with leprosy.[64] It has been suggested that local treatment with recombinant NGF may also improve nociception.[65]

Principles of therapy

First, it is essential to attempt to diagnose the cause of peripheral neuropathy and to treat the underlying cause if possible. The symptoms are often troublesome and disabling, and symptomatic relief is needed. Pain from neuropathy can be severe, and can produce greater disability than the primary disease process. It is important to understand, as far as possible, the mechanisms that underlie the pain symptoms to plan rational treatment. Full and sympathetic communication with the patient is necessary to maximize the therapeutic benefit.

Specific therapy

Apart from the symptomatic treatment, every attempt must be made to find the underlying cause of neuropathy and to treat it accordingly. Discussion of specific therapy for each category of neuropathy is beyond the scope of this book. Readers are referred to *Peripheral neuropathy*[66] for a comprehensive discussion of peripheral nerve disorders.

Symptomatic therapy

The various treatment options in patients with neuropathic pain are summarized in **Tables 25.2** and **25.3.** Current pharmacological treatment regimens for pain in neuropathy mainly include antidepressant or anticonvulsant drugs.

ANTIDEPRESSANTS

Tricyclic antidepressants are widely used in the treatment of neuropathic pain and have been tested in both experimental and clinical conditions.[67][I] The mechanisms of action in pain relief are not completely understood, but it is assumed that antidepressants are especially effective in pain relief through the descending inhibitory serotoninergic nociceptive system.[68] They inhibit pain transmission in the spinal cord by increasing levels of norepinephrine (NE) and serotonin (5-HT), as a result of their ability to prevent the presynaptic reuptake of these amines. Tricyclic antidepressants (TCA) might also affect histaminergic, cholinergic, and glutamatergic neurotransmission, and they appear to block sodium channels.[69] The effect on pain is believed to be essentially independent of antidepressive and anxiolytic effects. Amitriptyline, imipramine, and clomipramine are widely used antidepressants in pain therapy, the best available clinical evidence being for amitriptyline.[70][I] The different tricyclics appear to have similar effects and the new antidepressants have yet to be shown to be effective or superior in controlled trials. The side effects of these agents include dizziness, drowsiness, dry mouth, tremor (with clomipramine), and blurred vision, and often determine the choice.[71] Amitriptyline and imipramine are the most commonly used tricyclic antidepressants. Treatment is usually started with 10–25 mg/day, and subsequently increased by 10–25 mg in steps until sufficient pain relief occurs. The efficacy of amitriptyline was compared with gabapentin in a randomized, double-blind, crossover study in diabetic patients with neuropathic pain.[72][II] No significant difference in pain relief was found between amitriptyline and gabapentin. If the side effects from amitriptyline are troublesome, the noradrenergic agent desipramine can be used. It has fewer anticholinergic side effects and causes less sedation.

Table 25.2 Treatment options for neuropathic pain: oral medications.

Drug	Starting dose	Maintenance dose	Mechanism
Amitriptyline/imipramine	10–25 mg at night	75–150 mg/day	NE/5-HT reuptake inhibition Sodium channel blockade
Duloxetine	60 mg/day	Up to 120 mg/day	5- HT and NE reuptake inhibition
Gabapentin	300 mg o.d.	2400–4500 mg/day	Calcium channel blockade? GABA-ergic mechanism?
Pregabalin	50 mg t.i.d.	150–300 mg/day	Calcium channel blockade? GABA-ergic mechanism?
Clonazepam	0.5 mg at night	2 mg/day	GABA-ergic mechanism
Phenytoin	50 mg b.d.	300 mg/day	Sodium channel blocker
Clonidine	50 μg b.d.	75 μg b.d.	α_2-Adrenoreceptor agonist
Tramadol	50–100 mg q.i.d.	200–400 mg/day	Centrally acting opioid Nonopioid analgesic
Dextromethorphan	60 mg	60 mg b.d.	NMDA receptor antagonist

5-HT, 5-hydroxytryptamine; b.d., twice daily; q.i.d., four times daily; NE, norepinephrine; NMDA, *N*-methyl-D-aspartic acid; o.d., once daily.

Table 25.3 Treatment options for neuropathic pain: other therapies.

Therapy type	Details
Topical applications	Capsaicin cream (0.075% q.i.d., for 8 weeks) Local anesthetic, e.g. 5% lidocaine gel or lotion
Intravenous lidocaine infusion	5 mg/kg body weight over 30 minutes with electrocardiogram and blood pressure monitoring; useful for persistent paresthesiae; a response to lidocaine infusion may be a predictor of response to sodium channel blockers; epidural infusion with lidocaine
Sympathetic blocks	Intravenous guanethidine (1.25–30 mg in 20–50 mL saline solution) can be used for treatment of continuous burning pain and to test whether the sympathetic system is involved in the generation of pain; stellate ganglion blocks
Neuromodulation	TENS Spinal cord stimulation
Cognitive–behavioral rehabilitation	Pain management programs Relaxation therapy
Surgery	Decompression/neurolysis/neurotization DREZ lesions (for deafferentation pain)

5-HT, 5-hydroxytryptamine; b.d., twice daily; DREZ, dorsal root entry zone; q.i.d., four times daily; NE, norepinephrine; NMDA, *N*-methyl-D-aspartic acid; o.d., once daily; TENS, transcutaneous electrical nerve stimulation.

Selective serotonin reuptake inhibitors (SSRI) like citalopram, fluoxetine, and fluvoxamine inhibit serotonin reuptake without action on NE reuptake.[73] There are limited data on the effectiveness of SSRI on neuropathic pain other than painful diabetic peripheral neuropathy, where paroxetine and citalopram have been reported to be effective.[74][II], [75][II]

Another related class of drugs, the serotonin noradrenaline reuptake inhibitors (SNRI), such as venlafaxine, milnacipran, and duloxetine, cause a balanced inhibition of serotonin and noradrenaline.[73] Duloxetine and venlafaxine have been shown to be effective in treating and preventing postmastectomy pain syndrome, diabetic peripheral neuropathy (DPN), and painful polyneuropathy.[76][II], [77][II], [78][II], [79][II], [80][II] Duloxetine is indicated in the management of painful diabetic polyneuropathy. It has been shown to be significantly better than placebo with a number needed to treat (NNT) of 4.1.[80][II]

For further discussion of this topic, see Chapter 18, Chronic pain and depression.

ANTICONVULSANTS

Carbamazepine, an anticonvulsant, was reported to have an analgesic effect on trigeminal neuralgia in 1962.[81] Since then various other anticonvulsants have been studied for their analgesic action. Phenytoin, sodium valproate, gabapentin, clonazepam, or lamotrigine are often used for neuropathic pain. Phenytoin exerts its membrane-stabilizing effect by blocking sodium channels and reduces neuronal excitability in pain. It has been proposed that these drugs show antihyperalgesic activity in chronic pain by counteracting the hyperexcitability generated by the pathological expression and redistribution of Na^+ channels.[82] Gabapentin and pregabalin are considered to bind to the α2-δ subunit of voltage-gated calcium channels.[83, 84, 85] These channels are shown to be up-regulated in the spinal cord and dorsal root ganglia of a rat neuropathic pain model and are thought to play an important role in modulating neuropathic pain.[86] Pregabalin has a greater efficacy and longer half-life than gabapentin necessitating a lower dose, thus reducing the side effects of gabapentin. It has been licensed by the FDA for treatment of pain associated with PHN and DPN. Clinical trials have shown this drug to be effective in dental pain,[87][II] PHN,[88][II], [89][II] and painful DPN.[90][II], [91][II], [92][II], [93][II] Topiramate, a newer anticonvulsant, acts on neuronal transmission in at least five ways, by modulating voltage-gated sodium ion channels, potentiating gamma-aminobutyric acid inhibition, blocking excitatory glutamate neurotransmission, modulating voltage-gated calcium ion channels, and by inhibiting carbonic anhydrase. It has been shown to have a role in controlling pain in neuropathic pain syndromes.[94][V], [95][V], [96][V], [97][V] However, its role in treatment of painful diabetic neuropathy has been less certain.[98]

For further discussion of this topic, see Chapter 19, Antiepileptic and antiarrhythmic agents.

There are few data comparing the efficacy of antidepressants and anticonvulsants.[72][II], [99][II] A recent meta-analysis has addressed the effectiveness of both classes of drugs in comparison with a placebo. For both classes of drugs across syndromes of painful DPN and PHN, the NNT indicated that for every three patients receiving an antidepressant or anticonvulsant, one experienced over 50 percent pain relief that they would not have experienced with placebo. No difference in efficacy was demonstrated between gabapentin and the older anticonvulsants phenytoin and carbamazepine. The adverse effect rates were also similar across both classes of drugs.[100][I]

OTHER AGENTS

Capsaicin

Capsaicin is the active constituent of hot chilli peppers, responsible for eliciting the symptoms of heat, burning, and erythema. Capsaicin is a potent activator of the TRPV1 receptor, which is also activated by noxious heat above 43°C.[101] Capsaicin has been advocated as a topical agent for the therapy of PHN and painful DPN.[44][III], [102][III], [103, 104][II], [105][II] The underlying mechanisms may include depletion of substance P via activation of the TRPV1 receptor or desensitization of nerve terminals. The degeneration of epidermal nerve fibers, which is reversible on discontinuing capsaicin, is also postulated to contribute to analgesia.[106] The burning induced by capsaicin can be significantly reduced by pretreatment with a topical anesthetic.[107][III] Recently, capsaicin was shown in a preliminary study to relieve intractable neuropathic pain when used in very high doses (5–10 percent) in association with regional anesthesia.[108][III] High concentrations of capsaicin (8 percent) applied as a patch for 60 minutes have been shown to mimic the degeneration of epidermal nerve fibers seen with prolonged exposure to low-dose capsaicin and may provide an alternative treatment for neuropathic pain.[109][III]

Topical lidocaine patch

A 5 percent lidocaine patch has been approved by the FDA for PHN. Trials have demonstrated its effectiveness in reducing allodynia and pain.[47][II], [110][II]

Other topical agents

Eutectic mixture of local anesthetics (EMLA) and topical aspirin/diethyl ether mixture have been shown to be useful in painful conditions like herpes zoster and PHN.[111][V], [112][II]

Tramadol

Tramadol is a centrally acting analgesic. It is a weak opiate, modulates central serotoninergic and noradrenergic inhibition of pain, and has a very low risk of addiction.[113][V] It was shown to reduce pain in patients with diabetic neuropathy.[114][II] The side effects commonly seen are nausea, constipation, headache, and somnolence.[114][II]

Opioids

Severe pain may be relieved by opioids, which are predominantly centrally acting analgesics. The prototype is morphine. Opioids are generally reserved for severe acute pain states and for chronic pain due to malignancy with poor prognosis, in which they usually provide satisfactory pain relief with adequate doses. The application of opioids in diseases of nonmalignant origin is restricted by the potential risk of development of dependence. It is difficult to predict whether a neuropathic pain syndrome would respond to opioids, and it may be helpful to undertake a short trial in severe refractory pain states to see whether the patient is opioid sensitive. Opioids were not traditionally considered to be effective in neuropathic pain, but have a role where this is intractable; they are less likely to work if pain is in a numb area.[115][V] Recent trials have demonstrated the effectiveness of controlled-release oxycodone in pain secondary to PHN and diabetic neuropathy.[116][II], [117][II], [118][II]

Using the number needed to treat method (numbers of patients needed to treat to obtain one with more than 50 percent pain relief), Finnerup *et al.*[119] reviewed the efficacy of different pharmacological agents used in the treatment of painful neuropathy. For antidepressants of all types combined, an NNT of 3.3 was observed with a slightly better NNT for tricyclic antidepressants of serotoninergic type. Duloxetine had a NNT of 4.1 in painful diabetic neuropathy. For the ion channel blockers, the NNT values were: gabapentin and pregabalin 4.7, phenytoin 2.1, and topiramate 7.4. The values for other agents, such as dextromethorphan, tramadol, and capsaicin, were 4.4, 3.9, and 6.7, respectively.

For further discussion of this topic, see Chapter 16, Opioids and chronic noncancer pain.

OTHER THERAPIES

Transcutaneous electrical nerve stimulation

Transcutaneous electrical nerve stimulation (TENS) is based on the gate control theory, and involves selective activation of non-nociceptor fibers. It may be helpful, if correctly administered, in some patients with neuropathic pain[120][III], [121][II] and needs persistence to find the optimum conditions of stimulation.

Spinal cord stimulation

Spinal cord stimulation was based on the gate control theory of pain, and is now linked to many mechanisms. It is thought to activate spinal inhibitory circuits, mainly those concerned with γ-aminobutyric acid (GABA)-ergic mechanisms,[122][V], [123] and may have a suppressive action on dorsal horn neuronal hyperexcitability.[124] Before permanent implantation of a stimulation device, a trial period with temporary external stimulation is strongly recommended. Spinal cord stimulation has been shown to have long-term benefit in various conditions associated with neuropathic pain, including diabetic painful neuropathy, complex regional pain syndromes, and failed back syndrome.[125][III], [126][III], [127][III], [128][III], [129][III], [130][III], [131] Postherpetic pain and intercostal neuralgia seem to respond less favorably over the long term,[126][III] as do pain due to cauda equina injury and phantom limb pain.[127][III] Strict criteria need to be applied to the selection of a patient, and all therapeutic modalities should be exhausted before the decision to implant a stimulator is made.

REFERENCES

* 1. Attal N, Bouhassira D. Mechanisms of pain in peripheral neuropathy. *Acta Neurologica Scandinavica. Supplementum.* 1999; **173**: 12–24; discussion 48-52.
* 2. Woolf CJ, Mannion RJ. Neuropathic pain: aetiology, symptoms, mechanisms, and management. *Lancet.* 1999; **353**: 1959–64.
* 3. Bennett GJ. Neuropathic pain. In: Wall PD, Melzack R, Bonica JJ (eds). *Textbook of pain.* London: Churchill Livingstone, 1994: 201–24.
4. England JD, Happel LT, Kline DG *et al.* Sodium channel accumulation in humans with painful neuromas. *Neurology.* 1996; **47**: 272–6.
5. Coward K, Plumpton C, Facer P *et al.* Immunolocalization of SNS/PN3 and NaN/SNS2 sodium channels in human pain states. *Pain.* 2000; **85**: 41–50.
6. Novakovic SD, Tzoumaka E, McGivern JG *et al.* Distribution of the tetrodotoxin-resistant sodium channel PN3 in rat sensory neurons in normal and neuropathic conditions. *Journal of Neuroscience.* 1998; **18**: 2174–87.
7. Porreca F, Lai J, Bian D *et al.* A comparison of the potential role of the tetrodotoxin-insensitive sodium channels, PN3/SNS and NaN/SNS2, in rat models of chronic pain. *Proceedings of the National Academy of Sciences of the United States of America.* 1999; **96**: 7640–4.
8. Ishikawa K, Tanaka M, Black JA, Waxman SG. Changes in expression of voltage-gated potassium channels in dorsal root ganglion neurons following axotomy. *Muscle and Nerve.* 1999; **22**: 502–07.
9. Wall PD, Woolf CJ. The brief and the prolonged facilitatory effects of unmyelinated afferent input on the rat spinal cord are independently influenced by peripheral nerve section. *Neuroscience.* 1986; **17**: 1199–205.
10. Woolf CJ. Evidence for a central component of post-injury pain hypersensitivity. *Nature.* 1983; **306**: 686–8.
* 11. Dotson RM. Clinical neurophysiology laboratory tests to assess the nociceptive system in humans. *Journal of Clinical Neurophysiology.* 1997; **14**: 32–45.
12. Dyck PJ, O'Brien PC. Quantitative sensation testing in epidemiological and therapeutic studies of peripheral neuropathy. *Muscle and Nerve.* 1999; **22**: 659–62.
* 13. Quarles RH, Weiss MD. Autoantibodies associated with peripheral neuropathy. *Muscle and Nerve.* 1999; **22**: 800–22.
14. Said G. Indications and value of nerve biopsy. *Muscle and Nerve.* 1999; **22**: 1617–19.
* 15. Asbury AK, Bird SJ. Disorders of peripheral nerves. In: Asbury AK, McKhann GM, McDonald WI (eds). *Diseases of the nervous system: clinical neurobiology,* 2nd edn. Philadelphia: WB Saunders, 1992: 252–69.
* 16. Johnson PC, Doll SC, Cromey DW. Pathogenesis of diabetic neuropathy. *Annals of Neurology.* 1986; **19**: 450–7.
17. Thomas PK, Tomlinson DR. Diabetic and hypoglycemic neuropathy. In: Dyck PJ, Thomas PK, Griffin JW *et al.* (eds). *Peripheral neuropathy.* Philadelphia: WB Saunders, 1993: 1219–50.
* 18. Dyck PJ, Norell JE. Microvasculitis and ischemia in diabetic lumbosacral radiculoplexus neuropathy. *Neurology.* 1999; **53**: 2113–21.
19. Said G, Slama G, Selva J. Progressive centripetal degeneration of axons in small fibre diabetic polyneuropathy. *Brain.* 1983; **106**: 791–807.
20. Llewelyn JG, Gilbey SG, Thomas PK *et al.* Sural nerve morphometry in diabetic autonomic and painful sensory neuropathy. A clinicopathological study. *Brain.* 1991; **114**: 867–92.
* 21. Feldman EL, Russell JW, Sullivan KA, Golovoy D. New insights into the pathogenesis of diabetic neuropathy. *Current Opinion in Neurology.* 1999; **12**: 553–63.
* 22. Thomas PK. Diabetic neuropathy: mechanisms and future treatment options. *Journal of Neurology, Neurosurgery, and Psychiatry.* 1999; **67**: 277–9.
* 23. Windebank AJ. Polyneuropathy due to nutritional deficiency and alcoholism. In: Dyck PJ, Thomas PK, Griffin JW *et al.* (eds). *Peripheral neuropathy.* Philadelphia: WB Saunders, 1993: 1311–21.
24. Schaumburg H, Kaplan J, Windebank A *et al.* Sensory neuropathy from pyridoxine abuse. A new megavitamin syndrome. *New England Journal of Medicine.* 1983; **309**: 445–8.
* 25. Windebank AJ. Metal neuropathy. In: Dyck PJ, Thomas PK, Griffin JW *et al.* (eds). *Peripheral neuropathy.* Philadelphia: WB Saunders, 1993: 1549–70.
26. Agocs MM, Etzel RA, Parrish RG *et al.* Mercury exposure from interior latex paint. *New England Journal of Medicine.* 1990; **323**: 1096–101.
27. Clarkson TW. Mercury – an element of mystery. *New England Journal of Medicine.* 1990; **323**: 1137–9.
28. Windebank AJ. Chemotherapeutic neuropathy. *Current Opinion in Neurology.* 1999; **12**: 565–71.
29. Moyle GJ, Sadler M. Peripheral neuropathy with nucleoside antiretrovirals: risk factors, incidence and management. *Drug Safety.* 1998; **19**: 481–94.
30. Berger AR, Arezzo JC, Schaumburg HH *et al.* 2′,3′-dideoxycytidine (ddC) toxic neuropathy: a study of 52 patients. *Neurology.* 1993; **43**: 358–62.
31. Famularo G, Moretti S, Marcellini S *et al.* Acetyl-carnitine deficiency in AIDS patients with neurotoxicity on treatment with antiretroviral nucleoside analogues. *AIDS.* 1997; **11**: 185–90.
* 32. Simmons Z. Paraproteinemia and neuropathy. *Current Opinion in Neurology.* 1999; **12**: 589–95.
* 33. Brady RO. Fabry disease. In: Dyck PJ, Thomas PK, Griffin JW *et al.* (eds). *Peripheral neuropathy.* Philadelphia: WB Saunders, 1993: 1169–78.
34. Dyck PJ. Neuronal atrophy and degeneration predominantly affecting peripheral sensory and autonomic

neurons. In: Dyck PJ, Thomas PK, Griffin JW *et al.* (eds). *Peripheral neuropathy.* Philadelphia: WB Saunders, 1993: 1065–92.

35. Cummins TR, Dib-Hajj SD, Waxman SG. Electrophysiological properties of mutant Nav1.7 sodium channels in a painful inherited neuropathy. *Journal of Neuroscience.* 2004; **24**: 8232–6.
36. Dib-Hajj SD, Rush AM, Cummins TR *et al.* Gain-of-function mutation in Nav1.7 in familial erythromelalgia induces bursting of sensory neurons. *Brain.* 2005; **128**: 1847–54.
37. Rizzuto N, Cavallaro T, Monaco S *et al.* Role of HIV in the pathogenesis of distal symmetrical peripheral neuropathy. *Acta Neuropathologica.* 1995; **90**: 244–50.
38. Simpson DM, Olney RK. Peripheral neuropathies associated with human immunodeficiency virus infection. *Neurologic Clinics.* 1992; **10**: 685–711.
39. Ozawa A, Sasao Y, Iwashita K *et al.* HLA-A33 and -B44 and susceptibility to postherpetic neuralgia (PHN). *Tissue Antigens.* 1999; **53**: 263–8.
40. Wood MJ, Kay R, Dworkin RH *et al.* Oral acyclovir therapy accelerates pain resolution in patients with herpes zoster: a meta-analysis of placebo-controlled trials. *Clinical Infectious Diseases.* 1996; **22**: 341–7.
41. Jackson JL, Gibbons R, Meyer G, Inouye L. The effect of treating herpes zoster with oral acyclovir in preventing postherpetic neuralgia. A meta-analysis. *Archives of Internal Medicine.* 1997; **157**: 909–12.
42. Dworkin RH, Boon RJ, Griffin DR, Phung D. Postherpetic neuralgia: impact of famciclovir, age, rash severity, and acute pain in herpes zoster patients. *Journal of Infectious Diseases.* 1998; **178** (Suppl. 1): S76–80.
43. Ernst ME, Santee JA, Klepser TB. Oral corticosteroids for pain associated with herpes zoster. *Annals of Pharmacotherapy.* 1998; **32**: 1099–103.
44. Watson CP, Evans RJ, Watt VR. Post-herpetic neuralgia and topical capsaicin. *Pain.* 1988; **33**: 333–40.
45. Peikert A, Hentrich M, Ochs G. Topical 0.025% capsaicin in chronic post-herpetic neuralgia: efficacy, predictors of response and long-term course. *Journal of Neurology.* 1991; **238**: 452–6.
46. Frucht-Pery J, Feldman ST, Brown SI. The use of capsaicin in herpes zoster ophthalmicus neuralgia. *Acta Ophthalmologica Scandinavica.* 1997; **75**: 311–13.
47. Galer BS, Rowbotham MC, Perander J, Friedman E. Topical lidocaine patch relieves postherpetic neuralgia more effectively than a vehicle topical patch: results of an enriched enrollment study. *Pain.* 1999; **80**: 533–8.
48. Davies PS, Galer BS. Review of lidocaine patch 5% studies in the treatment of postherpetic neuralgia. *Drugs.* 2004; **64**: 937–47.
49. Oxman MN, Levin MJ, Johnson GR *et al.* A vaccine to prevent herpes zoster and postherpetic neuralgia in older adults. *New England Journal of Medicine.* 2005; **352**: 2271–84.
50. ✻ Devor M. Nerve pathophysiology and mechanisms of pain in causalgia. *Journal of the Autonomic Nervous System.* 1983; **7**: 371–84.
51. Chen Y, Michaelis M, Janig W, Devor M. Adrenoreceptor subtype mediating sympathetic-sensory coupling in injured sensory neurons. *Journal of Neurophysiology.* 1996; **76**: 3721–30.
52. McLachlan EM, Janig W, Devor M, Michaelis M. Peripheral nerve injury triggers noradrenergic sprouting within dorsal root ganglia. *Nature.* 1993; **363**: 543–6.
53. Berman JS, Birch R, Anand P. Pain following human brachial plexus injury with spinal cord root avulsion and the effect of surgery. *Pain.* 1998; **75**: 199–207.
54. Smith BE. Inflammatory sensory polyganglionopathies. *Neurologic Clinics.* 1992; **10**: 735–59.
55. ✻ Grisold W, Drlicek M. Paraneoplastic neuropathy. *Current Opinion in Neurology.* 1999; **12**: 617–25.
56. ✻ Holland NR, Crawford TO, Hauer P *et al.* Small-fiber sensory neuropathies: clinical course and neuropathology of idiopathic cases. *Annals of Neurology.* 1998; **44**: 47–59.
57. Larner AJ, Moss J, Rossi ML, Anderson M. Congenital insensitivity to pain: a 20 year follow up. *Journal of Neurology, Neurosurgery, and Psychiatry.* 1994; **57**: 973–4.
58. ✻ Dyck PJ, Mellinger JF, Reagan TJ *et al.* Not 'indifference to pain' but varieties of hereditary sensory and autonomic neuropathy. *Brain.* 1983; **106**: 373–90.
59. Rosemberg S, Marie SK, Kliemann S. Congenital insensitivity to pain with anhidrosis (hereditary sensory and autonomic neuropathy type IV). *Pediatric Neurology.* 1994; **11**: 50–6.
60. Mardy S, Miura Y, Endo F *et al.* Congenital insensitivity to pain with anhidrosis: novel mutations in the TRKA (NTRK1) gene encoding a high-affinity receptor for nerve growth factor. *American Journal of Human Genetics.* 1999; **64**: 1570–9.
61. Yotsumoto S, Setoyama M, Hozumi H *et al.* A novel point mutation affecting the tyrosine kinase domain of the TRKA gene in a family with congenital insensitivity to pain with anhidrosis. *Journal of Investigative Dermatology.* 1999; **112**: 810–14.
62. ✻ Ginsberg L. Specific painful neuropathies. In: Cervero F, Jensen TS (eds). *Handbook of clinical neurology.* Edinburgh: Elsevier, 2006: 635–52.
63. Hietaharju A, Croft R, Alam R *et al.* Chronic neuropathic pain in treated leprosy. *Lancet.* 2000; **356**: 1080–1.
64. Anand P, Pandya S, Ladiwala U *et al.* Depletion of nerve growth factor in leprosy. *Lancet.* 1994; **344**: 129–30.
65. Facer P, Mathur R, Pandya SS *et al.* Correlation of quantitative tests of nerve and target organ dysfunction with skin immunohistology in leprosy. *Brain.* 1998; **121**: 2239–47.
66. ✻ Dyck PJ, Thomas PK, Griffin JW *et al.* *Peripheral neuropathy.* Philadelphia: WB Saunders, 1993: 1311–21.
67. Fishbain DA, Cutler R, Rosomoff HL, Rosomoff RS. Evidence-based data from animal and human experimental studies on pain relief with antidepressants: a structured review. *Pain Medicine.* 2000; **1**: 310–16.

68. Dubner R, Bennett GJ. Spinal and trigeminal mechanisms of nociception. *Annual Review of Neuroscience*. 1983; **6**: 381–418.
69. Guay DR. Adjunctive agents in the management of chronic pain. *Pharmacotherapy*. 2001; **21**: 1070–81.
* 70. Saarto T, Wiffen PJ. Antidepressants for neuropathic pain. *Cochrane Database of Systematic Reviews*. 2005; **CD005454**.
71. Fields HL. Pain II: new approaches to management. *Annals of Neurology*. 1981; **9**: 101–06.
72. Morello CM, Leckband SG, Stoner CP *et al*. Randomized double-blind study comparing the efficacy of gabapentin with amitriptyline on diabetic peripheral neuropathy pain. *Archives of Internal Medicine*. 1999; **159**: 1931–7.
* 73. Baldessarini RJ. Drugs for the treatment of psychiatric disorders. In: Hardman JG, Limbird LE, Gilman AG (eds). *Goodman & Gilman's the pharmacological basis of therapeutics*, 10th edn. New York, USA: McGraw-Hill, 2001: 447–83.
74. Sindrup SH, Bjerre U, Dejgaard A *et al*. The selective serotonin reuptake inhibitor citalopram relieves the symptoms of diabetic neuropathy. *Clinical Pharmacology and Therapeutics*. 1992; **52**: 547–52.
75. Sindrup SH, Gram LF, Brosen K *et al*. The selective serotonin reuptake inhibitor paroxetine is effective in the treatment of diabetic neuropathy symptoms. *Pain*. 1990; **42**: 135–44.
76. Reuben SS, Makari-Judson G, Lurie SD. Evaluation of efficacy of the perioperative administration of venlafaxine XR in the prevention of postmastectomy pain syndrome. *Journal of Pain and Symptom Management*. 2004; **27**: 133–9.
77. Rowbotham MC, Goli V, Kunz NR, Lei D. Venlafaxine extended release in the treatment of painful diabetic neuropathy: a double-blind, placebo-controlled study. *Pain*. 2004; **110**: 697–706.
78. Sindrup SH, Bach FW, Madsen C *et al*. Venlafaxine versus imipramine in painful polyneuropathy: a randomized, controlled trial. *Neurology*. 2003; **60**: 1284–9.
79. Raskin J, Pritchett YL, Wang F *et al*. A double-blind, randomized multicenter trial comparing duloxetine with placebo in the management of diabetic peripheral neuropathic pain. *Pain Medicine*. 2005; **6**: 346–56.
80. Goldstein DJ, Lu Y, Detke MJ *et al*. Duloxetine vs. placebo in patients with painful diabetic neuropathy. *Pain*. 2005; **116**: 109–18.
81. Blom S. Trigeminal neuralgia: its treatment with a new anticonvulsant drug (G-32883). *Lancet*. 1962; **1**: 839–40.
82. Rizzo MA. Successful treatment of painful traumatic mononeuropathy with carbamazepine: insights into a possible molecular pain mechanism. *Journal of the Neurological Sciences*. 1997; **152**: 103–06.
83. Suman-Chauhan N, Webdale L, Hill DR, Woodruff GN. Characterisation of [3H]gabapentin binding to a novel site in rat brain: homogenate binding studies. *European Journal of Pharmacology*. 1993; **244**: 293–301.
84. Gee NS, Brown JP, Dissanayake VU *et al*. The novel anticonvulsant drug, gabapentin (Neurontin), binds to the alpha2delta subunit of a calcium channel. *Journal of Biological Chemistry*. 1996; **271**: 5768–76.
85. Gong HC, Hang J, Kohler W *et al*. Tissue-specific expression and gabapentin-binding properties of calcium channel alpha2delta subunit subtypes. *Journal of Membrane Biology*. 2001; **184**: 35–43.
86. Luo ZD, Chaplan SR, Higuera ES *et al*. Upregulation of dorsal root ganglion (alpha)2(delta) calcium channel subunit and its correlation with allodynia in spinal nerve-injured rats. *Journal of Neuroscience*. 2001; **21**: 1868–75.
87. Hill CM, Balkenohl M, Thomas DW *et al*. Pregabalin in patients with postoperative dental pain. *European Journal of Pain*. 2001; **5**: 119–24.
88. Sabatowski R, Galvez R, Cherry DA *et al*. Pregabalin reduces pain and improves sleep and mood disturbances in patients with post-herpetic neuralgia: results of a randomised, placebo-controlled clinical trial. *Pain*. 2004; **109**: 26–35.
89. Dworkin RH, Corbin AE, Young Jr JP *et al*. Pregabalin for the treatment of postherpetic neuralgia: a randomized, placebo-controlled trial. *Neurology*. 2003; **60**: 1274–83.
90. Rosenstock J, Tuchman M, LaMoreaux L, Sharma U. Pregabalin for the treatment of painful diabetic peripheral neuropathy: a double-blind, placebo-controlled trial. *Pain*. 2004; **110**: 628–38.
91. Lesser H, Sharma U, LaMoreaux L, Poole RM. Pregabalin relieves symptoms of painful diabetic neuropathy: a randomized controlled trial. *Neurology*. 2004; **63**: 2104–10.
92. Richter RW, Portenoy R, Sharma U *et al*. Relief of painful diabetic peripheral neuropathy with pregabalin: a randomized, placebo-controlled trial. *Journal of Pain*. 2005; **6**: 253–60.
93. Freynhagen R, Strojek K, Griesing T *et al*. Efficacy of pregabalin in neuropathic pain evaluated in a 12-week, randomised, double-blind, multicentre, placebo-controlled trial of flexible- and fixed-dose regimens. *Pain*. 2005; **115**: 254–63.
94. Solaro C, Uccelli MM, Brichetto G *et al*. Topiramate relieves idiopathic and symptomatic trigeminal neuralgia. *Journal of Pain and Symptom Management*. 2001; **21**: 367–8.
95. Potter D. Potential role of topiramate in relief of neuropathic pain. *Neurology*. 1998; **50**: A255.
96. Zvartau-Hind M, Din MU, Gilani A *et al*. Topiramate relieves refractory trigeminal neuralgia in MS patients. *Neurology*. 2000; **55**: 1587–8.
97. Bajwa ZH, Sami N, Warfield CA, Wootton J. Topiramate relieves refractory intercostal neuralgia. *Neurology*. 1999; **52**: 1917.
98. Edwards KR, Glanz MJ, Button J *et al*. Efficacy and safety of topiramate in the treatment of painful diabetic neuropathy: a double-blind, placebo-controlled study. *Neurology*. 2000; **54**: A81.

99. Dallocchio C, Buffa C, Mazzarello P, Chiroli S. Gabapentin vs. amitriptyline in painful diabetic neuropathy: an open-label pilot study. *Journal of Pain and Symptom Management.* 2000; **20**: 280–5.
100. McQuay HJ. Neuropathic pain: evidence matters. *European Journal of Pain.* 2002; **6** (Suppl. A): 11–18.
*101. Caterina MJ, Schumacher MA, Tominaga M *et al.* The capsaicin receptor: a heat-activated ion channel in the pain pathway. *Nature.* 1997; **389**: 816–24.
102. Westerman RA, Roberts RG, Kotzmann RR *et al.* Effects of topical capsaicin on normal skin and affected dermatomes in herpes zoster. *Clinical and Experimental Neurology.* 1988; **25**: 71–84.
103. Lynn B. Capsaicin: actions on nociceptive C-fibres and therapeutic potential. *Pain.* 1990; **41**: 61–9.
104. Anonymous. Treatment of painful diabetic neuropathy with topical capsaicin. A multicenter, double-blind, vehicle-controlled study. The Capsaicin Study Group. *Archives of Internal Medicine.* 1991; **151**: 2225–9.
*105. Rains C, Bryson HM. Topical capsaicin. A review of its pharmacological properties and therapeutic potential in post-herpetic neuralgia, diabetic neuropathy and osteoarthritis. *Drugs and Aging.* 1995; **7**: 317–28.
106. Nolano M, Simone DA, Wendelschafer-Crabb G *et al.* Topical capsaicin in humans: parallel loss of epidermal nerve fibers and pain sensation. *Pain.* 1999; **81**: 135–45.
107. Yosipovitch G, Maibach HI, Rowbotham MC. Effect of EMLA pre-treatment on capsaicin-induced burning and hyperalgesia. *Acta Dermato-venereologica.* 1999; **79**: 118–21.
108. Robbins WR, Staats PS, Levine J *et al.* Treatment of intractable pain with topical large-dose capsaicin: preliminary report. *Anesthesia and Analgesia.* 1998; **86**: 579–83.
109. Malmberg AB, Mizisin AP, Calcutt NA *et al.* Reduced heat sensitivity and epidermal nerve fiber immunostaining following single applications of a high-concentration capsaicin patch. *Pain.* 2004; **111**: 360–7.
110. Rowbotham MC, Davies PS, Verkempinck C, Galer BS. Lidocaine patch: double-blind controlled study of a new treatment method for post-herpetic neuralgia. *Pain.* 1996; **65**: 39–44.
111. Litman SJ, Vitkun SA, Poppers PJ. Use of EMLA cream in the treatment of post-herpetic neuralgia. *Journal of Clinical Anesthesia.* 1996; **8**: 54–7.
112. De Benedittis G, Lorenzetti A. Topical aspirin/diethyl ether mixture versus indomethacin and diclofenac/diethyl ether mixtures for acute herpetic neuralgia and postherpetic neuralgia: a double-blind crossover placebo-controlled study. *Pain.* 1996; **65**: 45–51.
*113. Nurmikko TJ, Nash TP, Wiles JR. Recent advances: control of chronic pain. *British Medical Journal.* 1998; **317**: 1438–41.
114. Harati Y, Gooch C, Swenson M *et al.* Double-blind randomized trial of tramadol for the treatment of the pain of diabetic neuropathy. *Neurology.* 1998; **50**: 1842–6.
*115. McQuay H. Opioids in pain management. *Lancet.* 1999; **353**: 2229–32.
116. Watson CP, Babul N. Efficacy of oxycodone in neuropathic pain: a randomized trial in postherpetic neuralgia. *Neurology.* 1998; **50**: 1837–41.
117. Gimbel JS, Richards P, Portenoy RK. Controlled-release oxycodone for pain in diabetic neuropathy: a randomized controlled trial. *Neurology.* 2003; **60**: 927–34.
118. Watson CP, Moulin D, Watt-Watson J *et al.* Controlled-release oxycodone relieves neuropathic pain: a randomized controlled trial in painful diabetic neuropathy. *Pain.* 2003; **105**: 71–8.
*119. Finnerup NB, Otto M, McQuay HJ *et al.* Algorithm for neuropathic pain treatment: an evidence based proposal. *Pain.* 2005; **118**: 289–305.
120. Meyer GA, Fields HL. Causalgia treated by selective large fibre stimulation of peripheral nerve. *Brain.* 1972; **95**: 163–8.
121. Kumar D, Marshall HJ. Diabetic peripheral neuropathy: amelioration of pain with transcutaneous electrostimulation. *Diabetes Care.* 1997; **20**: 1702–05.
*122. Stanton-Hicks M, Salamon J. Stimulation of the central and peripheral nervous system for the control of pain. *Journal of Clinical Neurophysiology.* 1997; **14**: 46–62.
123. Cui JG, O'Connor WT, Ungerstedt U *et al.* Spinal cord stimulation attenuates augmented dorsal horn release of excitatory amino acids in mononeuropathy via a GABAergic mechanism. *Pain.* 1997; **73**: 87–95.
124. Yakhnitsa V, Linderoth B, Meyerson BA. Spinal cord stimulation attenuates dorsal horn neuronal hyperexcitability in a rat model of mononeuropathy. *Pain.* 1999; **79**: 223–33.
125. Tesfaye S, Watt J, Benbow SJ *et al.* Electrical spinal-cord stimulation for painful diabetic peripheral neuropathy. *Lancet.* 1996; **348**: 1698–701.
126. Kumar K, Toth C, Nath RK. Spinal cord stimulation for chronic pain in peripheral neuropathy. *Surgical Neurology.* 1996; **46**: 363–9.
127. Lang P. The treatment of chronic pain by epidural spinal cord stimulation – a 15 year follow up; present status. *Axone (Dartmouth, N.S.)* 1997; **18**: 71–3.
*128. Kumar K, Toth C, Nath RK, Laing P. Epidural spinal cord stimulation for treatment of chronic pain – some predictors of success. A 15-year experience. *Surgical Neurology.* 1998; **50**: 110–20; discussion 20–1.
*129. Segal R, Stacey BR, Rudy TE *et al.* Spinal cord stimulation revisited. *Neurological Research.* 1998; **20**: 391–6.
130. Kemler MA, Barendse GA, Van Kleef M *et al.* Electrical spinal cord stimulation in reflex sympathetic dystrophy: retrospective analysis of 23 patients. *Journal of Neurosurgery.* 1999; **90**: 79–83.
131. Murphy D, Laffy J, O'Keeffe D. Electrical spinal cord stimulation for painful peripheral neuropathy secondary to coeliac disease. *Gut.* 1998; **42**: 448–9.

26

HIV and AIDS

SARAH COX AND ANDREW SC RICE

KEY LEARNING POINTS

- Human immunodeficiency virus (HIV) is a retrovirus which causes serious disease by progressive damage to the immune system of the human host.
- Antiretroviral treatment can result in long-term restoration of immune function. However, the therapeutic decisions inherent in antiretroviral therapy are complex, so such therapy must be managed by HIV clinicians.
- HIV/acquired immunodeficiency syndrome (AIDS) is associated with pain in a number of different contexts.
- Antiretroviral treatments are liable to interactions with other medications, so due diligence is required when prescribing analgesics and other drugs.
- Both HIV infection and antiretroviral therapy can be complicated by predominantly small fiber polyneuropathies, which are sometimes a cause of neuropathic pain.

INTRODUCTION

HIV is a retrovirus causing progressive cell-mediated immunodeficiency. Humans are susceptible to infection by two types of HIV: HIV-1 and HIV-2. Worldwide, HIV-1 is the most common virus associated with progressive disease, whilst HIV-2 is found predominantly in West Africa, is less infectious, and causes immunodeficiency more slowly than HIV-1.[1] Untreated HIV disease has a prognosis of approximately ten years with death from wasting disease, malignancy, and/or infections. Some of these conditions are AIDS-defining illnesses (**Box 26.1**).[2] The case definition for AIDS was developed for surveillance purposes, but the implications of such a diagnosis depend on whether effective highly active antiretroviral treatment (HAART) is available. Even after experiencing an AIDS defining illness an individual's prognosis depends on whether it is possible to restore or stabilize immune function.

HIV infection is a pandemic that represents one of the ten major causes of death worldwide. The Joint United Nations Programme on HIV/AIDS reported that in 2007 there were between 1.9 and 2.4 million deaths from HIV/AIDS and 30–36 million individuals living with the infection (see www.unaids.org).

The extent of immunosuppression in HIV disease is reflected in the clinical picture and is monitored in the laboratory by a combination of CD4 T-cell count and

Box 26.1 Communicable Disease Council AIDS indicator conditions for adolescents and adults[2]

- Candidiasis of esophagus, trachea, bronchi, or lungs
- Cervical cancer, invasive
- Coccidioidomycosis, extrapulmonary
- Cryptococcosis, extrapulmonary
- Cryptosporidiosis with diarrhea for more than one month
- Cytomegalovirus of any organ other than liver, spleen, or lymph nodes
- Herpes simplex with mucocutaneous ulcer for more than a month or bronchitis, pneumonitis, or esophagitis
- Histoplasmosis, extrapulmonary
- HIV-associated dementia; disabling cognitive and/or motor dysfunction interfering with occupation or activities of daily living
- HIV-associated wasting; involuntary weight loss of >10 percent of baseline plus chronic diarrhea (>2 loose stools/day for >30 days), or chronic weakness and documented enigmatic fever for >30 days
- Isoporosis with diarrhea for more than a month
- Kaposi's sarcoma
- Lymphoma of brain
- Lymphoma, non-Hodgkin's of B-cell, or unknown immunological phenotype and histology showing small, noncleaved lymphoma or immunoblastic sarcoma
- *Mycobacterium avium* or *M. kansasii*, disseminated
- *Mycobacterium tuberculosis*, pulmonary or disseminated
- Nocardiosis
- *Pneumocystis carinii* pneumonia
- Pneumonia, recurrent-bacterial
- Progressive multifocal leukoencephalopathy
- Salmonella septicemia (nontyphoid), recurrent
- Strongylosis, extraintestinal
- Toxoplasmosis of internal organ

HIV viral load measurements. A CD4 T-cell count of less than 200×10^6/L is associated with the appearance of opportunistic infections, diseases of the central nervous system and malignancies.

Although there is no cure for HIV, effective suppressive antiretroviral treatment has been available since the mid-1990s. Antiretroviral treatment is associated with considerable adverse effects and a propensity for drug interactions. HIV is a rapidly evolving virus with a tendency to mutate; hence combinations of at least three drugs are required.[3] Adherence to suppressive treatment has to be unusually good to reduce the risk of treatment failure. There are currently five classes of drugs available (**Table 26.1**, and see www.tthhivclinic.com), but options can still be limited for switching between various antiretroviral drugs since choices are dictated by prior exposure and resistance. Worldwide, only 20 percent of infected individuals who need antiretroviral treatment are receiving it. Funding is improving as is the coordination of approaches to prevention and treatment. HIV remains a stigmatizing illness because of associations with sexual activity and intravenous drug use. This affects the ability to access and comply with effective antiretroviral treatment and also symptom control.

Despite the availability of antiretroviral therapy, illness and pain occur as a direct consequence of the viral toxicity, concurrent illness, drug adverse effects, and immune recovery. Pain is frequently reported in HIV disease and the experience of pain increases with advancing disease.[4] Principles of pain management in the context of HIV are similar in many ways to those of pain management in other scenarios. However, painful peripheral neuropathy is common in HIV and requires particular attention, as does the potential for serious drug interactions with HIV therapy.

PAIN PREVALENCE, LOCALITY, AND TREATMENT IN HIV/AIDS

Published pain surveys in HIV disease mostly date from before the availability of effective antiretroviral therapy and there is some evidence of worsening pain with advancing disease. A report in 1993 compared the pain reports of patients with different stages of HIV disease. Pain was reported in 28 percent of asymptomatic patients, 56 percent of intermediate stage patients, and 80 percent of those with an AIDS diagnosis.[4]

In a survey of 438 ambulatory patients with AIDS diagnoses, 62 percent reported pain in the previous two weeks that was persistent and/or severe. Significant associations were found between presence of pain and psychological distress and depression.[5]

Table 26.1 Current classes of antiretroviral drugs.

Class	Example
Nucleoside reverse transcriptase inhibitors	Didanosine, zidovudine
Nucleotide reverse transcriptase inhibitors	Tenofovir
Non-nucleoside reverse transcriptase inhibitors	Efavirenz, nevirapine
Protease inhibitors	Ritonavir, lopinavir,
Fusion inhibitors	Enfuvirtide

See www.tthhivclinic.com.

Another prospective survey followed 95 patients with AIDS diagnoses for two years. The initial prevalence of pain was 74 percent and incidence of pain over the two years was 88 percent. Within this group 69 percent suffered constant pain interfering with daily living to a degree described as moderate or severe.[6]

Pain was categorized in terms of locality and occurred in the extremities in 41 percent of cases (with over half being described as "neuropathic"). Pain occurred in the head in 32 percent, upper gastrointestinal tract in 27 percent, and lower gastrointestinal tract in 34 percent. Muscular or joint pain was experienced by 31 percent of patients. Pain at entry to the study was associated with a shorter prognosis and the number of pains increased as death approached.

The impact of antiretroviral therapy on pain is complicated. Starting effective antiviral therapy helps to restore immune function and suppresses HIV viral load, but does not seem to be associated with pain relief or an improvement in overall quality of life.[7]

An online survey recruited homosexual men with HIV and compared symptom experience between those taking effective antiretroviral therapy and those currently off treatment. Of those on treatment 51 percent reported pain compared to 32 percent of those not currently taking therapy. The on-treatment group experienced higher symptom prevalence generally, even when degree of immunosuppression and year of diagnosis were taken into account.[8]

There is evidence that pain in the clinical context of HIV disease is poorly recognized by clinicians. In one multicenter study, out of 135 patients reporting pain, 52 percent had more severe pain than their doctors estimated.[9] Doctors were more likely to underestimate pain intensity when it was moderate or severe or when the source of the pain could not be identified. Most patients in pain received no analgesia and, using the pain management index, 85 percent were undermedicated according to the World Health Organization (WHO) guidelines. This undertreatment of pain in HIV is also well documented in other studies.[10, 11]

Barriers to adequate pain management may arise from cultural, political, patient, and/or clinician factors, which bear some similarities to those seen in the cancer population. For example, in terms of opioid therapy, both patients and healthcare professionals have been shown to have concerns regarding the psychological dependence potential of opioid analgesia and fear of unpleasant side effects.[12, 13] However, compared to the cancer pain population, the population of those infected with HIV are younger, have a higher incidence of past or present substance use, and also a higher incidence of social deprivation, which may influence attitudes to pain management.[5] Patients who reported a history of injecting drug use as their risk factor for transmission of HIV were compared with patients with other risk factors. Those with a history of injected drug use were more likely to receive inadequate analgesia and had lower levels of pain relief.[11] HIV physicians are more reluctant to prescribe opioids than oncologists.[14] A survey of 492 AIDS care providers identified lack of knowledge about pain management, lack of access to pain management experts, reluctance to prescribe opioids, and concerns regarding drug addiction or abuse as the most frequent barriers to adequate pain treatment.

CAUSES OF PAIN IN HIV

Pain may be caused by:[1]

- damage by HIV itself, for example HIV enteritis, HIV distal sensory polyneuropathy;
- disease arising because of immunosuppression, for example cerebral lymphoma causing headache, acute zoster pain;
- consequent on HIV treatment or drugs used for concomitant illness, for example antiretroviral toxic neuropathy;
- immune reconstitution inflammatory syndrome (IRIS). A result of restoration of immune function and unmasking of the symptoms from previous illness, for example herpes simplex and zoster infections;
- causes unrelated to HIV.

Knowledge of the degree of immunosuppression is vital when diagnosing pain in an HIV-infected individual. Monitoring CD4 count and viral load, the "surrogate markers" of progression of HIV, can help predict whether infective or neoplastic complications are likely. The antiretroviral drug history is also essential to suggest causes of pain and predict potential drug interactions. HIV therapy should only be changed or interrupted by HIV specialist clinicians because of the limited options for treatment and the propensity for the virus to mutate, resulting in resistance. Drug interactions can be serious as they can result in reduced efficacy of one of the antiretroviral drugs and subsequent development of resistant virus (see www.tthhivclinic.com).

NEUROPATHIC PAIN IN HIV INFECTION

HIV disease is associated with a number of painful neuropathies (**Box 26.2**), some of which have overlapping clinical features. Electrophysiological studies can reveal changes in the peripheral nervous system even in asymptomatic individuals with HIV.[18] Of the painful neuropathies, the most common are distal symmetrical polyneuropathy (DSP) and antiretroviral toxic neuropathy (ATN).[15, 16, 17] These two sensory neuropathies are found in over 40 percent of HIV-positive individuals. This figure has not changed in the era of HAART.[19]

Box 26.2 Painful neuropathies associated with HIV[15, 16, 17]

- Distal sensory polyneuropathy
- Antiretroviral toxic neuropathy
- Acute zoster pain
- Postherpetic neuropathy
- Mononeuritis multiplex
- Diffuse inflammatory lymphocytosis syndrome (DILS)
- Radiculopathy

HIV DSP

HIV causes a distal sensory neuropathy in about one-third of those with AIDS.[19] The pathogenesis is unclear. There is some evidence for an interaction between an HIV coat glycoprotein (gp120) and sensory neurons.[20] Neurotoxic cytokines released by activated macrophages have also been implicated[21] (see also Chapter 1, Applied physiology: neuropathic pain). The incidence of DSP is related to the degree of immunosuppression.[22, 23] DSP is a distal symmetrical axonal sensorimotor polyneuropathy, predominantly effecting small fibers. Sensory loss, paresthesiae, dysesthesiae, and pain are frequent features. Large fiber symptoms such as motor weakness of the intrinsic muscles of the feet are minimal but can complicate advanced DSP. Quantitative sensory testing, the preferred investigation for assessment of small fiber function, reveals sensory loss usually without evidence of hypersensory phenomena such as allodynia or hyperalgesia.[24] As with other predominantly small fiber neuropathies, the absence of abnormal findings in nerve conduction studies is frequent and does not necessarily exclude a peripheral neuropathy (see Chapter 4, Sensory testing and clinical neurophysiology in the *Practice and Procedures* volume of this series).

Assessment of epidermal innervation in 3 mm skin biopsies is also useful in the assessment of small fiber neuropathies[25, 26] (see Chapter 7, Diagnostic algorithms for painful peripheral neuropathy in the *Practice and Procedures* volume of this series). In a prospective study, epidermal nerve fiber density was significantly associated with the subsequent development of DSP.[27]

ATN

ATN is a distal sensory neuropathy, difficult to distinguish from DSP on clinical examination or investigation, which is associated with the use of antiretroviral medication, particularly some of the nucleoside reverse transcriptase inhibitors (NRTIs). ATN is thought to result from NRTI-induced mitochondrial toxicity in sensory neurones.[17] Although it is difficult to distinguish between DSP and ATN on the basis of clinical examination or the above investigations, it may be clear from the drug history and timing of onset of neuropathic symptoms that drug toxicity is the likely cause. Stavudine (d4T), didanosine (ddI), and zalcitabine (ddC) have all been implicated and typically result in neuropathic symptoms after one week to six months in 10–20 percent of patients treated with them.[17, 21] Combinations of ddI and d4T appear to be synergistic in their risk of ATN. Other risk factors include low CD4 count, previous AIDS-defining illness, and preexisting neuropathy from any other cause.[16] Indeed, it has been suggested that antiretroviral drugs may unmask subclinical neuropathies including DSP.[17]

Discontinuing or reducing implicated NRTIs may lead to improvement in some of those affected, but will reduce therapeutic options for virological control. Some patients experience a worsening of symptoms for four to eight weeks after stopping relevant NRTIs and others report that their painful symptoms persist in the long term despite changing therapy.[17]

Treatment of pain in DSP and ATN

There are still only a small number of robust randomized controlled trials which specifically assessed peripheral neuropathic pain therapies in the context of HIV. Most include patients with both DSP and ATN as they are clinically indistinguishable. In the absence of trials specific to HIV, the practice has been to extrapolate from the wider body of evidence in the treatment of non-HIV peripheral neuropathic pain.[28, 29, 30] Care must be taken to avoid drugs which exhibit significant known interactions with antiretroviral drugs. The most obvious example is carbamazepine which should be avoided in all patients on treatment as it interacts with protease inhibitors and some NNRTIs (see www.tthhivclinic.com).

Two randomized, double-blind studies found no significant difference in efficacy between amitriptyline and placebo in HIV-related peripheral neuropathy.[31, 32][I] Both studies were of sufficient quality to be included in a systematic review.[28] Both studies involved comparisons between several different treatments. Kieburtz *et al.*[31] compared amitriptyline, mexiletine, and placebo in 145 patients. Neither active treatment was superior to placebo in terms of efficacy. The authors comment that the study sample size was smaller than originally planned. Study enrolment was discontinued on the recommendation of the safety committee that suggested that even with full enrolment the trial would not be able to demonstrate a statistically significant benefit of either intervention. The study by Shlay *et al.*[32] was an unusual design in that it compared acupuncture to amitriptyline or placebo, acupuncture versus sham acupuncture, or amitriptyline versus placebo. The study design was modified during recruitment to improve accrual. A total of 250 patients was recruited of whom 71 received amitriptyline. Power calculations suggested 260 patients needed to be randomized to each group to detect a significant difference. We were unable to locate any published trials which indicate efficacy of amitriptyline or other tricyclic antidepressants in HIV neuropathy, a feature which stands in marked contrast to the broad efficacy of tricyclic antidepressants in other neuropathic pain scenarios.[28, 29, 30][I] We could locate no reports evaluating the use of other antidepressants including duloxetine or opioids in DSP or ATN.

Gabapentin and pregabalin are yet to be adequately tested for effectiveness in the symptomatic treatment of DSP and ATN. One very small placebo-controlled trial showed an initial modest efficacy for gabapentin compared to placebo, but this difference was not significant at the end of the four-week treatment period.[33][III] However, given the grade I evidence for the efficacy of gabapentin and pregabalin in other peripheral neuropathic pain conditions,[28, 29, 30][I] a reasoned argument might be made for their continued use in HIV-related peripheral neuropathic pain, pending the publication of substantive evidence supporting or refuting this practice.

Lamotrigine appeared to show promise in the relief of DSP and ATN in a small randomized trial,[34][II] but superiority over placebo was not demonstrated in a larger trial.[35][II]

Recombinant human growth factor (rhNGF) appeared to be effective at improving symptoms of HIV-related neuropathy in a phase II clinical study,[36][II] and two-year follow up in an open label design showed sustained benefit.[37][IV] However, adverse effects were problematic with rhNGF and it would appear that rhNGF is not being further developed for this indication.

A systematic review revealed that, on the basis of available evidence, mexilitine, capsaicin cream, and lidocaine gel are not efficacious in HIV peripheral neuropathic pain.[28][I] There is also no efficacy for intranasal peptide T[38][II] or memantidine.[39][II]

GUIDELINES FOR THE MANAGEMENT OF DSP AND ATN

New patient assessment

New patient assessment begins with a full history to include analgesic, antiretroviral, alcohol, and recreational drug use. Physical assessment includes neurological examination, including measurement of pinprick hyperalgesia, brush-evoked dynamic allodynia, and also vibration sense. A record should be made of pain sites on a body chart, with pain intensity recorded on a visual analog intensity scale. Sleep interference and other pain comorbidities should also be assessed (see Chapter 11, Assessment of the patient with neuropathic pain; and Chapter 1, History taking and examination of the patient with chronic pain; Chapter 2, Practical methods for pain intensity measurements and Chapter 3, Selecting and applying pain measures in the *Practice and Procedures* volume of this series).

Investigations should be conducted with the aim of excluding other causes for sensory neuropathies including diabetes, deficiencies of B vitamins, syphilis, and thyroid dysfunction. The immunological status of the individual can be estimated using recent HIV viral load and CD4 counts. Nerve conduction studies may be performed as baseline evaluations, but do not necessarily exclude DSP or ATN if normal, because of their lack of sensitivity in assessing small fiber function. If available, quantitative sensory testing (QST) and epidermal innervation assessment provide useful diagnostic information in the assessment of HIV and other small fiber neuropathies (see Chapter 4, Sensory testing and clinical neurophysiology and Chapter 7, Diagnostic algorithms for painful and nonpainful peripheral neuropathy in the *Practice and Procedures* volume of this series).

If the picture is not one of classical symmetrical distal sensory neuropathy, further investigations may be required and the opinion of a peripheral nerve neurologist should be sought. Alteration of antiretroviral therapy should only be executed by HIV specialists.

As will be seen from the above discussion, there is a paucity of direct positive evidence supporting the use of any analgesic therapy in the context of DSP and ATN. However, the current evidence base does make it reasonable to exclude treatment with amitriptyline, mexilitene, lamotrigine, peptide T, topical capsaicin cream, and topical lidocaine gel on the basis of lack of efficacy. Similarly, because of interactions with antiretroviral drugs, carbamazepine and related drugs should not be used (see www.tthhivclinic.com).

Until more direct evidence for analgesic therapies in DSP and ATN exist, then it is reasonable to extrapolate from the algorithm proposed by Finnerup *et al.*[28][I] for peripheral nonfocal neuropathies, providing there are no interactions with antiretroviral drugs. Thus, gabapentin/pregabalin might be used as first line (although the limited available evidence argues against a sustained analgesic efficacy in the case of gabapentin[33][III]), with opioids being reserved for second-line therapy. A caveat is that as the evidence base in this area builds, the reader is advised to consult resources such as the Cochrane database of systematic reviews and Bandolier (www.jr2.ox.ac.uk/bandolier) for up to date information. On the basis of the available grade I evidence, amitriptyline does not have efficacy in HIV-associated ATN and DSP[28, 30, 31, 32] and therefore tricyclic antidepressants cannot be recommended as a class for these conditions, at present. However, the efficacy of other tricyclic antidepressants or duloxetine has not yet been tested in ATN and DSP and this recommendation may change as more evidence emerges.

Guidelines for the use of strong opioids in nonmalignant pain should be adhered to[40][V] (see also Chapter 16, Opioids and chronic noncancer pain and Chapter 10, Treatment protocols for opioids in chronic nonmalignant pain in the *Practice and Procedures* volume of this series). Due caution should be exercised in patients with a history of substance use, although the use of opioids in such individuals is only a relative contraindication and should be considered on a case by case basis (see Chapter 46, Pain management and substance misuse for more details).

OTHER PAINFUL NEUROPATHIES IN HIV

Herpes zoster virus and neuropathic pain

Herpes zoster virus (HZV) is up to ten times more common in the HIV-positive population, increasing in frequency as CD4 counts fall.[41] Those with a CD4 count $<200 \times 10^6$/L are most at risk of major ocular or neurological complications. Patients with HIV demonstrate more complicated HZV infections with multidermatomal involvement, recurrent episodes, and systemic disease being more common.[42] Pain from HZV infection is more likely in advanced HIV infection.[4] The development of postherpetic neuralgia (PHN) is proportional to baseline pain severity and duration of zoster lesions[43][III] and occurs in a surprising proportion of young patients. In one retrospective study where all patients were less than 43 years of age, 18 percent of those who experienced HZV went on to develop PHN.[41][IV] Symptoms of herpes simplex and zoster infections also occur as part of the immune reconstitution syndrome. It is estimated to occur in 10–25 percent of patients commencing HAART and represents a recovering immune system responding to prior infections.[44]

Symptomatic treatment of PHN is as for the non-HIV population,[29][I] with evidence (number needed to treat (NNT) for 50 percent pain reduction <5.0) to support the use of orally administered tricyclic antidepressants, strong opioids, gabapentin, tramadol, and pregabalin. Topical therapies associated with efficacy were lidocaine 5 percent patch and capsaicin (see also Chapter 32, Herpes zoster pain including shingles and postherpetic neuralgia).

Mononeuritis multiplex

Mononeuritis mulitplex can present with sensory or motor deficits in the distribution of a single or multiple cranial, spinal, or peripheral nerve. Mononeuritis multiplex may occur early in HIV infection as a result of immune mechanisms or vasculitis. In advanced HIV infection, coinfection with cytomegalovirus (CMV) or HZV can produce a similar picture. Lymphomatous infiltration of cerebrospinal fluid or meninges can also present in this way. Establishing the diagnosis may be complicated by an overlapping clinical picture with other neuropathies.

Diffuse infiltrative lymphocytosis

Diffuse infiltrative lymphocytosis (DILS) is a disorder resembling Sjögren's syndrome and is associated with CD8 T-cell infiltration into glands, organs, and peripheral nerves. The neuropathy associated with DILS may be sensory or sensorimotor and symmetrical or asymmetric. In addition, it can mimic mononeuritis multiplex and demyelinating polyneuropathy.

Radiculopathy

Painful radiculopathy can occur secondary to nerve damage from HIV itself or coinfection with CMV or, less commonly, HZV, tuberculosis, or syphilis. Coinfection with CMV will usually require profound immunosuppression with a CD4 count of 50×10^6/L or less. This typically presents with cauda equina radicular pain, numbness, rapidly progressive flaccid paraparesis, and sphincter disturbance. If the adjacent spinal cord is involved, there can be a concurrent myelopathy and evidence of a "sensory level" on examination.

MUSCULOSKELETAL PAIN

Musculoskeletal symptoms are common in HIV-infected individuals, especially considering the younger age of his group. Joints are affected in various forms of oligo or polyarticular arthritides and arthralgias. In individuals coinfected with hepatitis C, approximately one-third experience arthritis or arthralgia,[45] psoriatic arthritis is seen more commonly in the context of HIV infection as is Reiter's syndrome. Avascular necrosis of the hip is an unusual but disabling complication of HIV disease.[46][V] Septic complications was the most frequent reason for referral of HIV patients to a rheumatology clinic. These included septic arthritis, cellulites, osteomyelitis, vertebral discitis, and pyomyositis. Fibromyalgia is seen frequently in HIV, with incidence up to 10 percent in certain series.[47][V] HIV infection may be associated with myopathies as a result of HIV itself, drugs such as zidovudine, HIV wasting syndrome, and opportunistic infections or malignant infiltrations.[48]

HEADACHE

Headache occurs in up to 50 percent of HIV-positive individuals during the course of their disease.[49] Patients with uncomplicated headaches and CD4 counts above

200×10^6/L have a low likelihood of having an abnormality discovered on computed tomography (CT) scanning.[50] Patients with a significant degree of immunosuppression should have brain imaging and lumbar puncture performed (**Table 26.2**).

In general, headaches are less common with diffuse brain lesions where changes in mental state predominate. Patients with focal brain lesions often complain of headache, but focal neurology is more common. Symptoms, including headache, can be mild or absent with opportunistic infections.[51]

GASTROENTEROLOGICAL PAIN

Oral and esophageal pain

Several studies have shown the prevalence of oral lesions to be decreased in the era of HAART. The prevalence remains high, however, with over 50 percent of patients experiencing oral pain.[52, 53] These studies also report an increase in oral lesions with more advanced HIV disease. Pain due to oral lesions can interfere with nutritional intake and hence contribute to the HIV wasting syndrome. Xerostomia occurs commonly in HIV-infected individuals and there is evidence for an increase in HIV salivary gland disease (**Table 26.3**).

Treatment is of the underlying cause together with appropriate symptomatic therapy. A double-blind, randomized controlled study compared the use of thalidomide 200 mg once daily with placebo for oral aphthous ulcers in HIV.[54][II] This found a significant improvement in both ulcer healing and discomfort whilst eating in the thalidomide group. Symptomatic treatment for oral and esophageal pain may follow the WHO analgesic ladder, but may also involve local measures. Coating agents such as sucralfate have been shown to be useful in oral ulceration from other causes.[55][II] Topical analgesia such as cocaine 2 percent mouthwash and topical anesthetic gels are commonly used, although there is no direct evidence to support this practice in HIV disease.

Abdominal pain

Pancreatitis is an adverse effect of antiretroviral therapy (ddI) and therapy for hepatitis C (ribovirin), so is seen more frequently in HIV-infected individuals than in the general population.

The biliary tree is also a source of abdominal pain in HIV with acalculous cholecystitis and AIDS-related sclerosing cholangitis. There may be associated secondary infections with CMV or cryptosporidium.[56]

Renal colic is also seen more commonly in patients taking the protease inhibitor indinavir as drug crystals can obstruct the renal tract if insufficient fluids are taken.

Lactic acidosis is a potentially serious metabolic complication of some antiretroviral therapies presenting with abdominal pain, nausea, vomiting, and diarrhea.

Tumors of the small and large bowel causing abdominal pain include Kaposi's sarcoma and non-Hodgkin's lymphoma (NHL). NHL can occur even when patients have relatively well-preserved immunity and in HIV can present in unusual sites such as the mouth or anus.[57] Abdominal colic can accompany infections such as HIV or CMV colitis, cryptosporidium, or *Mycobacterium avium* complex. Patients are likely to be relatively immunocompromised, experiencing severe diarrhea and anorexia. An acute presentation of colic may be caused by intussusception as a result of enlarged mesenteric lymph nodes.

Table 26.2 Causes of headache in HIV disease.[1]

Causes of headache in HIV disease		
1	Effects of HIV	HIV encephalopathy or AIDS dementia complex
		HIV meningitis
2	Opportunistic infections	CMV encephalitis
		Cryptococcal meningitis
		Cerebral toxoplasmosis
		Herpes encephalitis
		TB meningitis
		Progressive multifocal leukoencephalopathy (JC virus)
		Neurosyphillis
		Bacterial sinusitis
3	Malignancies	Cerebral lymphoma
		Cerebral metastases from systemic lymphoma
4	Drug induced, for example AZT induced	
5	Other	Tension headache
		Migraine

Table 26.3 Causes of oral and esophageal pain in HIV disease.[1]

Causes of oral and esophageal pain in HIV disease		
1	Opportunistic infections	Oral or esophageal candida
		Herpes infections
		CMV ulceration
		Oral hairy leukoplakia
		Histoplasmosis
		Cryptococcus neoformans
		Necrotizing ulcerative gingivitis
		Tuberculosis
		Primary chancre of syphilis
2	Malignancy	Lymphoma
		Kaposi's sarcoma
3	Aphthous ulceration	
4	Drug-induced ulceration	Mucositis post chemotherapy or radiotherapy
		ddC or Foscarnet

Anorectal pain

One study of 180 HIV-positive patients with anorectal symptoms showed that 57 percent complained of pain, mainly due to anal ulceration.[58] One-third had anal ulcers, mostly idiopathic but some secondary to HSV or CMV infection. Other causes of pain included fistulae, abscesses, hemorrhoids, and malignancy (Kaposi's sarcoma, NHL, and squamous cell carcinoma). In addition, 43 percent had anal warts.

Squamous cell carcinoma of the anus occurs with increased frequency in the HIV population due to coinfection with the oncogenic virus, human papilloma virus 8 (HPV8) and there is no evidence that its incidence has reduced since the introduction of HAART.[59] As well as the pain that can be caused by the primary lesion, the standard treatment of chemoradiation is often associated with very significant local reaction and pain.

GYNECOLOGICAL PAIN

Gynecological disease is prevalent among hospitalized women with HIV. A study of 67 HIV-positive women inpatients revealed lower pelvic pain in 19 percent, and dyspareunia in 16 percent.[60] Genital ulceration was found in 25 percent of these women. HSV genital ulceration is a frequent finding in HIV-seropositive women and, if present for more than four weeks, is AIDS defining. Other causes of genital ulceration include other sexually transmitted infections including syphilis and CMV. HIV-infected women have a higher incidence of cervical intraepithelial neoplasia (CIN) and invasive cervical cancer, an AIDS-defining disorder. HIV-positive women are also at an increased risk of developing other HPV-associated lesions including vulval intraepithelial neoplasia and possibly invasive vulval cancer.

There are high rates of pelvic inflammatory disease (PID) in HIV-positive women. In the USA, HIV seroprevalence among women with PID is reported to range from 6.7 to 27 percent.[61] Regular gynecological screening and surveillance is of prime importance in HIV-seropositive women.

REFERENCES

* 1. Marshall SJ, Cox S, Rice ASC. Pain in human immunodeficiency virus and acquired immunodeficiency syndrome. In: Ballentyne JC (ed.). *Massachusetts general hospital handbook of pain management*, 3rd edn. Philadelphia: Lippincott Williams & Wilkins, 2005: 446–60.

* 2. Centers for Disease Control. 1993 revised classification system for HIV infection and expanded case definition for AIDS among adolescents and adults. *MMWR*. 1992; **41**: 1–19.

* 3. Deeks SG. Antiretroviral treatment of HIV infected adults. *British Medical Journal*. 2006; **332**: 1489–93.

4. Singer EJ, Zorilla C, Fahy-Chandon B *et al*. Painful symptoms reported by ambulatory HIV-infected men in a longitudinal study. *Pain*. 1993; **54**: 15–19.

5. Breitbart W, McDonald MV, Rosenfeld B *et al*. Pain in ambulatory AIDS patients. 1: Pain characteristics and medical correlates. *Pain*. 1996; **68**: 315–21.

* 6. Frich LM, Borgbjerg FM. Pain and pain treatment in AIDS patients: a longitudinal study. *Journal of Pain and Symptom Management*. 2000; **19**: 339–47.

7. Brechtl JR, Breitbart W, Galietta M *et al*. The use of highly active antiretroviral therapy (HAART) in patients with advanced HIV infection: impact on medical, palliative care and quality of life outcomes. *Journal of Pain and Symptom Management*. 2001; **21**: 41–51.

8. Harding R, Molloy T, Easterbrook P *et al*. Is antiretroviral therapy associated with symptom prevalence and

burden? *International Journal of STD and AIDS*. 2006; **17**: 400–05.
9. Larue F, Fontaine A, Colleau S. Underestimation and undertreatment of pain in HIV disease: multicentre study. *British Medical Journal*. 1997; **314**: 23–28.
10. Fantoni M, Ricci F, Del Borgo C *et al*. Multicentre study on the prevalence of symptoms and symptomatic treatment in HIV infection. *Journal of Palliative Care*. 1997; **13**: 9–13.
11. Breitbart W, Rosenfeld B, Passik S *et al*. A comparison of pain report and adequacy of analgesic therapy in ambulatory AIDS patients with and without a history of substance abuse. *Pain*. 1997; **72**: 235–43.
12. Breitbart W, Passik S, McDonald MV *et al*. Patient-related barriers to pain management in ambulatory AIDS patients. *Pain*. 1998; **76**: 9–16.
13. Cleeland CS. Documenting barriers to cancer pain management. In: Chapman CR, Foley KM (eds). *Current and emerging isuues in cancer pain: research and practice*. New York: Raven Press, 1993: 321–30.
14. Peretti-Watel P, Bendiane MK, Galinier A *et al*. Opinions toward pain management and palliative care: comparison between HIV specialists and oncologists. *AIDS Care*. 2004; **16**: 619–27.
* 15. Verma A. Epidemiology and clinical features of HIV-1 associated neuropathies. *Journal of the Peripheral Nervous System*. 2001; **6**: 8–13.
* 16. Wulff EA, Wang AK, Simpson DM. HIV-associated peripheral neuropathy; epidemiology, pathophysiology and treatment. *Drugs*. 2000; **59**: 1251–60.
* 17. Keswani SC, Pardo CA, Cherry CL *et al*. HIV-associated sensory neuropathies. *AIDS*. 2002; **16**: 2105–17.
18. Farizo KM, Buehler JW, Chamberland ME *et al*. Spectrum of disease in persons with human immunodeficiency virus infection in the United States. *Journal of the American Medical Association*. 1992; **267**: 1798–805.
19. Smyth K, Affandi JS, McArthur JC *et al*. Prevalence of and risk factors for HIV-associated neuropathy in Melbourne, Australia 1993–2006. *HIV Medicine*. 2007; **8**: 367–73.
20. Wallace VCJ, Blackbeard J, Pheby T *et al*. Pharmacological, behavioural and mechanistic analysis of HIV-I gp120 induced painful neuropathy. *Pain*. 2007; **133**: 47–63.
21. Cherry CL, McArthur JC, Hoy JF, Wesslingh SL. Nucleoside analogues and neuropathy in the era of HAART. *Journal of Clinical Neurology*. 2003; **26**: 195–207.
22. Schifitto G, McDermott MP, McArthur JC *et al*. Incidence of and risk factors for HIV-associated distal sensory polyneuropathy. *Neurology*. 2002; **58**: 1764–8.
* 23. Tagliati M, Grinnell J, Godbold J, Simpson DM. Peripheral nerve function in HIV infection: clinical, electrophysiologic, and laboratory findings. *Archives of Neurology*. 1999; **56**: 84–9.
* 24. Martin C, Solders G, Sonnerborg A, Hansson P. Painful and non-painful neuropathy in HIV-infected patients: an analysis of somatosensory nerve function. *European Journal of Pain*. 2003; **7**: 23–31.
* 25. Lauria G, Cornblath DR, Johansson O *et al*. EFNS guidelines on the use of skin biopsy in the diagnosis of peripheral neuropathy. *European Journal of Neurology*. 2005; **12**: 747–58.
* 26. Griffin JW, McArthur JC, Polydefkis M. Assessment of cutaneous innervation by skin biopsies. *Current Opinion in Neurology*. 2001; **14**: 655–9.
27. Herrman DN, McDermott MP, Sowden JE *et al*. Is skin biopsy a predictor of transition to symptomatic HIV neuropathy? A longitudinal study. *Neurology*. 2006; **66**: 857–61.
* 28. Finnerup NB, Otto M, McQuay HJ *et al*. Algorithm for neuropathic pain treatment: An evidence based proposal. *Pain*. 2005; **118**: 289–305.
* 29. Hempenstall K, Nurmikko TJ, Johnson RW *et al*. Analgesic therapy in postherpetic neuralgia: a quantitative systematic review. *PLoS Medicine*. 2005; **2**: e164.
* 30. Dworkin RH, O'Connor AB, Backonja M *et al*. Pharmacologic management of neuropathic pain: evidence-based recommendations. *Pain*. 2007; **132**: 237–51.
31. Kieburtz K, Simpson D, Yiannoutsos C *et al*. A randomized trial of amitriptyline and mexiletine for painful neuropathy in HIV infection. *Neurology*. 1998; **51**: 1682–8.
32. Shlay JC, Chaloner K, Max M *et al*. Acupuncture and amitriptyline for pain due to HIV-related peripheral neuropathy. *Journal of the American Medical Association*. 1998; **280**: 1590–5.
33. Hahn K, Arendt G, Braun JS *et al*. A placebo-controlled trial of gabapentin for painful HIV-associated sensory neuropathies. *Journal of Neurology*. 2004; **251**: 1260–6.
34. Simpson DM, Olney R, McArthur JC *et al*. A placebo-controlled trial of lamotrigine for painful HIV-associated neuropathy. *Neurology*. 2000; **54**: 2115–19.
35. Simpson DM, McArthur JC, Olney R *et al*. Lamotrigine for HIV-associated painful sensory neuropathies. *Neurology*. 2003; **60**: 1508–14.
36. McArthur JC, Yiannoutsos C, Simpson DM *et al*. A phase II trial of nerve growth factor for sensory neuropathy associated with HIV infection. *Neurology*. 2000; **54**: 1080–8.
37. Schifitto G, Yiannoutsos C, Simpson DM *et al*. Long-term treatment with recombinant nerve growth factor for HIV-associated sensory neuropathy. *Neurology*. 2001; **57**: 1313–16.
38. Simpson DM, Dorfman D, Olney RK *et al*. Peptide T in the treatment of painful distal neuropathy associated with AIDS. *Neurology*. 1996; **47**: 1254–9.
39. Schifitto G, Yiannoutsos CT, Simpson DM *et al*. A placebo-controlled study of memantidine for the treatment of human immunodeficiency virus-associated sensory neuropathy. *Journal of Neurovirology*. 2006; **12**: 328–31.
* 40. The British Pain Society. Recommendations for the appropriate use of opioids for persistent non-cancer pain. A consensus statement prepared on behalf of the Pain Society, the Royal College of Anaesthetists, the Royal College of General Practitioners and the Royal College of

Psychiatrists. Last updated 2004; cited December 2007. Available from: www.britishpainsociety.org.
41. Gebo KA, Kalyani R, Moore R, Polydefkis MJ. The incidence of, risk factors for, and sequelae of herpes zoster among HIV patients in the highly active antiretroviral therapy era. *Journal of Acquired Immune Deficiency Syndromes*. 2005; **40**: 169–74.
* 42. Cohen PR, Grossman ME. Clinical features of human immunodeficiency virus-associated disseminated herpes zoster virus infection – a review of the literature. *Clinical and Experimental Dermatology*. 1989; **14**: 273–6.
43. Harrison RA, Soong S-J, Weiss H *et al.* A mixed model for factors predictive of pain in AIDS patients with herpes zoster. *Journal of Pain and Symptom Management*. 1999; **17**: 410–17.
44. Ratnam I, Chiu C, Kandal NB, Easterbrook PJ. Incidence and risk factors for immune reconstitution inflammatory syndrome in an ethnically diverse HIV type 1-infected cohort. *Clinical Infectious Diseases*. 2006; **42**: 418–27.
45. Lee YH, Ji JD, Yeon JE *et al.* Cryoglobulinaemia and rheumatic manifestations in patients with hepatitis C virus infection. *Annals of the Rheumatic Diseases*. 1998; **57**: 728–31.
46. Marquez J, Restrepo CS, Candia L *et al.* Human immunodeficiency virus-associated rheumatic disorders in the HAART era. *Journal of Rheumatology*. 2004; **31**: 741–6.
47. Simms RW, Zerbini CA, Ferrante N *et al.* Fibromyalgia syndrome in patients infected with human immunodeficiency virus. The Boston Hospital Clinical AIDS Team. *American Journal of Medicine*. 1992; **92**: 368–74.
* 48. Chariot P, Gheradi R. Myopathy and HIV infection. *Current Opinion in Rheumatology*. 1995; **7**: 497–502.
* 49. Hewitt DJ, McDonald M, Portenoy RK *et al.* Pain syndromes and aetiologies in ambulatory AIDS patients. *Pain*. 1997; **70**: 117–23.
50. Singer EJ, Kim J, Fahy-Chandon B *et al.* Headache in ambulatory HIV-1 infected men enrolled in a longitudinal study. *Neurology*. 1996; **47**: 487–94.
* 51. Holloway RG, Kieburtz KD. Headache and the human immunodeficiency virus type 1 infection. *Headache*. 1995; **35**: 245–55.
52. Eyeson JD, Tenant-Flowers M, Cooper DJ *et al.* Oral manifestations of an HIV positive cohort in the era of highly active anti-retroviral therapy (HAART) in South London. *Journal of Oral Pathology and Medicine*. 2002; **31**: 169–74.
53. Ceballos-Salobrena A, Gaitan-Cepeda LA, Ceballos-Garcia L, Lezama-Del Valle D. Oral lesions in HIV/AIDS patients undergoing highly active antiretroviral treatment including protease inhibitors: a new face of oral AIDS? *AIDS Patient Care and STDS*. 2000; **14**: 627–35.
54. Jacobson JM, Greenspan JS, Spritzler J *et al.* Thalidomide for the treatment of oral aphthous ulcers in patients with human immunodeficiency virus infection. National Institute of Allergy and Infectious Diseases AIDS Clinical Trials Group. *New England Journal of Medicine*. 1997; **336**: 1487–93.
55. Alpsoy E, Er H, Durusoy C, Yilmaz E. The use of sulcrafate suspension in the treatment of oral and genital ulceration of Behcet disease: a randomised, placebo-controlled, double-blind study. *Archives of Dermatology*. 1999; **135**: 529–32.
* 56. Keaveny AP, Karasik MS. Hepatobiliary and pancreatic infections in AIDS: Part II. *AIDS Patient Care and STDs*. 1998; **12**: 451–6.
57. Palmieri C, Treibel T, Large O, Bower M. AIDS-related non-Hodgkin's lymphoma in the first decade of highly active antiretroviral therapy. *QJM*. 2006; **99**: 811–26.
58. Yuhan R, Orsay C, Delpino A *et al.* Anorectal disease in HIV-infected patients. *Diseases of the Colon and Rectum*. 1998; **41**: 1367–70.
* 59. Bower M, Palmieri C, Dhillon T. AIDS-related malignancies: changing epidemiology and the impact of highly active antiretroviral therapy. *Current Opinion in Infectious Diseases*. 2006; **19**: 14–19.
60. Frankel RE, Selwyn PA, Mezger J, Andrews S. High prevalence of gynaecological disease among hospitalized women with human immunodeficiency virus infection. *Clinical Infectious Diseases*. 1997; **25**: 706–12.
61. Hankins CA, Handley MA. HIV disease and AIDS in women. Current knowledge and research agenda. *Journal of Acquired Immune Deficiency Syndromes*. 1992; **5**: 957–68.

27

Complex regional pain syndromes

PETER R WILSON

KEY LEARNING POINTS

- Complex regional pain syndrome (CRPS) is a pain syndrome diagnosed clinically, not in the laboratory.
- CRPS occurs in the extremities and limbs.
- The prevalence and incidence of CRPS in communities is not known.
- Clinical diagnosis is made with four factors.
- Sensory changes include hyperalgesia and allodynia.
- Vasomotor changes include asymmetrical vasodilatation and vasoconstriction.
- Sudomotor changes include asymmetrical sweating.
- Edema is variably present.
- Movement disorders include tremor, weakness, and dystonia.
- Treatment is by multidisciplinary functional restoration.
- Pain relief by any modality may be required to facilitate functional restoration.

INTRODUCTION

This chapter is organized in the same way as a recent publication on CRPS,[1] but updated as appropriate with relevant references. The subject is controversial in all aspects.[2] There has been no formal acceptance by the International Association for the Study of Pain (IASP) Taxonomy Committee for the diagnostic criteria proposed by Harden *et al.*[3] No mention will be made in this chapter of animal models of neuropathic pain.

History

"Complex regional pain syndrome" is the term recommended to the IASP to replace the term "reflex sympathetic dystrophy" (RSD) on the grounds that it does not represent a reflex, it does not need a sympathetic component, and there is not necessarily dystrophy. However, RSD is still the search term used by the National Library for Medicine/Medline and a patient support group (www.rsds.org). One of the best historical perspectives of pain related to nerve damage was provided by Sunderland.[4] This consisted of clinical observations from a senior and experienced neurologist rather than scientific data. They included observations relevant to CRPS, as well as causalgia. He noted:

- greatest incidence after lesions of the medial cord of the brachial plexus, median, sciatic, and intercostal nerves;
- immediate onset of pain;
- hyperesthesia and allodynia;
- spread to neighboring uninjured areas;
- gradual resolution;
- failure to relieve pain by neural blockade.

Sympathetic blockade sometimes provided temporary relief. It is implied that CRPS is a disorder of a single extremity, although there are case reports of migratory CRPS[5, 6] and whole-body CRPS.[7]

Taxonomy

The absence of generally agreed upon taxonomy makes all studies difficult or impossible to evaluate and compare. Many previous papers have used circular reasoning: for example, a case of RSD responded to sympathetic block, so response to sympathetic block became a diagnostic criterion.[8]

Diagnostic criteria were addressed in a very thoughtful paper by Veldman *et al.*[9] Their suggestions were based on more than 800 consecutive cases of RSD. They suggested that the general categories of criteria should include:

- inflammatory;
- neurologic;
- atrophy; and
- sympathetic.

They divided RSD into primarily warm and cold varieties, but could not define stages. This paper also points out that the absence of validated diagnostic criteria is the fundamental problem of all retrospective or meta-analyses to date.

Epidemiology

Two recent papers have addressed the epidemiology of CRPS in different populations. Sandroni *et al.*[10] reviewed the Mayo Clinic/Olmsted County, Minnesota, USA records to estimate the prevalence of RSD/CRPS, causalgia, sympathetically maintained pain, and chronic regional pain between 1989 and 1999. They found an incidence rate of 5.46 per 100,000 person years at risk (74 cases) and a period prevalence of 20.57 per 100,000. Female:male ratio was 4:1 and upper:lower limb ratio was 2:1. Bennett and Harden[11] questioned the methodology and findings of the study. Problems may have included the exclusion of patients with sympathetically independent pain, the composition of the Olmsted County population, search strategy, and the question of "spontaneous resolution."

Another retrospective study found a higher incidence in a different population.[12] A retrospective cohort study was conducted during the decade 1996–2005 in the Integrated Primary Care Information project in the Netherlands. This study also examined case records by wide diagnosis, but also by dimethyl sulfoxide (DMSO) prescription (exclusively for CRPS). Case records were subjected to analysis and the diagnostic criteria of the IASP, Bruehl *et al.*,[13] and Veldman *et al.*[9] Although there were significant methodological differences, this study found an incidence rate 4.2 times higher than Sandroni *et al.*[10] for all diagnosed cases. If cases diagnosed by specialists were used, the incidence rate was 2.7 times higher. Both studies rely on the patient attending for medical care, so cannot include minor cases that resolve spontaneously. Bruehl and Chung[14] provided editorial commentary and raised additional questions. It should be noted that DMSO is not approved for external human use in the USA (www.dmso.org), but only for interstitial cystitis and organ preservation.

It must be concluded that the incidence of CRPS is very difficult to estimate and that neither of these papers might be correct.

CLINICAL DIAGNOSIS

Criterion factors

CRPS was meant to be a descriptive term, not implying etiology or pathology. The initial IASP diagnostic criteria were developed as the result of a consensus conference (**Box 27.1**).[15] Empirical validation of these criteria was achieved by Bruehl *et al.*[13] and Harden *et al.*,[16] and explored in greater detail since then (**Table 27.1**).[3] They initially used cluster analysis of patients who satisfied IASP criteria for CRPS. This showed three subgroups of patients:

1. a relatively limited syndrome with vasomotor involvement predominating;
2. a relatively limited syndrome with neuropathic pain and sensory changes predominating; and
3. "florid" CRPS/RSD.

They defined four factors that appeared to be independent: sensory, vasomotor/edema, sudomotor, and motor. Three levels of diagnostic sensitivity and specificity were suggested. The most stringent was for research purposes, somewhat less (one symptom fewer) for clinical use, and a

Box 27.1 IASP diagnostic criteria for CRPS

1. Presence of an initiating noxious event or immobilization.
2. Continuing disproportionate pain, allodynia, or hyperalgesia.
3. Evidence at some time of edema, changes in skin blood flow, or sweating.
4. Diagnosis excluded by any other explanation.

Type I: without evidence of major nerve damage.
Type II: with evidence of major nerve damage.

Table 27.1 Proposed changes to the diagnostic criteria.

Proposed changes		
General definition of the syndrome		
CRPS describes an array of painful conditions characterized by:	Continuing spontaneous or evoked regional pain Disproportionate in duration and degree to the inciting process No specific nerve or dermatomal territory or distribution Distal predominance of abnormal sensory, motor, sudomotor, vasomotor, and/or trophic changes Variable progression over time	
Clinical diagnostic criteria (proposed)		
Sensitivity 0.85, specificity 0.69	1. Continuing pain, disproportionate in duration and degree	
	2. Report of at least one symptom in three of the following four symptom categories:	Sensory: hyperesthesia and/or allodynia Vasomotor: temperature and/or skin color asymmetry Sudomotor/edema: edema and/or sweating asymmetry Motor/trophic: decreased range of motion, motor dysfunction (weakness, tremor, dystonia), and/or trophic changes (skin, nails, hair)
	3. Display evidence of at least one sign at the time of evaluation in two of the following four objective (observable) categories:	Sensory: hyperalgesia (to pinprick) and/or allodynia (light touch, deep pressure, joint movement) Vasomotor: temperature and/or skin color asymmetry Sudomotor/edema: edema and/or sweating asymmetry Motor: decreased range of motion and/or motor dysfunction (weakness, tremor, dystonia) and/or trophic changes (skin, nails, hair)
	4. There is no other diagnosis that better explains the signs and symptoms (e.g. painful diabetic mononeuropathy)	
Research diagnostic criteria (proposed) Sensitivity 0.70, specificity 0.94	Identical to clinical criteria, except that there must be a report of one symptom in each of the four symptom groups (instead of three of the four)	
CRPS-NOS Partially meets CRPS criteria, pain state not better explained by any other condition		

CRPS, complex regional pain syndrome; NOS, not otherwise specified.
Adapted from Harden *et al.*[3, 16]

"not otherwise specified" for cases that did not satisfy the first two, but which behaved like CRPS clinically.

The concepts of sympathetically maintained pain and sympathetically independent pain were not included, as these are concepts that only might have some utility in guiding therapy. Sympathetically maintained pain is no longer (if it ever was) a diagnostic criterion. The terms CRPS I (without major nerve injury) and II ("causalgia") were not included because they generally have not contributed significantly to diagnosis or to guide therapy.

The definition of a major nerve injury is not helpful: what constitutes major? For example, if CRPS follows injury to the dorsal radial nerve (by any definition a minor nerve) from wrist fracture or surgery, is the condition type I or II?

FACTOR I: SENSORY CHANGES

Pain and peripheral somatosensory changes are the *sine qua non* of CRPS.[17] They have been described in detail by a number of authors.[18, 19] The nature of the pain and sensory evaluation are listed in **Table 27.2**.

Quantitative sensory testing

Results of computer-driven quantitative sensory testing (QST) are sparse because there are few clinical laboratories with this capability. However, it is essential to test for the function of large and small peripheral sensory fibers with the usual bedside modalities. Light touch, pinprick/von Frey, cold/heat, vibration, and proprioception should be recorded. In addition, a qualitative estimate should be made of allodynia and hyperesthesia to pinprick, light touch, deep pressure, and temperature, comparing the affected and unaffected limbs. Painful joint movement should also be noted.[17] Unfortunately, changes are not specific for CRPS.

Table 27.2 Incidence of sensory symptoms in CRPS I and II.

Sensory symptoms		Incidence (%)
Spontaneous pain		75–91
Hyperalgesia		93–96
	Cold	32–61[a]
Allodynia	Brush	26
Quality	Tearing	25–30
	Burning	16–26
	Stinging	17–22
	Squeezing	9–12
Location	Deep	63–65
	Superficial	30
Dysesthesia		28–52[a]
Distribution	Stocking/glove	30–37
	Palms/soles	30–52
Pinprick	Hypoalgesia	42–60
	Hyperalgesia	22–39
	No change	13–19
Touch	Hypoesthesia	50–70
	Hyperesthesia	9–18
	No change	22–32

CRPS, complex regional pain syndrome.
[a]Significantly higher in CRPS II.
Adapted from Oaklander AL, Birklein F. Factor I: sensory changes – pathophysiology and measurement. *CRPS: current diagnosis and therapy.* In: Wilson PR, Stanton-Hicks M, Harden RN (eds). *Progress in Pain Research and Management.* Seattle: IASP Press, 2005: 59–79.

FACTOR II: VASOMOTOR CHANGES

CRPS typically has pathological changes in the regulation of skin blood flow that is observed by the patient and medical attendants.[20] Vasodilatation and/or vasoconstriction occur, and are significant subjective and objective measures. The tone of the cutaneous vessels is maintained by both tonic and phasic activity in the sympathetic system in addition to antidromic vasodilatation. Changes in the blood flow of deeper structures, such as muscle and bone, are much more difficult to observe.[21]

Estimation of skin perfusion in real time may be obtained with laser Doppler flowmetry or by measurement of skin temperature. Simultaneous (or contemporaneous) measures must be obtained symmetrically from the unaffected extremity for four reasons.[20]

1. Cutaneous perfusion is usually symmetric.
2. Skin blood flow and temperature change in response to a variety of external and internal influences.
3. Laser Doppler measures relative flows.
4. Antidromic vasodilatation shows significant interindividual differences.

Vasomotor instability in acute CRPS may be related to changes in sympathetic tone, antidromic activity, as well as to neurogenic inflammation.[22] These changes, in addition to central changes, are capable of producing "warm" CRPS, as well as "cold" CRPS.[23] Evidence has suggested that cutaneous sympathetic vasoconstrictor tone may be reduced in the acute period, and skin blood flow may be increased. It is therefore not likely that sympathetic blockade will have any therapeutic effect during this phase.

Chronic CRPS has traditionally been regarded as cold. Sympathetic overactivity or supersensitivity to circulating catecholamines are the putative explanations for this phenomenon. Some studies indicate that the affected limb is always cooler than the contralateral side during whole-body heating (for example, during a thermoregulatory sweat test). Microneurography studies suggested that sympathetic efferent activity was reduced, and assays of circulating catechols showed reduced venous levels in the affected extremity. It is suggested that adrenergic supersensitivity to circulating catechols might be the culprit.

There are, of course, other influences on vasomotor control. For example, endothelial-derived nitric oxide or prostacyclins might be involved in vasodilatation.

Diagnostic value of vasomotor disturbance in the diagnosis of CRPS has been difficult to evaluate.[24] Dynamic changes in skin blood flow reduce the diagnostic value of skin temperature differences in CRPS. There are both short-term changes related to sympathetic control and long-term changes related to the underlying pathology and disuse.

It has been suggested that temperature asymmetry under stable baseline conditions (20 minutes at rest with environmental temperature of 20°C) can be used. A difference of 0.6°C (infrared thermometry) discriminated between CRPS and other conditions with a sensitivity of 68 percent and specificity of 67 percent. More complex measurements, for example with computerized thermography, have not entirely clarified the problem.[25]

Other pathologies also cause differences in skin temperatures of the affected and unaffected extremities. Acute arthritides, inflammatory disorders, vascular disorders, and peripheral neuropathies are all capable of producing significant temperature asymmetries.

FACTOR III: SUDOMOTOR CHANGES AND EDEMA

Differential sweating between the affected and unaffected side is regarded as one of the diagnostic criteria for CRPS.[26] Sweat production is a sympathetic cholinergic function, and variations occur in response to a wide variety of stimuli. Physiological variations are typically symmetric, and usually involve both hands and feet, as well as the head and trunk. These changes can occur apparently spontaneously or be induced by external or internal factors. These may include environmental temperature, physical activity, or psychological stress. If there is reduced sympathetic efferent activity in CRPS or other conditions, the affected extremity is likely to be warm and dry compared to the unaffected side. However, increased sympathetic efferent activity is likely to be associated with a cold, sweaty extremity compared to the unaffected side.

Measurement of sudomotor activity is difficult and not generally available. The quantitative sudomotor axon reflex test (QSART) is a validated test for CRPS. It measures resting sweat output and response to iontophoretically applied acetyl choline, comparing the affected and unaffected sides.

The thermoregulatory sweat test gives most information in small fiber neuropathy and autonomic failure, and has not been rigorously evaluated in CRPS. It is complicated and expensive, and not generally performed, even in tertiary centers. Some insurance companies restrict the use of such tests (**Table 27.3**).

Sympathetic skin responses may be of some value in the diagnosis of CRPS, if asymmetric.[27] The clinical observation that one hand or foot appears moist may be the only objective evidence of this factor. This change might only be present on occasions of physical or emotional stress, or may accompany a severe episode of pain.

Peripheral edema is a common clinical finding in many conditions. However, it is unilateral, localized edema that is of diagnostic significance in CRPS. This is not like the dependent, pitting ankle edema of congestive cardiac failure or the brawny lymphedema of the arm after axillary node dissection. This localized edema has been described by several authors (reviewed in Ref. 26), and is possibly neurogenic in origin.[28]

Edema is often not measured at all, but the patient may comment that there is too much swelling to wear customary rings or the veins cannot be seen. Quantitative measures, such as volume displacement of the hand or foot, or finger diameter, are rarely recorded. Patients and clinicians often note, however, that the sweating and edema resolve when the CRPS resolves. They could theoretically be used to monitor severity and progress. There are therefore no specific treatments that can be directed at these factors.

There are no studies of interrater reliability or of the reliability of self-observation of either sweating or edema. Both are very difficult to measure and the framers of the

Table 27.3 Aetna Clinical Policy Bulletin: autonomic testing/sudomotor tests.

Test		
I	Aetna considers autonomic testing such as quantitative sudomotor axon reflex test (QSART), thermoregulatory sweat test (TST), and silastic sweat imprint medically necessary for use as a diagnostic tool for any of the following conditions/disorders:	A Diabetic autonomic neuropathy; or B Amyloid neuropathy; or C Sjögren's syndrome; or D Idiopathic neuropathy; or E Pure autonomic failure; or F Multiple system atrophy; or G Distal small fiber neuropathy; or H Reflex sympathetic dystrophy or causalgia (sympathetically maintained pain)
	Aetna considers autonomic testing experimental and investigational for all other indications	
II	Aetna considers sympathetic skin response testing experimental and investigational for any indications because it has a relatively low sensitivity and uncertain specificity, and the peer-reviewed medical literature does not support its effectiveness	

www.aetna.com/cpb/medical/data/400_499/0485.html.

factors were well aware of this dilemma. The criteria require that these changes be observed at some time during the course of the condition, but prospective studies are lacking.

FACTOR IV: MOVEMENT DISORDERS AND DYSTROPHY

Motor and movement disorders[29] occur in as many as 95 percent of patients with CRPS[30] and include weakness, bradykinesia, dystonia, myoclonus, and tremor. The pathophysiology appears to be of central origin when studied with functional magnetic resonance imaging (fMRI). It is difficult to measure, but activity monitors are likely more accurate that questionnaires.[31, 32]

The picture is complicated because it has been shown that both immobility and disuse can affect motor function. Such changes might not be specific for CRPS and probably represent interactions between peripheral, spinal, and supraspinal mechanisms. It will be necessary to determine which of the motor abnormalities are generated by which particular pathologic process.

Unfortunately, there are no prospective studies of the cause of motor or movement disorders, or adequate studies of physical therapies or pharmacotherapies.

LABORATORY TESTS FOR CRPS

The four factors were derived from clinical symptoms and clinical signs that can be obtained at the bedside.[33] CRPS is therefore a clinical, not a laboratory, diagnosis. Inter-rater reliability is poor. For any test to be validated, the underlying condition must also be validated. The criteria listed above are the first to be validated for CRPS, albeit in a somewhat circular fashion. It has to be noted that there are three levels of confidence in the diagnosis. The most stringent is "research", less so is "clinical", and there is a gestalt category of "not otherwise specified."

Laboratory tests are subject to the same problems and circular arguments. For example, response to sympathetic block was once considered pathognomonic of RSD until it became apparent that pain did not necessarily involve the sympathetic nervous system.

Electrodiagnosis

Electrophysiological evaluation of the CRPS patient may involve estimation of nerve conduction velocity, somatosensory evoked potentials (including laser-evoked potentials[34]), and electromyography. Changes in these variables may indicate underlying neurological disorders. It is difficult to determine whether minor variations are the cause or consequence of the CRPS. Major abnormalities are likely to be of etiologic significance. These tests might some indication of possible therapies – release of entrapped nerves is sometimes carried out on the basis of electrodiagnostic studies, for example, carpal tunnel release after wrist fracture.

Diagnostic imaging

Diagnostic imaging has been used for diagnosis of CRPS since the description of Sudeck's atrophy. It is not clear whether any technique or combination has enough specificity and sensitivity to replace clinical evaluation.[35][I]

PLAIN RADIOGRAPHY

CRPS may be accompanied by demineralization of the extremity in later stages. Unfortunately, disuse, without CRPS, may also be accompanied by the same signs. CRPS can occur without demineralization, so this sign is not of diagnostic significance. It is not known whether and at what rate the demineralization reverses with successful treatment of the underlying condition.

THREE PHASE BONE SCAN

Bone scan after technetium 99 has been used for more than 25 years in the evaluation of painful extremities as an aid to diagnosis. Criteria for CRPS include (1) arterial hypoperfusion of the affected extremity, and increased periarticular uptake of wrist, carpal, metacarpal, and finger joints on blood pool (120 seconds) and delayed (three hour) images. It was proposed as the gold standard, but has come under some scrutiny recently, and its place redefined. Schurmann *et al.*[35][I] showed that three-phase bone scan (TPBS) eight weeks after distal radial fracture had 19 percent sensitivity and 96 percent specificity, with 53 percent positive predictive value (PPV) and 83 percent negative predictive value (NPV). At 16 weeks, these values had improved to 14 percent sensitivity, 100 percent specificity, 100 percent PPV, and 83 percent NPV. Unfortunately, inter-observer reliability for this test may not be good.[36]

MAGNETIC RESONANCE IMAGING

Changes in the magnetic resonance imaging (MRI) of the wrist attributed to CRPS include: (1) spotty bone marrow edema of the carpal bones; (2) skin edema; (3) gadolinium uptake of the skin and intra-articular structures; and (4) joint effusion. Sensitivity and specificity were somewhat less than TPBS.

FUNCTIONAL MAGNETIC RESONANCE IMAGING/REGIONAL CEREBRAL BLOOD FLOW

Changes have been described in the functional MRI and regional cerebral blood flow (rCBF)[37] related to CRPS. It is not yet known how specific and sensitive these changes are, or their diagnostic utility.

MANAGEMENT

CRPS represents a very complicated pathophysiological disturbance, further complicated by its biopsychosocial complications.[38] The pain is disproportionate to the initiating stimulus, and the consequences are likewise disproportionate. The specific initiating factor is often unknown, and the specific pathophysiological changes are also unknown. Prevention is therefore difficult or impossible.[39] Specific therapy is therefore not possible, so generalized functional restoration must occur. This is itself a difficult concept, as there are few studies that have been able to define the active modality or combination in overall successful comprehensive pain rehabilitation programs. General principles are necessarily espoused on reasonable empiric bases which sound logical.[40][III] If there is acceptance by both practitioner and patient, then positive results might occur. If one or both do not subscribe to the treatment premise, then no improvement will occur, or the situation might become even worse. It is an article of faith in the chronic pain and rehabilitation communities that interdisciplinary collaboration is essential for production of optimal outcomes. This is evident at the community level where the total expenditure on complementary and alternative medicine may exceed that on allopathic medicine.

An implicit assumption in CRPS treatment algorithms is that the precipitating or maintaining factors will be removed, or at least minimized. Unfortunately, there are no epidemiological data regarding this aspect of the condition. It could be argued that the Olmsted County study showed a high rate of "spontaneous" recovery because the underlying pathology was treated, without addressing the CRPS component. Clearly, more attention needs to be paid to this aspect of the problem. This author has seen patients who have not responded to conventional treatment of CRPS but who have recovered when an underlying problem was successfully treated. One case was referred after her insurance company declined further treatment after 49 stellate ganglion blocks. It was clear that she had carpal tunnel involvement, and she recovered after a surgeon could be prevailed upon to operate in the face of severe CRPS.

Integrated therapy has to address four interrelated aspects of functional restoration in CRPS. These aspects have been suggested as the result of thought experiments and not on the basis of evidence-based recommendations. The goal of therapy is to return the patient to pre-CRPS function at home, work, and community, with minimal ongoing involvement of the medical system. All aspects are ideally addressed simultaneously, continuing faith-based hope, rather than evidence-based outcomes.

Management of underlying pathology

It is difficult and sometimes impossible to identify the precipitating factors in CRPS. It would seem reasonable to treat these factors to the maximum possible extent, although there are virtually no data to suggest this. Unfortunately, some of the interventions, such as immobilization[41] for fractures, might contribute to CRPS. It is also logical that complications of CRPS should be prevented lest they exacerbate the syndrome. For example, if CRPS of the hand is not thoughtfully managed, the resulting frozen shoulder will make rehabilitation even more painful and difficult. Prolonged reflex ischemia (vasoconstriction) can produce nerve ischemia and additional pain.

Prevention of CRPS after injury or surgery would be the preferred route, but few studies have indicated the optimal method. The traditional advice seems reasonable: if acute post-operative pain is prevented, it cannot become chronic.[42] There has been a single study of prevention suggesting that 500 mg per day of vitamin C will reduce the prevalence of CRPS after wrist fracture.[43]

No rules or evidence-based recommendations can be given for this section. Prudent medical practice must dictate therapy of any underlying condition.

Treatment of pain and related dysfunction

CRPS is a pain syndrome and much attention has been given elsewhere to basic studies of mechanisms and treatment of the pain itself. This section will not address animal models, but clinical practice.

EVIDENCE-BASED PHARMACOTHERAPY

Several aspects of CRPS lend themselves to pharmacologic interventions.[44][I], [45][I] These include the pain itself, the inflammatory response, and the vasoconstriction. As with most other CRPS therapies, there are few good studies on which to base recommendations. There is no medication or treatment approved for CRPS. Indeed, guanethidine was withdrawn from the market as an orphan drug because it was shown to have been ineffective in Bier blocks.

The methodological problems of reviewing published studies have been discussed by Oaklander.[44] She also found it necessary to extrapolate from studies of other neuropathic pain states, such as postherpetic neuralgia (PHN) and painful diabetic neuropathy (PDN). It is only relatively recently that studies have been powered to estimate numbers needed to treat (NNT) to obtain a particular statistical response.

Topical agents

Local anesthetics, in the form of lidocaine patches, or with prilocaine (eutectic mixture of local anesthetics) have level II evidence in PHN, but only open-label studies in CRPS.

A gel containing amitriptyline 1 percent and ketamine 0.5 percent has anecdotal support.[46][V], [47][V] The National Cancer Institute has approved a phase III trial of baclofen/amitriptyline/ketamine gel (www.clinicaltrials.gov/ct2/show/NCT00516503).

Capsaicin is approved for painful diabetic peripheral neuropathy, but is usually not tolerated by CRPS patients with surface allodynia and hyperalgesia. It is sometimes tolerated if applied immediately on removal of a lidocaine patch.

Patent 20050095277 for neuropathy cream includes ketamine, clonidine, gabapentin, and amitriptyline.

Antidepressants

Tricyclic antidepressants, especially amitriptyline, have efficacy in PHN and are widely used in CRPS. Duloxetine is approved for use in PDN, so is being used in CRPS.

Antiepileptic/antineuropathic agents

Carbamazepine is the gold standard treatment for the pain of trigeminal neuralgia and is sometimes used off label for CRPS. Gabapentin has been extensively studied in many pain states, and is approved for PDN. It appears to be effective for pain management in CRPS,[48][II] but does not seem to improve function *per se*. Pregabalin is also approved for PDN and is being used for CRPS in similar doses. Lamotrigine is effective in PHN, but has been reported to produce Stevens–Johnson syndrome.

Local anesthetics

There are anecdotes of the use of intravenous lidocaine and oral mexiletine for pain management in neuropathic pain, including CRPS.

Anti-inflammatory agents

Inflammation is a common feature of CRPS,[49] so the use of any tolerated nonsteroidal anti-inflammatory drugs would seem to have a rational basis. There are anecdotes of the use of corticosteroids systemically or locally via intravenous regional administration (Bier block).

Opioids

Long-term use of opioids is controversial, but effective in some cases (see Chapter 16, Opioids and chronic non-cancer pain). The fundamental purpose of any intervention, particularly of invasive or scheduled modalities, must be to reduce pain to an extent that comprehensive rehabilitation can occur.

Placebo

The role of the placebo or nocebo effects in management of CRPS are impossible to measure. They are extremely important issues and relate closely to the interactions between the patient and therapists. There are placebo effects that can be obtained by medications, invasive modalities, and rehabilitation therapies. It is intuitively more beneficial to obtain a placebo effect in addition to the particular manipulation in the clinical situation. Placebo is discussed in Chapter 41, Placebo and nocebo in the *Practice and Procedures* volume of this series.

- Ineffective agents:
  - calcitonin;[50][II]
  - lorazepam;
  - mexilitene;
  - thalidomide;
  - electromagnetic fields.[51][II]
- Marginally effective agents:
  - gabapentin;[52][II]
  - alendronate;[53][II]
  - anti-TNF;[54][V]
  - DMSO;[55, 56][II]
  - acetylcysteine;[55, 56][II]
  - thalidomide.[57]

TRADITIONAL INTERVENTIONAL THERAPIES

Traditional interventions,[58][I] such as sympathetic blockade, were the mainstay of CRPS/RSD therapy for decades. These were interventions easily (and profitably) carried out by an anesthesiologist, and not subjected to any serious scrutiny until relatively recently.

Sympathetic nerve block

Critical analysis of published studies of sympathetic blockade at the stellate or lumbar ganglia levels[59] indicated that there were few, if any, published data, and success rate was dismal. There is a significant placebo effect which might explain the "success." However, sympathetic ganglion blockade still retains its historical place in diagnostic and treatment algorithms to define sympathetically maintained pain. It is not clear what to do with this information. The long-term outcomes of repeated sympathetic blockade or surgical, chemical, or radiofrequency sympathectomy are not encouraging (except, perhaps, for axillary hyperhidrosis).

Sympathectomy via intravenous regional (IVR) (Bier block) with guanethidine, reserpine, or bretylium, have usually reported negative outcomes in CRPS. There are anecdotal successes from an IVR combination of bretylium, phentolamine, and hydrocortisone, and also lidocaine with ketorolac.

Intravenous phentolamine has been suggested as a diagnostic tool, but the high cost, low specificity, and low sensitivity have led to its general abandonment.

Somatic nerve blockade

It has long been clinical practice to precede physical therapy with dilute axillary or interscalene blocks to produce some analgesia and sympathetic blockade with minimal motor block. However, data for this practice are sparse.

Epidural blockade

There are better data for the use of continuous epidural infusion of local anesthetic alone or in combination with opioids or clonidine in CRPS rehabilitation. Again, the intention is to produce analgesia and sympathetic blockade so that rehabilitation can be more effective.

Spinal cord stimulation

Some 40 years has elapsed since the first spinal cord stimulator was implanted, but it is relatively recently that its place in the management of CRPS has been validated. Grabow *et al.*[60][I] reviewed the available literature and concluded that spinal cord stimulation (SCS) is effective in the management of CRPS. However, they were unable to answer relevant questions, such as selection criteria and outcome measurement.

A recent meta-analysis concluded that SCS was an effective therapy for CRPS, and there was also evidence of cost-effectiveness. This study also noted the paucity of usable data in the literature, recommending additional properly designed studies.[61][I] There are few long-term studies of SCS efficacy.[62][II] It is discouraging to note that a clinical trial of SCS, previously registered at www.clinicaltrials.gov/ct2/show/NCT00414804, has been withdrawn.

Intrathecal drug delivery

There are no randomized prospective clinical trials of intrathecal medication for CRPS. Reported indications are for pain management and the usual pharmacology has been employed singly or, more commonly, in combination. Agents named in case reports and series include local anesthetics (usually bupivacaine), opioids (morphine, hydromorphone, fentanyl), adjuvants (clonidine, baclofen[63][V]), sodium channel blockers (ziconotide),[64][V] and botulinum toxins.[65][V] This route is discussed in more detail in Chapter 31, Intrathecal drug delivery in the *Practice and Procedures* volume of this series.

Reversal of disuse effects

Physical and occupational therapies form the basis of rehabilitation from the adverse effects of CRPS. Once again, there are few data regarding the most effective modality or combination. Harden *et al.*[3] reports a functional restoration algorithm using four stages (**Table 27.4**). Although this is not strictly an algorithm, it is a useful addition to the CRPS armamentarium. Patients can enter the process at whatever stage they are in the severity spectrum and progress to subsequent levels according to functional recovery.

This process assumes that any symptoms that prevent patient cooperation are optimized. For example, if pain or muscle spasm prevents joint mobilization, the pain should be treated before each formal therapy session. This might require breakthrough pain medication or temporary neural blockade. If the patient is depressed, anxious, or hostile, efforts should be made to optimize her/his mental status and attitude. If there are external factors, such as worker compensation or other legal issues, considerable ingenuity may need to be applied because of the conflicting vested interests of potentially adversarial stakeholders.

Table 27.4 Functional restoration algorithm: physical/occupational therapy; physiatry.

	Stage
1	Reactivation
	Contrast baths
	Desensitization
	Exposure therapy
2	Flexibility
	Edema control
	Isometric strengthening
	Postural correction
	Secondary myofascial pain diagnosis and treatment
3	Range of movement
	Stress loading
	Isotonic strengthening
	Aerobic conditioning
	Postural normalization/balanced use
4	Ergonomic principles
	Movement therapies
	Normalization of use
	Vocational/functional restoration

Management of biopsychosocial consequences

PSYCHOLOGICAL INTERVENTIONS

CRPS shares with all chronic pain states the problems inherent in a condition that adversely affects the individual's own psyche and self-image, role in the family, work status, financial status, and involvement in the legal system. It is apparent that CRPS does not have any predictable psychological precursor,[66] but equally apparent is that it produces severe psychological adverse effects. These are not only distressing for the patient and family, but also produce secondary adverse physiological and functional changes.

Pain and the accompanying allodynia and hyperalgesia produce learned disuse (illustrated by Bruehl[67]). There is significant kinesophobia as the patient adopts a protective posture and minimizes movement that is expected to increase the pain. Pain itself can increase circulating catecholamine, aggravating the vasospasm. Dysphoric states such as anger, anxiety, and depression are common and perpetuate the pain state. It is postulated that these vicious cycles eventually maintain the CRPS. Successful treatment therefore must address symptoms beyond the vasospasm.

It is therefore not surprising that cognitive/behavioral treatments are reported to be effective in the management of chronic pain states, including CRPS.[68][I] There are, of course, no randomized controlled studies of these methods in CRPS, but the published reports, as usual, are supportive (reviewed by Bruehl[67]).

The paucity of data in this area suggests that therapy should be in a comprehensive, integrated interdisciplinary model.

MANAGEMENT OF PEDIATRIC CRPS

There are increasing reports of CRPS in children,[69, 70] and there may be differences from the "adult" variety. The female:male ratio may be 4:1, with a lower:upper extremity ratio of 5:1. Diagnostic criteria remain the same in pediatric patients.

Management is anchored by effective physical therapy. Relief of spontaneous and evoked pain must occur to allow this, and follows the principles outlined for adults. Pharmacologic relief of pain may be necessary and neural blockade may also be needed.[71][III] Unfortunately, there are no randomized clinical trials of any interventions in the pediatric literature.

Cognitive/behavioral and psychological interventions are usually included. There is often significant psychological investment in the child's illness by the parent and other caregivers.

Wilder[69] therefore recommends a stepwise multidisciplinary program, with simple, noninvasive interventions first. Should these prove ineffective, more potent medications (including opioids) and invasive therapies may be needed to facilitate the required physical therapy.

REFERENCES

* 1. Wilson PR, Stanton-Hicks M, Harden RN (eds). CRPS: current diagnosis and therapy. In: *Progress in Pain Research and Management 32.* Seattle: IASP Press, 2005: 316.
* 2. Jänig W, Baron R. Is CRPS I a neuropathic pain syndrome? *Pain.* 2006; **120**: 227–9.
* 3. Harden RN, Bruehl S, Stanton-Hicks M, Wilson PR. Proposed new diagnostic criteria for complex regional pain syndrome. *Pain Medicine.* 2007; **8**: 326–31.
4. Sunderland S. Pain mechanisms in causalgia. *Journal of Neurology, Neurosurgery, and Psychiatry.* 1976; **39**: 471–80.
5. Akkus S, Yorgancigil H, Yener M. A case of recurrent and migratory complex regional pain syndrome type. I: Prevention by gabapentin. *Rheumatology International.* 2006; **26**: 852–4.
6. Agarwal V, Joseph B. Recurrent migratory sympathetically maintained pain syndrome in a child: a case report. *Journal of Pediatric Orthopaedics, Part B.* 2006; **15**: 73–4.
7. Chen Y, Kelly J. Reflex sympathetic dystrophy: a case of total body pain. *Nurse Practitioner.* 2007; **32**: 8–10.
8. Bandyk DF. Surgical sympathectomy for reflex sympathetic dystrophy syndromes. *Journal of Vascular Surgery.* 2002; **35**: 269–77.
* 9. Veldman PH, Reynen HM, Arntz IE, Goris RJ. Signs and symptoms of reflex sympathetic dystrophy: prospective study of 829 patients. *Lancet.* 1993; **342**: 1012–16.
10. Sandroni P, Benrud-Larson LM, McClelland RL, Low PA. Complex regional pain syndrome type I: incidence and prevalence in Olmsted county, a population-based study. *Pain.* 2003; **103**: 199–207.
11. Bennett GJ, Harden RN. Questions concerning the incidence and prevalence of complex regional pain syndrome type I (RSD). *Pain.* 2003; **106**: 209–10; author reply 210–11.
12. Duman I, Dincer U, Taskaynatan M *et al.* Reflex sympathetic dystrophy: a retrospective epidemiological study of 168 patients. *Clinical Rheumatology.* 2007; **26**: 1433–7.
* 13. Bruehl S, Harden RN, Galer BS *et al.* External validation of IASP diagnostic criteria for Complex Regional Pain Syndrome and proposed research diagnostic criteria. International Association for the Study of Pain. *Pain.* 1999; **81**: 147–54.
14. Bruehl S, Chung OY. How common is complex regional pain syndrome-type I? *Pain.* 2007; **129**: 1–2.
15. Stanton-Hicks M, Janig W, Hassenbusch S *et al.* Reflex sympathetic dystrophy: changing concepts and taxonomy. *Pain.* 1995; **63**: 127–33.
* 16. Harden RN, Bruehl S, Galer BS *et al.* Complex regional pain syndrome: are the IASP diagnostic criteria valid and sufficiently comprehensive? *Pain.* 1999; **83**: 211–19.
17. Oaklander AL, Birklein F. Factor I: sensory changes – pathophysiology and measurement. *CRPS: current diagnosis and therapy.* In: Wilson PR, Stanton-Hicks M, Harden RN (eds). *Progress in Pain Research and Management.* Seattle: IASP Press, 2005: 59–79.
18. Birklein F, Riedl B, Sieweke N *et al.* Neurological findings in complex regional pain syndromes – analysis of 145 cases. *Acta Neurologica Scandinavica.* 2000; **101**: 262–9.
* 19. Oaklander AL, Rissmiller JG, Gelman JB *et al.* Evidence of focal small-fiber axonal degeneration in complex regional pain syndrome-I (reflex sympathetic dystrophy). *Pain.* 2006; **120**: 235–43.
20. Wasner G, Baron R (eds). Factor II: Vasomotor changes – pathophysiology and measurement. *CRPS: current diagnosis and therapy.* In: Stanton-Hicks M, Wilson PR, Harden RN (eds). *Progress in Pain Research and Management, 32.* Seattle: IASP Press, 2005: 81–106.
21. Schattschneider J, Binder A, Siebrecht D *et al.* Complex regional pain syndromes: the influence of cutaneous and deep somatic sympathetic innervation on pain. *Clinical Journal of Pain.* 2006; **22**: 240–4.

* 22. Albrecht PJ, Hines S, Eisenberg E *et al.* Pathologic alterations of cutaneous innervation and vasculature in affected limbs from patients with complex regional pain syndrome. *Pain.* 2006; **120**: 244–66.
23. Vaneker M, Wilder-Smith OH, Schrombges P *et al.* Patients initially diagnosed as 'warm' or 'cold' CRPS 1 show differences in central sensory processing some eight years after diagnosis: a quantitative sensory testing study. *Pain.* 2005; **115**: 204–11.
24. Niehof SP, Huygen FJ, van der Weerd RW *et al.* Thermography imaging during static and controlled thermoregulation in complex regional pain syndrome type 1: diagnostic value and involvement of the central sympathetic system. *Biomedical Engineering Online.* 2006; **5**: 30.
25. Niehof SP, Huygen FJ, Stronks DL *et al.* Reliability of observer assessment of thermographic images in complex regional pain syndrome type 1. *Acta Orthopaedica Belgica.* 2007; **73**: 31–7.
26. Sandroni P, Wilson P. Factor III: Sudomotor changes and edema – pathophysiology and measurement. *CRPS: current diagnosis and therapy.* In: Stanton-Hicks M, Wilson PR, Harden RN (eds). *Progress in Pain Research and Management, 32.* Seattle: IASP Press, 2005: 107–18.
27. Bolel K, Hizmetli S, Akyuz A. Sympathetic skin responses in reflex sympathetic dystrophy. *Rheumatology International.* 2006; **26**: 788–91.
28. Heijmans-Antonissen C, Wesseldijk FD, Munnikes RJ *et al.* Multiplex bead array assay for detection of 25 soluble cytokines in blister fluid of patients with complex regional pain syndrome type 1. *Mediators of Inflammation.* 2006; **2006**: 28398.
29. van Hilten JJ, Blumberg H, Schwartzman RJ. Factor IV: Movement disorders – pathophysiology and measurement. *CRPS: current diagnosis and therapy.* In: Stanton-Hicks M, Wilson PR, Harden RN (eds). *Progress in Pain Research and Management, 32.* Seattle: IASP Press, 2005: 119–37.
30. Schasfoort FC, Bussmann JB, Krijnen HJ, Stam HJ. Upper limb activity over time in complex regional pain syndrome type 1 as objectively measured with an upper limb-activity monitor: an explorative multiple case study. *European Journal of Pain.* 2006; **10**: 31–9.
31. Schasfoort FC, Bussmann JB, Stam HJ. Correlation between a novel upper limb activity monitor and four other instruments to determine functioning in upper limb complex regional pain syndrome type I. *Journal of Rehabilitation Medicine.* 2005; **37**: 108–14.
32. Roorda LD, Milenaar IW, Lankhorst GJ, Bouter LM. Measuring Mobility Study Group. Improvement of a questionnaire measuring activity limitations in rising and sitting down in patients with lower-extremity disorders living at home. *Archives of Physical Medicine and Rehabilitation.* 2005; **86**: 2204–10.
33. Rommel O, Habler H-J, Schuermann M. Laboratory tests for complex regional pain syndrome. *CRPS: current diagnosis and therapy.* In: Stanton-Hicks M, Wilson PR, Harden RN (eds). *Progress in Pain Research and Management, 32.* Seattle: IASP Press, 2005: 139–59.
34. Moreau V, Berquin AD, Plaghki L. Laser-evoked potentials correlate with clinical evolution in a case of spontaneous and recurrent complex regional pain syndrome type I. *Clinical Journal of Pain.* 2007; **23**: 375–9.
* 35. Schurmann M, Zaspel J, Lohr P *et al.* Imaging in early posttraumatic complex regional pain syndrome: a comparison of diagnostic methods. *Clinical Journal of Pain.* 2007; **23**: 449–57.
36. Tondeur M, Sand A, Ham H. Interobserver reproducibility in the interpretation of bone scans from patients suspected of having reflex sympathetic dystrophy. *Clinical Nuclear Medicine.* 2005; **30**: 4–10.
37. Wu C-T, Fan YM, Sun CM *et al.* Correlation between changes in regional cerebral blood flow and pain relief in complex regional pain syndrome type 1. *Clinical Nuclear Medicine.* 2006; **31**: 317–20.
* 38. Harden RN, Swan M, King A *et al.* Treatment of complex regional pain syndrome: functional restoration. *Clinical Journal of Pain.* 2006; **22**: 420–4.
39. Zyluk A. Complex regional pain syndrome type I. Risk factors, prevention and risk of recurrence. *Journal of Hand Surgery, British Volume.* 2004; **29**: 334–7.
40. Acerra NE, Souvlis T, Moseley GL. Stroke, complex regional pain syndrome and phantom limb pain: can commonalities direct future management? *Journal of Rehabilitation Medicine.* 2007; **39**: 109–14.
41. Singh HP, Davis TRC. The effect of short-term dependency and immobility on skin temperature and colour in the hand. *Journal of Hand Surgery, British Volume.* 2006; **31**: 611–15.
42. Reuben SS. Chronic pain after surgery: what can we do to prevent it. *Current Pain and Headache Reports.* 2007; **11**: 5–13.
43. Zollinger PE, Tuinebreijer WE, Breederveld RS, Kreis W. Can vitamin C prevent complex regional pain syndrome in patients with wrist fractures? A randomized, controlled, multicenter dose-response study. *Journal of Bone and Joint Surgery, American Volume.* 2007; **89**: 1424–31.
44. Oaklander A. Evidence-based pharmacotherapy for CRPS and related conditions. *CRPS: current diagnosis and therapy.* In: Stanton-Hicks M, Wilson PR, Harden RN (eds). *Progress in Pain Research and Management, 32.* Seattle: IASP Press, 2005: 181–200.
* 45. Rowbotham MC. Pharmacologic management of complex regional pain syndrome. *Clinical Journal of Pain.* 2006; **22**: 425–9.
46. Sandroni P, Davis M. Combination gel of 1% amitriptyline and 0.5% ketamine to treat refractory erythromelalgia pain. *Archives of Dermatology.* 2006; **142**: 283–6.
47. Ushida T, Tani T, Kanbara T *et al.* Analgesic effects of ketamine ointment in patients with complex regional pain syndrome type 1. *Regional Anesthesia and Pain Medicine.* 2002; **27**: 524–8.

48. Tan AK, Duman I, Taşkaynatan MA *et al.* The effect of gabapentin in earlier stage of reflex sympathetic dystrophy. *Clinical Rheumatology.* 2007; **26**: 561–5.
49. Schinkel C, Gaertner A, Zaspel J *et al.* Inflammatory mediators are altered in the acute phase of posttraumatic complex regional pain syndrome. *Clinical Journal of Pain.* 2006; **22**: 235–9.
50. Sahin F, Yilmaz F, Kotevoglu N, Kuran B. Efficacy of salmon calcitonin in complex regional pain syndrome (type 1) in addition to physical therapy. *Clinical Rheumatology.* 2006; **25**: 143–8.
51. Durmus A, Cakmak K, Disci R, Muslumoglu L. The efficiency of electromagnetic field treatment in complex regional pain syndrome type I. *Disability and Rehabilitation.* 2004; **26**: 537–45.
52. van de Vusse AC, Stomp-van den Berg G, Kessels AH, Weber WE. Randomised controlled trial of gabapentin in complex regional pain syndrome type 1 (ISRCTN84121379). *BMC Neurology.* 2004; **4**: 13.
53. Manicourt D-H, Brasseur JP, Boutsen Y *et al.* Role of alendronate in therapy for posttraumatic complex regional pain syndrome type I of the lower extremity. *Arthritis and Rheumatism.* 2004; **50**: 3690–7.
54. Huygen FJ, Niehof S, Zijlstra J *et al.* Successful treatment of CRPS 1 with anti-TNF. *Journal of Pain and Symptom Management.* 2004; **27**: 101–03.
55. van Dieten HE, Perez RS, van Tulder MW *et al.* Cost effectiveness and cost utility of acetylcysteine versus dimethyl sulfoxide for reflex sympathetic dystrophy. *Pharmacoeconomics.* 2003; **21**: 139–48.
56. Perez RS, Zuurmond WW, Bezemer PD *et al.* The treatment of complex regional pain syndrome type I with free radical scavengers: a randomized controlled study. *Pain.* 2003; **102**: 297–307.
57. Schwartzman RJ, Chevlen E, Bengtson K. Thalidomide has activity in treating complex regional pain syndrome. *Archives of Internal Medicine.* 2003; **163**: 1487–8.
58. Nelson DV, Stacey BR. Interventional therapies in the management of complex regional pain syndrome. *Clinical Journal of Pain.* 2006; **22**: 438–42.
* 59. Cepeda MS, Carr DB, Lau J. Local anesthetic sympathetic blockade for complex regional pain syndrome. *Cochrane Database of Systematic Reviews.* 2005; **CD004598**.
60. Grabow TS, Tella PK, Raja SN. Spinal cord stimulation for complex regional pain syndrome: an evidence-based medicine review of the literature. *Clinical Journal of Pain.* 2003; **19**: 371–83.
61. Taylor RS, van Buyten J-P, Buchser E. Spinal cord stimulation for complex regional pain syndrome: a systematic review of the clinical and cost-effectiveness literature and assessment of prognostic factors. *European Journal of Pain.* 2006; **10**: 91–101.
* 62. Kemler MA, de Vet HCW, Barendse GA *et al.* Spinal cord stimulation for chronic reflex sympathetic dystrophy – five-year follow-up. *New England Journal of Medicine.* 2006; **354**: 2394–6.
63. Zuniga RE, Perera S, Abram SE. Intrathecal baclofen: a useful agent in the treatment of well-established complex regional pain syndrome. *Regional Anesthesia and Pain Medicine.* 2002; **27**: 90–3.
64. Stanton-Hicks M, Kapural L. An effective treatment of severe complex regional pain syndrome type 1 in a child using high doses of intrathecal ziconotide. *Journal of Pain and Symptom Management.* 2006; **32**: 509–11.
65. Argoff CE. A focused review on the use of botulinum toxins for neuropathic pain. *Clinical Journal of Pain.* 2002; **18**: S177–81.
66. Puchalski P, Zyluk A. Complex regional pain syndrome type 1 after fractures of the distal radius: a prospective study of the role of psychological factors. *Journal of Hand Surgery, British Volume.* 2005; **30**: 574–80.
67. Bruehl S. Psychological interventions. *CRPS: current diagnosis and therapy.* In: Stanton-Hicks M, Wilson PR, Harden RN (eds). *Progress in Pain Research and Management, 32.* Seattle: IASP Press, 2005: 201–16.
68. Geertzen JHB, Van Wilgen CP, Schrier E, Dijkstra PU. Chronic pain in rehabilitation medicine. *Disability and Rehabilitation.* 2006; **28**: 363–7.
* 69. Wilder RT. Management of pediatric patients with complex regional pain syndrome. *Clinical Journal of Pain.* 2006; **22**: 443–8.
70. Wilder RT, Olsson G. Management of pediatric CRPS. *CRPS: current diagnosis and therapy.* In: Stanton-Hicks M, Wilson PR, Harden RN (eds). *Progress in Pain Research and Management, 32.* Seattle: IASP Press, 2005: 275–89.
71. Dadure C, Motais F, Ricard C *et al.* Continuous peripheral nerve blocks at home for treatment of recurrent complex regional pain syndrome I in children. *Anesthesiology.* 2005; **102**: 387–91.

28

Central neuropathic pain: syndromes, pathophysiology, and treatments

JAMES C WATSON

KEY LEARNING POINTS

- A lesion anywhere in the central nervous system can cause neuropathic pain.
- Involvement of the spinothalamic tract pathways is critical, although not sufficient, to the development of central neuropathic pain.
- Non-neuropathic pain types are a common concomitant feature in patients with central neuropathic pain.
- Central neuropathic pain is generally severe, often debilitating, and difficult to treat.
- Pain is common with multiple sclerosis (40–70 percent any pain type; ~30 percent central neuropathic pain).
- Central poststroke pain is most common after lateral medullary and thalamic infarctions and occurs in 2–8 percent of those with strokes in other locations.
- The literature most strongly supports the following medications for the treatment of at least one central neuropathic pain subtype: gabapentin, pregabalin, lamotrigine, amitriptyline, and cannabinoids.

INTRODUCTION AND DEFINITIONS

Central neuropathic pain represents one of the most challenging clinical pain syndromes to treat and remains incompletely understood. The International Association for the Study of Pain (IASP) defines neuropathic pain as that which is initiated or caused by a lesion or dysfunction of the nervous system and can stem from either the peripheral or central nervous system. Central neuropathic pain arises from dysfunction within the central nervous system at any level (supratentorial, infratentorial/brain stem, and/or spinal cord) or combination of levels.[1] It is important to recognize that there are well recognized central neuroplastic changes ("central sensitization" or "wind up") that occur as a consequence of peripherally generated neurogenic, pain-producing, lesions. However, central neuropathic pain is a label reserved for processes in which the primary lesion or dysfunction (not the secondary effects of it) occur within the central nervous system.

Neuropathic pain has a number of well-recognized descriptors suggesting a neuropathic rather than nociceptive pathophysiology (**Box 28.1**). However, the sensitivity and specificity of these descriptors alone or when incorporated into questionnaires to identify neuropathic pain (Neuropathic Pain Questionnaire, Leeds Assessment of Neuropathic Symptoms and Signs (LANSS); and for categorizing subtypes of neuropathic pain (the Neuropathic Pain Symptom Inventory and Neuropathic Pain Scale) is limited, generally in the 70–85 percent range,[2, 3, 4, 5] and therefore verbal pain descriptors are insufficient alone to

> **Box 28.1 Common neuropathic descriptors**
>
> - Hot/burning/scalding
> - Cold (painful)/freezing
> - Prickling, tingling
> - Pins and needles
> - Electrical
> - Shock-like
> - Shooting/stabbing/lancinating
> - Itching
> - Stimulus evoked pain (Sensitive to light touch, brush-up, cold)
>
> Compiled from Störmer *et al.*,[7] Galer and Jensen,[5] Bennett,[4] Krause and Backonja,[3] and Bouhassira *et al.*[2]

make the diagnosis of neuropathic pain. Specifically in spinal cord injury patients, a central pain population highly prone to concomitant non-neuropathic (e.g. musculoskeletal nociceptive) pain, pain descriptors failed to effectively distinguish between neuropathic and non-neuropathic pain types.[6] Similarly, the character of the neuropathic pain is not specific in distinguishing between a peripheral and central neuropathic etiology.A number of IASP definitions are important for neuropathic pain processes, whether central or peripheral:[1]

- **paresthesia** – an abnormal sensation, spontaneous or evoked;
- **dysesthesia** – an abnormal, unpleasant sensation, spontaneous or evoked;
- **allodynia** – pain caused by a generally non-noxious stimulus (e.g. light touch);
- **hyperalgesia** – an increased painful response to a normally painful stimulus (e.g. pin prick);
- **hyperesthesia** – increased sensitivity to stimulation (noxious or not), excluding the special senses;
- **hyperpathia** – a painful syndrome characterized by an abnormally painful reaction to a stimulus, especially a repetitive stimulus, as well as an increased threshold;
- **anesthesia dolorosa** – pain in an area or region that is anesthetic.

General points and assumptions

There have been a number of comprehensive reviews on the subject of central neuropathic pain.[8, 9, 10] There are four major points that need to be recognized:

1. Central neuropathic pain can stem from a lesion anywhere in the central nervous system, but the clinical presentation and pain phenotype may be nondiagnostic.
2. Neuropathic pain can be persistent, paroxysmal, evoked, or some combination of these, independent of where the lesion exists.
3. Treatment efficacy, or lack thereof, may have as much to do with what the pain subtype is as it does to the site and etiology of the lesions. Age, metabolism, and coping/life skills, and comorbidities (depression, nonrestorative sleep, functional limitations) may affect medication response. In a field with few gold standard data to guide evidence-based recommendations, it would seem reasonable to consider a medication or interventional treatment trial for one central pain syndrome if it had shown promise or efficacy in another.
4. Non-neuropathic pain types are a common concomitant feature in patients with central neuropathic pain. Patients with central nervous system dysfunction are often neurologically and thus functionally impaired (para- or hemiparesis for example), placing a greater burden on nonimmobilized segments. The clinician needs to be aware that common processes, such as rotator cuff pathology, degenerative joint disease, or a peripheral neuropathic process (radiculopathy or ulnar neuropathy at the elbow for example), are prevalent and need to be considered when evaluating a pain disorder in a patient with a central nervous system disease.

More recent incidence and prevalence studies have attempted to identify pain subtypes (neuropathic, nociceptive, visceral) in their analysis. Many older studies did not specify whether the chronic pain associated with a central neurologic process was neuropathic or not.

CENTRAL PAIN SUBTYPES

The three most commonly studied central pain syndromes include spinal cord injury (SCI), central poststroke pain (CPSP), and multiple sclerosis (MS)-related pain.

Pain in spinal cord injury

Spinal cord injury pain is addressed in Chapter 29, Spinal cord injury.

Pain in multiple sclerosis

MS is a disorder of the central nervous system white matter, usually presenting first in young adulthood. It is most commonly in a relapsing and remitting form, although for many it eventually becomes a progressive disorder. Even for those for whom it does not become progressive, there is often an accumulation of functional deficits. While the prognosis is variable, 50 percent will require ambulatory assistance within 15 years of disease onset.[11] The median estimate of the prevalence of MS is reported as 0.9 per 1000 overall and 2 per 1000 in North America.[12] That would mean that based on estimated May 2007 population numbers, in the United States alone 270,000–600,000 people are afflicted with MS.

As MS lesions can occur supratentorially, infratentorially (in the brain stem), or in the spinal cord, their associated clinical picture can be quite varied. Estimates of the prevalence of pain in MS, like other central pain syndromes, is complicated by poor delineation in most studies between types of pain. Estimates range from 29 percent[13] to ~80 percent.[14, 15] However, most prevalence estimates (for all pain) fall within the 43–70 percent range.[16, 17, 18, 19, 20, 21, 22, 23, 24, 25] Variations in reported prevalence estimates can be attributed to the definition of MS-related pain (most studies exclude headache), patient populations assessed (MS rehabilitation center inpatients[22] to outpatient MS clinics[16, 17] to population-based studies[14]), and survey methods used.[18, 21]

Pain has been noted to be one of the cardinal presenting features of MS (either alone or in combination with other symptoms) in 5.5–10 percent of all MS patients.[13, 16, 19, 21] It has been suggested that of those who would later be definitively identified as having central neuropathic or chronic pain (~20 percent), a higher percentage have pain as a presenting feature of their MS – i.e. when pain is part of the presenting complex of MS, chronic and central pain are more likely in the future.[16, 20]

Few studies have delineated nociceptive pain from central neuropathic pain and neuropathic pain subtypes in these estimates. Those that have are important.

Osterberg *et al.*[16] were thorough in their assessment of pain subtypes. Of their cohort of 364 MS patients, 57.5 percent reported pain during the course of their disease, 27.5 percent had central neuropathic pain (including 5 percent with trigeminal neuralgia). This most commonly affected the lower extremities (87 percent) (upper extremities in 31 percent) and was bilateral and constant (76 percent) (these data are very similar to Moulin *et al.*[19]). Interestingly, only 2 percent had paroxysmal pain and only 1 percent had spasticity-related pain. Others have found higher prevalences of paroxysmal pains identifying Lhermitte's sign as a bothersome pain in 9 percent[17] and painful tonic leg spasms in 10 percent.[17, 19] One-third of those with central pain in Osterberg's series reported multiple central pain loci with different onsets, modalities, and severity. Others have also found multiple pain types in MS to be not uncommon[14, 17] and in fact it may be more the rule than the exception.[18] Nociceptive pain was evident in 21 percent in Osterberg's series,[16] while back pain was seen in 14–18 percent of Solaro's and Moulin's series[17, 19] and 40 percent (similar to that in the general population) of Svendsen's population-based study.[14] Joint pain was more common in MS patients than in the general Danish population.[14]

As in the other central pain syndromes, pain in MS was often severe (one-quarter of those reporting pain in one study[18] and, in another study, one-third reported it as one of the worst symptoms of MS[20]). In a population-based study from Denmark, while the prevalence of pain in the previous month did not differ in a MS cohort from the general population, MS patients had higher pain intensity levels and were more likely to report pain that interfered with their daily life.[14] In comparison with other chronic pain types, Ehde *et al.*[18] found MS pain to be more severe than in a US population sample, although less severe than pain problems in SCI cohorts. MS pain severity was similar to that in rheumatoid and osteoarthritis cohorts and MS-related neuropathic pain was more severe than MS-related nociceptive pain.[21] One-quarter of MS patients use daily analgesics (versus 9 percent of the general Danish population),[14] yet it has also been shown that relative to pain severity and frequency, MS related pain is un- or undertreated.[21] In keeping with other chronic pain states, pain in MS interferes with sleep, recreational activities, and work inside and outside the home.[18]

Osterberg *et al.* found central neuropathic pain to have the highest prevalence in the first 20 years of MS, thereafter decreasing. This differs from many other studies that have suggested chronic pain increases in prevalence with increasing disease duration.[13, 17, 19, 20] Others have not found this correlation.[14, 18, 21, 25] Most of these other studies have not defined specific pain types in assessing this correlation. Over time, MS patients often have accumulating functional deficits and it is in this setting that one would anticipate increasing prevalence of nociceptive/musculoskeletal pain complaints. Musculoskeletal pain prevalence has been shown to increase as soon as ambulatory assistance became necessary in MS patients.[22] This apparent discrepancy – higher likelihood of central neuropathic pain in the first two decades of MS, and likely higher prevalence of musculoskeletal pain in latter years with increasing functional burdens – may be the result of prior study limitations and failure to delineate pain types.

Multiple studies have reported a correlation with the prevalence of MS-related pain with clinical spasticity or myelopathy,[19, 20] even if pain directly from the spasticity is uncommon in MS.[16] This speaks to the pathogenesis of central neuropathic pain where most cases seem to have evidence of spinothalamic tract dysfunction (98 percent of those with MS-related central neuropathic pain).[16] Hence spasticity and myelopathy are indicators of a disease process localizing to the spinal cord and with higher likelihood of also affecting the spinothalamic tracts which are etiologically important for central pain.

Central poststroke pain

The median annual incidence of first stroke for all ages is 183 per 100,000 with the risk of stroke roughly doubling with each decade during adulthood.[12] In the United States in 2007, the incidence of first stroke would be estimated at approximately 551,000 cases per year (based on 301 million US population). Stroke is the third leading cause of death in the United States and a leading cause of disability.[26] Based on the prevalence of stroke in the population (compared with that of SCI or MS), CPSP is the most common cause of central neuropathic pain.[9, 27] Interestingly, the median age of patients who develop CPSP appears to be younger than the median age of patients having strokes.[27, 28, 29, 30, 31, 32, 33] However, Andersen *et al.*[34] found no statistically significant difference in age between those with and without somatosensory deficits or pain.

The classic CPSP example is the thalamic pain syndrome described by Dejérine and Roussy.[35] However, CPSP can occur with both ischemic and hemorrhagic lesions at any level: infratentorial/brain stem, thalamic, or various supratentorial, extra-thalamic sites. It does not appear that either ischemic or hemorrhagic insult is more likely to induce CPSP.[8, 27, 30, 36] Reported percentages of patients with CPSP in these series are in keeping with the relative proportion of ischemic versus hemorrhagic strokes in the population. As such, given that ~80 percent of strokes are ischemic,[12] more patients have CPSP from ischemic strokes. A pain series focusing on CPSP in lenticulo-capsular hemorrhages has been published.[37]

More important than what causes the lesion is where the lesion occurs and what deficits are associated. The incidence of CPSP varies based on the location of the stroke. Lateral medullary infarctions (Wallenberg's syndrome – i.e. the loss of pain and temperature function of the face ipsilateral and body contralateral to the lateral medullary stroke, vestibular dysfunction, hoarseness and dysphagia, and an ipsilateral Horner's syndrome), which selectively affect the spino- and trigeminothalamic pathways and spare lemniscal ("large fiber") pathways, has one of the highest incidences of CPSP at 25 percent within six months of the stroke.[31] The incidence of CPSP after thalamic infarction also appears to be high, particularly when it involves the ventral posterior nuclei. One literature review noted the frequency of pain after any thalamic stroke to be 11 percent (range, 8–16 percent), but confining analysis to strokes in the geniculothalamic arterial territory (the ventral posterior thalamus) the frequency was 24 percent (range, 13–59 percent).[28] However, in a study evaluating the clinical syndromes associated with 40 thalamic infarcts, only three patients developed CPSP, suggesting a lower incidence.[38] Thalamic infarcts are well represented in most unselected CPSP series (25–33 percent of CPSP cases),[34, 36] but importantly do not represent the majority of CPSP cases, stressing that while thalamic pain is the quintessential CPSP syndrome, strokes elsewhere can have the same consequences. A CPSP-MRI correlation study found a high percentage of CPSP patients had thalamic lesions (~60 percent), particularly involving the ventroposterior thalamus, although most patients had multiple lesions and were imaged well after the stroke making it impossible to know if this was the CPSP-causing lesion.[30]

Unselected prospective stroke series have demonstrated a lower incidence of CPSP when all patients with stroke are considered. The most cited study of CPSP is that of Anderson *et al.*[34] which prospectively evaluated an unselected stroke population for the first year poststroke (within the first week, at one month, six months, and one year poststroke). Of 267 patients, 207 were still alive and could communicate at six months and an additional seven patients were lost to follow up over the next year leaving the final cohort at 200 patients. Sixteen patients (8 percent) had developed CPSP by the end of one year (only 4/16 had thalamic infarcts, clearly demonstrating that CPSP can occur with lesions at many levels). Interestingly, the incidence of CPSP in this cohort of those whose stroke deficits included somatosensory deficits was 18 percent. Bowsher[39] retrospectively reviewed the experience with 400 patients with stroke of various types and found ~25 percent had somatosensory deficits, but only ~2 percent developed CPSP. He acknowledged that poor documentation of clinical encounters poststroke may have underestimated the frequency of CPSP. Based on these studies, the incidence of CPSP from non-lateral medullary, non-thalamic strokes is commonly cited at 2–8 percent.

Stroke-related pain can occur at stroke onset, but more commonly begins over the coming months, with most evident in the first month. In thalamic strokes, 18 percent had pain from stroke onset, 18 percent within the first week, 20 percent between one week and one month (in total 56 percent occurred within the first month), 15 percent between one and three months, 12 percent between four and six months, 6 percent between six and twelve months, and 11 percent greater than one year after the stroke.[28] Looking at CPSP in a prospective, unselected stroke population, onset within the first month was seen in 63 percent, one to six months in 19 percent, and six to twelve months in 19 percent (series limited follow up to one year and therefore would have missed those taking more one year to present).[34] Seventy-five percent of those developing CPSP after a lateral medullary infarct do so within the first month.[31] It has been reported, however, that CPSP may present up to three years after stroke.[36] Given patients with cerebrovascular disease are at risk for future, sometimes silent, events, one might wonder whether these seemingly rarer late presentations of CPSP are related to new, otherwise clinically silent, strokes. Modern imaging has not addressed this, but may be useful in further assessing these cases.

An interesting phenomenon, not reported with other central neuropathic pain types, has been noted in some forms of CPSP. In thalamic infarcts, CPSP appears to be more commonly associated with right-sided lesions. One hundred and eighty cases were pulled via a review of the literature with imaging or autopsy confirmed evidence of a thalamic infarction and clinical evidence of contralateral pain. Of these, 114 (63 percent) had right thalamic lesions, whereas only 66 (37 percent) had left-sided lesions. This laterality predominance was greatest among males. It was speculated that this is in keeping with interesting experimental evidence demonstrating right-hemisphere specialization for mediation of pain and internal representation of body image.[28] These retrospective results need to be confirmed prospectively and evaluated in nonthalamic pain types. Notably, there was no significant difference in the stroke side in relationship to development of CPSP in the lateral medullary infarct study[31] or the prospective, unselected stroke cohort of Andersen *et al.*[34]

As in other central neuropathic pain types, pain severity in CPSP can be significant and dysfunctioning. Of those with CPSP in Andersen's series, 10/16 (63 percent) reported their pain as moderate to severe.[34] All of the lateral medullary infarct cohort reported their pain severe and required treatment.[31] Allodynia is common to cold and to light touch (generally ~25–75 percent of CPSP patients).[27, 29, 34, 40, 41] Approximately 50 percent of CPSP patients report disturbed sleep, fatigue, and/or stress in relationships and 87 percent report mood changes.[42]

CENTRAL NEUROPATHIC PAIN PATHOPHYSIOLOGY

Further discussion of the applied physiology of neuropathic pain can be found in Chapter 1, Applied physiology: neuropathic pain and Chapter 24, Pain in neurological disease.

The pathogenesis of the various central neuropathic pain syndromes may or may not be the same. However, it appears that the site of the lesion and the affected pathways are more important than the etiology of the lesion (ischemia, hemorrhage, demyelination, trauma). Much of the work in humans has been carried out in CPSP, but the results appear to be largely applicable to post-SCI pain and MS-related central pain.

It is clear and widely reproduced that dysfunction of spinal-thalamic-cortical pathways (clinically evident as impaired pain (pinprick) and temperature) is almost universally prevalent[27, 28, 29, 31, 36, 43] and essential for the development of CPSP.[44, 45] Some have found that abnormal thermal sensation (cold especially) is more critical, and that pain (pinprick) pathway dysfunction may not discriminate poststroke pain and no-pain groups.[34] This cold-signaling pathway has been thought to project to the insula through the ventral medial posterior (VMpo) nucleus of the thalamus and when lesioned leads to cold hypoesthesia and disinhibition of pathways to the anterior cingulated cortex driving CPSP.[46, 47] However, Lenz *et al.*[47] found that lesions of the ventral caudalis (Vc or ventral posterior) nucleus are sufficient to impair cold and tactile sensations (and be associated with CPSP) without involvement of the VMpo. This is in keeping with thalamic pain syndrome cohorts which have shown that those regions involved in spinothalamic-cortical pathways – the ventral posterior thalamus in the region of the geniculothalamic arterial distribution – are particularly common (75–85 percent) with high incidences of CPSP.[28]

Importantly, in patients with stroke, large percentages that do not go on to develop CPSP still have somatosensory disturbances. For example, in Andersen *et al.*'s[34] series 42 percent had evidence of somatosensory deficits, but only 18 percent of these developed CPSP. Therefore, while spino-thalamic-cortical pathway dysfunction appears necessary for the development of central post-stroke pain, it is not sufficient to explain the development of CPSP.[44, 45]

The integrity (or lack thereof) of the lemniscal (large fiber, posterior column) sensory pathway (carrying the modalities of light touch, vibration, and proprioception) does not appear to be fundamentally involved in/vital to the development of CPSP. CPSP can occur when lemniscal pathways are intact or impaired.[29, 31, 44, 48] Interestingly, there is evidence that in those that develop CPSP, however, preserved dorsal column function is important in the setting of spinothalamic tract dysfunction for the development of tactile allodynia.[43]

Involvement of the spinothalamic pathways also appears critical, although not sufficient in and of itself, for the development of MS-related pain and post-SCI below-level central neuropathic pain.[8, 16, 49, 50, 51, 52, 53]

Given spinothalamic tract dysfunction appears necessary, although not necessarily sufficient independently, to cause central neuropathic pain; the concept of an associated denervation hypersensitivity has been proposed to be the required cofactor for development of central neuropathic pain. Spontaneous pain in CPSP is linked to hypersensitivity or spontaneous discharges in thalamic and central neurons that have lost part of their normal (inhibitory) input. This hyperexcitability of thalamic neurons has been shown post-SCI and with phantom limb pain.[44] MacGowan *et al.*,[31] in their CPSP associated with lateral medullary infarct series, noted that infarctions that extended medially to include the ventral trigeminothalamic tract did not develop CPSP, while those where this tract was spared were more prone to develop CPSP. Lying in close proximity to the trigeminothalamic tract is the medullary reticular formation with reticulothalamic projections. It is hypothesized that the spinoreticulothalamic system is tonically inhibited by spinothalamic tract input. Therefore a lesion of the spinothalamic tract that spares the spinoreticulothalamic system would lead to denervation hypersensitivity (loss of inhibitory input) of the spinoreticulothalamic system which could lead to "wind up" and abnormal activation of the reticular formation itself or of its thalamic projections, whereas including the reticulothalamic pathways in the lesion removes the possible affected "wound up" system that could drive the central pain and central pain does not develop.[31, 54] Lenz also noted that some thalamic cells which lose the sensory input of spinothalamic tract pathways show increased burst firing which may signal the sensation of pain.[45, 55, 56]

Some anatomical and temporal correlates, as well as implications from pharmacological studies, are also telling.

Pertinent to thalamic pain syndromes caused by lenticulo-capsular hemorrhages (and one would presume lacunar ischemic infarcts in posterior limb of the internal capsule damaging thalamo-cortical pathways), it is notable that pain has been reported to disproportionately (or solely) affect the leg despite more widespread motor and sensory deficits. The somatotopic arrangement of the ventral posterior nucleus of the thalamus in primates from medial to lateral is face, arm, and leg most laterally (i.e. adjacent to the posterior limb of the internal capsule). This arrangement also appears to hold in thalamocortical projections from this nucleus and hence a lesion (hemorrhagic or presumably lacunar) could affect these projections or the most lateral portions of the ventral-posterior thalamus explaining this leg predominant clinical central pain picture.[37]

Implications of pharmacologic treatment trials have led to hypotheses regarding which neurotransmitter systems and/or channels are important in central neuropathic pain. Efficacy of intravenous lidocaine (for SCI pain and CPSP),[57] lamotrigine (for CPSP and SCI pain),[58, 59] and amitriptyline and carbamazepine (for CPSP)[60] suggests that sodium channels are important in mediating central pain states. The authors point out that sodium channels are increased in the central nervous system demyelinating lesions of MS patients, while acknowledging studies of sodium channel expression in humans or animal models of central pain are lacking.[61] The effect of clonidine administered epidurally with an efficacy similar, and in some cases superior, to morphine in a spinal cord injury central neuropathic pain cohort suggested the importance of noradrenergic systems in pain transmission in this pain population.[62] Intravenous infusion of ketamine, an *N*-methyl-D-aspartic acid (NMDA) antagonist, significantly reduced continuous and evoked pain in SCI central pain patients suggesting the importance of activation of central NMDA receptors in this syndrome (which has also been shown to be important in central sensitization of peripheral neuropathic pain).[63]

TREATMENT OF CENTRAL NEUROPATHIC PAIN

If one were to include case studies and small, nonrandomized series, there may appear a wide breadth of experience on the treatment of central neuropathic pain. Unfortunately, prospective cohort series and randomized, double-blind, placebo-controlled trials are limited. Systemic reviews of multiple grade II studies and subsequent recommendations do not exist. While the mechanisms of action may vary in the various central neuropathic pain states, the evidence suggests overall that there is considerable overlap in the end pathways leading to below level SCI, MS-related, and CPSP central neuropathic pain states. Therefore, particularly in the context of limited high quality studies for low prevalence pain syndromes, it is rational to extrapolate data suggesting efficacy in one central pain state to justify clinically treating a patient with another central pain state.

Some general principles apply to treating central neuropathic pain, as to all types of neuropathic pain.

- Start with a low dosage and increase the dosage slowly, but give an adequate trial – get to a high enough dose and treat long enough – to be able to assess efficacy.
- Recognize that all medications have side effects. A patient with physical, cognitive, language, and sometimes emotional and/or behavioral issues as a consequence of the disorder leading to the central pain syndrome may be more prone and/or intolerant of these side effects.
- Recognize that patients with disorders leading to a central pain syndrome (particularly MS and CPSP) likely require multiple other medications. Polypharmacy and drug interactions are a constant challenge for the treating physician.
- Set realistic expectations. Central neuropathic pain states are one of the most challenging pain conditions to treat. Resolution of the pain is generally not a realistic expectation. Farrar *et al.*[64] found that a numerical pain scale score improvement of two points or 30 percent correlated with what pain patients felt was a significant improvement on global impression of change scores. The number needed to treat (NNT) is generally based on the number of patients in a study with at least 30 percent pain improvement. Some studies provide number of patients with 50 percent pain improvement. Regardless, this defines a realistic and good outcome – 30–50 percent pain improvement is a good pain outcome for any individual medication.
- Rational polypharmacy, utilizing multiple medications concomitantly with different mechanisms of action, may provide additive pain relief benefit, but needs to be weighed against the invariable cumulative side effects.

Pharmacologic management

The majority of the literature is made up of case presentations and prospective and retrospective series. These have suggested efficacy of gabapentin,[65, 66, 67, 68, 69, 70, 71] lamotrigine,[72, 73, 74, 75] topiramate,[76] levetiracetam,[77, 78, 79] oxcarbazepine,[80] carbamazepine combined with amitriptyline,[81] phenytoin,[82, 83] valproate,[84] nortriptyline (although this study is listed as for central pain, most are from peripheral nerve generators),[85] mexiletine,[86] and acupuncture.[87] A small open label trial of topiramate for various central pain states ($n = 7$) showed no efficacy.[88]

Table 28.1 lists the grade II evidence (randomized, double-blind, placebo-controlled) for the pharmacologic treatment of central neuropathic pain. Included is a randomized, controlled, blinded, dose-response, but no placebo-controlled study on opioids for central pain.[97] A couple of newer studies of cannabinoids for MS-related pain are included giving the level of the study structure and/or notable sample size, despite pain measurements being a secondary outcome.[98, 99] Unfortunately, most of these high quality studies stand alone (either as a positive or negative study) without further confirmatory or dose-ranging studies. Hence there is no grade I evidence (i.e. strong evidence from a systemic review of multiple grade II studies) for any of the pharmacologic treatments of central neuropathic pain.

In summary, the literature provides good support for the use of gabapentin (at least 1800 mg/day)[91] and pregabalin (mean dosage 460 mg/day)[92][II] for SCI central pain, lamotrigine (mean dosages 200–400 mg/day) for CPSP[58][II] and incomplete SCI related at- and below-level central pain,[59][II] amitriptyline (goal at least 75 mg/day) for CPSP,[60][II] (a study for SCI central pain with median dosages of 50 mg/day was negative[94]) and cannabinoids for MS-related central pain.[100, 101][II] The data for carbamazepine for central pain states are mixed, but the positive study was poorly powered and, while supportive of probable efficacy, limited in the strength of its conclusions.[89] As noted previously, given limited high quality data for these notoriously difficult to treat pain processes, it seems rational to extrapolate data suggesting efficacy in one central pain state to justify clinically treating a patient with another central pain state.

Parenteral and intrathecal treatments

Several well-designed, blinded, placebo-controlled trials of parenteral lidocaine have been performed with many showing a positive effect on central pain.[57, 105, 106][I] Unfortunately, the effects are short lived and this is not a viable long-term treatment option. These studies provide more information on pathogenesis than on treating a central pain patient in your office. They suggest the importance of central sodium channels and hence the rationale behind clinical trials of mexiletine and multiple anticonvulsants (carbamazepine, phenytoin, lamotrigine, for example). Intravenous propofol, a gamma-aminobutyric acid A (GABA-A) agonist, at subhypnotic doses has been reported to decrease central pain, but not peripheral neuropathic pain. This is hypothesized to be secondary to its strong effect on thalamic metabolic depression as well as on spinal cord gray matter, the somatosensory, frontal and cingulate cortex.[107, 108][III] Intravenous ketamine, an NMDA receptor antagonist, and alfentanil, a mu-opioid receptor agonist, have been shown in a randomized, placebo-controlled trial to decrease both continuous and evoked central neuropathic pain, highlighting the importance of NMDA receptors in central pain (whereas they have been long recognized as important in peripheral neuropathic pain states) and of the mu receptor systems in central pain modulation.[109][II] Unfortunately, dextromethorphan, an oral NMDA antagonist, was not effective for central pain.[96][II]

Parenteral opioid trials have suggested that intravenous morphine has analgesic effects on only some components of central neuropathic pain and in only a minority of patients and suggest long-term opioid therapy will be useful in only a small subset of central pain patients.[110, 111] Rowbotham *et al.*[97][II] have shown that oral opioids are effective in central pain states, however, long-term opioid trials in central pain are lacking.

Intrathecal (IT) trials are important as drugs can be administered through an intrathecal drug delivery system. IT baclofen has been shown in an open trial to reduce musculoskeletal, but not neuropathic, pain associated with spasticity following spinal cord injury.[112][III] In contradistinction, a controlled IT baclofen trial found it suppressed dysesthesias as well as spasm-related pain in a myelopathy cohort.[113][II] A blinded, randomized, placebo-controlled trial demonstrated efficacy of a combination of morphine and clonidine intrathecally in SCI central pain, although it was less efficacious for below level than at-level neuropathic pain. Interestingly, administered alone, morphine or clonidine were not superior to placebo, suggesting a synergistic effect of the two used in combination.[114][II] Finally, intrathecal (subarachnoid) lidocaine has been shown in a double-blind, placebo-controlled study to be effective in some patients with SCI central pain, although predicting that response is difficult. Spinal obstruction secondary to the SCI may prevent set up of a sensory level above the level of the injury and producing anesthesia above the level of a cervical SCI would be unsafe secondary to risk to the respiratory neurons.[115]

Surgical treatments

Numerous surgical remedies have been attempted and reported. Tasker,[9] a neurosurgeon, provides one of the most comprehensive reviews intermixed with his own extensive, generally published, observations. Interventional procedures can be broken into destructive lesions and stimulation procedures (neuromodulation).

Destructive lesions generally are applied to the spinal cord above the level of the lesion responsible for

Table 28.1 Randomized, controlled trials of oral treatments for central neuropathic pain.

Drug	Study	Type of central neuropathic pain	Dose	Design	Number of patients (n =)	Results	Number needed to treat for positive trials (95% confidence interval)
Carbamazepine	Espir *et al.*[89]	MS – paroxysmal disorders (14/21 painful – paresthesia 3, limb pain 6, trigeminal neuralgia 5)	200–800 mg/day (mean 540 mg/day)	Crossover ($n = 6$); remaining group ($n = 15$) case series	21 (only 6 compared w/ placebo)	*CBZ > placebo*	Cannot calculate
	Leijon *et al.*[60]	CPSP	800 mg/day	Crossover (3 phase: CBZ versus placebo and amitriptyline)	14	CBZ = placebo	–
Gabapentin	Tai *et al.*[90]	SCI – mixed neuropathic	1800 mg/day	Crossover	7	*GBP > placebo only for pain "unpleasantness"* GBP = placebo for all other (multiple) measures	Cannot calculate
	Levendoglu *et al.*[91]	SCI (complete) – all neuropathic (not further defined)	Up to 3600 mg/day (signif. pain relief not seen until 1800 mg/day; mean max tolerated dose 2850 mg/day)	Crossover	20	*GBP > placebo*	Cannot calculate
Pregabalin	Siddal *et al.*[92]	SCI – mostly below level pain	150–600 mg/day, bid dosing (mean: 460 mg/day)	Parallel	137	*PGB > placebo*	3.9 (2.2–5.8) 30% pain relief; 7.1 (3.9–43) 50% pain relief
Lamotrigine	Vestergaard *et al.*[58]	CPSP	200 mg/day	Crossover	27	*LTG > placebo*	3 (1.8–9)
	Finnerup *et al.*[59]	SCI – mixed neuropathic	200–400 mg/day	Crossover	22	LTG = placebo overall and complete SCI subset; *LTG > placebo incomplete SCI at or below level pain*	– 12 (2–∞)
Valproate	Drewes *et al.*[93]	SCI – below level pain	600–2400 mg/day	Crossover	20	Valproate = placebo	–
Amitriptyline	Leijon *et al.*[60]	CPSP	75 mg/day	Crossover (3 phase versus placebo and carbamazepine)	15	*Ami > placebo*	1.7 (1.1–3)

(Continued over)

Table 28.1 Randomized, controlled trials of oral treatments for central neuropathic pain (continued).

Drug	Study	Type of central neuropathic pain	Dose	Design	Number of patients (n =)	Results	Number needed to treat for positive trials (95% confidence interval)
	Cardenas *et al.*[94]	SCI – mixed nociceptive and neuropathic	10–125 mg/day (median 50 mg/day)	Parallel	84	Amitriptyline = active placebo (benztropine)	–
Trazodone	Davidoff *et al.* 1987[95]	SCI – below level neuropathic	150 mg/day	Parallel	18	Trazodone = placebo	–
Dextromethorphan	McQuay *et al.*[96]	Various neuropathic pain (some CPSP)	40.5–81 mg/day, TID dosing	Crossover	19 (only 9 central - CPSP)	Dextromethorphan = placebo	–
Levorphanol	Rowbotham *et al.*[97]	Mixed neuropathic (23/81 central pain)	Upto: 3.15 mg/day low dose cohort (mean 2.7 mg/day); 15.75 mg/day high dose cohort (mean: 8.9 mg/day)	Double blind, randomized, dose-response, NON-placebo controlled (high dose versus low dose)	23/81 central pain: 10 CPSP, 8 MS, 5 SCI	High dose > low dose (no placebo used); all subsets had pain reduced (all CPSP 10% from baseline; MS 27%; SCI 23%; but higher % in high dose groups)	–
Cannabis extract and Δ^9-THC (tetra-hydrocannabinol – Marinol)	Zajicek *et al.*[98]	MS – spasticity (1° outcome) and pain (2° outcome)	Variable (flexible based on tolerance, body-weight)	Parallel 3-way: (cannabis extract versus Δ^9-THC versus placebo)	630	Cannabis extract and Δ^9-THC = placebo for spasticity, *but > placebo for pain*	Cannot calculate
Cannabis extract (cannabidiol and Δ^9-THC)	Wade *et al.*[99]	MS – multiple symptoms including pain (ill defined type)	Variable	Parallel	160 (37 pain)	Cannabis extract = placebo overall and pain subset	–
Dronabinol (cannabinoid)	Svendsen *et al.*[100]	MS	10 mg/day	Crossover	24	Dronabinol > placebo	3 (1.7–13.8) 30% pain relief; 3.5 (1.9–24.8) 50% pain relief
Cannabis extract (cannabidiol and Δ^9-THC)	Rog *et al.*[101]	MS – 59/66 dysesthesias; 7/66 painful spasms	Variable – self titrated (mean 9.6 sprays – 2.7 mg THC, 2.5 mg CBD per spray)	Parallel	66	Cannabis extract > placebo	3.7 (2.2–13.0) 50% pain relief

CPSP, central post-stroke pain; MS, multiple sclerosis related pain; SCI, spinal cord injury related pain. Extrapolated from the individual cited studies, Sidall *et al.*,[10] Finnerup *et al.*,[102, 103] and Frese *et al.*[104]
Entries in italic in the Results column represent positive results.

the pain: cordotomy (selective lesioning of the lateral spinothalamic tract pain pathways in the anterolateral cord contralateral to the side of pain (as spinothalamic pathways decussate two to five segments above the level of input into the system) – open and percutaneous methods have been described), cordectomy (transaction of the spinal cord), dorsal root entry zone (DREZ) lesioning, commissurotomy (i.e. midline myelotomy – transection of the midline crossing fibers).[116, 117] Given variable, often disappointing long-term results and associated risks, destructive interventions are less commonly practiced with today's pain management alternatives.[8, 10, 116] Pertinent to all destructive spinal cord interventions, pain tends to recur over time (generally years) and it is paroxysmal, neuralgiform shooting pain (generally into the legs from SCI) and evoked pain/allodynia/hyperalgesia from peripheral nerve lesions (as opposed to steady constant pain) that appear most amenable to these destructive therapies.[9, 118, 119] Cordectomy has been reported to be most beneficial for lesions below T10.[9] Cordotomy is directed at contralateral pain below the level of the lesion (although bilateral lesions can be performed for bilateral pain).[120] Tasker notes that of those with neuralgiform or evoked pain, more than 50 percent receive good and more than 25 percent receive fair relief from cordotomy, although pain eventually returns.[9] There is a risk of ipsilateral arm paresis or respiratory compromise with cervical cordotomy which is avoided with DREZ lesions which also can be performed open or percutaneously. DREZ lesions would best targeted at level, segmental spinal cord pain.[9, 10, 118] Destructive lesions of the brain have been described for CPSP including mesencephalic tractotomy and medial thalamotomy (various targets reported, but all include the spinoreticulothalamic pathways), but their outcomes have been disappointing[8, 9] and seem rarely practiced today.

Neuromodulation relevant to central pain syndromes includes spinal cord stimulation (SCS), motor cortex stimulation, and deep brain stimulation. SCS involves placement of a wire electrode array epidurally in line with the dorsal columns. It has no role for supra-spinal cord central pain states. Its use is limited in spinal cord central pain secondary to wallerian degeneration of the posterior columns with a lower cord lesion. When this occurs, the dorsal columns cannot be stimulated to "capture" and create non-noxious paresthesias over the area of pain. Complete or near-complete lesions have little chance of successful stimulation because of this, whereas some incomplete lesions may be amendable.[121] It has been suggested that because of wallerian degeneration, SCS may be more useful for at-level, segmental pain than below-level pain after SCI.[10] Second, when related to trauma, safe access to the epidural space or ability to position the electrode appropriately may be impaired by skeletal injuries or prior surgical intervention addressing these injuries. Finally, when related to a cord neoplasm, magnetic resonance imaging (MRI) is contraindicated with an SCS system in place, thus eliminating the ability for serial imaging follow up or assessment for tumor recurrence. All of these factors and published reports suggest that SCS has a limited role for central pain syndromes and, even when effective, initially becomes less so over time.[9, 10, 119, 121, 122][III], [IV]

Motor cortex stimulation (MCS) involves surgical placement of an electrode array somatotopically oriented in the epidural space to overlie the primary motor cortex representing the area of primary pain. Given the relative proportional and more superficial representation of face and hand/arm portions of the homunculus in the cortical somatotopic organization (compared with foot/leg), one might anticipate pain in these regions may be better addressed with MCS than lower extremity pain. Indeed, atypical facial pain syndromes seem most amenable to MCS neuromodulation, although other central pain types have been reported to respond as well.[123, 124][III] Deep brain stimulation (DBS) has been reported with stimulation of the peri-aqueductal and ventricular gray matter (PAG, PVG – the primary targets for nociceptive pain) as well as sensory thalamus and medial lemniscus (the primary targets for neuropathic pain) with the goal (like spinal cord stimulation) of producing a distracting, non-noxious paresthesia in the area of pain. It has been reported that DBS with some sensory thalamus targets may promote (as opposed to relieve) pain in some CPSP patients with allodynia.[9] Reported success rates are variable but generally in the region of 20–50 percent.[9, 125, 126]

CONCLUSIONS

Central neuropathic pain states can stem from variable pathologies affecting various levels of the central nervous system, but invariably are severe, dysfunctioning, and all too often humbling in their response to treatment.

REFERENCES

1. Merskey H, Lindblom U, Mumford JM *et al.* Pain terms: A current list with definitions and notes on usage. In: Merskey H, Bogduk N (eds). *Classification of chronic pain: Descriptions of chronic pain syndromes and definitions of pain terms*, 2nd edn. Seattle: IASP Press, 1994 (reprinted 2002).
2. Bouhassira D, Attal N, Fermanian J *et al.* Development and validation of the Neuropathic Pain Symptom Inventory. *Pain.* 2004; **108**: 248–57.
3. Krause SJ, Backonja MM. Development of a neuropathic pain questionnaire. *Clinical Journal of Pain.* 2003; **19**: 306–14.
4. Bennett M. The LANSS Pain Scale: the Leeds assessment of neuropathic symptoms and signs. *Pain.* 2001; **92**: 147–57.
5. Galer BS, Jensen MP. Development and preliminary validation of a pain measure specific to neuropathic

pain: the Neuropathic Pain Scale. *Neurology.* 1997; **48**: 332–8.

6. Putzke JD, Richards JS, Hicken BL *et al.* Pain classification following spinal cord injury: the utility of verbal descriptors. *Spinal Cord.* 2002; **40**: 118–27.
7. Störmer S, Gerner HJ, Gruninger W *et al.* Chronic pain/dysaesthesiae in spinal cord injury patients: results of a multicentre study. *Spinal Cord.* 1997; **35**: 446–55.
* 8. Boivie J. Central pain. In: McMahon SB, Koltzenburg M (eds). *Wall and Melzack's textbook of pain*, 5th edn. Elsevier Churchill Livingstone, 2006: 1057–74.
* 9. Tasker RR. Central pain states. In: Warfield CA, Bajwa ZH (eds). *Principles and practice of pain medicine*, 2nd edn. New York: McGraw-Hill Medical Publishing Division, 2004: 394–404.
* 10. Siddall PJ. Pain following spinal cord injury. In: McMahon SB, Koltzenburg M (eds). *Wall and Melzack's textbook of pain*, 5th edn. Elsevier Churchill Livingstone, 2005: 1043–55.
11. Noseworthy JH, Lucchinetti C, Rodriguez M, Weinshenker BG. Multiple sclerosis. *New England Journal of Medicine.* 2000; **343**: 938–52.
12. Hirtz D, Thurman DJ, Gwinn-Hardy K *et al.* How common are the "common" neurologic disorders? *Neurology.* 2007; **68**: 326–37.
13. Clifford DB, Trotter JL. Pain in multiple sclerosis. *Archives of Neurology.* 1984; **41**: 1270–2.
14. Svendsen KB, Jensen TS, Overvad K *et al.* Pain in patients with multiple sclerosis. *Archives of Neurology.* 2003; **60**: 1089–94.
15. Kassirer MR, Osterberg DH. Pain in chronic multiple sclerosis. *Journal of Pain and Symptom Management.* 1987; **2**: 95–7.
* 16. Osterberg A, Boivie J, Thuomas K-A. Central pain in multiple sclerosis – prevalence and clinical characteristics. *European Journal of Pain.* 2005; **9**: 531–42.
17. Solaro C, Brichetto G, Amato MP *et al.* The prevalence of pain in multiple sclerosis. A multicenter cross-sectional study. *Neurology.* 2004; **63**: 919–21.
18. Ehde DM, Osborne TL, Hanley MA *et al.* The scope and nature of pain in persons with multiple sclerosis. *Multiple Sclerosis.* 2006; **12**: 629–38.
* 19. Moulin DE, Foley KM, Ebers GC. Pain syndromes in multiple sclerosis. *Neurology.* 1988; **38**: 1830–4.
20. Stenager E, Knudsen L, Jensen K. Acute and chronic pain syndromes in multiple sclerosis. *Acta Neurologica Scandinavica.* 1991; **84**: 197–200.
21. Kalia LV, O'Connor PW. Severity of chronic pain and its relationship to quality of life in multiple sclerosis. *Multiple Sclerosis.* 2005; **11**: 322–7.
22. Vermote R, Ketelaer P, Carton H. Pain in multiple sclerosis patients. A prospective study using the McGill Pain Questionnaire. *Clinical Neurology and Neurosurgery.* 1986; **88**: 87–93.
23. Beiske AG, Pedersen ED, Czujko B, Myhr KM. Pain and sensory complaints in multiple sclerosis. *European Journal of Neurology.* 2004; **11**: 479–82.
24. Ehde DM, Gibbons LE, Chwastiak L *et al.* Chronic pain in a large community sample of persons with multiple sclerosis. *Multiple Sclerosis.* 2003; **9**: 605–11.
25. Archibald CJ, McGrath PJ, Ritvo PG. Pain prevalence, severity, and impact in a clinic sample of multiple sclerosis patients. *Pain.* 1994; **58**: 89–93.
26. Statistics. CfDCNCfH. Death – leading causes and stroke/cerebrovascular disease. 2007.
27. Bowsher D. Central pain: clinical and physiological characteristics. *Journal of Neurology, Neurosurgery, and Psychiatry.* 1996; **61**: 62–9.
* 28. Nasreddine ZS, Saver JL. Pain after thalamic stroke: Right diencephalic predominance and clinical features in 180 patients. *Neurology.* 1997; **48**: 1196–9.
29. Boivie J, Leijon G, Johansson I. Central post-stroke pain – a study of the mechanisms through analysis of the sensory abnormalities. *Pain.* 1989; **37**: 173–85.
30. Bowsher D, Leijon G, Thuomas KA. Central poststroke pain: Correlation of MRI with clinical pain characteristics and sensory abnormalities. *Neurology.* 1998; **51**: 1352–8.
* 31. MacGowan DJ, Janal MN, Clark WC *et al.* Central poststroke pain and Wallenberg's lateral medullary infarction: frequency, character, and determinants in 63 patients. *Neurology.* 1997; **49**: 120–5.
32. Rosamond W, Flegal K, Friday G *et al.* Heart disease and stroke statistics – 2007 update: a report from the American Heart Association Statistics Committee and Stroke Statistics Subcommittee. *Circulation.* 2007; **115**: e69–171.
33. American Heart Association. Statistics. Cited December 2007. Available from: www.americanheart.org/statistics/05stroke.html.
* 34. Andersen G, Vestergaard K, Ingeman-Nielsen M, Jensen TS. Incidence of central post-stroke pain. *Pain.* 1995; **61**: 187–93.
35. Dejérine J, Roussy G. La syndrome thalamique. *Revue Neurologique.* 1906; **14**: 521–32.
36. Leijon G, Boivie J, Johansson I. Central post-stroke pain – neurological symptoms and pain characteristics. *Pain.* 1989; **36**: 13–25.
37. Kim JS. Central post-stroke pain or paresthesia in lenticulo-capsular hemorrhages. *Neurology.* 2003; **61**: 679–82.
38. Bogousslavsky J, Regli F, Uske A. Thalamic infarcts: Clinical syndromes, etiology, and prognosis. *Neurology.* 1988; **38**: 837–48.
39. Bowsher D. Sensory consequences of stroke. *Lancet.* 1993; **341**: 156.
40. Leijon G, Bowsher D. Somatosensory finding in central post-stroke pain and controls. *Pain.* 1990; (Suppl. 5): 468.
41. Bowsher D. Allodynia in relation to lesion site in central post-stroke pain. *Journal of Pain.* 2005; **6**: 736–40.
42. Widar M, Ek AC, Ahlstrom G. Coping with long-term pain after a stroke. *Journal of Pain and Symptom Management.* 2004; **27**: 215–25.
43. Greenspan JD, Ohara S, Sarlani E, Lenz FA. Allodynia in patients with post-stroke central pain (CPSP) studied by

statistical quantitative sensory testing within individuals. *Pain*. 2004; **109**: 357–66.
44. Vestergaard K, Nielsen J, Andersen G *et al*. Sensory abnormalities in consecutive, unselected patients with central post-stroke pain. *Pain*. 1995; **61**: 177–86.
45. Jensen TS, Lenz FA. Central post-stroke pain: a challenge for the scientist and the clinician. *Pain*. 1995; **61**: 161–4.
46. Craig AD, Reiman EM, Evans A, Bushnell MC. Functional imaging of an illusion of pain. *Nature*. 1996; **384**: 258–60.
47. Kim JS, Greenspan JD, Coghill RC *et al*. Lesions limited to the human thalamic prinicpal somatosensory nucleus (ventral caudal) are associated with loss of cold sensations and central pain. *Journal of Neuroscience*. 2007; **27**: 4995–5005.
48. Wessel K, Vieregge P, Kessler C, Kompf D. Thalamic stroke: Correlation of clinical symptoms, somatosensory evoked potentials, and CT findings. *Acta Neurologica Scandinavica*. 1994; **90**: 167–73.
49. Finnerup NB, Gyldensted C, Nielsen E *et al*. MRI in chronic spinal cord injury patients with and without central pain. *Neurology*. 2003; **61**: 1569–75.
50. Finnerup NB, Johannesen IL, Fuglsang-Frederiksen FW *et al*. Sensory function in spinal cord injury patients with and without central pain. *Brain*. 2003; **126**: 57–70.
51. Defrin R, Ohry A, Blumen N, Urca G. Characterization of chronic pain and somatosensory function in spinal cord injury subjects. *Pain*. 2001; **89**: 253–63.
52. Eide P, Jorum E, Stenehjem AE. Somatosensory findings in patients with spinal cord injury and central dysesthesia pain. *Journal of Neurology, Neurosurgery, and Psychiatry*. 1996; **60**: 411–15.
53. Siddall PJ, McClelland JM, Rutkowski SB, Cousins MJ. A longitudinal study of the prevalence and characteristics of pain in the first 5 years following spinal cord injury. *Pain*. 2003; **103**: 249–57.
54. Spillane W. Pain syndromes in selected neurological disorders. In: Raj PR (ed). *Practical management of pain*, 3rd edn. St Louis: Mosby, Inc., 2000.
55. Lenz FA, Seike M, Lin YC *et al*. Thermal and pain sensations evoked by microstimulation in the area of the human ventrocaudal nucleus (Vc). *Journal of Neurophysiology*. 1993; **70**: 200–12.
56. Lenz FA, Kwan HC, Martin R *et al*. Characteristics of somatotopic organization and spontaneous neuronal activity in the region of the thalamic principal sensory nucleus in patients with spinal cord transection. *Journal of Neurophysiology*. 1994; **72**: 1570–87.
57. Attal N, Gaude V, Brasseur L *et al*. Intravenous lidocaine in central pain: a double-blind, placebo-controlled, psychophysical study. *Neurology*. 2000; **54**: 564–74.
* 58. Vestergaard K, Andersen G, Gottrup H *et al*. Lamotrigine for central post-stroke pain. A randomized controlled trial. *Neurology*. 2001; **56**: 184–90.
* 59. Finnerup NB, Sindrup SH, Bach FW *et al*. Lamotrigine in spinal cord injury pain: a randomized controlled trial. *Pain*. 2002; **96**: 375–83.
* 60. Leijon G, Boivie J. Central post-stroke pain – a controlled trial of amitriptyline and carbamazepine. *Pain*. 1989; **36**: 27–36.
61. Max MB, Hagen NA. Do changes in brain sodium channels cause central pain? *Neurology*. 2000; **54**: 544.
62. Glynn CJ, Teddy PJ, Jamous MA *et al*. Role of spinal noradrenergic system in transmission of pain in patients with spinal cord injury. *Lancet*. 1986; **2**: 1249–50.
63. Eide P, Stubhaug A, Stenehjem AE. Central dysesthesia pain after traumatic spinal cord injury is dependent on N-methyl-D-aspartate receptor activation. *Neurosurgery*. 1995; **37**: 1080–7.
64. Farrar JT, Young JP, LaMoreaux L *et al*. Clinical importance of changes in chronic pain intensity measured on an 11-point numerical pain rating scale. *Pain*. 2001; **94**: 149–58.
65. Chen B, Stitik TP, Foye PM *et al*. Central post-stroke pain syndrome: yet another use for gabapentin? *American Journal of Physical Medicine*. 2002; **81**: 718–20.
66. To TP, Lim TC, Hill ST *et al*. Gabapentin for neuropathic pain following spinal cord injury. *Spinal Cord*. 2002; **40**: 282–5.
67. Putzke JD, Richards JS, Kezar L *et al*. Long-term use of gabapentin for treatment of pain after traumatic spinal cord injury. *Clinical Journal of Pain*. 2002; **18**: 116–21.
68. Kapadia NP, Harden N. Gabapentin for chronic pain in spinal cord injury: a case report. *Archives of Physical Medicine and Rehabilitation*. 2000; **81**: 1439–41.
69. Solaro C, Uccelli MM, Guglieri P *et al*. Gabapentin is effective in treating nocturnal painful spasms in multiple sclerosis. *Multiple Sclerosis*. 2000; **6**: 192–3.
70. Houtchens MK, Richert JR, Sami A, Rose JW. Open label gabapentin treatment for pain in multiple sclerosis. *Multiple Sclerosis*. 1997; **3**: 250–3.
71. Ness TJ, San Pedro EC, Richards JS *et al*. A case of spinal cord injury-related pain with baseline rCBF brain SPECT imaging and beneficial response to gabapentin. *Pain*. 1998; **78**: 139–43.
72. Leandri M, Lundardi G, Inglese M *et al*. Lamotrigine in trigeminal neuralgia secondary to multiple sclerosis. *Journal of Neurology*. 2000; **247**: 556–8.
73. Cianchetti C, Zuddas A, Randazzo AP *et al*. Lamotrigine adjunctive therapy in painful phenomena in MS: preliminary observations. *Neurology*. 1999; **53**: 433.
74. McCleane G. Lamotrigine can reduce neurogenic pain associated with multiple sclerosis. *Clinical Journal of Pain*. 1998; **14**: 269–70.
75. Canavero S, Bonicalzi V. Lamotrigine control of central pain. *Pain*. 1996; **68**: 179–81.
76. Dinoff BL, Richards JS, Ness TJ. Use of topiramate for spinal cord injury-related pain. *Journal of Spinal Cord Medicine*. 2003; **26**: 401–03.
77. Rizzo M. Adjunctive levetiracetam therapy for myelopathic pain and paresthesias. In: *Program and abstracts of the 22nd Annual Meeting of the American Pain Society* Chicago, IL. March 20–23, 2003, Abstract 911.
78. Guay DRP. Oxcarbazepine, topiramate, zonisamide, and levetiracetam: Potential uses in neuropathic pain.

American Journal of Geriatric Pharmacotherapy. 2003; **1**: 18–37.
79. Hawker K, Frohman E, Racke M. Levetiracetam for phasic spasticity in multiple sclerosis. *Archives of Neurology.* 2003; **60**: 1772–4.
80. Solaro C, Restivo D, Mancardi GL, Tanganelli P. Oxcarbazepine for treating paroxysmal painful symptoms in multiple sclerosis: a pilot study. *Neurological Sciences.* 2007; **28**: 156–8.
81. Sandford PR, Lindblom LB, Haddox JD. Amitriptyline and carbamazepine in the treatment of dysesthetic pain in spinal cord injury. *Archives of Physical Medicine and Rehabilitation.* 1992; **73**: 300–01.
82. Agnew DC, Goldberg VD. A brief trial of phenytoin therapy for thalamic pain. *Bulletin of the Los Angeles Neurological Societies.* 1976; **41**: 9–12.
83. Cantor FK. Phenytoin treatment of thalamic pain. *British Medical Journal.* 1972; **4**: 590.
84. Zachariah SB, Borges EF, Varghese R *et al.* Positive response to oral divalproex sodium (Depakote) in patients with spasticity and pain. *American Journal of the Medical Sciences.* 1994; **308**: 38–40.
85. Panerai AE, Monza G, Movilia P *et al.* A randomized, within-patient, cross-over, placebo-controlled trial on the efficacy and tolerability of the tricyclic antidepressants chlorimipramine and nortriptyline in central pain. *Acta Neurologica Scandinavica.* 1991; **82**: 34–8.
86. Awerbuch GI. Mexiletine for thalamic pain syndrome. *International Journal of Neuroscience.* 1990; **55**: 129–33.
87. Yen HL, Chan W. An East-West approach to the management of central post-stroke pain. *Cerebrovascular Diseases.* 2003; **16**: 27–30.
88. Caverno S, Bonicalzi V, Paolotti R. Lack of effect of topiramate for central pain. *Neurology.* 2002; **58**: 831–2.
* 89. Espir MLE, Millac P. Treatment of paroxysmal disorders in multiple sclerosis with carbamazepine (Tegretol). *Journal of Neurology, Neurosurgery, and Psychiatry.* 1970; **33**: 528–31.
* 90. Tai Q, Kirshblum S, Chen B *et al.* Gabapentin in the treatment of neuropathic pain after spinal cord injury: a prospective, randomized, double-blind, crossover trial. *Journal of Spinal Cord Medicine.* 2002; **25**: 100–05.
* 91. Levendoglu F, Ogun CO, Ozerbil O *et al.* Gabapentin is a first line drug for treatment of neuropathic pain in spinal cord injury. *Spine.* 2004; **29**: 743–51.
* 92. Siddall PJ, Cousins MJ, Otte A *et al.* Pregabalin in central neuropathic pain associated with spinal cord injury: A placebo-controlled trial. *Neurology.* 2006; **67**: 1792–800.
93. Drewes AM, Andreasen A, Poulsen LH. Valproate for treatment of chronic central pain after spinal cord injury. A double-blind cross-over study. *Paraplegia.* 1994; **32**: 565–9.
94. Cardenas DD, Warms CA, Turner JA *et al.* Efficacy of amitriptyline for relief of pain in spinal cord injury: results of a randomized controlled trial. *Pain.* 2002; **96**: 365–73.
95. Davidoff G, Guarracini M, Roth E *et al.* Trazodone hydrochloride in the treatment of dysesthetic pain in traumatic myelopathy: a randomized, double-blind, placebo-controlled study. *Pain.* 1987; **29**: 151–61.
96. McQuay HJ, Carroll D, Jadad AR *et al.* Dextromethorphan for the treatment of neuropathic pain: a double-blind randomised controlled crossover trial with integral n-of-1 design. *Pain.* 1994; **59**: 127–33.
* 97. Rowbotham M, Twilling L, Davies PS *et al.* Oral opioid therapy for chronic peripheral and central neuropathic pain. *New England Journal of Medicine.* 2003; **348**: 1223–32.
* 98. Zajicek J, Fox P, Sanders H *et al.* Cannabinoids for treatment of spasticity and other symptoms related to multiple sclerosis (CAMS study): multicentre randomised placebo-controlled trial. *Lancet.* 2003; **362**: 1517–26.
99. Wade DT, Makela P, Robson P *et al.* Do cannabis-based medicinal extracts have general or specific effects on symptoms in multiple sclerosis? A double-blind, randomized, placebo-controlled study on 160 patients. *Multiple Sclerosis.* 2004; **10**: 434–41.
*100. Svendsen KB, Jensen TS, Bach FW. Does the cannabinoid dronabinol reduce central pain in multiple sclerosis? Randomised double blind placebo controlled crossover trial. *British Medical Journal.* 2004; **329**: 253–60.
*101. Rog DJ, Nurmikko TJ, Friede T, Young CA. Randomized, controlled trial of cannabis-based medicine in central pain in multiple sclerosis. *Neurology.* 2005; **65**: 812–9.
102. Finnerup NB, Yezierski RP, Sang CN *et al.* Treatment of spinal cord injury pain. *Pain: Clinical Updates.* 2001; **IX**: 1–12.
103. Finnerup NB, Otto M, McQuay HJ *et al.* Algorithm for neuropathic pain treatment: An evidence based proposal. *Pain.* 2005; **118**: 289–305.
104. Frese A, Husstedt IW, Ringelstein EB, Evers S. Pharmacologic treatment of central post-stroke pain. *Clinical Journal of Pain.* 2006; **22**: 252–60.
105. Backonja MM, Gombar KA. Response of central pain syndromes to intravenous lidocaine. *Journal of Pain and Symptom Management.* 1992; **7**: 172–8.
106. Finnerup NB, Biering-Sorensen F, Johannesen IL *et al.* Intravenous lidocaine relieves spinal cord injury pain: a randomized controlled trial. *Anesthesiology.* 2005; **102**: 1023–30.
107. Canavero S, Bonicalzi V, Pagni CA *et al.* Propofol analgesia in central pain: preliminary clinical observations. *Journal of Neurology.* 1995; **242**: 561–7.
108. Canavero S, Bonicalzi V. Intravenous subhypnotic propofol in central pain: a double-blind, placebo-controlled, crossover study. *Clinical Neuropharmacology.* 2004; **27**: 182–6.
109. Eide PK, Stubhaug A, Stenehjem AE. Central dysesthesia pain after traumatic spinal cord injury is dependent on N-methyl-D-aspartate receptor activation. *Neurosurgery.* 1995; **37**: 1080–7.
110. Attal N, Guirimand F, Brasseur L *et al.* Effects of IV morphine in central pain: A randomized placebo-controlled study. *Neurology.* 2002; **58**: 554–63.

111. Kalman S, Osterberg A, Sorensen J *et al.* Morphine responsiveness in a group of well-defined multiple sclerosis patients: A study with IV morphine. *European Journal of Pain.* 2002; **6**: 69–80.
112. Loubser PG, Akman NM. Effects of intrathecal baclofen on chronic spinal cord injury pain. *Journal of Pain and Symptom Management.* 1996; **12**: 241–7.
113. Herman RM, D'Luzansky SC, Ippolito R. Intrathecal baclofen suppressed central pain in patients with spinal lesions: A pilot study. *Clinical Journal of Pain.* 1992; **8**: 338–45.
114. Siddall PJ, Molloy AR, Walker S, Rutkowski SB. The efficacy of intrathecal morphine and clonidine in the treatment of pain after spinal cord injury. *Anesthesia and Analgesia.* 2000; **91**: 1493–8.
115. Loubser PG, Donovan WH. Diagnostic spinal anesthesia in chronic spinal cord injury pain. *Paraplegia.* 1991; **29**: 25–36.
116. Kanpolat Y. Percutaneous cordotomy, tractotomy, and midline myelotomy: Minimally invasive stereotactic pain procedures. *Seminars in Neurosurgery.* 2004; **15**: 203–19.
117. Kanpolat Y. The surgical treatment of chronic pain: destructive therapies in the spinal cord. *Neurosurgery Clinics of North America.* 2004; **15**: 307–17.
118. Sindou M, Mertens P, Wael M. Microsurgical DREZotomy for pain due to spinal cord and/or cauda equina injuries: long-term results in a series of 44 patients. *Pain.* 2001; **92**: 159–71.
119. Tasker RR, DeCarvalho GTC, Dolan EJ. Intractable pain of spinal cord origin. Clinical features and implications for surgery. *Journal of Neurosurgery.* 1992; **77**: 373–8.
120. Kanpolat Y, Savas A, Caglar S *et al.* Computerized tomography-guided percutaneous bilateral selective cordotomy. *Neurosurgical Focus.* 1997; **2**: e4.
121. Cioni B, Meglio M, Plentimalli L, Visocchi M. Spinal cord stimulation in the treatment of paraplegic pain. *Journal of Neurosurgery.* 1995; **82**: 35–9.
122. Richardson RR, Meyer PR, Cerullo LJ. Neurostimulation in the modulation of intractable paraplegic and traumatic neuroma pains. *Pain.* 1980; **8**: 75–84.
123. Rasche D, Ruppolt M, Stippich C *et al.* Motor cortex stimulation for long-term relief of chronic neuropathic pain: A 10 year experience. *Pain.* 2006; **121**: 43–52.
124. Brown JA, Pilitsis JG. Motor cortex stimulation for central and neuropathic facial pain: A prospective study of 10 patients and observations of enhanced sensory and motor function during stimulation. *Neurosurg.* 2005; **56**: 290–7.
125. Levy RM, Lamb S, Adams JE. Treatment of chronic pain by deep brain stimulation: Long-term follow-up and review of the literature. *Neurosurgery.* 1987; **21**: 885–93.
126. Kumar K, Toth C, Nath RK. Deep brain stimulation for intractable pain: a 15 year experience. *Neursurgery.* 1997; **40**: 736–46.

29

Spinal cord injury

PHILIP J SIDDALL AND PAUL J WRIGLEY

KEY LEARNING POINTS

- Pain following spinal cord injury (SCI) is common and often severe, even in the acute phase.
- Pain following spinal cord injury is not a single entity.
- Neuropathic pain is the most difficult type of pain to treat following SCI.
- Different mechanisms are responsible for the various types of pain seen following SCI.
- Assessment and management of SCI pain requires a broad approach addressing biological, psychological, and social contributing factors.

INTRODUCTION

Although loss of mobility is often considered the most serious consequence of spinal cord injury, people with spinal cord injury (SCI) consistently rate pain as one of the most difficult problems.[1] A large number of studies demonstrate that around two-thirds of people following SCI experience persistent pain and approximately one-third of those, report their pain as severe.[2, 3, 4] Pain following SCI has a significant impact on quality of life and can contribute to disability by limiting participation in rehabilitation and return to work.[5, 6, 7, 8]

TYPES OF SCI PAIN

Towards a pain taxonomy

Before examining treatments, consideration should be given to the classification of SCI pain. Achieving optimal relief of pain relies on accurate identification of the type of pain present. A large number of SCI pain classification systems have been proposed[9, 10, 11, 12] and recent efforts have been made to achieve some consensus in the terminology used to describe the different types of pain seen following SCI. As part of this effort, the Spinal Cord Injury Pain Task Force of the International Association of the Study of Pain has proposed a taxonomy of pain that attempts to provide a structure for systematically identifying the different types of SCI pain.[13] Although efforts are continuing to develop a universally accepted taxonomy, this classification is at present cited most frequently and will be used in this chapter. This taxonomy proposes a tiered classification in which pain types are divided into nociceptive (musculoskeletal or visceral) and neuropathic (either above-level, at-level, or below-level) pain types (**Table 29.1**). For clinical purposes, the second tier classification outlines the five common types of pain encountered following SCI (described in more detail below under Musculoskeletal pain, Visceral pain, Above-level neuropathic pain, At-level neuropathic pain, and

Table 29.1 Proposed classification of pain related to spinal cord injury.[13]

Broad type (tier 1)	Broad system (tier 2)	Specific structures/pathology (tier 3)
Nociceptive	Musculoskeletal	Bone, joint, muscle trauma, or inflammation
		Mechanical instability
		Muscle spasm
		Secondary overuse syndromes
	Visceral	Renal calculus, bowel, sphincter dysfunction, etc.
		Dysreflexic headache
Neuropathic	Above level	Compressive mononeuropathies
		Complex regional pain syndromes
	At level	Nerve root compression (including cauda equina)
		Syringomyelia
		Spinal cord trauma/ischemia (transitional zone, etc.)
		Dual level cord and root trauma (double lesion syndrome)
	Below level	Spinal cord trauma/ischemia

Below-level neuropathic pain). Where neurological level of injury is used, this refers to the most caudal segment of the spinal cord with normal sensory and motor function bilaterally.[14]

MUSCULOSKELETAL PAIN

In the acute setting following injury, nociceptive pain arises from damage to structures including bone, ligaments, muscles, intervertebral disks, and facet joints. The pain is generally located in the region of preserved sensation close to the site of spinal injury, although it may radiate. People with incomplete SCI (where spinal cord pathways remain partially intact) also experience musculoskeletal pain below the neurological level. Chronic musculoskeletal pain may occur with overuse or abnormal use of structures, such as the arm and shoulder.[15, 16] For mobility reasons, this type of nociceptive pain is very common in people with paraplegia and much less common in people with tetraplegia.[17] Muscle spasm pain is another type of musculoskeletal pain commonly seen in people with incomplete injuries. For a full discussion of painful spasticity, please refer to Chapter 33, Management of painful spasticity.

VISCERAL PAIN

Pathology in visceral structures, such as urinary tract infections, bowel impaction, and renal calculi, will generally give rise to nociceptive pain, although the level of the injury will affect the quality of the pain. Individuals with paraplegia may experience visceral pain that is identical to those who have no spinal cord damage. Individuals with tetraplegia, however, may experience less well-defined, generalized unpleasant symptoms that are difficult to interpret. For a full discussion of the applied physiology of visceral pain, see Chapter 3, Applied physiology: persistent visceral pain.

ABOVE-LEVEL NEUROPATHIC PAIN

Neuropathic pain can occur above the neurological level of injury and includes pains that are not specific to SCI, such as complex regional pain syndrome (previously referred to as reflex sympathetic dystrophy, causalgia, or shoulder hand syndrome) and pain due to peripheral nerve injury. Although present in the general population, people with SCI may be more susceptible to some of these pains because of activities associated with wheelchair use or transfers.

AT-LEVEL NEUROPATHIC PAIN

At-level neuropathic pain refers to pain with the features typical of neuropathic pain and present in a band or segmental pattern within the dermatome at, and two dermatomes above or below, the neurological level of injury. This type of pain has also been referred to as segmental, transitional zone, border zone, end zone, and girdle zone pain, names that reflect its characteristic location in the dermatomes adjacent to the neurological level of injury. It is often associated with allodynia (pain from a normally nonpainful stimulus) or hyperalgesia (an exaggerated pain response) in the affected dermatomes. At-level neuropathic pain may be due to damage to either nerve roots (including the cauda equina) or the spinal cord itself. Syringomyelia (cyst formation within the spinal cord) must always be considered in the person who has delayed onset of at-level neuropathic pain, especially where there is a rising level of sensory loss. Loss of pain and temperature sensation is typical, but all sensory and motor functions can be affected.

BELOW-LEVEL NEUROPATHIC PAIN

This type of pain, which is also referred to as central dysesthesia syndrome, central pain, phantom pain, or deafferentation pain, presents with spontaneous and/or evoked pain which is present often diffusely caudal to the neurological level of SCI. It is characterized by sensations of burning, aching, stabbing, or electric shocks, often with hypersensitivity and it may develop some time after the initial injury. It is typically constant, varying with mood, distraction, and physical pathology (e.g. infections) and is not usually related to position or movement. Sudden noises or jarring movements may trigger this type of pain. Differences in the nature of below-level neuropathic pain may be apparent between those with complete and incomplete spinal cord lesions. Both complete and incomplete spinal cord injuries may be associated with the diffuse, burning pain that appears to be associated with spinothalamic tract damage. However, incomplete injuries are more likely to have an allodynic component due to sparing of tracts conveying touch sensations.

Psychological aspects of pain

Some classification systems have included psychological or psychogenic as a type of pain that occurs following SCI. However, applying a psychological label to the pain may be unhelpful. There is no doubt, however, that psychological issues significantly modify and potentially maintain the pain experience.[18, 19, 20] Persistent pain following SCI is associated with more depressive symptoms and greater perceived stress.[21, 22] There is also a strong relationship between pain, spasticity, abnormal nonpainful sensations, and sadness.[1] Therefore, efforts should be directed at elucidating the underlying psychological contributors and consequences associated with the pain, rather than simply labeling the pain as "all in their head."

MECHANISMS

As expected, the different types of pain observed following SCI have a range of possible generators and contributing factors.[23] Although regarded as a distinct type of pain, neuropathic SCI pain is not a single entity and may present in different ways that may reflect different underlying pathophysiological processes. The focus of this section will be on the mechanisms that may be responsible for the development of neuropathic SCI pain and in particular at-level and below-level neuropathic pain. As with all types of pain, abnormal processes may occur at peripheral, spinal, and supraspinal levels and it may be helpful to consider pathophysiological mechanisms using this broad framework.

Peripheral generator

Damage to spinal structures may result in impingement of nerve roots entering the spinal cord. This may lead to the generation of impulses within primary afferents and the production of radicular at-level neuropathic pain. The mechanisms responsible for this type of pain are similar, if not identical, to the mechanisms underlying other conditions in which peripheral neuropathic pain occurs following trauma to nerve roots (see Chapter 1, Applied physiology: neuropathic pain, which outlines neuropathic pain mechanisms).

Spinal generator

As mentioned above, at-level neuropathic pain may also be dependent on the presence of a spinal generator or amplifier. Several case reports of spinal local anesthetic blockade in people with SCI pain describe complete (although temporary) abolition of pain with sensory block up to and above the level of injury.[24] This ability of spinal local anesthetic blockade to relieve neuropathic pain following SCI led to the proposition that there was an "irritated focus" located at or above the rostral end of the spinal cord injury.

These clinical observations have, to some extent, been supported by subsequent investigations using animal models of SCI pain.[23] In spinal dorsal horn neurons above the site of injury, these models demonstrate an increased neuronal responsiveness to peripheral stimuli, an increase in the level of background neuronal activity and the presence of neuronal after-discharges following a stimulus.[25, 26, 27] This increase in neuronal excitability may be a result of either increased excitation or reduced inhibition. In addition, SCI results in glial activation and increased cytokine release,[28, 29] as well as structural reorganization of inputs in the dorsal horn of the spinal cord.[30]

Below-level neuropathic pain may also be dependent on the presence of a spinal generator. A higher proportion of patients with below-level neuropathic SCI pain have sensory hypersensitivity in dermatomes at the neurological level of injury than pain-free SCI patients.[31] This suggests that neuronal hyperexcitability at the level of the injury may play a role in below-level neuropathic pain. Below-level neuropathic pain may therefore be a result of a supraspinal neuroplastic changes in response to a spinothalamic lesion together with neuronal hyperexcitability due to gray matter lesions at the rostral end of the injury.

Supraspinal generator

A number of observations suggest that changes at more rostral levels of the central nervous system may also be important in the development of pain. Spinal local anesthetic blockade does not always result in relief of pain despite the presence of a demonstrated sensory block above the level of injury.[32] In addition, peripheral, sympathetic, and spinal blockade, and even surgical cordotomy above the level of injury does not reliably reduce neuropathic pain following SCI.[33]

The question then remains as to which supraspinal structures may be involved. Loss of inputs to the thalamus may lead to alterations in function which are associated with the presence of neuropathic pain. Electrophysiological studies in humans have demonstrated that deafferented thalamic neurons have abnormal patterns of activity including high rates of spontaneous bursting,[34, 35] although thalamic neuronal bursting alone may not be sufficient to explain the presence of pain.[36] Further evidence supporting the thalamus as a key supraspinal site of importance in SCI neuropathic pain includes research demonstrating alterations in the expression of sodium channels,[37] electrophysiological,[38] biochemical,[39] and blood flow[40] changes in the thalamus of people with SCI pain, and the demonstration of abnormal spontaneous and evoked activity of thalamic neurons in contusive SCI animal models.[41, 42]

Changes in other supraspinal sites, beyond the thalamus, are also likely to be important in the development of persistent neuropathic pain following SCI. The extent to which these supraspinal changes are dependent on ongoing abnormal ascending inputs is unclear. However, there is increasing evidence that pathophysiological changes occur at peripheral, spinal, and supraspinal levels and may contribute in varying degrees to the development of neuropathic SCI pain.

PATIENT ASSESSMENT

The primary aim of patient assessment is to identify the main contributors to pain through a careful history, physical examination, and appropriate further investigations or diagnostic procedures. A useful way of categorizing contributors is to use three broad categories: biological (nociceptive and neuropathic), psychological, and social. Although psychosocial factors rarely act as pain generators, they invariably impact on an individual's pain experience and need to be considered as part of any pain assessment.[1, 22] Psychological contributors modifying and maintaining pain include mood (e.g. anxiety and depression), pain behaviors (e.g. fear avoidance), and cognitions (e.g. catastrophizing). Social contributors include physical factors, such as wheelchair use and seating, workplace ergonomics, and other factors, such as relationships with family, friends, colleagues, and superiors at work, and injury compensation. For a full discussion of psychological assessment, see Chapter 10, The psychological assessment of pain in patients with chronic pain.

Musculoskeletal pain

If musculoskeletal pain is present, physical examination (site of tenderness, limitation of movement, muscle tone) will help to determine the structures that may be affected and the presence of inflammation or muscle spasm. There is often a relationship with activity or position. Particularly in the acute phase, if skeletal damage is suspected, investigations such as x-rays, computerized tomography (CT), and magnetic resonance imaging (MRI) may help to identify pathology, such as a fracture, dislocation, spinal misalignment, or instability. In the chronic phase, restriction in range of movement of the upper limb may suggest an overuse syndrome. The pain is described as aching in the area of pressure or overuse and is worse with use of involved joints or pressure on the part. For a full discussion of musculoskeletal pain, see Chapter 2, Applied physiology: persistent musculoskeletal pain.

Visceral pain

Visceral pain may be identified by location (pelvis, abdomen, or thorax) and by pain features (dull, poorly localized, bloating, and cramping in nature). The presence of visceral pain requires a standard diagnostic approach similar to that used in the person without SCI. However, in the person with SCI, particular attention should be paid to conditions that are more common in this population. These include infection of the urinary tract, obstruction from ureteric calculi, and bowel impaction. Other relatively common conditions to consider include cholelithiasis and esophagitis.

Physical examination and the appropriate tests (full blood count, electrolytes, urea and creatinine, liver function tests, inflammatory markers, urine culture) and imaging (ultrasound, x-rays, CT scan and MRI) or other special investigations (e.g. endoscopy) will help to localize the source of pain. However, diagnosis is often difficult when sensory inputs from visceral structures are disturbed. If investigations fail to find evidence of visceral pathology, and treatments directed at visceral pathology do not relieve the pain, then consideration must be given to classifying the pain as neuropathic rather than visceral. The onset of headache in a person with an upper thoracic or cervical SCI should alert the clinician to the possibility of a visceral disturbance, such as bladder distension or bowel impaction, producing autonomic dysreflexia. Autonomic dysreflexia may pose a medical emergency. For a full discussion of visceral pain, see Chapter 3, Applied physiology: persistent visceral pain.

Above-level neuropathic pain

Above-level neuropathic pain is located in the region above the neurological level of injury. Assessment depends on the description of the pain, the use of physical examination to detect the nature of any sensory disturbance, the presence of other features, such as autonomic dysfunction, and the use of diagnostic techniques, such as nerve conduction studies, CT scan, and MRI.

At-level and below-level neuropathic pain

At-level neuropathic pain is located adjacent to the neurological level of injury and has neuropathic pain descriptors, e.g. burning, tingling, evoked by brushing.[43] Below-level neuropathic pain is located diffusely below the neurological level of injury, but does not include the dermatomes immediately caudal (see **Figure 29.1**). At-level neuropathic pain may be due to peripheral nerve injury and nerve root impingement. This may be suggested by a pattern of pain in the region of a nerve or dermatomes that correspond to suspected trauma. Although not definitive, nerve root pain may be suggested by a unilateral distribution. Diagnosis is assisted by radiographic, CT, or MRI evidence of compression of the nerve root in the foramen by bone or disk that correlates with the location of the pain. If investigations fail to find evidence of a peripheral nerve lesion, the pain is possibly due to central changes and further assessment is unlikely to be helpful or provide further benefit in deciding on appropriate treatment. If there has been a recent change in the location or characteristics of the pain, magnetic resonance imaging may be useful to determine the formation or progression of syringomyelia.

Psychological and environmental contributors

As mentioned earlier, psychological and environmental contributors to the experience of pain need to be identified. These may include mood dysfunction, such as depression and anxiety, maladaptive coping strategies, such as fear avoidance and catastrophizing, and social reinforcers, such as over-solicitous family members. This entails careful observation and listening, obtaining input from family, friends, and other team members and may require assistance from other professionals with formal training in psychological or psychiatric medicine.

PAIN MANAGEMENT

Having identified the most likely cause of the pain, the next step is to, where possible, treat the underlying cause of the pain. However, in many situations, elimination of the cause of the pain either in the short- or long-term may not be possible. The focus of treatment then becomes symptomatic relief or helping the patient to manage their pain. There are a large number of treatments that are used for symptom relief, often with little evidence of efficacy. Treatments for each type of pain are described with the level of supporting evidence indicated.

Musculoskeletal pain

Acute inflammatory musculoskeletal pain often follows direct trauma to musculoskeletal structures and there is

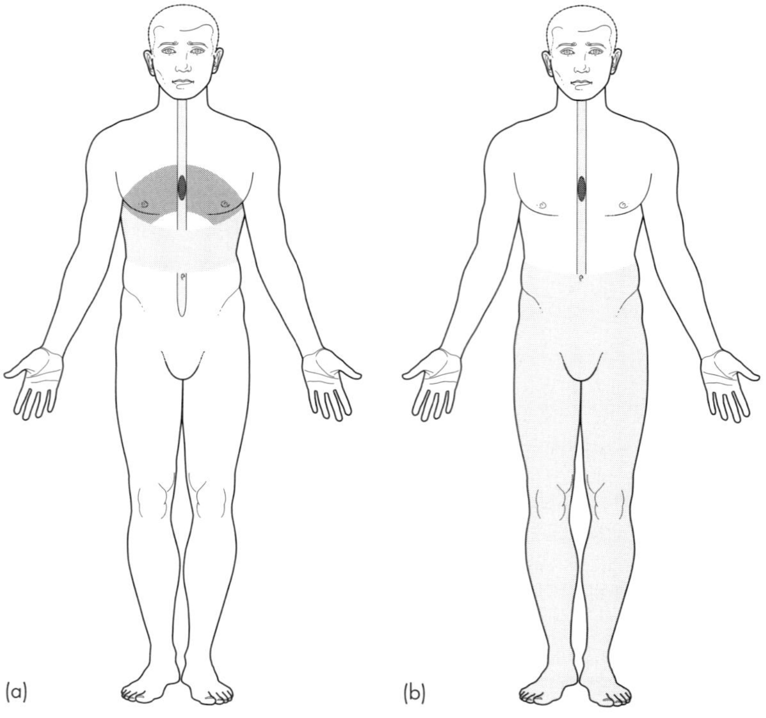

Figure 29.1 Typical patterns of (a) at- and (b) below-level neuropathic pain following SCI.

little that can be done to remove the cause. Pain usually resolves, however, as healing occurs. Damage due to unstable skeletal structures requires stabilization using external devices or internal fixation. Symptomatic pain management, as described below, may be required during the tissue-healing phase.

Chronic inflammatory musculoskeletal pain may be due to factors such as abnormal posture, abnormal gait, and overuse, related to transfers and wheelchair use. These factors may be corrected via education, retraining, and environmental modifications (e.g. adaptive equipment, seating modification, and attendant care prescription) and may be sufficient to eliminate the problem. In the short term, or if it is not possible to completely address the causative factors, symptomatic treatment may also be required.

In addition to correcting abnormal mechanical stresses, managing active disease processes, and modifying unhelpful psychosocial contributing factors, symptomatic pharmacological treatment of inflammatory musculoskeletal pain may be indicated. Similar principles can be used as those employed in the treatment of other degenerative and inflammatory joint conditions.[44] [V] Pharmacological management includes the use of simple analgesics, nonsteroidal anti-inflammatory drugs (NSAIDs), opioids, and local corticosteroid injections. Analgesic use will follow the usual stepwise approach of simple analgesics, such as paracetamol (acetaminophen), compound or "weak" opioids, such as codeine and dextropropoxyphene, and "strong" opioids such as oxycodone, morphine, and methadone. However, several considerations apply in the person with SCI. Opioid analgesics may exacerbate bowel dysfunction, as well as the usual considerations of tolerance and dependence. NSAIDs may cause gastric erosion that is more prevalent and harder to detect in those with high spinal cord lesions. Therefore, paracetamol is the safest first step in the treatment of musculoskeletal pain associated with SCI. If there is no response to paracetamol, the use of tramadol may be considered. While use of opioids for acute inflammatory pain is reasonable, continued use in persistent pain remains controversial.[45] There is general agreement that opioids should be considered for use in noncancer pain if they are the only effective treatment.[46] Unfortunately, conclusive data supporting the long-term efficacy of opioids remains lacking.[47] The use of opioids may be considered on a case-by-case basis in a manner consistent with published guidelines.[48]

Muscle spasm is also a common problem following SCI, associated with tissue trauma and altered inhibitory control. In addition to impairing function, spasm may also cause pain. Muscle spasm may be due to underlying pathology that is maintaining a heightened reflex arc. If so, this needs to be treated appropriately. More commonly, there is no underlying pathology that can be addressed and treatment once again focuses on symptomatic relief. At present, there is insufficient evidence to guide clinicians in a rational approach to anti-spastic treatment for SCI.[49][I] A number of approaches are traditionally used. Oral baclofen may be sufficient to control the symptoms and is the first-line approach. Alternatively, diazepam may be used, but consideration must be given to the side effects associated with benzodiazepine use. Injection of botulinum toxin has also been suggested to be effective in the management of localized spasticity.[50] Insertion of an intrathecal infusion device is invasive and is considered a second-line approach. However, there is good evidence to support the effectiveness of intrathecal baclofen administered in this way for the relief of muscle spasm where there is poor control with oral administration.[51, 52, 53][I]

Visceral pain

Identification of symptomatic urinary tract infection requires treatment with antibiotics. Obstruction from ureteric calculi may require surgical removal or lithotripsy. Bowel impaction may require disimpaction in the short term and adjustment of bowel regimen/routine in the long term. The presence of autonomic dysreflexia may constitute a medical emergency and requires immediate blood pressure reduction and treatment of the triggering stimulus.

Above-level neuropathic pain

The treatment of complex regional pain syndromes is itself complex and the reader is referred to other texts that deal with this condition in more detail.[54] Sympathetic blockade may provide complete relief of pain in some individuals, but effectiveness is unpredictable.[55] Physical rehabilitation may also be helpful in some people with complex regional pain syndromes. Nerve root or peripheral nerve compression may require surgical decompression. Syringomyelia may require drainage and shunting or a detethering procedure.

At-level and below-level neuropathic pain

Apart from treatment of a syrinx and surgical decompression of a compromised nerve root, there are no current treatments available that can treat the cause of at-level or below-level neuropathic pain. Treatments are therefore largely symptomatic. Unfortunately, there are few controlled trials that have been performed specifically examining the efficacy of treatments for at-level and below-level neuropathic pain. Available studies often have small numbers and therefore conclusions may not be reliable. Treatment is therefore often dependent on extrapolation from other neuropathic pain conditions. A summary of the evidence available on the treatment of at- and below-level neuropathic pain is listed below according to treatment category.

OPIOIDS

Two randomized controlled trials involving intravenous morphine[56][II] and alfentanil[57][II] demonstrate a short-term reduction in neuropathic pain following SCI. Intravenous morphine failed to relieve spontaneous pain, but reduced brush-evoked allodynia in central post-stroke and SCI pain patients.[56][II] However, intravenous opioid treatment is not suitable for the long-term management of neuropathic SCI pain. There is evidence to support the use of oral opioid analgesics, such as oxycodone,[58, 59][II] methadone,[60][II] and morphine,[61][II] in other neuropathic pain states. However, there is little direct evidence regarding efficacy in the treatment of neuropathic SCI pain. Side effects, tolerance, and dependence are also issues that need to be considered. If opioids are used, controlled-release preparations provide more stable analgesia and are preferred for long-term use. Tramadol may be less sedating and less constipating and because of its additional serotonergic and noradrenergic effects may be effective in some people with neuropathic pain.[62][I] Therefore it may be a useful first step if opioid agents are being considered.

ANTICONVULSANT DRUGS

Anticonvulsant drugs are often used in the treatment of neuropathic SCI pain. Although numbers are small, two cross-over studies indicate that gabapentin is effective in treating neuropathic SCI pain.[63, 64][II] More recently, pregabalin has been demonstrated to be efficacious in a larger randomized controlled trial.[65][II] Side effects of gabapentin and pregabalin include dizziness, sedation, ataxia, constipation, dryness of the mouth, and peripheral edema.

In a group of subjects with neuropathic SCI pain, lamotrigine 200–400 mg daily had no statistically significant pain-relieving effect. However, a subgroup of patients with incomplete injury and evoked pain demonstrated relief of spontaneous pain.[66][II] Side effects include diplopia, dizziness, ataxia, headache, somnolence, and nausea. The risk of rash (Stevens–Johnson syndrome) and potentially life-threatening hypersensitivity reactions and hepatic effects requires careful dose escalation.

Topiramate has also been administered in a randomized controlled trial, but numbers were small.[67][II] The efficacy of topiramate 800 mg daily in four different neuropathic pain diagnoses was examined with nine patients receiving topiramate and four receiving placebo. Topiramate was significantly better than placebo in the final two weeks of treatment, but only on one of the two primary outcome measures (present pain index) and not on the other primary outcome measure (visual analog scale). Topiramate treatment may cause anorexia, weight loss, drowsiness, dizziness, ataxia, fatigue, and gastrointestinal upset. Less commonly, it may also be associated with renal calculi, leukopenia, glaucoma, and metabolic acidosis.

Valproic acid is commonly used for the treatment of neuropathic SCI pain, but in a controlled trial 600–2400 mg daily was not statistically significantly better than placebo in relieving pain.[68][II] However, the small number involved in the study means there is a risk of type II error. Valproic acid treatment may be associated with skin reactions, gastrointestinal upset, weight gain, tremor, hair loss, liver dysfunction, and hematologic and teratogenic effects.

Carbamazepine has been used for many years for the treatment of neuropathic SCI pain, but evidence is limited to case reports in combination with other drugs.[69] [IV] More recently, oxcarbazepine has become available. However, neither carbamazepine nor oxcarbazepine have been tested in controlled trials in this condition.

ANTIDEPRESSANTS

Antidepressants, and in particular tricyclic antidepressants, are widely used in the management of neuropathic pain conditions, although there is little direct evidence for effectiveness in neuropathic SCI pain. Nevertheless, given the lack of effective agents and supportive evidence from other neuropathic pain conditions, a trial of tricyclic antidepressants is often part of clinical practice.

Traditionally, the mechanism of action of tricyclic antidepressants in treating pain has been attributed to inhibition of the reuptake of norepinephrine and serotonin. However, they also have other actions including *N*-methyl-D-aspartic acid (NMDA)-receptor antagonism[70] and sodium channel blockade that may contribute to their effect in neuropathic pain conditions.[71, 72] Amitriptyline (10–125 mg daily) has been studied in one controlled trial in patients with a mixture of musculoskeletal and neuropathic pains following SCI and was found to be not significantly better than placebo.[73][II] Tricyclic antidepressants are contraindicated in patients with ischemic heart disease, heart failure, cardiac conduction disturbances, and a history of seizures. Sedation and anticholinergic side effects, such as constipation, dry mouth, and urinary retention, may result in poor patient tolerance. The use of tricyclic antidepressants may also be associated with increased spasticity and disturbance of bladder function.[73]

Mixed serotonin and noradrenaline reuptake inhibitors, such as venlafaxine and duloxetine, selective serotonin reuptake inhibitors, and bupropion, a noradrenaline and dopamine reuptake inhibitor have been developed more recently and may be effective agents and better tolerated than the tricyclic antidepressants. However, evidence to support their use is largely anecdotal and they have not been studied in SCI pain. The exception to this is the serotonin reuptake inhibitor and 5HT receptor antagonist, trazodone, which has been studied in a randomized controlled trial, but with a lack of group effect when compared with placebo.[74][II]

LOCAL ANESTHETICS

In the acute, in-patient setting, systemic administration of the sodium channel blocker, lidocaine can result in effective relief of neuropathic pain.[75][III] Intravenous lidocaine failed to relieve pain in ten SCI patients in doses of 2.5 mg/kg intravenously over 40 minutes.[76][II] However, in another study, lidocaine at a higher dose (5 mg/kg over 30 minutes) significantly decreased spontaneous ongoing pain, brush-evoked allodynia, and static mechanical hyperalgesia in patients with post-stroke or SCI pain.[77][II] Lidocaine also decreased spontaneous at- and below-level pain in SCI patients with and without evoked pain.[78][II]

Although there is a report of long-term effectiveness with the use of lidocaine,[79] systemic administration is generally not practical as an ongoing treatment. Mexiletine, which is an oral congener of lidocaine with a similar action, has not demonstrated to be effective in a small trial of 11 patients using a dose of 450 mg/day.[80][II] Mexiletine may result in cardiac conduction disturbances and needs to be used with caution in those with a history of coronary artery disease and prior myocardial infarction.[81] Gastrointestinal upset may affect patient tolerance.

NMDA ANTAGONISTS

There is some evidence that drugs that target increased excitation by blocking NMDA receptor function may be effective. In the acute, in-patient setting, systemic administration of the NMDA receptor antagonist ketamine was shown to be better than placebo and similar to fentanyl in reducing below-level neuropathic pain.[57][II] However, there are currently no oral NMDA antagonists that have been demonstrated to be effective in the long-term management of neuropathic SCI pain.

DRUG COMBINATIONS

There are reports that combinations of anticonvulsants and tricyclic antidepressants are more effective than when either is administered alone.[69, 82][V] Therefore, if a single agent is ineffective, a combination of an anticonvulsant with either a tricyclic antidepressant or an opioid may produce additional relief.

OTHER MEDICATIONS

The effect of the anesthetic agent and $GABA_A$-receptor agonist propofol on neuropathic SCI pain has also been examined. A subhypnotic dose of propofol, injected as a single intravenous bolus (0.2 mg/kg) provided brief relief (less than one hour) of spontaneous pain and allodynia in approximately half of 44 patients with SCI and post-stroke pain.[83][II]

SPINAL DRUG ADMINISTRATION

If oral administration of agents fails to provide adequate analgesia, spinal administration can be considered, although this is an inherently more invasive approach supported by case series and limited controlled trials. Spinal administration of drugs such as morphine and clonidine[84][V] has been found to be effective in some individuals. Combinations of morphine or clonidine with baclofen in those with spasm may confer additional benefit.[85][V] In a controlled study, intrathecal administration of a mixture of morphine and clonidine was found to be effective in a group of people with chronic at-level and below-level neuropathic SCI pain.[86][II] Intrathecal drug administration with morphine and clonidine was associated with nausea, sedation, respiratory depression, and hypotension,[86] and there is little information available on patient tolerance and long-term side effects.

Intrathecal baclofen is effective in managing spasticity and spasm-related pain secondary to SCI.[51, 52] However, the effect on neuropathic SCI is less clear.[87] A positive outcome in relieving neuropathic pain was found with intrathecal baclofen in a small ($n=9$) randomized controlled trial,[53][II] but other reports have been less supportive.[88][III]

Spinal anesthesia with subarachnoid lidocaine was also studied in 21 patients with SCI and had a significantly greater analgesic effect than placebo.[32][V] However, the effect of spinal anesthesia is only temporary and therefore limits its usefulness. Adequate spinal anesthesia proximal to the sensory level of SCI seemed to be a positive predictor of response. This observation is similar to the study of intrathecal morphine and clonidine in which a positive response was associated with adequate drug availability above the level of SCI. Both studies provide clues as to the mechanisms underlying neuropathic SCI pain.

STIMULATION TECHNIQUES

Stimulation techniques, such as transcutaneous electrical nerve stimulation (TENS) and acupuncture may be effective for some people with neuropathic pain and may work by activating inhibitory mechanisms.[89][V] However, positive evidence of efficacy is limited, particularly with below-level neuropathic pain and most studies report a decline in efficacy over time (reviewed in Ref. 90[V]). Acupuncture appeared to have a sustained effect in 10 of 22 SCI patients with various types of pain, but was ineffective in those with pain below the injury level.[91][V] However, retrospective data from another study suggested

Table 29.2 Pharmacological treatments for persistent at- and below-level neuropathic SCI pain: level of evidence, limitations, and specific indications for third-line treatments.

Pharmacological treatment	Level of evidence for efficacy	Disadvantages or side effects[a]	Specific indications
Opioids			
Acute management (intravenous)	+ve RCTs[56, 57][II]	Short-term relief, invasive, respiratory depression, sedation, hypotension, nausea, vomiting	Mechanical allodynia
Ongoing management (oral)	Refer to text	Constipation, drowsiness, tolerance, dependence	
Anticonvulsants			
Gabapentin	+ve RCTs[63, 64][II]	Somnolence, dizziness	
Pregabalin	+ve RCT[65][II]	Somnolence, dizziness, asthenia, dry mouth, edema, constipation	
Topiramate	+ve RCT[67][II]	Drowsiness, dizziness, ataxia, anorexia, fatigue, gastrointestinal upset	
Lamotrigine	–ve RCT[66][II]	Potentially life-threatening skin rash, hepatic effects, diplopia, blurred vision, dizziness	
Valproic acid	–ve RCT[68][II]	Drowsiness, dizziness, liver dysfunction, hematological effects	
Antidepressants			
Amitriptyline	–ve RCT[73][II]	Sedative and anticholinergic actions	
Mixed serotonin/noradrenaline reuptake inhibitors (venlafaxine, duloxetine)	Refer to text	Hypertensive effects, gastrointestinal disturbance, dry mouth, reduced appetite, sweating	
Trazodone	–ve RCT[74][II]	Drowsiness, dry mouth, dizziness and increased spasticity	
Local anesthetics			
Lidocaine parenterally (5 mg/kg)	+ve RCTs[77, 78][II]	CNS excitation/depression, cardiovascular depression	
Mexiletine	–ve RCT[80][II]	Gastrointestinal upset, cardiovascular, hematological disturbance, skin reactions	
Spinal drug delivery			
Morphine and clonidine	+ve RCT[86][II]	Invasive, tolerance, hypotension, respiratory depression, drowsiness	
Baclofen	Unclear +ve RCT[53][II] –ve trial[88][III]	Invasive, reports of increased neuropathic pain	Stronger evidence for spasm related pain[51, 52, 53][I]
Lidocaine	+ve RCT[32][II]	Invasive, central nervous system disturbance	
Miscellaneous			
Intravenous ketamine	+ve RCT[57][II]	Short-term relief, invasive, dysphoria	
Intravenous propofol	+ve RCT[83][II]	Short-term relief, invasive, hypotension, arrhythmias, bradycardia	

CNS, central nervous system; RCT, randomized controlled trials.
[a]Commonly listed side effects. For further details consult prescribing information.

Table 29.3 Nonpharmacological treatments for persistent at- and below-level neuropathic SCI pain: level of evidence, limitations, and specific indications for third-line treatments.

Nonpharmacological treatment	Level of evidence for efficacy	Disadvantages or side effects	Specific indications
Physical therapy			
Exercise	+ve RCT[102][II]	Indirect influence on neuropathic SCI pain	
Stimulation			
TENS			
Acupuncture	+ve cases[91, 92][V]	Invasive	
Spinal cord stimulation	+ve cases[93][V]	Invasive	At-level neuropathic pain, incomplete injuries
Deep brain stimulation	+ve cases[90][V]	Invasive, intracranial hemorrhage, lack of long-term benefit	
Transcranial motor cortex	+ve RCT[95][II]	Short-term effect	
Epidural motor cortex	+ve cases[94][V]	Invasive	
Surgery			
DREZ	+ve cases[98, 99, 100, 101][V]	Invasive, risk of further deficits	At-level neuropathic pain
Cordotomy	+ve cases[96, 97][V]	Invasive, risk of further deficits	
Psychological therapy			
Cognitive behavioral program	+ve studies[104, 105][III]	Positive effect on mood and sleep, but not pain intensity	

DREZ, dorsal root entry zone; RCT, randomized controlled trials; TENS, transcutaneous electrical nerve stimulation.

an effect also on below-level neuropathic pain.[92][V] Spinal cord stimulation may also provide relief, although greater effect is obtained in those with at-level neuropathic pain and incomplete lesions.[93][V] Other available treatments are very invasive with limited evidence of efficacy. These include deep brain stimulation and motor cortex stimulation. Deep brain stimulation seems not to provide long-term pain relief in SCI pain.[90][V] Transcranial or epidural motor cortex stimulation[94][V] has been tested in a few SCI pain patients with varying results. A recent study using transcranial direct current stimulation (tDCS) demonstrated short-term reduction in pain following a five-day treatment trial.[95][II]

SURGICAL APPROACHES

Surgical approaches are often designed to relieve pain by reversing any structural problems giving rise to pain. For example, nerve root or peripheral nerve compression may require surgical decompression and a syrinx may require drainage and shunting. A detethering procedure may relieve pain caused by scarring around nerve roots.

If it is not possible to address a structural problem, surgical approaches attempt to deal with the pain by destroying or disconnecting the site of abnormal activity or disconnecting it from the brain. Several uncontrolled studies have been performed to examine efficacy of surgical approaches with variability in outcomes. Cordotomy or cordomyelotomy has been used to a limited extent and has been reported to be effective in some patients.[96, 97][V] Dorsal root entry zone (DREZ) lesioning is a procedure that destroys nerve cells in the dorsal horn close to the level of injury. It is less destructive than cordotomy and can be effective in providing relief of neuropathic pain, although best results are obtained in those with at-level neuropathic pain.[98, 99][V] DREZ lesioning guided by intramedullary recordings of spontaneous and C-fiber-evoked electrical hyperactivity is suggested to relieve both at- and below-level SCI pain.[100, 101][V] On the whole, however, surgical approaches are relatively invasive, may cause additional neurological deficits and may fail to address supraspinal changes and therefore provide only temporary or incomplete relief.

PHYSICAL APPROACHES

Physical approaches may help to improve pain associated with chronic musculoskeletal pain and may indirectly influence neuropathic SCI pain. Abnormal posture, gait, and overuse with transfers and wheelchair use may all contribute to the presence of pain and may be addressed by physiotherapy, exercise,[102][II] retraining, and environmental modifications, such as the use of specialized adaptive equipment, wheelchair adjustment and positioning, and assistance from carers.

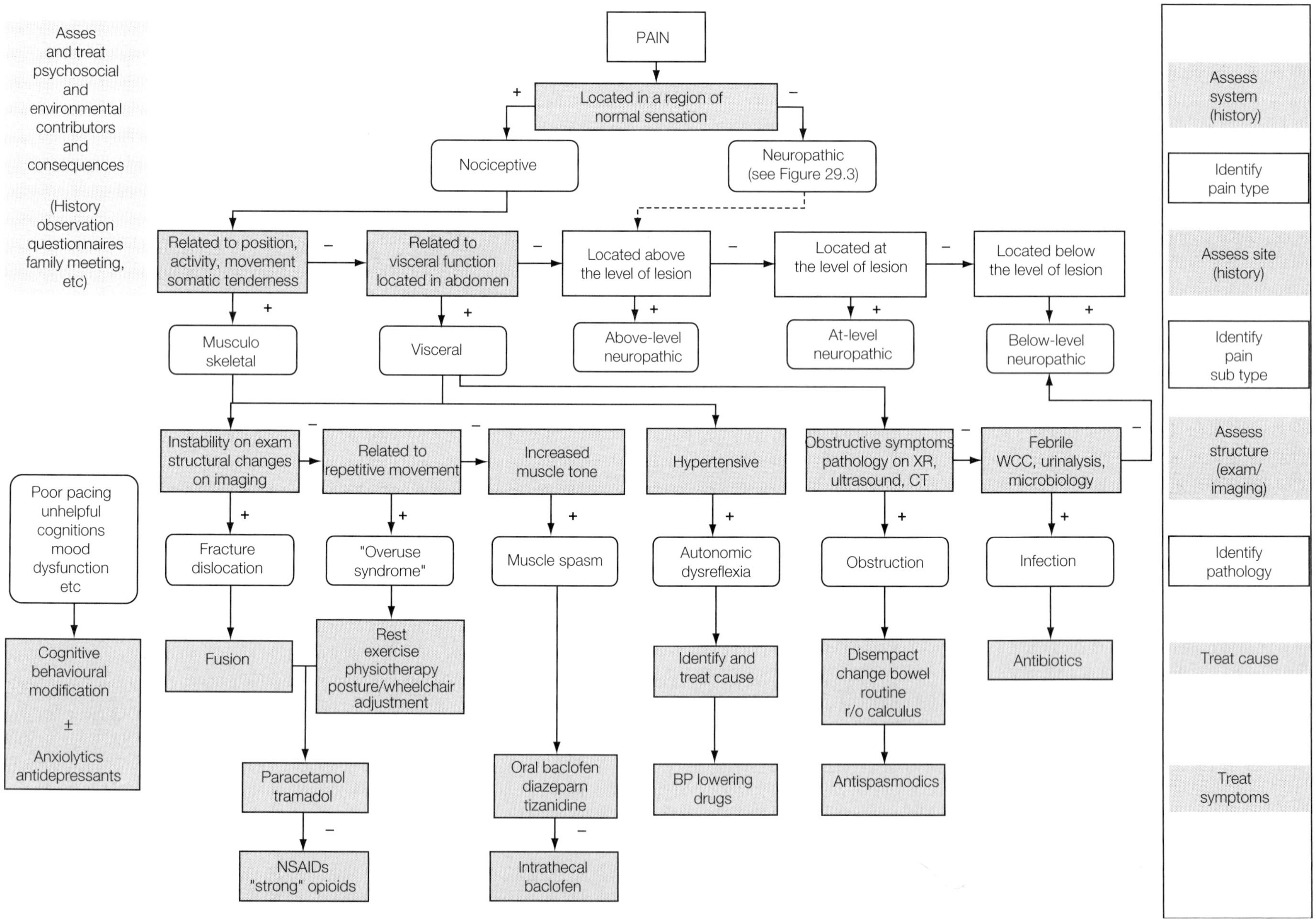

Figure 29.2 Proposed algorithm for the assessment and treatment of nociceptive pain following spinal cord injury (from Ref. 107).

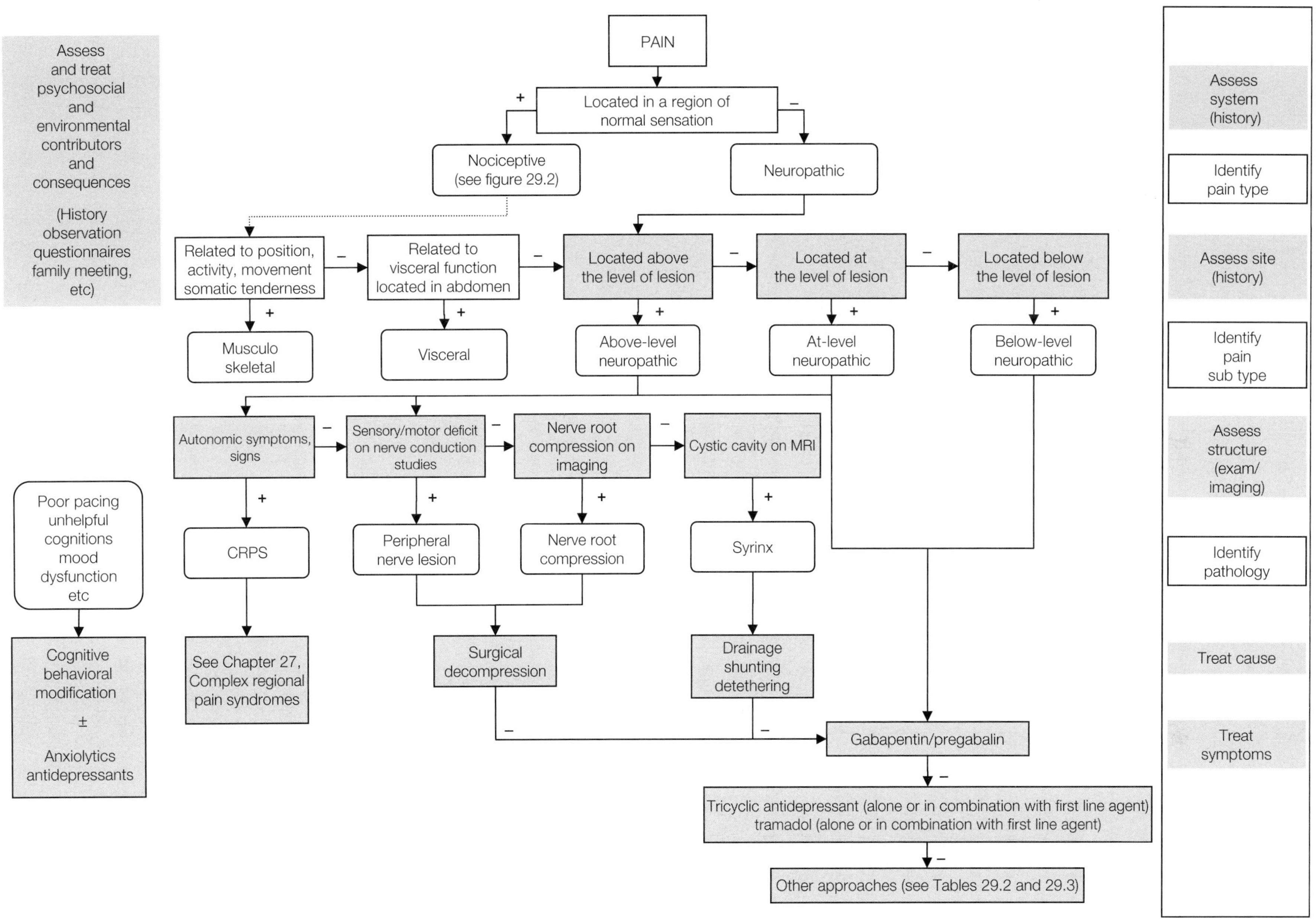

Figure 29.3 Proposed algorithm for the assessment and treatment of neuropathic pain following spinal cord injury (from Ref. 107).

Psychological and environmental aspects

The person with SCI undergoes a huge adjustment in relationships, lifestyle, vocation, and self-image that need to be addressed and people with a severe SCI often have significant psychological distress, particularly in the acute post injury period.[103][V] The presence of chronic pain may be an additional factor that prevents expected rehabilitation and return to employment and function in domestic life.[5, 6, 22, 104][V] Anxiety and depression are both normal responses to injury and often improve with time and the implementation of the person's inherent coping skills. In these people, formal intervention may not be required. However, for the minority who experience severe or chronic mood dysfunction that is having an impact on their ability to function and contributing to pain, intervention should be offered.

There are a variety of approaches for dealing with psychological and environmental contributors. These may include the use of anxiolytic and antidepressant medications and/or cognitive–behavioral treatment.[105][III], [106][III] It may also be necessary to address other external factors that are believed to be contributing to the pain. It is evident that psychological factors influence the experience of pain, and therefore it is likely that cognitive–behavioral interventions may improve the quality of life in pain patients. Relaxation techniques are suggested to be of benefit in SCI pain and may alter the attitude towards pain. Well-designed studies are needed to determine the effects of the nonpharmacological treatment of SCI pain.

Treatment summary

It is difficult to summarize the treatments options for pain associated with SCI succinctly. Guidelines need to take into consideration a broad range of issues including pain, other medical and psychological issues, personal preference, side effects, treatment availability, and cost. As mentioned, the evidence to support many interventions in the management of SCI pain is limited, making definitive recommendations difficult to formulate (**Tables 29.2** and **29.3**). Therefore, it is not possible to provide a prescriptive approach to the management of SCI pain. Nevertheless, it still may be helpful to consider guidelines that can provide a general approach that can be tailored to the individual. An assessment and treatment algorithm has been published which recognizes these limitations, and attempts to provide some direction for treatment (**Figures 29.2** and **29.3**).[107]

In this algorithm, a number of pharmacological options for SCI neuropathic pain are presented. In the acute, in-patient setting, parenteral lidocaine is suggested as a first-line agent and gabapentin in the subacute or chronic setting. With the recent evidence for the efficacy of pregabalin,[65] this is an alternative to the use of gabapentin. If gabapentin or pregabalin fail to provide adequate relief, the use of a tricyclic antidepressant, such as amitriptyline or nortriptyline, or a weak opioid, such as tramadol, are suggested as a second-line treatment. Although there is limited and even negative evidence with tricyclic antidepressants alone in the treatment of SCI pain,[73] there is strong evidence of efficacy in other neuropathic pain conditions, as well as reports that combinations of anticonvulsants and tricyclic antidepressants are more effective than when either is administered alone.[69, 82][V] Therefore, if a single agent is ineffective, a combination of an anticonvulsant with either a tricyclic antidepressant or an opioid may produce additional relief. Tricyclic antidepressants should generally not be combined with tramadol because of the increased potential to develop serotonergic syndrome. There are a number of third-line treatments that may be considered if the first- and second-line treatments fail. However, evidence is limited or negative, they may be indicated for specific populations or have disadvantages that make it difficult to recommend them as first- or second-line treatments.

REFERENCES

* 1. Widerström-Noga EG, Felipe-Cuervo E, Broton JG *et al.* Perceived difficulty in dealing with consequences of spinal cord injury. *Archives of Physical Medicine and Rehabilitation.* 1999; **80**: 580–6.
2. Bonica JJ. Introduction: semantic, epidemiologic, and educational issues. In: Casey KL (ed.). *Pain and central nervous system disease: the central pain sydromes.* New York: Raven Press, 1991: 13–29.
3. Siddall PJ, Taylor DA, McClelland JM *et al.* Pain report and the relationship of pain to physical factors in the first 6 months following spinal cord injury. *Pain.* 1999; **81**: 187–97.
4. Störmer S, Gerner HJ, Grüninger W *et al.* Chronic pain/dysaesthesiae in spinal cord injury patients: results of a multicentre study. *Spinal Cord.* 1997; **35**: 446–55.
5. Widerström-Noga EG, Duncan R, Felipe-Cuervo E, Turk DC. Assessment of the impact of pain and impairments associated with spinal cord injuries. *Archives of Physical Medicine and Rehabilitation.* 2002; **83**: 395–404.
6. Westgren N, Levi R. Quality of life and traumatic spinal cord injury. *Archives of Physical Medicine and Rehabilitation.* 1998; **79**: 1433–9.
7. Putzke JD, Richards JS, Hicken BL, DeVivo MJ. Interference due to pain following spinal cord injury: important predictors and impact on quality of life. *Pain.* 2002; **100**: 231–42.
8. Anke AGW, Stenehjem AE, Stanghelle JK. Pain and life quality within 2 years of spinal cord injury. *Paraplegia.* 1995; **33**: 555–9.
9. Bryce TN, Ragnarsson KT. Epidemiology and classification of pain after spinal cord injury. *Topics in Spinal Cord Injury and Rehabilitation.* 2001; **7**: 1–17.

10. Cardenas DA, Turner JA, Warms CA, Marshall HM. Classification of chronic pain associated with spinal cord injuries. *Archives of Physical Medicine and Rehabilitation.* 2002; **83**: 1708–14.
11. Donovan WH, Dimitrijevic MR, Dahm L, Dimitrijevic M. Neurophysiological approaches to chronic pain following spinal cord injury. *Paraplegia.* 1982; **20**: 135–46.
12. Siddall PJ, Taylor DA, Cousins MJ. Classification of pain following spinal cord injury. *Spinal Cord.* 1997; **35**: 69–75.
13. * Siddall PJ, Yezierski RP, Loeser JD. Taxonomy and epidemiology of spinal cord injury pain. In: Yezierski RP, Burchiel KJ (eds). *Spinal cord injury pain: assessment, mechanisms, management. Progress in Pain Research and Management.* Seattle: IASP Press, 2002: 9–24.
14. Marino RJ, Barros T, Biering-Sorensen F *et al.* International standards for neurological classification of spinal cord injury. *Journal of Spinal Cord Medicine.* 2003; **26**: S50–6.
15. Dalyan M, Cardenas DD, Gerard B. Upper extremity pain after spinal cord injury. *Spinal Cord.* 1999; **37**: 191–5.
16. van Drongelen S, de Groot S, Veeger HEJ *et al.* Upper extremity musculoskeletal pain during and after rehabilitation in wheelchair-using persons with a spinal cord injury. *Spinal Cord.* 2006; **44**: 152–9.
17. Curtis KA, Drysdale GA, Lanza D *et al.* Shoulder pain in wheelchair users with tetraplegia and paraplegia. *Archives of Physical Medicine and Rehabilitation.* 1999; **80**: 453–7.
18. Richards JS, Meredith RL, Nepomuceno C *et al.* Psychosocial aspects of chronic pain in spinal cord injury. *Pain.* 1980; **8**: 355–66.
19. Haythornthwaite JA, Benrud-Larson LM. Psychological aspects of neuropathic pain. *Clinical Journal of Pain.* 2000; **16**: S101–05.
20. Kennedy P, Frankel H, Gardner B, Nuseibeh I. Factors associated with acute and chronic pain following traumatic spinal cord injuries. *Spinal Cord.* 1997; **35**: 814–7.
21. Cairns MD, Adkins RH, Scott MD. Pain and depression in acute traumatic spinal cord injury – origins of chronic problematic pain. *Archives of Physical Medicine and Rehabilitation.* 1996; **77**: 329–35.
22. Rintala DH, Loubser PG, Castro J *et al.* Chronic pain in a community-based sample of men with spinal cord injury: prevalence, severity, and relationship with impairment, disability, handicap, and subjective well-being. *Archives of Physical Medicine and Rehabilitation.* 1998; **79**: 604–14.
23. * Vierck CJ, Siddall PJ, Yezierski RP. Pain following spinal cord injury: animal models and mechanistic studies. *Pain.* 2000; **89**: 1–5.
24. Loubser PG, Clearman RR. Evaluation of central spinal cord injury pain with diagnostic spinal anesthesia. *Anesthesiology.* 1993; **79**: 376–8.
25. Hao JX, Xu XJ, Yu YX *et al.* Transient spinal cord ischaemia induces temporary hypersensitivity of dorsal horn wide dynamic range neurons to myelinated, but not unmyelinated, fiber input. *Journal of Neurophysiology.* 1992; **68**: 384–91.
26. Yezierski RP, Park SH. The mechanosensitivity of spinal sensory neurons following intraspinal injections of quisqualic acid in the rat. *Neuroscience Letters.* 1993; **157**: 115–9.
27. Christensen MD, Everhart AW, Pickelman JT, Hulsebosch CE. Mechanical and thermal allodynia in chronic central pain following spinal cord injury. *Pain.* 1996; **68**: 97–107.
28. Plunkett JA, Yu CG, Easton JM *et al.* Effects of interleukin-10 (IL-10) on pain behavior and gene expression following excitotoxic spinal cord injury in the rat. *Experimental Neurology.* 2001; **168**: 144–54.
29. Peng XM, Zhou ZG, Glorioso JC *et al.* Tumor necrosis factor-alpha contributes to below-level neuropathic pain after spinal cord injury. *Annals of Neurology.* 2006; **59**: 843–51.
30. Christensen MD, Hulsebosch CE. Spinal cord injury and anti-NGF treatment results in changes in CGRP density and distribution in the dorsal horn of the rat. *Experimental Neurology.* 1997; **147**: 463–75.
31. Finnerup NB, Johannesen IL, Fuglsang-Frederiksen A *et al.* Sensory function in spinal cord injury patients with and without central pain. *Brain.* 2003; **126**: 57–70.
32. * Loubser PG, Donovan WH. Diagnostic spinal anaesthesia in chronic spinal cord injury pain. *Paraplegia.* 1991; **29**: 25–36.
33. * Melzack R, Loeser JD. Phantom body pain in paraplegics: evidence for a central "pattern generating mechanism" for pain. *Pain.* 1978; **4**: 195–210.
34. Jeanmonod D, Magnin M, Morel A. Thalamus and neurogenic pain: physiological, anatomical and clinical data. *Neuroreport.* 1993; **4**: 475–8.
35. * Lenz FA, Kwan HC, Dostrovsky JO, Tasker RR. Characteristics of the bursting pattern of action potentials that occurs in the thalamus of patients with central pain. *Brain Research.* 1989; **496**: 357–60.
36. Radhakrishnan V, Tsoukatos J, Davis KD *et al.* A comparison of the burst activity of lateral thalamic neurons in chronic pain and non-pain patients. *Pain.* 1999; **80**: 567–75.
37. * Hains BC, Saab CY, Waxman SG. Changes in electrophysiological properties and sodium channel Na(v)1.3 expression in thalamic neurons after spinal cord injury. *Brain.* 2005; **128**: 2359–71.
38. Llinas RR, Ribary U, Jeanmonod D *et al.* Thalamocortical dysrhythmia: A neurological and neuropsychiatric syndrome characterized by magnetoencephalography. *Proceedings of the National Academy of Sciences of USA.* 1999; **96**: 15222–7.
39. Pattany PM, Yezierski RP, Widerström-Noga EG *et al.* Proton magnetic resonance spectroscopy of the thalamus in patients with chronic neuropathic pain after spinal cord injury. *American Journal of Neuroradiology.* 2002; **23**: 901–05.
40. Ness TJ, San Pedro EC, Richards JS *et al.* A case of spinal cord injury-related pain with baseline rCBF brain SPECT imaging and beneficial response to gabapentin. *Pain.* 1998; **78**: 139–43.

41. Gerke MB, Duggan AW, Xu L, Siddall PJ. Thalamic neuronal activity in rats with mechanical allodynia following contusive spinal cord injury. *Neuroscience.* 2003; **117**: 715–22.
42. Koyama S, Katayama Y, Maejima S *et al.* Thalamic neuronal hyperactivity following transection of the spinothalamic tract in the cat: involvement of N-methyl-D-aspartate receptor. *Brain Research.* 1993; **612**: 345–50.
43. Bouhassira D, Attal N, Fermanian J *et al.* Development and validation of the Neuropathic Pain Symptom Inventory. *Pain.* 2004; **108**: 248–57.
44. American College of Rheumatology. American College of Rheumatology Subcommittee on Osteoarthritis Guidelines 2000 recommendations for the medical management of osteoarthritis of hip and knee: 2000 update. *Arthritis and Rheumatism.* 2000; **43**: 1905–15.
45. Large RG, Schug SA. Opioids for chronic pain of non-malignant origin – caring or crippling. *Health Care Analysis.* 1995; **3**: 5–11.
46. McQuay HJ. How should we measure the outcome? In: Kalso E, McQuay HJ, Wiesenfeld-Hallin Z (eds). *Opioid sensitivity of chronic noncancer pain.* Progress in Pain Research and Management. Seattle: IASP Press, 1999: 371–83.
47. Rowbotham MC. The debate over opioids and neuropathic pain. In: Kalso E, McQuay HJ, Wiesenfeld-Hallin Z (eds). *Opioid sensitivity of chronic noncancer pain.* Progress in Pain Research and Management. Seattle: IASP Press, 1999: 307–17.
48. Nicholas MK, Molloy AR, Brooker C. Using opioids with persisting noncancer pain: a biopsychosocial perspective. *Clinical Journal of Pain.* 2006; **22**: 137–46.
49. Taricco M, Pagliacci MC, Telaro E, Adone R. Pharmacological interventions for spasticity following spinal cord injury: results of a Cochrane systematic review. *Europa Medicophysica.* 2006; **42**: 5–15.
50. O'Brien CF. Treatment of spasticity with botulinum toxin. *Clinical Journal of Pain.* 2002; **18**: S182–90.
51. Penn RD, Kroin JS. Long-term intrathecal baclofen infusion for treatment of spasticity. *Journal of Neurosurgery.* 1987; **66**: 181–5.
52. Lewis KS, Mueller WM. Intrathecal baclofen for severe spasticity secondary to spinal cord injury. *Annals of Pharmacotherapy.* 1993; **27**: 767–74.
53. Herman RM, D'Luzansky SC, Ippolito R. Intrathecal baclofen suppresses central pain in patients with spinal lesions. A pilot study. *Clinical Journal of Pain.* 1992; **8**: 338–45.
54. Wilson PR, Stanton-Hicks M, Harden RN (eds). *CRPS: Current diagnosis and therapy.* Progress in Pain Research and Management 32. Seattle: IASP Press, 2005.
55. Kingery WS. A critical review of controlled clinical trials for peripheral neuropathic pain and complex regional pain syndromes. *Pain.* 1997; **73**: 123–39.
56. Attal N, Guirimand F, Brasseur L *et al.* Effects of IV morphine in central pain – a randomized placebo-controlled study. *Neurology.* 2002; **58**: 554–63.
57. Eide PK, Stubhaug A, Stenehjem AE. Central dysesthesia pain after traumatic spinal cord injury is dependent on N-methyl-D-aspartate receptor activation. *Neurosurgery.* 1995; **37**: 1080–7.
58. Watson CP, Babul N. Efficacy of oxycodone in neuropathic pain: a randomized trial in postherpetic neuralgia. *Neurology.* 1998; **50**: 1837–41.
59. Watson CP, Moulin D, Watt-Watson J *et al.* Controlled-release oxycodone relieves neuropathic pain: a randomized controlled trial in painful diabetic neuropathy. *Pain.* 2003; **105**: 71–8.
60. Raja SN, Haythornthwaite JA, Pappagallo M *et al.* Opioids versus antidepressants in postherpetic neuralgia: a randomized, placebo-controlled trial. *Neurology.* 2002; **59**: 1015–21.
61. Huse E, Larbig W, Flor H, Birbaumer N. The effect of opioids on phantom limb pain and cortical reorganization. *Pain.* 2001; **90**: 47–55.
62. Hollingshead J, Duhmke RM, Cornblath DR. Tramadol for neuropathic pain. *Cochrane Database of Systematic Reviews.* 2006; **CD003726**.
63. Levendoglu F, Ogun CO, Ozerbil O *et al.* Gabapentin is a first line drug for the treatment of neuropathic pain in spinal cord injury. *Spine.* 2004; **29**: 743–51.
64. Tai Q, Kirshblum S, Chen B *et al.* Gabapentin in the treatment of neuropathic pain after spinal cord injury: a prospective, randomized, double-blind, crossover trial. *Journal of Spinal Cord Medicine.* 2002; **25**: 100–05.
* 65. Siddall PJ, Cousins MJ, Otte A *et al.* Pregabalin in central neuropathic pain associated with spinal cord injury: A placebo-controlled trial. *Neurology.* 2007; **68**: 2158–9.
* 66. Finnerup NB, Sindrup SH, Flemming WB *et al.* Lamotrigine in spinal cord injury pain: a randomized controlled trial. *Pain.* 2002; **96**: 375–83.
67. Harden RN, Brenman E, Saltz S *et al.* Topiramate in the management of spinal cord injury pain: a double-blind, randomized, placebo-controlled pilot study. In: Burchiel KJ, Yezierski RP (eds). *Spinal cord injury pain: assessment, mechanisms, management.* Progress in Pain Research and Management 23. Seattle: IASP Press, 2002: 393–407.
68. Drewes AM, Andreasen A, Poulsen LH. Valproate for treatment of chronic central pain after spinal cord injury. A double-blind cross-over study. *Paraplegia.* 1994; **32**: 565–9.
69. Erzurumlu A, Dursun H, Gunduz S *et al.* The management of chronic pain at spinal cord injured patients: The comparison of effectiveness of amitryptyline and carbamazepine combination and electroacupuncture application. *Journal of Rheumatology and Medical Rehabilitation.* 1996; **7**: 176–80.
70. Eisenach JC, Gebhart GF. Intrathecal amitriptyline acts as an N-methyl-D-aspartate receptor antagonist in the presence of inflammatory hyperalgesia in rats. *Anesthesiology.* 1995; **83**: 1046–54.
71. Pancrazio JJ, Kamatchi GL, Lynch C. Does Na+ channel blockade underlie the analgesic property of antidepressants? *Anesthesiology.* 1996; **85**: A787.

72. Wang GK, Russell C, Wang SY. State-dependent block of voltage-gated Na+ channels by amitriptyline via the local anesthetic receptor and its implication for neuropathic pain. *Pain*. 2004; **110**: 166–74.
* 73. Cardenas DD, Warms CA, Turner JA *et al.* Efficacy of amitriptyline for relief of pain in spinal cord injury: results of a randomized controlled trial. *Pain*. 2002; **96**: 365–73.
74. Davidoff G, Guarracini M, Roth E *et al.* Trazodone hydrochloride in the treatment of dysesthetic pain in traumatic myelopathy: a randomized, double-blind, placebo-controlled study. *Pain*. 1987; **29**: 151–61.
75. Backonja M, Gombar KA. Response of central pain syndromes to intravenous lidocaine. *Journal of Pain and Symptom Management*. 1992; **7**: 172–8.
76. Kvarnstrom A, Karlsten R, Quiding H, Gordh T. The analgesic effect of intravenous ketamine and lidocaine on pain after spinal cord injury. *Acta Anaesthesiologica Scandinavica*. 2004; **48**: 498–506.
77. Attal N, Gaud V, Brasseur L *et al.* Intravenous lidocaine in central pain: a double-blind, placebo-controlled, psychophysical study. *Neurology*. 2000; **54**: 564–74.
78. Finnerup NB, Biering-Sorensen F, Johannesen IL *et al.* Intravenous lidocaine relieves spinal cord injury pain: a randomized controlled trial. *Anesthesiology*. 2005; **102**: 1023–30.
79. Cahana A, Carota A, Montadon ML, Annoni JM. The long-term effect of repeated intravenous lidocaine on central pain and possible correlation in positron emission tomography measurements. *Anesthesia and Analgesia*. 2004; **98**: 1581–4.
80. Chiou-Tan FY, Tuel SM, Johnson JC *et al.* Effect of mexiletine on spinal cord injury dysesthetic pain. *American Journal of Physical Medicine and Rehabilitation*. 1996; **75**: 84–7.
81. Vlay SC. Lessons from the past and reflections on the Cardiac Arrhythmia Suppression Trial. *American Journal of Cardiology*. 1990; **65**: 112–3.
82. Sandford PR, Lindblom LB, Haddox JD. Amitriptyline and carbamazepine in the treatment of dysesthetic pain in spinal cord injury. *Archives of Physical Medicine and Rehabilitation*. 1992; **73**: 300–01.
83. Canavero S, Bonicalzi V. Intravenous subhypnotic propofol in central pain: a double-blind, placebo-controlled, crossover study. *Clinical Neuropharmacology*. 2004; **27**: 182–6.
84. Glynn CJ, Jamous MA, Teddy PJ *et al.* Role of spinal noradrenergic system in transmission of pain in patients with spinal cord injury. *Lancet*. 1986; **2**: 1249–50.
85. Middleton JW, Siddall PJ, Walker S *et al.* Intrathecal clonidine and baclofen in the management of spasticity and neuropathic pain following spinal cord injury: a case study. *Archives of Physical Medicine and Rehabilitation*. 1996; **77**: 824–6.
86. Siddall PJ, Molloy AR, Walker S *et al.* The efficacy of intrathecal morphine and clonidine in the treatment of pain after spinal cord injury. *Anesthesia and Analgesia*. 2000; **91**: 1493–8.
87. Siddall PJ. Spinal drug administration in the treatment of spinal cord injury pain. In: Yezierski RP, Burchiel K (eds). *Spinal cord injury pain: assessment, mechanisms, management*. Seattle: IASP Press, 2002: 353–64.
88. Loubser PG, Akman NM. Effects of intrathecal baclofen on chronic spinal cord injury pain. *Journal of Pain and Symptom Management*. 1996; **12**: 241–7.
89. Norrbrink Budh C, Lundeberg T. Non-pharmacological pain-relieving therapies in individuals with spinal cord injury: a patient perspective. *Complementary Therapies in Medicine*. 2004; **12**: 189–97.
* 90. Finnerup NB, Yezierski RP, Sang CN *et al.* Treatment of spinal cord injury pain. *Pain: Clinical Updates*. 2001; **9**: 1–6. Available from: http://www.iasp-pain.org/PCU01-2.html.
91. Nayak S, Shiflett SC, Schoenberger NE *et al.* Is acupuncture effective in treating chronic pain after spinal cord injury? *Archives of Physical Medicine and Rehabilitation*. 2001; **82**: 1578–86.
92. Rapson LM, Wells N, Pepper J *et al.* Acupuncture as a promising treatment for below-level central neuropathic pain: a retrospective study. *Journal of Spinal Cord Medicine*. 2003; **26**: 21–6.
93. Cioni B, Meglio M, Pentimalli L, Visocchi M. Spinal cord stimulation in the treatment of paraplegic pain. *Journal of Neurosurgery*. 1995; **82**: 35–9.
94. Nguyen JP, Lefaucheur JP, Decq P *et al.* Chronic motor cortex stimulation in the treatment of central and neuropathic pain. Correlations between clinical, electrophysiological and anatomical data. *Pain*. 1999; **82**: 245–51.
95. Fregni F, Boggio PS, Lima MC *et al.* A sham-controlled, phase II trial of transcranial direct current stimulation for the treatment of central pain in traumatic spinal cord injury. *Pain*. 2006; **122**: 197–209.
96. Tasker RR, DeCarvalho GTC, Dolan EJ. Intractable pain of spinal cord origin: clinical features and implications for surgery. *Journal of Neurosurgery*. 1992; **77**: 373–8.
97. Pagni CA, Canavero S. Cordomyelotomy in the treatment of paraplegia pain – experience in two cases with long-term results. *Acta Neurologica Belgica*. 1995; **95**: 33–6.
98. Nashold Jr BS, Bullitt E. Dorsal root entry zone lesions to control central pain in paraplegics. *Journal of Neurosurgery*. 1981; **55**: 414–9.
99. Sindou M, Mertens P, Wael M. Microsurgical DREZotomy for pain due to spinal cord and/or cauda equina injuries: long-term results in a series of 44 patients. *Pain*. 2001; **92**: 159–71.
100. Edgar RE, Best LG, Quail PA, Obert AD. Computer-assisted DREZ microcoagulation: posttraumatic spinal deafferentation pain. *Journal of Spinal Disorders*. 1993; **6**: 48–56.
101. Falci S, Best L, Bayles R *et al.* Dorsal root entry zone microcoagulation for spinal cord injury-related central pain: operative intramedullary electrophysiological guidance and clinical outcome. *Journal of Neurosurgery*. 2002; **97**: 193–200.

102. Hicks AL, Martin KA, Ditor DS *et al.* Long-term exercise training in persons with spinal cord injury: effects on strength, arm ergometry performance and psychological well-being. *Spinal Cord.* 2003; **41**: 34–43.
103. Summers JD, Rapoff MA, Varghese G *et al.* Psychosocial factors in chronic spinal cord injury pain. *Pain.* 1991; **47**: 183–9.
104. Lundqvist C, Siosteen A, Blomstrand C *et al.* Spinal cord injuries: clinical, functional, and emotional status. *Spine.* 1991; **16**: 78–83.
105. Craig AR, Hancock K, Dickson H, Chang E. Long-term psychological outcomes in spinal cord injured persons: results of a controlled trial using cognitive behavior therapy. *Archives of Physical Medicine and Rehabilitation.* 1997; **78**: 33–8.
*106. Budh CN, Kowalski J, Lundeberg T. A comprehensive pain management programme comprising educational, cognitive and behavioural interventions for neuropathic pain following spinal cord injury. *Journal of Rehabilitation Medicine.* 2006; **38**: 172–80.
107. Siddall PJ, Middleton JW. A proposed algorithm for the management of pain following spinal cord injury. *Spinal Cord.* 2006; **44**: 67–77.

30

Chronic pain after surgery

WILLIAM MACRAE AND JULIE BRUCE

KEY LEARNING POINTS

- Chronic pain after surgery is common.
- Definition is difficult at a clinical level, but essential for research purposes.
- Chronic pain may occur after any operation.
- The severity and frequency of pain are not proportional to the size of the surgical operation.
- There are many different types of pain syndrome after surgery.
- The mechanisms are ill understood and complex.
- In most cases, it is inappropriate and unhelpful to blame the surgeon.

INTRODUCTION

Chronic pain after surgery is now a well-recognized phenomenon and there are several review articles dealing with the subject in general.[1, 2, 3, 4] There is also a wealth of publications on pain after individual operations, and this chapter will only briefly review the prevalence and demographic data on the subject, given that this has been covered extensively in these other publications. Chapter 31, Preventing chronic pain after surgery in the *Acute Pain* volume in this series covers the risk factors and prevention of chronic pain after surgery.

On reviewing the literature, it is interesting to note that certain operations are well represented (e.g. hernia, limb amputation, and breast surgery), but there is less information about others (e.g. cholecystectomy, gynecological, and orthopedic procedures). Although the fact that many patients suffer chronic pain after surgery is well documented, it has not yet reached all doctors, the general public, or the media. Postsurgical pain is mentioned as a potential complication on some websites dealing with recovery from breast cancer surgery, but is not commonly discussed in surgical textbooks. When obtaining consent prior for surgery, chronic postsurgical pain (CPSP) should be discussed, along with other possible adverse events, complications, and side effects of operations. Future studies on outcomes of surgery should include chronic pain as an outcome measure.

PROBLEM OF DEFINITION

It is difficult to define when a pain becomes chronic. Pain lasting longer than the usual period of healing, or pain that is unlikely to resolve have been suggested, as well as various time scales, for example three or six months.[5]

These time scales are all arbitrary and in practice it may not be possible to be exact. As the mechanisms of the changes that occur after injury and surgery become better understood, details of definition, such as the time scale, will become less important. To illustrate this point, if a patient has an operation for varicose veins and the saphenous nerve is injured, then they will probably have pain immediately after the operation. This may persist from the time of the operation and possibly be permanent, as it is a neuropathic pain. When does it become chronic? In chronic pain after surgery, the difficulty is compounded because pain may have been one of the symptoms that the patient was complaining of prior to surgery, and in fact may have been the main reason for seeking medical help. For example, in patients who have had a cholecystectomy for right upper quadrant pain, the preexisting pain will confuse the issue and complicate understanding the process of development. Is the pain merely a continuation of the presurgical problem or is it a new problem? If it is new, was it caused by the surgery? In some cases, it is obvious that there is a new problem; for example, if there is nerve injury following open cholecystectomy the description of the pain will be quite different from the pain of gallstones and will be accompanied by sensory changes. Unfortunately, in many cases it is difficult to disentangle the pains, especially if the pain that the patient complained of prior to surgery was not helped by the operation. In many patients with abdominal pain, no obvious cause can be found, despite exhaustive investigations. Surgeons are often put under pressure by patients and their relatives, that "something must be done." Sometimes an incidental finding in one of the investigations may serve as a focus for an unfounded belief about the cause, which then leads to surgery. In cases where visceral hyperalgesia is part of the mechanism, surgery is likely to make the pain worse.[6]

A working definition of chronic postsurgical pain has been proposed,[3] which suggests the following criteria:

- the pain developed after a surgical procedure;
- the pain is of at least two months duration;
- other causes for the pain should have been excluded (e.g. continuing malignancy or chronic infection);
- the possibility that the pain is continuing from a preexisting problem must be explored and exclusion attempted. (There is an obvious gray area here in that surgery may simply exacerbate a preexisting condition, but attributing escalating pain to the surgery is clearly not possible as natural deterioration cannot be ruled out.)

Unfortunately, most published studies do not attempt to define chronic pain after surgery, and in the studies where a definition is attempted, there are differences in timing and criteria used.[7] Although the above definition is arbitrary, it is a starting point.

RANGE OF SYNDROMES

There is no single entity "chronic pain after surgery," it may present with several different types of pain syndrome. Even one operation, such as open thoracotomy, can cause chronic pain in several different ways; the surgeon has to either resect a piece of rib or spread the ribs in order to gain access to the chest. This causes skeletal trauma to the ribs or to the joints at the posterior and anterior articulations which may result in a nociceptive, musculoskeletal pain. The intercostal nerves, lying just deep to the inferior border of the ribs, are vulnerable to injury, which may cause neuropathic pain. Surgery involving the lungs, heart, or other organs may contribute to a chronic visceral pain. Chest drains can be a source of pain.[8] After breast surgery, patients may experience several types of pain: phantom pain,[9, 10] neuropathic pain caused by damage to the intercostobrachial nerve,[11] or scar pain.[12] In addition to pain, patients report a wide diversity of symptoms including numbness, tingling, swelling, or sensitivity which they report as unpleasant and distressing.[13, 14] These symptoms also cause morbidity and can severely impact upon quality of life. It is obvious therefore that even after a single operation there may be a diverse group of sensations felt in the postoperative period. This can also present a challenge for accurate classification of CPSP syndromes as the majority of the studies are epidemiological, thus population-based, relying on questionnaires to gather data. Few studies have used clinical assessment, which is understandable because of resource implications, but inevitably calls into question the quality and reliability of the findings. Studies on pain after amputation have stressed how difficult patients find it to differentiate between stump pain, phantom pain, and other unpleasant sensations,[15] and it is probable that patients with other postsurgical pain syndromes have similar difficulties.

MECHANISMS OF CHRONIC POSTSURGICAL PAIN

Most people expect to have some pain after an operation. This represents the same process within the organism as pain after any injury. The pain caused by an injury does not bear a simple relationship to the severity or "size" of the injury and in the same way the size of the operation does not neatly correlate to the severity of the chronic pain that follows. An example would be to compare vasectomy with total hip replacement or sternotomy. Vasectomy is an operation carried out for social rather than medical reasons, on fit men, and is minimally traumatic. However, in a proportion of men, the pain suffered after surgery can be severe and cause considerable disability. The prevalence of chronic pain after vasectomy varies between studies from 5[16] to 15 percent.[17, 18] In contrast, total hip replacement is a major operation on patients who have normally long-standing and painful pathology. This is a lengthy procedure that involves cutting and reaming bone, injury to muscles and other soft tissues, and a large incision which must inevitably cut some nerves. Nikolajsen *et al.*[19] found a prevalence of chronic pain of 28 percent at 12–18 months following total hip arthroplasty, which caused sleep disturbance in 9 percent and moderate, severe, or very severe impact on daily life in 12 percent. In this group of 1048 patients, only one did not have pain prior to the operation, the majority had severe pain. After sternotomy, another traumatic procedure, about 28 percent of patients report chronic pain, with about 13 percent overall experiencing moderate or severe pain.[20, 21]

In a recent paper, Peters *et al.*[22] explored somatic and psychological predictors of outcome after surgery. This interesting study found that operations lasting more than three hours were associated with more chronic pain, as well as increased functional limitation, poor global recovery, and poorer quality of life at six months postoperatively. Fear of surgery and severe postoperative pain were also associated with a worse outcome. The authors suggest that the prolonged and intense nociceptive barrage may increase central sensitizations. Recent work on the role of the brain stem in influencing spinal cord amplification may help to explain the role of emotions and psychological factors.[23]

Clearly, the mechanisms involved in the etiology of chronic pain are complex and any operation has the potential to cause chronic pain, but changes in the nervous system are probably the most important factor.

Changes to the nervous system after injury and surgery

Neuropathic pain has many etiologies and mechanisms.[24] Nerve injury, such as transection, stretching, or constriction, will obviously cause structural and functional changes. However, it is important to appreciate that injury to other tissues changes the pain system as well.[25] A good example is sunburn, a thermal injury to the skin. To explain the pain after sunburn simply in terms of "damage to the skin" is an illogical and inadequate explanation; thermal injury to the skin initiates a cascade of changes, including the release of inflammatory mediators from the damaged cells. These change the nociceptors by reducing their thresholds and increasing excitability, both at the periphery and in the spinal cord. This hyperexcitability results in allodynia and hyperalgesia. It is this sensitization in the sensory nerves to the skin (caused by the damage) that causes the ongoing pain, not the damage to the skin itself. In the same way, the injuries involved in surgery can also cause changes, both peripheral and central, resulting in sensitization and hyperalgesia. Many postsurgical pain syndromes are in fact allodynic and hyperalgesic syndromes.

Neuronal plasticity after injury occurs not only at the periphery and the spinal cord, but also in the brain. Pons *et al.*[26] first described remapping of the sensory cortex after deafferentation. Cortical remapping is now known to occur in humans after limb amputation[27] and may be evident soon after injury.[28] It has been shown to change with time.[29] Plasticity can also occur in the thalamus.[30] In an interesting case described by Halligan *et al.*,[31] a patient developed the sensation of a third arm following a stroke, suggesting that this may be a two-way process – injury to the brain can cause misperceptions at the periphery. The changes in the brain after amputation contribute to the reason why amputees have phantom sensations and pain.

EVOLUTIONARY PERSPECTIVE

As described above, the nervous system changes following injury. The injured part becomes painful and sensitive because the peripheral receptor thresholds are decreased and central amplification occurs, making any signals "louder." This hypersensitivity following injury probably confers an evolutionary benefit by encouraging rest, preventing further damage, and allowing healing. The abnormal "settings" of the nervous system should return to normal after the injury has healed. Failure to return to normal would leave the nervous system in a sensitized state and this is probably one of the causes of chronic pain after surgery. Why the nervous system does not readjust is unknown, but animal work suggests that there is a genetic component to the development of neuropathic pain after injury.[32, 33] There are many similarities between memory and chronic pain; long-term potentiation (LTP) is a mechanism common to both.[34, 35] In many ways, chronic pain represents a failure to forget.

POSTSURGICAL PAIN SYNDROMES

As stated earlier, there are several different types of pain syndromes which may develop after surgery. Most studies of chronic pain after surgery focus on patient cohorts undergoing one surgical procedure, such as mastectomy or chest surgery, rather than assessment of large, diverse surgical populations. In this chapter, it is not possible to review all the literature on postsurgical conditions. We will review the pain syndromes associated with three types of surgery, amputation, hernia surgery, and breast surgery. These are the three areas that have received the most attention and in which there are sufficient good quality publications to draw valid conclusions. The review articles mentioned in the Introduction above cover pain syndromes after some other types of surgery, but it has to be emphasized that for many types of surgery there is little or no published evidence and often the studies are of poor quality.

Pain after amputation

Pain after limb amputation was undoubtedly the first of all the postsurgical pain syndromes to be recognized. Silas Weir Mitchell described phantom limbs and pain syndromes caused by gunshot wounds following the American Civil War.[36] Pain following limb amputation falls into two broad categories, phantom pain and stump pain (also called residual limb pain). Many lower limb amputees also report back pain.[37] For a detailed review of phantom pain, see the excellent article by Nikolajsen and Jensen, and Chapter 31, Postamputation pain.[38]

The incidence of phantom limb pain varies from around 50 to 85 percent.[39, 40, 41, 42] In a study of amputees from the Yom Kippur war, Carlen *et al.*[43] reported an incidence of phantom pain of 67 percent. The onset of the phantom pain was immediate in 12 percent of patients, during the first day in 10 percent, during the first week in 12 percent, in the second week in 5 percent, third week in 16 percent, and longer than three weeks in 2 percent. The remaining patients had no pain or were uncertain about the date of onset. A study of upper limb amputees from the Iran–Iraq War found an incidence of phantom pain of 32 percent.[44] In general, phantom pain seems to be less common after upper limb amputation than lower limb amputation.[45, 46] The severity of phantom pain varies between studies, from 59 percent with mostly mild or moderate pain,[41] to 40 percent of amputees with severe pain.[47] Although several studies have shown that phantom pain can improve or resolve in individuals, in a population of amputees the prevalence of phantom limb pain changes little; some patients improve, while others become worse. Overall, the literature does suggest that the duration and frequency of phantom limb episodes tends to decrease in the first six months, but remain stable thereafter.[40] Several studies have investigated risk factors for phantom limb pain, but areas of controversy remain.[48, 49, 50]

In the past it was thought that young children rarely suffer phantom limb pain and that those with congenital absence of limbs do not experience phantom limbs or phantom limb pain. However, a study of children by Smith and Thompson[51] found a pain prevalence of 12 percent for amputation following trauma and 48 percent for amputations because of cancer. Interestingly, in this subgroup of cancer patients the incidence rose to 74 percent if the children had chemotherapy at or before the time of amputation, but the incidence was 44 percent if the chemotherapy was given after the amputation. The prevalence was only 12 percent if chemotherapy was not used. Melzack *et al.*[52] have shown that children with congenital absence of limbs can indeed suffer phantom pain.

The prevalence of stump pain varies in different studies. In a survey of US Army veterans, Sherman *et al.*[39] found an incidence of 62 percent and Richardson *et al.*[42] reported 51 percent, in a prospective study of patients with peripheral vascular disease. However, Pohjolainen[41] found a prevalence of stump pain in only 5 percent in a study of amputees attending a prosthetics factory. The differences in prevalence between these studies probably reflect methodological rather than real differences.

Phantom pain can occur after removal of other body parts as well as limbs, such as breast,[9, 10] eye,[53] rectum,[54, 55] tongue,[56] teeth,[57] and genitals.[58] Despite the fact that circumcision is the most common operation carried out on males, there are no reports of phantom foreskin in the literature.

Chronic pain after hernia surgery

The epidemiology of chronic pain after inguinal hernia surgery is well documented. Indeed, the volume of literature reporting CPSP after hernia surgery has increased dramatically in the last two decades. Many studies have been specifically designed to investigate persistent pain as an outcome rather than the traditional outcomes of hernia recurrence, wound infection, or return to work. Guidance on laparoscopic and open hernia surgery published by the UK National Institute for Clinical Excellence (NICE) acknowledged chronic pain as a common postoperative adverse event and recommended that future studies assess persistent pain along with recurrence and other adverse outcomes.[59]

Two systematic reviews of the epidemiology of chronic pain after inguinal herniorrhaphy have been published since 2003. First, Poobalan *et al.*[7] reviewed data on chronic pain from 40 experimental and epidemiological studies published up to the year 2000. Using strict inclusion criteria, with chronic pain defined as that at or beyond three months, 40 of 101 potential studies were eligible for inclusion. The frequency of chronic pain after herniorrhaphy ranged from 0 to 53 percent depending upon timing and method of follow up, with moderate to severe pain in about 10 percent of patients. An updated systematic review only included studies published between 2000 and 2004, with sample sizes of at least 100 patients and a rigorous definition of chronicity of pain at or beyond six months of surgery.[60] Despite these strict limiting criteria, the search still yielded over 100 potential studies, although many were rejected because of lack of follow up beyond six months. Chronic pain was the primary outcome in 16 studies. Both reviews found higher pain prevalence rates where chronic pain was the primary outcome of interest, with rates being three times higher compared to studies where pain was the secondary outcome.[7, 60] These systematic reviews indicate the increase in volume of literature, from both epidemiological and experimental studies.

Hernia surgery provides a good model for studying the mechanisms of chronic pain, given it is a common elective procedure for a benign condition in a relatively healthy and active population. The condition can be uncomplicated by extensive comorbidity or by confounding treatment variables, such as chemotherapy and radiotherapy. It is a common surgical procedure, with approximately 70,000 procedures being conducted in England per annum and 700,000 in the USA.[59, 61] Therefore, the potential burden of illness is high given the population exposed to surgery and given that 10 percent will be expected to develop chronic pain after surgery.

Chronic pain after breast surgery

In the UK alone, 42,000 new patients are diagnosed with primary breast cancer each year and most undergo surgery, either mastectomy or breast conservation surgery with sentinel node sample or clearance. Chronic pain was initially reported in the 1970s as a rare consequence of breast cancer treatment.[62] There are now many epidemiological and clinical studies reporting the prevalence and characteristics of persistent pain which suggest that it occurs commonly, with subsequent impact upon quality of life. There are several types of pain suffered by women after breast surgery.[9, 63, 64] Although prevalence varies by methodology used and timing of follow up,[10] postmastectomy pain is thought to affect up to half of women undergoing surgery up to one year after their surgery.[12] Chronic pain is also common after breast reduction and augmentation operations.[63, 65] It is also important to recognize that pain is not the only symptom that may be bothersome for patients after breast surgery; swelling, tingling, numbness, and other symptoms are commonly reported.[14, 66, 67]

The cause of pain following breast surgery is complex and various etiologies have been postulated. Early theories mostly attributed the cause to peripheral nerve damage and traumatic neuroma. Although predominantly referred to as "postmastectomy pain syndrome" in the past, it has been suggested that this term be changed to intercostobrachial neuralgia (ICN) to describe the neuropathic pain syndromes, regardless of operative procedure, whether radical mastectomy or lumpectomy with axillary clearance.[12] Damage may occur to nerves during surgery, particularly to the intercostobrachial nerve which arises from the second and/or third thoracic intercostal nerve and crosses the axilla supplying sensation to the upper half of the arm and axillary region. The intercostobrachial nerve is often sacrificed to accomplish complete removal of axillary lymph nodes. It was reported that sacrifice of the intercostobrachial nerve led to persistent discomfort, resultant numbness, and paraesthesia and that the nerve should be preserved wherever possible.[68] However, preservation may not be possible because of tumor spread or anatomical variations in its course. The situation is complicated because throughout the 1990s, studies of breast conservation surgery reported that chronic pain and abnormal sensations persisted even where the nerve was preserved.[69] Carpenter *et al.*[70] state, "the generally accepted risk factor of damage to the intercostobrachial nerve is mostly anecdotal." Axillary hematoma has been reported as a possible and treatable cause of postmastectomy pain syndrome.[71] Chronic pain and persistent upper arm symptoms have been reported after lumpectomy, sentinel node biopsy procedures, and also breast augmentation or reduction surgery.[63, 65, 70, 72, 73] As the surgical procedure is quite different in these procedures, and the intercostobrachial nerve may not be affected, clearly other factors in addition to nerve injury contribute to the development of pain. The risk factors for CPSP after breast surgery are examined in more detail in Chapter 31, Preventing chronic pain after surgery in the *Acute Pain* volume in this series.

A comprehensive review article proposed a classification system for postoperative neuropathic pain after breast cancer surgery.[12] The authors described nociceptive chronic pain after surgery as that resulting from injury to ligament or muscle, and neuropathic pain as that initiated or caused by a primary lesion or dysfunction in the nervous system. They suggest classifying the neuropathic pain syndromes into four groups: (1) phantom breast pain, (2) intercostobrachial neuralgia, (3) neuroma pain, and (4) other nerve injury pain. Although comprehensive in that it included 17 primary studies, the review was unsystematic in methodology and failed to describe bibliographic databases or search strategy, or the criteria for study inclusion or exclusion. The timing of pain chronicity ranged from two to six months after breast surgery. The review presents prevalence rates by pain syndrome: phantom breast pain (13–44 percent), ICN (13–61 percent), and neuroma pain (23–49 percent).[12] This is the first attempt at syndrome classification; however, it fails to account for variation or misclassification within patient samples from individual studies, particularly because most primary studies have used postal methodology rather than detailed clinical assessment. Many patients may have mixed pain syndromes and may be troubled by other symptoms, not usually described as painful.[14, 66, 67] The need for clean distinctions between syndromes for research purposes is not reflected in the clinical reality. Many patients present at pain clinics with complex problems and many different symptoms, and the challenge is to develop valid and reliable data collection tools to improve upon accuracy of detection and classification of syndromes.

IMPLICATIONS OF THE COMPLEXITY OF MECHANISMS

Understanding the scale of the changes to the nervous system and the mechanisms that predispose to chronic pain after surgery is important for many reasons. It can change the climate of blame that exists when patients have pain after an operation. Because people expect the pain after injury or an operation to resolve as the injury heals, it is natural that they should imagine that something must have gone wrong with the operation if the pain persists. It is not possible to perform surgery without some damage to tissues, and therefore a hyperalgesic state will be induced after any operation, regardless of how it is done. Usually this will revert to normal as healing occurs, but not always. Whether a patient experiences chronic pain after surgery or not is therefore more likely to depend on the "set" of their nervous system than on precisely what the surgeon did. For patients who have chronic pain after surgery, it is inappropriate to assume that the surgeon has necessarily done anything wrong or that it is anyone's fault.

Patients who believe that someone was to blame for their chronic pain report more distress and behavioral disturbance, as well as poor response to treatments and lower expectations of future benefits.[74] Cognitive mechanisms of symptom perception in chronic pain may be affected by a patient's belief that they were injured,[75] leading to lower pain threshold and tolerance, decreased activity, and general deconditioning. It is therefore clear that removing the climate of blame would help both patients and surgeons. By accepting that chronic pain is, for a proportion of patients, an inevitable consequence of surgery, like a wound infection, and openly discussing it before surgery, much subsequent grief could be avoided.

The complexity also has implications for clinical practice. The extent of the changes in the nervous system suggests that pharmacological, psychological, and behavioral therapies may be more beneficial to patients than invasive treatments. Simplistic notions about treatment, for example simple nerve blocks, or further surgery are unlikely to help, and may well do harm, by causing further damage. If surgery has the potential to cause chronic pain, then caution is needed before embarking on operations. This is of particular relevance for cosmetic surgery, or for other procedures that are performed out of choice rather than need. It also raises important questions about surgery in conditions where the evidence for efficacy is lacking, for example some types of surgery for back pain, producing the post laminectomy syndrome.[76]

Lastly, acknowledging the complexity of chronic pain after surgery, especially the changes in the nervous system, should help to guide the directions of future research, in particular by taking into account the mechanisms that lead to the development of chronic pain.

FUTURE DIRECTIONS

Many of the studies on this topic from the past are of poor quality. There are papers in which the methods section describes how to perform the surgical operation, but does not clearly identify the sample size, the definitions used, the follow-up time, or outcome measures. The problem of definition has been ignored by many authors. Many studies report pain incidence but without preoperative data, making it hard to draw valid conclusions about incidence. Some studies are described as cohort studies when they are in fact cross-sectional studies reporting point or period prevalence. There are many papers, which in the title purport to look at outcomes of surgery, but do not mention pain, despite previously published evidence that chronic pain is a recognized sequela of that type of surgery. Fortunately, there is evidence of a large increase in literature on CPSP in the last few decades and that the quality of literature is improving. Studies which are designed specifically to investigate the incidence of chronic pain usually find a higher incidence than studies in which chronic pain is only studied as part of a broader investigation. These broader studies can be less well conducted, often with methodological flaws.

Most previous research has concentrated on the epidemiology of CPSP after different procedures, the surgery, and patient demographics. While this is understandable and useful, we need to move beyond studies of prevalence which merely draw attention to the frequency of the problem. In future clinical studies, researchers should be concentrating on risk factors, prevention, and management. Good quality prospective studies are required that record baseline preoperative data, in order to identify subgroups of patients who may be at higher risk of developing CPSP. There is a need to broaden the scientific approach, acknowledging the complex interactions between the "patient" factors, such as genotype, previous medical history, and psychosocial factors, and the "surgical" factors, such as type of surgery, type of anesthesia, concomitant treatments, and perioperative analgesia. These wider investigative approaches have been used to identify risk factors for other types of nonsurgical chronic pain syndromes, such as fibromyalgia and chronic widespread pain.[77] Therefore, we argue for a multidisciplinary approach, to design new studies with experts from chronic pain, epidemiology, health psychology, brain imaging, neurosciences, genetics, and probably other disciplines as well.

Many questions remain unanswered. Why is it that only a proportion of patients have chronic pain after a standardized operation, why not everyone or nobody? What is different about this group of patients? Why are the results of studies examining nerve transection so contradictory? In order to begin to understand these questions, we need to investigate the mechanisms of pain after surgery, which is in essence the same as that of pain after any injury. Castillo *et al.*[78] have shown that after lower limb trauma, the numbers of patients demonstrating high levels of long-term pain are similar to chronic postsurgical pain syndromes. This highlights the importance of relevant basic science research into the mechanisms of pain after injury. It is only by bringing together basic scientists and clinicians that we will understand and solve the problem of chronic pain after surgery, and work to prevent it.

REFERENCES

* 1. Crombie IK, Davies HTO, Macrae WA. Cut and thrust: antecedent surgery and trauma among patients attending a chronic pain clinic. *Pain.* 1998; **76**: 167–71.
* 2. Macrae WA. Chronic pain after surgery. *British Journal of Anaesthesia.* 2001; **87**: 88–98.
* 3. Macrae WA, Davies HTO. Chronic postsurgical pain. In: Crombie IK, Linton S, Croft P *et al.* (eds). *Epidemiology of pain.* Seattle: International Association for the Study of Pain, 1999: 125–42.
* 4. Perkins FM, Kehlet H. Chronic pain as an outcome of surgery. *Anesthesiology.* 2000; **93**: 1123–33.

5. Merskey H, Bogduk N (eds). *Classification of chronic pain. Descriptions of chronic pain syndromes and definitions of pain terms*, 2nd edn. Seattle: IASP Press, 1994.
6. Wilder-Smith OH, Tassonyi E, Senly C *et al.* Surgical pain is followed not only by spinal sensitization but also by supraspinal antinociception. *British Journal of Anaesthesiology.* 1996; **76**: 816–21.

* 7. Poobalan AS, Bruce J, Smith WC *et al.* A review of chronic pain after inguinal herniorrhaphy. *Clinical Journal of Pain.* 2003; **19**: 48–54.

8. Richardson J, Sabanathan S, Mearns AJ *et al.* Post-thoracotomy neuralgia. *Pain Clinic.* 1994; **7**: 87–97.
9. Kroner K, Knudsen UB, Lundby L, Hvid H. Long term phantom breast syndrome after mastectomy. *Clinical Journal of Pain.* 1992; **8**: 346–50.

* 10. Dijkstra PU, Rietman JS, Geertzen JHB. Phantom breast sensations and phantom breast pain: A 2-year prospective study and a methodological analysis of literature. *European Journal of Pain.* 2007; **11**: 99–108.

11. Vecht CJ, Van der Brand HJ, Wajer OJM. Post-axillary dissection pain in breast cancer due to a lesion of the intercostobrachial nerve. *Pain.* 1989; **38**: 171–6.

* 12. Jung BF, Ahrendt GM, Oaklander AL, Dworkin RH. Neuropathic pain following breast cancer surgery: proposed classification and research update. *Pain.* 2003; **104**: 1–13.

13. Polinsky ML. Functional status of long-term breast cancer survivors. *Health and Social Work.* 1994; **19**: 165–73.
14. Tasmuth T, Blomqvist C, Kalso E. Chronic post-treatment symptoms in patients with breast cancer operated in different surgical units. *European Journal of Surgical Oncology.* 1999; **25**: 38–43.
15. Hill A. Phantom limb pain: a review of the literature on attributes and potential mechanisms. *Journal of Pain and Symptom Management.* 1999; **17**: 125–42.
16. Ahmed I, Rasheed S, White C, Shaikh NA. The incidence of post-vasectomy chronic testicular pain and the role of nerve stripping (denervation) of the spermatic cord in its management. *British Journal of Urology.* 1997; **79**: 269–70.
17. Manikandan R, Srirangam SJ, Pearson E, Collins GN. Early and late morbidity after vasectomy: a comparison of chronic scrotal pain at 1 and 10 years. *BJU International.* 2004; **93**: 571–4.
18. McMahon AJ, Buckley J, Taylor A *et al.* Chronic testicular pain following vasectomy. *British Journal of Urology.* 1992; **69**: 188–91.
19. Nikolajsen L, Brandsborg B, Lucht U *et al.* Chronic pain following total hip arthroplasty: a nationwide questionnaire study. *Acta Anaesthesiologica Scandinavica.* 2006; **50**: 495–500.
20. Kalso E, Mennander S, Tasmuth T, Nilsson E. Chronic post-sternotomy pain. *Acta Anaesthesiologica Scandinavica.* 2001; **45**: 935–9.
21. Meyerson J, Thelin S, Gordh T, Karlsten R. The incidence of chronic post-sternotomy pain after cardiac surgery – a prospective study. *Acta Anaesthesiologica Scandinavica.* 2001; **45**: 940–4.

* 22. Peters ML, Sommer M, Rijke JM *et al.* Somatic and psychologic predictors of long-term unfavourable outcome after surgical intervention. *Annals of Surgery.* 2007; **245**: 487–94.

23. Suzuki R, Rygh LJ, Dickenson AH. Bad news from the brain: descending 5-HT pathways that control spinal pain processing. *Trends in Pharmacological Sciences.* 2004; **25**: 613–7.
24. Woolf CJ, Mannion RJ. Neuropathic pain: Aetiology, symptoms, mechanisms and management. *Lancet.* 1999; **353**: 1959–64.
25. Villanueva L, Dickenson AH, Ollat H. *The pain system in normal and pathological states.* Seattle: IASP Press, 2004.
26. Pons TP, Preston E, Garraghty AK. Massive cortical reorganisation after sensory deafferentation in adult macaques. *Science.* 1991; **252**: 1857–60.
27. Ramachandran VS, Hirstein W. The perception of phantom limbs. *Brain.* 1998; **121**: 1603–30.
28. Borsook D, Becerra L, Fishman S *et al.* Acute plasticity in the human somatosensory cortex following amputation. *NeuroReport.* 1998; **9**: 1013–7.
29. Knecht S, Henningsen H, Hohling C *et al.* Plasticity of plasticity? Changes in the pattern of perceptual correlates of reorganisation after amputation. *Brain.* 1998; **121**: 717–24.
30. Dostrovsky JO. Immediate and long-term plasticity in human somatosensory thalamus and its involvement in phantom limbs. *Pain.* 1999; Suppl. 6: S37–43.
31. Halligan PW, Marshall JC, Wade DT. Three arms: a case study of supernumerary phantom limb after right hemisphere stroke. *Journal of Neurology, Neurosurgery and Psychiatry.* 1993; **56**: 159–66.
32. Devor M, Raber P. Heritability of symptoms in an experimental model of neuropathic pain. *Pain.* 1990; **42**: 51–67.
33. Seltzer Z, Wu T, Max MB, Diehl SR. Mapping a gene for neuropathic pain-related behaviour following peripheral neurectomy in the mouse. *Pain.* 2001; **93**: 101–6.
34. Ji RR, Kohno T, Moore KA, Woolf CJ. Central sensitization and LTP: do pain and memory share similar mechanisms? *Trends in Neurosciences.* 2003; **26**: 696–705.
35. Rygh LJ, Svendsen F, Fiska A *et al.* Long-term potentiation in spinal nociceptive systems – how acute pain may

become chronic. *Psychoneuroendocrinology.* 2005; **30**: 959–64.

36. Mitchell SW. *Injuries of nerves and their consequences.* Philadelphia, PA: JB Lippincott, 1872.
37. Kusljugic A, Kapidzic-Durakovic S, Kudumovic Z, Cickusic A. Chronic low back pain in individuals with lower-limb amputation. *Bosnian Journal of Basic Medical Sciences.* 2006; **6**: 67–70.
* 38. Nikolajsen L, Jensen TS. Phantom limb pain. *British Journal of Anaesthesia.* 2001; **87**: 107–16.
39. Sherman RA, Sherman CJ, Parker L. Chronic phantom and stump pain among American veterans: results of a survey. *Pain.* 1984; **18**: 83–95.
40. Jensen TS, Krebs B, Nielsen J, Rasmussen P. Immediate and long-term phantom limb pain in amputees: incidence, clinical characteristics and relationship to pre-amputation limb pain. *Pain.* 1985; **21**: 267–78.
41. Pohjolainen T. A clinical evaluation of stumps in lower limb amputees. *Prosthetics and Orthotics International.* 1991; **15**: 178–84.
42. Richardson C, Glenn S, Nurmikko T, Horgan M. Incidence of phantom phenomena including phantom limb pain 6 months after major lower limb amputation in patients with peripheral vascular disease. *Clinical Journal of Pain.* 2006; **22**: 353–8.
43. Carlen PL, Wall PD, Nadvorna H. Phantom limbs and related phenomena in recent traumatic amputations. *Neurology.* 1978; **28**: 211–7.
44. Ebrahimzadeh MH, Fattahi AS, Nejad AB. Long-term follow-up of Iranian veteran upper extremity amputees from the Iran-Iraq war (1980–1988). *Journal of Trauma.* 2006; **61**: 886–8.
45. Lacoux PA, Crombie IK, Macrae WA. Pain in traumatic upper limb amputees in Sierra Leone. *Pain.* 2002; **99**: 309–12.
46. Kooijman CM, Dijkstra PU, Geertzen JH *et al.* Phantom pain and phantom sensations in upper limb amputees: an epidemiological study. *Pain.* 2000; **87**: 33–41.
47. Smith DG, Ehde DM, Legro MW *et al.* Phantom pain, residual limb, and back pain after lower extremity amputations. *Clinical Orthopedics and Related Research.* 1999; **361**: 29–38.
48. Hanley MA, Jensen MP, Smith DG *et al.* Preamputation pain and acute pain predict chronic pain after lower extremity amputation. *Journal of Pain.* 2007; **8**: 102–09.
49. Dijkstra PU, Geertzen JH, Stewart R, van der Schans CP. Phantom pain and risk factors: a multivariate analysis. *Journal of Pain and Symptom Management.* 2002; **24**: 578–85.
50. Nikolajsen L, Ilkjaer S, Kroner K *et al.* The influence of preamputation pain on postamputation stump and phantom pain. *Pain.* 1997; **72**: 393–405.
51. Smith J, Thompson JM. Phantom limb pain and chemotherapy in pediatric amputees. *Mayo Clinic Proceedings.* 1995; **70**: 357–64.
52. Melzack R, Israel R, Lacroix R, Schultz G. Phantom limbs in people with congenital limb deficiency or amputation in early childhood. *Brain.* 1997; **120**: 1603–20.
53. Soros P, Vo O, Husstedt IW *et al.* Phantom eye syndrome: Its prevalence, phenomenology, and putative mechanisms. *Neurology.* 2003; **60**: 1542–3.
54. Ovesen P, Kroner K, Ornsholt J, Bach K. Phantom-related phenomena after rectal amputation: prevalence and clinical characteristics. *Pain.* 1991; **44**: 289–91.
55. Boas RA, Schug SA, Acland RH. Perineal pain after rectal amputation: a 5-year follow-up. *Pain.* 1993; **52**: 67–70.
56. Hanowell S, Kennedy SF. Phantom tongue pain and causalgia: case presentation and treatment. *Anesthesia and Analgesia.* 1979; **58**: 436–7.
57. Marbach JJ, Hulbrook J, Hohn C, Segal AG. Incidence of phantom tooth pain: an atypical facial neuralgia. *Oral Surgery, Oral Medicine, and Oral Pathology.* 1982; **53**: 190–3.
58. Heusner AP. Phantom genitalia. *Transactions of the American Neurological Association.* 1950; **75**: 128–34.
59. National Institute for Clinical Excellence. Laparoscopic surgery for inguinal hernia repair. In: *Technology appraisal guidance.* London: NICE, 2004.
* 60. Aasvang E, Kehlet H. Chronic postoperative pain: the case of inguinal herniorrhaphy. *British Journal of Anaesthesiology.* 2005; **95**: 69–76.
61. Neumayer L, Jonasson O, Fitzgibbons R *et al.* Tension-free inguinal hernia repair: the design of a trial to compare open and laparoscopic surgical techniques. *Journal of the American College of Surgeons.* 2003; **196**: 743–52.
62. Wood KM. Intercostobrachial nerve entrapment syndrome. *Southern Medical Journal.* 1978; **71**: 662–3.
63. Wallace MS, Wallace AM, Lee J, Dobke MK. Pain after breast surgery: a survey of 282 women. *Pain.* 1996; **66**: 195–205.
64. Stevens PE, Dibble SL, Miaskowski C. Prevalence, characteristics, and impact of postmastectomy pain syndrome: an investigation of women's experiences. *Pain.* 1995; **61**: 61–8.
65. Romundstad L, Breivik H, Roald H *et al.* Chronic pain and sensory changes after augmentation mammoplasty: long term effects of preincisional administration of methylprednisolone. *Pain.* 2006; **124**: 92–9.
66. Polinsky ML. Functional status of long-term breast cancer survivors: demonstrating chronicity. *Health and Social Work.* 1994; **19**: 165–73.
67. Tasmuth T, von Smitten K, Hietanen P *et al.* Pain and other symptoms after different treatment modalities of breast cancer. *Annals of Oncology.* 1995; **6**: 453–9.
68. Teicher I, Poulard B, Wise L. Preservation of the intercostobrachial nerve during axillary dissection for carcinoma of the breast. *Surgery, Gynecology and Obstetrics.* 1982; **155**: 891–2.
69. Salmon RJ, Ansquer Y, Asselain B. Preservation versus section of intercostal-brachial nerve (IBN) in axillary dissection for breast cancer – a prospective randomized

trial. *European Journal of Surgical Oncology.* 1998; **24**: 158–61.

70. Carpenter JS, Sloan P, Andrykowski MA *et al.* Risk factors for pain after mastectomy/lumpectomy. *Cancer Practice.* 1999; **7**: 66–70.
71. Blunt C, Schmiedel A. Some cases of severe post-mastectomy pain syndrome may be caused by an axillary haematoma. *Pain.* 2004; **108**: 294–6.
72. Peintinger F, Reitsamer R, Stranzl H, Ralph G. Comparison of quality of life and arm complaints after axillary lymph node dissection vs sentinel lymph node biopsy in breast cancer patients. *British Journal of Cancer.* 2003; **89**: 648–52.
73. Tasmuth T, Estlanderb A-M, Kalso E. Effects of present pain and mood on the memory of past postoperative pain in women treated surgically for breast cancer. *Pain.* 1996; **68**: 343–7.
74. DeGood DE, Kiernan B. Perception of fault in patients with chronic pain. *Pain.* 1996; **64**: 153–9.
75. Turk DC, Okifuji A. Perception of traumatic onset, compensation status, and physical findings: impact on pain severity, emotional distress, and disability in chronic pain patients. *Journal of Behavioural Medicine.* 1996; **19**: 435–53.
76. Turner JA, Ersek M, Herron L *et al.* Patient outcomes after lumbar spinal fusions. *Journal of the American Medical Association.* 1992; **268**: 907–11.
77. McBeth J, Silman AJ, Gupta A *et al.* Moderation of psychosocial risk factors through dysfunction of the hypothalamic–pituitary–adrenal stress axis in the onset of chronic widespread musculoskeletal pain: findings of a population-based prospective cohort study. *Arthritis and Rheumatism.* 2007; **56**: 360–71.
78. Castillo RC, MacKenzie EJ, Wegener ST, Bosse MJ. Prevalence of chronic pain seven years following limb threatening lower extremity trauma. *Pain.* 2006; **124**: 321–9.

31

Postamputation pain

LONE NIKOLAJSEN AND SIGNE KOCH

KEY LEARNING POINTS

- The present chapter focuses on clinical characteristics, mechanisms, treatment, and possible preventive measures for pain after limb amputation.
- The incidence of phantom pain, i.e. pain referred to the missing limb, is 60–80 percent. The number of amputees with severe phantom pain is substantially smaller and in the range of 10–15 percent.
- Phantom sensations, i.e. nonpainful sensations referred to the missing limb, are experienced by almost all amputees, but rarely pose any clinical problem.
- Pain located to the residual limb is frequent immediately after amputation. Residual limb pain, however, persists in 5–10 percent of amputees and is often associated with sensory abnormalities, such as hypoesthesia, hyperalgesia, or allodynia.
- The mechanisms underlying chronic pain in amputees are not fully known, but both peripheral and central mechanisms are involved.
- Chronic residual limb and phantom pain are difficult to treat. Treatment regimens used for other neuropathic pain conditions are probably the best approximation.
- It is not possible to prevent all postamputation pain from developing even by intense perioperative pain management.

INTRODUCTION

The first medical descriptions of postamputation phenomena were published in the sixteenth century by such authors as Ambroise Paré, René Descartes, Aaron Lemos, and Charles Bell. Historically, Silas Weir Mitchell is credited with coining the term "phantom limb." In *Injuries of Nerves and their Consequences* (1872) he presented results from clinical studies of amputees and approached phantom limbs physiologically, experimentally, and therapeutically (for historical review see Finger and Hustwit).[1]

In modern times, the Second World War, Vietnam, Israeli, and Iraqi wars have been responsible for many sad cases of traumatic amputations in otherwise healthy people. Landmine explosions in Cambodia still result in many amputations,[2] and during the recent civil war in Sierra Leone, the opposing sides performed limb amputations to terrorize the enemy.[3] Judicial amputations are still carried out in some societies (see www.amnesty.org.uk, www.hrweb.org/legal/cat.html). In western countries, the main reason for surgical amputation is peripheral vascular disease and, less often, tumors. Most of these patients are elderly and have often suffered from long-lasting preamputation pain.

Amputation is followed by phantom phenomena in virtually all amputees. The incidence and nature of phantom pain are probably similar in patients amputated for medical or traumatic reasons.[4] Most patients feel that the missing limb is still present, and some may have vivid sensations of shape, length, posture, and movement. Such nonpainful phantom sensations rarely pose any clinical problem, but 60–80 percent of all amputees also have painful sensations located to the missing limb. The intensity and frequency of both nonpainful and painful phantom sensations usually diminish in time, but in a substantial number of patients (5–10 percent) severe phantom pain persists. Residual limb pain is another consequence of trauma or surgery, but in most patients the pain subsides within a few weeks. However, some patients develop chronic pain located in the residual limb. Phantom sensation, phantom pain, and residual limb pain often coexist in the same patient and the elements may be difficult to separate.

The mechanisms underlying chronic pain in amputees are not fully known, despite extensive research in the area. The development of animal models mimicking neuropathic pain and research in other neuropathic pain conditions has, however, contributed significantly to the understanding of phantom pain. It is now clear that nerve injury is followed by a series of changes in the peripheral and central nervous system, and that these changes may play a role in the induction and maintenance of phantom pain.

Chronic residual limb and phantom pain may be exceedingly difficult to treat. Many different treatments have been proposed but the vast majority are based on small groups with no controls. Tricyclic antidepressants (TCAs) and anticonvulsants have proven effective in other neuropathic pain conditions.[5] These drugs are probably also effective in the treatment of chronic postamputation pain. Other medications may include opioids and perhaps *N*-methyl-D-aspartic acid (NMDA) receptor antagonists. Nonmedical treatments, for example physiotherapy and transcutaneous electrical nerve stimulation (TENS), should also be tried. Surgery must be avoided, except in cases with obvious stump pathology.

Although phantom pains may occur after the loss of other body parts, for example the breast[6] or the rectum,[7] the present chapter will focus on postamputation pain after limb amputation. The following definitions will be used:

- **phantom pain**: painful sensations referred to the missing limb;
- **phantom sensation**: any sensation of the missing limb, except pain;
- **residual limb pain**: pain referred to the amputation residual limb.

CLINICAL CHARACTERISTICS

Phantom pain

PREVALENCE

The reported prevalence of phantom pain varies much in the literature. Very early studies claimed that the prevalence was 2–4 percent,[8, 9] but today most studies agree that 60–80 percent of all amputees experience phantom pain following amputation (see **Table 31.1** for details).[3, 4, 8, 9, 10, 11, 12, 13, 14, 15, 16, 17, 18, 19, 20, 21, 22, 23, 24, 25, 26, 27] In a recent study including 914 amputees, 80 percent reported experiencing phantom pain.[24]

There are several explanations for this variation, including different methods of estimating pain. Studies based on patients' request for pain treatment are likely to underestimate the prevalence because many amputees – at least in the past – were reluctant to report pain to healthcare providers.[14] In a retrospective study of the methods of anesthesia and analgesia for 349 major lower limb amputations, there was a written record of only 18 percent patients experiencing phantom pain, although 37 percent were prescribed carbamazepine.[28]

The prevalence of phantom pain seems to be independent of age in adults, gender, side or level of amputation, and cause (nontraumatic versus traumatic) of amputation.[4, 13, 19, 24, 29] Interestingly, phantom limb pain is more frequent when the amputation occurs in adulthood, less frequent in child amputees, and virtually nonexistent in congenital amputees.[30, 31] In a study of 60 child and adolescent amputees who were missing a limb because of congenital limb deficiency ($n = 27$), trauma or surgery ($n = 33$), the prevalence of phantom pain was 3.7 percent in the congenital group and 48.5 percent in the surgical group.[13, 20, 26]

TIME COURSE OF PHANTOM PAIN

Prospective studies in patients amputated mainly because of peripheral vascular disease have shown that the onset of phantom pain is usually within the first week after amputation.[13, 20, 26] Amputees who do not experience phantom pain in the first days or weeks after amputation are less likely to develop phantom pain later in the course. Richardson *et al.*[26] prospectively examined the incidence of phantom pain in 52 amputees. Phantom pain was reported by 92.3 percent in the first week after amputation and by 78.8 percent after six months. In a retrospective study, however, of individuals who were either born limb-deficient or amputated before the age of six years, Melzack *et al.*[31] found that the mean time for onset of phantom pain was nine years in the group of congenital amputees and 2.3 years in the group with early amputations.

Case reports confirm that the onset of phantom pain can be delayed for months or even years.[32] In some cases a trauma to the residual limb can elicit phantom pain in a previously pain-free individual. Others have reported phantom pain after spinal neoplasia or spinal tuberculosis.[33, 34, 35]

The exact long-term course of phantom limb pain is unclear because no prospective studies with long-term (many years) follow up exist. Some prospective studies

Table 31.1 Reported prevalence of phantom pain, phantom sensation, and residual limb pain.

Authors	Year	No. of amputees	Phantom pain (%)	Phantom sensations (%)	Residual limb pain (%)
Ewalt *et al.*[8]	1947	2284	2	–	–
Henderson and Smyth[9]	1948	300	4	–	–
Parkes[10]	1973	46	61	–	13
Carlen *et al.*[11]	1978	73	67	100	43
Finch *et al.*[12]	1980	133	30	54	17
Jensen *et al.*[13]	1983	58	72	84	57
Sherman and Sherman[14]	1983	764	85	–	58
Wall *et al.*[15]	1985	25	88	100	–
Pohjolainen[16]	1991	124	59	41	5
Houghton *et al.*[4]	1994	176	78	82	–
Krane and Heller[17]	1995	24	83	100	–
Wartan *et al.*[18]	1997	526	55	66	56
Montoya *et al.*[19]	1997	32	50	81	44
Nikolajsen *et al.*[20]	1997	56	75	–	6
Wilkins *et al.*[21]	1998	33	49	70	70
Ehde *et al.*[22]	2000	255	72	79	74
Kooijman *et al.*[23]	2000	72	51	76	49
Lacoux *et al.*[3]	2002	40	33	93	100
Ephraim *et al.*[24]	2005	914	80	–	68
Desmond *et al.*[25]	2005	582	70	–	77
Richardson *et al.*[26]	2006	52	79	100	52
Hanley *et al.*[27]	2006	57	62	–	57

with a maximum follow-up period of two years have reported a slight decline in the proportion of patients affected over time.[10, 20, 36] In the study by Nikolajsen *et al.*,[20] the incidence and intensity of pain remained constant during the six months follow up, but both frequency and duration of phantom pain attacks decreased significantly. In a survey of 526 veterans with long-standing amputations, phantom pain had disappeared in 16 percent, decreased markedly in 37 percent, remained similar in 44 percent, and increased in 3 percent of the respondents reporting phantom pain.[18]

FREQUENCY, INTENSITY, CHARACTER, AND POSITION OF PHANTOM PAIN

Phantom pain is episodic in nature, and only few amputees are in constant pain.[37] Diary studies have shown that most amputees report pain attacks occur daily or at daily or weekly intervals.[38] Kooijman *et al.*[23] studied 99 upper limb amputees; among patients with phantom pain, 24 percent had pain constantly, 24 percent experienced pain a few times a day, 16 percent had pain a few times per week, and the rest had less frequent pain. In a survey of 255 lower limb amputees, Ehde *et al.*[22] found that the duration of pain attacks was a few minutes in 52 percent of patients, several minutes to an hour in 26 percent of patients, and even longer in the rest of the patients.

The mean intensity of pain on a visual analog scale (VAS, 0–100) was 22 (range 3–82) six months after amputation in a prospective study of mainly vascular amputees.[20] Houghton *et al.*[4] retrospectively asked 176 amputees to specify intensity of phantom pain on a VAS (0–10) at six months and one, two, and five years after amputation; the mean scores were 4, 3, 3, 2, and 1, respectively. In a survey of 526 veterans with a median time of 50 years since amputation, patients with phantom pain graded the intensity of pain as 5.6 on a numeric rating scale (NRS) from 0 to 10 (0 = no pain; 10 = unbearable pain).[18] In a recent study by Hanley *et al.*,[27] the average phantom pain intensity was 2.05 on an NRS at 24 months after amputation among 57 amputees. In another recent study of 914 amputees, pain was classified into three categories: 38.9 percent experienced severe pain intensity (rating 7–10), 26.4 percent experienced moderate pain intensity (rating 5–6), and 34.7 percent experienced mild pain intensity (rating 1–4).[24]

Phantom pain can have several different qualities and is often described as shooting, pricking, stabbing, throbbing, burning, pin and needles, tingling, crushing, or cramping.[18, 19, 20, 21, 22, 38]

Phantom pain seems to be more intense in the distal portions of the missing limb: fingers and palm in upper-limb amputees; toes, foot, and ankle in lower limb amputees. In a prospective study of 52 amputees, the position of phantom pain within the phantom limb was in the toes or foot in 66.7 percent of cases.[26] These distal parts of the limbs are represented by a larger area in the sensory cortex compared to more proximal parts, and this may play a role for the more frequent phantom experience of hands and feet.

The following example illustrates some of the clinical characteristics of phantom pain. A middle-aged man had his left arm amputated because of a malignant tumor. After the amputation, he suffered from severe phantom pain located to his hand and fingers. The pain was present constantly and described as cramping, burning, and shooting. The phantom arm was located in front of the chest and the hand was clenched in a painful fist. Light touch of a trigger point in front of the ear resulted in exacerbation of phantom pain. Occasionally, massage of the residual limb loosened the fingers and allowed for voluntary movements. TCAs, anticonvulsants, and opioids had been tried, but the patient either experienced a lack of effect or intolerable side effects.

PREAMPUTATION PAIN AND PHANTOM PAIN

Both retrospective[4, 15, 17] and prospective studies[13, 20, 27, 36] have pointed to preamputation pain as a risk factor for phantom pain. The hypothesis is that preoperative pain may sensitize the nervous system, thus making the individual very susceptible to the development of phantom pain.

In a study by Houghton *et al.*[4] there was a significant relationship in vascular amputees between preamputation pain and phantom pain in the first two years after amputation. In traumatic amputees, phantom pain was only related to preamputation pain immediately after the amputation. In a study by Nikolajsen *et al.*[20] of mostly vascular amputees, a correlation was found between preoperative pain and phantom pain one week and three months after the amputation, but not after six months. However, some patients with severe preoperative pain never developed phantom pain, while others with traumatic amputations who never experienced pain before the amputation developed phantom pain to the same extent as patients with longstanding preamputation pain amputated for medical reasons. In a recent prospective study by Hanley *et al.*,[27] the associations of preamputation pain and acute postoperative pain with chronic amputation-related pain in 57 lower-limb amputees were examined. Acute postamputation pain intensity was the only significant independent predictor of chronic phantom pain at 6 and 12 months after amputation, whereas preamputation pain intensity was the only significant predictor of chronic phantom at 24 months.

Lacoux *et al.*[3] examined 40 upper-limb amputees who had lost their limbs following injury during the civil war in Sierra Leone. Some amputees lost their limbs at the time of the initial injury (immediate, 56 percent); others suffered a severe injury and had a subsequent limb amputation at hospital on average ten days after the injury (delayed, 44 percent). It is reasonable to assume that the latter group suffered from severe pain between the two events. There was, however, no relation between the development of phantom pain and whether the amputation was immediate or delayed.

Another issue concerns to what extent phantom pain is a revivification of pain experienced before the amputation. Remarkable case reports show that phantom pain may mimic the pain experienced before the amputation in both character and localization.[20, 39, 40] For example, Hill *et al.*[39] described a woman who had her left leg amputated because of recurrent wound infection. The most distressing preoperative pain was invoked by the treatment carried out on the open drainage site on the calf, which required cleaning and repacking twice daily. Immediately after the amputation, the patient experienced phantom pain localized to the open drainage site that was no longer there.[39]

In a retrospective study by Katz and Melzack,[40] 68 patients were questioned about preamputation pain and phantom pain from 20 days to 46 years after amputation. A very large proportion (57 percent) of amputees who had preamputation pain claimed that their present phantom pain resembled the pain they had before the amputation. Prospective studies, however, in which pain is described before and at intervals after the amputation, suggest that preamputation pain only persists as phantom pain in very few cases.[13, 20] In a study by Nikolajsen *et al.*,[20] 56 patients were interviewed before and at specific time intervals after the amputation about the character and localization of pain. This was done using different word descriptors: the McGill Pain Questionnaire and their own words. About 42 percent of the patients reported that their phantom pain resembled the pain they had experienced at the time of the amputation. There was, however, no relation between the patients' own opinion about similarity between preamputation pain and phantom pain and the actual similarity found when comparing pre- and postoperative recordings of pain. Patients significantly overestimated the preamputation pain intensity after six months. Thus, retrospective memories about pain should be judged carefully because of the type of assessment and potential errors in retrospective reports. It is likely that pain experienced preoperatively may survive as phantom pain in some patients, but this is not the case in the vast majority of patients.

PSYCHOLOGICAL FACTORS AND IMPACT ON DAILY LIFE

Losing a limb is a traumatic experience and amputees often exhibit a range of psychological symptoms such as depression, anxiety, self-pity, and isolation. It has previously been proposed that complaints of persisting pain were related to patients with a rigid, self-reliant personality and to unemployment or retirement.[10] There is, however, no evidence that phantom pain represents a psychological disturbance.[40, 41] It has been shown that coping strategies are important for the experience of phantom pain,[42] and as in other chronic pain conditions, phantom pain may be triggered and exacerbated by psychosocial factors.[43] In a study by Jensen *et al.*,[44] biopsychosocial factors such as catastrophizing and a coping response of resting were shown to play an important role in the adjustment to phantom pain.

Desmond *et al.*[25] recently investigated psychological distress among 582 amputees with long-term amputations and showed that distress was related to residual limb pain. In another recent study, depressive symptoms were found to be a significant predictor of level of pain intensity and bothersomeness.[24]

Others have looked at pain-related disability and rehabilitation.[22, 45, 46] A study in the Netherlands examining the occupational situation of people with lower limb amputations found that amputees experiencing a long delay between the amputation and their return to work had difficulty in finding suitable jobs and had fewer opportunities for promotion.[47]

OTHER FACTORS

Evidence is growing that the individual's genetic predisposition to develop neuropathic pain may be important. Seltzer *et al.*[48] suggested several candidate genes on chromosome 15 that could be involved in the autotomy that follows peripheral neurectomy in rodents, an animal model of phantom pain. On the other hand, Schott[49] described an interesting case in which five members of a family sustained traumatic amputations of their limbs. The development of phantom pain was unpredictable despite their being first-degree relatives. An inherited component is not always a feature of phantom pain.

It has been claimed that phantom pain may recur in lower-limb amputees undergoing spinal anesthesia.[50] Tessler and Kleiman,[51] however, prospectively investigated 23 spinal anesthetics in 17 patients and only one patient developed phantom pain that resolved in ten minutes.

Phantom pain may also be related to several internal and external factors, such as attention, emotional stress, anxiety, and autonomic reflexes, such as coughing and urination. A certain position or movement of the phantom and manipulation of the residual limb can affect the phantom pain, and pain may also be elicited or exacerbated by a range of physical factors, for example weather changes.[37, 38] Phantom pain may decrease by the use of a prosthesis that allows extensive use of the affected limb as opposed to using a cosmetic prosthesis.[52, 53] A list of modulating factors is shown in **Table 31.2**.

Phantom sensation

Phantom sensation is experienced by almost everyone who undergoes limb amputation, but it rarely represents a clinical problem. Immediately after the amputation, the phantom limb often resembles the preamputation limb in shape, size, and volume.[11, 19, 22, 23, 54] The sensation can be very vivid and often includes feelings of posture and movement. The phantom sensation may fade over time. Richardsen *et al.*[26] prospectively studied phantom phenomena in 52 lower amputees. At six-months follow up, nonpainful phantom sensations were present in 100 percent, spontaneous movements occurred in 65.4 percent, and 58 percent stated that they were able to move the phantom themselves. In another study, amputees were asked about the frequency of phantom sensations a median time of 19 years after amputation. Twenty-two percent experienced phantom sensations always, another 11 percent had phantom sensations daily, and the rest had sensations with intervals of weeks, months, or even years.[23]

In some patients, a phenomenon called telescoping occurs when the distal parts of the phantom are gradually felt to approach the residual limb and eventually they may even be experienced within the residual limb (**Figure 31.1**). It has been suggested that phantom pain prevents telescoping, but Montoya *et al.*[19] failed to find such a relation: 12 of 16 patients with phantom pain and 5 of 10 patients without pain reported telescoping. The following case illustrates telescoping: A 54-year-old man had his right arm crushed in a machine at work. The arm was subsequently amputated at hospital. Immediately after the operation, the patient had a vivid sensation that the arm was still present. The phantom arm felt as if it had the same size and shape as before the amputation. Gradually, the phantom arm underwent shrinkage, and

Table 31.2 Factors that may modulate the experience of phantom pain.

Internal factors	External factors
Genetic predisposition	Weather change
Anxiety/emotional distress	Touching the residual limb
Attention/distraction	Use of prosthesis
Urination/defecation	Spinal anesthesia
Coping strategies	Rehabilitation
Other disease (prolapsed intervertebral disk, spinal neoplasia)	Treatment

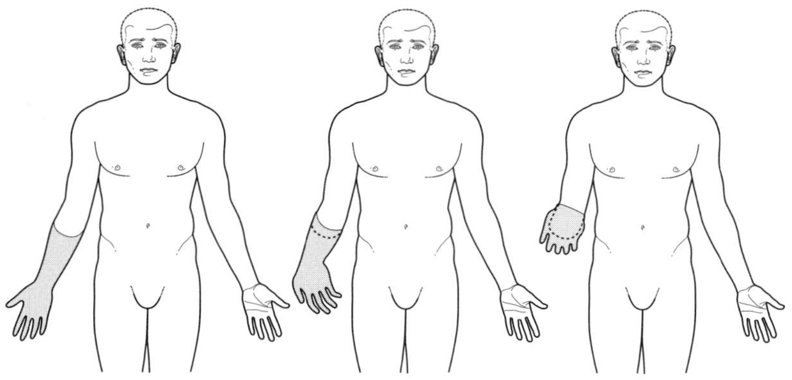

Figure 31.1 Telescoping: a gradual shrinkage of the phantom limb. In upper limb amputees, the hand may eventually become located within the residual limb.

the phantom hand eventually became located within the residual limb. Telescoping may in some cases resolve. The patient reported that the phantom arm resumed its genuine size and shape during the use of an artificial prosthesis.

Phantom pain and phantom sensation are strongly correlated. In a study by Kooijmann *et al.*,[23] phantom pain was present in 36 out of 37 upper limb amputees with phantom sensations, but only in one out of 17 without phantom sensations. Phantom sensations are less frequent in congenital amputees and in patients who underwent amputation before the age of six years.[31]

Residual limb pain

Not surprisingly, residual limb pain is common in the early postoperative period, but in most patients it subsides with healing. The prevalence of chronic residual limb pain is reported to vary between 5 and 100 percent (**Table 31.1**). Variations in the literature may reflect different methods of estimating pain and the fact that some amputees find it difficult to distinguish between residual limb and phantom pain. In a survey of 78 traumatic amputees, Pezzin *et al.*[46] found that 14.1 percent suffered from severe and constant pain in the residual limb. Similar results have been found by others in patients who have undergone amputation for different reasons, including medical.[16, 22, 23] In two recent studies, the mean prevalence of residual limb pain was reported to be 51.2 and 67.7 percent, respectively.[24, 26] In the latter study, mean intensity of residual limb pain among those reporting pain was 5.1 (NRS, 0–10).[24] Chronic residual limb pain is more likely to be present in war zones.[2, 3]

Residual limb pain may be described as pressing, throbbing, burning, squeezing, or stabbing.[36] Some patients have spontaneous movements of the residual limb, ranging from slight, hardly visible jerks to severe contractions.

Residual limb pain and phantom pain are strongly correlated. Carlen *et al.*[11] noted that phantom pain was decreased by the resolution of stump-end pathology. In a survey of 648 amputees, Sherman and Sherman[14] found that residual limb pain was present in 61 percent of amputees with phantom pain, but in only 39 percent of those without phantom pain. Similar results have been found in at least four prospective studies.[11, 20, 26, 36]

Other clinical studies have shown that temperature and muscle activity at the residual limb are related to phantom pain.[41, 55, 56] Nikolajsen *et al.*[57] studied 35 amputees and found that low mechanical thresholds (pressure algometry) at the residual limb were associated with residual limb and phantom pain one week after amputation.

The association between residual limb and phantom pain is consistent with experimental studies in amputees. Nyström and Hagbarth[58] observed abnormal activity in the peroneal and median nerve fibers of two amputees with ongoing pain in their phantom foot and hand, respectively. Percussion of neuromas in these two patients produced increased nerve fiber discharges and an augmentation of their phantom pain.

Careful sensory examination of amputation residual limbs may reveal areas with sensory abnormalities, such as hypoesthesia, hyperalgesia, or allodynia.[59] However, it is not clear whether there is any correlation between phantom pain and the extent and degree of sensory abnormalities in the residual limb. Hunter *et al.*[60] carefully examined the residual limb in 12 traumatic upper-limb amputees, but failed to find any simple relation between psychophysical thresholds and phantom phenomena.

Chronic residual limb pain can be very severe as illustrated by the following case study. A 48-year-old woman fractured her ankle in 1999. Healing was difficult and two years later the osteosynthesic material was removed because of infection. Physiotherapy was not possible due to pain, and the foot became fixed in an extended and pronated posture. Signs of chronic regional pain syndrome (CRPS) were evident. A below-knee amputation was performed in 2003 because of ulcers resistant to treatment. The patient subsequently developed severe residual limb pain. The pain was present constantly and described as shooting, burning, and scalding. The intensity of pain was 4–10 on a VAS. In addition to residual limb pain, the patient also experienced phantom pain. Medical treatment (TCAs, antiepileptic drugs, slow-release opioids) had only a modest effect on the pain. Physical examination of the residual limb revealed allodynia and hyperalgesia (**Figure 31.2**). In 2006, an epidural electrode was implanted for spinal cord stimulation (SCS). Within the first week after the implantation, the intensity of residual limb pain decreased to 2 on the VAS, and the allodynia at the residual limb was replaced by a feeling of numbness.

MECHANISMS

The mechanisms underlying chronic postamputation pain have not been completely clarified, but both peripheral and central mechanisms are likely to play a role. Nerve section is associated with clear changes in the periphery, which represents an obvious origin for pain. It is clear, however, that the phantom limb with its complex perceptual qualities is ultimately integrated in the brain. An extensive experimental and clinical literature documents that nerve injury induces a number of morphological, physiological, and chemical changes in both the peripheral and central nervous system (for review, see Flor *et al.*[61]). These changes will be described briefly in the following. An understanding of the underlying mechanisms is likely to lead to new and rational-founded types of treatment.

Peripheral factors

Several clinical studies support the notion that mechanisms in the periphery (i.e. in the residual limb or in central parts of sectioned afferents) play a role for the phantom limb concept.

- Phantom pain is significantly more frequent in amputees with long-term residual limb pain than in those without persistent pain.[23]

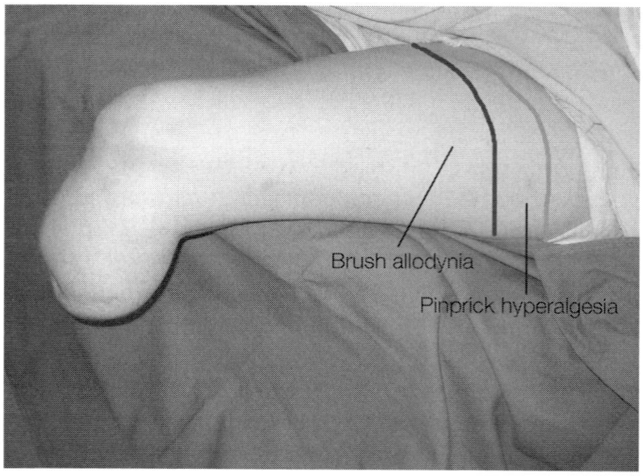

Figure 31.2 Patient with severe residual limb pain. Areas of allodynia and hyperalgesia are indicated.

- Residual limb pathology with altered residual limb sensibility is a common feature.[13]
- Phantom pain and pressure pain thresholds at the residual limb are inversely correlated early after amputation.[57]
- Phantom sensations can be modulated by various residual limb manipulations.[62]
- Tapping neuromas may increase phantom pain.[58]
- Phantom limb sensations are temporarily abolished after local residual limb anesthesia.[63]
- Changes in blood flow may alter the phantom limb perception.[41]

These clinical observations are supported by experimental studies. Following a nerve transection, formation of neuromas is seen universally. Such neuromas show spontaneous and abnormal evoked activity following mechanical or chemical stimulation (for review, see Devor[64]). The ectopic and increased spontaneous and evoked activity from the periphery is assumed to be the result of an increased expression of sodium channels.[65] In the dorsal root ganglion (DRG) cells, changes also occur following a complete nerve cut. Cell bodies in the DRG show abnormal spontaneous activity and increased sensitivity to mechanical and neurochemical stimulation.[66]

The sympathetic nervous system may also play an important role. From animal studies it is known that application of norepinephrine (noradrenaline) at the residual limb or activation of the postganglionic sympathetic fibers excites and sensitizes damaged, but not normal, nerve fibers.[67] Sympathetic–sensory coupling at the level of the DRG may also contribute to the increased pain response following changes in sympathetic activity.[64]

Spinal factors

The increased barrage from neuromas and from DRG cells is thought to induce long-term changes in central projecting neurons in the dorsal horn, including spontaneous neuronal activity, induction of immediate–early genes, increases in spinal metabolic activity,[68] and expansion of receptive fields.[69]

The pharmacology of spinal sensitization involves an increased activity in NMDA receptor-operated systems, and many aspects of the central sensitization can be reduced by NMDA receptor antagonists.[70] In human amputees, the evoked residual limb or phantom pain caused by repetitively stimulating the residual limb can be reduced by the NMDA antagonist ketamine.[71]

Another type of anatomical reorganization may also be present and contribute to central sensitization. Substance P is normally expressed in small afferent fibers, but following nerve injury, substance P may be expressed in large Aβ fibers; this phenotypic switch of large Aβ fibers into nociceptive-like nerve fibers may be one of the reasons why nonnoxious stimuli can be perceived as painful.[72]

Clinical observations confirm that spinal factors are involved in the generation of phantom pain. For example, phantom pain may appear or disappear following spinal cord neoplasia[33] and spinal analgesia may modulate phantom pain.[50, 51]

Supraspinal factors

Amputation produces a cascade of events in the periphery and in the spinal cord. It is reasonable to assume that these changes will eventually sweep more centrally and alter the neuronal activity in cortical and subcortical structures.

Animal studies have demonstrated functional plasticity of the primary somatosensory cortex after amputation. After dorsal rhizotomy, a lowered threshold to evoked activity in the thalamus and cortex can be demonstrated, and adult monkeys display cortical reorganization in which the mouth and chin invade cortices corresponding to the representation of the arm and digits that have lost their normal afferent input.[73, 74]

Studies in humans have also documented a cortical reorganization after amputation using different cerebral imaging techniques. In a series of studies, Flor *et al.*[75, 76] showed a correlation between phantom pain and the amount of reorganization in the somatosensory cortex. Birbaumer *et al.*[77] studied the effect of regional anesthesia on cortical reorganization in upper limb amputees and found that a brachial plexus blockade abolished pain and reorganization in three out of six amputees. Huse *et al.*[78] showed in a small group of amputees that cortical reorganization and pain were reduced during treatment with morphine.

At more subcortical levels, changes have also been observed. Using neuronal recording and stimulation techniques, thalamic neurons that normally do not respond to stimulation in amputees begin to respond and show enlarged somatotopic maps.[79, 80] In addition to functional plasticity, structural alterations also follow amputation. Draganski *et al.*[81] recently demonstrated a decrease in the gray matter of the thalamus in 28 amputees. The decrease was correlated with the time span after the amputation and explained as a structural correlate of the loss of afferent input.

Summary

The findings described here indicate that a series of mechanisms are involved in generating phantom pains, and that these include elements in the periphery, spinal cord, thalamus, and cerebral cortex. It is likely that the first events occur in the periphery, which subsequently generates a cascade of events that sweeps more centrally, finally recruiting cortical brain structures. The latter may be responsible for the complex and vivid sensations that characterize certain phantom pain sensations. **Figure 31.3** shows a proposed model for the development of phantom pain.

TREATMENT

Acute postamputation pain

Immediate postoperative residual limb pain can usually be successfully treated with conventional analgesics (paracetamol, nonsteroidal anti-inflammatory drugs (NSAIDs), opioids), perhaps in combination with various blocks (e.g. epidurals, and axillary, femoral, or sciatic nerve blocks).

It is the first author's personal impression that acute phantom pain can in some cases be attenuated or delayed by a well-functioning regional blockade in the immediate postoperative period. There is no evidence, however, that a short-lasting regional block has any long-term effect on phantom pain. For example, Pinzur *et al.*[82] prospectively randomized 21 patients to continuous postoperative infusion of either bupivacaine or saline, but failed to find any difference between the two groups with regard to the prevalence of phantom pain after three and six months.[82][II]

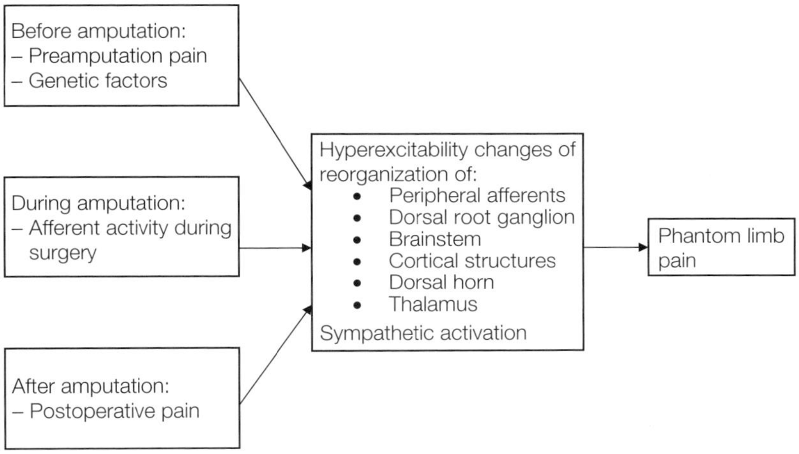

Figure 31.3 Proposed model of the development of phantom pain.

Chronic postamputation pain

Treatment of chronic postamputation pain represents a major challenge to the clinician and in particular the treatment of phantom pain. There is only little evidence from randomized trials to guide clinicians with treatment, and most studies dealing with phantom pain suffer from major methodological errors: samples are small, randomization and blinding are either absent or inappropriate, controls are often lacking, and follow-up periods are short. Halbert *et al.*[83] performed a systematic literature search to determine the optimal management of phantom pain. The authors identified 186 articles, but after exclusion of letters, reviews, descriptive trials without intervention, case reports, and trials with major methodological errors, only 12 articles were left for review. Since then, some well-designed studies have been published.[78, 84, 85, 86, 87, 88, 89, 90, 91, 92] Until more clinical data become available, guidelines in analogy with treatment regimens used for other neuropathic pain conditions are probably the best approximation, especially for the treatment of residual limb pain. A combination of medical and non-medical treatment may be advantageous. In general, treatment should be noninvasive. Surgery on the peripheral or central nervous system always implicates further deafferentation and thereby an increased risk of persistent pain. Suggestions for treatment of postamputation pain are presented in **Table 31.3**.

MEDICAL TREATMENT

A large number of randomized controlled trials have shown a beneficial effect of tricyclic antidepressants and sodium channel blockers in different neuropathic pain conditions.[5][I] Only few controlled data are available for phantom pain, but the drugs are generally believed to be effective, at least in some patients.

A recent study examined the effect of tricyclic antidepressants on phantom pain.[88][II] Thirty-nine patients were randomized to receive either amitriptyline or active placebo during a six-week trial period. The dosage of amitriptyline was increased until the patient reached the maximum tolerated dose or 125 mg/day. Unfortunately, this study showed no effect of amitriptyline on pain intensity or secondary outcome measures, such as satisfaction with life. In contrast, Wilder-Smith *et al.*[89] found excellent pain relief of amitriptyline (mean dose, 55 mg) on both residual limb and phantom pain. Ninety-four posttraumatic amputees were randomized to receive

Table 31.3 Suggestions for treatment of postamputation pain (not evidence-based).

Postamputation pain
Early postoperative pain
Residual limb pain: Conventional analgesics (paracetamol, NSAIDs, opioids), perhaps combined with regional blocks
Residual limb and phantom pain: In case of clear neuropathic pain signs – paroxyms or abnormal residual limb sensitivity – tricyclic antidepressants or anticonvulsants can be tried
Chronic pain
Local residual limb surgery: If obvious stump pathology is present, residual limb revision should be considered. Surgery should be avoided in chronic regional pain syndrome
Local medical treatment: Topical lidocaine/capsaicin can be tried in cases with residual limb pain without clear stump pathology
Residual limb and phantom pain (medical treatment, listed in order of preference)
1. Tricyclic antidepressants (imipramine, amitriptyline, nortriptyline) 10–100 mg/day, start dose 10–25 mg/day, weekly increments of 25 mg. Check ECG before start. Monitor plasma levels with dose > 100 mg/day. Amitriptyline should be preferred if sedation is wanted
2. Gabapentin 1200–2400 mg/day, start dose 300 mg, increments of 300 mg every 3rd day, maximum dose 3600 mg/day
Pregabalin 75–600 mg/day, start dose 25–75 mg, increments of 75 mg/day every 3rd day, maximum dose 600 mg/day
3. Serotonin noradrenaline reuptake inhibitors
Venlafaxine 175–225 mg/day, start dose 75 mg
Duloxetine 30–60 mg/day, start dose 30 mg
4. In cases of mainly radiating, lancinating or paroxysmal pain:
(a) Oxcarbazepine 600–900 mg/day, start dose 300 mg, weekly increments of 300 mg
(b) Carbamazepine 200–400 mg/day, start dose 100 mg, weekly increments of 100 mg. Monitor plasma levels after 10 days on maximum dose
(c) Lamotrigine 100–200 mg/day, start dose 25 mg/day, slow titration with increments of 25 mg/14 days (to avoid rash)
5. Opioids (long-acting or sustained-release preparations) or tramadol
6. No effect of the above: Consider referral to pain clinic

ECG, electrocardiogram; NSAID, nonsteroidal anti-inflammatory drugs.

amitriptyline, tramadol, or placebo for one month. The administration of tramadol and placebo was blinded, amitriptyline was given nonblinded as open comparison. Nonresponders (less than 10 mm pain relief on a VAS from baseline on day three) were switched to the alternative active treatment, e.g. tramadol to amitriptyline treatment and vice versa. Placebo nonresponders were switched to tramadol or amitriptyline. Both tramadol and amitriptyline almost abolished residual limb and phantom pain at the end of the treatment period.[89][II]

Bone *et al.*[84][II] examined the effect of gabapentin in a well-designed crossover study including 19 patients with phantom pain. The dose of gabapentin was titrated in increments of 300 mg to a maximum dosage of 2400 mg per day. After six weeks of treatment, gabapentin was better than placebo in reducing phantom pain. A similar effect of gabapentin was described in an open study by Rusy *et al.*[93][V] Two other studies have recently examined the effect of gabapentin on postamputation residual limb and phantom pain. Smith *et al.*[90][II] administered gabapentin or placebo for six weeks to 24 amputees in a double-blind crossover fashion. The maximum dose given was 3600 mg. Gabapentin did not decrease intensity of pain significantly, but the participants rated the decrease of pain as more meaningful during the treatment period with gabapentin. All the above-mentioned studies examined the effect of gabapentin on established phantom pain. Nikolajsen *et al.*[91][II] randomized 46 lower-limb amputees to receive either gabapentin or placebo for the first 30 days after amputation. The first dose of 300 mg gabapentin/placebo was given on the first postoperative day, and the dosage was gradually increased until a maximum of 2400 mg was reached. Intensity, frequency, and duration of phantom pain attacks were recorded daily in the first 30 days and after three and six months. Intensity of residual limb pain was also recorded and sensory testing of the residual limb was performed. The two treatment groups were similar as regards all outcome parameters. Thus, early treatment with gabapentin started before the phantom pain becomes established does not seem to affect outcome.

Failure to provide efficient pain relief should not be accepted until opioids have been tried. Opioids can probably be used safely – with a limited risk of dependence – for several years.[94][I] In a randomized, double-blind, crossover study with active placebo, 31 amputees received a 40-minute infusion of lidocaine (lignocaine), morphine, or diphenhydramine. Compared with placebo, morphine reduced both residual limb and phantom pain, whereas lidocaine decreased only residual limb pain.[87][II] In another placebo-controlled, crossover study including 12 patients, Huse *et al.* found a significant reduction of phantom pain during treatment with oral morphine.[78][II] Case reports have suggested that methadone may reduce phantom pain.[95][V]

The effect of NMDA receptor antagonists has been examined in different studies. In a double-blind, placebo-controlled study, intravenous ketamine reduced pain, hyperalgesia, and wind up-like pain in 11 amputees with residual limb and phantom pain.[71][II] Two other trials have examined the effect of memantine, an NMDA receptor antagonist available for oral use. In both studies, memantine was administered in a blinded, placebo-controlled, crossover fashion to patients with established residual limb and phantom pain. Memantine at doses of 20 or 30 mg per day, respectively, failed to have any effect on spontaneous pain, allodynia, and hyperalgesia.[85][II], [86][II] Schley *et al.*[92][II] recently randomized 19 patients with traumatic amputations to receive either memantine or placebo in combination with a continuous brachial plexus blockade in the immediate postoperative phase. The dose of memantine was increased from 10 to 30 mg during the four-week treatment period. Treatment with memantine resulted in a decrease of phantom pain at four-week and six-month follow up, but not at 12-month follow up. Dextromethorphan, another NMDA receptor antagonist, was suggested to be effective in a study including ten patients with phantom pain.[96][III]

Calcitonin significantly reduced phantom pain when used intravenously in the early postoperative phase.[97][II] A large number of other treatments, for example β-blockers,[98, 99][V] the oral congener of lidocaine,[100][V] topical application of capsaicin,[101][V] intrathecal opioids,[102][III], [103][V] various anesthetic blocks,[104, 105][V] injection of botulinum toxin,[106][V] and topiramate[107][V] have been claimed to be effective in phantom pain, but none of them have proved to be effective in well-controlled trials with a sufficient number of patients.

NONMEDICAL TREATMENT

A recent survey of treatments used for phantom pain revealed that after pharmacological treatments physical therapy was the treatment modality most often used.[108] Physical therapy involving massage, manipulation, and passive movements may prevent trophic changes and vascular congestion in the residual limb. Other treatments, such as TENS, acupuncture,[109][V] ultrasound, and hypnosis,[110][V] may in some cases have a beneficial effect on residual limb and phantom pain. At least three studies have examined the effect of TENS on phantom pain, but the results are not consistent.[111][II], [112][III], [113][III] One study showed an effect of a Farabloc, a metal-threaded sock to be worn over the residual limb.[114] Ramachandran and Rogers-Ramachandran[115][V] used visual feedback with a mirror to eliminate painful phantom limb spasms. In a larger clinical trial of 80 amputees, Brodie *et al.*[116][II] failed to find any significant effect of mirror treatment on phantom limb pain, sensation, and movement. Flor *et al.* demonstrated that sensory discrimination training obtained by applying stimuli at the residual limb reduced pain in five upper limb amputees.[62][III] The advantage of most of the above-mentioned methods is the absence of side effects and complications, and the fact that the treatment can be easily repeated. However, most of these studies are uncontrolled observations.

SURGICAL TREATMENT

Surgery on amputation neuromas and more extensive amputation previously played important roles in the treatment of residual limb and phantom pain. Today, residual limb revision is probably performed only in cases of obvious stump pathology, and in properly healed residual limbs there is almost never any indication for proximal extension of the amputation because of pain. The results of other invasive techniques, such as, for example, dorsal root entry zone lesions,[117][V] sympathetectomy, and cordotomy have generally been unfavorable, and most of them have been abandoned. Surgery may produce short-term pain relief, but the pain often reappears. Spinal cord stimulation[118][III] and deep brain stimulation[119][V], [120][V] are methods that may be used for carefully selected patients.

PREVENTION

The idea of a preemptive analgesic effect in postamputation pain was prompted by observations that the phantom pain in some cases seemed to be similar to pain experienced before the amputation, and that the presence of severe pain before the amputation was associated with a higher risk of postamputation phantom pain. These observations led to the theory that preamputation pain created an imprint in memorizing structures of the central nervous system, and that such an imprint could be responsible for persistent pain after amputation.

Inspired by this, Bach *et al.* carried out the first study on the prevention of phantom pain.[121][III] Twenty-five patients were randomized by birth year to either epidural pain treatment 72 hours before the amputation or conventional analgesics. All patients had spinal or epidural analgesia for the amputation, and both groups received conventional analgesics to treat postoperative pain. Blinding was not described. After six months, the incidence of phantom pain was lower among patients who had received the preoperative epidural blockade.

At that time, the findings of Bach *et al.* were supported by a growing body of work in animal and other clinical settings, showing an effect of preemptive treatment on the subsequent development of pain.[122] Since then, a few trials have examined the short- and long-term impact of regional analgesia (epidural and peri- or intraneural nerve blocks) on phantom pain. Some of these studies,[123][III], [124][III], [125][III], [126][III] but not all,[82][II], [127][II], [128][II], [129][III]have confirmed that regional analgesia may be effective in reducing chronic postamputation pain. Unfortunately, some of the studies are of very poor methodological quality.

Nikolajsen *et al.*[127][II] carried out a randomized, double-blind, and placebo-controlled study in which 60 patients scheduled for lower limb amputation were randomly assigned to one of two groups: a blockade group that received epidural bupivacaine and morphine before the amputation and during the operation (29 patients) and a control group that received epidural saline and oral or intramuscular morphine (31 patients). Both groups had general anesthesia for the amputation and all patients received epidural analgesics for postoperative pain management. Patients were interviewed about preamputation pain on the day before the amputation and about residual limb and phantom pain after one week and 3, 6, and 12 months. The median duration of preoperative epidural blockade was 18 hours. After one week, the percentage of patients with phantom pain was 51.9 percent in the blockade group and 55.6 percent in the control group. Subsequently, the percentages were (blockade/control): at three months, 82.4/50 percent; at six months, 81.3/55 percent; and at 12 months, 75/68.8 percent. The intensity of residual limb and phantom pain and the consumption of opioids were similar in the two groups at all four postoperative interviews.

The aim of preemptive treatment is to avert spinal sensitization by blocking, in advance, the cascade of intraneuronal responses that takes place after peripheral nerve injury. A true preemptive approach is probably not possible in patients scheduled for amputation. Many have suffered from ischemic pain for months or years and are likely to present with preexisting neuronal hyperexcitability. It cannot be excluded that a preoperative regional blockade for a longer period would prevent phantom pain from developing. However, this would be very inconvenient from a practical point of view as the decision to amputate is often not taken until the day before.

In conclusion, regional blocks are effective in the treatment of preoperative ischemic pain and postoperative residual limb pain. At present, no studies of sufficient methodological quality have provided evidence that regional blocks have any beneficial effect in preventing phantom pain. It cannot be excluded that other approaches may be effective. For example, it has been suggested that peri- and postamputation administration of NMDA receptor antagonists as ketamine[130][III] and memantine[92][II] reduces phantom pain.

REFERENCES

* 1. Finger S, Hustwit MP. Five early accounts of phantom limb in context: Paré, Descartes, Lemos, Bell, and Mitchell. *Neurosurgery.* 2003; **52**: 675–86.

2. Husum H, Resell K, Vorren G *et al.* Chronic pain in land mine accident survivors in Cambodia and Kurdistan. *Social Science and Medicine.* 2002; **55**: 1813–16.

3. Lacoux PA, Crombie IK, Macrae WA. Pain in traumatic upper limb amputees in Sierra Leone. *Pain*. 2002; **99**: 309–12.
4. Houghton AD, Nicholls G, Houghton AL *et al*. Phantom pain: natural history and association with rehabilitation. *Annals of the Royal College of Surgeons of England*. 1994; **76**: 22–5.
5. * Finnerup NB, Otto M, Mcquay HJ *et al*. Algorithm for neuropathic pain treatment: An evidence based proposal. *Pain*. 2005; **118**: 289–305.
6. Rothemund Y, Grüsser SM, Liebeskind U *et al*. Phantom phenomena in mastectomized patients and their relation to chronic and acute pre-mastectomy pain. *Pain*. 2004; **107**: 140–6.
7. Ovesen P, Krøner K, Ørnsholt J, Bach K. Phantom-related phenomena after rectal amputation: prevalence and clinical characteristics. *Pain*. 1991; **44**: 289–91.
8. Ewalt JR, Randall GC, Morris H. The phantom limb. *Psychosomatic Medicine*. 1947; **9**: 118–23.
9. Henderson WR, Smyth GE. Phantom limbs. *Journal of Neurology, Neurosurgery, and Psychiatry*. 1948; **11**: 88–112.
10. Parkes CM. Factors determining the persistence of phantom pain in the amputee. *Journal of Psychosomatic Research*. 1973; **17**: 97–108.
11. * Carlen PL, Wall PD, Nadvorna H *et al*. Phantom limbs and related phenomena in recent traumatic amputations. *Neurology*. 1978; **28**: 211–17.
12. Finch DRA, MacDougal M, Tibbs DJ *et al*. Amputation for vascular disease: the experience of a peripheral vascular unit. *British Journal of Surgery*. 1980; **67**: 233–7.
13. Jensen TS, Krebs B, Nielsen J *et al*. Phantom limb, phantom pain and stump pain in amputees during the first 6 months following limb amputation. *Pain*. 1983; **17**: 243–56.
14. Sherman R, Sherman C. Prevalence and characteristics of chronic phantom limb pain among American veterans: results of a trial survey. *American Journal of Physical Medicine*. 1983; **62**: 227–38.
15. Wall R, Novotny-Joseph P, Macnamara TE. Does preamputation pain influence phantom limb pain in cancer patients? *Southern Medical Journal*. 1985; **78**: 34–6.
16. Pohjolainen T. A clinical evaluation of stumps in lower limb amputees. *Prosthetics and Orthotics International*. 1991; **15**: 178–84.
17. Krane EJ, Heller LB. The prevalence of phantom sensation and pain in pediatric amputees. *Journal of Pain and Symptom Management*. 1995; **10**: 21–9.
18. Wartan SW, Hamann W, Wedley JR *et al*. Phantom pain and sensation among British veteran amputees. *British Journal of Anaesthesia*. 1997; **78**: 652–9.
19. Montoya P, Larbig W, Grulke N. Relationship of phantom limb pain to other phantom limb phenomena in upper extremity amputees. *Pain*. 1997; **72**: 87–93.
20. Nikolajsen L, Ilkjær S, Krøner K *et al*. The influence of preamputation pain on postamputation stump and phantom pain. *Pain*. 1997; **72**: 393–405.
21. Wilkins KL, McGrath PJ, Finley GA *et al*. Phantom limb sensations and phantom limb pain in child and adolescent amputees. *Pain*. 1998; **78**: 7–12.
22. Ehde DM, Czerniecki JM, Smith DG *et al*. Chronic phantom sensations, phantom pain, residual limb pain, and other regional pain after lower limb amputation. *Archives of Physical Medicine and Rehabilitation*. 2000; **81**: 1039–44.
23. * Kooijman CM, Dijkstra PU, Geertzen JHB *et al*. Phantom pain and phantom sensations in upper limb amputees: an epidemiological study. *Pain*. 2000; **87**: 33–41.
24. Ephraim PL, Wegener ST, MacKenzie EJ *et al*. Phantom pain, residual limb pain, and back pain in amputees: Results of a national survey. *Archives of Physical Medicine and Rehabilitation*. 2005; **86**: 1910–19.
25. Desmond DM, Maclachlan M. Affective distress and amputation-related pain among older men with long-term, traumatic limb amputations. *Journal of Pain and Symptom Management*. 2006; **31**: 362–8.
26. Richardson C, Glenn S, Nurmikko T, Horgan M. Incidence of phantom phenomena including phantom limb pain 6 months after major lower limb amputation in patients with peripheral vascular disease. *Clinical Journal of Pain*. 2006; **22**: 353–8.
27. * Hanley MA, Jensen MP, Smith DG *et al*. Preamputation pain and acute pain predict chronic pain after lower extremity amputation. *Journal of Pain*. 2007; **8**: 102–09.
28. Campbell WB, Marriott S, Eve R *et al*. Anaesthesia and analgesia for major lower limb amputation. *Cardiovascular Surgery*. 2000; **8**: 572–5.
29. Sherman RA, Sherman CJ. A comparison of phantom sensations among amputees whose amputations were of civilian and military origins. *Pain*. 1985; **21**: 91–7.
30. Saadahl ESM, Melzack R. Phantom limb experiences in congenital limb-deficient adults. *Cortex*. 1994; **30**: 479–85.
31. Melzack R, Israel R, Lacroix R *et al*. Phantom limbs in people with congenital limb deficiency or amputation in early childhood. *Brain*. 1997; **120**: 1603–20.
32. Rajbhandari SM, Jarett JA, Griffiths PD *et al*. Diabetic neuropathic pain in a leg amputated 44 years previously. *Pain*. 1999; **83**: 627–9.
33. Chang VT, Tunkel RS, Pattillo BA, Lachmann EA. Increased phantom limb pain as an initial symptom of spinal neoplasia. *Journal of Pain and Symptom Management*. 1997; **13**: 362–4.
34. Pithwa YK, Rajasekaran S. Phantom-limb pain due to cervical spinal tuberculosis. *Journal of Bone and Joint Surgery*. 2004; **86A**: 1289–91.
35. Aydin MD, Cesur M, Aydin N, Alici HA. Disappearance of phantom limb pain during cauda euina compression by spinal meningioma and gradual reactivation after decompression. *Anesthesia and Analgesia*. 2005; **101**: 1123–6.
36. Jensen TS, Krebs B, Nielsen J *et al*. Immediate and long-term phantom limb pain in amputees: incidence, clinical characteristics and relationship to preamputation limb pain. *Pain*. 1985; **21**: 267–78.

37. Whyte AS, Niven CA. Variation in phantom limb pain: results of a diary study. *Journal of Pain and Symptom Management*. 2001; **22**: 947–53.
38. Wilkins KL, McGrath PJ, Allen Finley G, Katz J. Prospective diary study of nonpainful and painful phantom sensations in a preselected sample of child and adolescent amputees reporting phantom limbs. *Clinical Journal of Pain*. 2004; **20**: 293–301.
39. Hill A, Niven CA, Knussen C. Pain memories in phantom limbs: a case story. *Pain*. 1996; **66**: 381–4.
* 40. Katz J, Melzack R. Pain 'memories' in phantom limbs: review and clinical observations. *Pain*. 1990; **43**: 319–36.
41. Sherman RA, Glenda GM. Concurrent variation of burning phantom limb and stump pain with near surface blood flow in the stump. *Orthopedics*. 1987; **10**: 1395–402.
42. Hill A, Niven CA, Knussen C. The role of coping in adjustment to phantom limb pain. *Pain*. 1995; **62**: 79–86.
43. Arena JG, Sherman RA, Bruno GM *et al*. The relationship between situational stress and phantom limb pain: cross-lagged correlational data from six month pain logs. *Journal of Psychosomatic Research*. 1990; **34**: 71–7.
44. Jensen MP, Ehde DM, Hoffman AJ *et al*. Cognitions, coping and social environment predict adjustment to phantom pain. *Pain*. 2002; **95**: 133–42.
45. Ide M, Obayashi T, Toyonaga T. Association of pain with employment status and satisfaction among amputees in Japan. *Archives of Physical Medicine and Rehabilitation*. 2002; **83**: 1394–8.
46. Pezzin LE, Dillingham TR, Mackenzie EJ. Rehabilitation and the long-term outcomes of persons with trauma-related amputations. *Archives of Physical Medicine and Rehabilitation*. 2000; **81**: 292–300.
47. Schoppen T, Boonstra A, Groothoff JW *et al*. Employment status, job characteristics, and work-related health experience of people with a lower limb amputation in The Netherlands. *Archives of Physical Medicine and Rehabilitation*. 2002; **82**: 239–45.
48. Seltzer Z, Wu T, Max MB *et al*. Mapping a gene for neuropathic pain-related behavior following peripheral neurectomy in the mouse. *Pain*. 2001; **93**: 101–06.
49. Schott G D. Pain and its absence in an unfortunate family of amputees. *Pain*. 1986; **25**: 229–31.
50. Mackenzie N. Phantom limb pain during spinal anaesthesia. Recurrence in amputees. *Anaesthesia*. 1983; **38**: 886–7.
51. Tessler MJ, Kleiman SJ. Spinal anaesthesia for patients with previous lower limb amputations. *Anaesthesia*. 1994; **49**: 439–41.
52. Lotze M, Grodd W, Birbaumer N *et al*. Does use of a myoelectric prosthesis prevent cortical reorganization and phantom limb pain? *Nature Neuroscience*. 1999; **2**: 501–02.
53. Weiss T, Miltner WH, Adler T *et al*. Decrease in phantom limb pain associated with prosthesis-induced increased use of an amputation stump in humans. *Neuroscience Letters*. 1999; **272**: 131–4.
54. Jensen TS, Krebs B, Nielsen J *et al*. Non-painful phantom limb phenomena in amputees: incidence, clinical characteristics and temporal course. *Acta Neurologica Scandinavica*. 1984; **70**: 407–14.
55. Katz J. Psychophysical correlates of phantom limb experience. *Journal of Neurology, Neurosurgery, and Psychiatry*. 1992; **55**: 811–21.
56. Sherman RA, Griffin VD, Evans CB, Grana AS. Temporal relationship between changes in phantom limb pain intensity and changes in surface electromyogram of the residual limb. *International Journal of Psychophysiology*. 1992; **13**: 71–7.
57. Nikolajsen L, Ilkjær S, Jensen TS. Relationship between mechanical sensitivity and postamputation pain: a prospective study. *European Journal of Pain*. 2000; **4**: 327–34.
* 58. Nyström B, Hagbarth KE. Microelectrode recordings from transected nerves in amputees with phantom limb pain. *Neuroscience Letters*. 1981; **27**: 211–6.
59. Nikolajsen L, Ilkjær S, Jensen TS. Effect of preoperative epidural bupivacaine and morphine on stump sensations in lower limb amputees. *British Journal of Anaesthesia*. 1998; **81**: 348–54.
* 60. Hunter JP, Katz J, Davis KD. Dissociation of phantom limb phenomena from stump tactile spatial acuity and sensory thresholds. *Brain*. 2005; **128**: 308–20.
* 61. Flor H, Nikolajsen L, Staehelin Jensen T. Phantom limb pain: a case of maladaptive CNS plasticity? *Nature Reviews Neuroscience*. 2006; **7**: 873–81.
62. Flor H, Denke C, Schaefer M *et al*. Effect of sensory discrimination training on cortical reorganisation and phantom limb pain. *Lancet*. 2001; **357**: 1763–4.
63. Chabal C, Jacobson L, Russell LC *et al*. Pain responses to perineuromal injection of normal saline, gallamine, and lidocaine in humans. *Pain*. 1989; **36**: 321–5.
64. Devor M. Response of nerves to injury in relation to neuropathic pain. In: McMahon SB, Koltzenburg M (eds). *Wall & Melzack's textbook of pain*, 5th edn. London: Elsevier Churchill Livingstone, 2006: 905–28.
65. Novakovic SD, Tzoumaka E, McGivern JG *et al*. Distribution of the tetrodotoxin-resistant sodium channel PN3 in rat sensory neurons in normal and neuropathic pain conditions. *Journal of Neuroscience*. 1998; **18**: 2174–87.
66. Kajander KC, Wakisaka S, Bennett GJ. Spontaneous discharge originates in the dorsal root ganglion at the onset of a painful peripheral neuropathy in the rat. *Neuroscience Letters*. 1992; **138**: 225–8.
67. Koltzenburg M, McMahon SB. The enigmatic role for the sympathetic nervous system in chronic pain. *Trends in Pharmacological Sciences*. 1991; **12**: 399–402.
68. Woolf CJ, Salter MW. Plasticity and pain: role of the dorsal horn. In: McMahon SB, Koltzenburg M (eds). *Wall & Melzack's textbook of pain*, 5th edn. London: Elsevier Churchill Livingstone, 2006: 91–106.
69. Cook AJ, Woolf CJ, Wall PD, McMahon SB. Dynamic receptive field plasticity in rat spinal cord dorsal horn

following C-primary afferent input. *Nature*. 1987; **325**: 151–3.

70. Eide PK. Wind-up and the NMDA receptor complex from a clinical perspective. *European Journal of Pain*. 2000; **4**: 5–15.
71. Nikolajsen L, Hansen CL, Nielsen J *et al.* The effect of ketamine on phantom pain: a central neuropathic disorder maintained by peripheral input. *Pain*. 1996; **67**: 69–77.
72. Hökfelt T, Zhang X, Xu Z-Q *et al.* Phenotypic regulation in dorsal root ganglion neurons after nerve injury: focus on peptides and their receptors. In: Borsook D (ed.). *Molecular neurobiology of pain*. Progress in Pain Research and Management, 9. Seattle: IASP Press, 1997: 115–43.

* 73. Florence SL, Kaas JH. Large-scale reorganization at multiple levels of the somatosensory pathway follows therapeutic amputation of the hand in monkeys. *Journal of Neuroscience*. 1995; **15**: 8083–95.

* 74. Pons TP, Garraghty PE, Ommaya AK *et al.* Massive cortical reorganization after sensory deafferentation in adult macaques. *Science*. 1991; **252**: 1857–60.

* 75. Flor H, Elbert T, Knecht S. Phantom limb pain as a perceptual correlate of cortical reorganization following arm amputation. *Nature*. 1995; **375**: 482–4.

76. Flor H, Elbert T, Mühlnickel W. Cortical reorganization and phantom phenomena in congenital and traumatic upper-extremity amputees. *Experimental Brain Research*. 1998; **119**: 205–12.
77. Birbaumer N, Lutzenberger W, Montoya P *et al.* Effects of regional anesthesia on phantom limb are mirrored in changes in cortical reorganization in upper limb amputees. *Journal of Neuroscience*. 1997; **17**: 5503–08.
78. Huse E, Larbig W, Flor H *et al.* The effect of opioids on phantom limb pain and cortical reorganization. *Pain*. 2001; **90**: 47–55.

* 79. Davis KD, Kiss ZH, Luo L. Phantom sensations generated by thalamic microstimulation. *Nature*. 1998; **391**: 385–7.

80. Dostrovsky JO. Immediate and long-term plasticity in human somatosensory thalamus and its involvement in phantom limbs. *Pain Supplement*. 1999; **6**: 37–43.
81. Draganski B, Moser T, Lummel N *et al.* Decrease of thalamic gray matter following limb amputation. *NeuroImage*. 2006; **31**: 951–7.
82. Pinzur MS, Garla PGN, Pluth T *et al.* Continuous postoperative infusion of a regional anaesthetic after an amputation of the lower extremity. *Journal of Bone and Joint Surgery*. 1996; **78**: 1501–05.

* 83. Halbert J, Crotty M, Cameron ID. Evidence for the optimal management of acute and chronic phantom pain: a systematic review. *Clinical Journal of Pain*. 2002; **18**: 84–92.

84. Bone M, Critchley P, Buggy DJ. Gabapentin in postamputation phantom limb pain: a randomized, double-blind, placebo-controlled, cross-over study. *Regional Anesthesia and Pain Medicine*. 2002; **27**: 481–6.
85. Maier C, Dertwinkel R, Mansourian N *et al.* Efficacy of the NMDA-receptor antagonist memantine in patients with chronic phantom limb pain – results of a randomized double-blinded, placebo-controlled trial. *Pain*. 2003; **103**: 277–83.
86. Nikolajsen L, Gottrup H, Kristensen AGD *et al.* Memantine (a N-methyl D-aspartate receptor antagonist) in the treatment of neuropathic pain following amputation or surgery: a randomised, double-blind, cross-over study. *Anesthesia and Analgesia*. 2000; **91**: 960–6.
87. Wu CL, Tella P, Staats PS *et al.* Analgesic effects of intravenous lidocaine and morphine on postamputation pain. *Anesthesiology*. 2002; **96**: 841–8.
88. Robinson LR, Czerniecki JM, Ehde DM *et al.* Trial of amitriptyline for relief of pain in amputees: results of a randomized controlled study. *Archives of Physical Medicine and Rehabilitation*. 2004; **85**: 1–6.
89. Wilder-Smith CH, Hill LT, Laurent S. Postamputation pain and sensory changes in treatment-naive patients: characteristics and responses to treatment with tramadol, amitriptyline, and placebo. *Anesthesiology*. 2005; **103**: 619–28.
90. Smith DG, Ehde DM, Hanley MA *et al.* Efficacy of gabapentin in treating chronic phantom limb and residual limb pain. *Journal of Rehabilitation Research and Development*. 2005; **42**: 645–54.
91. Nikolajsen L, Finnerup NB, Kramp S *et al.* A randomized study of the effects of gabapentin on postamputation pain. *Anesthesiology*. 2006; **105**: 1008–15.
92. Schley M, Topfner S, Wiech K *et al.* Continuous brachial plexus blockade in combination with the NMDA receptor antagonist memantine prevents phantom pain in acute traumatic upper limb amputees. *European Journal of Pain*. 2006; **11**: 299–308.
93. Rusy LM, Troshynski TJ, Weisman SJ. Gabapentin in phantom limb pain management in children and young adults: report of seven cases. *Journal of Pain and Symptom Management*. 2001; **21**: 78–82.
94. Dellemijn P. Are opioids effective in relieving neuropathic pain? *Pain*. 1999; **80**: 453–62.
95. Bergmans L, Snijdelaar DG, Katz J *et al.* Methadone for phantom limb pain. *Clinical Journal of Pain*. 2002; **18**: 203–5.
96. Abraham RB, Marouani N, Weinbroum AA. Dextromethorphan mitigates phantom pain in cancer amputees. *Annals of Surgical Oncology*. 2003; **10**: 268–74.
97. Jaeger H, Maier C. Calcitonin in phantom limb pain: a double-blind study. *Pain*. 1992; **48**: 21–7.
98. Ahmad S. Phantom limb pain and propranolol. *British Medical Journal*. 1979; **1**: 415.
99. Marsland AR, Weekes JWN, Atkinson RL *et al.* Phantom limb pain: a case for beta blockers? *Pain*. 1982; **12**: 295–7.
100. Davis RW. Successful treatment for phantom pain. *Orthopedics*. 1993; **16**: 691–5.
101. Rayner HC, Atkins RC, Westerman RA. Relief of local stump pain by capsaicin cream. *Lancet*. 1989; **2**: 1276–7.
102. Jacobsen L, Chabal C, Brody MC. A comparison of the effects of intrathecal fentanyl and lidocaine on established postamputation stump pain. *Pain*. 1990; **40**: 137–41.

103. Omote K, Ohmori H, Kawamata M *et al.* Intrathecal buprenorphine in the treatment of phantom limb pain. *Anesthesia and Analgesia.* 1995; **80**: 1030–2.
104. Lierz P, Schroegendorfer K, Choi S *et al.* Continuous blockade of both brachial plexus with ropivacaine in phantom pain: a case report. *Pain.* 1998; **78**: 135–7.
105. Wassef MR. Phantom pain with probable reflex sympathetic dystrophy. Efficacy of fentanyl infiltration of the stellate ganglion. *Regional Anesthesia.* 1997; **22**: 287–90.
106. Kern U, Martin C, Scheicher S *et al.* Botulinum-Toxin-A in der Behandlung von Phantomschmerzen. *Schmerz.* 2003; **17**: 117–24.
107. Harden RN, Houle TT, Remble TA *et al.* Topiramate for phantom limb pain: A time-series analysis. *Pain Medicine.* 2005; **6**: 375–8.
108. Hanley MA, Ehde DM, Campbell KM *et al.* Self-reported treatments used for lower-limb phantom pain: Descriptive findings. *Archives of Physical Medicine and Rehabilitation.* 2006; **87**: 270–7.
109. Bradbrook D. Acupuncture treatment of phantom limb pain and phantom limb sensation in amputees. *Acupuncture in Medicine.* 2004; **22**: 93–7.
110. Oakley DA, Whitman LG, Halligan PW. Hypnotic imagery as a treatment for phantom pain: two case reports and a review. *Clinical Rehabilitation.* 2002; **16**: 368–77.
111. Finsen V, Persen L, Lovlien M *et al.* Transcutaneous electrical nerve stimulation after major amputation. *Journal of Bone and Joint Surgery: British Volume.* 1988; **70**: 109–12.
112. Katz J, Melzack R. Auricular transcutaneous electrical nerve stimulation (TENS) reduces phantom limb pain. *Journal of Pain and Symptom Management.* 1991; **6**: 73–83.
113. Lundeberg T. Relief of pain from a phantom limb by peripheral stimulation. *Journal of Neurology.* 1985; **232**: 79–82.
*114. Conine TA, Herschler C, Alexander ST *et al.* The efficacy of Farabloc in the treatment of phantom limb pain. *Canadian Journal of Rehabilitation.* 1993; **6**: 155–61.
115. Ramachandran VS, Rogers-Ramachandran D. Phantom limbs and neural plasticity. *Archives of Neurology.* 2000; **57**: 317–20.
116. Brodie EE, Whyte A, Niven CA. Analgesia through the looking-glass? A randomized controlled trial investigating the effect of viewing a 'virtual' limb upon phantom limb pain, sensation and movement. *European Journal Pain.* 2007; **11**: 428–36.
117. Prestor B. Microsurgical junctional DREZ coagulation for treatment of deafferentation pain syndromes. *Surgical Neurology.* 2001; **56**: 259–65.
118. Krainick JU, Thoden U, Riechert T. Pain reduction in amputees by long-term spinal cord stimulation. Long-term follow-up study over 5 years. *Journal of Neurosurgery.* 1980; **52**: 346–50.
119. Bittar RG, Otero S, Carter H, Aziz TZ. Deep brain stimulation for phantom limb pain. *Journal of Clinical Neuroscience.* 2005; **12**: 399–404.
120. Yamamoto T, Katayama Y, Obuchi T *et al.* Thalamic sensory relay nucleus stimulation for the treatment of peripheral deafferentation pain. *Stereotactic and Functional Neurosurgery.* 2006; **84**: 180–3.
*121. Bach S, Noreng MF, Tjéllden NU. Phantom limb pain in amputees during the first 12 months following limb amputation after preoperative lumbar epidural blockade. *Pain.* 1988; **33**: 297–301.
122. Woolf CJ, Chong MS. Preemptive analgesia – treating postoperative pain by preventing the establishment of central sensitization. *Anesthesia Analgesia.* 1993; **77**: 362–79.
123. Jahangiri M, Jayatunga AP, Bradley JWP *et al.* Prevention of phantom pain after major lower limb amputation by epidural infusion of diamorphine, clonidine and bupivacaine. *Annals of the Royal College of Surgeons of England.* 1994; **76**: 324–6.
124. Schug SA, Burell R, Payne J *et al.* Pre-emptive epidural analgesia may prevent phantom limb pain. *Regional Anesthesia.* 1995; **20**: 256.
125. Katsuly Liapis I, Georgakis P, Tierry C. Preemptive extradural analgesia reduces the incidence of phantom pain in lower limb amputees. *British Journal of Anaesthesia.* 1996; **76**: 125.
126. Fischer A, Meller Y. Continuous postoperative regional analgesia by nerve sheath block for amputation surgery – a pilot study. *Anesthesia and Analgesia.* 1991; **72**: 300–03.
*127. Nikolajsen L, Ilkjær S, Krøner K *et al.* Randomised trial of epidural bupivacaine and morphine in prevention of stump and phantom pain in lower-limb amputation. *Lancet.* 1997; **350**: 1353–7.
128. Lambert AW, Dashfield AK, Cosgrove C *et al.* Randomised prospective study comparing preoperative epidural and intraoperative perineural analgesia for the prevention of postoperative stump and phantom limb pain following major amputation. *Regional Anesthesia and Pain Medicine.* 2001; **26**: 316–21.
129. Elizaga AM, Smith DG, Sharar SR *et al.* Continuous regional analgesia by intraneural block: effect on postoperative opioid requirements and phantom limb pain following amputation. *Journal of Rehabilitation Research and Development.* 1994; **31**: 179–87.
130. Dertwinkel R, Heinrichs C, Senne I *et al.* Prevention of severe phantom limb pain by perioperative administration of ketamine – an observational study. *Acute Pain.* 2002; **4**: 9–13.

32

Herpes zoster pain including shingles and postherpetic neuralgia

ROBERT W JOHNSON

KEY LEARNING POINTS

- Herpes zoster (HZ) results from reactivation of varicella zoster virus (VZV) clinically latent since primary infection with varicella. Incidence increases with age.
- Although other serious complications such as encephalitis may occur, postherpetic neuralgia (PHN) is the most common complication and is predicted by greater age, acute pain, and rash, as well as more painful or prolonged prodrome.
- PHN is a neuropathic pain and the precise pathology, signs, and symptoms vary between individuals. It has central and peripheral components and may involve deafferentation, peripheral or central sensitization, or a combination.
- Although antiviral drugs, prolonged neural blockade, and effective analgesia may reduce the duration of pain following HZ, there is no practical strategy for preventing PHN, except vaccination, which reduces HZ incidence and severity with resultant reduction in PHN and burden of illness (BOI).
- Established PHN may be treated with tricyclic antidepressants, alpha 2 delta ligands, opioids, topical lidocaine, and topical capsaicin. Numbers needed to treat (NNT) range from ~2 to ~5 and numbers needed to harm (NNH) indicate that the therapeutic index is poor.
- Intrathecal methylprednisolone has been shown in a single study to effectively manage established and intractable PHN. To date, there has been no confirmatory study and there are concerns that serious adverse events could follow this treatment.

WHAT IS HERPES ZOSTER?

Herpes zoster (HZ), also known as shingles, results from reactivation of varicella zoster virus (VZV), an α herpes virus, which has been persistent in a clinically latent state in spinal and cranial sensory ganglia since primary infection with varicella (chickenpox), often several decades earlier. Varicella is usually a childhood disease in temperate climates, but more often affects adolescents and adults in tropical areas. Latency is maintained by competent VZV-specific cell-mediated immunity (CMI), which declines as a normal function of aging (immunesenescence)[1] (**Figure 32.1**). VZV-specific CMI may also fall below a threshold necessary to prevent clinical virus reactivation as a result of disease (e.g. lymphoma, human immunodeficiency virus (HIV)), therapeutic immune suppression (e.g. after organ transplant, for autoimmune disease), or as a result of treatment of malignancy (e.g. radiotherapy, chemotherapy). However, younger individuals may develop HZ with no coexisting disease process. Prodromal pain usually lasting three to five days is followed by a typical unilateral rash in a dermatomal distribution. The rash progresses from erythematous patches to vesicles, pustules, and scabs. Healing occurs typically within three weeks, often leaving hyper- or hypopigmented scars and sensory changes. HZ cannot be contracted from contact with varicella, but varicella may occur after contact with HZ although the force of infection is low (~0.1 percent)[3] compared with that for contracting varicella from another person with varicella (~20 percent for varicella affecting children two to four years of age).

DEFINITIONS

Defined in the IASP Classification on Chronic Pain (2nd edition) as "chronic pain with skin changes in the distribution of (one or more cranial/spinal sensory roots) subsequent to herpes zoster," PHN has no universally accepted definition and the term may refer to any pain after HZ rash healing or may specify various time intervals after rash appearance or healing and/or a requirement that average or worst pain exceeds a certain value: usually three on a zero to ten scale. The rationale for including a pain severity qualification of ≥ 3 arises from work showing that pain below this level has little effect on activities of daily living (ADL).[4] However, there is no evidence that pain <3 may not result in distress. Such distress may be poorly assessed by standard instruments for quality of life and ADL. Although multiple definitions of PHN have been used, the results of recent studies suggest that pain persisting for at least 120 days after rash onset may be considered a validated definition of PHN for research purposes.[5, 6, 7]

COMPLICATIONS OF HZ

Although PHN is numerically the most common complication by far, other adverse events may result and some are serious or life threatening. These occur most frequently in immunocompromised and frail, elderly individuals and include secondary bacterial infection, ophthalmic sequelae ranging from conjunctivitis to retinal necrosis, encephalitis, and myelitis.[8] Two to three percent of HZ cases are hospitalized and more than 10 percent of patients >65 years. Annual mortality of HZ is estimated to be 0.6–1 per million of the population.[9, 10]

Motor nerves may be involved in 5–15 percent of cases where these can be adequately examined (especially muscles in the extremities). Using an electromyogram (EMG), it is possible to show that muscles are involved in 50 percent of cases.[11] VZV is frequently involved in cases of Bell's palsy.

EPIDEMIOLOGY

Any seropositive individual (i.e. has had primary infection in the form of varicella) is a potential HZ sufferer. Approximately 3.4 per 1000 of the population per year develop HZ with up to 11/1000 per year above the age of 80 years.[12, 13] Those living beyond 80 years have a 50 percent lifetime risk of having HZ. It is believed that VZV-specific CMI is enhanced at intervals during life by two mechanisms. First by exposure of seropositive individuals to children with varicella (exogenous boosting)

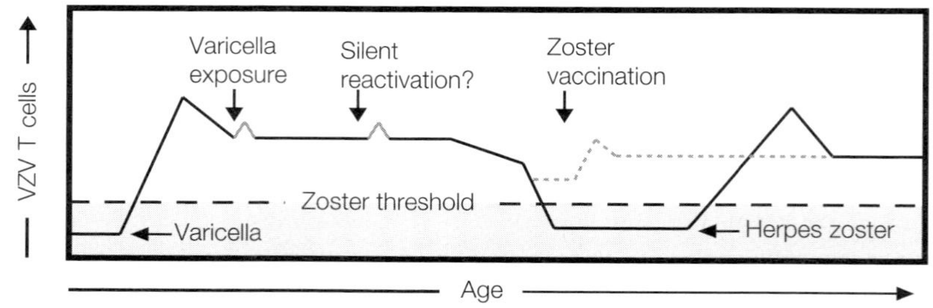

Figure 32.1 Lifetime changes in cell-mediated immunity to varicella zoster virus (VZV). Varicella is the primary infection caused by VZV, and its resolution is associated with the induction of memory T cells specific for VZV (black line). Memory immunity to VZV may be boosted periodically by exposure to varicella or silent reactivation from latency (gray peaks). Memory T cells specific for VZV decline with age. The decline below a threshold (dashed black line) correlates with an increased risk of zoster. The occurrence of zoster, in turn, is associated with an increase in T cells specific for VZV. Administering zoster vaccine to older people may prevent T cells specific for VZV from dropping below the threshold for zoster occurrence (dashed gray line). Published with permission from Arvin A. Aging, immunity, and the varicella-zoster virus. *New England Journal of Medicine*. 2005; **352**: 2266-7.[2]

and second by immune response to subclinical, contained reactivations of latent virus occurring periodically after primary infection (endogenous boosting).[2] There are theoretical reasons to believe that HZ incidence will increase as a result of universal childhood vaccination against varicella because seropositive adults will be deprived of CMI exogenous boosting resulting from decreased incidence of varicella.[14] To date, more than ten years after the introduction of childhood varicella vaccination in the USA, there is no available evidence of this effect.

Increases in HZ, and therefore PHN, from increasing longevity and greater numbers of therapeutically immunocompromised individuals are inevitable. Second cases of HZ are uncommon (5 percent or less) in the immunocompetent individual, presumably because an episode of HZ will boost immunity thereby preventing subsequent symptomatic VZV reactivations.[12, 15, 16]

There is interest in the concept of VZV reactivation causing dermatomal pain in the absence of skin lesions, termed "zoster sine herpete." This concept is controversial but has been supported by virological evidence of concurrent VZV reactivation during some acute pain syndromes.[17]

The epidemiology of PHN is less easy to detail as so many definitions have been used. However, pain at defined time intervals after HZ has been the subject of a number of studies and it is clear that PHN is extremely rare in younger subjects (<50) and that incidence rises sharply above the age of 60. In the shingles prevention study, incidence of PHN (pain ≥ 3 at 90 days after rash appearance) was 5.1 percent in the placebo group.[18]

The cost of HZ and PHN has been addressed in a number of studies. Scott *et al.*[19] followed 70 patients of all ages recruited from primary care in London for six months from diagnosis. In those aged <65 (45 patients), the combined median costs to the patient, society, and the National Health Service (NHS) were £173 (min 20, max 3578). For patients ≥ 65 (25 patients) combined median costs were £138 (min 48, max 4218). Societal costs considerably exceeded costs to the NHS in younger patients with the position reversed in older patients.[19] Davies *et al.*[20] estimated the 1994 cost of PHN in the UK to be between £4.8 and 17.9 million.

PHASES OF HZ PAIN

Clinical observation and mathematical modeling suggest that HZ pain may be divided into an acute phase (including prodromal) lasting 30 days, subacute (30–120 days) and chronic phases (PHN) from three months after rash healing or four months from onset of prodrome. It is likely that the contributions of inflammation, viral activity, immune response, neuronal damage, and peripheral and central sensitization explain the differing characteristics between and within the three phases.[5]

Approximately 70–80 percent of patients with HZ describe prodromal pain in the dermatome where skin lesions subsequently appear. It may be constant or intermittent, and may or may not interfere with sleep. Pain varies between patients and is commonly described as burning, shooting, stabbing, or throbbing. Some patients describe only allodynia and others complain primarily of pruritus. The prodrome typically lasts two to three days but longer durations of one week or more are not uncommon. Significant prodromal pain may lead to expensive and potentially hazardous medical investigation for diseases characterized by pain in the area of the prodrome (e.g. angina, cholecystitis, glaucoma, nephrolithiasis, spinal nerve compression).

The diagnosis becomes obvious when the characteristic rash appears.[21] The prodrome represents the time required for reactivated VZV to replicate in the ganglion and to traverse cutaneous nerve to the skin where VZV induces sufficient necrosis and inflammatory response to cause the rash.

In some patients, pain does not resolve following the subacute phase but continues for months or years as PHN when patients describe different types of pain, including continuous burning or throbbing pain, intermittent sharp or electric shock-like pain, and allodynia.[22] There have been no systematic attempts to investigate the prevalence of PHN and estimates of the number of cases have ranged up to one million in the United States.[23]

PATHOPHYSIOLOGY OF PHN

Both peripheral and central processes contribute to PHN and their contributions vary widely between patients from minimal deafferentation and severe allodynia to severe sensory loss but no allodynia.[24] Patients with prominent allodynia often have minimal sensory loss and gain pain relief following local application of some analgesic agents. This suggests that preserved, and possibly sensitized, primary afferent nociceptors and their chronically sensitized central connections are responsible for initiating and maintaining pain and allodynia in these patients.[25] Pathological findings in PHN include degeneration of affected primary afferent neuronal cell bodies and axons, atrophy of the spinal cord dorsal horn, scarring of the dorsal root ganglion, and loss of epidermal innervations.[26, 27, 28, 29]

It is possible that the senescent nervous system is more vulnerable to the effects of VZV infection facilitating development of PHN.[30, 31]

PREVENTION OF HZ AND PHN

At this time the use of an effective live attenuated, Oka strain, varicella vaccine given during childhood is standard in some geographic areas, notably the USA, and it seems likely that vaccinated populations will not develop varicella to a large extent (protection of the individual combined with a herd immunity effect) and are therefore not subject to HZ from wild-type (natural) VZV. Reactivation of Oka strain virus appears to be infrequent and mild. The same attenuated virus has been utilized in a higher dose form for vaccination of seropositive adults to prevent HZ and its complications. The greater strength is required because older adults have a reduced immune response compared with younger persons. The Shingles Prevention Study (SPS) investigated 38,546 subjects of $\geq$60 years of age who were injected either with the active vaccine or placebo. They were followed for a median of 3.12 years and the incidence of HZ was reduced by 51.3 percent, PHN (defined as pain rating $\geq$3 90 days after rash onset) by 66.5 percent, and BOI (an area under the curve construct of incidence, severity, and duration of pain and discomfort over six months from onset of HZ) by 61.1 percent in the vaccine group, indicating that where HZ occurred despite vaccination, its course was attenuated.[18] The vaccine has been licensed in the USA and Europe and long-term surveillance will be required to assess its overall benefit. Unfortunately, the vaccine is not appropriate for use in immunocompromised individuals; in the future a vaccine may be developed offering safe protection to such patients.

Reviews of significant available data show that greater age is the most significant predictor of PHN but greater acute pain and rash are also predictive as are longer and more severe prodromal symptoms. Although some studies have suggested that trigeminal distribution and female gender are predictive, others have not confirmed this.[7, 32, 33, 34]

Antiviral drugs, apart from providing good control of acute pain and rash progression, reduce the duration of pain following HZ. Because of study design, it is difficult to say to what extent they may prevent PHN.[35, 36][I] It is certain that PHN occurs and persists in many patients despite appropriate use of antiviral drugs. Interpretation of pain data from the studies suggests that the number of patients with pain at six months may be approximately halved with the prodrugs valaciclovir and famciclovir given t.d.s being more effective than acyclovir given 5 × daily. Brivudin has recently been licensed in some countries for once daily use and appears equivalent to famciclovir but with the disadvantage of a serious, sometimes fatal, interaction with 5 fluorouracil should the drugs be coadministered. With this exception the antiviral drugs, which have their effect by inhibition of VZV viral DNA replication, are specific and remarkably safe. Evidence-based guidelines suggest that antiviral drugs, preferably the prodrugs valaciclovir or famciclovir, are given to all patients of 50 years or greater and to patients with ophthalmic zoster. They are also indicated for patients less than 50 years when acute pain and/or rash are severe. All immunocompromised patients should be given antivirals; the route of administration will depend on the degree of immune suppression.

The addition of oral steroids to acyclovir has been shown to offer better control of acute pain and quicker return to normal ADL and sleep pattern over acyclovir alone, but it has no effect in preventing PHN.[37, 38][I]

Local anesthetic blocks, with or without the addition of steroids, have been investigated. Single epidural injection of local anesthetic and steroid in the acute phase of herpes zoster has failed to prevent PHN in a randomized multicenter clinical trial although acute symptoms were reduced when compared with standard antiviral therapy.[39]

More prolonged epidural administration of local anesthetic and steroid was effective in one study although the incidence of PHN in the control group was remarkably high.[40] Local anesthetic drugs alone, by sustained epidural injection or repeated stellate ganglion blocks, have also be shown to reduce duration of pain.[41]

It is thought likely that the administration of drugs providing good control of acute pain may reduce the incidence of PHN. An indicative study of amitriptyline adds support to this belief as does animal work utilizing gabapentin. The results of a placebo-controlled trial of amitriptyline 25 mg once daily for three months beginning within 48 hours of rash onset and a reanalysis examining the subgroup of patients also treated with an antiviral suggested that amitriptyline reduced the prevalence of PHN at six months by at least 50 percent.[42, 43] [V] The effect of amitriptyline on acute pain was not assessed in this study, and because treatment continued for three months after rash onset, it cannot be determined whether the reduction in PHN was the result of early treatment.

In addition, acute pain should be treated effectively. Evidence for which drug class is most effective is lacking but paracetamol and weak opioids may be escalated to strong opioids such as tramadol, oxycodone, or morphine. α_2-δ ligands and tricyclic antidepressants, such as nortriptyline, may be effective for acute pain control and, possibly, PHN prevention and their use can be justified.

MANAGEMENT OF HZ ACUTE PHASE AND PHN

Prodrome

Although presentation of an elderly person with dermatomal unilateral onset of pain and tingling might lead to the suspicion that the classic skin rash of HZ will follow, it has been shown not to have sufficient specificity to justify initiation of antiviral therapy.[44] However, this combination of symptoms, in the absence of an objective diagnosis, should lead to advice from healthcare workers that the patient should look out for a shingles rash over subsequent days and seek medical advice promptly should this occur.

Acute HZ

Although the classic combination of unilateral dermatomal rash and pain often leads to prompt and correct diagnosis, studies have shown significant incorrect clinical diagnosis rates in up to 20 percent of cases. The most common confusing diagnoses are herpes simplex type 1 (labial), type 2 (genital), or allergy. Pain accompanies acute HZ in over 90 percent of cases. Antiviral drugs (acyclovir, valaciclovir, famciclovir, and brivudin) control viral DNA replication and significantly reduce acute pain, hasten rash healing, and shorten the period of viral shedding (infectivity).[45, 46][I] The effectiveness of analgesic drugs has not been well studied with regard to whether paracetamol, paracetamol with opioid, or non-steroidal anti-inflammatory drugs (NSAIDs) are the drugs of choice. Some patients require strong opioid medication. The place of drugs more commonly associated with PHN management is unproven but there is expert consensus that they have a place in the management of acute pain. Such drugs would include strong opioids, α_2-δ ligands, and tricyclic antidepressant drugs. Topical modalities probably have no place during acute HZ other than to maintain cleanliness and provide additional comfort (cold packs for instance). Treatment of HZ should occur in conjunction with careful explanation of the disease, including the risk of viral transmission to individuals who have not had chickenpox, and of the proposed treatment plan. Encouragement, reassurance, and advice on quality of life are important and include supporting adequate nutrition and optimal levels of mental, physical, and social activity. Patients should be advised to keep the rash clean and dry to reduce the risk of bacterial superinfection (~2 percent).[8][V]

TREATMENT OF PHN

At the present time there is no category 1 evidence to provide a rationale for mechanism-based therapy of PHN. However, there does exist good evidence for treating PHN as a single clinical entity. Guidance for use of drugs for PHN is given in **Table 32.1**. Clinical trials of pain-modifying drugs have been subjected to strict systematic review, providing a clear picture of their efficacy and adverse effects. Effectiveness is more difficult to judge as agents have been studied under clinical trial conditions and for relatively short periods of only a few weeks.[47, 48, 49][I]

Recent systematic reviews give a clear overview and evaluation of current drug treatment in PHN[50, 51][I] and neuropathic pain in general.[52] Most studies compare single drugs with placebo, a few are of cross-over design and one examines drug combinations. Direct comparisons of one drug with another, for both efficacy and adverse effects, would provide valuable information but few have been reported. Calculations of NNT and NNH provide a useful method for comparing therapeutic indices at this time[53] (**Table 32.2**). Usually an NNT for >50 percent pain relief is used because it is seems to indicate a useful clinical effect. Treatments discussed below have all been demonstrated to provide statistically significant benefits compared with placebo in multiple randomized controlled trials. However, the sample size of investigated patients varies, which also has to be considered when comparing drug efficacy.[52]

Tricyclic antidepressants

Tricyclic antidepressants (TCAs, e.g. amitriptyline, desipramine, nortriptyline) are effective in the treatment of PHN.[49][I] These compounds inhibit reuptake of monoaminergic transmitters and are believed to potentiate the effects of biogenic amines in descending central nervous system pain modulating pathways. In addition, they block voltage-dependent sodium channels and alpha adrenergic receptors. TCAs, of which amitriptyline is the most widely prescribed, have significant side effects limiting their use, especially in the elderly and those with comorbidities. They can produce orthostatic hypotension, sedation, urinary retention, memory loss, dry mouth, constipation, and cardiac conduction abnormalities. Higher doses of tricyclic antidepressants may even be associated with the risk of sudden cardiac death.[54] It is considered that the relatively selective noradrenaline reuptake inhibitors, such as desipramine and nortriptyline, cause less anticholinergic side effects as compared to the unselective serotonin and noradrenaline reuptake inhibitor, amitriptyline.[55]

Anticonvulsants

Gabapentin and pregabalin act at the $\alpha 2\delta$-subunit of presynaptic calcium channels on primary nociceptive endings.[56, 57] Dizziness and drowsiness are the most commonly reported adverse events, especially during upward titration to targeted doses. Both drugs have a low potential for drug interactions, and no negative impact on cardiac function. Peripheral edema occurs in some patients. Both drugs have been shown to be effective in the management of PHN. Pregabalin has superior bioavailability and dose titration-to-effect seems to produce fewer side effects than gabapentin.[58] Gabapentin and pregabalin improve sleep disturbance, overall mood, and other measures of quality of life in neuropathic pain patients.[56, 59][I]

These features make the $\alpha 2\delta$-subunit ligands suitable for first-line therapy especially for the elderly, a population very often suffering from several comorbidities that need multiple drug therapies. In most situations they are a more costly option than TCAs but their perceived greater safety may overcome this limitation, particularly in elderly or frail patients. Abrupt discontinuation should

Table 32.1 Guidance for use of drugs for postherpetic neuralgia.

Medication	Start dosage	Titration	Maximum dosage	Duration of adequate trial
Gabapentin	100–300 mg every night or 100 mg 3 × times daily	Increase by 100–300 mg 3 × daily every 1–7 days as tolerated	1800 mg/day (600 mg 3 × daily); reduce if low creatinine clearance[a]	3–6 weeks for titration plus 1–2 weeks at maximum tolerated dosage
Pregabalin	50 mg 3 × daily	Increase to 100 mg 3 × daily within one week	600 mg/day (200 mg 3 × daily) reduce if low creatinine clearance	2 weeks for titration plus 1–2 weeks at maximum tolerated dosage
Tricyclic antidepressants (e.g. nortriptyline, amitriptyline)	10–25 mg every night	Increase by 10–25 mg/day every 3–7 days as tolerated	75–150 mg/day; if blood level of active drug and its metabolite is > 100 ng/mL, continue titration with caution	6–8 weeks with at least 1–2 weeks at maximum tolerated dosage
Opioid analgesics (morphine)	5–15 mg every 4 hours as needed	After 1–2 weeks convert total daily dosage to long-acting opioid analgesic and continue short-acting medication as rescue medication	No maximum with careful titration over time	4–6 weeks
Tramadol	50 mg once or twice daily	Increase by 50–100 mg/day in divided doses every 3–7 days as tolerated	400 mg/day (100 mg 4 times daily); in patients older than 75 years, 300 mg/day in divided doses	4 weeks
5% Lidocaine patch	Maximum of 3 patches daily for a maximum of 12 hours	None needed	Maximum of 3 patches daily for a maximum of 12 hours	2 weeks

[a]This dose is frequently exceeded in specialist clinical practice.

Table 32.2 Number needed to treat (NNT) and number needed to harm (NNH) for effective treatments for postherpetic neuralgia.

Active treatment	Number of patient episodes	Number of studies	NNT (95% CI)	NNH (95% CI) minor harm	NNH (95% CI) major harm
Combined tricyclic antidepressants	248	4	2.64 (2.1–3.54)	5.67 (3.34–18.58)	16.9 (8.85–178)
Combined gabapentin	559	3	4.39 (3.34–6.07)	3.93 (2.64–7.66)	12.25 (7.69–30.2)
Combined pregabalin	411	3	4.93 (3.66–7.58)	4.27 (2.78–9.18)[a]	–
Combined opioids	211	2	2.67 (2.07–3.77)	3.57 (2.16–10.23)[a]	6.29 (4.16–12.8)
Tramadol	108	1	4.76 (2.61–26.97)	–	–
Topical lidocaine (5% patch)	64	1	2 (1.43–3.31)	–	–

[a]Data from Ref. 50.

be avoided after a case study reporting encephalopathic changes following sudden pregabalin withdrawal.[60] There is no convincing evidence for efficacy of sodium-blocker anticonvulsants, such as carbamazepine, in PHN.[61]

Opioid analgesics

Double-blind placebo-controlled studies have demonstrated that intravenous infusions of morphine or fentanyl give significant pain relief in PHN.[62][II] Controlled trials have demonstrated sustained efficacy for several weeks of oral oxycodone[63][II] and tramadol.[64][II] Additionally, in a nonplacebo-controlled parallel group study of neuropathic pain management comparing two doses of levorphanol, significant dose-dependent pain relief was found in PHN patients.[65][II] In one study, oral morphine was analyzed in a group of PHN patients comparing the effect of tricyclic antidepressants in the same cohort. Both drugs were similarly effective. However, there was no correlation in the response rate between both drugs, indicating that different mechanisms are active in these PHN patients.[66] The use of opioids requires caution in elderly patients and those with a history of chemical dependence or pulmonary disease. Standard guidelines for use of strong opioids in nonterminal pain should be followed. After dose titration with a short-acting agent, conversion to long-acting opioid analgesics (e.g. sustained release morphine or oxycodone preparation) is desirable. Prophylactic treatment of common side effects, nausea and constipation, is necessary and improves patient compliance. Further common adverse effects are dizziness, sedation, and pruritus. Psychotic symptoms may occur, in particular in elderly patients. Withdrawal should be by gradual reduction in dosage.

Topical medications

Topical capsaicin 0.075 percent reduces pain in PHN.[67][II] Capsaicin is an agonist of the vanilloid receptor which is present on the terminals of primary nociceptive afferents. On initial application it has an excitatory action and produces burning pain and hyperalgesia, often leading to discontinuation of its use. However, with perseverance and repeated and prolonged application, it inactivates the receptive terminals of nociceptors. Recent work investigating the use of high-concentration topical capsaicin (8 percent) following topical local anesthetic pretreatment gives some cause for hope that this therapy may prove useful.[68][V] Therefore, this approach is reasonable for those patients whose pain is maintained by anatomically intact sensitized nociceptors and in whom long-term side effects do not exceed benefit. Topical lidocaine patches (5 percent) placed over the painful area for approximately 12 hours each day may provide significant pain relief in PHN.[69, 70][II] Blood levels of lidocaine are very low and do not explain the analgesic effect. Minor side effects, such as local irritation or rash, occur in some patients. Lidocaine patch therapy is a safe and well-tolerated supplemental modality for PHN pain relief. Because of fewer side effects it is generally preferred over topical capsaicin.

Miscellaneous treatments

If this treatment strategy fails, further drugs should be considered that have been effective in animal models, smaller studies, or other neuropathic pain conditions but for which neither category 1 or 2 evidence exists. Intrathecal administration of lidocaine and methyl prednisolone combined appears to be associated with remarkable benefit in PHN patients.[71][II] However, the therapy has potentially dangerous short- and long-term side effects and the trial has not yet been replicated.[72] Therefore, further high-quality controlled trials of this therapy are required before definite recommendations can be made.[50] Based on pathophysiological pain mechanisms and animal studies, *N*-methyl-D-aspartic acid (NMDA) receptor antagonists are pain-relieving candidates. However, data from three controlled studies did not demonstrate a superior efficacy over placebo in humans.[50, 73, 74, 75, 76] The anticonvulsant valproate was effective in one controlled study on 48 PHN patients.[77] Anticonvulsants such as lamotrigine, the selective serotonin and noradrenaline reuptake inhibitors venlafaxine and duloxetine, and cannabinoids might be considered as they have been effective in neuropathic pain conditions other than PHN.[52] Transcutaneous electrical nerve stimulation (TENS) may be effective in some cases and has minimal side effects. In particular cases, invasive stimulation techniques, such as epidural spinal cord stimulation, may be indicated.

However, beyond these treatment approaches the importance of the biopsychosocial model of chronic pain should be considered and management of psychological and social aspects of PHN is invaluable.[50, 78]

TREATMENT GUIDELINES

In summary, the proportion of seropositive individuals in the population will decline as a result of childhood varicella vaccination. In time, this will reduce the incidence of HZ. Adult vaccination has been shown to be effective for the prevention of shingles and PHN.[18][II] In acute HZ, early antiviral therapy is recommended and pain treatment with strong opioids, tricyclic antidepressants, or gabapentin should be considered in addition to conventional analgesics. The pharmacological management of PHN consists of three main classes of oral medication (tricyclic antidepressants, anticonvulsants [calcium channel], opioids), and two categories of topical medications (lidocaine and capsaicin). Possibly because more than one mechanism of PHN operates in most patients, a combination of two or more analgesic agents may produce greater pain relief and fewer side effects. In a recent controlled four-period crossover trial, gabapentin and morphine combined achieved better analgesia at lower doses of each drug than either as a single agent with constipation, sedation, and dry mouth as the most frequent adverse effects.[79] A treatment plan for pain associated with HZ is shown in **Table 32.3**.

Table 32.3 Treatment plan for pain associated with herpes zoster (HZ).

Treatment plan		
Prevention of varicella	Varicella vaccination	As child "Catch-up" as adult
Prevention of HZ and PHN	HZ vaccination	Age $\geq$60 Immunocompetent
Management of HZ	Psychosocial support	
	Prompt antiviral drug treatment	
	Analgesia	Paracetamol, NSAID
	Early neuropathic pain treatment	e.g. TCA, opioid or $\alpha2\delta$ ligand
Management of PHN	Tricyclic antidepressant drugs (TCA)	Nortriptyline Amitriptyline Desipramine
	Anticonvulsants ($\alpha2\delta$ ligands)	Pregabalin Gabapentin
	Opioids	Tramadol Oxycodone Morphine
	Topical agents	Lidocaine Capsaicin
	Combinations	TCA+topical $\alpha2\delta$ ligand+topical Opioid+topical Opioid+$\alpha2\delta$ ligand Opioid+$\alpha2\delta$ ligand+topical

Vulnerable and frail elderly patients

The health status of older adults varies widely from well elders who have no diseases or functional problems to chronically ill elders who have multiple comorbidities and disabilities. Increased longevity of the population indicates that "years are being added to life": however, evidence that "life has been added to years" is not convincing. These individuals have markedly diminished physiologic reserves to respond to stressors, including acute illnesses such as HZ. Cutaneous dissemination and possibly visceral dissemination seem to be more common in elderly individuals as is the need for hospitalization. Short periods of reduced competence may lead to long-term inability for self-care, thus jeopardizing independence.[80, 81] Drug absorption, binding, and elimination may be affected thereby increasing the risks of drug therapy. These individuals experience significant age- and disease-related declines in glomerular filtration rate so dosages of renally excreted medications must be adjusted (e.g. antiviral agents, gabapentin, pregabalin). Hence, when HZ occurs in this population, it is important to modify pharmacotherapeutic and augment non-pharmacotherapeutic approaches to management. Starting dosages of medications should be lower than those recommended for younger individuals and the dosage titrated more slowly, particularly for opioid analgesics, gabapentin, pregabalin, TCAs, and NSAIDs.[82]

The clinical course of vulnerable and frail elders needs to be monitored more closely than well elders to detect inadequate compliance, response to therapy and early functional decline, and to step up interventions if needed. The management of HZ pain is more complicated in demented patients because of the risk for adverse cognitive effects of opioid analgesics, gabapentin, pregabalin, and TCAs. In addition, traditional pain measures (e.g. 0–10 numerical rating scale) to track response to analgesics are not useful in patients with advanced dementia.[83]

REFERENCES

1. Weksler ME. Immune senescence. *Annals of Neurology.* 1994; **35**: S35–7.
2. Arvin A. Aging, immunity, and the varicella-zoster virus. *New England Journal of Medicine.* 2005; **352**: 2266–7.
3. Brisson M, Edmunds WJ, Gay NJ *et al.* Modelling the impact of immunization on the epidemiology of varicella zoster virus. *Epidemiology and Infection.* 2000; **125**: 651–69.
4. Lydick E, Epstein RS, Himmelberger D, White CJ. Herpes zoster and quality of life: a self-limited disease with severe impact. *Neurology.* 1995; **45**: S52–3.
* 5. Arani RB, Soong SJ, Weiss HL *et al.* Phase specific analysis of herpes zoster associated pain data: a new

statistical approach. *Statistics in Medicine*. 2001; **20**: 2429–39.
6. Desmond RA, Weiss HL, Arani RB *et al*. Clinical applications for change-point analysis of herpes zoster pain. *Journal of Pain and Symptom Management*. 2002; **23**: 510–6.
7. Jung BF, Johnson RW, Griffin DR, Dworkin RH. Risk factors for postherpetic neuralgia in patients with herpes zoster. *Neurology*. 2004; **62**: 1545–51.
* 8. Dworkin R, Johnson R, Breuer J *et al*. Recommendations for the management of herpes zoster. *Clinical Infectious Diseases*. 2007; **44**: S1–26.
* 9. Brisson M, Edmunds WJ, Law B *et al*. Epidemiology of varicella zoster virus infection in Canada and the United Kingdom. *Epidemiology and Infection*. 2001; **127**: 305–14.
10. MacIntyre CR, Chu CP, Burgess MA. Use of hospitalization and pharmaceutical prescribing data to compare the prevaccination burden of varicella and herpes zoster in Australia. *Epidemiology and Infection*. 2003; **131**: 675–82.
11. Haanpaa M, Hakkinen V, Nurmikko T. Motor involvement in acute herpes zoster. *Muscle and Nerve*. 1997; **20**: 1433–8.
* 12. Hope-Simpson RE. The nature of herpes zoster: a long-term study and a new hypothesis. *Proceedings of the Royal Society of Medicine*. 1965; **58**: 9–20.
13. Hope-Simpson RE. Postherpetic neuralgia. *Journal of the Royal College of General Practitioners*. 1975; **25**: 571–5.
14. Brisson M, Edmunds WJ, Gay NJ. Varicella vaccination: impact of vaccine efficacy on the epidemiology of VZV. *Journal of Medical Virology*. 2003; **70**: S31–7.
15. Ragozzino MW, Melton LJ, Kurland 3rd LT *et al*. Population-based study of herpes zoster and its sequelae. *Medicine*. 1982; **61**: 310–6.
16. Donahue JG, Choo PW, Manson JE, Platt R. The incidence of herpes zoster. *Archives of Internal Medicine*. 1995; **155**: 1605–9.
17. Gilden DH, Wright RR, Schneck SA *et al*. Zoster sine herpete, a clinical variant. *Annals of Neurology*. 1994; **35**: 530–3.
* 18. Oxman MN, Levin MJ, Johnson GR *et al*. A vaccine to prevent herpes zoster and postherpetic neuralgia in older adults. *New England Journal of Medicine*. 2005; **352**: 2271–84.
* 19. Scott FT, Johnson RW, Leedham-Green M *et al*. The burden of herpes zoster: a prospective population based study. *Vaccine*. 2006; **24**: 1308–14.
20. Davies D, Cossins L, Bowsher D, Drummond M. The cost of treatment for post-herpetic neuralgia in the UK. *Pharmacoeconomics*. 1994; **6**: 142–8.
21. Gnann Jr JW, Whitley RJ. Clinical practice. Herpes zoster. *New England Journal of Medicine*. 2002; **347**: 340–6.
22. Dworkin RH, Portenoy RK. Pain and its persistence in herpes zoster. *Pain*. 1996; **67**: 241–51.
23. Bowsher D. The lifetime occurrence of Herpes zoster and prevalence of post-herpetic neuralgia: A retrospective survey in an elderly population. *European Journal of Pain*. 1999; **3**: 335–42.
* 24. Woolf CJ. Pain: moving from symptom control toward mechanism-specific pharmacologic management. *Annals of Internal Medicine*. 2004; **140**: 441–51.
25. Petersen KL, Fields HL, Brennum J *et al*. Capsaicin evoked pain and allodynia in post-herpetic neuralgia. *Pain*. 2000; **88**: 125–33.
26. Head H, Cempbell AW. The pathology of herpes zoster and its bearing on sensory localisation. *Brain*. 1900; **23**: 354–439.
27. Watson CPN, Deck JH, Morshead C *et al*. Post-herpetic neuralgia: further post-mortem studies of cases with and without pain. *Pain*. 1991; **44**: 105–17.
28. Rowbotham MC, Yosipovitch G, Connolly MK *et al*. Cutaneous innervation density in the allodynic form of postherpetic neuralgia. *Neurobiology of Disease*. 1996; **3**: 205–14.
29. Oaklander AL, Romans K, Horasek S *et al*. Unilateral postherpetic neuralgia is associated with bilateral sensory neuron damage. *Annals of Neurology*. 1998; **44**: 789–95.
30. Whitton TL, Johnson RW, Lovell AT. Use of the Rydel-Seiffer graduated tuning fork in the assessment of vibration threshold in postherpetic neuralgia patients and healthy controls. *European Journal of Pain*. 2005; **9**: 167–71.
31. Baron R, Haendler G, Schulte H. Afferent large fiber polyneuropathy predicts the development of postherpetic neuralgia. *Pain*. 1997; **73**: 231–8.
32. McKendrick MW, Wood MJ. Acyclovir and post-herpetic neuralgia. Two other participating study centres report different results. *British Medical Journal*. 1995; **310**: 1005.
33. Meister W, Neiss A, Gross G *et al*. A prognostic score for postherpetic neuralgia in ambulatory patients. *Infection*. 1998; **26**: 359–63.
34. Whitley RJ, Weiss HL, Soong SJ, Gnann JW. Herpes zoster: risk categories for persistent pain. *Journal of Infectious Diseases*. 1999; **179**: 9–15.
35. McKendrick MW, McGill JI, Wood MJ. Lack of effect of acyclovir on postherpetic neuralgia. *British Medical Journal*. 1989; **298**: 431.
36. Wood M, Kay R. Efficacy of oral aciclovir in herpes zoster – a meta-analysis. published from the EADV, Brussels, 1995.
37. Wood MJ, Johnson RW, McKendrick MW *et al*. A randomized trial of acyclovir for 7 days or 21 days with and without prednisolone for treatment of acute herpes zoster. *New England Journal of Medicine*. 1994; **330**: 896–900.
38. Whitley RJ, Weiss H, Gnann Jr JW *et al*. Acyclovir with and without prednisone for the treatment of herpes zoster. A randomized, placebo-controlled trial. The National Institute of Allergy and Infectious Diseases Collaborative Antiviral Study Group. *Annals of Internal Medicine*. 1996; **125**: 376–83.
39. van Wijck AJ, Opstelten W, Moons KG *et al*. The PINE study of epidural steroids and local anaesthetics to prevent postherpetic neuralgia: a randomised controlled trial. *Lancet*. 2006; **367**: 219–24.

40. Pasqualucci A, Pasqualucci V, Galla F *et al.* Prevention of post-herpetic neuralgia: acyclovir and prednisolone versus epidural local anesthetic and methylprednisolone. *Acta Anaesthesiologica Scandinavica.* 2000; **44**: 910–8.
41. Higa K, Dan K, Manabe H, Noda B. Factors influencing the duration of treatment of acute herpetic pain with sympathetic nerve block: importance of severity of herpes zoster assessed by the maximum antibody titers to varicella-zoster virus in otherwise healthy patients. *Pain.* 1988; **32**: 147–57.
42. Bowsher D. The effects of pre-emptive treatment of postherpetic neuralgia with amitriptyline: a randomized, double-blind, placebo-controlled trial. *Journal of Pain and Symptom Management.* 1997; **13**: 327–31.
43. Dworkin RH. Prevention of postherpetic neuralgia. *Lancet.* 1999; **353**: 1636–7.
44. McKendrick MW, Care CC, Kudesia G *et al.* Is VZV reactivation a common cause of unexplained unilateral pain? Results of a prospective study of 57 patients. *Journal of Infection.* 1999; **39**: 209–12.
* 45. Wood MJ, Kay R, Dworkin RH *et al.* Oral acyclovir therapy accelerates pain resolution in patients with herpes zoster: a meta-analysis of placebo-controlled trials. *Clinical Infectious Diseases.* 1996; **22**: 341–7.
46. Jackson JL, Gibbons R, Meyer G, Inouye L. The effect of treating herpes zoster with oral acyclovir in preventing postherpetic neuralgia. A meta-analysis. *Archives of Internal Medicine.* 1997; **157**: 909–12.
47. Dworkin RH, Schmader KE. Treatment and prevention of postherpetic neuralgia. *Clinical Infectious Diseases.* 2003; **36**: 877–82.
48. Sindrup SH, Jensen TS. Efficacy of pharmacological treatments of neuropathic pain: an update and effect related to mechanism of drug action. *Pain.* 1999; **83**: 389–400.
49. Sindrup SH, Otto M, Finnerup NB, Jensen TS. Antidepressants in the treatment of neuropathic pain. *Basic and Clinical Pharmacology and Toxicology.* 2005; **96**: 399–409.
* 50. Hempenstall K, Nurmikko TJ, Johnson RW *et al.* Analgesic therapy in postherpetic neuralgia: a quantitative systematic review. *PLoS Medicine.* 2005; **2**: e164.
51. Dubinsky RM, Kabbani H, El-Chami Z *et al.* Practice parameter: treatment of postherpetic neuralgia: an evidence-based report of the Quality Standards Subcommittee of the American Academy of Neurology. *Neurology.* 2004; **63**: 959–65.
* 52. Finnerup NB, Otto M, McQuay HJ *et al.* Algorithm for neuropathic pain treatment: an evidence based proposal. *Pain.* 2005; **118**: 289–305.
53. McQuay HJ, Tramer M, Nye BA *et al.* A systematic review of antidepressants in neuropathic pain. *Pain.* 1996; **68**: 217–27.
54. Ray WA, Meredith S, Thapa PB *et al.* Cyclic antidepressants and the risk of sudden cardiac death. *Clinical Pharmacology and Therapeutics.* 2004; **75**: 234–41.
55. Watson CP, Vernich L, Chipman M, Reed K. Nortriptyline versus amitriptyline in postherpetic neuralgia: a randomized trial. *Neurology.* 1998; **51**: 1166–71.
56. Rowbotham M, Harden N, Stacey B *et al.* Gabapentin for the treatment of postherpetic neuralgia: a randomized controlled trial. *Journal of American Medical Association.* 1998; **280**: 1837–42.
57. Garry EM, Delaney A, Anderson HA *et al.* Varicella zoster virus induces neuropathic changes in rat dorsal root ganglia and behavioral reflex sensitisation that is attenuated by gabapentin or sodium channel blocking drugs. *Pain.* 2005; **118**: 97–111.
* 58. Dworkin RH, Corbin AE, Young Jr JP *et al.* Pregabalin for the treatment of postherpetic neuralgia: a randomized, placebo-controlled trial. *Neurology.* 2003; **60**: 1274–83.
59. Sabatowski R, Galvez R, Cherry DA *et al.* Pregabalin reduces pain and improves sleep and mood disturbances in patients with post-herpetic neuralgia: results of a randomised, placebo-controlled clinical trial. *Pain.* 2004; **109**: 26–35.
60. Oaklander AL, Buchbinder BR. Pregabalin-withdrawal encephalopathy and splenial edema: a link to high-altitude illness? *Annals of Neurology.* 2005; **58**: 309–12.
61. Bowsher D. The management of postherpetic neuralgia. *Postgraduate Medical Journal.* 1997; **73**: 623–9.
62. Rowbotham MC, Reisner-Keller LA, Fields HL. Both intravenous lidocaine and morphine reduce the pain of postherpetic neuralgia. *Neurology.* 1991; **41**: 1024–8.
* 63. Watson CP, Babul N. Efficacy of oxycodone in neuropathic pain: a randomized trial in postherpetic neuralgia. *Neurology.* 1998; **50**: 1837–41.
64. Boureau F, Legallicier P, Kabir-Ahmadi M. Tramadol in post-herpetic neuralgia: a randomized, double-blind, placebo-controlled trial. *Pain.* 2003; **104**: 323–31.
65. Rowbotham MC, Twilling L, Davies PS *et al.* Oral opioid therapy for chronic peripheral and central neuropathic pain. *New England Journal of Medicine.* 2003; **348**: 1223–32.
66. Raja SN, Haythornthwaite JA, Pappagallo M *et al.* Opioids versus antidepressants in postherpetic neuralgia: a randomized, placebo-controlled trial. *Neurology.* 2002; **59**: 1015–21.
67. Watson CP, Tyler KL, Bickers DR *et al.* A randomized vehicle-controlled trial of topical capsaicin in the treatment of postherpetic neuralgia. *Clinical Therapeutics.* 1993; **15**: 510–26.
68. Backonja M. High-concentration capsaicin for treatment of PHN and HIV neuropathy pain. *European Journal of Pain.* 2007; **11** (Suppl. 1): S40.
69. Galer BS, Rowbotham MC, Perander J, Friedman E. Topical lidocaine patch relieves postherpetic neuralgia more effectively than a vehicle topical patch: results of an enriched enrollment study. *Pain.* 1999; **80**: 533–8.
70. Meier T, Wasner G, Faust M *et al.* Efficacy of lidocaine patch 5% in the treatment of focal peripheral neuropathic pain syndromes: a randomized, double-blind, placebo-controlled study. *Pain.* 2003; **106**: 151–8.

* 71. Kotani N, Kushikata T, Hashimoto H *et al.* Intrathecal methylprednisolone for intractable postherpetic neuralgia. *New England Journal of Medicine.* 2000; **343**: 1514–9.
72. Nelson DA, Landau WM. Intrathecal methylprednisolone for postherpetic neuralgia. *New England Journal of Medicine.* 2001; **344**: 1019; author reply 21–2.
73. Nelson KA, Park KM, Robinovitz E *et al.* High-dose oral dextromethorphan versus placebo in painful diabetic neuropathy and postherpetic neuralgia. *Neurology.* 1997; **48**: 1212–8.
74. Wallace MS, Rowbotham MC, Katz NP *et al.* A randomized, double-blind, placebo-controlled trial of a glycine antagonist in neuropathic pain. *Neurology.* 2002; **59**: 1694–700.
75. Sang CN, Booher S, Gilron I *et al.* Dextromethorphan and memantine in painful diabetic neuropathy and postherpetic neuralgia: efficacy and dose-response trials. *Anesthesiology.* 2002; **96**: 1053–61.
* 76. Baron R, Wasner G. Prevention and treatment of postherpetic neuralgia. *Lancet.* 2006; **367**: 186–8.
77. Kochar DK, Garg P, Bumb RA *et al.* Divalproex sodium in the management of post-herpetic neuralgia: a randomized double-blind placebo-controlled study. *QJM.* 2005; **98**: 29–34.
78. Haythornthwaite JA, Benrud-Larson LM. Psychological aspects of neuropathic pain. *Clinical Journal of Pain.* 2000; **16**: S101–5.
* 79. Gilron I, Bailey JM, Tu D *et al.* Morphine, gabapentin, or their combination for neuropathic pain. *New England Journal of Medicine.* 2005; **352**: 1324–34.
80. Gill TM, Allore HG, Holford TR, Guo Z. Hospitalization, restricted activity, and the development of disability among older persons. *Journal of the American Medical Association.* 2004; **292**: 2115–24.
81. Gill TM, Allore H, Guo Z. The deleterious effects of bed rest among community-living older persons. *Journals of Gerontology. Series B, Psychological Sciences and Social Sciences.* 2004; **59**: 755–61.
82. Rochon PA, Gurwitz JH. Drug therapy. *Lancet.* 1995; **346**: 32–6.
83. Weiner D, Peterson B, Ladd K *et al.* Pain in nursing home residents: an exploration of prevalence, staff perspectives, and practical aspects of measurement. *Clinical Journal of Pain.* 1999; **15**: 92–101.

33

Management of painful spasticity

BARRY RAWICKI

KEY LEARNING POINTS

- Spasticity needs to be considered by its origin (spinal or cerebral).
- Spasticity is focal or general in nature.
- The mainstay of spasticity management is appropriate physical treatment.
- The management of the pain of spasticity is the management of the underlying spasticity.
- Systemic treatments are generally not indicated for the management of focal spasticity.
- Oral baclofen is the most important oral antispasticity agent, but it must be used in an effective regime and dose.
- Intrathecal baclofen treatment is effective in the management of otherwise resistant general spasticity.
- Botulinum toxin is the most important medical treatment for focal spasticity.

INTRODUCTION

Pain is a common feature of people suffering spasticity following a lesion of the central nervous system (CNS). There are a number of mechanisms whereby spasticity can lead to or directly cause pain, and these will be discussed in this chapter. There is a lack of good data on the mechanisms of spasticity producing pain,[1] although some mechanisms will be discussed. In considering the relationships between pain and spasticity, it is necessary to have a general understanding of the pathophysiology of spasticity and the mechanisms of the production of spasticity.

PATHOPHYSIOLOGY OF SPASTICITY

Spasticity has been described as "a disorder of the sensorimotor system characterised by a velocity-dependent increase in muscle tone with exaggerated tendon jerks (deep tendon reflexes) resulting from hyperexcitability of the stretch reflex as one component of the upper motor neuron syndrome (UMNS)."[2] The UMNS is the result of the changes to the normal functioning motor system following lesions to the CNS. These changes can be considered as both negative (i.e. things taken away from normal control) and positive (i.e. superimposed on normal motor control, not positive as "good"). The negative components include weakness, loss of dexterity, and fatigability. The positive components include velocity-dependent increase in tone and changes in deep tendon reflexes as described above. They also include changes in cutaneous-mediated reflexes (via disinhibition of flexor reflex afferents (FRA)), increased spread of cutaneous and deep tendon reflexes (via disinhibition of propriospinal pathways), abnormal reflexes (e.g. Babinski, Hoffmann), and flexor and extensor spasms.[3] Many clinicians consider spasticity as not just the velocity-dependent increase in muscle tone, but the total picture of the positive component of the UMNS. These changes are summarized in **Table 33.1**.

It is also important to appreciate that in addition to the neurological changes there are also considerable muscle changes following lesions of the CNS. These changes include a relative increase in collagen compared to elastin, with an increase in tissue stiffness plus possible changes in muscle fiber type,[4] contributing to the increase in stiffness.[5]

It is axiomatic that in spasticity there is hyperexcitability or disinhibition of the alpha motor neuron pool.[6] The mechanism for this excitation is different for spasticity following lesions of the brain (cerebral origin spasticity) and for lesions of the spinal cord (spinal origin spasticity) (**Table 33.2**).

Cerebral origin spasticity has a rapid build up of reflex activity consistent with loss of inhibition of mono- and oligosynaptic pathways between brain stem nuclei, in particular rubro- and vestibulospinal pathways[7] and the alpha motor neuron pool. Cerebral origin spasticity also differs from spinal origin spasticity in the expression of hemiplegic, or in the case of bilateral brain damage, double hemiplegic posturing with the typical features of shoulder adduction, elbow, wrist, and finger flexion and forearm pronation (flexor posturing), and hip adduction, knee extension, and ankle and foot plantar flexion (extensor posturing).

Spinal origin spasticity, on the other hand, has a relatively slow rise in reflex activity which is consistent with disinhibition of polysynaptic pathways between the dorsal column and the alpha motor neuron pool.[3,7,8] This occurs particularly in Rexed laminae III and IV, where the FRA and C- and Aδ-fibers have their primary synapses. Spinal origin spasticity is also marked by disinhibition of propriospinal pathways resulting in longitudinal spread of reflexes. Consequently, a muscle response may occur many segments from the muscle stimulus. Unlike cerebral origin spasticity, flexor pattern spasticity and spasms tend to dominate the presentation, although, especially in severe spasticity, extensor patterning particularly of the trunk and lower limbs may dominate the clinical picture. Spasms are much more common in spinal origin spasticity[9] than cerebral due to disinhibition of FRA.

Table 33.1 Components of the upper motor neuron syndrome.

Positive	Negative
Spontaneous spasms	Paresis
Increased sensitivity to cutaneous mediated reflexes	Loss of dexterity beyond the degree of weakness
Increased sensitivity and spread of deep tendon reflexes	Fatigability
Abnormal reflexes, e.g. pantar, adductor, etc.	Poor isolated movements
Increased tone velocity independent, i.e. spastic dystonia, as well as velocity dependent, i.e."spasticity"	

FOCAL VERSUS GENERAL SPASTICITY

In considering the management of spasticity and hence, as will be discussed, spasticity-associated pain, it is necessary to look at the clinical presentation of spasticity in terms of focal and general presentations.

Focal or regional spasticity typically results from cerebral origin.[7] This refers to spasticity primarily affecting one limb, e.g. upper limb with the flexion/pronation/adduction patterning described above or lower limb with the extension/adduction patterning. However, flexion spasticity of the hamstrings and sometimes the psoas

Table 33.2 Spinal versus cerebral origin spasticity.

Spinal origin spasticity	Cerebral origin spasticity
Loss of supraspinal control of spinal pathways	Interruption to corticoreticular and corticovestibular pathways
Loss of interneuron inhibition from flexor reflex afferents	Loss of cortical inhibition to ipsilateral vestibulospinal and reticulospinal pathways
Loss of propriospinal inhibition	Oligo- and monosynaptic connections from vestibular and reticular nuclei to α and γ motor neurones
Loss of descending catecholamines and rubrospinal inhibition of interneurons	Movement patterning common
Limb flexor and extensor spasms common	Rigidity (velocity independent), as well as spasticity
Trunk extensor spasms	Spasms less common
Marked increase in cutaneous mediated reflexes	Relatively drug resistant
Abnormal spread and sensitivity of reflexes	
Polysynaptic pathways, relatively drug sensitive	

may also occur. Clearly, upper and lower limb spasticity resulting from a cerebral lesion often occur together.

General spasticity typically results from spinal origin UMNS.[10] It depends on the level of the spinal cord lesion. Lumbar and thoracic spasticity will affect both legs and possibly the trunk, depending on the level and nature of the lesion. The upper limbs are likely to be involved with cervical lesions.

PAIN AND SPASTICITY

There are a number of ways that spasticity can result in chronic pain. These will be considered as follows:

- abnormal posture;
- muscle spasm and spasticity;
- contracture and pain;
- hygiene and pain;
- musculoskeletal pain;
- neuropathic pain.

Abnormal posture

Spasticity, particularly cerebral origin spasticity, will often result in abnormal posturing, most usually with flexion/pronation/adduction of the upper limb and extension/adduction of the lower limb. The resulting muscle imbalances of this posturing will often result in pain as a direct consequence of the prolonged muscle tightness of the affected prime mover muscles and the corresponding stretching of the antagonists. It is usually the tighter contracted muscles that cause more pain than the chronically stretched antagonists.

Abnormal posture will also result in changes in normal weight bearing and weight distribution, once again often resulting in pain. The most common example of this is the equinovarus foot and associated knee hyperextension during standing and walking. The knee hyperextension itself is usually due to a combination of plantar flexion/knee hyperextension coupling, quadriceps weakness, and quadriceps spasticity. The consequence, with respect to pain is two-fold.

1. The abnormal posturing of the foot in equinovarus (plantar flexed and inverted) means that during standing and walking the anterolateral border of the foot becomes the primary weight-bearing portion of the foot. This will lead to pain in the foot and ankle on weight bearing and often to skin breakdown.
2. Chronic knee hyperextension in gait will often lead to stretching of the posterior cruciate ligament and the knee capsule leading to chronic knee joint pain and eventual instability and arthritis of the knee.

A common problem that often requires intervention is foot and toe pain related to toe flexor spasticity. The great toe often displays extensor pattern spasticity, although may join the other toes in a generally flexor pattern. This patterning frequently results in forefoot pain, pain on the balls of the toes as they are forced into the floor or footwear, and pain over the proximal metatarsophalangeal joints which will rub against footwear. In the frequent situation where the great toe is extended rather than flexed, this will often result in pain on the dorsum of the foot and the toe catching on footwear once again resulting in pain and discomfort.

Similar problems will occur in the upper limb, although the weight-bearing issues are clearly not as important or frequent. Forearm pain arises due to spasticity of finger flexors and, to a lesser extent, wrist flexors. Supination, whether active or passive, is frequently painful. Where weight bearing does occur, such as in the use of a walking aid, the inability or difficulty in supination can result in pain.

Muscle spasm and spasticity

Muscle spasm is a particular feature of spinal (including brain stem) origin spasticity as described above under Pathophysiology of spasticity.[10, 11] Mass extensor spasms affect lower limbs, trunk and, in higher lesions, the upper limbs (**Figure 33.1**). In severe spasticity, flexor spasms of the lower limbs also occur (**Figure 33.2**) and may be associated with pain in those people with preserved sensation. These sorts of spasms frequently occur in people with poor or absent sensation where the typical muscle pain cannot be expressed. It is often the spasms themselves rather than the pain that require treatment.[12] Even so, pain not infrequently accompanies these spasms and can be very severe. Chronic muscle spasticity will

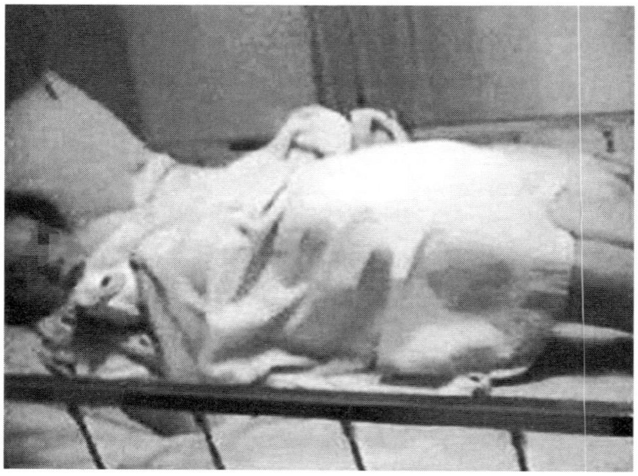

Figure 33.1 Severe generalized spasticity with opisthotonus posturing and pain following a traumatic brain injury.

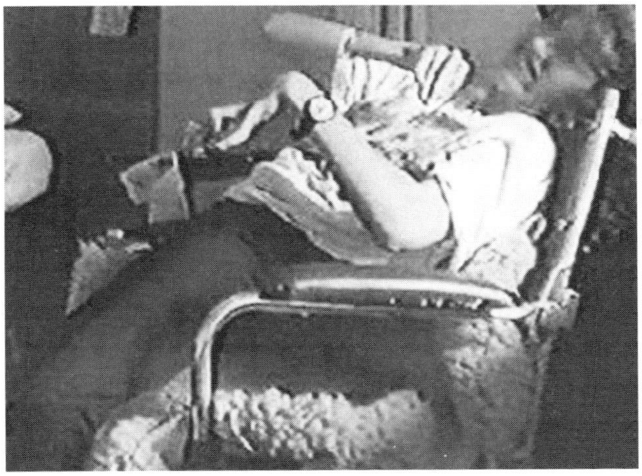

Figure 33.2 Severe generalized spasticity preventing sitting.

frequently be felt as tightness or discomfort or pain, even in the absence of spasms.

Contracture and pain

Contracture associated with chronic spasticity involves the remodelling of soft tissues including muscles, connective tissue, and joint capsule around joints, so that there is loss of range of movement almost invariably with the joint in an abnormal posture. Severe contracture, especially flexion contracture of the distal upper limb, is more a feature of cerebral origin spasticity than of spinal origin spasticity. Severe wrist and finger flexor spasticity can lead to carpal subluxation and pain.

Contractures can affect just about any joint in the body. Shoulder adduction, elbow flexion, wrist and finger flexion (**Figure 33.3**) and thumb in palm contractures (adduction, flexion of the metacarpophalangeal joint, with or without flexion of the interphalangeal joint) all occur in the upper limb. Hip flexion, knee flexion, ankle equinus and equinovarus, and forefoot and toe flexion contractures occur in the lower limb.

Contractures lead to pain associated with joints and soft tissues and with skin breakdown in flexures or the development of pressure decubiti.

Hygiene and pain

Skin hygiene can be significantly compromised when there is the development of contractures or when spasticity is high. Both result in difficulty of access to skin flexures, in particular in the distal upper limb, but also at the elbow (**Figure 33.4**) or less commonly behind the knee. This may lead to skin breakdown with pain, maceration, infection, and malodorous flexures.

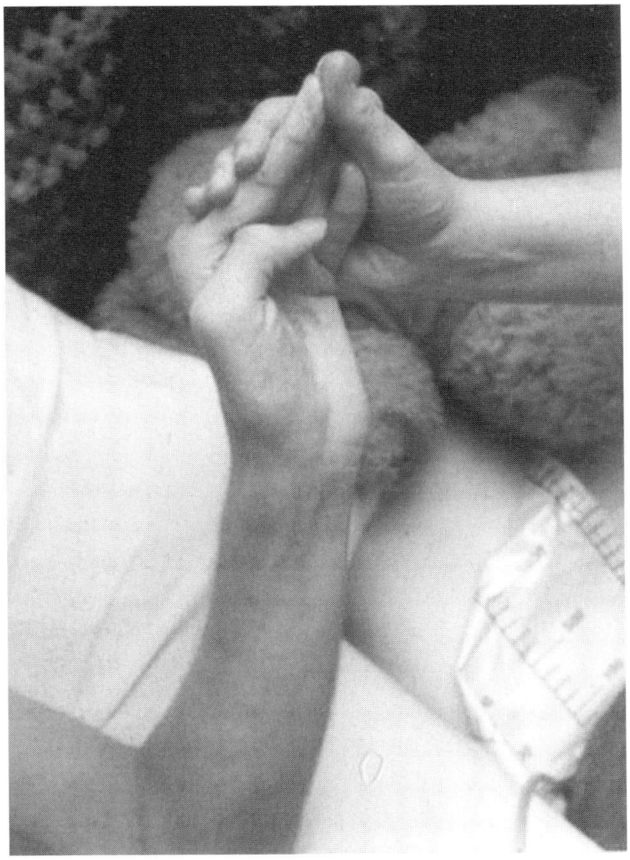

Figure 33.3 Palmar skin breakdown following hypoxic brain injury.

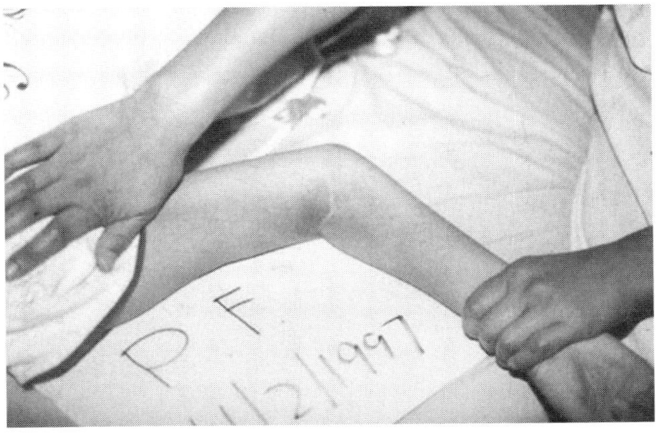

Figure 33.4 Elbow flexor spasticity and flexure breakdown following traumatic brain injury.

Hip adductor spasticity may lead to difficulties with perineal access and the development of painful excoriation and skin maceration in the groin area. Infections, either fungal or bacterial, may accompany this skin breakdown. Shoulder adductor spasticity may lead to similar problems of access to and breakdown of skin in the axilla.

Musculoskeletal pain

Musculoskeletal pain is a frequent problem in people with spasticity. Poor seating posture as a result of trunk or lower limb spasticity will result in postural muscle pain, particularly back and trunk pain. Paralytic scoliosis, particularly in children and adolescents, may result from either high paraplegia or tetraplegia or from a double hemiplegia. This will result in significant back and trunk musculoskeletal pain. Skin and soft tissue breakdown can occur, particularly over the major deformity. Paralytic scoliosis may be progressive and very difficult to control.

Musculoskeletal pain may also occur in the upper trunk, neck, and shoulder as a result of shoulder and arm paralysis and spasticity.

Neuropathic pain

Neuropathic or deafferentation type pain may occur following lesions of the central nervous system. Neuropathic pain is usually independent of spasticity and is considered in Chapter 28, Central neuropathic pain: syndromes, pathophysiology, and treatments.

TREATMENT OF THE PAIN OF SPASTICITY

The treatment of pain resulting from spasticity is primarily the treatment of the underlying spasticity itself. This section will discuss spasticity management. Clearly, in considering pain management, simple (or complex) analgesics will often be an integral part of the treatment, but will not be considered in detail in this section. It will examine pertinent pain management issues and modalities.

General principles of spasticity management

The management of spasticity is determined by whether you are dealing with focal or general spasticity. Treatment decisions will for the most part be predicated on this. Before considering specific interventions, it is essential that factors that can exacerbate the spasticity be treated or managed. Potentially, nociceptive stimulus can exacerbate spasticity. These include factors such as pressure areas, ingrown toenails, heterotopic ossification, fractures, bladder or bowel distention, and postural abnormalities.[7, 11] Once the decision to treat the spasticity has been made, then irrespective of the nature of the spasticity, the mainstay of management is good and appropriate physical treatment.[13, 14, 15] Expert physical therapy is essential and forms the basis of management. The most important physical approach is muscle stretching and, where appropriate, muscle and joint splinting[16] to maintain range of movement and to prevent the development of contractures.[9, 17] Physical modalities, including ultrasound diathermy and local heat and local cold therapy, may assist in joint and muscle flexibility. Passive stretch to assist in spasticity management and the prevention of contractures is essential. Hydrotherapy is often beneficial in spasticity management allowing a combination of supported weight bearing and local heat.

MANAGEMENT OF GENERAL AND REGIONAL SPASTICITY

Oral medications

Oral medications are the mainstay of medical treatment of mild to moderate general or regional spasticity of spinal origin not controlled by physical management. Oral medications are far less useful in the management of cerebral origin spasticity, although it is often reasonable to trial them in appropriate patients. Cerebral origin spasticity is marked by disinhibition of oligosynaptic pathway, making specific pharmacological management very difficult. There are few sites at which oral medications can act to modify this type of spasticity. In spinal origin spasticity, which is mediated by polysynaptic pathways, there are many synapses available for medication to act upon.[18] Thus, there are strong theoretical reasons, often borne out clinically, for the differential use of oral systemic antispasticity medications. Four medications are commonly used in spasticity management.

BACLOFEN

The most commonly used oral medication is baclofen. Baclofen is a GABA-B agonist that acts pre- and postsynaptically to inhibit the release of excitatory neurotransmitters.[14, 19][I] In addition to its antispasticity effect, baclofen has also been shown to be antinociceptive.[20] This may also be useful in the management of spasticity-associated pain. Baclofen is considered more useful for the management of spinal origin spasticity than for cerebral origin spasticity.[21] Because of its relatively short half-life, baclofen should be administered in divided doses at least three times a day. Doses are usually between 40 and 120 mg/day. The most common side effects include drowsiness and a feeling of detachment. Oral baclofen may lower the seizure threshold in people with epilepsy, and therefore care must be exercised (Novartis product information for Baclofen), especially when it is used in people with cerebral origin spasticity.

DIAZEPAM

Diazepam has long been used for spasticity management for both cerebral[4, 22][II] and spinal origin.[23, 24][II]

Diazepam acts on the benzodiazepine (BZD) site of the GABA-A receptor to increase the inhibitory effects of endogenous GABA.[25, 26] Although there are no formal data or studies confirming the advantage of diazepam over baclofen in cerebral origin spasticity, many physicians believe that there are some advantages. As with baclofen, diazepam is generally considered to be more effective in spinal origin spasticity than cerebral origin spasticity.[16] The common side effects of diazepam are drowsiness, sedation, and CNS depression. Diazepam can also cause addiction.[27] Doses of between 4 and 50 mg/day can be used, titrating the clinical effect against side effects.

ALPHA-2 AGONISTS

The $\alpha 2$ receptor agonists,[28] most notably tizanidine and clonidine, can be useful. Their antispasticity activity may be related to the presynaptic inhibition of normal catecholamine release.[29, 30] These medications may be used in combination with baclofen. Clonidine can be used in doses up to 500 µg/day. It does have some $\alpha 1$ activity and may cause an increase in spasms at high doses. Side effects include hypotension, drowsiness, sedation, and constipation. Once again these medications are more useful in spinal than cerebral origin spasticity.[21, 31][II] Tizanidine is not available in Australia and is reported to have a lower side-effect profile than clonidine.

DANTROLENE

Dantrolene sodium is the last of the commonly used oral medications. Unlike the three medications discussed briefly above, dantrolene acts peripherally in skeletal muscle to inhibit calcium release from the endoplasmic reticulum. It blocks excitation contraction coupling in skeletal muscle.[32][II] The primary effect of dantrolene is muscle weakness,[18, 24] but because it acts on intrafusal as well as extrafusal fibers, it has a true antispasticity effect.[16] The most notable side effect of dantrolene is an idiosyncratic hepatotoxicity, and liver function needs to be monitored, particularly over the first few months of treatment. Because dantrolene causes muscle weakness, it is rarely used where motor function is important.[14, 23] Some authors feel it is the medication of choice in cerebral origin spasticity.[33]

There are a number of other oral medications that can be used, usually in addition to the above medications. These include, but are not limited to, cyproheptadine,[34] some of the newer GABAergic anticonvulsants such as piracetam, lamotrigine, and progabide[34] and the cannabinoids,[35] either medically prescribed or otherwise obtained. In general, these other medications show level III or IV evidence for effectiveness in the management of chronic spasticity.

Intrathecal baclofen therapy

When general or regional spasticity is severe and cannot be managed by physical or oral pharmacological means, continuous delivery of intrathecal medication should be considered. Intrathecal baclofen (ITB) therapy follows the same principles as intrathecal therapy for chronic pain as discussed elsewhere in this volume. Baclofen does not easily cross the blood–brain barrier.[36] Administering this medication directly into the subarachnoid space means that very low doses of medication can be delivered directly to the spinal cord at high local concentrations. This results in good clinical effects with very low systemic absorption and hence a low incidence of side effects. A typical dose of oral baclofen is 60–80 mg/day in divided doses. A typical intrathecal baclofen dose is 350 µg/day (1/2000th of the oral dose) as a continuous infusion. Some patients like a bolus dose in the early hours of the morning to assist them when getting out of bed.

ITB therapy has been shown to be effective in both cerebral origin[17, 28, 37, 38][I] and in spinal origin spasticity.[15, 18, 39][I] ITB is much more useful for trunk and lower limb spasticity than for upper limb spasticity. ITB is

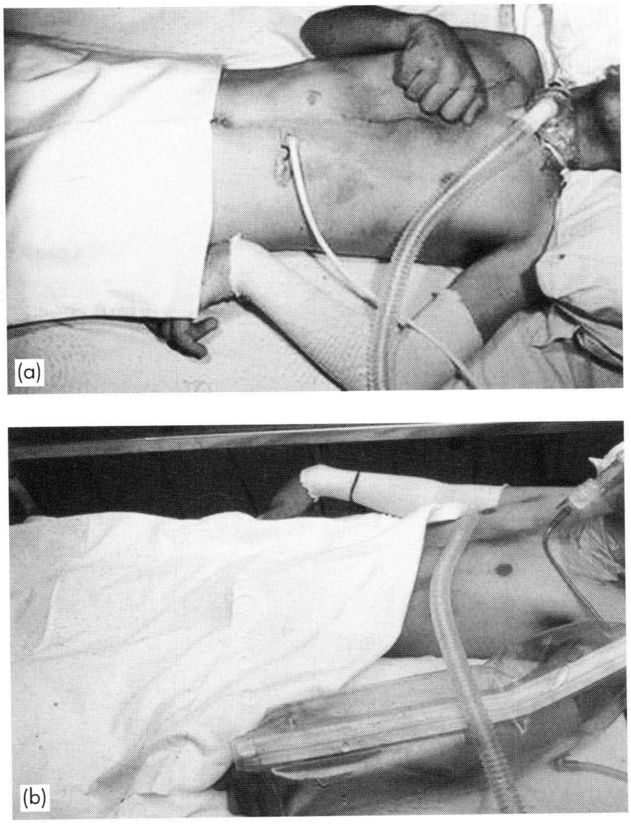

Figure 33.5 Severe traumatic brain injury. (a) The patient has had botulinum toxin injections to left biceps and brachialis. (b) The patient has had botulinum toxin to biceps and brachialis of both arms plus musculocutaneous nerve phenolization.

particularly effective for the management of flexor and extensor spasms which are a frequent cause of pain, as well as for hypertonus. Some authors have recorded better upper limb effects with a higher placement of the catheter in the cervical or upper thoracic spine. However, these reports are inconsistent, and there are theoretical reasons why high placement of the catheter does not improve upper limb effects.[40]

Surgical management

Surgical management of general or regional spasticity is usually neurosurgical.[41] There are a number of operations that have been described. Selective dorsal rhizotomy (SDR)[23, 24][I] is an occasional but useful procedure in children with cerebral palsy. The advent of ITB therapy has made the surgical approach to general or regional spasticity a rarity.

MANAGEMENT OF FOCAL SPASTICITY

Physical therapy is the mainstay of all spasticity management. When this is not effective then botulinum neurotoxin, most commonly type A (BoNT-A), or phenolization of selected peripheral nerves can provide effective treatment for focal spasticity. Neither of these techniques is permanent, but may be helpful in selected cases.

Botulinum toxin

Apart from its well-known cosmetic uses, there are many clinical noncosmetic indications for the use of BoNT-A. There are at least 30 proposed or accepted uses for botulinum toxin. Some of the well-accepted indications include the management of hyperhydrosis,[42] hemifacial spasm,[43] detrusor overactivity,[44] cervical[45] and other focal

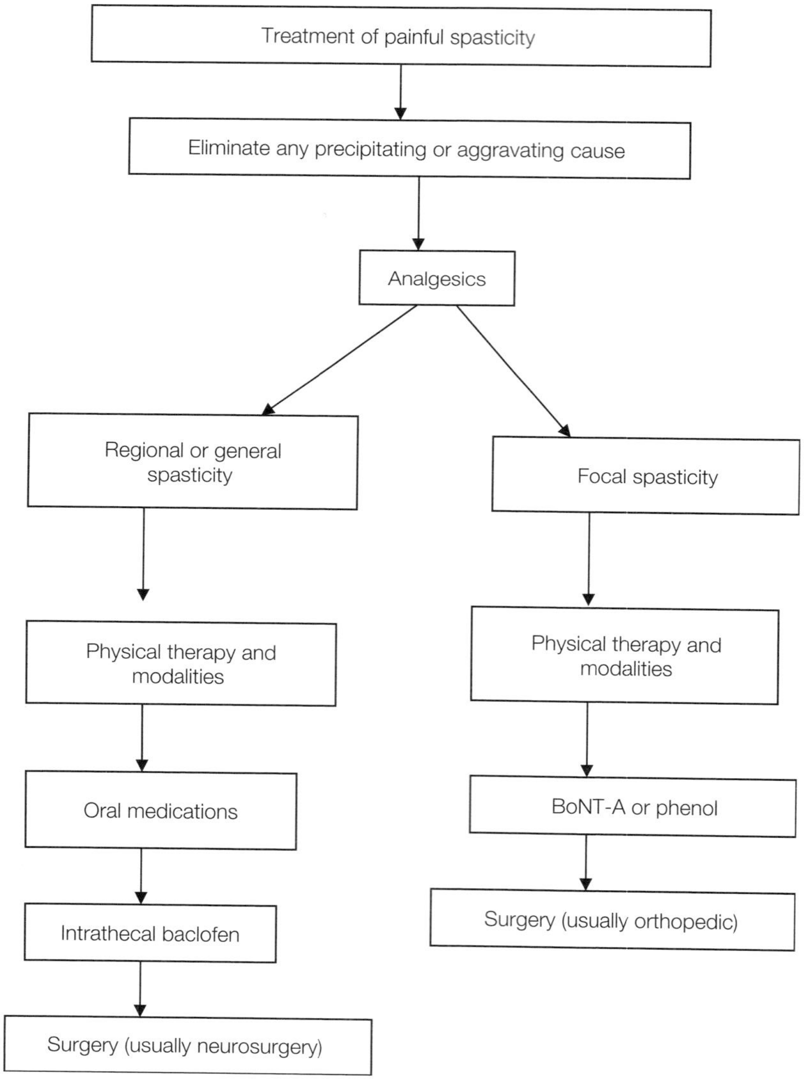

Figure 33.6 Treatment algorithm for spasticity management.

dystonias,[26] spasmodic dysphonia,[46] and anal fissure. BoNT-A blocks the release of acetylcholine (Ach) at the neuromuscular junction of injected muscles, thus causing focal weakness by the action on extrafusal fibers, and decrease in spasticity by its action on intrafusal fibers. In addition to its antispasticity effect on pain, there is a growing evidence of a separate antinociceptive effect.[47, 48, 49, 50]

There is a very large body of evidence showing that BoNT-A injected directly into spastic muscles is effective in the treatment of focal spasticity of cerebral[1, 51, 52, 53, 54, 55][I] and, to a lesser extent, spinal origin,[56, 57][II] but it is not useful for the management of established contractures. BoNT-A has duration of benefit of around three months and injections can be repeated. Side effects are uncommon and usually very minor. Antibodies may occasionally develop and render subsequent injections less effective.

Phenol injections

Phenol injected perineurally on to mixed motor/sensory or motor nerves results in patchy demyelination of those nerves with a slowing of nerve conduction and a resulting decrease in spasticity.[24, 58][III] Phenol can be moderately useful in focal spasticity. Whereas BoNT-A affects the individual muscle into which it is injected, phenol affects all muscles supplied by the injected nerve (**Figure 33.5**). The main disadvantage of phenol is the relatively high rate of late dysesthesia in the sensory distribution of the injected nerve. Phenol injected intravascularly can cause seizures, and if injected intramuscularly can lead to the development of sterile abscess.

Surgery

Surgery for focal spasticity usually involves orthopedic-type procedures with muscle lengthening, transfers, excision of bone, or joint reconstruction.[41, 58] Surgery of this type can be useful and is often the only available medical treatment for established contractures. Surgery is not usually indicated in the management of the pain of spasticity unless there are also contractures.

CONCLUSIONS

There are many ways for spasticity to cause pain, both directly related to the spasticity itself or to the consequences of the spasticity. Management of spasticity-related pain is essentially the management of the spasticity. There are major differences in the etiology, pathogenesis, and treatment of spinal as compared to cerebral origin spasticity, and treatment decisions will be based to a large extent on the nature of the spasticity (**Figure 33.6**).

REFERENCES

1. Tsui J, Bhatt M, Calne S, Calne DB. Botulinum toxin in the treatment of writer's cramp: a double blind study. *Neurology.* 1993; **43**: 183–5.
2. Lance JW. Symposium synopsis. In: Feldman RG, Young RR, Koella WP (eds). *Spasticity: disordered motor control.* Chicago: Year Book Medical Publishers, 1980: 23.
3. Mayer N. Clinicophysiologic concepts of spasticity and motor dysfunction in adults with an upper motorneuron lesion. *Muscle and Nerve.* 1997; **6** (Suppl.): S1–13.
4. Katz RT. Management of spasticity. *American Journal of Physical Medicine and Rehabilitation.* 1988; **67**: 108–16.
5. * Morris S. Ashworth and Tardieu scales: their clinical relevance for measuring spasticity in adult and paediatric neurological populations. *Physical Therapy Reviews.* 2002; **7**: 53–62.
6. Burke D. Spasticity as an adaptation to pyramidal tract injury. *Advances in Neurology.* 1988; **47**: 401–23.
7. Herman R, Freedman W, Meeks S. Physiological aspects of hemiplegic and paraplegic spasticity. In: Desmedt JE (ed.). *New developments in electromyography and clinical neurophysiology: human reflexes, pathophysiology of motor systems, methodology of human reflexes.* Basel: Karger, 1973: 579–89.
8. * Decq P. Pathophysiology of spasticity. *Neurochirurgie.* 2003; **49**: 163–84.
9. Ada L, Canning C. Anticipating and avoiding muscle shortening. In: Ada L, Canning C (eds). *Key issues in neurological physiotherapy.* Stoneham, MA: Butterworth-Heinemann, 1990: 219–36.
10. Sköld C, Levi R, Seiger A. Spasticity after traumatic spinal cord injury: nature, severity, and location. *Archives of Physical Medicine and Rehabilitation.* 1999; **80**: 1548–57.
11. * Adams MM, Hicks AL. Spasticity after spinal cord injury. *Spinal Cord.* 2005; **43**: 577–86.
12. Maynard FM, Karunas RS, Waring 3rd WP. Epidemiology of spasticity following traumatic spinal cord injury. *Archives of Physical Medicine and Rehabilitation.* 1990; **71**: 566–9.
13. Dietz V. Spinal cord lesion: effects of and perspectives for treatment. *Neural Plasticity.* 2001; **8**: 83–90.
14. Kita M, Goodkin DE. Drugs used to treat spasticity. *Drugs.* 2000; **59**: 487–95.
15. Ward AB. Long-term modification of spasticity. *Journal of Rehabilitation Medicine.* 2003; **35** (Suppl.): 60–5.
16. Elovic E. Principles of pharmaceutical management of spastic hypertonia. *Physical Medicine and Rehabilitation Clinics of North America.* 2001; **12**: 793–816.
17. Campbell SK, Almeida GL, Penn RD, Corcos DM. The effects of intrathecally administered baclofen on function in patients with spasticity. *Physical Therapy.* 1995; **75**: 352–62.

* 18. Gracies JM, Nance P, Elovic E *et al.* Traditional pharmacological treatments for spasticity. Part II: General and regional treatments. *Muscle and Nerve.* 1997; **6** (Suppl.): S92–120.
19. Potashner SJ. Baclofen: effects on amino acid release. *Canadian Journal of Physiology and Pharmacology.* 1978; **56**: 150–4.
20. Lund S, Lundberg A, Vyklicky L. Inhibitatory action from the flexor reflex afferents on transmission to Ia afferents. *Acta Physiologica Scandinavica.* 1965; **64**: 345–55.
21. Norman KE, Pepin A, Barbeau H. Effects of drugs on walking after spinal cord injury. *Spinal Cord.* 1998; **36**: 699–715.
22. Cocchiarella A, Downey JA, Darling RC. Evaluation of the effect of diazepam on spasticity. *Archives of Physical Medicine and Rehabilitation.* 1967; **48**: 393–6.
23. Burchiel KJ, Hsu FP. Pain and spasticity after spinal cord injury: mechanisms and treatment. *Spine.* 2001; **26**: S146–60.
24. Kirshblum S. Treatment alternatives for spinal cord injury related spasticity. *Journal of Spinal Cord Medicine.* 1999; **22**: 199–217.
25. Olsen RW. GABA-benzodiazepine-barbiturate receptor interactions. *Journal of Neurochemistry.* 1981; **37**: 1–13.
26. Tseng TC, Wang SC. Locus of action of centrally acting muscle relaxants, diazepam and tybamate. *Journal of Pharmacology and Experimental Therapeutics.* 1971; **178**: 350–60.
* 27. Gallichio JE. Pharmacologic management of spasticity following stroke. *Physical Therapy.* 2004; **84**: 973–81.
28. Verrotti A, Greco R, Spalice A *et al.* Pharmacotherapy of spasticity in children with cerebral palsy. *Pediatric Neurology.* 2006; **34**: 1–6.
29. Nance PW, Shears AH, Nance DM. Reflex changes induced by clonidine in spinal cord injured patients. *Paraplegia.* 1989; **27**: 296–301.
30. Stein R, Nordal HJ, Oftedal SI, Slettebo M. The treatment of spasticity in multiple sclerosis. *Acta Neurologica Scandinavica.* 1987; **75**: 190–4.
* 31. Gracies JM, Elovic E, McGuire J, Simpson DM. Traditional pharmacological treatments for spasticity. Part I: Local treatments. *Muscle and Nerve.* 1997; **6** (Suppl.): S61–91.
32. Young RR, Delwaide PJ. Drug therapy: spasticity (first of 2 parts). *New England Journal of Medicine.* 1981; **304**: 28–33.
33. Ward AB, Kadies M. The management of pain in spasticity. *Disability and Rehabilitation.* 2002; **24**: 443–53.
34. Barbeau H, Richards CL, Bedard BJ. Action of cyproheptadine in spastic paraparetic patients. *Journal of Neurology, Neurosurgery, and Psychiatry.* 1982; **45**: 923–6.
35. Brooks JW, Pryce G, Bisogno T *et al.* Arvanil-induced inhibition of spasticity and persistent pain: evidence for therapeutic sites of action different from the vanilloid VR1 receptor and cannabinoid CB(1)/CB(2) receptors. *European Journal of Pharmacology.* 2002; **439**: 83–92.
36. Francisco GE, Boake C. Improvement in walking speed in poststroke spastic hemiplegia after intrathecal baclofen therapy: a preliminary study. *Archives of Physical Medicine and Rehabilitation.* 2003; **84**: 1194–9.
37. Meythaler JM, Guin-Renfroe S, Brunner RC, Hadley MN. Intrathecal baclofen for spastic hypertonia from stroke. *Stroke.* 2001; **32**: 2099–109.
38. Rawicki HB. Treatment of cerebral origin spasticity with continuous intrathecal baclofen delivered via an implantable pump: long term follow-up and review of 18 patients. *Journal of Neurosurgery.* 1999; **91**: 733–6.
39. Korenkov AI, Niendorf WR, Darwish N *et al.* Continuous intrathecal infusion of baclofen in patients with spasticity caused by spinal cord injuries. *Neurosurgical Review.* 2002; **25**: 228–30.
40. Kroin JS, Ali A, York M, Penn RD. The distribution of medication along the spinal canal after chronic intrathecal administration. *Neurosurgery.* 1993; **33**: 226–30.
* 41. Chambers HG. The surgical treatment of spasticity. *Muscle and Nerve.* 1997; **6** (Suppl.): S121–8.
42. Naumann N, Flachenecher P, Brocker E. Botulinum toxin for palmar hyperhydrosis. *Lancet.* 1997; **349**: 252.
43. Geller BD, Hallett M, Ravits L. Botulinum toxin therapy in hemifacial spasm: clinical and electrophysiological studies. *Muscle and Nerve.* 1989; **12**: 716–22.
44. Dykstra DD, Sidi AA. Treatment of detrusor sphincter dyssinergia with botulinum A toxin: a double blind study. *Archives of Physical Medicine and Rehabilitation.* 1990; **71**: 24–6.
45. Blackie JD, Lees AJ. Botulinum toxin treatment in spasmodic torticollis. *Journal of Neurology, Neurosurgery, and Psychiatry.* 1990; **53**: 640–3.
46. Blitzer A, Brin MF. Laryngeal dystonia a series with botulinum toxin therapy. *Annals of Otology, Rhinology, and Laryngology.* 1991; **100**: 85–9.
47. Cui M, Khanijoi S, Aoki JR. Subcutaneous administration of botulinum toxin A reduces formalin-induced pain. *Pain.* 2004; **107**: 125–33.
48. Freund BJ, Schwartz M. Treatment of chronic cervical-associated headache with botulinum toxin A: a pilot study. *Headache.* 2000; **40**: 231–6.
49. Lane A. Botulinum toxin type a for the management of cervicothoracic and cervicobrachial pain: treatment rationale and open-label results in 25 patients. *American Journal of Pain Management.* 2004; **14**: 13–23.
50. Porta M. A comparative trial of botulinum toxin type A and methylprednisolone for the treatment of myofascial pain syndrome and pain from chronic muscle spasm. *Pain.* 2000; **85**: 101–05.
51. Bakheit AM, Thilmann AF, Ward AB *et al.* A randomized, double-blind, placebo-controlled, dose-ranging study to compare the efficacy and safety of three doses of botulinum toxin type A (Dysport) with placebo in upper limb spasticity after stroke. *Stroke.* 2000; **31**: 2402–06.
52. Bhakta BB, Cozens JA, Bamford JM, Chamberlain MA. Use of botulinum toxin in stroke patients with severe upper

limb spasticity. *Journal of Neurology, Neurosurgery, and Psychiatry.* 1996; **61**: 30–5.

53. Fock J, Galea MP, Stillman BC *et al.* Botulinum toxin A injection to reduce spastic equinus in adults with traumatic brain injury. *Brain Injury.* 2004; **18**: 57–63.
54. Hesse S, Lucke D, Malezic M *et al.* Botulinum toxin treatment for lower limb extensor spasticity in chronic hemiparetic patients. *Journal of Neurology, Neurosurgery, and Psychiatry.* 1994; **57**: 1321–4.
55. Remy-Neris O, Tiffreau V, Bouilland S, Bussel B. Intrathecal baclofen in subjects with spastic hemiplegia: assessment of the anti-spastic effect during gait. *Archives of Physical Medicine and Rehabilitation.* 2003; **84**: 643–50.
56. Al Khodairy AT, Gobelet C, Rossier AB. Has botulinum toxin type A a place in the treatment of spasticity in spinal cord injury patients? *Spinal Cord.* 1998; **36**: 854–8.
57. Barnes M. Botulinum toxin – mechanisms of action and clinical use in spasticity. *Journal of Rehabilitation Medicine.* 2003; **41** (Suppl.): 56–9.
58. Jozefczyk PB. The management of focal spasticity. *Clinical Neuropharmacology.* 2002; **25**: 158–73.

34

Headache

PEER TFELT-HANSEN AND RIGMOR JENSEN

KEY LEARNING POINTS

- Migraine has a lifetime prevalence of 16 percent.
- The prevalence of chronic tension-type headache is 2–3 percent.
- Migraine is a neurovascular headache with associated symptoms.
- Migraine can be treated with acute or preventive treatment.
- The specific antimigraine drugs, the triptans, are new treatment options.
- For prevention, beta-blockers and antiepileptics can be used.

INTRODUCTION AND CLASSIFICATION

Headache is the most frequent pain disorder and has been experienced by almost everyone. Despite the widespread prevalence, the pathophysiology behind the primary headache disorders is widely unknown. Treatment strategies are still nonspecific in most cases, although acute migraine therapy with the advent of the triptans (5-HT$_{1B/1D}$ receptor agonists) has improved considerably in the last decade.

Headache disorders are classified as primary and secondary headaches on the basis of their clinical symptoms and by means of a hierarchical and operational diagnostic system. This classification system[1] is used and accepted worldwide and has improved headache research considerably.

Migraine and tension-type headache (TTH) are the most prevalent primary headaches. Migraine is classified as either migraine with or without aura (**Table 34.1**). Tension-type headache is divided into infrequent episodic tension-type headache (ETTH) (less than one day per month), frequent tension-type headache (less than one, but not more than 15 days per month), and chronic tension-type headache (CTTH) ($\geq$15 days per month) (**Table 34.2**).[1] Distinguishing episodic from chronic tension-type headache and episodic tension-type headache from migraine without aura has practical implications in management strategies. Chronic tension-type headache is often associated with more severe pain, with more accompanying symptoms, is often combined with medication overuse, and is less influenced by daily hassle and stress. It can be difficult to distinguish between

Table 34.1 Operational diagnostic criteria for migraine without aura.[1]

Headache characteristics	
At least five headache attacks of 4–72 hours duration (untreated or unsuccessfully treated)	
The attacks should fulfil at least two out of four characteristics:	Unilateral location
	Pulsating quality
	Moderate or severe pain intensity
	Aggravation by or causing avoidance of routine physical activity (e.g. walking or climbing stairs)
During headache, at least one of the following:	Nausea and/or vomiting
	Photophobia and phonophobia
Not attributed to another disorder	

Table 34.2 International Headache Society (IHS) diagnostic criteria for tension-type headache.[1]

Diagnostic criteria		
Episodic tension-type headache (IHS 2.1) IHCD-II		
A.	At least ten previous headache episodes fulfilling criteria B–D listed below Number of days with such headache < 180/year (< 15/month)	
B.	Headache lasting from 30 minutes to 7 days	
C.	At least two of the following pain characteristics:	1. Pressing/tightening (nonpulsating quality) 2. Mild or moderate severity 3. Bilateral location 4. No aggravation by walking stairs or similar routine physical activity
D.	Both of the following:	1. No nausea or vomiting (anorexia may occur) 2. Photophobia and phonophobia are absent, one but not the other is present
E.	At least one of the following:	1. History, physical and neurological examinations do not suggest one of the disorders listed in group 5–11 (secondary headache disorders) (IHCD-II)[1] 2. History, physical and neurological examinations do suggest such disorder, but is ruled out by appropriate investigations 3. Such disorder is present, but tension-type does not occur for the first time in close temporal relation to the disorder
Chronic tension-type headache (IHS 2.2)		
A.	Average headache frequency 15 days/month or more (180 days/year) for six months or more fulfilling criteria B–D listed below	
B.	As listed in episodic tension-type headache	
C.	Both of the following:	1. No vomiting 2. No more than one of the following: nausea, photophobia, or phonophobia
D.	As (E) in episodic TTH above	

various headache disorders in the severely affected patients with very frequent attacks and a diagnostic headache diary and a long-term follow up are therefore mandatory.[2]

EPIDEMIOLOGY

Migraine has a quite uniform worldwide prevalence with a lifetime prevalence at 16 percent and a one year prevalence at 10 percent.[3,4,5,6] The male/female ratio varies from 1:2 to 1:3 with a more pronounced female preponderance in migraine without aura than in migraine with aura.[6]

The prevalence of migraine increases with age until peak prevalence is reached during the fourth decade of life and thereafter declines again. It is more pronounced in females than in males[3,6] and the most common age at onset is in the second or third decade of life.[3,6]

In its milder and infrequent forms, tension-type headache is a nuisance, not a disease, but in its frequent forms, it becomes distressing and socially disturbing like other primary headaches. The prevalence of episodic tension-type headache varies considerably among population-based studies, and ranges from 38 percent in the most recent American study[7] to 74 percent in a Danish cross-sectional study.[3] In contrast, the prevalence of chronic tension-type headache is quite uniform, 2–3 percent in most studies.[3,4,7]

The male:female ratio of tension-type headache is 4:5 indicating that, unlike migraine, females are only slightly more affected.[3,4,7] The median frequency of the frequent episodic form varies from 2 to 6 days per month,[4,8] whereas the vast majority of patients with chronic tension-type headache suffer from a daily almost constant headache. In contrast to migraine, there is no consistent decline in prevalence with increasing age.[3]

Cluster headache is also a primary headache, but far less prevalent than migraine and tension-type headache with a prevalence between 0.5 and 1 per thousand and with an almost inverse male/female ratio at 4–5/1 compared to migraine.[9] The male preponderance, the very severe pain attacks, the clustering of attacks in one to two months, and the highly characteristic features are very clear, but nevertheless there is still an unacceptable long mean diagnostic delay of nine years (Jensen RM, personal communication).

CLINICAL FEATURES

The typical migraine attack is often dominated by a severe and pulsating, unilateral pain which is intensely aggravated by physical activity,[1,10] although various clinical manifestations are described. The prominent associated symptoms (photophobia, phonophobia, and nausea, sometimes with vomiting) are often just as incapacitating as the pain itself.

In tension-type headache, the patients usually describe their pain as a dull, nonpulsating headache. Terms such as a sensation of "tightness," "pressure," or "soreness" are often employed. Some patients refer to a "band" or a "cap" compressing their head, while others mention a big "weight" over their head and/or shoulders.[11,12,13,14] The headache of tension-type headache is typically bilateral. Thus 90 percent of subjects in one population-based study reported bilateral pain.[13]

At 12-years follow up of a general population, Lyngberg *et al.*[15] found that 42 percent of migraineurs had remission with a lower attack frequency, 38 percent had unchanged infrequent migraine, while 20 percent had developed increased migraine frequency. Some 47 percent of subjects with chronic TTH had remission, while 12 percent with episodic TTH had developed the chronic form.[15]

In cluster headache, there is a severe orbital or periorbital pain lasting 15–180 minutes with accompanying symptoms such as Horner's syndrome, lacrimation, rhinorrhea, and restlessness and agitation. The attacks occur in clusters of weeks to months duration, and in a minority of 15 percent the condition is chronic, lasting for years.

PATHOPHYSIOLOGY

Migraine

Several pathophysiological mechanisms of migraine have been suggested: genetic, neurogenic, vascular, inflammatory, or combinations of these (an update appears in Ref. 16).

Very exciting data have been published in the field of genetics.[17,18] In the very rare condition of familial hemiplegic migraine, mutations in the P/Q calcium channel complex have been described. However, this gene has so far not been linked to migraine with and without aura.[19] A genetic mechanism is undoubtedly involved as Russell *et al.*[20] have found an increased familial risk in first-degree relatives of migraineurs. The risk appears to vary from 1.9 in migraine without aura to 3.8 in migraine with aura, and to 14 in cluster headache.[20] These data indicate that the mode of inheritance is multifactorial and that the primary headache disorders have somewhat different pathophysiological mechanisms. The prevalence of tension-type headache was the same in monozygotic and dizogotic twins and it was concluded that environmental factors were more important than genetic factors in tension-type headache.[21]

Can the precipitating factors provide any important clues to the pathophysiology? The factors, such as stress, mental tension, certain foods, wine and spirits,[10,22] are quite nonspecific. They can only be identified in some patients and vary considerably between and within patients. Precipitating factors are therefore only of limited guidance, although the frequent reports of mental and biochemical stressors along with the accompanying symptoms, such as nausea, photo- and phonophobia, indicate central mechanisms.

For years, the migraine aura has been linked to a cortical hyperexcitability, but neurophysiological evidence for this very likely mechanism has actually been scarce and results are conflicting. Application of more advanced methods, such as transcranial magnetic stimulation has demonstrated consistently and significantly lowered thresholds (44 versus 69). Recorded visual symptoms, such as phosphenes, occur in all migraine patients in contrast to only 27 percent of the controls[23] favoring an increased excitability explanation.

The previous theory of cortical spreading depression of Leao was demonstrated in animal models and recently in man after brain injury[24] and during migraine aura.[25] It is very likely to play a role in the migraine aura where a slowly spreading decrease in regional cerebral blood flow (rCBF) has been observed.[26] Whether this cortical and neuronal hyperexcitability is a factor in both migraine with and without aura and whether it is the causative mechanism for the entire attack, or just a triggering factor, is not yet known.

Positron emission tomography (PET) scanning showed an increase in rCBF in median brain stem structures during migraine attacks. This increase was also observed after relief of symptoms after sumatriptan.[27] These changes in the brain stem have been suggested as a "migraine generator."

The cranial vessels have been extensively studied as peripheral factors. The patients never doubt that their pain is a vascular pain due to the throbbing, pulsating quality and the transient comfort experienced by a minority of patients by compressing the temporal artery on the painful site. Simple dilatation of the large intracranial arteries can play a role in the pain process, as dilation of various segments of the middle cerebral artery can produce referred pain in relevant areas, but the pain is transient and not a migraine. A strictly unilateral dilation of the temporal artery on the painful site has been demonstrated during an episode.[28] There is also indirect evidence of dilatation of the middle cerebral artery on the migraine site by means of transcranial Doppler measurements in some,[29] but not in all studies.[30] Infusion of the nitric oxide (NO)-donor nitroglycerin (NTG) also gives rise to a dilation of the cephalic arteries and a delayed headache indistinguishable from genuine migraine attack. It is elicited in most migraine patients after five to six hours.[31, 32] The NO molecule acts, however, on multiple systems, including the cortical and the brain stem neurons, and the vascular effect may therefore represent another epiphenomenon. Nevertheless, the NTG model is a very useful human model for the study of various aspects of the entire migraine episode.[31, 32, 33] The highly prominent vasoconstrictor effect of specific and effective acute migraine drugs, such as the triptans, ergotamine, and dihydroergotamine (DHE), also supports a prominent vascular mechanism.

Activation of the trigeminal ganglion and the trigeminal nucleus by neurogenic inflammation has been intensively studied in animal models[34, 35] and may be involved in the migraine attack leading to the concept of migraine being a trigeminovascular disease. Whether the activation of the trigeminal system is primary or secondary to the migraine pain is yet unknown, but these models have also been very useful for the study of pain-producing mechanisms and for the screening procedure of possible therapeutic agents. Calcitonin gene-related peptide (CGRP) in the external jugular venous blood was increased in one study,[36] but in a recent, controlled study[37] no such increase was found. However, CGRP infusion induces headache in migraine patients[38] and a CGRP antagonist BIBN4096BS has been shown to be effective in the treatment of migraine attacks.[39]

In conclusion, migraine is a transient, complex disorder in otherwise healthy individuals. The most likely mechanism that can unify the numerous existing hypotheses is a spreading regional neuronal depolarization. This depolarization is probably due to a genetically inherited membrane channel dysfunction in the neurons, either as increased excitability or lack of inhibitory transmitters. If a certain number and combination of idiosyncratic external triggers are present, a migraine attack can be initiated. In the intervals between attacks, there are no clinical signs of the underlying neuronal dysfunction. Similarly, the trigger factors alone cannot initiate the migraine attack, as a genetic disposition also appears to be required. Activation of the trigeminal and the vascular system is most likely to be secondary to the basic migraine process, although highly involved in the elicited central–peripheral–central migraine cascade. Future studies applying more advanced neurophysiological and neuroimaging techniques and genetic studies will hopefully shed more light on the basic mechanisms of migraine.

Tension-type headache

The pathophysiology of tension-type headache is far from elucidated. Headaches of tension-type generally are reported to occur with emotional conflict and psychosocial stress, but the cause–effect relation is not clear. Stress and mental tension are thus the most frequently reported precipitating factors, but occurred with similar frequency in tension-type headache and migraine.[10, 22] Widely normal personality profiles are found in subjects with episodic tension-type headache, whereas studies of subjects with the chronic form often reveal higher frequency of depression and anxiety.[13, 40] In a controlled study, Holroyd *et al.*[41] reported that depression, anxiety, and somatization were highly abnormal during ongoing pain and normalized when patients were retested outside the pain period. However, it was recently demonstrated that depression increases vulnerability to TTH in patients with frequent headaches during and following a laboratory stress test and that the induced headache was associated with elevated pericranial muscle tenderness.[42] The authors suggested that depression may aggravate existing central sensitization (see below under Prophylactic treatment) in patients with frequent headaches.[42] Thus, there may be a bidirectional relationship between depression and frequent TTH.

Peripheral factors have traditionally been considered of major importance in TTH. Numerous studies have reported increased tenderness of pericranial myofascial tissues in these patients.[43, 44] Moreover, TTH patients are more liable to develop shoulder and neck pain in response to static exercise than healthy controls.[45] The increased myofascial pain sensitivity in TTH could be due to release of inflammatory mediators resulting in excitation and sensitization of peripheral sensory afferents.[43, 44] A recent study demonstrated normal *in vivo* interstitial concentrations of inflammatory mediators and metabolites in a tender point of patients with CTTH.[46] Concomitant psychophysical measures indicated that a peripheral sensitization of myofascial sensory afferents was responsible for the muscular hypersensitivity in these patients,[47] but firm evidence is still lacking.

Central factors also play an important role in CTTH and increased suprathreshold pain sensitivity, both in skin and muscle and in cephalic and extracephalic regions, was confirmed in a recent study of patients with CTTH.[48] The fact that the hyperalgesia is generalized, i.e. found in all the examined tissues, makes it highly unlikely that the hyperalgesia is caused by peripheral sensitization of nociceptors in muscle and skin or by abnormal pain modulation in the central nervous system. A recent study demonstrated a decrease in volume of gray matter brain structures involved in pain processing in patients with CTTH.[49] This decrease was positively correlated with duration of headache and the authors interpreted the data as being the consequence of central sensitization. Thus, present knowledge strongly suggests that the central nervous system is sensitized both at the level of the spinal dorsal horn/trigeminal nucleus and supraspinally in patients with CTTH, while the central pain processing seems to be normal in patients with ETTH.

A recent longitudinal population study demonstrated that pain sensitivity is inversely related to headache frequency in both migraine and tension-type headache. Frequent pain did not appear to be a causative factor as pain thresholds were normal before the headache became frequent.[50]

Cluster headache

Cluster headache is a chronobiological headache with a tendency for the attacks to occur at a certain time of the day. The attacks are most likely generated from the hypothalamus where activation has been observed during attacks.[51] The pain is most likely a trigeminovascular pain with dilation of large cerebral arteries.

DIAGNOSIS

A diagnosis of primary headaches as migraine or tension-type headache requires exclusion of other organic disorders. The differential diagnoses for primary headaches are listed in **Table 34.3**. If an intracranial lesion is suspected on the basis of a clinical history and/or examination a computed tomography (CT) or magnetic resonance (MR) scan should be performed. At present, there are no reliable clinical or laboratory tests that are useful in the differential diagnosis. Therefore, a careful history and neurological examination, as well as a prospective follow up using diagnostic headache diaries, are of utmost importance to reach the diagnosis.

A migraine attack should be treated quite differently from an episode of tension-type headache and a separation between these disorders is therefore important. The intensity of pain, the aggravation by physical activity, and the pronounced accompanying symptoms are some of the main features of migraine, although recall bias often influences the history. It has to be kept in mind that tension-type headache and migraine often coexist in the same patient, and an exact diagnosis can only seldom be applied at the initial consultation.

Chronic sinusitis cannot be accepted as a cause of headache on the basis of a simple radiological thickening of sinus mucosa. At least intermittent radiological or clinical signs of ongoing sinus disease have to be present. Similarly, radiological evidence of cervical spondylosis is rarely a satisfactory explanation for a headache since it can be found with equal prevalence in age-matched nonheadache subjects and in other headache patients.[52, 53] The relation between oromandibular dysfunction and headache also remains controversial as a similar prevalence of oromandibular dysfunction in subjects from the general population, suffering from tension-type headache, migraine, or devoid of headache, suggests that a causal relationship with primary headaches must be rare.[54]

Table 34.3 Most frequent differential diagnosis for primary headaches.

Differential diagnosis
Medication overuse headache
Transient ischemic attack
Intracranial tumors
Meningitis
Encephalitis
Subarachnoid hemorrhage
Subdural hematoma
Venous sinus thrombosis
Stroke
Temporal arteritis
Arterial dissection
Primary angle-closure glaucoma
Idiopathic intracranial hypertension
Carbon monoxide poisoning

Each of the primary headaches is in the differential diagnosis of each of the others.

Changes in intracranial pressure are well-known causes of headache. While spontaneous or symptomatic intracranial hypotension is most often distinguishable from other headache types by its clear-cut accentuation in the erect position ("orthostatic headache"), the syndrome of idiopathic intracranial hypertension, also known as "pseudotumor cerebri" or "benign intracranial hypertension," may mimic chronic migraine or chronic tension-type headache. It is vital to remember that idiopathic intracranial hypertension may occur without papilledema and especially young female patients with obesity and pulsatile tinnitus may suggest this diagnosis.[55, 56]

Although brain tumors represent only a very small minority among the causes of headache, they obviously are a major concern to patients and clinicians. Headache awakening the patient from sleep or present on awakening, and/or associated with vomiting, are frequent characteristics with brain tumors, but may also occur in some migraineurs and in subjects with medication overuse.

In clinical practice, the most frequent cause for chronic daily headache is medication overuse headache (MOH) due to chronic analgesic and/or ergotamine or triptan overuse, to which patients may evolve after having presented initially with migraine or episodic/chronic tension-type headache.[57] The prevalence of MOH is as high as 30–50 percent in headache clinic populations.[57, 58, 59] Recognizing this condition is of crucial importance, since the outcome in general is very positive after withdrawal.[58] Likewise, migraineurs become responsive to prophylactic drugs after a successful detoxification, despite prior prophylactic failures in combination with acute medication overuse.[60]

TREATMENT

It is important to establish an accurate diagnosis, where the individual headache episode is identified and separated from a secondary headache, most frequently drug-induced headache. The treatment of primary headache disorders consists primarily of prevention by avoidance of any possible trigger factors. Treatment of the acute attack and prophylaxis is typically by pharmacological methods. One of the most important elements in treating headache patients in general is to take their complaints seriously, show empathy, and examine them.

THE ACUTE EPISODE

Migraine

Migraine attacks can be treated with nonspecific drugs, such as analgesics and nonsteroidal anti-inflammatory drugs (NSAIDs),[61][II] which have an effect on headaches generally, or with specific antimigraine drugs, such as triptans (5-$HT_{1B/1D}$ receptor agonists),[62][I] and ergot alkaloids (ergotamine and dihydroergotamine), which only are effective in migraine.[63][II] The absorption of orally administered drugs is delayed during migraine attacks.[64] If nonspecific drugs are used, it is recommended therefore that they are combined with a prokinetic antiemetic drug, such as metoclopramide, in order to optimize absorption.[64] Nonspecific drugs, often combined with metoclopramide,[64][II] were comparable to sumatriptan in several randomized clinical trials (RCTs) (see **Table 34.4**). An exception is tolfenamic acid (58 percent headache relief) which was inferior to sumatriptan (75 percent headache relief).[69] Oral ergotamine[70] [II] has a very low bioavailability ($<$1 percent)[71] and, as expected, was inferior to oral triptans (sumatriptan, rizatriptan, eletriptan, and almotriptan) in four RCTs (**Table 34.4**). In contrast, rectal ergotamine[70][II] was superior to rectal sumatriptan [I] (**Table 34.4**), but because it also acts on dopamine and 5-HT_2 receptors, it causes more side effects than triptans. The benefit/tolerability ratio for effective doses of ergotamine is thus less than that for triptans. Ergotamine was recently only recommended in patients who already use it, are responding satisfactorily to the drug, with no contraindications to its use, and with no signs of dose escalation.[72] Long-lasting migraine attacks ($>$48 hours) may be usefully treated with ergotamine, since headache recurrence (primary successful treatment within two hours with subsequent increase to moderate or severe headache within 24 hours) is probably less likely with ergotamine.[72] If ergotamine is used, the rectal route, provided it is acceptable to the patient, should be used.[72]

TRIPTANS

The triptans are a new class of compounds which act as agonists on the-$HT_{1B/1D}$ receptor. The first of this family, sumatriptan, was undoubtedly a significant advance in migraine therapy.[73, 74][I]

The mechanisms of action of triptans in migraine are mainly constriction of dilated cranial extracerebral blood vessels,[75] reduction of neuropeptide release and plasma protein extravasation across dural vessels,[34] and inhibition impulse transmission centrally within the trigeminovascular system.[76] However, the possible contribution of the neuronal effect of triptans, mediated via 5-HT_{1D} receptor, has been put in doubt because PNU142633, a selective 5-HT_{1D} receptor agonist, has not proved effective in the acute treatment of migraine.[77]

Efficacy of triptans in randomized clinical trials

The relative efficacy of the different triptans has only been investigated in 15 comparative, randomized clinical trials (**Table 34.5**).[62, 65] In addition to direct comparative trials, more information on the efficacy of different drugs can be obtained by meta-analyses of the drugs.[65, 78] An extensive meta-analysis of oral triptans is shown in **Figure 34.1**. The efficacy measure recommended by the International

Table 34.4 Randomized clinical trials comparing triptans with nontriptan drugs.

Drug	Dose	Headache relief (%)[a]	Difference (%)	95% CI
Sumatriptan	Oral 100 mg	66	**+18**	**+9 to +27**
Ergotamine and caffeine	Oral 2+200 mg	48		
Sumatriptan	Oral 50 mg	56	+3	-5 to +13
Aspirin	1000 mg	53		
Ibuprofen	400 mg	60	-4	-14 to+5
Sumatriptan	Oral 50 mg	49	0	-11 to +12
Aspirin	Oral 1000 mg	49		
Sumatriptan	Oral 100 mg	56	+11	-1 to +23
Aspirin and metoclopramide	Oral 900+10 mg	45		
Sumatriptan	Oral 100 mg	53	-4	-17 to +8
L-ASA and metoclopramide	Oral 1620+10 mg	57		
Sumatriptan	Oral 100 mg	79	+2	-17 to +20
Tolfenamic acid (rapid release formulation)	Oral 200+200 mg	77		
Sumatriptan	Oral 100 mg	75	**+17**	**+5 to +28**
Tolfenamic acid (rapid release formulation)	Oral 200+200 mg	58		
Placebo		47		
Sumatriptan	6 mg s.c.	80	**+30**	**+19 to +41**
Didydroergotamine	Nasal 1+1 mg	50		
Sumatriptan	6 mg s.c.	85 (83)[b]	**+12** (-3)[b]	**+3 to +21** (-11 to +5)[b]
Dihydroergotamine	1+1 mg s.c.	73 (86)[b]		
Sumatriptan	Nasal 20 mg	63	**+12**	**+4 to +20**
Dihydroergotamine	1+1 mg	51		
Sumatriptan	6 mg s.c.	91	**+17**	**+8 to +27**
L-ASA	1800 mg i.v.	74		
Sumatriptan	Rectal 25 mg	63	**-10**	**-18 to -2**
Ergotamine and caffeine	Rectal 2+200 mg	73		
Eletriptan	80 mg	68	**+35**	**+26 to +44**
Ergotamine and caffeine	2+200 mg	33		
Eletriptan	40 mg	54	**+21**	**+11 to +30**
Ergotamine and caffeine	2+200 mg	33		
Rizatriptan	10 mg	76	**+29**	**+19 to +38**
Ergotamine and caffeine	2+200 mg	47		
Almotriptan	12.5 mg	58	**+13**	**+6 to +25**
Ergotamine and caffeine	2+200 mg	45		

[a]A decrease from severe or moderate headache to none or mild after two hours.
[b]After four hours.
CI, confidence intervals; L-ASA, lysine acetylsalicylate.
Significant differences are shown in bold.
For further details see Refs 62, 65, 66, 67, 68.

Headache Society, rizatriptan (10 mg), eletriptan (80 mg), and almotriptan, were superior to the standard drug sumatriptan (100 mg). Naratriptan (2.5 mg) was inferior to sumatriptan.[78, 79][I] In later comparative randomized trials, eletriptan (40 mg) was superior to sumatriptan (100 mg),[80][I] whereas almotriptan (12.5 mg) was inferior to sumatriptan (50 mg) for this variable.[66][II] Rizatriptan (10 mg) was superior for pain relief to sumatriptan (100 mg);[62, 66][II] naratriptan (2.5 mg) was inferior to 100 mg sumatriptan and 10 mg rizatriptan.[62, 65][II]

How do the triptans compare with other drugs for acute migraine treatment? As shown in **Table 34.4**, sumatriptan (100 mg), eletriptan (40 and 80 mg), almotriptan (12.5 mg), and rizatriptan (10 mg) were superior to oral ergotamine plus caffeine (2 mg+200 mg).[62][II] Oral sumatriptan (100 mg) was not superior to aspirin with metoclopramide for the first treated attack (but superior for the second and third attacks),[62][II] and was comparable to lysine acetylsalicylate plus metoclopramide (1620 mg (~900 mg aspirin)+10 mg).[81][II] Sumatriptan (50 mg) was equivalent to effervescent aspirin (1000 mg) in two trials.[82, 83][II] Sumatriptan was superior to tolfenamic acid rapid release in a randomized clinical trial, 75 versus 58 percent.[69] Rectal sumatriptan (25 mg) was

Table 34.5 Mean therapeutic gain[a] for different triptans and forms of administration based on published papers and abstracts.

Drug	Dose	Mean therapeutic gain (%)[b]	95% confidence intervals (%)
Sumatriptan	6 mg s.c.	51	48–51
	Oral 100 mg	32	29–34
	Oral 50 mg	29	25–34
	Oral 25 mg	24	18–29
	Nasal 20 mg	30	25–34
	Rectal 25 mg	31	25–37
Zolmitriptan	Oral 2.5 mg	32	26–38
Naratriptan	Oral 2.5 mg	22	18–26
Rizatriptan	Oral 10 mg	37	34–40
	Oral 5 mg	28	23–34
	Wafer 10 mg[c]	37	29–45
Eletriptan	Oral 80 mg	42	37–47
	Oral 40 mg	37	32–42
Almotriptan	Oral 12.5 mg	26	20–32
Frovatriptan	Oral 2.5 mg	16	8–25

[a]Percentage headache relief after active drug minus percentage headache relief after placebo.
[b]Based on headache relief (a decrease from severe or moderate headache to none or mild after two hours (for subcutaneous sumatriptan after one hour)).
[c]A rapidly dissolving wafer.
For references and number of patients, see Refs 62, 65.

inferior to rectal ergotamine plus caffeine (2 mg+200 mg), but caused fewer adverse events (8 versus 27 percent).[62][II] In four out of five RCTs where a triptan and an ergot alkaloid were compared, there were less recurrences after the ergot alkaloid than after the triptan.[62, 67][II]

In one RCT, not shown in **Table 34.4** because of a difference in design from the other RCTs listed, diclofenac–potassium (50 and 100 mg) was equivalent to 100 mg sumatriptan.[62][II]

Therapeutic use of triptans

The contraindications to the use of triptans[62] are shown in **Table 34.6**, together with the recommended doses. In the RCTs mentioned above under Efficacy of triptans in randomized clinical trials, migraine was treated when the headache was moderate or severe. Recently, treatment in the mild phase of migraine was introduced. The efficacy measure used in these RCTs was pain relief after two hours. In these placebo-controlled RCTs a pain-free state after two hours was achieved in 70 percent with rizatriptan (10 mg),[84][II] 50 and 57 percent with sumatriptan tablets (50 and 100 mg, respectively),[85][II] and 51 and 66 percent with a fast-disintegrating/rapid-release tablet formulation of sumatriptan (50 and 100 mg, respectively).[86][II] As shown in **Figure 34.1b** the pain-free response is, as expected, much lower when treating moderate or severe migraine pain. If the patients are sure that they are experiencing a migraine attack, the use of triptans in the first mild phase can be recommended. The risk of this strategy is that the patients will treat all their headaches, including episodes of tension-type headache, with triptans, and careful instructions to the patients are therefore required.

Use of triptans should be limited to a maximum of nine days per month. A study using prescription data suggests that sumatriptan abuse is a real problem with 5 percent of sumatriptan users using a daily (or more) dose of sumatriptan and a total consumption of 44 percent of all the national use of sumatriptan in Denmark.[87, 88] Migraine patients should not be allowed such frequent use of triptans and other treatment strategies as detoxification and subsequent prophylactic strategies shoud be initiated. In previous drug overusers, it has been recommended to limit the use of triptans to one dose per week.[89]

It has been shown that if one triptan is not effective, another triptan can be used successfully;[62, 90] and it is our clinical experience that if one triptan is not effective, clinical success can sometimes be obtained with another triptan or another mode of administration.

The main problem with the triptans is the high cost. Currently, only 10 percent of migraine patients in a Danish county receive a prescription for any triptan (Jensen R, personal communication) and the corresponding figure for the UK is 15 percent (Steiner TJ, personal communication). Sumatriptan is now generic which has resulted in a considerable decrease in price.

TREATMENT OF TENSION-TYPE HEADACHE

The acute episode

Due to the lack of pathophysiological knowledge of tension-type headache there is no selective or specific therapy. Pharmacological treatment of the acute episode includes simple analgesics and NSAIDs. The efficacy of these drugs in treating tension-type headache has only been systematically tested using modern day methodology in a few cases.[91][II] In one study, aspirin (76 percent) was superior to placebo (56 percent) in episodic tension-type headache.[92][II]

The effect of solid aspirin was compared to effervescent aspirin in a placebo-controlled study and demonstrated that aspirin was significantly better than placebo, but that there was no significant difference between solid and effervescent aspirin.[93][II] In another placebo-controlled study, it was noted that paracetamol (acetaminophen) and aspirin were more effective than placebo, but not different from each other.[91][II] However, as the gastric side-effect profile is much better with paracetamol than with aspirin, paracetamol may be recommended as the first drug of choice for these mild or moderate headache episodes. Although simple over-the-counter drugs are the most commonly used drugs for headache, excessive and frequent use, particularly when combined with caffeine and/or sedatives, should clearly be avoided due to the high risk of drug-induced headache.[89] Therefore, thorough information and an upper daily/weekly limit of such drug consumption are essential to these patients.

The value of NSAIDs in treating tension-type headache is barely substantiated in randomized controlled trials. In one comparative study, ketoprofen was superior to paracetamol and placebo,[94][II] whereas ketoprofen was similar to paracetamol in another study.[95][II] When different doses of ketoprofen, ibuprofen, and naproxen sodium were compared to each other, no significant difference between the NSAIDs was demonstrated.[96, 97][II] Finally, the use of muscle relaxants is only on empirical basis and cannot be recommended.

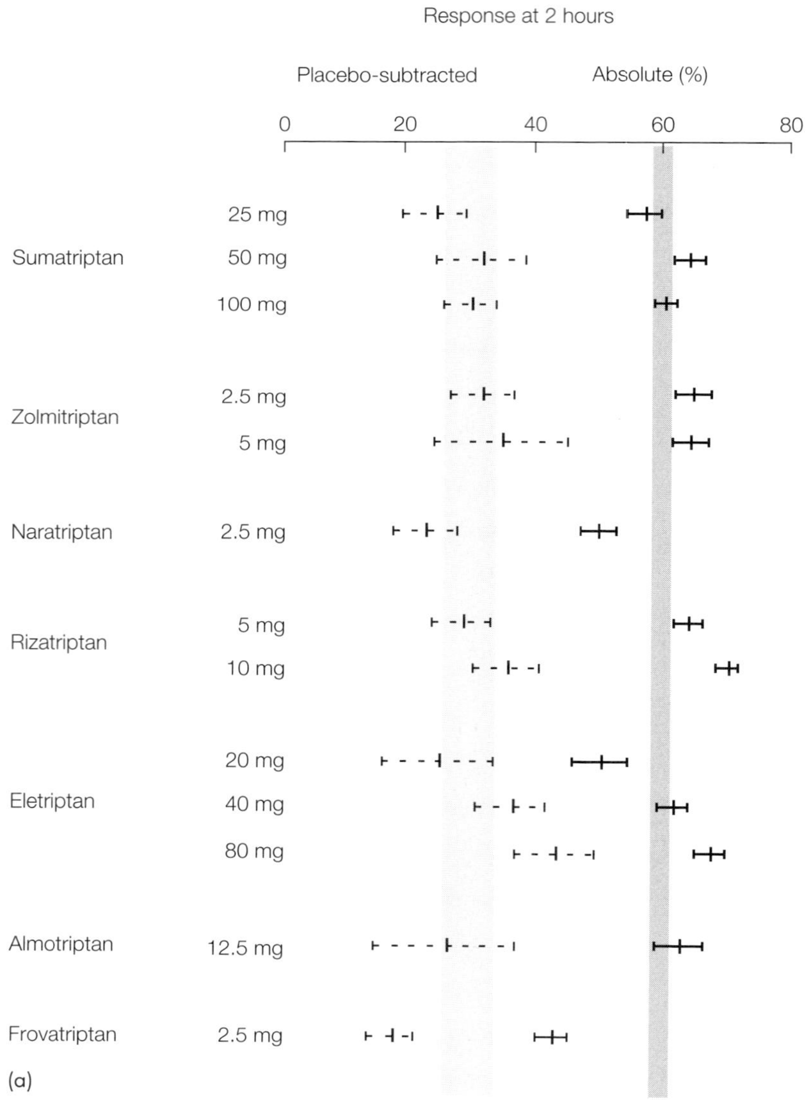

Figure 34.1 (a) Headache response after seven oral triptans. The shaded area indicates the 95% confidence intervals for sumatriptan (100 mg) both for absolute responses and placebo-subtracted results (continued over). Redrawn from Ferrari MD, Roon KI, Lipton RB, Goadsby PJ. Oral triptans (serotonin 5-$HT_{1B/1D}$ agonists) in acute migraine: a meta-analysis of 53 trials. *Lancet.* 2001; **358**: 1668–75, with permission from the publisher.

In conclusion, the mainstay of acute treatment of tension-type headache is simple analgesics and NSAIDs. Muscle relaxants and migraine-specific drugs are only empirically used. Combined drugs consisting of analgesics, tranquillizers, and sedatives should clearly be avoided because of the potential of habituation and subsequent MOH.[89] Clinical experience indicates a positive effect of combinations of nonpharmacological and pharmacological treatment, [V] but there are no formal studies to substantiate these impressions.[98]

PROPHYLACTIC TREATMENT

Migraine

Prioritizing prophylactic treatment of migraine can be a complex task and should be regarded as a joint venture between the doctor and the patient. The first priority is to use the drug with the highest benefit/tolerability ratio.[99]

The ranking of prophylactic drugs is summarized in **Table 34.7** and is based on a combination of the authors' judgment of the publications and personal experience.[66] The potential for side effects is an important factor in the choice of prophylactic drug because use may be prolonged over months to years. It is our clinical experience that migraine patients often have more side effects with these drugs than other patients. We therefore generally try to start out with small doses of prophylactic drugs (e.g. 40–60 mg propranolol daily) and then gradually increase the dose depending on side effects and effect.

In general, the drugs of first choice are the β-blockers,[102] [I] which are also, in practice, the most frequently used. There are no trials to show superiority of one of the effective β-blockers over another. When β-blockers are not effective or are contraindicated, the choice of a

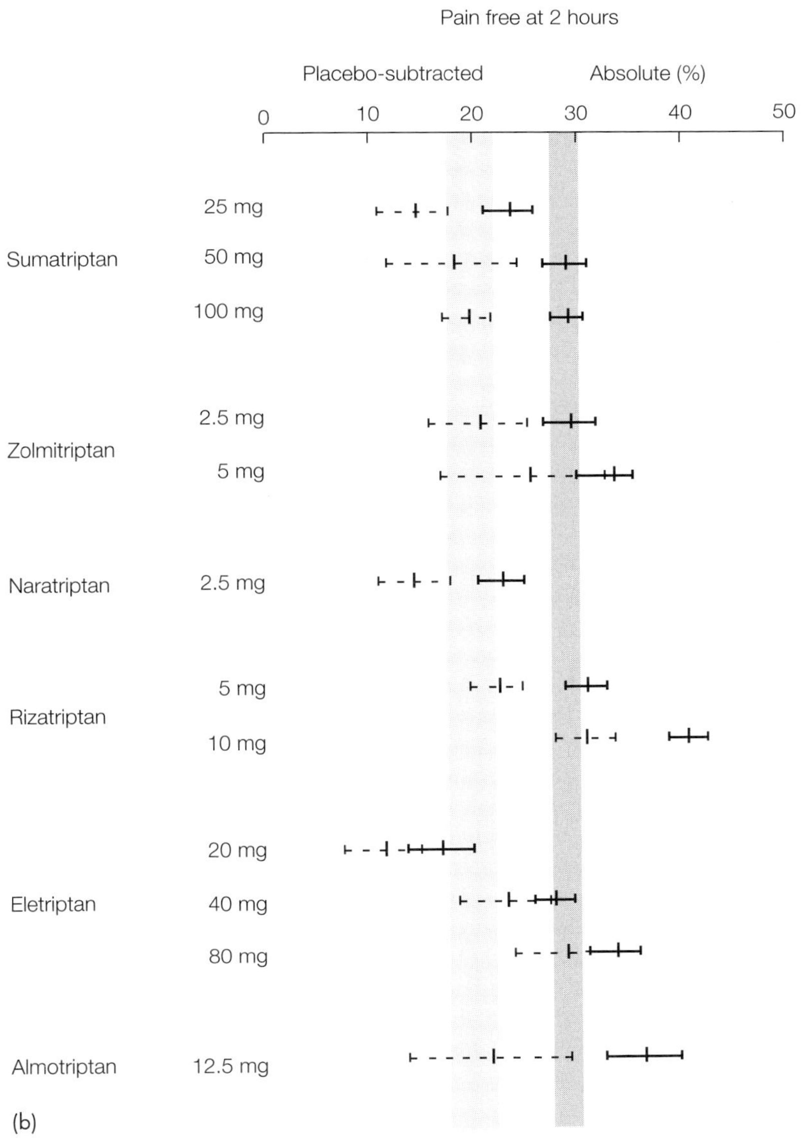

Figure 34.1 (b) Pain relief after two hours. The shaded area indicates the 95% confidence intervals for sumatriptan (100 mg) both for absolute responses and placebo-subtracted results (continued).

Table 34.6 Therapeutic use of marketed triptans in currently recommended doses.

Recommended doses of triptans	Maximum daily dosage
6 mg subcutaneous sumatriptan	12 mg
50–100 mg oral sumatriptan	300 mg
50 mg sumatriptan rapidly dissolving tablets	300 mg (25 mg tablets available in the USA)
20 mg intranasal sumatriptan	40 mg
25 mg sumatriptan as suppositories	50 mg
2.5–5 mg oral zolmitriptan	10 mg
2.5 mg orally melting tablets of zolmitriptan	10 mg
2.5 mg oral naratriptan	5 mg
10 mg oral rizatriptan[a]	20 mg
10 mg oral rizatriptan wafer[a]	20 mg
40 mg oral eletriptan	80 mg
12.5 mg oral almotriptan	25 mg
2.5 mg frovatriptan	5 mg?
Clinical efficacy in the treatment of migraine attacks	Subcutaneous sumatriptan (6 mg) > eletriptan (40 mg) ≥ oral sumatriptan (50–100 mg) = intranasal sumatriptan (20 mg) = rectal sumatriptan (25 mg) = oral zolmitriptan (2.5–5 mg) = oral rizatriptan (10 mg) > oral sumatriptan (25 mg), oral naratriptan (2.5 mg) = oral frovatriptan (2.5 mg)
Speed of onset of effect compared with placebo	Subcutaneous sumatriptan (10 min) > intranasal sumatriptan (15 min) > oral sumatriptan = oral eletriptan = oral rizatriptan (30 min) > rectal sumatriptan (30–60 min) > oral zolmitriptan and oral naratriptan (60 min). It should be noted, however, that these "early responses," apart from subcutaneous sumatriptan, are often of relatively small magnitude
Speed of onset of effect compared directly among two triptans or two administration forms of a triptan	Oral rizatriptan > oral sumatriptan Oral rizatriptan = oral zolmitriptan Oral rizatriptan > oral naratriptan Intranasal sumatriptan (>) oral sumatriptan
Adverse events with triptans	So-called "triptan" symptoms: tingling, numbness, warm/hot sensation, pressure or tightness in different part of the body, including chest and neck. Rarely regular chest pain. Dizziness and sedation. Naratriptan and almotriptan cause no more adverse events than placebo
Choice of form of administration	Tablets generally most convenient. If severe nausea/vomiting is present, the patient could alternatively use an injection, nasal spray, or a suppository
Additional dose if the first dose of a triptan is not effective	There is no evidence that a second dose of a triptan increases the efficacy. If the chosen dose of a triptan is ineffective, patients should instead try another dose or different forms of administration or another triptan
Recurrence or secondary treatment failure	Most triptans have the same recurrence rate of 20–40%. Naratriptan has a lower recurrence rate than sumatriptan in some trials and could be tried in recurrence-prone patients
Use of a second dose for the treatment of a recurrence when the first dose of a triptan is primarily effective	A second dose of a triptan will probably be effective, but with multiple recurrence, alternative drugs should probably be tried
Abuse or inappropriate use of triptans	Triptans should not be used on a daily basis (except in the treatment of chronic cluster headache). Set an upper limit of 9 days per month with triptan use. Use triptans with extreme caution in previous drug abusers
Breast feeding	Sumatriptan can be used if milk is expressed and discarded for eight hours after the dose. Not recommended with the other triptans
Possible drug interactions	In patients on propranolol 5 mg rizatriptan should be used. Eletriptan should not be used in patients on CYP3A4 inhibitors
Contraindications to triptans	Ischemic heart disease, variant angina, cerebral and peripheral vascular disease, and uncontrolled hypertension. Pregnancy. Use of ergot alkaloids within 24 hours. Current use or use of MAO-inhibitors within the last two weeks. Hypersensitivity to the triptan. Hemiplegic and basilar migraine
Cautious use	Patients on SSRIs can be treated with triptans, but should be warned about the symptoms of the serotonin syndrome

[a]5 mg rizatriptan in patients on propranolol.
For details, see above under Prophylactic treatment.

Table 34.7 Clinical efficacy,[a] scientific proof of efficacy,[b] and potential for side effects[a] rated on a scale from + to ++++ for some drugs used in migraine prophylaxis.

Drug	Clinical efficacy	Scientific proof for efficacy	Side-effect potential	Examples of side effects (examples of contraindications in brackets)
β-blockers (propranolol, metoprolol, atenolol, nadolol, timolol	++++	++++	++	Tiredness, cold extremities, vivid dreams, depression (asthma, brittle diabetes, A–V conduction defects)
Antiepileptics				
Sodium valproate (divalproex)	+++	+++	+++	Weight gain, tremor, hair loss, (thrombocytopenia, liver disease,[c] pregnancy)
Topiramate	+++	++++	+++	Sedation, paresthesia, weight loss (kidney stones)
Antiserotonin drugs				
Methysergide	++++	++	++++	Chronic use: fibrotic disorders (cardiovascular diseases)
Pizotifen	+++	++	+++	Weight gain, sedation (obesity)
Calcium antagonists				
Flunarizine	+++	++++	+++	Sedation, weight gain, depression (depression, parkinsonism)
Verapamil	+	+	+	Constipation (bradycardia, A–V conduction defects)
NSAIDs				Dyspepsia, peptic ulcers
Naproxen	++	+++	++	(Active peptic ulcers)
Tolfenamic acid	++	+++	++	
Miscellaneous				
Amitriptyline	++	++	++	Sedation, dry mouth, weight gain (glaucoma)
Candesartan	++	++	+	Dizziness (liver disease)
Clonidine	+	+	+	Dry mouth
Dihydroergotamine	++	+	++	Nausea, diarrhea (ischemic heart disease)

[a]The rating is based on a combination of the published literature and the authors' personal experience.
[b]As judged by the authors (apparently conflicting with the overwhelming majority of comparative trials claiming equipotency of two drugs. This claim of comparability is probably due to small trials, see above under Prophylactic treatment).
[c]In most countries, routine hematological screening and biochemical tests of liver function are considered necessary prior to starting and during valproate (divalproex) treatment.
DHE, dihydroergotamine; NSAIDs, nonsteroidal anti-inflammatory drugs.
For details and references, see Refs 100, 101, 102, 103, 104.

prophylactic drug will depend to some extent on local availability (for example, pizotifen and flunarizine are not available in the USA); but based on the ratios for efficacy/side effects, all of which should be discussed with the patient, the choice can be either topiramate,[100][II] valproate semisodium (divalproex),[100][II] one of the NSAIDs listed, pizotifen,[103][II] flunarizine,[101][II]amitriptyline,[101][II] or candesartan.[105][II] Amitriptyline is often useful in patients with a mixture of migraine and tension-type headache. Clonidine, dihydroergotamine, and methysergide[106][II] (in a headache specialist's hands) should probably only be used as the last resort. Finally, the physician should follow the patient at two- to three-month intervals. The patient should keep a simple headache diary for monitoring migraine attack frequency and side effects should always be recorded by and discussed with the patient. The patient can then decide together with the physician whether to continue with that particular prophylactic treatment or try another. Even with successful treatment, we recommend to try to taper it off after one year.

Tension-type headache

Tricyclic antidepressants have been extensively used, but only relatively few placebo-controlled studies have investigated their efficacy. Results are to some extent contradictory.[107] The effect of amitriptyline has been confirmed in a few placebo-controlled, double-blind studies where the most extensive study reported a significant reduction in the area under the headache curve during amitriptyline, compared with placebo, while the specific serotonin reuptake inhibitor citalopram had no significant effect.[108][II] The mechanism of action of amitriptyline in tension-type headache is independent of its antidepressant effect[109, 110] and the effective dosage in headache is usually much lower than used in the treatment of depression, namely 10–75 mg per day. The lack of significant effect of the selective serotonin reuptake inhibitors (SSRIs)[109, 111] indicates that serotonergic mechanisms are not of decisive importance. The antidepressant drug mirtazapine, which is both a serotonin and noradrenalin reuptake inhibitor, was found to be more effective in doses of 15–30 mg than placebo in one RCT,[107, 112][II] whereas a lower dose of 4.5 mg alone or combined with ibuprofen (ibumetin) had no prophylactic effect.[113][II] A few other tricyclic antidepressants have been reported to have a prophylactic effect in chronic tension-type headache, but unfortunately these studies have never been replicated. Valproate and NSAIDs cannot be recommended for prophylaxis of tension-type headache until properly designed trials have been conducted.

NONPHARMACOLOGICAL TREATMENT

Physical treatment modalities, such as hot and cold packs, ultrasound and electrical stimulation, improvement of posture, relaxation, and exercise programs, have all been used. However, the majority of these treatments have not been properly evaluated, and most of the reported studies are not controlled. In one open-label study, the beneficial long-term effect of physical therapy was excellent,[114][IV] whereas a controlled study reported only a minor effect on headache frequency after eight weeks of standardized treatment.[115, 116][II] A recent controlled study concluded that there was no significant effect of spinal manipulation on patients with episodic tension-type headache.[98][II] Likewise botulinum toxin plays no role in the treatment of tension-type headache or migraine.[117, 118][II]

TREATMENT OF CLUSTER HEADACHE

Attacks of cluster headache can be treated with oxygen or subcutaneous sumatriptan (6 mg).[119][II] For acute treatment, sumatriptan (20 mg) administered as a nasal spray was superior to placebo (57 versus 26 percent relief).[120][II] Intranasal zolmitriptan (10 mg) was superior to placebo (65 versus 21 percent relief) after 30 minutes.[121][II]

The prophylactic treatment is based on verapamil in doses of 360–720 mg daily. In addition, lithium, ergotamine, methysergide, valproate, and topiramate can be used together with verapamil, although the scientific evidence for most of these prophylactic drugs and their combinations is lacking.[122] A placebo-controlled trial has shown that infiltration of the greater occipital nerve with steroids on the side of the pain is an effective prophylactic treatment.[123][II] Invasive procedures, such as deep brain stimulation and occipital nerve stimulation, are under evaluation and there is no general consensus.

CONCLUSIONS

Primary headaches represent some of the most costly diseases in modern society and epidemiological studies indicate that tension-type headache and migraine represent two different diseases, although coexisting in many patients. Only limited knowledge of the underlying pathophysiology is yet available. Scientific interest in migraine over recent decades has increased and resulted in specific treatment for the acute attack, through the use of the triptans. These specific drugs are available worldwide but are still underused, most likely due to the high price. The majority of migraine attacks are treated with nonspecific drugs such as aspirin. Prophylactic treatment of migraine is still nonspecific and only more scientific evidence for the pathophysiology of the disease will result in specific prophylactic treatment.

Tension-type headache is the stepchild of headache research, but the burden of tension-type headache in its frequent and chronic forms is even higher than the burden of migraine. This fact should result in prioritizing research in the pathophysiology of this primary headache disorder.

One secondary chronic headache disorder which is preventable and treatable is medication overuse headache which occurs in 1 percent of the population.[89] Patients should be warned against daily or almost daily intake of any analgesic drugs, even over-the-counter drugs, and if they have MOH they can be treated satisfactorily by merely withdrawal of the drug for two months.[63]

REFERENCES

* 1. Headache Classification Committee of the International Headache Society. The International Classification of Headache Disorders. 2nd edn. *Cephalalgia.* 2004; **24**: 1–150.
2. Russell M, Rasmussen BK, Brennum J *et al.* Presentation of a new instrument. The diagnostic headache diary. *Cephalalgia.* 1992; **12**: 369–74.
3. Rasmussen BK, Jensen R, Schroll M, Olesen J. Epidemiology of headache in a general population – a prevalence study. *Journal of Clinical Epidemiology.* 1991; **44**: 1147–57.
4. Göbel H, Petersen-Braun M, Soyka D. The epidemiology of headache in Germany: a nationwide survey of a representative sample on the basis of the Headache Classification of the International Headache Society. *Cephalalgia.* 1994; **14**: 97–106.

5. Russell MB, Rasmussen BK, Thorvaldsen P, Olesen J. Prevalence and sex-ratio of subtypes of migraine. *International Journal of Epidemiology.* 1995; **24**: 612–18.
6. Rasmussen BK, Stewart WF. Epidemiology of migraine. In Olesen J, Tfelt-Hansen P, Welch KMA (eds). *The headaches*, 2nd edn. Philadelphia: Lippincott Williams & Wilkins, 2000: 227–33.
7. Schwartz BS, Stewart WF, Simon D, Lipton RB. Epidemiology of tension-type headache. *JAMA.* 1998; **279**: 381–3.
8. Iversen HK, Langemark M, Andersson PG *et al.* Clinical characteristics of migraine and tension-type headache in relation to new and old diagnostic criteria. *Headache.* 1990; **30**: 514–19.
* 9. Goadsby P, Tfelt-Hansen P. Cluster headache: introduction and epidemiology. In: Olesen J, Tfelt-Hansen P, Goadsby PJ *et al.* (eds). *The headaches*, 3rd edn. Philadelphia: Lippincott Williams & Wilkins, 2006: 743–5.
10. Rasmussen BK. Migraine and tension-type headache in a general population: Precipitating factors, female hormones, sleep pattern and relation to lifestyle. *Pain.* 1993; **53**: 65–72.
11. Kudrow L. Muscle contraction headaches. In: Clifford Rose F (ed.). *Handbook of clinical neurology.* Headache. Amsterdam: Elsevier Science, 1986. **4**: 343–52.
12. Langemark M, Olesen J, Poulsen DL, Bech P. Clinical characterization of patients with chronic tension headache. *Headache.* 1988; **28**: 590–6.
13. Rasmussen BK. Migraine and TTH in a general population: psychosocial factors. *International Journal of Epidemiology.* 1992; **21**: 1138–43.
14. Olesen J. Clinical characterization of tension headache. In: Olesen J, Edvinsson L (eds). *Basic mechanisms of headache.* Amsterdam: Elsevier Science, 1988: 9–14.
15. Lyngberg AC, Rasmussen BK, Jorgensen T, Jensen R. Prognosis of migraine and tension-type headache: a population-based follow-up study. *Neurology.* 2005; **65**: 580–5.
* 16. Olesen J, Goadsby PJ, Ramadan N *et al.* (eds). *The headaches*, 3rd edn. Philadelphia: Lippincott, Williams & Wilkins, 2006.
17. Ophoff RA, Terwindt GM, Vergouwe MN *et al.* Familial hemiplegic migraine and epidodic ataxia type-2 are caused by mutations in the Ca^{2+} channel gene CACNL1A4. *Cell.* 1996; **87**: 543–52.
18. Terwindt GM, Ophoff RA, Haan J *et al.* Migraine, ataxia and epilepsy: a challenging spectrum of genetic determined calcium channelopathies. *European Journal of Human Genetics.* 1998; **6**: 297–307.
19. Ferrari MD, Haan J, Palotie A. Genetic of migraine. In: Olesen J, Goadsby PJ, Ramadan NM *et al.* (eds). *The headaches*, 3rd edn. Philadelphia: Lippincott Williams & Wilkins, 2006: 251–68.
20. Russell M. Genetic epidemiology of migraine and cluster-headache. *Cephalalgia.* 1997; **17**: 683–701.
21. Ulrich V, Gervil M, Olesen J. The relative influence of environment and genes in episodic tension-type headache. *Neurology.* 2004; **62**: 2065–9.
22. Ulrich V, Russell MB, Jensen R, Olesen J. A comparison of tension-type headache in migraineurs and in non-migraineurs: a population-based study. *Pain.* 1996; **67**: 501–06.
23. Aurora SK, Welch KMA. Brain hyperexcitability in migraine: evidence from transcranial magnetic stimulation studies. *Current Opinion in Neurology.* 1998; **11**: 205–09.
24. Fabricius M, Fuhr S, Bhatia R *et al.* Cortical spreading depression and peri-infarct depolarization in acutely injured human cerebral cortex. *Brain.* 2006; **129**: 778–90.
25. Hadjikhani N, Sanchez Del Rio M, Wu O *et al.* Mechanisms of migraine aura revealed by functional MRI in human visual cortex. *Proceedings of the National Academy of Sciences of the United States of America.* 2001; **98**: 4687–92.
26. Olesen J, Larsen B, Lauritzen M. Focal hyperemia followed by spreading oligemia and impaired activation of rCBF in classic migraine. *Annals of Neurology.* 1981; **9**: 344–52.
27. Weiller C, May A, Limmroth V *et al.* Brain stem activation in spontaneous human migraine attacks. *Nature Medicine.* 1995; **1**: 658–60.
28. Iversen HK, Nielsen TH, Olesen J, Tfelt-Hansen P. Arterial responses during migraine headache. *Lancet.* 1990; **336**: 837–9.
29. Friberg L, Olesen J, Iversen HK, Sperling B. Migraine pain associated with middle cerebral artery dilatation: reversal by sumatriptan. *Lancet.* 1991; **338**: 13–17.
30. Zwetsloot CP, Caekebe JF, Ferrari MD. Lack of asymmetry of middle artery blood flow velocity in unilateral migraine. *Stroke.* 1993; **24**: 1335–8.
31. Iversen HK, Thomsen LL, Olesen J. Headache induced by a nitric oxide donor (nitroglycerin) responds to sumatriptan. A human model for development of migraine drugs. *Cephalalgia.* 1996; **16**: 412–18.
32. Thomsen LL, Kruuse C, Iversen HK, Olesen J. A nitric oxide donor (nitroglycerin) triggers genuine migraine attacks. *European Journal of Neurology.* 1994; **1**: 73–80.
33. Olesen J, Iversen HK, Thomsen LL. Nitric oxide hypersensitivity. A possible molecular mechanisms of migraine pain. *Neuroreport.* 1993; **4**: 1027–30.
34. Moskowitz MA. Neurogenic inflammation in the pathophysiology and treatment of migraine. *Neurology.* 1993; **43**: 242–6.
35. Buzzi MG, Carter WB, Shimizu T *et al.* Dihydroergotamine and sumatriptan attenuate levels of CGRP in plasma in rat superior sagittal sinus during electrical stimulation of the trigeminal ganglion. *Neuropharmacology.* 1991; **30**: 1193–200.
36. Goadsby PJ, Edvinsson L. The trigeminovascular system and migraine: studies characterizing cerebrovascular and neuropeptide changes in human and cats. *Annals of Neurology.* 1993; **33**: 48–56.

37. Tvedskov JF, Lipka K, Ashina M *et al.* No increase of calcitonin gene-related peptide in jugular blood during migraine. *Annals of Neurology.* 2005; **58**: 561–8.
38. Lassen LH, Haderslev PA, Jacobsen VB *et al.* CGRP may play a causative role in migraine. *Cephalalgia.* 2002; **22**: 54–61.
39. Olesen J, Diener HC, Hustedt IW *et al.* BIBN 4096 BS Clinical Proof of Concept Study Group. Calcitonin gene-related peptide receptor antagonist BIBN 4096 BS for the acute treatment of migraine. *New England Journal of Medicine.* 2005; **350**: 1104–10.
40. Mitsikostas DD, Thomas AM. Comorbidity of headache and depressive disorders. *Cephalagia.* 1999; **19**: 211–17.
41. Holroyd KA, France JL, Nash JM, Hursey KG. Pain state as artefact in the psychological assessment of recurrent headache sufferers. *Pain.* 1993; **53**: 229–35.
42. Janke EA, Holroyd KA, Romanek K. Depression increases onset of tension-type headache following laboratory stress. *Pain.* 2004; **111**: 230–8.
43. Bendtsen L, Treede RD. Sensitization of myofascial pain pathways in tension-type headaches. In: Olesen J, Goadsby PJ, Ramadan N (eds). *The headaches*, 3rd edn. Philadelphia: Lippincott Williams & Wilkins, 2005: 635–9.
44. Ashina S, Babenko L, Jensen R *et al.* Increased muscular and cutaneous pain sensitivity in cephalic region in patients with chronic tension-type headache. *European Journal of Neurology.* 2005; **12**: 543–9.
45. Christensen M, Bendtsen L, Ashina M, Jensen R. Experimental induction of muscle tenderness and headache in tension-type headache patients. *Cephalalgia.* 2005; **25**: 1061–7.
46. Ashina M, Stallknecht B, Bendtsen L *et al.* Tender points are not sites of ongoing inflammation – *in vivo* evidence in patients with chronic tension-type headache. *Cephalalgia.* 2003; **23**: 109–16.
47. Ashina S, Bendtsen L, Ashina M. Pathophysiology of tension-type headache. *Current Pain and Headache Reports.* 2005; **9**: 415–22.
48. Ashina S, Bendtsen L, Ashina M *et al.* Evidence for generalized muscular and cutaneous hyperalgesia in patients with chronic tension-type headache. *Cephalalgia.* 2006; **26**: 940–8.
49. Schmidt-Wilcke T, Leinisch E, Straube A *et al.* Gray matter decrease in patients with chronic tension type headache. *Neurology.* 2005; **65**: 1483–6.
50. Bendtsen L. Central sensitization in tension-type headache-possible pathophysiological mechanisms. *Cephalalgia.* 2000; **20**: 486–508.
51. May A, Bahra A, Buchel C *et al.* Hypothalamic activation in cluster headache attacks. *Lancet.* 1998; **352**: 275–8.
52. Wöber-Bingöl C, Wöber C, Zeiler K *et al.* Tension headache and the cervical spine – plain X-ray findings. *Cephalalgia.* 1992; **12**: 152–4.
53. Zwart JA. Neck mobility in different headache disorders. *Headache.* 1997; **37**: 6–11.
54. Jensen R, Bendtsen L, Olesen J. Muscular factors are of importance in tension-type headache. *Headache.* 1998; **38**: 10–17.
55. Wang SJ, Silberstein SD, Patterson S, Young WB. Idiopathic intracranial hypertension without papilledema: a case-control study in a headache centre. *Neurology.* 1998; **51**: 245–9.
56. Skau M, Brennum J, Gjerris F, Jensen R. What is new about idiopatic intracranial hypertension? An updated review of mechanism and treatment. *Cephalalgia.* 2006; **26**: 384–99.
57. Rapoport A, Stann P, Gutterman DL *et al.* Analgesic rebound headache in clinical practice: data from a physician survey. *Headache.* 1996; **36**: 14–19.
58. Schnieder P, Aull S, Baumgartner C *et al.* Long-term outcome of patients with headache and drug abuse after inpatient withdrawal: five year follow-up. *Cephalalgia.* 1996; **16**: 481–5.
59. Zeeberg P, Olesen J, Jensen R. Efficacy of multidisciplinary treatment in a tertiary referral headache centre. *Cephalalgia.* 2005; **25**: 1159–67.
60. Zeeberg P, Olesen J, Jensen R. Probable medication-overuse headache: effect of a 2-month drug-free period. *Neurology.* 2006; **66**: 1894–8.
61. Tfelt-Hansen P, Rolan P. Nonsteroidal antiinflammatory drugs in the acute treatment of migraine. In: Olesen J, Goadsby PJ, Ramadan NM *et al.* (eds). *The headaches*, 3rd edn. Philadelphia: Lippincott Williams & Wilkins, 2006: 449–57.
62. Saxena PR, Tfelt-Hansen P. Triptans, 5HT1B/1D agonists in the acute treatment of migraine. In: Olesen J, Goadsby PJ, Ramadan NM *et al.* (eds). *The headaches*, 3rd edn. Philadelphia: Lippincott Williams & Wilkins, 2006: 469–503.
63. Mathew N, Tfelt-Hansen P. General and pharmacological approach to management of migraine. In: Olesen J, Goadsby PJ, Ramadan NM *et al.* (eds). *The headaches*, 3rd edn. Philadelphia: Lippincott Williams & Wilkins, 2006: 433–40.
64. Tfelt-Hansen P, Young WB, Silberstein SD. Antiemetics, prokinetics, neuroleptic and miscellaneous drugs in the acute treatment of migraine. In: Olesen J, Goadsby PJ, Ramadan NM *et al.* (eds). *The headaches*, 3rd edn. Philadelphia: Lippincott Williams & Wilkins, 2006: 505–13.
65. Tfelt-Hansen P, De Vries P, Saxena PR. Triptans in migraine. A comparative review of pharmacology, pharmacokinetics and efficacy. *Drugs.* 2000; **60**: 1259–87.
66. Tfelt-Hansen P. A review of evidence-based medicine and meta-analytic reviews in migraine. *Cephalalgia.* 2006; **26**: 1265–74.
67. Lainez MJ, Galvan J, Heras J, Vila C. Crossover, double-blind clinical trial comparing almotriptan an ergotamine plus caffeine for acute migraine therapy. *European Journal of Neurology.* 2007; **14**: 269–75.
68. Diener HC, Bussone G, de Liang H *et al.* Placebo-controlled comparison of effervescent acetylsalicylic acid,

sumatriptan and ibuprofen in the treatment of migraine attacks. *Cephalalgia.* 2004; **24**: 947–54.

69. Tfelt-Hansen P. Triptans vs. other classes of migraine medication. *Cephalalgia.* 2006; **26**: 628.
70. Tfelt-Hansen P, Saxena PR. Ergot alkaloids in the acute treatment of migraine. In: Olesen J, Goadsby PJ, Ramadan NM *et al.* (eds). *The headaches*, 3rd edn. Philadelphia: Lippincott Williams & Wilkins, 2006: 459–67.
71. Ibraheem JJ, Paalzow L, Tfelt-Hansen P. Low bioavailability of ergotamine tartrate after oral and rectal administration in migraine patients. *British Journal of Clinical Pharmacology.* 1983; **16**: 695–9.
72. Tfelt-Hansen P, Saxena PR, Dahlof C *et al.* Ergotamine in the acute treatment of migraine – European Consensus. *Brain.* 2000; **123**: 9–18.
73. Humphrey PP, Feniuk W, Perren MJ *et al.* The pharmacology of the novel 5-HT1-like agonist GR43175. *Cephalalgia.* 1989; **9**: 23–33.
74. Plosker GL, McTavish D. Sumatriptan. A reappraisal of its pharmacology and therapeutic efficacy in the acute treatment of migraine and cluster headache. *Drugs.* 1994; **47**: 622–51.
75. Ferrari MD, Saxena PR. Clinical and experimental effect of sumatriptan in humans. *Trends in Pharmacological Sciences.* 1993; **14**: 129–33.
76. Ahn AH, Goadsby PJ. Animal models of headache. In: Olesen J, Goadsby PJ, Ramadan NM *et al.* (eds). *The headaches*, 3rd edn. Philadelphia: Lippincott Williams & Wilkins, 2006: 213–19.
77. Gomez-Mancilla B, Cutler NR, Leibowitz MT *et al.* Safety and efficacy of PNU-142633, a selective 5-HT1D agonist, in migraine. *Cephalalgia.* 2001; **21**: 727–32.
78. Ferrari MD, Roon KI, Lipton RB, Goadsby PJ. Oral triptans (serotonin 5-$HT_{1B/1D}$ agonists) in acute migraine: a meta-analysis of 53 trials. *Lancet.* 2001; **358**: 1668–75.
79. Ferrari MD, Goadsby PJ, Roon KI, Lipton RB. Triptans (serotonin, 5-$HT_{1B/1D}$ agonists) in migraine: detailed results and methods of a meta-analysis of 53 trials. *Cephalalgia.* 2002; **22**: 633–58.
80. Diener HC, Ryan R, Sun W, Hettiarachchi J. The 40-mg dose of eletriptan: comparative efficacy and tolerability versus sumatriptan 100 mg. *European Journal of Neurology.* 2004; **11**: 125–34.
81. Tfelt-Hansen P, Henry P, Mulder K *et al.* The effectiveness of combined oral lysine acetylsalicylate and metoclopramide compared with oral sumatriptan for migraine. *Lancet.* 1995; **346**: 923–6.
82. Diener HC, Bussone G, de Liano H *et al.* EMSASI Study Group. Placebo-controlled comparison of effervescent acetylsalicylic acid, sumatriptan and ibuprofen in the treatment of migraine attacks. *Cephalalgia.* 2004; **24**: 947–54.
83. Diener HC, Eikerman A, Gessner U *et al.* Efficacy of 1,000 mg effervescent acetylsalicylic acid and sumatriptan in treating associated migraine symptoms. *European Neurology.* 2004; **52**: 50–6.
84. Mathew NT, Kailasam J, Meadors L. Early treatment of migraine with rizatriptan: a placebo-controlled study. *Headache.* 2004; **44**: 669–73.
85. Winner P, Landy S, Richardson M, Ames M. Early intervention in migraine with sumatriptan tables 50 mg versus 100 mg: a pooled analysis of data from six clinical trials. *Clinical Therapeutics.* 2005; **27**: 1785–94.
86. Carpay J, Schoenen J, Ahmad F *et al.* Efficacy and tolerability of sumatriptan tablets in a fast-disintegrating, rapid-release formulation for the acute treatment of migraine: results of a multicenter, randomized, placebo-controlled study. *Clinical Therapeutics.* 2004; **26**: 214–23.
87. Gaist D, Andersen M, Aarup AL *et al.* Use of sumatriptan in Denmark in 1994–5: an epidemiological analysis of nationwide prescription data. *British Journal of Clinical Pharmacology.* 1997; **43**: 429–33.
88. Gaist D, Tsiropoulos, Sindrup SH *et al.* Inappropriate use of sumatriptan: population based register and interview study. *BMJ.* 1998; **316**: 1352–3.
89. Diener HC, Silberstein SD. Medication overuse headaches. In: Olesen J, Goadsby PJ, Ramadan NM *et al.* (eds). *The headaches*, 3rd edn. Philadelphia: Lippincott Williams & Wilkins, 2006: 971–80.
90. Färkilä M, Olesen J, Dahlöf C *et al.* Eletriptan for the treatment of migraine in patients with a previous poor response or tolerance to oral sumatriptan. *Cephalalgia.* 2003; **23**: 463–71.
91. Mathew N, Schoenen J. Acute pharmacotherapy of tension-type headache. In: Olesen J, Tfelt-Hansen P, Welch KMA (eds). *The headaches*, 2nd edn. Philadelphia: Lippincott, Williams & Wilkins, 2000: 661–6.
92. Steiner TJ, Lange R, Voelker M. Aspirin in episodic tension-type headache: a placebo-controlled dose-ranging comparison with paracetamol. *Cephalagia.* 2003; **23**: 59–66.
93. Langemark M, Olesen J. Effervescent ASA versus solid ASA in the treatment of TTH. A double blind, placebo controlled study. *Headache.* 1987; **27**: 90–5.
94. Dahlhöf CGH, Jacobs LD. Ketoprofen, paracetamol and placebo in the treatment of episodic tension-type headache. *Cephalalgia.* 1998; **16**: 117–23.
95. Steiner TJ, Lange R. Ketoprofen (25 mg) in the symptomatic treatment of episodic tension-type headache: double blind placebo-controlled comparison with acetaminophen (1000 mg). *Cephalalgia.* 1998; **18**: 38–43.
96. Van Gerven JMA, Schoemaker RC, Jacobs LD *et al.* Self-medication of a single episode of tension-type headache with ketoprofen, ibuprofen and placebo, home-monitored with an electronic patient diary. *British Journal of Clinical Pharmacology.* 1996; **42**: 475–81.
97. Harden RN, Rogers D, Fink K, Gracely RH. Controlled trial of ketorolac in tension-type headache. *Neurology.* 1998; **50**: 507–09.
98. Bove G, Nielsson N. Spinal manipulation in the treatment of episodic tension-type headache. A randomized controlled trial. *JAMA.* 1998; **280**: 1576–9.

99. Evers S, Afra J, Frese A *et al.* (Members of the task force). EFNS guidelines on the drug treatment of migraine – report of an EFNS task force. *European Journal of Neurology.* 2006; **13**: 560–72.
100. Silberstein SD, Tfelt-Hansen P. Antiepileptic drugs in migraine prophylaxis. In: Olesen J, Tfelt-Hansen P, Goadsby PJ *et al.* (eds). *The headaches*, 3rd edn. Philadelphia: Lippincott Williams & Wilkins, 2006: 545–51.
101. Toda N, Tfelt-Hansen P. Calcium antagonists in migraine prophylaxis. In: Olesen J, Goadsby PJ, Ramadan NM *et al.* (eds). *The headaches*, 3rd edn. Philadelphia: Lippincott Williams & Wilkins, 2006: 539–44.
102. Tfelt-Hansen P, Rolan P. β-Adrenoceptor blocking drugs in migraine prophylaxis. In: Olesen J, Goadsby PJ, Ramadan NM *et al.* (eds). *The headaches*, 3rd edn. Philadelphia: Lippincott Williams & Wilkins, 2006: 519–28.
103. Tfelt-Hansen P, Saxena PR. Antiserotonin drugs in migraine prophylaxis. In: Olesen J, Tfelt-Hansen P, Goadsby PJ *et al.* (eds). *The headaches*, 3rd edn. Philadelphia: Lippincott Williams & Wilkins, 2006: 529–37.
104. Tfelt-Hansen P. Prioritizing prophylactic treatment of migraines. In: Olesen J, Goadsby PJ, Ramadan NM *et al.* (eds). *The headaches*, 3rd edn. Philadelphia: Lippincott Williams & Wilkins, 2006: 567–8.
105. Tronvik E, Stovner LJ, Helde G *et al.* Prophylactic treatment of migraine with an angiotensin II receptor blocker: a randomized controlled trial. *JAMA.* 2003; **289**: 65–9.
106. Mylecharane EJ, Tfelt-Hansen P. Nonsteroidal antiinflammatory and miscellaneous drugs in migraine prophylaxis. In: Olesen J, Tfelt-Hansen P, Welch KMA (eds). *The headaches*, 2nd edn. Philadelphia: Lippincott Williams & Wilkins, 2000: 489–98.
107. Bendtsen L, Mathew N. Prophylactic pharmacotherapy of tension-type headache. In: Olesen J, Goadsby PJ, Ramadan NM *et al.* (eds). *The headaches*, 3rd edn. Philadelphia: Lippincott Williams & Wilkins, 2006: 735–42.
108. Bendtsen L, Jensen R, Olesen J. A nonselective (amitriptyline), but not a selective (citalopram), serotonin reuptake inhibitor is effective in the prophylactic treatment of chronic tension-type headache. *Journal of Neurology, Neurosurgery, and Psychiatry.* 1996; **61**: 285–90.
109. Bendtsen L. Efficacy of antidepressants in headache prophylaxis. In: Olesen J, Silberstein P (eds). *Preventive pharmacotherapy of headache disorders*, 12th edn. New York: Oxford University Press, 2004: 103–11.
110. Cerbo R, Barbananti P, Fabbrini G *et al.* Amitriptyline is effective in chronic but not in episodic tension-type headache: pathogenic implications. *Headache.* 1998; **38**: 453–7.
111. Oguzhanoglu A, Sahiner T, Kurt T, Akalin O. Use of amitriptyline and fluoxetine in the prophylaxis of migraine and tension-type headaches. *Cephalalgia.* 1999; **19**: 531–2.
112. Bendtsen L, Jensen R. Mirtazapine is effective in the prophylactic treatment treatment of chronic tension-type headache. *Neurology.* 2004; **62**: 1706–11.
113. Bendtsen L, Buchgreitz L Ashina S, Jensen R. Combination of low-dose mirtazapine and ibuprofen for prophylaxis of chronic tension-type headache. *European Journal of Neurology.* 2007; **14**: 187–93.
114. Hammill JM, Cook TM, Rosecrane JC. Effectiveness of a physical therapy regimen in the treatment of tension-type headache. *Headache.* 1996; **36**: 149–53.
115. Jensen R, Olesen J. Is there an effect of physiotherapy in tension-type headache? *Cephalalgia.* 1995; **15**: 152.
116. Torelli P, Jensen R, Olesen J. Physiotherapy for tension-type headache: a controlled study. *Cephalalgia.* 2004; **24**: 29–36.
117. Evers S, Olesen J. Botulinum toxin in headache treatment: the end of the road? *Cephalalgia.* 2006; **26**: 769–71.
118. Silberstein SD, Göbel H, Jensen R *et al.* Botulinum toxin type A in the prophylactic treatment of chronic tension-type headache: a multicentre, double-blind, randomized, placebo-controlled, parallel-group study. *Cephalalgia.* 2006; **26**: 790–800.
119. Sandrini G, Ward TN. Acute treatment of cluster headaches. In: Olesen J, Goadsby PJ, Ramadan NM *et al.* (eds). *The headaches*, 3rd edn. Philadelphia: Lippincott Williams & Wilkins, 2006: 803–07.
120. van Vielt JA, Bahra A, Martin V *et al.* Intranasal sumatriptan in cluster headache: randomized, double-blind placebo-controlled study. *Neurology.* 2003; **60**: 630–3.
121. Cittadini E, May A, Straube A *et al.* Effectiveness of intranasal zolmitriptan in acute cluster headache: a randomized, placebo-controlled, double-blind crossover study. *Archives of Neurology.* 2006; **63**: 1537–42.
122. Leone M, Rapoport A. Preventive and surgical management of cluster headache. In: Olesen J, Goadsby PJ, Ramadan NM *et al.* (eds). *The headaches*, 3rd edn. Philadelphia: Lippincott Williams & Wilkins, 2006: 809–14.
123. Ambrosini A, Vandenheede M, Rossi P *et al.* Suboccipital injection with a mixture of rapid-and long-acting steroids in cluster headache: a double-blind placebo-controlled study. *Pain.* 2005; **118**: 92–6.

35

Facial pain

PETER SVENSSON AND LENE BAAD-HANSEN

KEY LEARNING POINTS

- Facial pain problems are common and cover a wide variety of chronic pain problems.
- Facial pain problems share many of the same pathophysiological mechanisms with chronic pain in other parts of the body, but there are some salient differences.
- Diagnosis of facial pain should always include a comprehensive examination of the orofacial region to exclude dental pain conditions.
- Management of facial pain follows similar guidelines as for other chronic pain problems, except for some specific dental procedures and treatment of trigeminal neuralgia.

INTRODUCTION

Facial pain is encountered by a high percentage of the population and has special biological, emotional, and psychological meaning to the patient because of the special role of the orofacial region in vital functions, such as chewing, swallowing, talking, and expression of emotions. In addition, facial pain may lead to emotional and social consequences for the patient and others and represent an increasing socioeconomic burden as the population changes with more people being middle-aged or elderly, the age span in which many chronic facial pain conditions are prevalent. This chapter will describe the most common facial pain conditions that general practitioners and dentists will encounter in their clinic. Thus, the chapter is not an exhaustive review of all chronic facial pain conditions and the reader is referred to more specialized textbooks for more detailed information.[1, 2, 3]

TEMPOROMANDIBULAR DISORDERS

Temporomandibular disorders (TMD) are not a single entity but rather a cluster of related pain conditions in the masticatory muscles, temporomandibular joint (TMJ), and associated structures, i.e. an orofacial musculoskeletal pain condition. A nonhierarchical classification scheme based on operationalized and systematic criteria has been developed and extensively tested for reliability and validity.[4, 5, 6] These research diagnostic criteria (RDC/TMD) (**Table 35.1**) have indeed been essential for the initiation of extensive international collaborations and new clinical research in TMD pain and can also rationally be applied in daily clinical practice.

Diagnoses of, for example, muscle contracture, muscle spasm, myositis and other less frequent painful conditions in the masticatory muscles, are not possible in this classification scheme. In a similar way, various mechanical problems in the TMJ, for example ankylosis, disk–condyle

Table 35.1 Axis I of the RDC/TMD.

Axis I. Biomedical/physical status
I. Muscle diagnoses
a. Myofascial pain
b. Myofascial pain with limited opening
II. Disk displacements
a. Disk displacement with reduction
b. Disk displacement without reduction, with limited opening
c. Disk displacement without reduction, without limited opening
III. Arthralgia, arthritis, arthrosis
a. Arthralgia
b. Osteoarthritis of the TMJ
c. Osteoarthrosis of the TMJ

There is also an axis II which describes pain-related disability and psychological status. Modified from Ref. 4.

derangements, hypermobility, and capsular fibrosis, have not been included in the RDC/TMD mainly because such conditions are rare.[7]

Epidemiology

Epidemiological studies have indicated that between 3 and 15 percent of the population will qualify for a TMD pain diagnosis.[8, 9] Few studies have tried to separate TMJ pain from myofascial TMD pain, but the latter appears to be less prevalent than the former.[9] Most studies have, however, found that TMD pain is 1.5–2 times more prevalent in women, but it is critical to distinguish between the number of TMD cases presenting in the clinic and the number of TMD cases in the community, because treatment-seeking patterns and use of health services may bias a biological sex difference.[10, 11] The prevalence of TMD across the lifetime is still debated but there seems to be a peak around 20–45 years for women, although elderly people may also suffer from TMD pain.[12, 13] For some types of TMD problems such as osteoarthrosis, there seems to be an increase over the life span. There are few good studies on the incidence of TMD pain problems, but there is some evidence that the incidence is in the range of 2–4 percent with the persistent types being around 0.1 percent.[9] Some longitudinal studies have shown substantial variations in the time course of myofascial TMD[14] with 31 percent being persistent over a five-year period, 33 percent being remittent, and 36 percent recurring. Asymptomatic clicks in the TMJ (disk displacement with reduction (DDwR)) are very common (10–35 percent),[8, 15] but have been shown to very rarely progress to disk displacement without reduction (DDwoR), in fact none of the 114 adolescents that were followed over a nine year period progressed from DDwR to DDwoR.[15] Interestingly, this study also indicated major fluctuations in the presence and absence of a DDwR so that only 2 percent of the examined population had a consistent click at all examination points during the nine year study period.[15] This strongly indicates that asymptomatic DDwR should be managed by conservative techniques. Other studies have shown that patients with combined diagnosis of DDwR and arthralgia may have a higher risk to progress to a DDwoR.[16, 17]

Symptomatology

Classicially, three cardinal symptoms of TMD are mentioned: (1) pain in the masticatory muscle and/or joints; (2) sounds from the TMJ (clicks, crepitation); and (3) changes in mandibular movements, usually as restriction in jaw-opening capacity. Pain is moderate to intense, can vary during the day, often with exacerbations during jaw-movements such as chewing and wide opening.[18] The quality of myofascial TMD pain is a deep ache, tender and taut, which can be diffuse and difficult for the patient to pinpoint. The pain is often associated with referred pains to the TMJ, ear, temple, and teeth.[19] TMJ pain is more localized around the TMJ with a sharp component and pain referrals to the ear region. Both the masticatory muscles and the TMJ will be painful on manual palpation. Clicking in the TMJ is not a problem in itself but can sometimes be unpleasant for the patient and cause irregularities during jaw-opening and closing. The disk in the TMJ can also cause a limitation in the maximal opening-capacity, in particular in acute conditions. In addition, the oral health-related quality of life is impaired in most TMD pain patients.[20]

There are no specific diagnostic tests for TMD pain and electronic measures of jaw movements and sounds cannot be recommended in clinical settings.[21] Thus, the diagnosis is based on a systematic history and clinical examination, e.g. with the use of the RDC/TMD.

Pathophysiology

The exact pathophysiology of TMD pain is not known, given the fact that multiple factors related to anatomical, psychological-psychosocial, and neurobiological components seem to be involved.[22] Thus, on a population basis, TMD may still be viewed as multifactorial conditions, which in the individual patient actually means an idiopathic pain condition.[11, 23]

One of the most prominent features of painful TMDs is the report of pain on palpation of jaw muscles or TMJ. Several studies have, indeed, reported lower pressure pain thresholds in the jaw muscles of patients with TMD pain compared to normal subjects.[24, 25, 26, 27] The pathophysiological mechanism responsible for lower pain thresholds in deep tissues could be a sensitization of peripheral nociceptors. Animal data have documented that deep noxious inputs cause sensitization of the peripheral receptors.[28, 29] Thus, endogenous substances released by tissue trauma such as bradykinin, serotonin, prostaglandins, adrenaline, and hypoxia, in addition to the excitatory amino acid glutamate, lower the mechanical threshold of nociceptors into the innocuous range making weak stimuli able to excite nociceptors and elicit pain.[30, 31, 32]

Patients with myofascial TMD pain have also been found to have hyperalgesic responses to segmental, as well as extrasegmental, application of thermal heat, although this may less often be a clinical problem.[27] Temporal summation mechanisms and wind-up phenomena in central neurons could be strongly related to the development of central hyperexcitability.[33, 34] This indicates that patients with persistent TMD pain are in a state of generalized central hyperexcitability. Dysfunction of the nociceptive system is also implicated by the finding of suppression of cortical responses and brain stem reflexes elicited by painful laser stimulation of the skin in TMD patients.[35] Furthermore, ischemic pain models have been used to demonstrate a less effective activation of endogenous pain-inhibitory systems in TMD patients.[36] In particular, female TMD patients appear unable to effectively engage the normal pain-inhibitory systems[37] and it has been suggested that opioid receptor desensitization and/or down-regulation could be involved.[38] Catechol-O-methyl transferase (COMT) activity has been linked to experimental pain sensitivity, and it appears that the three major haplotypes which determine COMT activity in humans are inversely correlated with pain sensitivity and the risk of developing TMD.[39, 40] Recently, variations in the adrenergic receptor beta (2) (ADRB2) has also been suggested to be a genetic risk factor for the development of TMD pain.[41, 42] Taken together, the pain studies cited above suggest that a more generalized state of neuronal hyperexcitability is likely to play an important role in TMD patients.[43] Thus, peripheral sensitization of deep craniofacial tissues alone may not be adequate to explain persistent TMD pain.

Differential diagnosis

Spontaneous pain or pain on jaw movement is a characteristic and necessary feature for the diagnosis of myofascial TMD pain. Patient-based drawings of their typical pain patterns demonstrate a concentration around the masseter muscle and spreading towards the anterior part of the temporalis muscle.[44] When patients with episodic or chronic tension-type headache (TTH) draw the location of their typical pain, the lower part of the face, including the masseter muscle, is usually spared, whereas there is a significant occurrence of pain in the neck and pericranial regions.[45] These findings imply that different muscles and structures are involved in myofascial TMD pain and TTH. TMD and TTH disorders do overlap and appear to share many of the same pathophysiological mechanisms; however, it would be premature to consider them as identical entities since the importance of, for example, the affected muscles and associated function in addition to genetic background factors need to be further examined.[44]

Rheumatoid arthritis and other systemic manifestations of arthritis (psoriatic or infectious arthritis) may also affect the TMJ. Differential diagnosis will be based on history, blood tests, and magnetic resonance imaging (MRI) of the TMJ.

A number of more generalized pain conditions such as fibromyalgia, whiplash-associated disorders, low-back pain, and general joint laxity have been found to be comorbid with TMD pain conditions.[46, 47] These conditions should be taken into consideration in the management strategy and calls for the involvement of healthcare providers other than dentists.

Management and prognosis

When the underlying mechanisms and etiology of TMD pain are only known in part (see under Differential diagnosis) it is difficult to perform causal therapy and cure the pain and dysfunction. Instead, a more realistic goal will be to alleviate TMD pain and restore function.

It is a common clinical experience that various physical strategies (e.g. stretching, relaxation, etc.) can be effective for the management of different types of TMD pain. Unfortunately, it has been much more difficult to support this with proper research data adhering to randomized controlled trial (RCT) principles. Critical reviews and meta-analysis have, however, started to appear to evaluate the claimed efficacy of the procedures.[48, 49][III] There have been attempts to calculate the number needed to treat (NNT) values for oral splints. The available NNT estimates range between three and four for management of myofascial TMD patients and around five and six for TMJ arthralgia patients,[50] suggesting a moderate efficacy of oral splints.[51, 52][I] Very recently, another controlled study compared the conventional hard splint with a soft splint and a usual self-care-based treatment approach.[53] This study failed to show any significant differences between the three different treatment groups and all patients improved over time which suggests that oral splints are not essential in the management of most TMD patients and that low-cost nonsplint self-care therapy should be considered as an initial step in the management.

Nonsteroidal anti-inflammatory drugs (NSAIDs) such as ibuprofen in combination with diazepam have been shown to provide significantly better pain relief compared to ibuprofen alone and placebo in myofascial TMD pain patients.[54][II] However, naproxen (500 mg twice a day) is significantly better than celecoxib (100 mg twice a day) and placebo for the management of TMJ arthralgia.[55][II] A short-acting benzodiazepine (triazolam) has also been shown to improve sleep but failed to provide significant pain relief in myofascial TMD patients.[56][II] Cyclobenzaprine (a muscle relaxant) has been shown to have a minor but significant effect on jaw-muscle pain upon awakening[57][II] and it has been suggested that flupirtine (another muscle relaxant), with its additional effects on potassium channels and membrane-stabilizing actions, may be useful in management of myofascial TMD pain.[58] [V] A combination of paracetamol, codeine, and doxylamine succinate (antihistamine) provided significantly greater pain relief than placebo in another study on mixed TMD patients.[59][III] Also, low doses of tricyclic antidepressants (TCA) have been shown to provide significantly better pain relief than placebo.[60][III] Open studies later supported the usefulness of TCAs in the management of persistent TMD pain.[61][IV] Intra-articular morphine (0.1–1.0 mg) administered as a single dose has been shown to increase the pressure pain thresholds and mouth opening capacity and to reduce the visual analog scale (VAS) pain intensity. However, the clinical relevance of these findings was not impressive.[62] [II] The use of botulinum toxin for myofascial TMD pain cannot be recommended at present due to inconclusive evidence.[63, 64][II] Recently, evidence was presented in favor of gabapentin in the management of myofascial TMD pain and tenderness.[65][II] There is clearly a need for more research before firm recommendations of specific pharmacological procedures in the management of TMD pain conditions can be given since there is only scattered, reliable information on the efficacy of most of the suggested drugs.[66]

There is nevertheless good evidence that self-care instructions and monitoring can provide at least as good pain relief as usual dental approaches to TMD pain and that in more severely affected patients the inclusion of comprehensive care provided by a clinical psychologist will provide a significant advantage compared to the usual dental treatment.[67, 68][II] It appears to be important to tailor the treatment to each individual patient and not consider psychological interventions of TMD pain as a treatment of last resort, but rather use it concurrently with biomedical/dental treatments.[69] Recently, it was shown that a brief cognitive-behavioral treatment program was, indeed, able to significantly reduce catastrophizing and increase perceived control over pain and improve activity interferences and jaw use limitations.[70] [II] The current guidelines recommend reversible and noninvasive management of TMD pain.

NEUROPATHIC OROFACIAL PAIN

Traumatic stimuli, such as mechanical, thermal, or chemical, to trigeminal nerve branches can lead to primary lesions which may, on rare occasions, be associated with neuropathic orofacial pain (NOP). In fact, the trigeminal system seems to have unique features compared to the spinal system with respect to its propensity to develop neuropathic pain following a nerve injury.[71] There are unfortunately no operationalized criteria for the diagnosis of NOP, but a hierarchical system for general neuropathic pain conditions has been proposed[72] and is currently being adjusted for NOP and tested.[73] In this paragraph, emphasis is on procedures and trauma which potentially may induce NOP, although many other diseases can also cause lesions to the nervous system, for example autoimmune diseases, metabolic diseases, infections, vascular diseases, and cancer.

Epidemiology

Extraction of a tooth or a root canal treatment is in fact a deafferentation of the nerve supply to the tooth pulp. Fortunately, these procedures, which are still common in dental practice due to advanced caries and periodontitis,[74, 75] only carry a very small risk for development of NOP. It can be speculated that the presence of chronic infections and inflammatory reactions in the tooth pulp or periapical region may in some cases increase the risk but there are no systematic data available on this topic.

Third molar surgery is another very common procedure in dental practice and it has been estimated that between 4 and 6 percent of patients undergoing third molar surgery will have sensory disturbances in the inferior alveolar or lingual nerves after one week, but these numbers drop down to 0.7–1 percent after two years.[76] Other reports suggest that only about 1 per 2500 lower third molar extractions will be associated with permanent injuries to the inferior alveolar nerve.[77] Thus, most trigeminal nerve injuries are reversible and do not necessarily lead to NOP but stringent criteria for assessment of neurosensory deficits and NOP need to be applied.

Orthognathic surgery is increasingly used for corrections of the basal relationships between the jaws and for alignment of the occlusion in younger adults (20–30 years). It is a well-established fact that a significant proportion of the patients undergoing osteotomies on either the maxilla or mandible suffer injuries to the maxillary or mandibular divisions of the trigeminal nerve. Depending on the specific type of osteotomy, age of the patients, intraoperative variables such as magnitude of movements of bony segments, and assessment techniques of somatosensory disturbances, prevalence data vary between 10 and 85 percent.[78] However, it is important that only a small percentage (~5 percent) of all the patients will eventually develop NOP.[79]

Dental injections also carry a risk for the development of NOP. The proposed mechanisms of nerve lesions are direct trauma from the injection needle, formation of hematoma, or neurotoxicity of the local anesthetics.[80] The risk is, however, very low and estimates predict 1 out of 26,762 mandibular blocks with approximately one-third experiencing dysesthesia or NOP symptoms. On the other hand, since dental injections are so frequently used to control procedural-related pains in clinical dentistry, every dentist working full-time can expect to see one or two patients with this kind of complication.[81]

Zygomatico-orbital fractures are one of the most common facial injuries and occur in about 1 in 10,000 people with frequent (~50 percent) involvement of the sensory function of the infraorbital nerve.[82] However, only a small proportion (<3–4 percent) of patients with zygomatic arch fractures appears to develop chronic NOP.[82]

In addition, the frequent use of oral implants and other surgical procedures, for example on the salivary glands, may also contribute to risk for trigeminal nerve injuries.[83]

In summary, although a great number of dental procedures and facial injuries carry a significant risk to impede the trigeminal nerve branches, it seems that only relatively few patients will end up with a manifest NOP condition.

Symptomatology

Patients with NOP often complain of a constant burning pain starting with a clear traumatic onset. Although burning is a frequent word used to describe the pain, other words like dull aching or sharp and shooting are commonly reported. In addition to the spontaneous pain, there is frequently stimulus-evoked pain triggered mainly by mechanical stimuli, for example touching the skin or oral mucosa or intensified by normal oral functions, such as chewing, talking, and jaw-opening. Unfortunately, there are no universal criteria for NOP which significantly hampers the description of clinical characteristics.[84]

Clinical findings are rare. There are no visible signs of inflammation and only in very rare cases may there be swelling and reddening of the facial skin or oral mucosa possibly mimicking complex regional pain syndromes.[85]

One of the hallmark findings in NOP may be changes in somatosensory function. The use of quantitative sensory testing (QST) has revealed a number of somatosensory disturbances with both hypo- and hyperesthesia. According to the criteria suggested, there should be complete or partial sensory loss in the painful area, but these areas could potentially be masked by hyperphenomona from the surrounding areas.[86] It should be noted that although a number of QST techniques are available for intraoral use, there are no widely accepted guidelines for the standardized assessment of intraoral sensitivity which varies substantially from region to region and with type, thickness, and vascularization of the tissues. However, in the painful facial areas of patients with NOP, increased temperature and tactile thresholds have been demonstrated in addition to abnormal temporal summation of painful stimuli.[87] Relatively few QST studies are available,[83, 88] but there seems to be a trend that not all NOP patients have sensory disturbances and that there can be modality-specific differences.[73] This therefore suggests that a comprehensive battery of QST techniques should be used.[89, 90]

Advanced electrophysiological tests may be of help. For example, the blink reflex and recording of sensory nerve action potentials may provide important diagnostic information about the integrity of the trigeminal nerve fibers[83] (**Figure 35.1**). In addition, laser-evoked potentials and other brain stem reflexes can be used.[91]

Pathophysiology

The underlying pathophysiology of NOP involves the same basic mechanisms linked with lesions of the spinal nerves.[86, 92, 93] In brief, the mechanisms involved in an injury to a peripheral nerve can be summarized as sensitization of the primary afferent due to up-regulation of sodium-channels and ectopic activity. As a consequence there is an increased release of glutamate and activation of *N*-methyl-D-aspartic acid (NMDA) receptors and metabotropic glutamate receptors on second order neurons. A cascade of intracellular events will lead to spontaneous discharges and reduced thresholds, increased responses to peripheral stimuli, and expansion of receptive fields, i.e. central sensitization. In addition, loss of inhibitory control can be a consequence of the altered trafficking of impulses.[86] Evidence also points to the importance of microglia and the interaction between somatic afferent fibers and sympathetic activity.[94, 95] Despite the similarities in the responses to damage of trigeminal and spinal nerve fibers, there are a few noticeable differences. For example, the time course of recovery appears to be faster in the trigeminal system, autonomic responses differ so there is no sprouting of sympathetic terminals on the trigeminal ganglion cells, and the neuropeptide content and the specific patterns of up- and down-regulation of the sodium channel family appear to be different between the trigeminal and spinal system.[96, 97, 98] The importance of these differences is not established, but could contribute to the apparent higher resistance of the trigeminal system to develop a manifest NOP.

Differential diagnosis

First of all, dental types of pain must be ruled out (see under Dental pain). Also, inflammatory conditions such as sinusitis or sialoadenitis must be excluded. The most troublesome differential diagnosis is atypical odontalgia and atypical facial pain. The discriminating factor has been suggested to be disturbances in somatosensory

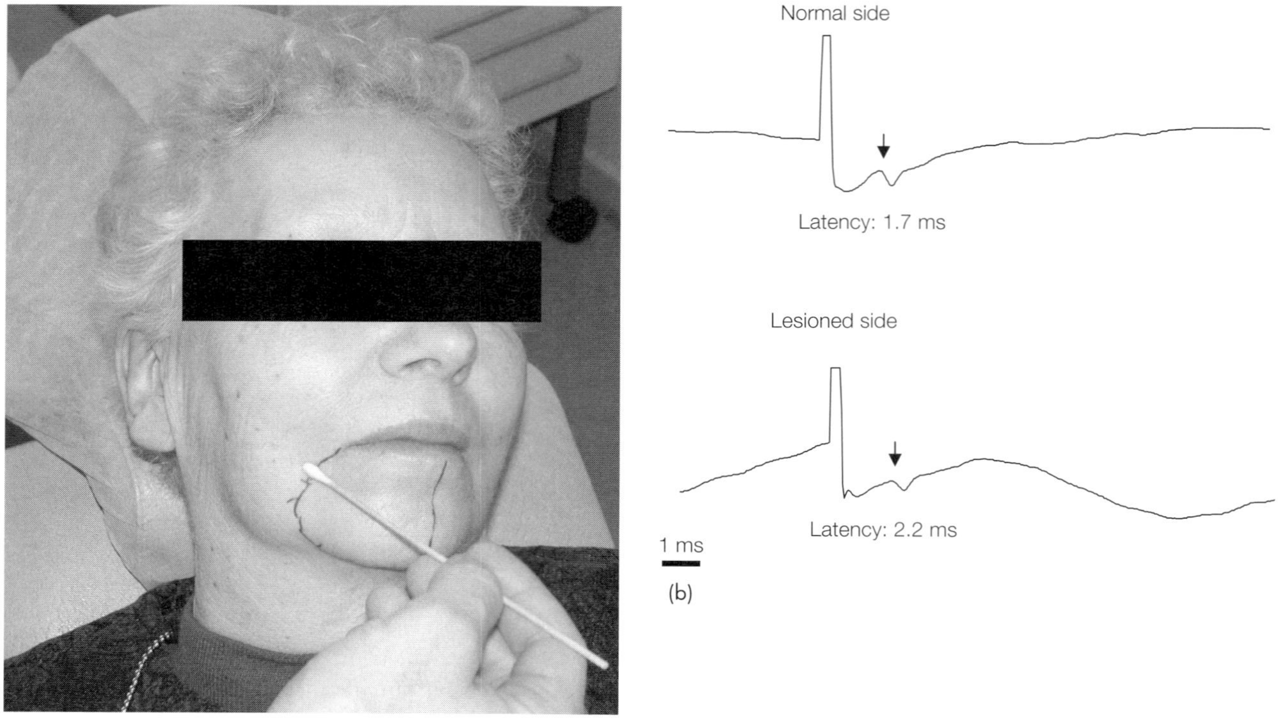

(a)

Figure 35.1 (a) Patient with definite neuropathic orofacial pain after injection trauma to the inferior alveolar nerve. One year after the injection there is a discrete area with loss of sensation and a paradoxical hypersensitivity to light tactile stimuli (allodynia) (marked area). (b) Recording of sensory nerve action potentials from the inferior alveolar nerve revealed longer latency on the ipsilateral side compared to the contralateral normal side (Reference values: mean 1.5 ± 0.2 ms; 95 percent confidence interval 1.3–1.9 ms; from Jaaskelainen *et al.*[83]).

function, but recent studies have indeed suggested disturbances in atypical odontalgia.[99] Trigeminal neuralgia must also be considered but the symptomatology is usually very different.

Management and prognosis

There are relatively few controlled clinical trials on the specific management of NOP, but generally the same principles and guidelines for other neuropathic pain conditions should be followed. Thus, low doses of tricyclic antidepressants would be the first choice.[100][I] Antiepileptics, such as gabapentin and pregabalin, would be second choices followed by opioids and tramadol and selective serotonin reuptake inhibitors.[100][I] Capsaicin and other topical formulations such as lidocaine patches have been reported to be efficient in some NOP conditions, but mainly in open trials. The advantage of topical medication is the potential to reduce the side effects but so far there is only relatively limited evidence for their efficacy.[85, 101][III] An important point is to avoid further trauma to the area, for example by avoiding further explorative oral surgery.

TRIGEMINAL NEURALGIA

Trigeminal neuralgia (TN) is defined by the International Association for the Study of Pain (IASP) as a sudden, usually unilateral, brief stabbing recurrent pain in the distribution of one of more branches of the trigeminal nerve. TN is usually divided into classical or idiopathic TN and symptomatic or secondary TN. For classical trigeminal neuralgia (CTN), there is no apparent cause other than vascular compression (see under Pathophysiology), whereas for symptomatic trigeminal neuralgia (STN) there are structural lesions, for example multiple sclerosis or compression of the posterior fossa.[102]

Epidemiology

CTN is considered a rare facial pain conditions with a prevalence of around 0.7–1/1000. Women are more often affected than men, F:M ratio = 1.7–2.2:1, and the annual incidence is between two and six people per 100,000. Typically, CTN is diagnosed in elderly patients with a peak incidence around 50–60 years. In contrast, there seems to be no sex-related differences for STN and the onset age is slightly younger. An intriguing finding without explanation is the fact that the right side is more often affected than the left side, both in CTN and STN.[102, 103]

Symptomatology

The diagnosis of TN can often be derived from the patient history alone. The intensity of the pain is severe, lasting a few seconds and with pain-free intervals in which the pain cannot be provoked (refractory period). Multiple attacks (paroxysms) can be evoked by gently touching the facial skin or oral mucusa, for example during chewing or brushing teeth. It is characteristic that the paroxysmal pain can be provoked from distinct areas (trigger zones) located in one or more divisions of the trigeminal nerve and most often only ipsilateral.[103] There is some debate as to whether thermal stimuli are sufficient to provoke the pain, but light tactile and mechanical stimuli are usually described. There is also a periodicity to the pain so there can be pain-free intervals of weeks or months. Words like "shooting," "electric-shock-like," "sharp," and "stabbing" are often used and the McGill Pain Questionnaire can provide important information in this respect. In addition, TN is often associated with poor quality of life, weight loss, depression, and problems related to chewing.[104]

Somatosensory deficits are not characteristic in the clinical work up of patients, but quantitative sensory tests have been able to demonstrate damage of nerve fiber populations leading to hypoesthesia.[105] However, in the individual patient, the QST results do not have major diagnostic implications. Electrophysiological tests, such as laser-evoked potentials and trigeminal somatosensory tests, have also been used and have demonstrated subtle changes in the processing of sensory inputs.[91]

MRI techniques and angiography are now considered the best options to image the trigeminal ganglion and the adjacent vessels.[106] In approximately two-thirds of patients with CTN there is an intimate relationship between the ganglion and the vessels. However, it is also clear that the neurovascular contact is not always associated with TN.[107]

Pathophysiology

The classical explanation for CTN is the so-called neurovascular contact between the root entry zone of the trigeminal nerve and, in particular, the superior cerebellar artery.[107] In support of this explanation are biopsies from TN patients showing axonal swelling and demyelination. As a consequence of the loss of myelin, ephaptic activity and high-frequency discharges of touch-transmitting axons to nociceptive axons can lead to the paroxysms of pain. The fact that not all patients with CTN have a demonstrable neurovascular conflict and that patients who do appear to have a neurovascular conflict do not have CTN has led to some doubts about this as the universal explanation for TN.

Devor *et al.*[108] have promoted the "ignition hypothesis" based on an up-regulation of ion channels in response to an injury of the trigeminal nerve. Another possibility to be discussed is the involvement of the secondary neurons in the trigeminal sensory nuclear complex and that central sensitization may be part of the pathophysiological mechanisms.[102]

Differential diagnosis

The correct diagnosis of TN is important because there are specific treatments related to this condition (see under Management and prognosis). A number of orofacial pain conditions can be mistaken for TN. The most common will be dental types of pain in their acute stage. Therefore, it is mandatory to rule out dental pathology using clinical examination radiographs in order to avoid unnecessary tooth extractions. Atypical facial pain or atypical odontalgia (persistent idiopathic facial pain) can also mimic TN, but usually the pain is more constant/persistent without paroxysms characteristic for TN. Sinusitis and acute ear infections (otitis externa, otitis media) also need to be ruled out by the general history and examination.

Management and prognosis

Carbamazepine has been used extensively in the management of TN and with good success. Several meta-analyses are available and generally agree that about 70 percent of patients will benefit from therapeutic doses (100–2400 mg).[100][I] The NNT value is accordingly good in the range of 1.8 (1.3–2.2 95 percent confidence interval). However, side effects are frequently observed such as allergic rash, hyponatremia, and numerous drug interactions, so elderly patients in particular must be monitored carefully. A second choice may be oxcarbazepine which also has been documented to be effective in a number of RCT studies.[100][I] Other options are lamotrigene, baclofen, and topiramate.[103]

Surgery may be an option if pharmacological management provides insufficient pain relief. Microvascular decompression provides good pain relief in the majority of the patients over a longer period of time with approximately three-quarters of patients being pain-free three years after surgery.[107] A number of other ablative surgical techniques are available but generally do not provide similar long-term pain relief and are associated with significant disturbances in the facial sensory function.

PERSISTENT IDIOPATHIC FACIAL PAIN

A condition called persistent idiopathic facial pain has been described in *The International Classification of Headache Disorders*, 2nd edition, by The International Headache Society (IHS).[109] This term covers the diagnoses atypical facial pain (AFP) and atypical odontalgia (AO). Burning mouth syndrome (BMS) is separate from AFP and AO in the IHS classification but is often grouped together with these conditions and sometimes also with TMD as being so-called idiopathic, i.e. medically unexplained orofacial pain conditions.[84, 110, 111]

Atypical facial pain

The IHS describes AFP as a "persistent facial pain that does not have the characteristics of the cranial neuralgias... and is not attributed to another disorder."

EPIDEMIOLOGY

Reliable prevalence and incidence data on AFP are presently not available,[112] but it is believed to be more frequent than trigeminal neuralgia (0.7/100,000) and less common than temporomandibular disorders (10–12 percent).[110] A preponderance of middle-aged or older women is often reported in studies on AFP.

SYMPTOMATOLOGY

The symptoms of AFP are usually described by the patient as deep, poorly localized pain in the mid-face but the pain can also be superficial.[113] The pain is mostly unilateral but approximately one-third of the patients experience bilateral pain. At onset, the pain is confined to a defined zone of the face, e.g. the nasolabial groove. Later, the pain spreads in a way that often does not follow the distribution of a peripheral nerve.[114] The pain is present every day for most of the day and is not associated with somatosensory loss.[109] The pain quality of AFP has been reported to be diffuse, drawing, burning, stabbing, or throbbing and with emotional terms as vicious and excruciating.[113, 115, 116] The pain may debut after surgery or injury to the face but persists after healing without signs of pathology.

Importantly, it is a diagnostic criterion whereby investigations such as an x-ray of face and jaw and clinical examination do not demonstrate any relevant abnormality.[109] Hence, an AFP diagnosis is based on exclusion of local orofacial disease, neurological disorders, etc. Therefore, an AFP diagnosis can only follow a thorough clinical examination of the mouth including the teeth and nearby structures, palpation of the masticatory and cervical muscles, examination of the temporomandibular joints, examination of possible sinus pathology, and a cranial nerve examination.

A high level of comorbidity in AFP patients has been reported. Especially, psychiatric comorbidity has been emphasized but also the presence of additional pain conditions, for example headache and back pain.[111]

PATHOPHYSIOLOGY

The etiology of AFP is largely unknown, although some risk factors have been suggested.[117] These risk factors include psychological factors, hormonal factors, minor nerve trauma, and infection of the sinuses or teeth.[117] None of these risk factors can be considered the sole etiological factor. The high level of psychiatric comorbidity has led to the assumption that AFP is secondary to mental illness, for example depression.[111] However, whether AFP pain is secondary to mental illness, or *vice versa*, can be very difficult to determine. Furthermore, the large proportion of middle-aged women suffering from AFP has aroused the suspicion that AFP could be caused or worsened by a deficiency or imbalance in female sex hormones.[117] At present, a widely discussed hypothesis is that AFP is neuropathic in origin, which could explain the temporal relationship between debut of AFP and the history of trauma or surgery in or near the painful region.

DIFFERENTIAL DIAGNOSES

During examination of a patient with chronic facial pain, many different pain conditions, for example dental pain, must be ruled out in order for the patient to receive a diagnosis of AFP. Sometimes, diagnostic local anesthetic blocks can be useful when dental pathology is suspected to cause the facial pain. Pain originating from the maxillary sinuses often cause pain in the mid-facial region and can be ruled out by nasal endoscopy, x-ray, or computed tomography (CT) of the sinuses. Examination of the masticatory muscles and the temporomandibular joint with palpation over joint and muscles, as well as evaluation of jaw function can reveal the presence of TMD. TN can usually be distinguished from AFP by the symptomatology. Trigeminal neuralgia patients are pain-free most of the time and suffer from attacks with short-lasting, shock-like pain paroxysms (see under Trigeminal neuralgia), whereas AFP pain is constant and non-paroxysmal. Furthermore, TN, and not AFP, is characterized by the presence of trigger-points.[118] Some forms of primary headaches may also present with symptoms like AFP and, hence, must be excluded. As can be seen, the diagnostic process is multidisciplinary involving, for example, family practitioners, dentists, otorhinolaryngologists, and neurologists.

Examination of trigeminal sensory function with QST in combination with neurophysiological testing of sensory nerve conduction velocity or brain stem reflexes has been shown to increase the sensitivity to detect trigeminal neural pathology.[119] Also, MRI examination is recommended in order to exclude the possibility that the pain can be caused by intracranial pathology.[120]

MANAGEMENT AND PROGNOSIS

The management of AFP can be challenging. AFP patients are reported to consult multiple healthcare professionals in order to obtain pain relief.[113] Many unnecessary invasive treatments, which may possibly aggravate the symptoms, are performed because of this.

The first step in management of carefully diagnosed AFP is patient education. The patient may need help in order to accept the fact that there is no infection or "bad tooth" that can be easily treated or extracted. The next step is pharmacological treatment where the first choice is TCAs such as amitriptyline.[60, 117][V] Treatment with TCA must be continued for several months since the analgesic effect can take weeks to occur. When pain relief has been reached, TCA treatment can be phased out, but if the pain returns it may be necessary to continue TCA treatment.[121] Anticonvulsants such as gabapentin may also have some effect.[101, 117][V] Unfortunately, not many randomized controlled clinical trials have been performed. Surgery has been reported to cause pain aggravation and should only be performed after the confirmed presence of pathology, for example a periapical granuloma. Other types of treatments such as acupuncture, transcutaneous electric nerve stimulation (TENS), and biofeedback have been mentioned as possible treatment strategies, but the evidence in favor is scarce.[121][V]

Atypical odontalgia

The IHS considers AO as a subgroup of persistent idiopathic facial pain, i.e. "persistent facial pain that does not have the characteristics of the cranial neuralgias and is not attributed to another disorder."[109] The IHS states that "the term AO has been applied to a continuous pain in the teeth or in a tooth socket after extraction in the absence of any identifiable cause."[109] AO has also been called "phantom tooth pain"[122, 123] or idiopathic toothache.[124]

EPIDEMIOLOGY

As with AFP, no reliable data on incidence or prevalence exist in the literature but it has been estimated to occur in 3–6 percent of patients undergoing endodontic treatment.[125, 126] Both sexes and all adult ages can be affected with a predominance of women in their mid-40s.[127]

SYMPTOMATOLOGY

As mentioned under Atypical odontalgia, AO pain is perceived in a tooth or in a tooth socket after extraction of the tooth. Some diagnostic criteria for AO have been proposed as follows: pain has been ongoing for more than six months, is present every day during most of the day, and is not paroxysmal in character. No signs of pathology are present in clinical and radiological examinations.[110] The pain is often reported to occur after dental or surgical treatments and the patients have typically seen five to six different specialists before being referred to a specialized pain clinic.[122, 124]

PATHOPHYSIOLOGY

The precise pain mechanisms behind AO are presently unknown but hypotheses much like those of AFP have been put forward, i.e. psychogenic pain, vascular pain, or neuropathic pain.[127] As with AFP, many AO patients suffer from psychiatric or psychological comorbidity but it is not considered causal for AO pain. At present, the prevailing hypothesis is that AO is a neuropathic pain condition.[128, 129] Recently, some studies have aimed at investigating possible pain mechanisms behind AO. Fairly subtle changes in somatosensory sensitivity and the blink reflexes have been reported in AO patients compared with healthy controls, lending some support for the neuropathic hypothesis.[99, 130, 131]

DIFFERENTIAL DIAGNOSES

The differential diagnoses for AO are the same as for AFP.

MANAGEMENT AND PROGNOSIS

Management of AO is performed as management of AFP. Recently, an RCT was published evaluating the effect of fentanyl (a μ-opioid agonist) and S-ketamine (an NMDA-receptor antagonist) on AO pain and capsaicin-evoked pain in a placebo-controlled manner. Fentanyl effectively reduced evoked pain, but none of the two active drugs alleviated AO pain more effectively than placebo, indicating that opioid- and NMDA-receptors are not promising targets in the treatment of AO (**Figure 35.2**).[132][II]

Burning mouth syndrome

The IHS describes BMS as "an intraoral burning sensation for which no medical or dental cause can be found."[109] Other terms, such as glossodynia, glossopyrosis, stomatodynia, sore mouth, and oral dysesthesia, have been used in the past for this condition.

EPIDEMIOLOGY

Prevalence estimates on BMS range from 0.7[133] to 15 percent,[134] but the highest estimates may be due to

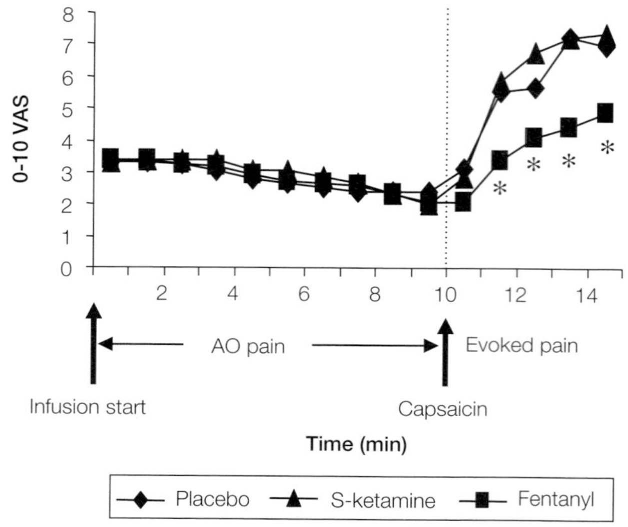

Figure 35.2 Mean effect of fentanyl and S-ketamine on atypical odontalgia (AO) pain and capsaicin-evoked pain ($n = 10$). *Indicate significant different from placebo and S-ketamine ($p \leq 0.05$).

including burning mouth as a symptom rather than a syndrome.[112] BMS prevalence increases with age and women aged 60–69 have the highest prevalence (12 percent).[135, 136]

SYMPTOMATOLOGY

BMS is characterized by daily pain in the mouth, sometimes with dysesthetic qualities, persisting for most of the day. Most often, BMS patients complain about a moderate to severe burning pain located to the tongue, palate, lips, or gingiva.[136, 137] The oral mucosa is of normal appearance and no pathology can be detected.[109] Symptoms are usually bilateral, but can be unilateral. This burning pain can be associated with taste changes and a subjective feeling of dry mouth.[136] Many patients wake up with negligible symptoms in the morning and experience a build up of symptoms during the day.[138] Others describe constant pain during the day and some only have intermittent symptoms.

The presence of emotional and psychological issues has been the focus of many of the earlier investigations on BMS and it has been shown that BMS patients have a high occurrence of depression, anxiety, somatization, and personality disorders.[138]

PATHOPHYSIOLOGY

The etiology and pathophysiology of BMS is presently unknown, although several hypotheses have been put forward. Hence, BMS belongs to the group of idiopathic orofacial pain conditions, although recent studies have demonstrated (subclinical) sensory changes and abnormal brain stem reflex responses,[137, 139, 140] which suggests a dysfunction in the peripheral or central nervous system, either in the form of a neuropathic or a "functional" pain condition.[137, 141] A psychogenic etiology has also been suggested, but is generally not accepted as a causal factor for BMS.

DIFFERENTIAL DIAGNOSES

Like AFP and AO, BMS is a diagnosis of exclusion. Burning pain symptoms in the oral mucosa can be caused by systemic or local conditions, including anemia, vitamin B, folic acid, or iron deficiency, untreated diabetes, hormonal disturbances (menopausal complaints, estrogen deficiency), oral candidiasis, hyposalivation, Sjögren's syndrome, oral lichen planus, or systemic lupus.[136, 142] Furthermore, burning symptoms can be a side effect to some medications such as angiotensin-converting enzyme (ACE) inhibitors and also allergy to dental materials, dentures, toothpaste, etc., must be considered and excluded before a BMS diagnosis can be given.[136, 142]

MANAGEMENT AND PROGNOSIS

When a BMS diagnosis has been reached after exclusion of local or systemic causes for the symptoms, the first management step is patient education and information. Avoidance of spicy and acidic foods is recommended and some patients experience pain relief while sucking pastilles.[142] In a recent Cochrane review, pharmacological treatment of BMS was evaluated with disappointing results.[143] Antidepressants (such as amitriptyline) or other systemic drugs (trazodone, paroxetine, clordemetildiazepam, amisulprid) were not found to be more effective in symptom alleviation than placebo. Topical clonazepam has been shown to be able to reduce pain in patients with BMS.[144][II]

DENTAL PAIN

Dental pain is very common and is usually an acute phenomenon. It rarely becomes chronic if treated appropriately. A short presentation of dental pain conditions will be provided in this chapter since it is a relevant differential diagnosis to most of the other facial pains.

Epidemiology

Prevalence estimates range from 7 to 66 percent, depending on the specific criteria used for the classification of dental pain and, importantly, the population studied.[145]

Symptomatology

Numerous conditions can produce dental pain. The most frequent local causes of dental pain are dental caries, dentine hypersensitivity, cracked-tooth-syndrome (dental infractions), reversible and irreversible pulpitis, apical periodontitis with and without abscess, postoperative dental pain, and transient pain from dental procedures. Pain can also quite frequently be referred from structures outside the mouth, for example the maxillary sinuses, the masticatory muscles, or the heart (during angina pectoris). Less frequently, dental pain can be part of the symptomatology of trigeminal neuralgia (see under Trigeminal neuralgia) and various headache conditions.[11]

Dentine hypersensitivity is a common clinical problem where patients experience sharp or shooting pain in a tooth as a result of mechanical or thermal stimulation of the dentinal surface. Dentine hypersensitivity most often occurs in the cervical and root areas of the tooth.[146] Cracked-tooth-syndrome refers to an incomplete fracture of a vital tooth that may extend into the pulp. The symptoms are a sharp pain evoked by chewing and is relieved by removing the pressure from the tooth.[147] The pain is poorly localized and the radiographic examination does not reveal pathology.

Patients with acute irreversible pulpitis complain about intense pain induced by temperature changes caused by ingestion of hot or cold drinks or food, or pain may occur spontaneously without any obvious provoking stimulus.[148] Pulpitis pain often disturbs sleep and over-the-counter analgesics may not be effective in relieving the pain. If there is no spontaneous pain, the pulpitis may be reversible.

Apical periodontitis is often asymptomatic, but symptoms when present are pain, tooth elevation, sensitivity to percussion, and swelling.[146]

Pathophysiology

Pulpitis pain is caused by inflammation in the tooth pulp. The inflammatory condition causes changes in the pulpal nociceptors and their central connections,[149] thereby resulting in changes in pain quality and response to external stimuli.[150] The inflammation can be a response to a deep carious lesion and the inflammatory mediators in the pulp cause sensitization of the pulpal nociceptors.[148] Furthermore, neurovascular reactions occur with branching and sprouting of nerve terminals, increased pulpal blood flow, increased vascular permeability, and extravasation of fluid and plasma proteins.[151, 152, 153]

Dentine hypersensitivity is believed to be caused by hydrodynamic activation of the intradental A-fibers.[148] This hydrodynamic activation is caused by any stimulus capable of removal of fluid from the outer part of the dentinal tubules, which results in an outward flow in the dentinal tubule due to capillary forces.[154]

Apical periodontitis is an inflammatory condition of the periapical periodontium, most often caused by necrosis of the tooth pulp, which leads to accumulation of bacteria, bacterial products, and inflammatory mediators in the root canal. This spreads into the periapical tissues.[146] A host defense is initiated with inflammatory cells, intercellular mediators, metabolites, effector molecules, and humoral antibodies.[155]

Differential diagnoses

A thorough dental examination is always performed if a patient presents with dental pain. If no pathological findings can be found in the clinical or radiological examination, alternative causes of the pain should be considered and diagnosed if present. One of the most frequent nonodontogenic conditions to present as dental pain is sinusitis, which may cause pain and sensitivity to percussion of one or more of the upper premolars and molars. Another common type pain, which can be referred to the teeth, is myofascial pain of the masticatory muscles.

Importantly, most pain of dental origin is acute and rarely persists for more than a few days or weeks at worst. This fact differentiates dental pain from the pain conditions, which are the main focus of this chapter.

Management and prognosis

Cracked-tooth-syndrome is managed by the application of a band around the tooth or a temporary crown. If this does not relieve the pain, endodontic treatment or extraction may be necessary.[147]

Reversible pulpitis can be treated by prescription of an NSAID for relief of the pain due to inflammation of the pulp. Definitive treatment consists of removal of the stimulus that is evoking the pain, such as treating the carious lesion. This condition does not require treatment with antibiotics or opioid analgesics.[147]

Treatment for irreversible pulpitis consists of endodontic treatment (removal of the inflamed pulp tissue) and prescription of analgesics, either NSAIDs or paracetamol with 30 mg of codeine, one to two tablets every four to six hours as needed for pain. Systemic administration of antibiotics is not indicated.[147][V]

Dentine hypersensitivity can be quite difficult to manage. Treatment consists mainly of application of fluoride gel or a desensitizing agent to the hypersensitive tooth surface.[147, 156][III]

Apical pariodontitis also requires endodontic treatment (removal of the necrotic tooth pulp and bacteria). If an abscess is present, it must be drained and systemic antibiotics may be indicated. Surgical removal of the periapical granuloma can be performed if proper healing is not obtained by endodontic treatment.

SUMMARY

The present chapter has highlighted some of the most common facial pain conditions which the general physician and dentist need to be aware of in order to reach the correct diagnosis and initiate the most rational therapy. Due to the complexity of many facial pain conditions and the special emotional and psychological meaning of the orofacial region, the diagnostic work up and management strategy will often require a substantial interdisciplinary approach between the medical profession, dentists, and specialists in orofacial pain, neurology, anesthesiology, and psychology. As for most chronic pain conditions, a careful history and standardized clinical examination must be performed, but attention has also been directed towards the application of additional diagnostic tests, such as QSTs and electrophysiological recordings. Evidence-based guidelines for the management of chronic facial pain conditions are relatively scarce but the general principles for documentation of efficacy are, more recently, also being applied to the facial pain conditions. Indeed, there will be the need in future studies to examine the efficacy of interventions tailored to the trigeminal system.

REFERENCES

* 1. Okeson JP. *Bell's orofacial pains*. Hanover Park, IL: Quintessence Books, 2005.

* 2. Zakrzewska JM, Harrison SD (eds). *Pain research and clinical management. Assessment and management of orofacial pain*. London: Elsevier, 2002.

3. Turp JC, Sommer C, Hugger A (eds). *The Puzzle of orofacial pain. Pain and headache*. Basel: Karger, 2007.

* 4. Dworkin SF, LeResche L. Research diagnostic criteria for temporomandibular disorders: review, criteria, examinations and specifications, critique. *Journal of Craniomandibular Disorders*. 1992; **6**: 301–55.

5. Pehling J, Schiffman E, Look J *et al.* Interexaminer reliability and clinical validity of the temporomandibular index: a new outcome measure for temporomandibular disorders. *Journal of Orofacial Pain*. 2002; **16**: 296–304.

6. John MT, Dworkin SF, Mancl LA. Reliability of clinical temporomandibular disorder diagnoses. *Pain*. 2005; **118**: 61–9.

7. Stegenga B. Osteoarthritis of the temporomandibular joint organ and its relationship to disc displacement. *Journal of Orofacial Pain*. 2001; **15**: 193–205.

8. LeResche L. Epidemiology of temporomandibular disorders: implications for the investigation of etiologic factors. *Critical Reviews in Oral Biology and Medicine*. 1997; **8**: 291–305.

9. Drangsholt M, LeResche L. Temporomandibular disorder pain. In: Crombie IK, Croft PR, Linton SJ (eds). *Epidemiology of pain*. Seattle: IASP Press, 1999: 203–33.

10. Warren MP, Fried JL. Temporomandibular disorders and hormones in women. *Cells, Tissues, Organs*. 2001; **169**: 187–92.

* 11. Svensson P, Sessle BJ. Orofacial pain. In: Miles TS, Nauntofte B, Svensson P (eds). *Clinical oral physiology*. Hanover Park, IL: Quintessence, 2004: 93–139.

12. Riley JL, Gilbert GH, Heft MW. Orofacial pain symptom prevalence: selective sex differences in the elderly? *Pain*. 1998; **76**: 97–104.

13. Schmitter M, Rammelsberg P, Hassel A. The prevalence of signs and symptoms of temporomandibular disorders in very old subjects. *Journal of Oral Rehabilitation*. 2005; **32**: 467–73.

14. Rammelsberg P, LeResche L, Dworkin S, Mancl L. Longitudinal outcome of temporomandibular disorders: a 5-year epidemiologic study of muscle disorders defined by research diagnostic criteria for temporomandibular disorders. *Journal of Orofacial Pain*. 2003; **17**: 9–20.

15. Kononen M, Waltimo A, Nystrom M. Does clicking in adolescence lead to painful temporomandibular joint locking? *Lancet*. 1996; **347**: 1080–1.

16. Lundh H, Westesson PL, Kopp S. A three-year follow-up of patients with reciprocal temporomandibular joint clicking. *Oral Surgery, Oral Medicine, Oral Pathology*. 1987; **63**: 530–3.

17. Sato S, Goto S, Nasu F, Motegi K. Natural course of disc displacement with reduction of the temporomandibular joint: changes in clinical signs and symptoms. *Journal of Oral and Maxillofacial Surgery*. 2003; **61**: 32–4.

18. van Grootel RJ, van der Glas HW, Buchner R *et al.* Patterns of pain variation related to myogenous temporomandibular disorders. *Clinical Journal of Pain*. 2005; **21**: 154–65.

19. Svensson P, Graven-Nielsen T. Craniofacial muscle pain: review of mechanisms and clinical manifestations. *Journal of Orofacial Pain*. 2001; **15**: 117–45.

20. John MT, Reissmann DR, Schierz O, Wassell RW. Oral health-related quality of life in patients with temporomandibular disorders. *Journal of Orofacial Pain*. 2007; **21**: 46–54.

21. Baba K, Tsukiyama Y, Yamazaki M, Clark GT. A review of temporomandibular disorder diagnostic techniques. *Journal of Prosthetic Dentistry*. 2001; **86**: 184–94.

22. De Boever JA, Carlsson GE. Etiology and differential diagnosis. In: Zarb GA, Carlsson GE, Sessle BJ, Mohl ND (eds). *Temporomandibular joint and masticatory muscle disorders*. Copenhagen: Munksgaard, 1994: 171–87.

23. Green CS. The etiology of temporomandibular disorders: implications for treatment. *Journal of Orofacial Pain*. 2001; **15**: 93–105.

24. Reid KI, Gracely RH, Dubner RA. The influence of time, facial side, and location on pain-pressure thresholds in chronic myogenous temporomandibular disorder. *Journal of Orofacial Pain*. 1994; **8**: 258–65.

25. Svensson P, List T, Hector G. Analysis of stimulus-evoked pain in patients with myofascial temporomandibular pain disorders. *Pain*. 2001; **92**: 399–409.

26. Maixner W, Fillingim R, Booker D, Sigurdsson A. Sensitivity of patients with painful temporomandibular disorders to experimentally evoked pain. *Pain.* 1995; **63**: 341–51.
27. Maixner W, Fillingim R, Sigurdsson A *et al.* Sensitivity of patients with painful temporomandibular disorders to experimentally evoked pain: evidence for altered temporal summation of pain. *Pain.* 1998; **76**: 71–81.
28. Berberich P, Hoheisel U, Mense S. Effects of carrageenan-induced myositis on the discharge properties of group III and IV muscle receptors in the cat. *Journal of Neurophysiology.* 1988; **59**: 1395–409.
29. Schaible HG. Basic mechanisms of deep somatic tissue. In: McMahon SB, Koltzenburg M (eds). *Wall and Melzack's textbook of pain.* Edinburgh: Churchill Livingstone, 2006: 621–34.
* 30. Graven-Nielsen T, Mense S. The peripheral apparatus of muscle pain: evidence from animal and human studies. *Clinical Journal of Pain.* 2001; **17**: 2–10.
31. Cairns BE, Hu JW, Arendt-Nielsen L *et al.* Sex-related differences in human pain perception and rat afferent discharge evoked by injection of glutamate into the masseter muscle. *Journal of Neurophysiology.* 2001; **86**: 782–91.
32. Cairns BE, Svensson P, Wang K *et al.* Activation of peripheral NMDA receptors contributes to human pain and rat afferent discharges evoked by injection of glutamate into the masseter muscle. *Journal of Neurophysiology.* 2003; **90**: 2098–105.
33. Arendt-Nielsen L. Induction and assessment of experimental pain from human skin, muscle, and viscera. In: Jensen TS, Turner JA, Wiesenfeld-Hallin Z (eds). *Proceedings of the 8th World Congress on Pain. Progress in Pain Research and Management*, Vol 8. Seattle: IASP Press, 1997: 393–425.
* 34. Woolf CJ, Salter MW. Plasticity and pain: role of the dorsal horn. In: McMahon SB, Koltzenburg M (eds). *Wall and Melzack's textbook of pain.* Edinburgh: Churchill Livingstone, 2006: 91–106.
35. Romaniello A, Cruccu G, Frisardi G *et al.* Assessment of nociceptive trigeminal pathways by laser-evoked potentials and laser silent periods in patients with painful temporomandibular disorders. *Pain.* 2003; **103**: 31–9.
36. Kashima K, Rahman OI, Sakoda S, Shiba R. Increased pain sensitivity of the upper extremities of TMD patients with myalgia to experimentally-evoked noxious stimulation: possibility of worsened endogenous opioid systems. *Cranio.* 1999; **17**: 241–6.
37. Zubieta JK, Smith YR, Bueller JA *et al.* mu-Opioid receptor-mediated antinociceptive responses differ in men and women. *Journal of Neuroscience.* 2002; **22**: 5100–07.
38. Bragdon EE, Light KC, Costello NL *et al.* Group differences in pain modulation: pain-free women compared to pain-free men and to women with TMD. *Pain.* 2002; **96**: 227–37.
* 39. Zubieta JK, Heitzeg MM, Smith YR *et al.* COMT val158met genotype affects mu-opioid neurotransmitter responses to a pain stressor. *Science.* 2003; **299**: 1240–3.
40. Diatchenko L, Slade GD, Nackley AG *et al.* Genetic basis for individual variations in pain perception and the development of a chronic pain condition. *Human Molecular Genetics.* 2005; **14**: 135–43.
41. Nackley AG, Tan KS, Fecho K *et al.* Catechol-O-methyltransferase inhibition increases pain sensitivity through activation of both beta2- and beta3-adrenergic receptors. *Pain.* 2007; **128**: 199–208.
* 42. Diatchenko L, Anderson AD, Slade GD *et al.* Three major haplotypes of the beta2 adrenergic receptor define psychological profile, blood pressure, and the risk for development of a common musculoskeletal pain disorder. *American Journal of Medical Genetics Part B Neuropsychiatric Genetics.* 2006; **141**: 449–62.
43. Sarlani E, Grace EG, Reynolds MA, Greenspan JD. Evidence for up-regulated central nociceptive processing in patients with masticatory myofascial pain. *Journal of Orofacial Pain.* 2004; **18**: 41–55.
44. Svensson P. Muscle pain in the head: overlap between temporomandibular disorders and tension-type headaches. *Current Opinion in Neurology.* 2007; **20**: 320–5.
45. Schmidt-Hansen PT, Svensson P, Bendtsen L *et al.* Increased muscle pain sensitivity in patients with tension-type headache. *Pain.* 2007; **129**: 113–21.
46. Aaron LA, Burke MM, Buchwald D. Overlapping conditions among patients with chronic fatigue syndrome, fibromyalgia, and temporomandibular disorder. *Archives of Internal Medicine.* 2000; **160**: 221–7.
47. John MT, Miglioretti DL, LeResche L *et al.* Widespread pain as a risk factor for dysfunctional temporomandibular disorder pain. *Pain.* 2003; **102**: 257–63.
* 48. Michelotti A, de Wijer A, Steenks M, Farella M. Home-exercise regimes for the management of non-specific temporomandibular disorders. *Journal of Oral Rehabilitation.* 2005; **32**: 779–85.
* 49. McNeely ML, Armijo Olivo S, Magee DJ. A systematic review of the effectiveness of physical therapy interventions for temporomandibular disorders. *Physical Therapy.* 2006; **86**: 710–25.
50. Forssell H, Kalso E. Application of principles of evidence-based medicine to occlusal treatment for temporomandibular disorders: are there lessons to be learned? *Journal of Orofacial Pain.* 2004; **18**: 9–22.
* 51. Forssell H, Kalso E, Koskela E *et al.* Occlusal treatments in temporomandibular disorders: a qualitative systematic review of randomized controlled trials. *Pain.* 1999; **83**: 549–60.
* 52. Al-Ani MZ, Davies SJ, Gray RJ *et al.* Stabilisation splint therapy for temporomandibular pain dysfunction syndrome. *Cochrane Database of Systematic Reviews.* 2004: **CD002778**.
53. Truelove E, Huggins KH, Mancl L, Dworkin SF. The efficacy of traditional, low-cost and nonsplint therapies for temporomandibular disorder: a randomized controlled trial. *Journal of the American Dental Association.* 2006; **137**: 1099–107.

54. Singer E, Dionne R. A controlled evaluation of ibuprofen and diazepam for chronic orofacial muscle pain. *Journal of Orofacial Pain.* 1997; **11**: 139–46.
55. Ta LE, Dionne RA. Treatment of painful temporomandibular joints with a cyclooxygenase-2 inhibitor: a randomized placebo-controlled comparison of celecoxib to naproxen. *Pain.* 2004; **111**: 13–21.
56. DeNucci DJ, Sobiski C, Dionne RA. Triazolam improves sleep but fails to alter pain in TMD patients. *Journal of Orofacial Pain.* 1998; **12**: 116–23.
57. Herman CR, Schiffman EL, Look JO, Rindal DB. The effectiveness of adding pharmacologic treatment with clonazepam or cyclobenzaprine to patient education and self-care for the treatment of jaw pain upon awakening: a randomized clinical trial. *Journal of Orofacial Pain.* 2002; **16**: 64–70.
58. Schindler H, Svensson P. Masticatory myofascial pain. In: Turp JC, Sommer C, Hugger A (eds). *The puzzle of orofacial pain. Pain and headache.* Basel: Karger, 2007.
59. Gerschman JA, Reade PD, Burrows GD. Evaluation of a proprietary analgesic/antihistamine in the management of pain associated with temporomandibular joint pain dysfunction syndrome. *Australian Dental Journal.* 1984; **29**: 300–04.
60. Sharav Y, Singer E, Schmidt E *et al.* The analgesic effect of amitriptyline on chronic facial pain. *Pain.* 1987; **31**: 199–209.
61. Plesh O, Curtis D, Levine J, McCall Jr WD. Amitriptyline treatment of chronic pain in patients with temporomandibular disorders. *Journal of Oral Rehabilitation.* 2000; **27**: 834–41.
62. List T, Tegelberg K, Haraldson T, Isacsson G. Intra-articular morphine as analgesic in temporomandibular joint arthralgia/osteoarthritis. *Pain.* 2001; **94**: 275–82.
63. Nixdorf DR, Heo G, Major PW. Randomized controlled trial of botulinum toxin A for chronic myogenous orofacial pain. *Pain.* 2002; **99**: 465–73.
64. von Lindern JJ, Niederhagen B, Berge S, Appel T. Type A botulinum toxin in the treatment of chronic facial pain associated with masticatory hyperactivity. *Journal of Oral and Maxillofacial Surgery.* 2003; **61**: 774–8.
65. Kimos P, Biggs C, Mah J *et al.* Analgesic action of gabapentin on chronic pain in the masticatory muscles: a randomized controlled trial. *Pain.* 2007; **127**: 151–60.
* 66. List T, Axelsson S, Leijon G. Pharmacologic interventions in the treatment of temporomandibular disorders, atypical facial pain, and burning mouth syndrome. A qualitative systematic review. *Journal of Orofacial Pain.* 2003; **17**: 301–10.
67. Dworkin SF, Turner JA, Mancl L *et al.* A randomized clinical trial of a tailored comprehensive care treatment program for temporomandibular disorders. *Journal of Orofacial Pain.* 2002; **16**: 259–76.
68. Dworkin SF, Huggins KH, Wilson L *et al.* A randomized clinical trial using research diagnostic criteria for temporomandibular disorders – axis II to target clinic cases for a tailored self-care TMD treatment program. *Journal of Orofacial Pain.* 2002; **16**: 48–63.
69. Sherman JJ, Turk DC. Nonpharmacologic approaches to the management of myofascial temporomandibular disorders. *Current Pain and Headache Reports.* 2001; **5**: 421–31.
70. Turner JA, Mancl L, Aaron LA. Brief cognitive-behavioral therapy for temporomandibular disorder pain: effects on daily electronic outcome and process measures. *Pain.* 2005; **117**: 377–87.
71. Bennett GJ. Neuropathic pain in the orofacial region: clinical and research challenges. *Journal of Orofacial Pain.* 2004; **18**: 281–6.
72. Kehlet H, Jensen TS, Woolf CJ. Persistent postsurgical pain: risk factors and prevention. *Lancet.* 2006; **367**: 1618–25.
73. Drangsholt M, Nguyen K, Svensson P. Systematic review of orofacial pain mechanisms: Which conditions are neuropathic? *Journal of Dental Research.* 2007: 261 (abstract).
74. Hiidenkari T, Parvinen T, Helenius H. Missing teeth and lost teeth of adults aged 30 years and over in south-western Finland. *Community Dental Health.* 1996; **13**: 215–22.
75. Baelum V, Van Palenstein Helderman W, Hugoson A *et al.* A global perspective on changes in the burden of caries and periodontitis: Implications for dentistry. *Journal of Oral Rehabilitation.* 2007; **34**: 872–906.
76. Jerjes W, Swinson B, Moles DR *et al.* Permanent sensory nerve impairment following third molar surgery: a prospective study. *Oral Surgery, Oral Medicine, Oral Pathology, Oral Radiology and Endodontics.* 2006; **102**: e1–7.
77. Robert RC, Bacchetti P, Pogrel MA. Frequency of trigeminal nerve injuries following third molar removal. *Journal of Oral and Maxillofacial Surgery.* 2005; **63**: 732–5.
78. Thygesen TH, Bardow A, Helleberg M *et al.* Risk factors affecting somatosensory function after sagittal split osteotomy. *Journal of Oral and Maxillofacial Surgery.* 2008; **66**: 469–74.
79. Jaaskelainen SK, Teerijoki-Oksa T, Virtanen A *et al.* Sensory regeneration following intraoperatively verified trigeminal nerve injury. *Neurology.* 2004; **62**: 1951–7.
80. Smith MH, Lung KE. Nerve injuries after dental injection: a review of the literature. *Journal of the Canadian Dental Association.* 2006; **72**: 559–64.
81. Pogrel MA, Thamby S. Permanent nerve involvement resulting from inferior alveolar nerve blocks. *Journal of the American Dental Association.* 2000; **131**: 901–07.
82. Benoliel R, Birenboim R, Regev E, Eliav E. Neurosensory changes in the infraorbital nerve following zygomatic fractures. *Oral Surgery, Oral Medicine, Oral Pathology, Oral Radiology and Endodontics.* 2005; **99**: 657–65.
* 83. Jaaskelainen SK, Teerijoki-Oksa T, Forssell H. Neurophysiologic and quantitative sensory testing in the diagnosis of trigeminal neuropathy and neuropathic pain. *Pain.* 2005; **117**: 349–57.
* 84. Woda A, Tubert-Jeannin S, Bouhassira D *et al.* Towards a new taxonomy of idiopathic orofacial pain. *Pain.* 2005; **116**: 396–406.

85. Lewis MA, Sankar V, De Laat A, Benoliel R. Management of neuropathic orofacial pain. *Oral Surgery, Oral Medicine, Oral Pathology, Oral Radiology and Endodontics.* 2007; **103** (Suppl. S32): e1–24.
86. Finnerup NB, Jensen TS. Mechanisms of disease: mechanism-based classification of neuropathic pain – a critical analysis. *Nature Clinical Practice Neurology.* 2006; **2**: 107–15.
87. Eide PK, Rabben T. Trigeminal neuropathic pain: pathophysiological mechanisms examined by quantitative assessment of abnormal pain and sensory perception. *Neurosurgery.* 1998; **43**: 1103–10.
88. Renton T, Thexton A, Crean SJ, Hankins M. Simplifying the assessment of the recovery from surgical injury to the lingual nerve. *British Dental Journal.* 2006; **200**: 569–73.
* 89. Svensson P, Baad-Hansen L, Thygesen T *et al.* Overview on tools and methods to assess neuropathic trigeminal pain. *Journal of Orofacial Pain.* 2004; **18**: 332–8.
90. Rolke R, Baron R, Maier C *et al.* Quantitative sensory testing in the German Research Network on Neuropathic Pain (DFNS): standardized protocol and reference values. *Pain.* 2006; **123**: 231–43.
91. Cruccu G, Biasiotta A, Galeotti F *et al.* Diagnosis of trigeminal neuralgia: a new appraisal based on clinical and neurophysiological findings. *Supplements to Clinical Neurophysiology.* 2006; **58**: 171–86.
92. Baron R. Mechanisms of disease: neuropathic pain – a clinical perspective. *Nature Clinical Practice Neurology.* 2006; **2**: 95–106.
93. Campbell JN, Meyer RA. Mechanisms of neuropathic pain. *Neuron.* 2006; **52**: 77–92.
94. Marchand F, Perretti M, McMahon SB. Role of the immune system in chronic pain. *Nature Reviews Neuroscience.* 2005; **6**: 521–32.
* 95. Devor M. Responses of nerves to injury in relation to neuropathic pain. In: McMahon SB, Koltzenburg M (eds). *Wall and Melzack's textbook of pain.* Edinburgh: Churchill Livingstone, 2006: 905–28.
96. Fried K, Bongenhielm U, Boissonade FM, Robinson PP. Nerve injury-induced pain in the trigeminal system. *Neuroscientist.* 2001; **7**: 155–65.
97. Eriksson J, Jablonski A, Persson AK *et al.* Behavioral changes and trigeminal ganglion sodium channel regulation in an orofacial neuropathic pain model. *Pain.* 2005; **119**: 82–94.
98. Davies SL, Loescher AR, Clayton NM *et al.* Changes in sodium channel expression following trigeminal nerve injury. *Experimental Neurology.* 2006; **202**: 207–16.
99. Baad-Hansen L, List T, Jensen TS, Svensson P. Increased pain sensitivity to intraoral capsaicin in patients with atypical odontalgia. *Journal of Orofacial Pain.* 2006; **20**: 107–14.
*100. Attal N, Cruccu G, Haanpaa M *et al.* EFNS guidelines on pharmacological treatment of neuropathic pain. *European Journal of Neurology.* 2006; **13**: 1153–69.
*101. Clark GT. Persistent orodental pain, atypical odontalgia, and phantom tooth pain: when are they neuropathic disorders? *Journal of the Californian Dental Association.* 2006; **34**: 599–609.
102. Truini A, Galeotti F, Cruccu G. New insight into trigeminal neuralgia. *Journal of Headache and Pain.* 2005; **6**: 237–9.
*103. Zakrzewska JM. Trigeminal neuralgia. In: Zakrzewska JM, Harrison SD (eds). *Pain research and clinical management. Assessment and management of orofacial pain.* London: Elsevier, 2002: 267–370.
104. de Siqueira SR, da Nobrega JC, Teixeira MJ, de Siqueira JT. Masticatory problems after balloon compression for trigeminal neuralgia: a longitudinal study. *Journal of Oral Rehabilitaion.* 2007; **34**: 88–96.
105. Nurmikko TJ. Altered cutaneous sensation in trigeminal neuralgia. *Archives of Neurology.* 1991; **48**: 523–7.
106. Satoh T, Onoda K, Date I. Fusion imaging of three-dimensional magnetic resonance cisternograms and angiograms for the assessment of microvascular decompression in patients with hemifacial spasms. *Journal of Neurosurgery.* 2007; **106**: 82–9.
107. Zakrzewska JM, Lopez BJ. Trigeminal and glossopharyngeal neuralgia. In: McMahon SB, Koltzenburg M (eds). *Wall and Melzack's textbook of pain.* Edinburgh: Churchill Livingstone, 2006: 1001–10.
108. Devor M, Amir R, Rappaport ZH. Pathophysiology of trigeminal neuralgia: the ignition hypothesis. *Clinical Journal of Pain.* 2002; **18**: 4–13.
*109. International Classification of Headache Disorders, 2nd edn. *Cephalalgia.* 2004; **24** (Suppl. 1): 9–160.
*110. Woda A, Pionchon P. A unified concept of idiopathic orofacial pain: clinical features. *Journal of Orofacial Pain.* 1999; **13**: 172–84.
*111. Woda A, Pionchon P. A unified concept of idiopathic orofacial pain: pathophysiologic features. *Journal of Orofacial Pain.* 2000; **14**: 196–212.
*112. Zakrzewska JM, Hamlyn PJ. Facial pain. In: Crombie IK (ed.). *Epidemiology of pain.* Seattle: IASP Press, 1999: 171–202.
113. Pfaffenrath V, Rath M, Pollmann W, Keeser W. Atypical facial pain – application of the IHS criteria in a clinical sample. *Cephalalgia.* 1993; **13** (Suppl. 12): 84–88.
114. Madland G, Feinmann C. Chronic facial pain: a multidisciplinary problem. *Journal of Neurology, Neurosurgery and Psychiatry.* 2001; **71**: 716–9.
115. Vickers ER, Cousins MJ, Woodhouse A. Pain description and severity of chronic orofacial pain conditions. *Australian Dental Journal.* 1998; **43**: 403–09.
116. Melzack R, Terrence C, Fromm G, Amsel R. Trigeminal neuralgia and atypical facial pain: use of the McGill Pain Questionnaire for discrimination and diagnosis. *Pain.* 1986; **27**: 297–302.
117. Agostoni E, Frigerio R, Santoro P. Atypical facial pain: clinical considerations and differential diagnosis. *Neurological Sciences.* 2005; **26**: 71–4.
118. Zakrzewska JM. Facial pain: neurological and non-neurological. *Journal of Neurology, Neurosurgery and Psychiatry.* 2002; **72**: ii27–ii32.

*119. Jaaskelainen SK. Clinical neurophysiology and quantitative sensory testing in the investigation of orofacial pain and sensory function. *Journal of Orofacial Pain*. 2004; **18**: 85–107.

120. Majoie CB, Hulsmans FJ, Castelijns JA *et al*. Symptoms and signs related to the trigeminal nerve: diagnostic yield of MR imaging. *Radiology*. 1998; **209**: 557–62.

121. Frediani F. Pharmacological therapy of atypical facial pain: actuality and perspective. *Neurological Sciences*. 2005; **26**: 92–4.

122. Turp JC. Atypical odontalgia – a little known phantom pain. *Schmerz*. 2001; **15**: 59–64.

123. Marbach JJ, Raphael KG. Phantom tooth pain: a new look at an old dilemma. *Pain Medicine*. 2000; **1**: 68–77.

*124. Graff-Radford SB, Solberg WK. Atypical odontalgia. *Journal of Craniomandibular Disorders*. 1992; **6**: 260–5.

125. Campbell RL, Parks KW, Dodds RN. Chronic facial pain associated with endodontic therapy. *Oral Surgery, Oral Medicine, Oral Pathology*. 1990; **69**: 287–90.

126. Marbach JJ, Hulbrock J, Hohn C, Segal AG. Incidence of phantom tooth pain: an atypical facial neuralgia. *Oral Surgery, Oral Medicine, Oral Pathology*. 1982; **53**: 190–3.

*127. Melis M, Lobo SL, Ceneviz C *et al*. Atypical odontalgia: a review of the literature. *Headache*. 2003; **43**: 1060–74.

128. Marbach JJ. Is phantom tooth pain a deafferentation (neuropathic) syndrome? Part I: Evidence derived from pathophysiology and treatment. *Oral Surgery, Oral Medicine, Oral Pathology*. 1993; **75**: 95–105.

129. Marbach JJ. Is phantom tooth pain a deafferentation (neuropathic) syndrome? Part II: Psychosocial considerations. *Oral Surgery, Oral Medicine, Oral Pathology*. 1993; **75**: 225–32.

130. Baad-Hansen L, List T, Kaube H *et al*. Blink reflexes in patients with atypical odontalgia and matched healthy controls. *Experimental Brain Research*. 2006; **172**: 498–506.

131. List T, Leijon G, Helkimo M *et al*. Effect of local anesthesia on atypical odontalgia – a randomized controlled trial. *Pain*. 2006; **122**: 306–14.

132. Baad-Hansen L, Juhl GI, Jensen TS *et al*. Differential effect of intravenous S-ketamine and fentanyl on atypical odontalgia and capsaicin-evoked pain. *Pain*. 2007; **129**: 46–54.

133. Lipton JA, Ship JA, Larach-Robinson D. Estimated prevalence and distribution of reported orofacial pain in the United States. *Journal of the American Dental Association*. 1993; **124**: 115–21.

134. Tammiala-Salonen T, Hiidenkari T, Parvinen T. Burning mouth in a Finnish adult population. *Community Dentistry and Oral Epidemiology*. 1993; **21**: 67–71.

135. Bergdahl J, Anneroth G, Perris H. Cognitive therapy in the treatment of patients with resistant burning mouth syndrome: a controlled study. *Journal of Oral Pathology and Medicine*. 1995; **24**: 213–5.

136. Grushka M, Ching V, Epstein J. Burning mouth syndrome. *Advances in Oto-Rhino-Laryngology*. 2006; **63**: 278–87.

137. Forssell H, Jaaskelainen S, Tenovuo O, Hinkka S. Sensory dysfunction in burning mouth syndrome. *Pain*. 2002; **99**: 41–7.

138. Grushka M, Sessle BJ, Howley TP. Psychophysical assessment of tactile, pain and thermal sensory functions in burning mouth syndrome. *Pain*. 1987; **28**: 169–84.

139. Svensson P, Bjerring P, Arendt-Nielsen L, Kaaber S. Sensory and pain thresholds to orofacial argon laser stimulation in patients with chronic burning mouth syndrome. *Clinical Journal of Pain*. 1993; **9**: 207–15.

140. Jaaskelainen SK, Forssell H, Tenovuo O. Abnormalities of the blink reflex in burning mouth syndrome. *Pain*. 1997; **73**: 455–60.

*141. Woolf CJ. Pain: moving from symptom control toward mechanism-specific pharmacologic management. *Annals of Internal Medicine*. 2004; **140**: 441–51.

142. Forssell H, Svensson P. Atypical facial pain and burning mouth syndrome. In: Cervero F, Jensen TS (eds). *Handbook of clinical neurology*, vol. 81. Amsterdam: Elsevier, 2006: 597–608.

143. Zakrzewska JM, Forssell H, Glenny AM. Interventions for the treatment of burning mouth syndrome. *Cochrane Database Systematic Reviews*. 2005; **CD002779**.

144. Gremeau-Richard C, Woda A, Navez ML *et al*. Topical clonazepam in stomatodynia: a randomised placebo-controlled study. *Pain*. 2004; **108**: 51–7.

145. Pau AK, Croucher R, Marcenes W. Prevalence estimates and associated factors for dental pain: a review. *Oral Health and Preventive Dentistry*. 2003; **1**: 209–20.

146. Nair PN. Pathogenesis of apical periodontitis and the causes of endodontic failures. *Critical Reviews in Oral Biology and Medicine*. 2004; **15**: 348–81.

*147. Rodriguez DS, Sarlani E. Decision making for the patient who presents with acute dental pain. *AACN Clinical Issues*. 2005; **16**: 359–72.

*148. Narhi M. Dentinal and pulpal pain. In: Hørsted-Bindslev P, Reit C (eds). *Textbook of endodontology*. Oxford: Blackwell-Munksgaard. 2005: 43–56.

*149. Sessle BJ. The neurobiology of facial and dental pain: present knowledge, future directions. *Journal of Dental Research*. 1987; **66**: 962–81.

150. Byers MR, Narhi MV. Dental injury models: experimental tools for understanding neuroinflammatory interactions and polymodal nociceptor functions. *Critical Reviews in Oral Biology and Medicine*. 1999; **10**: 4–39.

151. Knutsson G, Jontell M, Bergenholtz G. Determination of plasma proteins in dentinal fluid from cavities prepared in healthy young human teeth. *Archives of Oral Biology*. 1994; **39**: 185–90.

152. Matthews B, Vongsavan N. Interactions between neural and hydrodynamic mechanisms in dentine and pulp. *Archives of Oral Biology*. 1994; **39** (Suppl): 87–95.

153. Olgart L, Bergenholtz G. The dentine-pulp complex: responses to adverse influences. In: Bergenholtz G, Hørsted-Bindslev P, Reit C (eds). *Textbook of endodontology.* Oxford: Blackwell Munksgaard. 2003: 21–42.
154. Gysi A. An attempt to explain sensitiveness of dentine. *British Dental Journal.* 1900; **43**: 865–8.
155. Nair PN. Apical periodontitis: a dynamic encounter between root canal infection and host response. *Periodontology 2000.* 1997; **13**: 121–48.
156. Orchardson R, Gillam DG. Managing dentin hypersensitivity. *Journal of the American Dental Association.* 2006; **137**: 990–8.

36

Neck pain and whiplash

NIKOLAI BOGDUK

KEY LEARNING POINTS

- Neck pain and cervical radicular pain are different entities, and should not be confused.
- Patterns of cervical referred pain indicate the likely segmental location of the source of pain, but not its cause.
- Neck pain is common.
- The cardinal risk factors relate to the work environment.
- The natural history of neck pain is not always favorable.
- Tumors, infections, and aneurysms are serious causes of neck pain but are uncommon.
- Spondylosis and osteoarthrosis are not valid causes of neck pain.
- The natural history of neck pain after whiplash is generally favorable.
- Lesions of the disk and zygapophysial joints are the likely causes of the chronic neck pain after whiplash.
- History is the most important and most useful component of clinical assessment for neck pain.
- Imaging is indicated only if the history reveals indications of a possible serious disorder.
- Disk stimulation may be used to diagnose cervical discogenic pain.
- Cervical medial branch blocks can diagnose cervical zygapophysial joint pain.
- Evidence is lacking for most treatments of neck pain.
- For acute neck pain, the focus of management should be on explanation, reassurance, resuming activity, and simple exercises.
- For chronic neck pain, exercises may be palliative.
- Radiofrequency medial branch neurotomy is the only proven treatment for chronic neck pain.

INTRODUCTION

The foremost message that any pain physician should take from a chapter on neck pain is that neck pain and cervical radicular pain are not synonymous. The causes, mechanisms, investigations, and treatment of radicular pain differ from those of neck pain, and the two conditions have a different evidence base. Most emphatically, when a patient presents with just neck pain there is no justification for investigating and treating them as if they had radicular pain. Confusion in this regard has led to inappropriate investigations and therapeutic misadventure in the past and continues to do so. The topic of cervical radicular pain is covered elsewhere.[1, 2, 3] The present chapter deals exclusively with neck pain.

DEFINITION

Neck pain is pain perceived in a region bounded laterally by the margins of the neck, superiorly by the superior nuchal line, and inferiorly by an imaginary transverse line through the T1 spinous process.[4] This definition does not necessarily imply that the cause of pain lies within this region; it is based solely on where the patient perceives their pain.

According to this definition, neck pain is perceived in the back of the neck, and this is typically where patients indicate neck pain. It is unusual for a patient to indicate neck pain anteriorly. In such cases, neck pain needs to be distinguished from pain in the throat or elsewhere in the visceral column of the neck. If a patient complains of visceral pain it should be so described and recorded, and not confused with neck pain. Conceptually, anterior neck pain would be pain perceived behind the visceral structures of the neck. Accordingly, the term "anterior neck pain" should be reserved strictly for those patients who can identify pain at the front of their neck, but not in the pharynx, larynx, trachea, or esophagus, or their adnexae. Little has been published about this type of pain. The evidence base for neck pain pertains to pain perceived in the back of the neck.

REFERRED PAIN

Referred pain is pain perceived in a region that has a nerve supply different from that of the source of pain.[4] In the context of spinal pain, it is pain perceived in the territory of the ventral rami of the spinal nerves when the source of pain lies in the territory of the dorsal rami or other branches of the spinal nerves. The mechanism appears to be convergence, in that when afferents from deep spinal tissues innervated by certain branches of a spinal nerve converge on second-order neurones in the spinal cord that happen also to receive afferents from other branches of that spinal nerve. Referred pain may also arise when afferents from a particular spinal nerve converge within the spinal cord or thalamus with afferents from another spinal nerve.

By these mechanisms, pain arising in the cervical spine can be referred to a variety of regions. From upper cervical segments it can be referred to the head. From lower segments it can be referred to the shoulder girdle, upper limb, and chest wall. Although somatic referred pain has been evoked experimentally from the cervical spine to areas as remote as the forearm and hand,[5, 6] such patterns have not been reported in the clinical literature. Referred pain from the cervical spine tends to be localized proximally: around the shoulder girdle or chest wall, and in the arm rather than the forearm and hand.

Somatic referred pain tends to be felt deeply as an aching pain or expanding pressure. It occurs in patterns whose boundaries are hard to identify but whose centroids are readily identified. Furthermore, somatic referred pain is static or sessile: it rests in relatively fixed locations. Although its boundaries might fluctuate – becoming broader when the pain is more intense – its epicenter remains essentially the same. These features help to distinguish somatic referred pain from radicular pain.

Cervical radicular pain tends to radiate into the upper limb, being perceived in areas more like linear bands. In quality, the pain can be deep and aching, but when it is shooting or lancinating, its radicular origin is beyond doubt. Moreover, to be consistent with the mechanism of radicular pain, it should be associated with paresthesiae or other features of nerve root compromise, such as segmental numbness or weakness. Neurological features do not accompany somatic referred pain. Their presence is perhaps the cardinal distinguishing feature of radicular pain. Conversely, however, in the absence of neurological features, aching pain in the upper limb may be either somatic referred pain or early radicular pain, and the distinction may not readily be made clinically. However, aching pain in the upper limb, in the absence of any neck pain is far more likely to be radicular than somatic referred pain.

Patterns

Cervical referred pain tends to occur in distinctive patterns that can be depicted as pain maps. Previously, such maps had been derived using noxious stimulation of various structures in the cervical spine, either in normal volunteers[7, 8] or in patients undergoing procedures.[9, 10, 11] These maps provided an idealized and somewhat conservative picture of where pain can be referred to from different segments (**Figures 36.1** and **36.2**). More recent

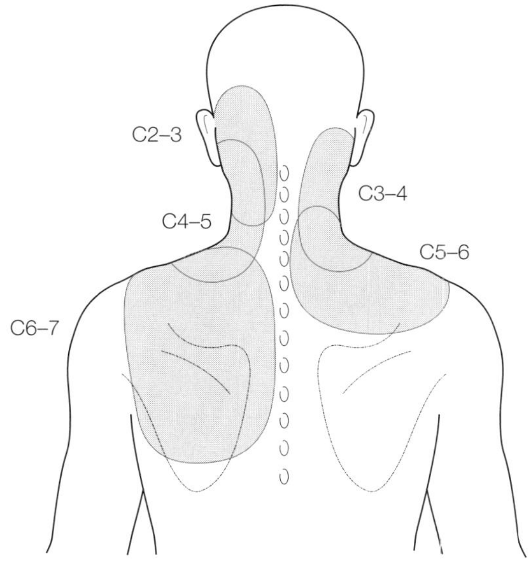

Figure 36.1 Patterns of referred pain evoked in normal volunteers by noxious stimulation of the vertebral segments indicated. Although these patterns were originally derived from stimulation of the zygapophysial joints in normal volunteers,[7] the same patterns have been shown to apply to stimulation of the intervertebral disks at the same segments.[11]

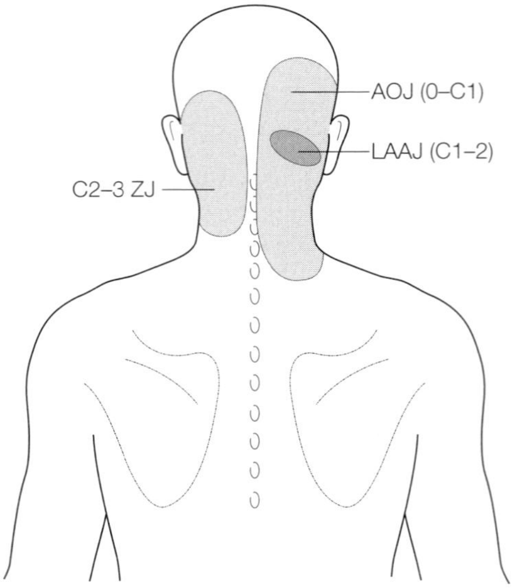

Figure 36.2 Patterms of referred pain evoked in normal volunteers by noxious stimulation of the C2–3 zygapophysial joint (ZJ),[7] the lateral atlanto-axial joint (LAAJ),[8] and the atlanto-occipital joint (AOJ).[8]

data are based on responses to controlled, diagnostic blocks in patients presenting with neck pain.[12] They show that pain from a given segment is concentric with areas evoked in normal volunteers, but can spread further afield (**Figure 36.3**).

Pain from the C1–2, C2–3, and C3–4 segments is often perceived in the suboccipital region but can spread to various other regions, or may present primarily in these other regions. From C1–2 and C2–3, pain can be referred caudally into the upper neck, but it tends to be referred, more often or more intensely into the head. Pain can be referred to the orbit from both C1–2 and C2–3, but pain from C1–2 tends to refer to the vertex and ear, whereas pain from C2–3 tends to cross the temporoparietal region. Although pain from C3–4 can radiate into the head, it tends more often, or more intensely, to refer caudally into the upper neck.

Pain from C4–5 typically occupies the lower neck, near its junction with the shoulder girdle. Pain from C5–6 or C6–7 also covers this region but typically radiates from it. Pain from C5–6 tends to radiate over the top of the shoulder girdle, into the deltoid region and upper arm. Pain from C6–7 typically radiates more medially over the scapula and particularly over its medial border.

Although these patterns have been derived largely from studies of the cervical zygapophysial joints, they do not imply the actual source of pain. Referred pain from interspinous muscles,[5, 6] from the cervical zygapophysial joints,[7, 9, 12] and from the cervical intervertebral disks[10, 11] follows similar patterns. Those patterns are dictated not by the structure stimulated but by its segmental nerve supply. Thus, any structure innervated by C5,6 will have a referred pain pattern like any other structure innervated by C5,6. Pain maps, therefore, cannot be used to diagnose the source of pain, but they do serve to indicate the likely segmental location of the source.

Epidemiology

Neck pain is a common complaint whose prevalence differs in different communities and amongst different occupations. The yearly prevalence of acute neck pain in the general community is approximately 10 percent; that of chronic neck pain is as high as 14 percent.[13, 14, 15] The prevalence increases with age, and is somewhat higher in women. Some 5 percent of the population are highly disabled by neck pain.[16]

Risk factors

Many factors have been studied as risk factors for the development of neck pain. Some have been refuted; others have only a weak or moderate association, with odds ratios less than 3.0 (**Table 36.1**).[17] The most pervasive risk factors for neck pain relate to the work environment. They include high job demands,[18, 19] low decision authority,[19, 20] little influence over the work situation[21] or low job control,[22] low coworker social support,[19, 22, 23] high psychological demand,[23] and low decision latitude.[23] Although psychosocial in nature, these factors stem from the patient's work circumstances, and do not constitute personal psychological factors.

Specific and classical psychological variables have failed to emerge as determinants of neck pain. Distinctly unrelated to neck pain are variables such as social support, depression, anxiety, coping ability, self-confidence, ability to solve problems, sense of humor, irritability, impatience, psychosis, extroversion, and lying, on the Eysenck Personality Questionnaire.[24] Factors found to be significantly related to neck pain upon univariate analysis disappear upon multivariate analysis.[24, 25] Upon multivariate analysis, psychological state accounts for only 2 percent of the variance in symptoms of neck pain.[26]

Natural history

Some 14 percent of the population experience a new episode of neck pain in a given year, with 0.6 percent experiencing disabling pain.[27] Approximately 37 percent of those affected progress to complete resolution, with the passage of time; and a further 33 percent experience improvement; but neck pain persists in the remainder.[27] Some 23 percent of individuals suffer a recurrence within the year. In effect, neck pain persists in about half of those initially afflicted.[28] Some 25 percent of patients have moderate symptoms after ten years, and some 7 percent remain or become severely disabled.[29, 30]

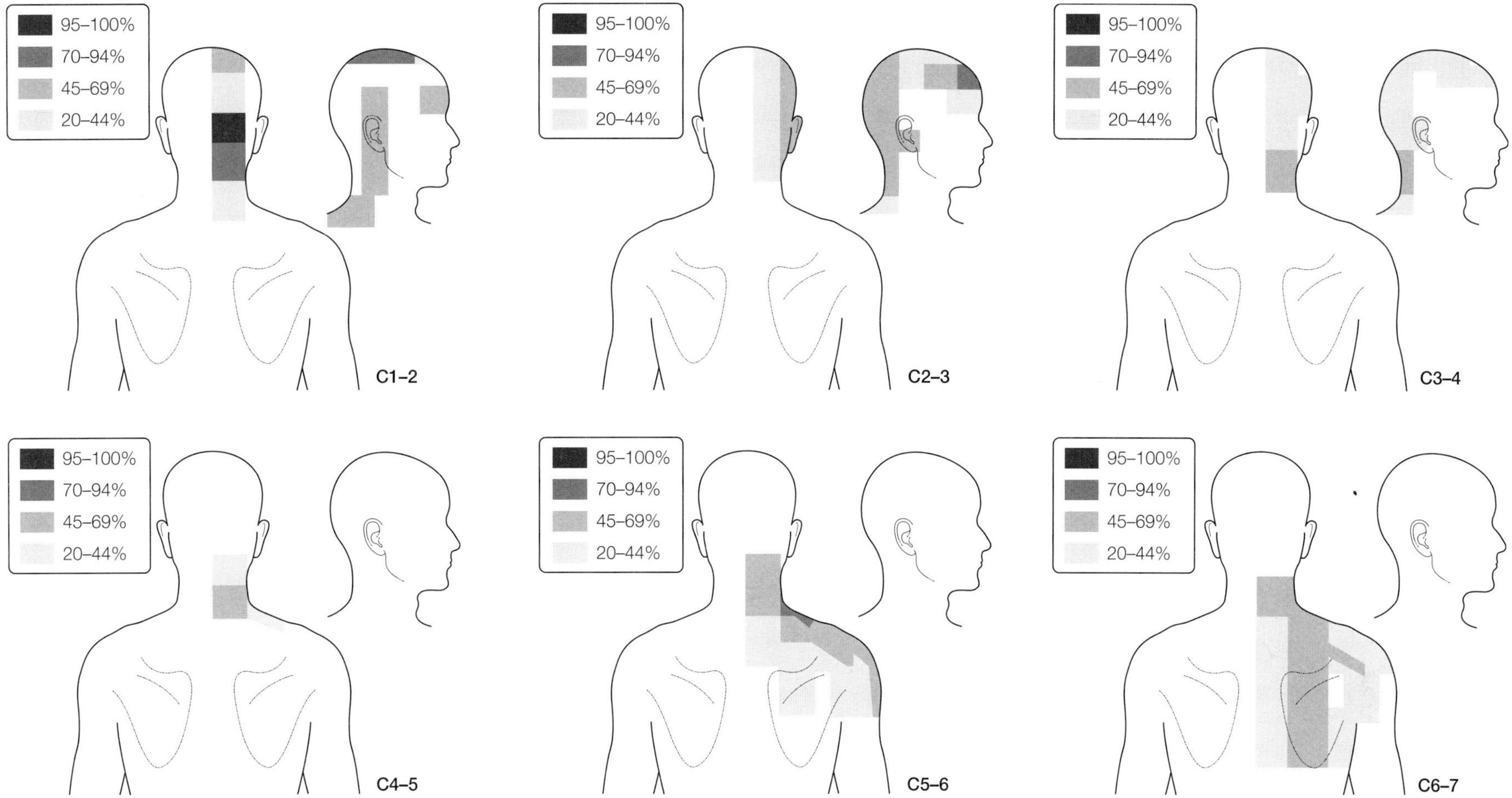

Figure 36.3 The distribution of referred pain relieved by anesthetizing the synovial joints at the segments indicated. The density of shading reflects the proportion of patients with pain from the segment indicated who reported pain in the area shaded. Adapted from Cooper *et al.*[12]

Table 36.1 Refuted and weak to moderate risk factors for the development of neck pain.[17]

Refuted as risk factors	Weak to moderate risk factors
Degenerative disk disease	Female gender
Zygapophysial osteoarthrosis	Previous injury
Smoking	Working with machines
Socioeconomic status	Occupation
Prolonged sitting at work station	Educational level

Prognostic factors

Systematic reviews have found few studies that reported on prognostic factors for neck pain.[31, 32] None provided a statistical analysis that yielded either the relative risk or odds ratio for any association. Consequently, there are no validated prognostic factors for neck pain.

Etiology

The taxonomy of the International Association for the Study of Pain (IASP) lists some 60 recognized causes of neck pain.[4] These, and others, can be grouped as shown in **Table 36.2**. Tumors, infections, and aneurysms constitute the "red flag" conditions of the neck because they threaten serious neurological or systemic sequelae.

Neck pain can occur in patients with known rheumatoid arthritis, but it is unlikely to be the sole presenting feature. Less than 2 percent of patients with rheumatoid arthritis have neck pain as their only feature.[33] Rheumatoid arthritis becomes potentially serious if it affects the C1–2 joints, but even then the prognosis is favorable.[34] Gout and the seronegative spondylarthropathies (ankylosing spondylitis, Reiter's syndrome, and psoriatic arthritis) can each involve the neck, but are rare causes of neck pain in patients without other manifestations of these conditions.

Tumors, infections, and metabolic disorders are very uncommon causes of neck pain. Although their prevalence has not been explicitly established, the failure of large radiological surveys to detect such conditions[35, 36] implies that their prevalence is less than 0.4 percent in primary care.

Headache is the most common presenting feature of internal carotid artery dissection, but neck pain has been the sole presenting feature in some 6 percent of cases.[37, 38] In 17 percent of patients, headache may occur in combination with neck pain.[38] Neck pain has been the initial presenting feature in 50–90 percent of patients with vertebral artery dissection, but is usually also accompanied by headache, typically in the occipital region although not exclusively so.[37, 39] Although the typical features of dissecting aneurysm of the aorta are chest pain and cardiovascular distress, neck pain has been reported as the presenting feature in some 6 percent of cases.[40, 41]

Although considered common and feared as a cause of neck pain (for medicolegal reasons), fractures of the neck are actually not common. In accident and emergency settings, only about 3 percent of patients suspected of having a fracture prove to have fractures upon cervical radiography.[42, 43, 44, 45, 46, 47]

Missing from **Table 36.2** are cervical spondylosis and cervical osteaoarthrosis. Although hallowed by tradition, these entities are not valid causes of neck pain. The radiological features of these conditions are normal age changes. They correlate poorly with neck pain.[35] Indeed, cervical osteoarthrosis is more common in subjects with no neck pain.[48]

For patients with neck pain whose cause is not apparent, the IASP recommends the rubric cervical spinal pain of unknown origin, as an honest diagnosis.[4] Zygapophysial joint pain and discogenic pain are specific subsets of what otherwise might be known as "mechanical" neck pain, but their diagnosis requires invasive procedures such as zygapophysial joint blocks and disk stimulation (see under Invasive techniques below).

Although favored by many, there is no evidence that trigger points are a cause of neck pain. Even in the hands

Table 36.2 The causes of neck pain grouped according to whether they are common and serious.

	Nonthreatening	Serious
Uncommon	Rheumatoid arthritis Ankylosing spondylitis Reiter's syndrome Psoriatic arthritis Crystal arthropathies	Fractures Tumors Spinal infections Dissecting aneurysms Spinal hematomas Metabolic disorders
Common	Cervical spinal pain of unknown origin Acceleration–deceleration injuries of the neck Zygapophysial joint pain Discogenic pain	

of experts, the diagnosis is unreliable,[49] and the absence of a criterion standard means that its validity cannot be tested. Furthermore, trigger points in the neck do not satisfy the prescribed criteria for a trigger point. They are characterized solely by tenderness and reproduction of pain, in which regard they cannot be distinguished from tenderness of underlying zygapophysial joints.[50]

Acceleration–deceleration injury, or whiplash, is perhaps the most common traumatic basis for neck pain. In population studies, a large proportion of patients attribute their neck pain to an injury incurred in a motor vehicle accident.[16]

WHIPLASH

There is no evidence that neck pain following whiplash differs physiologically from neck pain due to other causes. It is an entity defined by its circumstances of onset, and complicated by its social context. The onset is attributed to an inertial injury sustained in a motor vehicle accident. The complicating factor is that it may be subject to compensation.

Epidemiology

In western societies, the incidence of neck pain attributed to whiplash is about 1/1000 population per year,[51] but this figure may be larger or smaller in different countries, or different states or provinces, depending on the nature of the administrative system that applies, and depending on whether population samples or hospital samples are used to calculate the figure.

Risk factors

Being involved in a motor vehicle accident does not destine a victim to suffer neck pain. Many suffer no symptoms. Individuals who do not suffer neck pain at the time of being involved in a motor vehicle accident subsequently exhibit a prevalence of chronic neck pain that is no greater than that expressed by those who have never suffered an accident.[52] However, individuals who experience neck pain immediately or soon after an accident, are three times more likely to suffer persistent neck pain than is the general community.[52]

Natural history

The natural history of neck pain after whiplash is remarkably benign. The rate of recovery appears to be considerably better than that of neck pain in general. Within 12 months, some 75 percent of victims are asymptomatic, with the figure rising to 82 percent by two years. This leaves some 20 percent of patients still with symptoms, but only 4 percent are severely disabled.[53]

Prognostic factors

Persistence of neck pain after whiplash is not related to factors such as age, gender, psychological response, or compensation.[54] It is weakly related to sleep disturbance, cognitive impairments, poor concentration, neuroticism, past history of headache, and being unprepared for the collision.[54] The cardinal determinant of poor outcome is the initial intensity of pain and other symptoms.[54, 55, 56, 57] Patients least likely to recover exhibit hyperalgesia, both in the cervical region and in regions remote from the neck, as well as psychological distress in the face of their symptoms.[58, 59, 60, 61, 62] Evidence has also emerged that, independent of the initial intensity of pain, engaging a lawyer is a predictor of poor outcome.[56, 57]

Etiology

The favorable natural history of neck pain after whiplash indicates that most patients suffer no substantive injury. Perhaps they suffer a minor muscle strain, or a minor injury to a joint in the neck, which spontaneously resolves. A pathology is required only to explain the minority of cases in which pain becomes chronic.

Rare injuries include disruption of the alar ligaments, prevertebral hematoma, perforation of the esophagus, tears of the sympathetic trunk, damage to the recurrent laryngeal nerve, spinal cord injury, periplymph fistula, thrombosis or traumatic aneurysms of the vertebral or internal carotid arteries, retinal angiopathy, and anterior spinal artery syndrome.[51, 58] Fractures after whiplash are so uncommon as to be rare. Such fractures as have been attributed to whiplash have been reported only in case studies or small, descriptive series. These fractures may be difficult to detect on conventional investigations, and special attention needs to be paid to their possibility if they are to be detected. The majority involve the upper cervical spine, and include fractures of the odontoid process, the laminae and articular processes of C2, and the occipital condyles. In one study of 283 patients with acute neck pain after whiplash, however, no fractures were found on plain radiography.[46] This result implies a prevalence of less than 1.3 percent.

The most likely lesions that underlie chronic neck pain after whiplash are injuries to the intervertebral disks and zygapophysial joints. Cineradiography studies in normal volunteers undergoing simulated whiplash collisions reveal that at some 100 msec after impact, the cervical spine undergoes a sigmoid deformation, during which the lower cervical vertebrae undergo extension about an abnormal axis of rotation.[59] The movement is such that the anterior edges of the vertebral bodies separate and the zygapophysial joints impact (**Figure 36.4**). These movements indicate that the anterior anulus fibrosus can be sprained while the zygapophysial joints can suffer impaction fractures or contusions to their meniscoids.[59] These are the very lesions that have been demonstrated in post mortem studies of victims of motor vehicle accidents.[60, 61, 62]

Clinical assessment

A comprehensive history of neck pain can be recorded by noting the standard features of any type of pain, as listed in **Table 36.3**. Asking the duration of illness establishes if the condition is acute or chronic. The circumstances of onset identify if the cause was spontaneous or traumatic, or associated with an illness or intervention. The mode of onset is usually unremarkable, but a sudden, spontaneous onset of severe neck pain should warn of a red flag condition. The site of pain and its radiation may be helpful in indicating, *prima facie*, the likely segmental origin of pain, but widespread neck pain offers no localizing clue. Neck pain should be dull and aching in quality; lancinating or sharp pain suggests a possible neurogenic cause. Asking about frequency and duration establishes if the pain is episodic or constant, but lends little to establishing the cause, nor does the timing of the pain. Pain precipitated and aggravated by neck movement suggests an articular or muscular source of pain, as does pain relieved by rest.

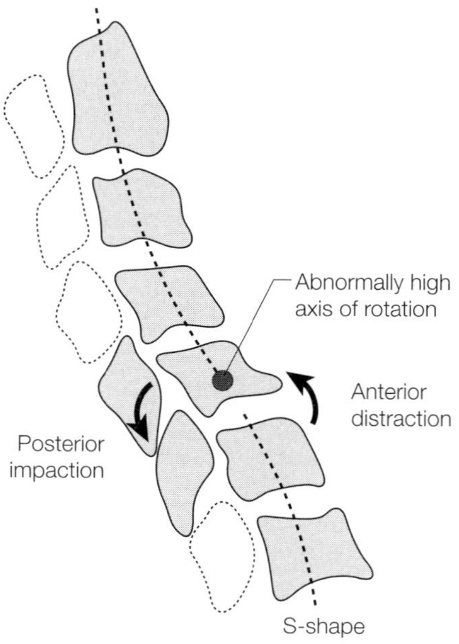

Figure 36.4 The mechanism of whiplash injury. The cervical spine is compressed from below and undergoes a sigmoid deformation. Lower cervical vertebra undergo posterior sagittal rotation about an abnormally high axis of rotation. This results in impaction of the zygapophysial joints posteriorly and distraction of the intervertebral disk anteriorly.

Table 36.3 Categories of enquiry for taking a history of neck pain.

Categories	
Duration of illness	Frequency
Circumstances of onset	Duration
Mode of onset	Time of onset
Site of pain	Precipitating factors
Radiation	Aggravating factors
Quality	Relieving factors
	Associated features

However, these features are not valid indicators of any particular source or cause of pain. More sinister is pain that is not affected by movement, and not relieved by rest. This suggests a possible red flag condition, affecting a nonarticular structure, but the likelihood ratio of this contention is low. The detection of red flag conditions relies on an index of suspicion, not on a specific finding or set of findings.

The most critical aspect of taking a history of neck pain is enquiry as to associated features. It is in this regard that the red flag conditions of the neck are most readily recognized. The enquiry can be rendered systematic by obtaining a systems review that asks both about current symptoms and past history of illness, as prompted by **Table 36.4**. If at any stage a response is positive, a more thorough enquiry and investigation of a possible medical disorder should be initiated.

A positive response with respect to neurological symptoms may indicate spinal tumor or cerebrovascular disorder. Cardiovascular risk factors prompt consideration of aneurysms. Respiratory features, genitourinary features, or a history of thyroid cancer warrant consideration of spinal metastases. Weight loss and anorexia suggest neoplasia. Diarrhea and skin lesions suggest spondylarthropathy, as do peripheral features of inflammatory arthropathy. Neck pain in the elderly warrants consideration of myeloma or other tumors. Hyperparathyroidism is a possible cause of spinal pain that is easily overlooked because of its rarity.

Infection of the cervical spine may be very difficult to identify clinically. Mercifully it is rare. However, the cardinal risk factors are diabetes, immunosuppresion, or a history of penetration, in the form of a surgical or other invasive procedure, catheterization, cannulation, or intravenous drug use.

Physical examination

Physical examination offers little towards the diagnosis of neck pain. Typically, the patient will be tender in the cervical spine, and will exhibit restriction of neck movements because of pain. Neither of these features, however, is a valid indicator of any particular source or cause of pain.

Table 36.4 A comprehensive checklist of associated features of neck pain that might indicate a red flag condition, if evident on systems review or past history of illness.

System	Feature or condition
Nervous	Weakness
	Numbness
	Bladder dysfunction
	Impaired balance
	Impaired vision
	Altered speech
	Disorientation
	Altered consciousness
Cardiovascular	Risk factors
	Chest pain
	Anticoagulants
	Transient ischemic attacks
Respiratory	Carcinoma
	Tuberculosis
	Cough
	Weight loss
Alimentary	Carcinoma
	Weight loss
	Loss of appetite
	Dysphagia
	Diarrhea
	Altered bowel habits
Urinary	Incontinence
	Obstruction
Reproductive	Breast lump
	Uterine dysfunction
Endocrine	Thyroid cancer
	Hyperparathyroidism
Reticulo-endothelial	Lymph nodes
Skin	Rash
Musculoskeletal	Other joint pain
	Other muscle pain
Age	Risk of Paget's disease
	Risk of myeloma

In this context, neurological examination is immaterial in the assessment of neck pain, for it is not a neurological disorder. Neurological examination is pertinent if the patient has neurological symptoms, but not if pain is the only presenting feature. In that event, a screening neurological examination, looking for weakness or numbness, is all that is justified.

Special techniques of examination, such as the detection of cervical intersegmental motion, have either not been shown to be valid, or have been found to lack reliability, validity, or both. For the detection of tenderness over the zygapophysial joints, inter-observer agreement has been shown to be good, with a kappa score of 0.68.[63] For other signs, particularly those espoused by chiropractors, observer agreement is poor.[64, 65, 66, 67, 68] Manual examination of passive intersegmental motion lacks validity for the diagnosis of zygapophysial joint pain.[69]

INVESTIGATIONS

Medical imaging is notoriously unhelpful for the diagnosis of neck pain. The common causes of pain cannot be detected by imaging. Particular investigations are indicated only if there are clinical grounds for suspecting particular lesions.

Plain radiography

The only valid indication for plain radiography in a patient with neck pain is a history of trauma. In that context, radiography is used as a screening test for fractures. However, the pretest likelihood of fracture is low, even in patients with a history of trauma.[70] The Canadian C-spine rules define the responsible use of radiography in such patients[71] (see Chapter 12, Diagnostic procedures in chronic pain). Radiography is indicated if the patient is older than 65; has suffered a dangerous injury, such as a fall or high speed collision; or expresses neurological symptoms. A simple rear-end motor vehicle collision does not qualify as a dangerous injury, and is not an indication for radiography. Otherwise, if the patient has been ambulatory and is able to rotate their neck by 45° to the left and right, radiography is not indicated. Under these rules, the chances of missing a significant fracture by failing to undertake radiography are essentially nil.

In patients with neck pain but no history of trauma, radiography is not indicated. Two large studies, each involving over 1000 patients, have found that no instances of unexpected malignancy or infection were found.[35, 36] The British study concluded that "the request for x-ray films of the cervical spine 'just in case' such a finding is present is probably unjustified".[35] The US study found that upon five-year follow up "no medically dangerous diagnoses would have been missed if the cervical spine series had not been done".[36] These results underscore the guideline that x-ray examination of the neck should be performed only if there is a clinical suspicion of infection or malignancy or after some instances of trauma.

What plain radiography is likely to reveal in a patient with neck pain is either a normal cervical spine or cervical spondylosis. The features of cervical spondylosis, however, are simply age-related changes. In some studies cervical spondylosis occurs somewhat more commonly in symptomatic individuals than in asymptomatic individuals,[35, 72] but the odds ratios for disk degeneration or osteoarthrosis as predictors of neck pain are only 1.1 and 0.97 respectively for women, and 1.7 and 1.8 for men.[72] In other studies, the prevalence of disk degeneration, at individual segments of the neck, is not significantly different between symptomatic patients and asymptomatic controls.[48] Indeed, uncovertebral osteophytes and osteoarthrosis are less prevalent in symptomatic individuals.[48]

Of significance is the false-positive impact of a report of cervical spondylosis. Such a report is more likely to lead to a referral to a hospital orthopedic department.[35] The reason for this is not evident, but presumably it is because of a belief that, somehow, spondylosis is diagnostic of neck pain and that orthopedic management, somehow, is indicated. Yet, the evidence indicates that cervical spondylosis is not diagnostic of neck pain, and there is no evidence that orthopedic management for neck pain ascribed to cervical spondylosis is superior to any other management for neck pain. There is also the risk that someone might choose to operate on a patient on the basis of having found spondylosis, thereby incurring the risks of failure and the production of iatrogenic disease.

Loss of lordosis is a feature sometimes reported in cervical spine films, but this phenomenon is a normal variant, and carries no diagnostic implication. It is equally prevalent amongst patients with acute neck pain, chronic neck pain, and no neck pain.[73] It is independent of age and symptoms, but is more common in females.

Computed tomography scanning

No data, and no studies, justify the use of computed tomography (CT) as a screening test for undiganosed neck pain. CT may be of use in better defining known or suspected pathology, such as fractures or tumors; but it offers no value in the pursuit of uncomplicated neck pain. Nothing that might be evident on CT has been shown to correlate with any known cause of neck pain.

Magnetic resonance imaging

In patients with acute neck pain, but with no clinical indicators of any serious cause, magnetic resonance imaging (MRI) offers little prospect of a positive diagnosis. The only indication for MRI is as a screening test for rare and clinically occult disorders in patients with persistent or chronic neck pain. Yet even in that context, the use of MRI is questionable. By definition, rare conditions are unlikely to be evident, and in the absence of clinical indicators they are even more unlikely. The cardinal indicators are a past history of cancer, risk factors for infection, or signs of systemic illness. In patients with risk factors for aneurysm (see Chapter 12, Diagnostic procedures in chronic pain), magnetic resonance angiography is indicated.

In the absence of clinical indicators, MRI will reveal a normal cervical spine or normal age changes. Disk degeneration, disk bulges, spinal stenosis, and even spinal cord impingement occur in asymptomatic individuals, and with increasing frequency with age.[74, 75] Finding such abnormalities does not provide a diagnosis. In patients with neck pain after whiplash, multiple studies have shown that MRI reveals nothing but normal age changes, with the same prevalence as in the general population.[76, 77, 78, 79, 80, 81]

Single-photon emission tomography scanning

A small study reported that single-photon emission tomography (SPECT) could reveal small articular fractures and avulsions of the vertebral rims, at about four to six weeks after whiplash.[82] The results of this study have not been corroborated.

Emerging prospects

It is possible that lesions responsible for neck pain can escape detection because of the limited resolution of conventional imaging techniques. Advanced technology has been explored for its ability to provide greater resolution. A case report illustrated that functional MRI could reveal lesions of the atlanto-axial joints and ligaments that had escaped detection by conventional means.[83] A pair of studies reported that MRI could demonstrate various grades of lesions in the alar and transverse ligaments, and that such lesions were significantly more common in patients with a history of whiplash than in control subjects.[84, 85] Others have not yet reproduced these observations. Nor have the lesions detected been shown to correlate with pain. A study in progress issued a preliminary report to the effect that lesions affecting the zygapophysial joints, disks, and other structures could be revealed in patients after whiplash, using MRI spectroscopy.[86]

Invasive techniques

It is not surprising that medical imaging lacks utility for the vast majority of patients with neck pain. Pain is a symptom. It cannot be seen on morphological tests. It requires physiological tests. In this regard, two such tests have been advocated.

DISK STIMULATION

Disk stimulation is a test designed to determine if an intervertebral disk is painful or not. It involves introducing a needle into the center of the suspected disk, through which contrast medium is injected in order to stress the disk by distending it from within.[87] The recommended criteria for a diagnosis of cervical discogenic pain are that stressing a particular disk reproduces the patient's pain, with an intensity of at least seven on a ten-point scale, but provided that stressing adjacent disks does not reproduce pain.[87]

Two phenomena complicate the interpretation of cervical disk stimulation. First, disk stimulation can be false-positive when the patient has zygapophysial joint pain at the same segment.[88] Therefore, in order to be valid, disk stimulation must be performed after zygapophysial joint pain has been excluded.[87] Second, it is uncommon for cervical disks to be symptomatic at one segmental level, or just at lower cervical levels. Positive responses are commonly encountered at two, three, and even four levels or more.[11] The assessment of the patient is, therefore, not complete unless and until all levels are studied, which makes cervical disk stimulation a demanding procedure. If disk stimulation is undertaken at only one, two, or three, preferred or habitual levels, the likelihood of an incomplete, and incorrect, diagnosis is high.

The one virtue of cervical disk stimulation is that, if multiple disks are found to be symptomatic, surgery is not indicated. Disk stimulation, therefore, plays an important role in reducing unnecessary and futile cervical surgery.[11]

MEDIAL BRANCH BLOCKS

Cervical medial branch blocks can be used to test if a zygapophysial joint is the source of a patient's neck pain. They involve anesthetizing, under fluoroscopic control, the small nerves that innervate the target joint, each with no more than 0.3 mL of local anesthetic[89] (**Figure 36.5**).

Cervical medial branch joint blocks have face-validity, in that they selectively anesthetize the target nerves, and do not anesthetize any nearby structures that realistically might be the source of pain.[90] Single diagnostic blocks, however, are not valid. They carry a false-positive rate of some 27 percent.[91] Controls are, therefore, required in each and every patient. When performed under controlled conditions, cervical medial branch blocks have proven construct validity.[92]

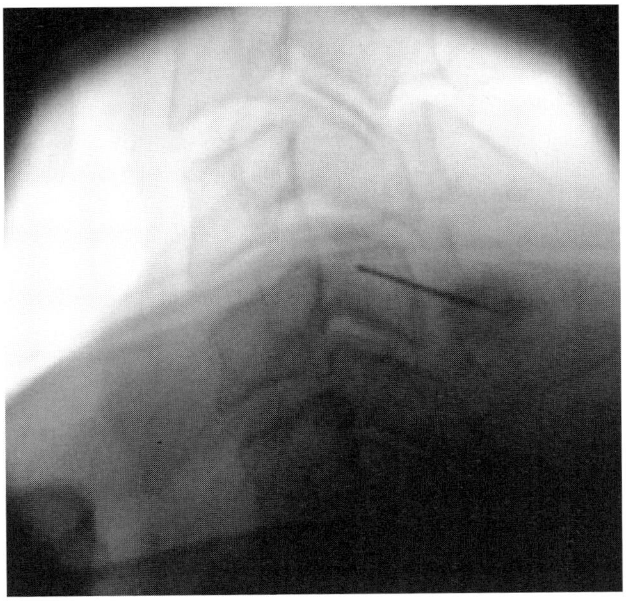

Figure 36.5 A lateral fluoroscopy view of a needle in place on the articular pillar of C5 in preparation for a C5 medial branch block.

Two types of control are available. Foremost, placebo controls can be used. However, this requires three blocks to be performed on separate occasions.[89] The first block must be with a local anesthetic in order to establish, *prima facie*, that the joint is painful. The second block cannot summarily be a local anesthetic agent, for a mischievous patient would know that they were expected to respond. Rather, in order to maintain chance, the second agent must be randomized as either a local anesthetic or a placebo. For the third block, the reciprocal agent should be used. A valid response would be relief of pain on each occasion that a local anesthetic was used, but no relief when placebo was administered. However, although they are stringent, placebo-controlled blocks are not practical in most clinical circumstances.

An alternative are comparative diagnostic blocks.[89, 92] Blocks are performed on separate occasions using different local anesthetic agents. A valid response is one in which the patient obtains a duration of relief concordant with the expected duration of action of the agent administered, i.e. long-lasting relief when a long-acting agent is used, and short-lasting relief when a short-acting agent is used. Controlled studies have shown that diagnostic decisions based on this paradigm are robust.[93]

Epidemiologic studies, using double-blind, controlled, diagnostic blocks, have shown that zygapophysial joint pain is the single most common basis of chronic neck pain, both after whiplash and in heterogeneous samples. In patients with a history of whiplash, prevalence figures (with 95 percent confidence intervals) of 54 percent (40–68 percent)[94] and 60 percent (46–73 percent)[95] have been reported. In patients with headache after whiplash, the prevalence of C2–3 zygapophysial joint pain was 53 percent (37–68 percent).[96] Amongst drivers involved in high-speed collisions, the prevalence was as high as 74 percent (65–83 percent).[97] In patients with neck pain not restricted to those with whiplash, the prevalence of cervical zygapophysial joint pain has been at least 36 percent (27–45 percent) in a rehabilitation practice,[98] and 60 percent (50–70 percent) in a pain clinic.[99]

Of all the possible diagnostic tests that might be applied to a patient with neck pain, cervical medial branch blocks are the only validated test. Of all the possible causes of chronic neck pain, zygapophysial joint pain is the only proven entity and is the most common cause of neck pain after whiplash.

TREATMENT

For the treatment of neck pain, the evidence differs according to whether the pain is acute or chronic. In both instances, the available evidence refutes or fails to support many traditional interventions that still continue to be used.

Acute neck pain

For the treatment of acute neck pain, the Australian Acute Musculoskeletal Pain Guidelines Group found evidence that collars were ineffective, and found evidence to be lacking or insufficient on the effectiveness of acupuncture, analgesics, manipulation, passive mobilization, electrotherapy, gymnastics, multidisciplinary biopsychosocial rehabilitation, muscle relaxants, neck school, nonsteroidal anti-inflammatory drugs, patient education, spray and stretch, traction, or transcutaneous electrical nerve stimulation (TENS).[100][I] The literature pertaining to this evidence is reviewed in detail elsewhere.[100, 101]

The Australian Guidelines Group recommended that the treatment of acute neck pain be based on explanation and reassurance, activation, and exercises.[100][I] These recommendations were consonant with the results of an earlier systematic review of conservative therapy for neck pain.[102, 103][I] In support of these recommendations, the literature is positive but limited.

In a randomized, controlled study, simply instructing patients to act as usual was at least as effective, or slightly more effective, in terms of recovery, than having sick-leave and using a collar and analgesics.[104][II] One controlled study found that keeping the neck active, by using simple home exercises, was more effective in the short term than rest and analgesia, and no less effective than physiotherapy.[105][II] In the long term, a greater proportion of patients who used home exercises were free of pain than in either of the other groups.[106][II] In another study, home exercises were compared with treatment with information, advice, postural correction, and a collar. It showed that patients who exercised had greater reductions in pain, and greater proportions were either pain-free or had only low levels of pain, at six months.[107][II] A subsequent report confirmed that these differences persisted at 12 months.[108][II]

The most recent Cochrane review still supports these recommendations but with less confidence.[109][I] The basis for this change is a more critical analysis of the literature. For example, in the revision, the studies of McKinney[105, 106] are rated as low quality, for a variety of technical reasons.

Contentious is how effective manual therapy is for acute neck pain. A systematic review found no evidence of efficacy for manual therapy used as a sole intervention.[110][I] Any attributable benefit of manual therapy lies in its combination with exercise therapy. Even so, the effect-sizes of combined therapy are small.[101, 111] The available data do not allow the attributable effect of manual therapy to be differentiated from that attributable to exercises.[101] The circumstantial evidence strongly implies that exercises are the cardinal active component of combined therapy.[101]

Of difficulty is the challenge for practitioners to modify their practice, by abjuring traditional, passive interventions and instead engaging the patient to provide explanation and reassurance, and promoting activation with simple exercises. Descriptions of how this can be achieved in practice are provided elsewhere.[111]

Chronic neck pain

For the treatment of chronic neck pain, the evidence is even more sparse than that for acute neck pain, and even less supportive of traditional approaches. There is no published evidence supporting the effectiveness of a collar, TENS, traction, trigger point therapy, or multimodal therapy for chronic neck pain.[112] There is no published evidence of any drugs being effective.

For acupuncture, the evidence is conflicting. While some studies have reported an effect greater than that of placebo,[113][II] others have found no difference from placebo,[114, 115, 116, 117, 118, 119][II] and one study found placebo to be more effective.[120][II] Injections of Botulinum toxin are not effective for chronic neck pain.[121][II] One study found trigger point injections to be as effective as ultrasound treatment[122][II] but another found ultrasound to be no more effective than placebo treatment.[123][II] Intra-articular injections of corticosteroids are not effective for cervical zygapophysial joint pain.[124][II]

A systematic review[110][I] found no evidence of benefit from manipulative therapy or cervical mobilization for chronic neck pain. Physiotherapy provides only small improvements in pain, and is not more effective than a brief session of advice.[125][II] No controlled trials have determined if multidisciplinary or behavioral therapy is effective for chronic neck pain.[112]

Of the conventional, conservative therapies, exercises are the mainstay of treatment for chronic neck pain. Exercises of various types can reduce pain by anywhere between 25 and 75 percent, but they are not demonstrably more effective than treatments with which they have been compared, which include manual therapy and ordinary activity (**Table 36.5**). In the most recent study, exercises were barely more effective than three sessions of advice.[134][II]

Surgical therapy

There is no compelling evidence of the efficacy of cervical fusion for neck pain. Such studies as have reported on this therapy claim success,[135, 136][IV] but outcome measures are few and lacking in rigor. Some studies report disheartening results,[137][IV] particularly for surgical therapy of neck pain after whiplash.[138][IV] Some 57 percent of patients report their pain as much better after surgery, but only 10 percent are rendered free of pain.[139][IV]

Table 36.5 The pain scores reported in various studies of exercises for chronic neck pain. All studies provide level II evidence.

Study	Treatment	Pain scores				
		Baseline	3M	4M	6M	12M
Randlov *et al.*[126]	Intensive exercises	60			40	45
	Light exercises	60	50		60	60
Jordan *et al.*[127]	Intensive exercises	40		10		15
	Physiotherapy+manual therapy	40		10		20
	Manual therapy	43		15		15
Taimela *et al.*[128]	Multimodal stabilization exercises	43	22			No difference
	Home exercises with instruction	31	23			
	Home exercises written	40	39			
Bronfort *et al.*[129, 130]	Manual therapy+exercises	57	30		30	31
	Exercises	57	25		30	30
	Manual therapy	57	37		36	37
Viljanen *et al.*[131]	Dynamic exercises	48	29		29	31
	Relaxation	48	29		30	33
	Ordinary activity	41	27		29	32
Ylinen *et al.*[132]	Strengthening exercises	50				18
	Endurance exercises	57				22
	Written advice	58				34
	Home stretching					
Chiu *et al.*[133]	Dynamic strengthening	46			31	
	Infrared heat	43			38	

Radiofrequency neurotomy

Percutaneous radiofrequency (RF) neurotomy is the one surgical procedure that has withstood scientific scrutiny. In this procedure, the nerves that innervate the cervical zygapophysial joints are coagulated in an effort to relieve pain stemming from these joints.[140] Under double-blind, controlled conditions, the procedure has proven not to be a placebo.[141][II] Moreover, it is the only treatment for neck pain that has been shown to achieve complete relief of pain, and restoration of activities of daily living.[141, 142] [II], [III] Furthermore, relief of pain is attended by complete resolution of psychological distress.[143][III]

A limitation of the procedure is that pain recurs as the treated nerves regenerate, but in that event, the procedure can be repeated and the pain once again completely relieved. Long-term studies have shown that continued, repeated relief can be sustained for up to 2000 days.[142][III]

In the context of whiplash, it has repeatedly been shown that the outcomes following RF neurotomy are not worse statistically in patients with litigation pending than in patients who have settled litigation or did not pursue litigation.[141][III], [142][III], [144][II], [145][III], [146][III]

RECOMMENDATIONS

For acute neck pain.

- A thorough history should look for possible red flag indicators.
- Imaging should be undertaken only if clinical indicators justify doing so.
- If a serious condition is evident or detected, management should follow conventional lines for that condition.
- If no serious causes are evident, the management should focus on explanation, reassurance, staying active, and using simple exercises.

For chronic neck pain.

- MRI serves as a screening test for occult serious causes, but conventional imaging is unlikely to be diagnostic.
- Cervical medial branch blocks are the only validated diagnostic tests, and are likely to provide a diagnosis in approximately 60 percent of patients.
- Cervical disk stimulation may be used in the remaining patients, but needs to be performed in a rigorous manner.
- Exercises may be palliative for some patients.
- The effectiveness of surgery is contentious.
- Radiofrequency medial branch neurotomy is the only validated treatment, and is the only treatment shown to be able to relieve neck pain completely.

REFERENCES

1. Bogduk N. *Medical management of acute cervical radicular pain: an evidence-based approach.* Newcastle: Newcastle Bone and Joint Institute, 1999.

2. Bogduk N. Cervical pain. In: Ashbury AK, McKhann GM, McDonald WI *et al.* (eds). *Disease of the nervous system. Clinical neuroscience and therapeutic principles.* Cambridge: Cambridge University Press, 2002: 742–59.
3. Bogduk N. Neck and arm pain. In: Aminoff MJ, Daroff RB (eds). *Encyclopedia of the neurological sciences*, Vol. 3. Amsterdam: Academic Press, 2003: 390–8.
4. Merskey H, Bogduk N (eds). *Classification of chronic pain. Descriptions of chronic pain syndromes and definition of pain terms*, 2nd edn. Seattle: IASP Press, 1994.
5. Feinstein B, Langton JNK, Jameson RM, Schiller F. Experiments on pain referred from deep somatic tissues. *Journal of Bone and Joint Surgery.* 1954; **36-A**: 981–7.
6. Kellgren JH. On the distribution of pain arising from deep somatic structures with charts of segmental pain areas. *Clinical Science.* 1939; **4**: 35–46.
7. Dwyer A, Aprill C, Bogduk N. Cervical zygapophyseal joint pain patterns I: a study in normal volunteers. *Spine.* 1990; **15**: 453–7.
8. Dreyfuss P, Michaelsen M, Fletcher D. Atlanto-occipital and lateral atlanto-axial joint pain patterns. *Spine.* 1994; **19**: 1125–31.
9. Fukui S, Ohseto K, Shiotani M *et al.* Referred pain distribution of the cervical zygapophyseal joints and cervical dorsal rami. *Pain.* 1996; **68**: 79–83.
10. Schellhas KP, Smith MD, Gundry CR, Pollei SR. Cervical discogenic pain: prospective correlation of magnetic resonance imaging and discography in asymptomatic subjects and pain sufferers. *Spine.* 1996; **21**: 300–12.
11. Grubb SA, Kelly CK. Cervical discography: clinical implications from 12 years of experience. *Spine.* 2000; **25**: 1382–9.
12. Cooper G, Bailey B, Bogduk N. Cervical zygapophysial joint pain maps. *Pain Medicine.* 2007; **8**: 344–53.
13. Bovim G, Schrader H, Sand T. Neck pain in the general population. *Spine.* 1994; **19**: 1307–09.
14. Mäkelä M, Heliövaara M, Sievers K *et al.* Prevalence, determinants and consequences of chronic neck pain in Finland. *American Journal of Epidemiology.* 1991; **134**: 1356–67.
15. Cassou B, Derriennic F, Mofrit C *et al.* Chronic neck and shoulder pain, age, and working conditions: longituinal results from a large random sample in France. *Occupational and Environmental Medicine.* 2002; **59**: 537–44.
16. Cote P, Cassidy JD, Corroll L. The factors associated with neck pain and its related disability in the Saskatchewan population. *Spine.* 2000; **25**: 1109–17.
17. Bogduk N, McGuirk B. *Medical management of acute and chronic neck pain. An evidence-based approach.* Amsterdam: Elsevier, 2006: 21–7.
18. Van den Heuvel SG, van der Beek AJ, Blatter BM *et al.* Psychosocial work characteristics in relation to neck and upper limb symptoms. *Pain.* 2005; **114**: 47–53.
19. Ariens GA, Bongers PM, Hoogendoorf WE *et al.* High quantitative job demands and low coworker support as risk factors for neck pain: results of a prospective cohort study. *Spine.* 2001; **26**: 1896–901.
20. Ariens GA, Bongers PM, Hoogendoorn WE *et al.* High physical and psychosocial load at work and sickness absence due to neck pain. *Scandinavian Journal of Work, Environment and Health.* 2002; **28**: 222–31.
21. Eriksen W, Natvig B, Knardahl S, Bruusgaard D. Job characteristics as predictors of neck pain. A 4.4-year prospective study. *Journal of Occupational and Environmental Medicine.* 1999; **41**: 893–902.
22. Ariens GA, van Mechelen W, Bongers PM *et al.* American Journal of Industrial Medicine. 2001; **39**: 180–93.
23. Rugulies R, Krause N. Job strain, iso-strain, and the incidence of low back and neck injuries. A 7.5-year prospective study of San Francisco transit operators. *Social Science and Medicine.* 2005; **61**: 27–39.
24. Vasseljen O, Westgaard RH, Larsen S. A case-control study of psychological and psychosocial risk factors for shoulder and neck pain at the workplace. *International Archives of Occupational and Environmental Health.* 1995; **66**: 375–82.
* 25. Pietri-Taleb F, Riihimaki H, Viikari-Juntura E, Lindstrom K. Longitudinal study on the role of personality characteristics and psychological distress in neck trouble among working men. *Pain.* 1994; **58**: 261–7.
26. Westgaard RH, Jansen T. Individual and work related factors associated with symptoms of musculoskeletal complaints. II Different risk factors among sewing machine operators. *British Journal of Industrial Medicine.* 1992; **49**: 154–62.
27. Cote P, Cassidy JD, Carroll LJ, Kritsman V. The annual incidence and course of neck pain in the general population: a population-based cohort study. *Pain.* 2004; **112**: 267–73.
28. Hill J, Lewis M, Papgeorgious AC *et al.* Predicting persistent neck pain: a 1-year follow-up of a population cohort. *Spine.* 2004; **29**: 1648–54.
29. Gore DR, Sepic SB, Garnder GM, Murray MP. Neck pain: a long-term follow-up of 205 patients. *Spine.* 1987; **12**: 1–5.
30. Lees F, Turner JWA. Natural history and prognosis of cervical spondylosis. *British Medical Journal.* 1963; **2**: 1607–10.
31. Ariens GAM, Borghouts AJ, Koes BW. Neck pain. In: Crombie IK (ed.). *Epidemiology of pain.* Seattle: IASP Press, 1999: 235–55.
32. Borghouts JAJ, Koes BW, Bouter LM. The clinical course and prognostic factors of non-specific neck pain: a systematic review. *Pain.* 1998; **77**: 1–13.
33. Sharp J, Purser DW, Lawrence JS. Rheumatoid arthritis of the cervical spine in the adult. *Annals of the Rheumatic Diseases.* 1958; **17**: 303–13.
34. Isdale IC, Conlon PW. Atlanto-axial subluxation. A six-year follow-up report. *Annals of the Rheumatic Diseases.* 1971; **30**: 387–9.
* 35. Heller CA, Stanley P, Lewis-Jones B, Heller RF. Value of x-ray examinations of the cervical spine. *British Medical Journal.* 1983; **287**: 1276–8.

* 36. Johnson MJ, Lucas GL. Value of cervical spine radiographs as a screening tool. *Clinical Orthopaedics and Related Research*. 1997; **340**: 102–08.
37. Silbert PL, Makri B, Schievink WI. Headache and neck pain in spontaneous internal carotid and vertebral artery dissections. *Neurology*. 1995; **45**: 1517–22.
38. Biousse V, D'Anglejan-Chatillon J, Massiou H, Bousser MG. Head pain in non-traumatic carotid artery dissection: a series of 65 patients. *Cephalalgia*. 1994; **14**: 33–6.
39. Sturzenegger M. Headache and neck pain: the warning symptoms of vertebral artery dissection. *Headache*. 1994; **34**: 187–93.
40. Garrard P, Barnes D. Aortic dissection presenting as a neurological emergency. *Journal of the Royal Society of Medicine*. 1996; **89**: 271–2.
41. Hirst AE, Johns VJ, Kime FW. Dissecting aneurysm of the aorta: a review of 505 cases. *Medicine*. 1958; **37**: 217–75.
42. McNamara RM. Post-traumatic neck pain: a prospective and follow-up study. *Annals of Emergency Medicine*. 1988; **17**: 906–11.
43. Bachulis BL, Long WB, Hynes GD, Johnson MC. Clinical indications for cervical spine radiographs in the traumatized patient. *American Journal of Surgery*. 1987; **153**: 473–7.
44. Roberge RJ, Wears RC, Kelly M *et al*. Selective application of cervical spine radiography in alert victims of blunt trauma: a prospective study. *Journal of Trauma*. 1988; **28**: 784–8.
45. Kreipke DL, Gillespie KR, McCarthy MC *et al*. Reliability of indications for cervical spine films in trauma patients. *Journal of Trauma*. 1989; **29**: 1438–9.
46. Hoffman JR, Schriger DL, Mower W *et al*. Low-risk criteria for cervical-spine radiography in blunt trauma: a prospective study. *Annals of Emergency Medicine*. 1992; **21**: 1454–60.
47. Gerrelts BD, Petersen EU, Mabry J, Petersen RSR. Delayed diagnosis of cervical spine injuries. *Journal of Trauma*. 1991; **31**: 1622–6.
* 48. Fridenberg ZB, Miller WT. Degenerative disc disease of the cervical spine. A comparative study of asymptomatic and symptomatic patients. *Journal of Bone and Joint Surgery*. 1963; **45**: 1171–8.
49. Wolfe F, Simons DG, Fricton J *et al*. The fibromyalgia and myofascial pain syndromes: A preliminary study of tender points and trigger points in persons with fibromyalgia, myofascial pain and no disease. *Journal of Rheumatology*. 1992; **19**: 944–51.
50. Bogduk N, Simons DG. Neck pain: joint pain or trigger points. In: Vaeroy H, Merskey H (eds). *Progress in fibromyalgia and myofascial pain*. Amsterdam: Elsevier, 1993: 267–73.
51. Barnsley L, Lord S, Bogduk N. Clinical review: whiplash injuries. *Pain*. 1994; **58**: 283–307.
* 52. Berglund A, Alfredsson L, Cassidy JD *et al*. The association between exposure to a rear-end collision and future neck or shoulder pain: a cohort study. *Journal of Clinical Epidemiology*. 2000; **53**: 1089–94.
53. Radanov BP, Sturzenegger M, Di Stefano G. Long-term outcome after whiplash injury: a 2-year follow-up considering features of injury mechanism and somatic, radiologic, and psychosocial findings. *Medicine*. 1995; **74**: 281–97.
* 54. Scholten-Peeters GGM, Verhagen AP, Bekkering GE *et al*. Prognostic factors of whiplash-associated disorders: a systematic review of prospective cohort studies. *Pain*. 2003; **104**: 303–22.
55. Hendriks EJ, Scholten-Peeters GGM, van der Windt DAWM *et al*. Prognostic factors for poor recovery in acute whiplash patients. *Pain*. 2005; **114**: 408–16.
56. Osti OL, Gun RT, Abraham G *et al*. Potential risk factors for prolonged recovery following whiplash injury. *European Spine Journal*. 2005; **14**: 90–4.
57. Gun RT, Osti AL, O'Riordan A *et al*. Risk factors for prolonged disability after whiplash injury: a prospective study. *Spine*. 2005; **30**: 386–91.
58. Bogduk N, McGuirk B. *Medical management of acute and chronic neck pain. An evidence-based approach*. Amsterdam: Elsevier, 2006: 127–31.
* 59. Kaneoka K, Ono K, Inami S, Hayashi K. Motion analysis of cervical vertebrae during whiplash loading. *Spine*. 1999; **24**: 763–70.
60. Jonsson H, Cesarini K, Sahlstedt B, Rauschning W. Findings and outcomes in whiplash-type neck distortions. *Spine*. 1994; **19**: 2733–43.
61. Taylor JR, Twomey LT. Acute injuries to cervical joints: An autopsy study of neck sprain. *Spine*. 1993; **18**: 1115–22.
62. Taylor JR, Taylor MM. Cervical spinal injuries: an autopsy study of 109 blunt injuries. *Journal of Musculoskeletal Pain*. 1996; **4**: 61–79.
63. Hubka MJ, Phelan SP. Interexaminer reliability of palpation for cervical spine tenderness. *Journal of Manipulative and Physiological Therapeutics*. 1994; **17**: 591–5.
64. Levoska S, Keinanen-Kiukaanniemi S, Bloigu R. Repeatability of measurement of tenderness in the neck-shoulder region by a dolorimeter and manual palpation. *Clinical Journal of Pain*. 1993; **9**: 229–35.
65. Sandmark H, Nisell R. Validity of five common manual neck pain provoking tests. *Scandinavian Journal of Rehabilitation Medicine*. 1995; **27**: 131–6.
66. De Boer KF, Harman R, Tuttle CD, Wallace H. Reliability study of detection of somatic dysfunctions in the cervical spine. *Journal of Manipulative and Physiological Therapeutics*. 1985; **8**: 9–16.
67. Nansel DD, Peneff AL, Jansen RD, Cooperstein R. Interexaminer concordance in detecting joint-play asymmetries in the cervical spines of otherwise asymptomatic subjects. *Journal of Manipulative and Physiological Therapeutics*. 1989; **12**: 428–33.
68. Mior SA, King RS, McGregor M, Bernard M. Intra and interexaminer reliability of motion palpation in the cervical spine. *Journal of the Canadian Chiropractic Association*. 1985; **29**: 195–8.

69. King W, Lau P, Lees R, Bogduk N. The validity of manual examination in assessing patients with neck pain. *The Spine Journal.* 2007; **7**: 22–6.
70. Bogduk N, McGuirk B. *Medical management of acute and chronic neck pain. An evidence-based approach.* Amsterdam: Elsevier, 2006: 51–66.
* 71. Stiell IG, Wells GA, Vandemheen KL *et al.* The Canadian C-spine rule for radiography in alert and stable trauma patients. *Journal of the American Medical Association.* 2001; **286**: 1841–8.
72. Van der Donk J, Schouten JSAG, Passchier J *et al.* The associations of neck pain with radiological abnormalities of the cervical spine and personality traits in a general population. *Journal of Rheumatology.* 1991; **18**: 1884–9.
73. Helliwell PS, Evans PF, Wright V. The straight cervical spine: does it indicate muscle spasm? *Journal of Bone and Joint Surgery.* 1994; **76B**: 103–06.
74. Boden SD, McCowin PR, Davis DG *et al.* Abnormal magnetic-resonance scans of the cervical spine in asymptomatic subjects: a prospective investigation. *Journal of Bone and Joint Surgery.* 1990; **72**: 1178–84.
75. Teresi LM, Lufkin RB, Reicher MA *et al.* Asymptomatic degenerative disk disease and spondylosis of the cervical spine: MR imaging. *Radiology.* 1987; **164**: 83–8.
76. Ellertsson AB, Sigurjonsson K, Thorsteinsson T. Clinical and radiographic study of 100 cases of whiplash injury. *Acta Neurologica Scandinavica.* 1978; **5**: 269.
77. Pettersson K, Hildingsson C, Toolanen G *et al.* MRI and neurology in acute whiplash trauma. *Acta Orthopaedica Scandinavica.* 1994; **65**: 525–8.
78. Fagerlund M, Bjornebrink J, Pettersson K, Hildingsson C. MRI in acute phase of whiplash injury. *European Radiology.* 1995; **5**: 297–301.
79. Borchgrevink GE, Smevik O, Nordby A *et al.* MR imaging and radiography of patients with cervical hyperextension-flexion injuries after car accidents. *Acta Radiologica.* 1995; **36**: 425–8.
80. Ronnen HR, de Korte PJ, Brink PRG *et al.* Acute whiplash injury: is there a role for MR imaging? A prospective study of 100 patients. *Radiology.* 1996; **201**: 93–6.
81. Voyvodic F, Dolinis J, Moore VM *et al.* MRI of car occupants with whiplash injury. *Neuroradiology.* 1997; **39**: 25–40.
82. Seitz JP, Unguez CE, Corbus HF, Wooten WW. SPECT of the cervical spine in the evaluation of neck pain after trauma. *Clinical Nuclear Medicine.* 1995; **20**: 667–73.
83. Johansson BH. Whiplash injuries can be visible by functional magnetic resonance imaging. *Pain Research and Management.* 2006; **11**: 197–9.
84. Krakenes J, Kaale BR, Moen G *et al.* MRI assessment of the alar ligaments in the late stage of whiplash injury – a study of structural abnormalities and observer agreement. *Neuroradiology.* 2002; **44**: 617–24.
85. Krakenes J, Kaale BR, Moen G *et al.* MR analysis of the transverse ligament in the late stage of whiplash injury. *Acta Radiologica.* 2003; **44**: 637–44.
86. Anderson SE, Bogduk N, Boesch C *et al.* Preliminary MRI findings in the cervical spine after whiplash injury. *Skeletal Radiology.* 2006; **35**: 322.
87. International Spine Intervention Society. Cervical disc stimulation. In: Bogduk N (ed.). *Practice guidelines for spinal diagnostic and treatment procedures.* San Francisco: International Spinal Intervention Society, 2004: 95–111.
88. Bogduk N, Aprill C. On the nature of neck pain, discography and cervical zygapophysial joint pain. *Pain.* 1993; **54**: 213–17.
89. International Spine Intervention Society. Cervical medial branch blocks. In: Bogduk N (ed.). *Practice guidelines for spinal diagnostic and treatment procedures.* San Francisco: International Spinal Intervention Society, 2004: 112–37.
90. Barnsley L, Bogduk N. Medial branch blocks are specific for the diagnosis of cervical zygapophysial joint pain. *Regional Anesthesia.* 1993; **18**: 343–50.
91. Barnsley L, Lord S, Wallis B, Bogduk N. False-positive rates of cervical zygapophysial joint blocks. *Clinical Journal of Pain.* 1993; **9**: 124–30.
92. Barnsley L, Lord S, Bogduk N. Comparative local anaesthetic blocks in the diagnosis of cervical zygapophysial joints pain. *Pain.* 1993; **55**: 99–106.
93. Lord SM, Barnsley L, Bogduk N. The utility of comparative local anaesthetic blocks versus placebo-controlled blocks for the diagnosis of cervical zygapophysial joint pain. *Clinical Journal of Pain.* 1995; **11**: 208–13.
94. Barnsley L, Lord SM, Wallis BJ, Bogduk N. The prevalence of chronic cervical zygapophysial joint pain after whiplash. *Spine.* 1995; **20**: 20–6.
95. Lord S, Barnsley L, Wallis BJ, Bogduk N. Chronic cervical zygapohysial joint pain after whiplash: a placebo-controlled prevalence study. *Spine.* 1996; **21**: 1737–45.
96. Lord S, Barnsley L, Wallis B, Bogduk N. Third occipital nerve headache: a prevalence study. *Journal of Neurology, Neurosurgery, and Psychiatry.* 1994; **57**: 1187–90.
97. Gibson T, Bogduk N, Macpherson J, McIntosh A. The accident characteristics of whiplash associated chronic neck pain. *Journal of Musculoskeletal Pain.* 2000; **8**: 87–95.
98. Speldewinde GC, Bashford GM, Davidson IR. Diagnostic cervical zygapophysial joint blocks for chronic cervical pain. *Medical Journal of Australia.* 2001; **174**: 174–6.
99. Manchikanti L, Singh V, Rivera J, Pampati V. Prevalence of cervical facet joint pain in chronic neck pain. *Pain Physician.* 2002; **5**: 243–9.
100. Australian Acute Musculoskeletal Pain Guidelines Group. Evidence-based management of acute musculoskeletal pain. Brisbane, Australia: Australian Academic Press, last updated 2003; cited December 2007. Available from: www.nhmrc.gov.au/publications/synopses/cp94syn.htm.
101. Bogduk N, McGuirk B. *Medical management of acute and chronic neck pain. An evidence-based approach.* Amsterdam: Elsevier, 2006: 79–90.

102. Peeters GGM, Verhagen AP, de Bie RA, Oostendorp RAB. The efficacy of conservative treatment in patients with whiplash injury. A systematic review of clinical trials. *Spine*. 2001; **26**: E64–73.
103. Verhagen AP, Peeters GGM, de Bie RA, Oostendorp RAB. Conservative treatment for whiplash. *Cochrane Library*. 2002; **2**. Oxford: Update Software.
104. Borchgrevink GE, Kaasa A, McDonagh D *et al*. Acute treatment of whiplash neck sprain injuries: a randomized trial of treatment during the first 14 days after a car accident. *Spine*. 1998; **23**: 25–31.
105. McKinney LA, Dornan JO, Ryan M. The role of physiotherapy in the management of acute neck sprains following road-traffic accidents. *Archives of Emergency Medicine*. 1989; **6**: 27–33.
106. McKinney LA. Early mobilisation and outcomes in acute sprains of the neck. *British Medical Journal*. 1989; **299**: 1006–08.
107. Rosenfeld M, Gunnarsson R, Borenstein P. Early intervention in whiplash-associated disorders. A comparison of two treatment protocols. *Spine*. 2000; **25**: 1782–7.
108. Rosenfeld M, Seferiadis A, Carlsson J, Gunnarsson R. Active intervention in patients with whiplash-associated disorders improves long-term prognosis. A randomized controlled trial. *Spine*. 2003; **28**: 2491–8.
109. Verhagen AP, Peeters GGM, de Bie RA, Bierma-Zeinstra SMA. Conservative treatment for whiplash. *Cochrane Database of Systematic Reviews*. 2004; CD003338.
110. Gross AR, Kay T, Hondras M *et al*. Manual therapy for mechanical neck disorders: a systematic review. *Manual Therapy*. 2002; **7**: 131–49.
111. Bogduk N, McGuirk B. *Medical management of acute and chronic neck pain. An evidence-based approach*. Amsterdam: Elsevier, 2006: 69–77.
112. Bogduk N, McGuirk B. *Medical management of acute and chronic neck pain. An evidence-based approach*. Amsterdam: Elsevier, 2006: 115–21.
113. Petrie JP, Langley GB. Acupuncture in the treatment of chronic cervical pain. A pilot study. *Clinical and Experimental Rheumatology*. 1983; **1**: 333–5.
114. Birch S, Jamison RB. Controlled trial of Japanese acupuncture for chronic myofascial neck pain: assessment of specific and non-specific effects of treatment. *Clinical Journal of Pain*. 1998; **14**: 248–55.
115. He D, Veiersted KB, Hostmark AT, Medbo JI. Effect of acupuncture treatment on chronic neck and shoulder pain in sedentary female workers: a 6-month and 3-year follow-up study. *Pain*. 2004; **109**: 299–307.
116. Thomas MM, Eriksson SV, Lundeberg T. A comparative study of diazepam and acupuncture in patients with osteoarthritis pain: a placebo controlled study. *American Journal of Chinese Medicine*. 1991; **19**: 95–100.
117. Irnich D, Behrens N, Molzen H *et al*. Randomised trial of acupuncture compared with conventional massage and "sham" laser acupuncture for treatment of chronic neck pain. *British Medical Journal*. 2001; **322**: 1–6.
118. Lewith GT, Machin D. A randomised trial to evaluate the effect of infra-red stimulation of local trigger points, versus placebo, on the pain caused by cervical osteoarthrosis. *Acupuncture and Electro-therapeutics Research*. 1981; **6**: 277–84.
119. Petrie JP, Hazleman BL. A controlled study of acupuncture in neck pain. *British Journal of Rheumatology*. 1986; **25**: 271–5.
120. Thorsen H, Gam AN, Svensson BH *et al*. Low level laser therapy for myofascial pain in the neck and shoulder girdle. A double-blind cross-over study. *Scandinavian Journal of Rheumatology*. 1992; **21**: 139–42.
121. Wheeler AH, Goolkasian P, Gretz SS. Botulinum toxin A for the treatment of chronic neck pain. *Pain*. 2001; **94**: 255–60.
122. Esenyel CZ, Caglar N, Aldemir T. Treatment of myofascial pain. *American Journal of Physical Medicine and Rehabilitation*. 2000; **79**: 48–52.
123. Gam AN, Warming S, Larsen LH *et al*. Treatment of myofascial trigger points with ultrasound combined with massage and exercise – a randomised controlled trial. *Pain*. 1998; **77**: 73–9.
124. Barnsley L, Lord SM, Wallis BJ, Bogduk N. Lack of effect of intraarticular corticosteroids for chronic pain in the cervical zygapophyseal joints. *New England Journal of Medicine*. 1994; **330**: 1047–50.
125. Klaber Moffett JA, Jackson DA, Richmond S *et al*. Randomised trial of a brief physiotherapy intervention compared with usual physiotherapy for neck pain patients: outcomes and patients' preference. *British Medical Journal*. 2005; **330**: 75–8.
126. Randlov A, Ostergaard M, Manniche C *et al*. Intensive dynamic training for females with chronic neck/shoulder pain. A randomised controlled trial. *Clinical Rehabilitation*. 1998; **12**: 200–10.
127. Jordan A, Bendix T, Nielsen H *et al*. Intensive training, physiotherapy, or manipulation for patients with chronic neck pain. A prospective, single-blinded, randomised clinical trial. *Spine*. 1998; **23**: 311–19.
128. Taimela S, Takala EP, Asklof T *et al*. Active treatment of chronic neck pain. A prospective randomised intervention. *Spine*. 2000; **25**: 1021–7.
129. Bronfort G, Evans R, Nelson B *et al*. A randomised clinical trial of exercise and spinal manipulation for patients with chronic neck pain. *Spine*. 2001; **26**: 788–99.
130. Evans R, Bronfort G, Nelson B, Goldmsith CH. Two-year follow-up of a randomised clinical trial of spinal manipulation and two types of exercise for patients with chronic neck pain. *Spine*. 2002; **27**: 2383–9.
131. Viljanen M, Malmivaara A, Uitti J *et al*. Effectiveness of dynamic muscle training, relaxation training, ordinary activity for chronic neck pain: randomised controlled trial. *British Medical Journal*. 2003; **327**: 475.
132. Ylinen J, Takala EP, Nykanen M *et al*. Active neck muscle training in the treatment of chronic neck pain in women. A randomized controlled trial. *Journal of the American Medical Association*. 2003; **289**: 2509–16.

133. Chiu TTW, Lam THL, Hedley AJ. A randomised controlled trial on the efficacy of exercise for patients with chronic neck pain. *Spine*. 2005; **30**: E1–7.

*134. Stewart MJ, Maher CG, Refshauge KM *et al.* Randomized controlled trial of exercise for chronic whiplash-associated disorders. *Pain*. 2007; **128**: 59–68.

135. Kikuchi S, Macnab I, Moreau P. Localisation of the level of symptomatic cervical disc degeneration. *Journal of Bone and Joint Surgery*. 1981; **63B**: 272–7.

136. Whitecloud TS, Seago RA. Cervical discogenic syndrome. Results of operative intervention in patients with positive discography. *Spine*. 1987; **12**: 313–16.

137. De Plama AF, Subin DK. Study of the cervical syndrome. *Clinical Orthopaedics and Related Research*. 1965; **38**: 135–42.

138. Algers G, Pettersson K, Hildingsson C, Toolanen G. Surgery for chronic symptoms after whiplash injury. Follow-up of 20 cases. *Acta Orthopaedica Scandinavica*. 1993; **64**: 654–6.

139. Garvey TA, Transfeldt EE, Malcolm JR, Kos P. Outcome of anterior cervical diskectomy and fusion as perceived by patients treated for dominant axial-mechanical cervical spine pain. *Spine*. 2002; **27**: 1887–94.

140. Lord SM, McDonald GJ, Bogduk N. Percutaneous radiofrequency neurotomy of the cervical medial branches: a validated treatment for cervical zygapophysial joint pain. *Neurosurgery Quarterly*. 1998; **8**: 288–308.

*141. Lord SM, Barnsley L, Wallis BJ *et al.* Percutaneous radio-frequency neurotomy for chronic cervical zygapophysial-joint pain. *New England Journal of Medicine*. 1996; **335**: 1721–6.

142. McDonald G, Lord SM, Bogduk N. Long-term follow-up of patients treated with cervical radiofrequency neurotomy for chronic neck pain. *Neurosurgery*. 1999; **45**: 61–8.

143. Wallis BJ, Lord SM, Bogduk N. Resolution of psychological distress of whiplash patients following treatment by radiofrequency neurotomy: a randomised, double-blind, placebo-controlled trial. *Pain*. 1997; **73**: 15–22.

144. Sapir DA, Gorup JM. Radiofrequency medial branch neurotomy in litigant and nonlitigant patients with cervical whiplash. *Spine*. 2001; **26**: E268–73.

145. Barnsley L. Percutaneous radiofrequency neurotomy for chronic neck pain: outcomes in a series of consecutive patients. *Pain Medicine*. 2005; **6**: 282–6.

146. Govind J, King W, Bailey B, Bogduk N. Radiofrequency neurotomy for the treatment of third occipital headache. *Journal of Neurology, Neurosurgery, and Psychiatry*. 2003; **74**: 88–93.

37

Chronic back pain

RANDY A SHELERUD

KEY LEARNING POINTS

- Understanding the chronic lower back pain (CLBP) patient's motivation for seeking care improves satisfaction, treatment compliance, outcomes, and saves time.
- Spine clinicians best serve as gatekeepers to the growing list of other local spine care specialists.
- Initial assessment emphasizes measuring pain, disability, red and yellow flags, and diagnostic subgroups.
- Several pitfalls for the initial assessment of the CLBP patient exist.
- History and examination are geared toward ruling out serious underlying diseases.
- Many theories exist for the causes of CLBP.
- CLBP treatment must emphasize maximizing function through rehabilitative exercise and return to work programs.
- Temporizing measures for treating pain also include medications, manipulation, massage, injections, and modalities.
- Multidisciplinary cognitive-behavioral therapy is perhaps one of the most useful treatment tools for chronic disabling CLBP.

INTRODUCTION

The medical management of the patient with chronic lower back pain (CLBP) is a process that has evolved over time. Prior evaluation and treatment recommendations using a bioanatomic model[1] of low back pain have given way to a newer biopsychosocial model.[2,3,4] This model is, as will be discussed, more multidimensional and patient-centric.[5] For example, treatment efficacy is higher when patient's thoughts, beliefs, attitudes, and expectations are taken into account.[6,7,8] Therefore, empathic listening is also a prerequisite for assessment and the development of a care plan.[9,10] The astute clinician will still want to assess pain, functional limitations or disability, work ability, and to screen for serious pathology. Care planning should strongly emphasize the concept of maximizing function.

The goals of this chapter are to review motivation for seeking medical care and the components of the initial assessment, including the details of the history and examination. In addition, discussion will be directed toward counseling patients with CLBP in the context of known literature, as well as to outline sound management programs for CLBP patients.

One needs to understand at the outset that CLBP is a symptom rather than a clinical entity with wide variations in severity of disability and duration.[2] The screening of prognostic factors for disability in this population (yellow flags) is therefore an essential component of the evaluative process.[11] Overall, there is limited literature support to guide the clinician in this patient population, and as a result, there is a paucity of guidelines available.

The approach to treatment should take into account the fact that no single treatment intervention is likely to be effective in isolation given the complexity of CLBP. For instance, using modalities and medications to control pain while progressing a back rehabilitation program with a cognitive-behavioral counseling style may be far more successful in a severely disabled patient than simply offering physical therapy. In addition, the effect sizes for the various treatments available for chronic low back pain are modest at best.[12] Reducing pain by 50 percent may be a more realistic goal than hoping to take most or all pain away. Reducing pain by 30 percent is actually used to define "efficacy" in drug efficacy research.[13]

Very few CLBP patients will have a "fixable" etiology for their pain. Therefore, to optimize care, the clinician should function as a gatekeeper partnering with the patient and utilizing the talents of various spine care providers as needed. The gatekeeper philosophy of spine care delivery allows the treating clinician to protect the CLBP patient from an expensive and often criticized trap of receiving unimodal treatment from one type of care provider over the long term.[14] It is essential then to also understand the spine care providers in the area in which one practices, so as to be an effective management gatekeeper.

WHY ARE THEY COMING TO SEE YOU?

The office evaluation of the CLBP patient should include, at a minimum, the assessment of pain severity, functional disability, and screening for underlying serious disease.[15] However, most of these issues carry little importance to the chronic low back pain patients as their reasons for seeking care may be entirely different.

Perhaps the most common reason for seeking care is to find the source of the back pain.[16] However, many other reasons exist (**Box 37.1**). Simply continuing to probe into the patient's reasons for seeking an evaluation will allow more meaningful counsel and is less time-consuming.[10] This can lead to improved outcomes of not only patient satisfaction, but compliance of treatment, self-rated improvement, and decreased desire for ordering further testing.[17]In addition, to the patient's reasons for seeking care for the CLBP, referring physicians have additional interests. They may hold some of the same expectations as their patients.[18] For example, low back pain myths shared by physician and patient may need to be addressed.[19] These myths include:

- if you have a slipped disk, you should have surgery;
- radiographs and newer imaging tests can always find the cause of pain;
- bed rest is the mainstay of therapy;
- if your back hurts you should take it easy until the pain goes away;
- most back pain is caused by injuries or heavy lifting;
- back pain is usually disabling;
- everyone with back pain should have a spine x-ray.

Box 37.1 Common reasons why patients seek medical care for low back pain

- To receive information regarding recovery time
- To find out the cause of their pain
- Advice on activity modification
- Advice regarding medication options
- Reassurance about the absence of serious pathology
- Opportunity to challenge misdiagnoses or inappropriate management
- Sickness certification
- To explore alternative management strategies

Primary care physicians may be uncomfortable making management decisions in this population[18] and may assume that you have better tools to treat these patients, or access to other spine care practitioners. There may be an assumption that you will provide ongoing care for the CLBP patient, prescribe opioids, or perform a more thorough evaluation. The management options outlined in this chapter will give the spine care provider a working feel for making reasonable choices for and with the CLBP patient.

THE SPINE CARE TEAM

The spine clinician, as gatekeeper, has a team of spine care providers to assist in patient management. Over recent decades, the spine care team has grown. For example, specialists who act as intermediaries between primary care providers and spine surgeons include physiatrists or physicians trained in the specialty of physical medicine and rehabilitation (www.aapmr.org). Many physiatrists have a special interest in medical management of musculoskeletal problems like CLBP. In addition, physicians of various specialties have additional board certification in pain medicine and deal with a large proportion of CLBP patients. Some, including anesthesiologists, physiatrists, and radiologists among others, may have taken fellowship training in interventional spine techniques (www.spinalinjection.com).

Physical therapists, chiropractors, as well as osteopathic-trained physicians, in many countries provide a significant amount of care for CLBP patients. Occupational therapists can be valuable particularly in assessing work or home ergonomic issues for CLBP patients as well. Complementary and alternative medicine practitioners, such as those who provide massage therapy, acupuncture, manipulation, or other manual medicine techniques, also have an increasingly large role in the care of patients with acute and chronic spine problems.

Other spine care service lines to be aware of include pain rehabilitation programs. These programs are intensive with two to four weeks of full day, multidisciplinary treatments for patients with chronic pain and chronic pain syndrome.[20, 21] These typically have a cognitive-behavioral approach to rehabilitation. Pain medicine physicians are trained in pharmacologic management options that include oral and pump delivery systems (www.painmed.org). Work rehabilitation facilities are thriving, offering rehabilitation geared toward specific work tasks, full return-to-work programs, and functional capacity evaluations.

Spine surgeons are most appropriately positioned as a third tier of expertise downstream from the primary care providers and the other subspecialists. Their expertise is required of only a small percentage of CLBP patients. Among spine surgeons, the neurosurgeons are participating in spine care to a larger extent as neurosurgical residency programs are increasingly offering training in spinal instrumentation techniques similar to their orthopedic spine colleagues.

Given the changes in the spine care team, it is imperative that clinicians caring for patients with CLBP get to know the various spine subspecialists in their geographic area. This will ensure appropriate referrals by allowing an understanding of the types of patients subspecialists can help and are interested in seeing, as well as treatments they can provide.

INITIAL ASSESSMENT

Goals of the initial assessment

The initial assessment of patients with CLBP needs to be thorough and systematic. The goals of the initial evaluation are as listed in **Box 37.2**. Part of the initial evaluation should include a screen for risk factors for chronicity.[11] These so-called "yellow flags" are psychosocial factors that increase the risk of developing or maintaining chronic pain and disability, and include:

- inappropriate attitudes and beliefs about back pain;
- inappropriate pain behavior, such as fear-avoidance;
- work satisfaction and related return-to-work issues;
- associated emotional issues, such as depression, anxiety, or stress.

Assessment for the presence of yellow flags and management suggestions are detailed elsewhere.[1]

Box 37.2 Goals of the initial assessment of chronic low back pain patients

- Identify the reason(s) why they are seeking care
- Identify patients with an evolving chronic pain syndrome
- Don't be fooled by certain subgroups of patients:
  - the chronic low back pain patient you have seen regularly over years;
  - the patient with psychological overlay;
  - the poor historian;
  - the patient who has been seen by everyone else;
  - the patient who has been sent with a diagnosis of "low back pain."
- Assessment of pain
- Assessment of disability
- Identify red flag medical issues by history and examination
- Identify yellow flag psychosocial issues
- Look for diagnostic subgroups

Chronic low back pain or chronic pain syndrome?

The International Association for the Study for Pain defines pain as an unpleasant sensory and emotional experience associated with actual or potential tissue damage or described in terms of such damage.[22] Chronic low back pain is defined and distinguished from acute pain by symptom duration, treatment responses, the concept of neuroplasticity (sensitization) of the central nervous system, and the relationship of symptoms to the initial noxious stimulus. In contrast, in chronic pain syndrome, the balance between the sensation of pain and the emotional experience associated with it is far out of balance in favor of the emotional side.[23] The criteria are as follows:

- chronic symptoms often severe;
- disproportionate to the pathology;
- atypical sensory features;
- "nonanatomic" location;
- associated symptoms (fatigue, sleep, memory, libido);
- psychological distress (depression, anxiety, posttraumatic stress disorder (PTSD));
- social role dysfunction (work, home, play);
- excessive healthcare utilization.

Don't be fooled by these patient populations

The evaluation of CLBP patients is often a search for the needle in a haystack with regard to the presence of serious underlying pathology or surgically correctable disease.[24, 25] There is a tendency, then, to be somewhat dismissive with regard to the evaluation of these patients in a busy practice. However, one must remain vigilant as to not miss the patient with real pathology (**Box 37.2**).[26]

The chronic low back pain patient, who has presented on numerous occasions, can subsequently develop a life-threatening reason for their pain. They may only complain of worsening symptoms over time or an additional area of pain, when indeed they are harboring a new cancer, infection, or fracture. The patient with psychological overlay or the possibility of chronic pain syndrome similarly can have a serious underlying reason for their pain.

The poor historian presents a unique challenge as many of the spine disease subcategories are defined best by their historical features. The challenge for the clinician is to dig deeper and spend the extra time to ensure that nothing is missed. Then there are those patients whose records indicate visits to many of your colleagues or other clinicians in the region and are now in your office with the same complaints. Clinicians can fall into the trap of assuming that a proper evaluation must have been completed by someone along the way. It is important to follow through on a meticulous and systematic evaluation, independent of previous diagnoses given in the past.

Assess the pain severity and disability

The Joint Commission for Hospital Accreditation (JCAHO) requires an assessment of pain severity on the initial and all follow-up visits. Pain assessment is described in detail in Chapter 8 Assessment, measurement, and history in the *Acute Pain* volume of this series. This can be documented by the patient on a simple 11-point numerical scale completed in the waiting room. The assessment of pain alone gives an incomplete picture as pain poorly correlates with the amount of impairment and disability in CLBP patients.[7, 27, 28, 29, 30, 31] Therefore, even if the patient's documented pain scores are improving, one cannot assume that their function is improving as well.

The impact of pain on the patient's function and quality of life should be assessed, by asking the patient what activity they enjoy and document how much of that activity they can do. This serves as a useful guide for initial assessment and follow-up progress over time. Additionally, assessment of the patient's sleep quality, work capabilities, and self-care skills all contribute to the understanding of disability.

Effective screening for red flag and yellow flag issues

Screening for serious underlying pathology includes screening for malignancy and/or benign tumor, infection, fracture, inflammatory arthropathy, and neurologic disease, such as radiculopathy, spinal stenosis, or the rare but serious cauda equina syndrome.[25] In all of these cases, with the exception of neurologic disorders, the examination is nonspecific.[32, 33] There is often very little difference in the appearance of someone with gardening-variety low back pain on examination and those with cancer, infection, or fracture. Therefore, the history is relied upon heavily to assess risk (**Table 37.1**).

Physical examination

The examination of a patient's chronic low back pain is best performed with the patient wearing garments that allow viewing of the spine, buttock region, and extremities. The examination is also geared towards screening for serious underlying disease processes. It is most heavily weighted towards neurologic conditions, most commonly radiculopathy or other diseases, involving the cauda

Table 37.1 Assessment for red flags.

Site	
Tumor or cancer	A history of cancer, unexplained fever, weight loss, night sweats, pain not relieved by rest (unremitting), or pain worse at night, progressively worsening pain over time, or pain refractory to treatment
Infection	As above, but also consider immunosuppression, intravenous drug use, foreign travel, recent trauma, or infection (urinary tract, pulmonary, skin, etc.)
Fracture	Recent significant trauma, fall, or lift, or trivial trauma in someone at risk for osteoporosis, disabling symptoms of sudden onset, or pain located in the sacrum instead of the usual low back location (sacral insufficiency fractures)
Inflammatory arthropathy	Younger ages (20s and 30s), prolonged morning stiffness >30 minutes, symptoms improved with exercise but not rest, significant inability to bend well, also possible lower extremity large joint involvement
Cauda equina syndrome	Typically abrupt onset of back pain with pain in one or both legs $\pm$ weakness, sensory changes, saddle distribution sensory changes, urinary retention or incontinence without warning, occasionally rectal sphincter dysfunction as well (a surgical emergency)

equina. However, it is also useful to screen for the range of motion of the spine, hips, and knees, as well as assessing for any asymmetry of flexibility and movement. Similarly, assessing the presence of significant muscle tenderness and spasm can help direct the patient towards treatment that may be of value for a muscular component of their symptoms. Finally, examination can also be useful in identifying pain behaviors that may alert the clinician to the presence of psychological distress[34] or evolving chronic pain syndrome, such as grimacing, vocalization, excessive rubbing of areas, or posturing during the examination.

Excellent resource texts are available to further define individual features of the physical examination.[35, 36] An outline of the comprehensive physical examination is given in **Table 37.2**. Essentially, the examination progresses from assessment in a standing position, sitting position, supine, side lying, and if needed, prone.

Patients can be potentially grouped together by findings on history and examination into several special subcategories, as follows.

CAUDA EQUINA SYNDROME

Cauda equina syndrome (CES) is the new onset of sacral nerve dysfunction manifested by initial urinary retention, then overflow incontinence, and unilateral or bilateral saddle distribution sensory loss with the possibility of rectal sphincter dysfunction. This is all in the context of typically abrupt onset of back pain and unilateral or bilateral leg pain, weakness, or paresthesias. While this is classically a bilateral leg problem different from radiculopathy, occasional patients will present with what otherwise looks like radiculopathy but have the sacral segment symptoms (incontinence) that make this syndrome a surgical emergency.[37, 38]

CHRONIC BACK PAIN OF POTENTIAL DISCOGENIC ORIGIN

Patients are typically younger than 50 years, often with acute injury and worsening pain in positions that load the spine to the greatest extent (i.e. sitting, twisting, and flexion), positive cough, sneeze, and strain effect. Examination is nonspecific with spasm, tightness, or segmental hypomobility.[39]

SYMPTOMATIC FACET JOINT DISEASE

Symptomatic facet joint disease accounts for 15–40 percent of CLBP.[40] This is often focal low back pain (LBP) frequently referring to the buttocks unilaterally or bilaterally. Examination may find increased pain with extension, stork test, or quadrant test[41] and focal tenderness in the periarticular regions.

SYMPTOMATIC SACROILIAC JOINT DISEASE

Studies vary, but patients are more often symptomatic in one buttock only and have no low back pain component. Examination findings with the most potential (controversial) include Faber's test, Gaenslen's test, shear test, and forced hip abduction.[42, 43, 44]

OVERLYING SIGNIFICANT FOCAL MYOFASCIAL PAIN

Patients with overlying significant focal myofascial pain present with a history of acute injury or repetitive overload with pain along the paraspinal muscles that occurs a day or two after significant or new labor. Examination may show tenderness, spasm, and guarding with segmental hypomobility.[45]

SYMPTOMATIC HIP JOINT DISEASE

Symptomatic hip joint disease is usually confused with upper lumbar radiculopathy as the hip can refer pain down the anterior thigh to the knee and occasionally further. Variable pain locations may also include the groin, buttock, or other areas in the thigh. The severity of arthritis demonstrated on x-ray only roughly correlates with pain which can be severe and often at night. Hip motion asymmetry is often diagnostic as is Trendelenberg gait, Faber's test, or Stinchfield's test compared to the well leg.[46]

SACRAL INSUFFICIENCY FRACTURES

Like those with a vertebral compression fracture, the only clue to sacral insufficiency fracture (SIF) may be the profile of someone with osteoporosis risks. SIF patients look different in that their pain may be predominantly in the buttocks compared to the typical CLBP patient. Palpatory examination of the sacrum or pain with sitting versus standing is highly variable and nondiagnostic. Bone scan is more sensitive than x-ray and lumbar magnetic resonance imaging (MRI).[47]

LUMBAR RADICULOPATHY

Ninety-five percent of patients have either L5 or S1 root symptoms. Leg pain typically dominates over back pain. L5 patients have pain down the posterolateral thigh and lateral calf. If the foot is involved, pain is on the top including the great toe. S1 patients have pain down the back of the thigh and back of the calf with foot symptoms on the bottom and/or outside of the foot. Sensory symptoms may or may not be present and can be localized to a dermatomal distribution. About half of patients are weak (usually mild) in the respective myotome.[48]

BAASTRUP'S DISEASE

Baastrup's disease is a radiographic finding more often than a clinical syndrome. Best seen on a lateral x-ray,

Table 37.2 Examination outline and rationale.

Criteria for assessment	
General assessment	
Global level of comfort	Assess how disabling the pain is or signs of pain behaviors suggesting chronic pain syndrome grimacing vocalizations, rubbing, over-reacting (Waddell's signs (W))[34]
General quality of movement	Look for guarding, posturing suggesting muscle spasm, or fear of movement
Assess pain location	Regionalization (W) of pain complaints or sensory changes
Standing	
Standing posture	Look for guarding, off-weighting a limb or atrophy; scoliosis may suggest mass lesion, iliac crest height asymmetry suggests a functional or anatomic leg length discrepancy
Gait	Antalgic, Trendelenberg; suggests hip disease or weak hip girdle weakness, steppage; compensating for foot drop, spastic; suggests central nervous system problem
Gross motor examination	Walking on heels and on toes; an extension of the muscle testing examination looking for L5 or S1 weakness, respectively
Spine range of motion	Look for quality and quantity of movement; Schober test can measure amount of flexion. Extension, stork, and quadrant test load the posterior elements (i.e. facet joints or spondylolysis if present)
Palpation	Look for muscular tenderness, possible bursitis (ischial or greater trochanteric), spinous process tenderness may suggest level of facet or disk pain
Simulation tests (of Waddell)	Simulated hip rotation, axial loading; nonanatomic tenderness (W); superficial skin rolling (W)
Sitting	
Muscle stretch reflex examination	Look for symmetry; heel jerk tests S1, internal hamstring test L5 and knee jerk tests L4, relaxation is important
Upper motor neuron signs	Babinski, clonus, hypertonicity, hyper-reflexia
Manual muscle testing	Must have 30–40% of strength loss to be able to see it on this part of the examination; L2, hip flexion; L3, knee extension; L4, ankle dorsiflexion; L5, great toe extension, foot inversion, and hip abduction; S1, ankle plantar flexion or foot eversion and hip extension; S2, knee flexion
Vascular examination	Screening for vascular disease, especially if claudication is suspected
Sensory examination	Pin examination discriminates best between dermatomes: look for dermatomal sensory loss if radiculopathy is suspected
Distraction (W)	Seated straight leg raise, while performing Babinski testing
Supine	
Straight leg raising	Look for reproduction of leg complaints if present below the knee up to 70° of hip flexion. Must have leg relaxed
Hip provocative maneuvers and range of motion	Look to reproduce pain complaints in the area of the hip and compare to well side (Faber's, Stinchfield's tests)
Knee joint examination	Look to reproduce pain complaints with joint line palpation, meniscal testing, full flexion or extension
Side lying	
Repeat palpatory examination	Look for reproducibility of tenderness found standing. Look for a potential muscular target for focal pain treatments
Rectal examination and perineal sensory examination	If cauda equine syndrome is suspected

generously sized adjacent spinous processes make contact creating degenerative changes and occasionally a pseudo bursa. Focal pain in the interspinous process region with tenderness would make this a potential clinical issue.[49]

BERTOLOTTI'S SYNDROME

Bertolotti's syndrome is also more often only an anatomic finding. Patients present with a transitional lumbosacral interval, such that one or both transverse processes of L5 create a false joint with the top of the sacrum. Degenerative changes can develop and patients may have focal mechanical pain at that location. Injection or surgery have been completed successfully.[50]

SPINAL INSTABILITY

This rare phenomenon is seen most often in those with spondylolisthesis or in the setting of previous spinal fusion surgery. Trauma without fracture, but with instability, would be rare. Flexion and extension lateral x-ray views showing >3.5 mm of translation suggest instability.

FIBROMYALGIA SYNDROME

Patients with fibromyalgia may complain of back pain predominantly and the two issues can coexist. Widespread pain complaints with poor sleep quality and deconditioning is typical. Classic tender points on examination help diagnostically.[51]

DOCTOR, WHAT IS CAUSING MY CHRONIC LOW BACK PAIN?

The issue of finding the source of pain is an important one on several levels. First, patients expect their practitioner to find the pain source and expect to discuss it in detail. Second, aside from rare and serious underlying disease screening, clinicians need to understand that there is a lack of diagnostic tools to indeed answer this question accurately. In other words, a meticulous history and examination along with judicious use of imaging studies all fail to localize the source of pain in most cases.[52, 53, 54] There are important exceptions that need to be considered (see above under Don't be fooled by these patient populations), therefore, one must not become complacent or dismissive. Third, the astute spine care provider will do well to understand the various etiologic theories currently espoused regarding chronic low back pain (see below under Setting up a sound treatment program) in order to provide meaningful counsel.

The patient's mindset regarding the causes of their pain is crucial for effective counseling and education. Their mindset may be colored by contrasting input from family members with previous spine issues, friends, coworkers, as well as other care providers. Additionally, there may have been miscommunication or overinterpretation of the findings on imaging studies such as "degenerative disk disease." Isolated data like these may allow the patient to "wed" themselves to a particular etiology which varies significantly (**Table 37.3**).[17] It is important to understand that patients will hold tightly to their concepts of chronic low back pain and will often do so in a cause and effect or bioanatomic way.[55] This will often conflict with the care provider's overarching biopsychosocial view and therefore result in treating clinician discomfort to attempt to try to resolve this conflict.[56, 57] Chronic low back pain disability can actually be decreased by effective education centered around the patient's beliefs, attitudes, and their expectations about their pain and activity.[58] As Dr RG Hazaard recommended in a recent review, "... it may be more effective to specifically address an individual's (spouse supported) fear of re-injury than to hand print a pamphlet describing clinical 'red flags' or a video on therapeutic options."[59] In CLBP, a complex interaction between the peripheral and central nervous system has occurred. Neurons, neurotransmitters, neuroplasticity in the context of wind up, can all contribute in theory to an overall long-standing change in the pain signal transmission, maintaining the signal chronically.[59]

Second, the literature is replete with contrasting theories regarding the etiology of low back pain. In a traditional, bioanatomic view, Kirkaldy-Willis *et al.*[60] and Andersson[61] have identified the disks, facet joints, or sacroiliac joints, as some of the main causes of chronic low back pain. These are often found with a "myofascial cycle" that explains a muscular component often seen in chronic low back pain patients and also allows for the interplay between "emotional factors" to contribute to the overall pain problem.[62] Diagnostic injection studies have supported this view,[40, 43] though it is unclear whether a

Table 37.3 Patient models regarding the etiology of low back pain.

Category	
Purely biological or mechanical terms	"I jumped from a height as a child and that's how it started"
Gender	Women associate childbirth, men associate military service
Environmental factors	Improper chair, exposure to wind, wrong shoes or car seat
Aging	"My muscles are not strong... decline in well being"
Overuse, misuse, or bad habits	
Psychosocial factors	Stress and unhappiness
Defective spine (congenital or acquired)	"It is obvious to me that there is some defect in my spine"

response to diagnostic blocks confirms the presence of a clinical entity.

In contrast, the osteopathic view of the etiology of CLBP suggests that a lesion defined as "somatic dysfunction"[63] is identified (see below under Spinal manipulation). Others have postulated that spinal manipulation treats lesions that may include the release of entrapped synovial folds or plica within facet joints, relaxation of hypertonic muscle by sudden stretching, disruption of articular or periarticular adhesion, or unbuckling of motion segments that have undergone disproportionate displacements.[64] Others have recently put forward an argument that atherosclerosis of the lumbar vessels is responsible for low back pain.[65]

These theories and others have to be understood in terms of a wider context. Historically, the orthopedic literature has been the most robust with regard to low back pain in general, and therefore, also theories regarding CLBP etiology have a strong orthopedic influence. This literature is dominated particularly from the 1940s to the 1980s by the assumption that the disk and disk disease is the primary cause of acute and chronic low back pain.[66] This assumption has driven much of the treatment decision-making and research of that time. Many other theories, such as gynecological, neuritis, or muscle rheumatism, have preceded the era of the disk and many other potential etiologies re-emerged at the end of the twentieth century.[66] All await definitive support.

SETTING UP A SOUND TREATMENT PROGRAM

The medical management of a typical CLBP patient is oriented toward maximizing function and quality of life. In the ideal setting, the patient would be taught the tools to self-manage their symptoms. Keep in mind that a realistic reduction in pain (~50 percent) is a secondary goal. The patient's main focus may be the treatment of pain, so setting expectations including full participation in the rehabilitation process while addressing pain is fundamental. Many options for pain control exist and there are few guides to assist in deciding which are best for any individual patient. Taking into account patient preferences, patient expectations, as well as weighing the risk/benefit ratio of a pain control treatment, aids in decision-making.

Medication

Medications (described in Chapter 15, The use of NSAIDs and paracetamol (acetaminophen) in chronic pain; Chapter 16, Opioids and chronic noncancer pain; Chapter 17, Topical analgesics for neuropathic pain; and Chapter 19, Antiepileptic and antiarrhythmic agents) are one of the most common treatments given for CLBP. However, there exist no data supporting longer-term (>2–16 weeks) use of any of these medications. Studies demonstrating short-term efficacy generally show only minor improvements in pain or function compared to placebo.

Literature supports the use of antidepressants including noradrenergic and mixed noradrenergic-serotonergic inhibitor types.[67, 68, 69][II] However, their consumption has failed to improve function or disability. Nonsteroidal anti-inflammatory drugs (NSAIDs), on the other hand, appear to have some literature support[70, 71, 72, 73, 74, 75][II] in improving pain and function, but side effects including potential cardiac risks are poorly understood for use for a period of over 12 weeks.

Opioid medications are also commonly prescribed for CLBP patients, although studies supporting their use are difficult to interpret given the heterogenicity of opioids studied and the small sample sizes.[76, 77, 78][II] These studies show no improvement in function even if effective at controlling pain and typically do not address sampling issues such as whether patients were opioid-naive or opioid-experienced. Systematic reviews find patients using opioids not uncommonly have histories of substance abuse.[79, 80] Finally, it has to be appreciated that significant variability exists in the metabolism of these drugs highlighted by examples that normal doses can be life-threatening in certain circumstances.[81] Overall, limiting use to short periods of time and favoring long-acting, scheduled opioids makes the most sense. If faced with longer-term prescribing of opioids, consider an opioid-use contract signed by the patient. It should include having one source for prescriptions, restriction of other medication use, frequent return visits, a plan for tapering if not effective, consequences of breaking the agreement, and the approval of urine drug screening when needed. Resources are available to assess candidacy for opioids and screening for addiction.[82, 83]

Muscle relaxants may be of some value in controlling CLBP, but their efficacy does not appear to be related to controlling muscle spasm. Therefore, other medications with fewer side effects may be preferred.[84, 85, 86][II] Tramadol, a mixed peripheral and centrally acting agent with weak central nervous system opioid receptor activity, improves pain in patients with CLBP[87, 88][II] given with or without paracetamol (acetaminophen). Paracetamol as a single agent has unproven efficacy for CLBP, but from a risk/benefit standpoint, it is perhaps the most appealing of all oral agents.

Other medications to consider based on safety include lidocaine patches[89] in those with focal pain, topical capsaicin plaster,[90] or topical menthol, camphor, or salicylates available over the counter.[91, 92, 93] Oral corticosteroids enjoy popularity as they are generally considered potent, safe, and address a presumptive inflammatory etiology to worsening pain. However, this empiric practice for axial pain is not supported by the literature and side effects are a very real issue to consider.[76]

Exercise therapy

Patients with CLBP have decreased general conditioning,[94] as well as reduced back support muscle strength, if not frank muscle inhibition,[95] decreased coordination of contraction, and decreased back muscle endurance.[96, 97, 98] Patients may fall into the trap of waiting for pain to significantly improve or resolve prior to addressing these issues.

Rehabilitation of the spine support muscles perhaps is one of the best studied and literature-supported treatments for CLBP patients.[99][I] In literature reviews, it appears that pain and function is improved best when therapy programs are supervised, individualized, intensive, and progressive.[99, 100][I] Specific exercises that appear to be the most efficacious include stretching or strengthening of the spine support muscles and they appear to be nonharmful.[101][II] Both pilates and yoga, which involve exercises that address these core muscle groups, may provide a comparable benefit.[102, 103][II]

Individualization of therapy programs may add to chances of success, therefore working with an experienced physical therapist is important. Long *et al.*[104] screened LBP patients for postural or repeated end range movements that decreased or eliminated pain. The presence of this directional preference was found in 230 (74 percent) of 312 patients. Those patients randomized to therapy who matched their individual directional preference had superior improvement in pain and patient satisfaction with decreased medication use.

In addition, programs that address fear-avoidance beliefs[105, 106][III] or have a motivational component added to the program[107][II] may be superior to exercise alone. **Box 37.3** outlines an example of a motivational program. It is generally believed that an aerobic program of 30–40 minutes at least five days per week should supplement a specific back muscle program.

Spinal manipulation

In the United States, manual medicine encompasses a variety of techniques. Thrusting techniques or mobilization with impulse referred to in layman's terms as "adjustments" are best known. The goal of this treatment is to restore the full active range of motion to a restricted joint or spinal segment which will secondarily decrease afferent neuronal signals into the central nervous system and consequentially decrease muscle spasm and pain. Most studies on the efficacy of manipulation utilize about two treatments per week for two to three weeks.

In CLBP, manipulation is superior to sham manipulation for pain and functional improvement.[108, 109, 110] [II] It also appears to be about as effective as back school, exercise therapy, or general practitioner care with analgesics.[111][II] The risk of serious side effects, such as cauda equine syndrome, disk herniation, or vertebrobasilar accidents (cervical manipulation), range from 1 in 2 million to 1 in 400,000 treatments.[112, 113][IV] Flexion distraction technique appears to compare favorably with exercise.[114][II]

Box 37.3 Example of a motivational component of a physical therapy program for chronic low back pain

- Counseling on the importance of regular and consistent exercise
- Exercise decreases the likelihood of recurrences
- Rehabilitation depends on the patient's behavior
- Problem-solving with the therapist
- Reinforcement techniques used
- A reward strategy can be used
- Oral agreements reinforced in writing
- Exercise diary used daily

Massage therapy

Massage therapy can be thought of as soft tissue manipulation using the hands.[115][II] Various types exist, but most have evolved out of traditional Swedish school massage popularized decades ago. The goals of massage therapy include sedation, adhesion reduction, fluid mobilization, muscular relaxation, and vascular changes. For chronic LBP, there is only limited evidence that suggests massage is superior to sham treatment, exercise and postural training, relaxation exercise, acupuncture, or self-care education. Combining massage therapy with education and exercises may be better than using massage therapy alone.[116][II]

Physical modalities

Physical modalities as management tools for CLBP have the potential advantage of independent use by the patient. This can help empower the patient to take responsibility for their CLBP. This advantage has to be tempered by the fact that these are generally passive treatments which can, if overused, contribute to deconditioning. Physical modalities often have a relaxing effect in addition to temporarily controlling pain which gives them the potential for abuse. Ideally, they should be used as adjuncts to the rehabilitative process and their efficacy assessed in terms of their contribution to the overall goals of maximizing function and quality of life.

HEAT

Much more is known about the physiological effects of heat on the body than its efficacy in CLBP or other painful musculoskeletal conditions. Local effects include increased blood flow, nerve conduction, tendon extensibility, and analgesia, in addition to elevating pain threshold and general relaxation.[117] Any condition where increased blood flow is of concern (tumors, edema, impaired circulation, bleeding diatheses) or situations with decreased ability to appreciate excessive heating (scars, decreased sensation, cognitive deficits) are contraindications to heat.[118]

Typical treatment duration of superficial heat, such as a heat pack, is 20–30 minutes. Electric heating pads are commonly used, but often poorly control temperatures. This, combined with use while lying down, have resulted in burns after patients fell asleep.[118] Short-term use has some supportive evidence[119, 120][III] and heat plus exercise may be superior to either alone for LBP.[121][III] It is often used prior to or after activities. Overall, the evidence to support this common practice for LBP is limited.[122] [III]

Deep heat modalities exist, but ultrasound is used almost exclusively in clinical practice. It heats at tissue interfaces where sound energy is converted to heat and therefore it is used best for focal issues that may accompany CLBP such as bursitis, tendonitis, or capsulitis.[123]

COLD

Similar to heat modalities, various cold treatments have well-understood physiological effects, but little clinical support. Vasoconstriction, decreased nerve conduction, decreased tendon extensibility, and increased joint stiffness add to an analgesic effect and general relaxation.[117] No studies have compared cold to placebo or to no cold treatment.[122] Two low quality studies have compared cold to heat for LBP and had conflicting results.[122] Treatments are typically 20 minutes, but frostbite can occur.[124] If the expected increased erythema at the site of cold application subsequently turns white, frostbite is beginning. Intermittent ice application (on for ten minutes, off for five minutes, on for ten minutes) may be superior to one 20-minute treatment.[125][III]

TRANSCUTANEOUS AND PERCUTANEOUS ELECTRICAL NERVE STIMULATION

Transcutaneous electrical nerve stimulation (TENS) has been used for CLBP for years based on the gate control theory of pain reduction by Melzack and Wall.[126] The attractiveness of TENS is that the units themselves are portable. They easily hang from a belt or fit in a pocket, with electrodes attached to the back. Many variations of treatment duration and stimulation settings exist. Typical treatment is 30 minutes, four times per day. Evidence of efficacy in CLBP is limited and inconsistent.[127][II] When combined with neuromuscular electrical stimulation, there is an increase in benefit compared to either modality alone.[128][III] Percutaneous electrical nerve stimulation (PENS) combines electrical stimulation with acupuncture-type needles placed in the skin and appears to be more effective than the TENS for CLBP.[129][III] Randomized, controlled trials have shown PENS superior to sham PENS for LBP.[130][II]

TRACTION

Traction is a traditional CLBP treatment that has fallen out of favor as better efficacy studies have become available.[131] Anatomically, spinal traction enlarges the intevertebral space (theoretically decreasing forces on the intervertebral disk), stretches muscles and ligaments, separates apophyseal (facet) joints, and enlarges the intervertebral foramen. For CLBP, it appears to be no more effective than placebo, sham, or no treatment.[131, 132] [III] However, intermittent and continuous traction studies have been combined in systematic reviews. Proponents of traction suggest that intermittent traction may be beneficial. Currently, heavily marketed elaborate systems, such as VAX-D (VAX-D Medical Technologies LLC, Oldsmar, FL, USA) or DRX-9000 (Axiom, Tampa, FL, USA), await studies to support their claims of benefit, but use intermittent traction. Candidates for traction include those with discogenic radiculopathy and an x-ray that reveals no evidence of serious spine disease. Reports of various systems "pulling" a herniated disk back into the disk space are unsubstantiated.

Return to work programs

Rehabilitation programs designed for workers with CLBP and other musculoskeletal conditions can be effective at reducing work absenteeism. These successful programs share several key components including intensive physical training. The training for these workers, who are typically either off work or in modified duties, is oriented to specific work tasks. In addition, there exists a significant cognitive-behavioral therapy (CBT) component. CBT involves attempting to change the CLBP patient's cognitions and behaviors consistent with the biopsychosocial model of Waddell.[2] In this model, the pain and secondary disability are influenced not only by the structure(s) in the back, but also the culture in which the patient experiences the pain. Therefore, the individual's beliefs, attitudes as well as psychological distress will play into how much illness behavior they display. Modifying maladaptive beliefs and attitudes, and addressing distress, changes behavior and thus disability. So called "work hardening" programs have support in the literature[20, 21] [II] and can be cost-effective.

Cognitive-behavioral treatment

CBT in the setting of a return to work program can be effective. In addition, these programs even outside the work-hardening arena are perhaps one of the most useful tools for the spine clinician.[133, 134, 135, 136][II] Programs can be as short as six educational sessions[137][II] or up to two to four weeks in the case of a multidisciplinary pain management program.[138][II] The more multidisciplinary the program, the more spine rehabilitation exercise is built into the program as well. Programs can vary considerably with regard to content, but ideally should contain pharmacologic treatment options, education, exercise, a vocational emphasis, and a large component of CBT.[20, 21]

Injection therapies

In moving the CLBP patient toward rehabilitation, whether it is with an experienced spine therapist, a work-hardening program, or a multidisciplinary CBT program, more aggressive pain control options may be considered. Various spine injections should be considered a stepping stone to one of these main treatments, not used in isolation. This is one example where the treating physician can be the patient's gatekeeper and help direct care. Many patients find such dramatic relief with a facet joint injection or sacroiliac joint block that they abandon all other treatments until pain returns weeks or months later. They invariably return to the treating clinician's office specifically asking for another "shot."

The attractiveness of corticosteroid injections lies in a systemic effect of the steroid causing decreased pain in multiple areas and mild euphoria. There may be a placebo effect of the injection as well. In addition, the injections are thought of as diagnostic tests since placing medication into a facet joint, for example, may lead one to conclude that pain reduction "proves" that the injected structure was a pain generator. This is a debatable issue as efficacy data in general are conflicting and of poor quality. Many suggest that variability of techniques used and in particular the lack of image-guidance for epidural injections, is a big factor behind these study results. Looking at the 15 randomized trials on the efficacy of epidural corticosteroid injections for discogenic radiculopathy, systematic reviews are conflicting.[139][I] However, all but two of these studies can be dismissed based on a lack of proper image-guided and contrast-controlled injection technique at the level of the targeted disk.

Overall, there are conflicting or poor quality studies to support the use of epidural, facet joint, sacroiliac joint, radiofrequency procedures, intradiscal electrothermotherapy (IDET), botulinum toxin injections, prolotherapy, trigger point injections, or spinal cord stimulation for patients with CLBP.[15][IV] Proper patient selection and wise counseling to set realistic expectations for these procedures is important. They should only be performed with the intent to move along the rehabilitation process, after proper screening for contraindications, and executed in experienced hands. Patients should assume that the effects of injection treatments are temporary (weeks to months).

LUMBAR RADICULOPATHY AND SPINAL STENOSIS PATIENTS

Patients with radiculopathy are approached with the same treatment tools in mind as the patient with only CLBP with some important additional considerations. First, the back pain and radicular leg pain component are approached as two different problems since they can act and respond to treatments in very different ways. For instance, the back pain component does not usually respond to the treatments that are helpful for the radicular component. Treatments, such as surgical discectomy, epidural steroid injections, or neuropathic drugs, can eliminate radicular leg pain, but have not shown efficacy for treating axial pain.[140] Most of these patients will have a discogenic or bony hypertrophic etiology for their radicular pain. Occasionally, the radicular pain comes from a synovial cyst, but serious underlying spine disease as a source of radiculopathy is extremely rare[32] and only investigated if the usual low back screening red flags are positive.

The natural history of discogenic radiculopathy is one of complete elimination of leg symptoms over time.[141, 142] However, someone with continued chronic and activity-limiting radicular pain can be approached with several treatment tools. The least invasive treatment options involve physical therapy combined with anlagesic oral medications. The therapy can generally consist of pain-control treatments via modalities like heat, ice, or electrical stimulation, foraminal opening maneuvers, a trial of McKenzie techniques, education on back care, sleeping positions, body mechanics, stretches, and possibly a trial of traction.[143][III] As the patient progresses, typical stabilization exercise can also be introduced.

Analgesics are similar to those discussed above under Medication, with the addition of medications specific for treating neuropathic pain, such as gabapentin, pregabalin, duloxetine, tramadol, or tricyclic antidepressants. For patients who have not responded adequately to these types of treatments over time, fluoroscopically guided and contrast-controlled injections into the epidural space may add additional pain control. Empirically, patients are limited to three injections a year to avoid steroid side effects. Injections are approached one at a time and efficacy is evaluated ten days to two weeks later before any repeat injections are considered.

For patients with predominantly leg pain and continued disability despite treatments as described, a surgical consultation could be offered.

Patients with classical spinal stenosis may well have significant back pain, but they usually present because of bilateral leg pain that limits their standing and walking (pseudoclaudication). Treatments worth pursuing include a trial of flexion-biased stabilization exercises which promote a posture that opens the stenotic or narrowed spinal canal areas. This is carried out in addition to the usual back pain treatments described above under Setting up a sound treatment program. Many patients find that using a walker to allow some forward flexion while walking, increases walking tolerance significantly. Oral analgesics or epidural corticosteroid injections may be of benefit especially if there is a significant discogenic component to the stenotic area of the spinal canal. Surgery is considered an elective procedure which should ultimately be offered based on disability and lack of medical contraindications.[144, 145][II]

WHO MAY BENEFIT FROM SPINAL SURGERY?

Patients with CLBP and their treating physicians need to approach the issue of spinal surgery with caution. It is important to understand that the spine surgical community is indeed split as to whether they believe spinal surgery is an option for the patient with CLBP. This is a controversial area of medicine highlighted by recent published expert opinion statements critical of spinal fusion surgery[146][V] and in response, supportive of surgery.[147][V]

Part of the controversy is centered around the assumption that CLBP is caused by a painful disk and therefore removing the disk surgically should alleviate the pain. This view fits well with the orthopedic model of CLBP which is arguably bioanatomically based. History, examination, and imaging or provocative discography studies do a poor job at differentiating patients with truly discogenic pain from others.

On the other hand, recent clinical trials using a biopsychosocial model of CLBP have shown evidence supporting conservative care for these patients. The first randomized trials comparing spinal fusion to an aggressive exercise therapy treatment approach within a CBT program have shown virtually identical results. Both groups showed improvement in pain and disability, but the surgical group had more morbidity in the interoperative and postoperative periods.[133, 148][II] Another similarly designed comparison published earlier showed an advantage to spinal fusion surgery. However, the conservative treatment group in that study was poorly defined and treatment was variable with little attempt at a formal therapy component.[149][II]

Probably the best candidate for spinal fusion surgery for CLBP is one in whom the imaging studies and discography define a single discogenic pain generator in a patient who is otherwise fit, motivated to get better, and continues to have disabling CLBP, despite all the reasonable medical treatments previously discussed. In addition, they need to have realistic expectations for and understand the risks of the surgery itself.

Radiculopathy patients are surgical candidates if they have predominantly leg pain, a clear corroborative disk on imaging studies, and have failed with aggressive medical management for at least six weeks. About 70 percent of patients will realize significant improvement within six weeks of symptom onset[150] without the need for surgery. Rarely, progressive neurological deficit (2–4 percent) or cauda equine syndrome (1–2 percent) will prompt urgent or emergency surgery, respectively. Otherwise, it does not appear that mild static weakness is an indication for surgery as patients will recover strength to the same extent and at the same rate, whether they are treated surgically or medically.[150, 151]

Spinal stenosis surgery is similar to radiculopathy as it is an elective procedure driven by patient function/disability. The natural history of typical degenerative central spinal canal stenosis is one of very little change over many months with 15 percent actually improving over time.[152]

CONCLUSIONS

The chronic low back pain patient can be effectively managed by clinicians if a biopsychosocial model of back pain is implemented. A thorough and systematic evaluation of red and yellow flag issues, as well as pain and disability, are the goals of all treating clinicians. Understanding the patient's motivations, beliefs, and preferences through empathic listening allows superior outcomes. Assuming the role of gatekeeper to mobilize the spine care neighborhood team when needed, will provide the best care possible. Setting patient expectations for self-management through effective and informed counsel, as well as emphasizing a return to function and work avoids the pitfalls of passive and temporizing treatment dead ends. Cognitive and behavioral programs hold the most promise for the future treatment of patients with CLBP.

REFERENCES

1. Waddell G, Main CJ. *The back pain revolution*, 2nd edn. Edinburgh: Churchill Livingstone, 2004.
* 2. Waddell G. A new clinical model for the treatment of low back pain. *Spine*. 1987; **12**: 632–44.
3. Flor H, Birbaumer N. Acquisition of chronic pain: psychophysiological mechanisms. *American Pain Society Journal*. 1994; **3**: 119–27.
4. Main CJ, Watson PJ. Guarded movements: development of chronicity. *Journal of Musculoskeletal Pain*. 1996; **4**: 163–70.
5. Waddell G, Main CJ. The biopsychosocial model. In: Waddell G (ed.). *The back pain revolution*, 2nd edn. London: Churchill Livingstone, 2004: 265–82.

6. Symonds T. Do attitudes and beliefs influence work loss die to low back trouble? *Occupational Medicine.* 1996; **46**: 25–32.
* 7. Waddell G, Newton M, Henderson I *et al.* A fear-avoidance beliefs questionnaire (FABQ) and the role of fear-avoidance beliefs in chronic low back pain and disability. *Pain.* 1993; **52**: 157–68.
8. Epstein R, Alper B, Quill T. Communicating evidence for participatory decision making. *Journal of the American Medical Association.* 2004; **291**: 2359–66.
9. Platt FW, Gaspar DL, Coulehan JL *et al.* "Tell me about yourself": the patient-centered interview. *Annals of Internal Medicine.* 2001; **134**: 1079–85.
* 10. Barrier PA, Li JT-C, Jensen NM. Two words to improve physician–patient communication: What else? *Mayo Clinic Proceedings.* 2003; **78**: 211–14.
* 11. Kendall NAS, Linton SJ, Main CJ. *Guide to assessing psychosocial yellow flags in acute low back pain: risk factors for long-term disability and work loss.* Wellington, NZ: Accident Rehabilitation and Compensation Insurance Corporation of New Zealand and the National Health Committee, 1997.
12. Deyo RA. Treatments for back pain: can we get past trivial effects? *Annals of Internal Medicine.* 2004; **141**: 957–8.
13. Farrar JT, Young Jr JP, LaMoreaux L *et al.* Clinical importance of changes in chronic pain intensity measured on an 11-point numerical pain rating scale. *Pain.* 2001; **94**: 149–58.
14. Cherkin DC, Deyo RA, Wheeler K, Ciol MA. Physician views about treating low back pain. The results of a national survey. *Spine.* 1995; **20**: 1–9; discussion 9-10.
* 15. Working Group on Guidelines for Prevention in Low Back Pain. COST B13: European guidelines for the management of low back pain. *European Spine Journal.* 2006; **15**: S125–300.
16. Dreyfuss P, Michaelsen M, Pauza K *et al.* The value of medical history and physical examination in diagnosing sacroiliac joint pain. *Spine.* 1996; **21**: 2594–602.
* 17. Borkan J, Reis S, Hermoni D, Biderman A. Talking about the pain: a patient-centered study of low back pain in primary care. *Social Science and Medicine.* 1995; **40**: 977–88.
18. Rainville J, Bagnall D, Phalen L. Health care providers' attitudes and beliefs about functional impairments and chronic back pain. *Clinical Journal of Pain.* 1995; **11**: 287–95.
19. Deyo RA. Low back pain. *Scientific American.* 1998; **279**: 29–33.
* 20. Guzman J, Esmail R, Karjalainen K *et al.* Multidisciplinary rehabilitation for chronic low back pain: systematic review. *BMJ.* 2001; **322**: 1511–16.
21. Schonstein E, Kenny D, Keating J *et al.* Physical conditioning programs for workers with back and neck pain: a Cochrane systematic review. *Spine.* 2003; **28**: E391–5.
22. International Association for the Study of Pain. 1979 pain terms: A list of definitions with notes on usage. *Pain.* 1979; **6**: 249–52.
23. Rome JD. Chronic pain: sensation, emotion and neuroplasticity. Paper presented at Pain Medicine: A State-of-the-Art Course in Pain Management for the Non-Pain Specialist, Key West, January 2007.
24. Carragee EJ, Hannibal M. Diagnostic evaluation of low back pain. *Orthopedic Clinics of North America.* 2004; **35**: 7–16.
25. Slipman CW, Patel RK, Botwin K *et al.* Epidemiology of spine tumors presenting to musculoskeletal physiatrists. *Archives of Physical Medicine and Rehabilitation.* 2003; **84**: 492–5.
26. Shelerud RA. Low back evaluation. Paper presented at the 1st Annual Pain Management for the Primary Care Practitioner Course. Key West, Florida, January 2007.
27. Strong J, Large R. Coping with chronic low back pain. In idiographic exploration through focus groups. *International Journal of Psychiatry in Medicine.* 1995; **25**: 371–87.
28. Hadler N. MRI for regional back pain: Need for less imaging, better understanding. *Journal of the American Medical Association.* 2003; **289**: 2863–4.
29. Leonard N, Beauvais L, Scholl R. A self concept-based model of work motivation. Paper presented at the Annual Meeting of the Academy of Management, Vancouver 1995.
30. Kalauokalani D, Cherkin D, Sherman K *et al.* Lessons from a trial of acupuncture and massage for low back pain. *Spine.* 2001; **26**: 1418–24.
31. Grahn B, Stigmar K, Ekdajl C. Motivation for change in patients with prolonged musculoskeletal disorders: A qualitative two-year follow-up study. *Physiotherapy Research International.* 1999; **4**: 170–89.
32. Shelerud RA, Paynter KS. Rarer causes of radiculopathy: spinal tumors, infections, and other unusual causes. *Physical Medicine and Rehabilitation Clinics of North America.* 2002; **13**: 645–96.
33. van den Hoogen HM, Koes BW, van Eijk JT, Bouter LM. On the accuracy of history, physical examination, and erythrocyte sedimentation rate in diagnosing low back pain in general practice. A criteria-based review of the literature. *Spine.* 1995; **20**: 318–27.
* 34. Waddell G, McCulloch JA, Kummel E, Venner RM. Nonorganic physical signs in low-back pain. *Spine.* 1980; **5**: 117–25.
* 35. Magee DJ. *Orthopedic physical assessment,* 3rd edn. Philadelphia: WB Saunders, 1997: 362–433.
36. Cole AJ, Herring SA. *The low back pain handbook. A guide for the practicing clinician,* 2nd edn. Philadelphia: Hanley and Belfus, 2003: 69–116.
* 37. McCarthy MJ, Aylott CE, Grevitt MP, Hegarty J. Cauda equina syndrome: factors affecting long-term functional and sphincteric outcome. *Spine.* 2007; **32**: 207–16.
38. Storm PB, Chou D, Tamargo RJ. Lumbar spinal stenosis, cauda equina syndrome, and multiple lumbosacral radiculopathies. *Physical Medicine and Rehabilitation Clinics of North America.* 2002; **13**: 713–33.

39. Cole AJ, Herring SA. *The low back pain handbook. A guide for the practicing clinician*, 2nd edn. Philadelphia: Hanley and Belfus, 2003: 57–101.
40. Schwarzer AC, Aprill CN, Dergy R *et al.* The relative contributions of the disc and zygapophyseal joint in chronic low back pain. *Spine.* 1994; **19**: 801–06.
41. Magee DJ. *Orthopedic physical assessment*, 3rd edn. Philadelphia: WB Saunders Company, 1997: 398–9.
42. Slipman CW, Sterenfeld EB, Chou LH *et al.* The predictive value of provocative sacroiliac joint stress maneuvers in the diagnosis of sacroiliac joint syndrome. *Archives of Physical Medicine and Rehabilitation.* 1998; **79**: 288–92.
43. Schwarzer AC, Aprill CN, Bogduk N. The sacroiliac joint in chromic low back pain. *Spine.* 1995; **20**: 31–7.
44. Laslett M, Williams M. The reliability of selected pain provocation tests for sacroiliac joint pathology. *Spine.* 1994; **19**: 1243–9.
45. Cole AJ, Herring SA. *The low back pain handbook. A guide for the practicing clinician*, 2nd edn. Philadelphia: Hanley and Belfus, 2003: 97.
46. Magee DJ. *Orthopedic physical assessment*, 3rd edn. Philadelphia: WB Saunders, 1997: 460–505.
47. Blake SP, Connors AM. Sacral insufficiency fracture. *British Journal of Radiology.* 2004; **77**: 891–6.
48. Lauder TD. Physical examination signs, clinical symptoms, and their relationship to electrodiagnostic findings and the presence of radiculopathy. *Physical Medicine and Rehabilitation Clinics of North America.* 2002; **13**: 451–67.
49. Rajasekaran S, Pithwa YK. Baastrup's disease as a cause of neurogenic claudication: a case report. *Spine.* 2003; **28**: E273–5.
50. Quinlan JF, Duke D, Eustace S. Bertolotti's syndrome. A cause of back pain in young people. *Journal of Bone and Joint Surgery, British Volume.* 2006; **88**: 1183–6.
51. Wolfe F, Smythe HA, Yunus MB *et al.* The American College of Rheumatology 1990 criteria for the classification of fibromyalgia: report of the multicenter criteria committee. *Arthritis and Rheumatism.* 1990; **33**: 160–72.
52. Carragee E, Tanner C, Khurana S *et al.* The rates of false-positive discography in select patients without low back symptoms. *Spine.* 2000; **25**: 1373–80.
53. Carragee E, Chen Y, Tanner C *et al.* Provocative discography in patient after limited lumbar discectomy: a controlled randomized study of pain response in symptomatic and asymptomatic subjects. *Spine.* 2000; **25**: 3065–71.
54. Carragee E, Tanner C, Yang B *et al.* False-positive findings on lumbar discography. Reliability of subjective concordance assessment during provocative disc injection. *Spine.* 1999; **24**: 2542–7.
* 55. May CR, Rose MJ, Johnstone FC. Dealing with doubt. How patients account for non-specific chronic low back pain. *Journal of Psychosomatic Research.* 2000; **49**: 223–5.
56. Chew-Graham C, May C. Chronic low back pain in general practice: the challenge of the consultation. *Family Practice.* 1999; **16**: 46–9.
57. Cedraschi C, Tobert J, Perrin E *et al.* The role of congruence between patient and therapist in chronic low back pain patients. *Journal of Manipulative and Physiological Therapeutics.* 1996; **19**: 244–9.
58. Phillips L. Patient education: Understanding the process to maximize time and outcomes. *Journal of Intravenous Nursing.* 1999; **22**: 19–35.
* 59. Hazard RG. Low-back and neck pain diagnosis and treatments. *American Journal of Physical Medicine and Rehabilitation.* 2007; **86** (Suppl.): S59–68.
* 60. Kirkaldy-Willis WH, Burton CV, Cassidy JD. *Managing low back pain*, 3rd edn. New York: Churchill Livingstone, 1992: 105–48.
61. Andersson GBJ. Lumbar spine pain generators – where are we in our understanding? Paper presented at the PASSOR Annual Scientific Session and Meeting: Current Concepts in Diagnosis and Management of Industrial Injuries in the Lumbar Spine. Vancouver, November 1996.
62. Vlaeyen JWS, Kole-Snijders AMJ, Boeren RGB *et al.* Fear of movement/(re)injury in chronic low back pain and its relation to behavioral performance. *Pain.* 1995; **62**: 363–72.
63. Kimberly PE. Formulating a prescription for osteopathic manipulative treatment. *Journal of the American Osteopathic Association.* 1980; **79**: 506–13.
64. Evans DW. Mechanisms and effects of spinal high-velocity, low-amplitude thrust manipulation: previous theories. *Journal of Manipulative and Physiologic Therapeutics.* 2002; **25**: 251–62.
65. Leino-Arjas P, Kaila-Kangas L, Solovieva S *et al.* Serum lipids and low back pain: An association? A follow-up study of a working population sample. *Spine.* 2006; **31**: 1032–7.
66. Lutz GK, Butzlaff M, Schultz-Venrath U. Looking back on back pain: trial and error of diagnoses in the 20th century. *Spine.* 2003; **28**: 1899–905.
67. Fishbain D. Evidence-based data on pain relief with antidepressants. *Annals of Medicine.* 2000; **32**: 305–16.
68. Salerno SM, Browining R, Jackson JL. The effect of antidepressant treatment on chronic back pain: a meta-analysis. *Archives of Internal Medicine.* 2002; **162**: 19–24.
69. Staiger TO, Gaster B, Sullivan MD, Deyo RA. Systematic review of antidepressants in the treatment of chronic low back pain. *Spine.* 2003; **28**: 2540–5.
70. Berry H, Bloom B, Hamilton EB *et al.* Naproxen sodium, diflunisal and placebo in the treatment of chronic back pain. *Annals of the Rheumatic Diseases.* 1982; **41**: 129–32.
71. Birbara CA, Puopolo AD, Munoz DR *et al.* Treatment of chronic low back pain with etoricoxib, a new cyclo-oxygenase-2 selective inhibitor: improvement in pain and disability – a randomized, placebo-controlled, 3-month trial. *Journal of Pain.* 2003; **4**: 307–15.
72. Hickey RF. Chronic low back pain: a comparison of diflunisal with paracetamol. *New Zealand Medical Journal.* 1982; **95**: 312–4.

73. Postacchini F, Facchini M, Palieri P. Efficacy of various forms of conservative treatment in low back pain: a comparative study. *Neuro-Orthopedics*. 1988; **6**: 113–6.
74. Vetter G, Bruggemenn G, Lettko M *et al.* Shortening diclofenac therapy by B vitamins. Results of a randomized double-blind study, diclofenac 50 mg versus diclofenac 50 mg plus B vitamins, in painful spinal diseases with degenerative changes. *Zeitschrift für Rheumatologie*. 1988; **47**: 351–62.
75. Videman T, Osterman K. Double-blind parallel study of piroxicam versus indomethacin in the treatment of low back pain. *Annals of Clinical Research*. 1984; **16**: 156–60.
76. Hart LG, Deyo RA, Cherkin DC. Physician office visits for low back pain. Frequency, clinical evaluation, and treatment patterns from a US national survey. *Spine*. 1995; **20**: 11–19.
77. Cherkin DC, Deyo RA, Wheeler K, Ciol MA. Physician views about treating low back pain. The results of a national survey. *Spine*. 1995; **20**: 1–9; discussion 9-10.
78. Maier C, Heodebrandt J, Klinger R *et al.* Morphine responsiveness, efficacy and tolerability in patients with chronic non-tumor associated pain – results a double-blind placebo-controlled trial (MONTAS). *Pain*. 2002; **97**: 223–33.
79. Hosted J. Addiction to opioids in chronic pain patients: A literature review. *European Journal of Pain*. 2007; **11**: 490–518.
* 80. Rome JD, Townsend CO, Bruce BK *et al.* Chronic noncancer pain rehabilitation with opioid withdrawal: comparison of treatment outcomes based on opioid use status at admission. *Mayo Clinic Proceedings*. 2004; **79**: 759–68.
81. Gasche Y, Daali Y, Fathi M *et al.* Codeine intoxication associated with ultrarapid CYP2D6 metabolism. *New England Journal of Medicine*. 2004; **351**: 2827–31.
82. Adams LL, Gatchel RJ, Robinson RC *et al.* Development of a self-report screening instrument for assessing potential opioid medication misuse in chronic pain patients. *Journal of Pain and Symptom Management*. 2004; **27**: 440–59.
83. Institute for Clinical Systems Improvements. Pain, chronic; assessment and management. Bloomington, MN: Institute for Clinical Systems Improvements. Last updated April 2007, cited February 2008. Available from: www.icsi.org/guidelines_and_more/gl_os_prot/musculo-skeletal/pain__chronic__assessment_and_management_of_14399/pain__chronic__assessment_and_management_of_14400.html.
84. Arbus L, Fajadet B, Aubert D *et al.* Activity of tetrazepam in low back pain. *Clinical Trials Journal*. 1990; **27**: 258–67.
85. Pratzel HG, Alken RG, Ramm S. Efficacy and tolerance of repeated oral doses of tolperisone hydrochloride in the treatment of painful reflex muscle spasm; results of a prospective placebo-controlled double-blind trial. *Pain*. 1996; **67**: 417–25.
86. Salzmann E, Pforringer W, Paal G, Gierend M. Treatment of chronic low-back syndrome with tetrazepam in a placebo controlled double-blind trial. *Journal of Drug Development*. 1992; **4**: 219–28.
87. Ruoff GE, Rosenthal N, Jordan D *et al.* Tramadol/acetaminophen combination tablets for the treatment of chronic lower back pain: a multicenter, randomized, double-blind, placebo-controlled outpatient study. *Clinical Therapy*. 2003; **25**: 1123–41.
88. Schnitzer TJ, Gray WL, Paster TZ, Kamin M. Efficacy of tramadol in treatment of chronic low back pain. *Journal of Rheumatology*. 2000; **27**: 772–8.
89. Gimbel J, Linn R, Hale M, Nicholson B. Lidocaine patch treatment in patients with low back pain: results of an open-label, nonrandomized pilot study. *American Journal of Therapeutics*. 2005; **12**: 311–19.
90. Frerick H, Keitel W, Kuhn U *et al.* Topical treatment of chronic low back pain with a capsicum plaster. *Pain*. 2003; **106**: 59–64.
91. Kraemer WJ, Ratamess NA, Maresh CM *et al.* Acetylated fatty acid topical cream with menthol reduces pain and improves functional performance in individuals with arthritis. *Journal of Strength and Conditioning Research*. 2005; **19**: 475–80.
92. Cohen M, Wolfe R, Mai T, Lewis D. A randomized, double blind, placebo controlled trial of a topical cream containing glucosamine sulfate, chondroitin sulfate, and camphor for osteoarthritis of the knee. *Journal of Rheumatology*. 2003; **30**: 523–8.
93. Mason L, Moore RA, Edwards JE *et al.* Systematic review of efficacy of topical rubefacients containing salicylates for the treatment of acute and chronic pain. *BMJ*. 2004; **328**: 995.
94. Smeets RJ, Wittink H, Hidding A, Knottnerus JA. Do patients with chronic low back pain have a lower level of aerobic fitness than healthy controls?: Are pain, disability, fear of injury, working status, or level of leisure time activity associated with the difference in aerobic fitness level? *Spine*. 2006; **31**: 90–7.
95. Hodges PW, Richardson CA. Inefficient muscular stabilization of the lumbar spine associated with low back pain. A motor control evaluation of transversus abdominis. *Spine*. 1996; **21**: 2640–50.
96. Hides JA, Richardson CA, Jull GA. Multifidus muscle recovery is not automatic after resolution of acute, first-episode low back pain. *Spine*. 1996; **21**: 2763–9.
97. Rantanen J, Hurme M, Falck B *et al.* The lumbar multifidus muscle five years after surgery for a lumbar intervertebral disc herniation. *Spine*. 1993; **18**: 568–74.
98. Roy SH, De Luca CJ, Emley M, Buijs RJ. Spectral electromyographic assessment of back muscles in patients with low back pain undergoing rehabilitation. *Spine*. 1995; **20**: 38–48.
* 99. Hayden JA, van Tulder MW, Malmivaara AV, Koes BW. Meta-analysis: Exercise therapy for nonspecific low back pain. *Annals of Internal Medicine*. 2005; **142**: 765–75.
100. Maul I, Laubli T, Oliveri M, Krueger H. Long-term effects of supervised physical training in secondary prevention of low back pain. *European Spine Journal*. 2005; **14**: 599–611.

101. Videman T, Sarna S, Battie MC *et al.* The long-term effects of physical loading and exercise lifestyles on back-related symptoms, disability and spinal pathology among men. *Spine.* 1995; **20**: 699–709.
102. Rydeard R, Leger A, Smith D. Pilates-based therapeutic exercise: effect on subjects with nonspecific chronic low back pain and functional disability: a randomized controlled trial. *Journal of Orthopaedic and Sports Physical Therapy.* 2006; **36**: 472–84.
103. Sherman KJ, Cherkin DC, Erro J *et al.* Comparing yoga, exercise, and a self-care book for chronic low back pain: a randomized, controlled trial. *Annals of Internal Medicine.* 2005; **143**: 849–56.
104. Long A, Donelson R, Fung T. Does it matter which exercise? A randomized control trial of exercise for low back pain. *Spine.* 2004; **29**: 2593–602.
105. George SZ, Fritz JM, Bialosky JE, Donald DA. The effect of a fear-avoidance-based physical therapy intervention for patient with acute low back pain: results of a randomized clinical trial. *Spine.* 2003; **28**: 2551–60.
106. Smeets RJ, Vlaeyen JW, Kester AD *et al.* Reduction of pain catastrophizing mediates the outcome of both physical and cognitive-behavioral treatment in chronic low back pain. *Journal of Pain.* 2006; **7**: 261–71.
*107. Friedrich M, Gitter G, Arendasy M *et al.* Long-term effect of a combined exercise and motivational program on the level of disability of patients with chronic low back pain. *Spine.* 2005; **30**: 995–1000.
108. Ongley MJ, Klein RG, Dorman TA *et al.* A new approach to the treatment of chronic low back pain. *Lancet.* 1987; **2**: 143–6.
109. Triano JJ, McGregor M, Hondras MA, Brennan PC. Manipulative therapy versus education programs in chronic low back pain. *Spine.* 1995; **20**: 948–55.
110. Waagen GN, Haldeman S, Cool G *et al.* Short term trial of chiropractic adjustments for the relief of chronic low back pain. *Manual Medicine.* 1986; **2**: 63–7.
*111. Assendelft WJ, Koes BW, van der Heijden GJ, Bouter LM. The effectiveness of chiropractic for treatment of low back pain: an update and attempt at statistical pooling. *Journal of Manipulative and Physiological Therapeutics.* 1996; **19**: 499–507.
112. Ernst E, Harkness E. Spinal manipulation: a systematic review of sham-controlled, double-blind, randomized clinical trials. *Journal of Pain and Symptom Management.* 2001; **22**: 879–89.
113. Stevinson C, Ernst E. Risks associated with spinal manipulation. *American Journal of Medicine.* 2002; **112**: 566–71.
114. Cambron JA, Gudavalli MR, Hedeker D *et al.* One-year follow-up of a randomized clinical trial comparing flexion distraction with an exercise program for chronic low back pain. *Journal of Alternative and Complementary Medicine.* 2006; **12**: 659–68.
*115. Furlan AD, Brosseau L, Imamura M, Irvin E. Massage for low-back pain: a systematic review within the framework of the Cochrane Collaboration Back Review Group. *Spine.* 2002; **27**: 1896–910.
116. Preyde M. Effectiveness of massage therapy for sub-acute low-back pain; a randomized controlled trial. *CMAJ.* 2000; **162**: 1815–20.
117. Lehman JF. *Therapeutic heat and cold*, 4th edn. Baltimore: Williams and Wilkins, 1990.
118. Weber DC, Brown AW. Physical agent modalities. In: Braddom RL (ed.). *Physical medicine and rehabilitation*, 2nd edn. Philadelphia: WB Saunders, 2000, 450–7.
119. Nadler SF, Steiner DJ, Erasala GN *et al.* Continuous low-level heat wrap therapy provides more efficacy than ibuprofen and acetaminophen for acute low back pain. *Spine.* 2002; **27**: 1012–7.
120. Nuhr M, Hoerauf K, Bertalanffy A *et al.* Active warming during emergency transport relieves acute low back pain. *Spine.* 2004; **29**: 1499–503.
121. Mayer JM, Ralph L, Look M *et al.* Treating acute low back pain with continuous low-level heat wrap therapy and/or exercise: a randomized controlled trial. *Spine Journal.* 2005; **5**: 395–403.
*122. French SD, Cameron M, Walker BF *et al.* A Cochrane review of superficial heat or cold for low back pain. *Spine.* 2006; **31**: 998–1006.
123. Falconer J, Hayes KW, Chang RW. Therapeutic ultrasound in the treatment of musculoskeletal conditions. *Arthritis Care and Research.* 1990; **3**: 85–91.
124. Keskin M, Tosun Z, Duymaz A, Savaci N. Frostbite injury due to improper usage of an ice pack. *Annals of Plastic Surgery.* 2005; **55**: 437–8.
125. Bleakley CM, McDonough SM, MacAuley DC, Bjordal J. Cryotherapy for acute ankle sprains: a randomised controlled study of two different icing protocols. *British Journal of Sports Medicine.* 2006; **40**: 700–5; discussion 705.
126. Melzack R, Wall PD. Pain mechanisms: a new theory. *Science.* 1965; **150**: 971–9.
127. Khadilkar A, Milne S, Brosseau L *et al.* Transcutaneous electrical nerve stimulation for the treatment of chronic low back pain: a systematic review. *Spine.* 2005; **30**: 2657–66.
128. Snyder-Mackler L, Delitto A, Stralka SW, Bailey SL. Use of electrical stimulation to enhance recovery of quadriceps femoris muscle force production in patients following anterior cruciate ligament reconstruction. *Physical Therapy.* 1994; **74**: 901–07.
129. Yokoyama M, Sun X, Oku S *et al.* Comparison of percutaneous electrical nerve stimulation with transcutaneous electrical nerve stimulation for long-term pain relief in patients with chronic low back pain. *Anesthesia and Analgesia.* 2004; **98**: 1552–6.
130. Ghoname EA, Craig WF, White PF *et al.* Percutaneous electrical nerve stimulation for low back pain: a randomized crossover study. *Journal of the American Medical Association.* 1999; **281**: 818–23.
131. Clarke J, van Tulder M, Blomberg S *et al.* Traction for low back pain with or without sciatica: an updated systematic

review within the framework of the Cochrane Collaboration. *Spine*. 2006; **31**: 1591–9.

132. van der Heijden GJ, Beurskens AJ, Koes BW *et al*. The efficacy of traction for back and neck pain: a systematic, blinded review of randomized clinical trial methods. *Physical Therapy*. 1995; **75**: 93–104.
133. Brox JI, Sorensen R, Friis A *et al*. Randomized clinical trial of lumbar instrumented fusion and cognitive intervention and exercises in patient with chronic low back pain and disc degeneration. *Spine*. 2003; **28**: 1913–21.
134. Spinhoven P, ter Kuile M, Kole-Snijders AM *et al*. Catastrophizing and internal pain control as mediators of outcome in the multidisciplinary treatment of chronic low back pain. *European Journal of Pain*. 2004; **8**: 211–19.
135. Staal JB, Hlobil H, Twisk JW *et al*. Graded activity for low back pain in occupational healthcare: a randomized, controlled trial. *Annals of Internal Medicine*. 2004; **140**: 77–84.
*136. van Tulder MW, Ostelo R, Vlaeyen JW *et al*. Behavioral treatment for chronic low back pain: a systematic review within the framework of the Cochrane Back Review Group. *Spine*. 2000; **25**: 2688–99.
*137. Linton SJ, Andersson T. Can chronic disability be prevented? A randomized trial of a cognitive-behavior intervention and two forms of information for patients with spinal pain. *Spine*. 2000; **25**: 2825–31; discussion 2824.
138. Turner JA, Jensen MP. Efficacy of cognitive therapy for chronic low back pain. *Pain*. 1993; **52**: 169–77.
139. Koes BW, Scholten RJ, Mens JM, Bouter LM. Efficacy of epidural steroid injections for low-back pain and sciatica: a systematic review of randomized clinical trials. *Pain*. 1995; **63**: 279–88.
140. Spangfort EV. The lumbar disc herniation; a computer-aided analysis of 2,504 operations. *Acta Orthopaedica Scandinavica. Supplementum*. 1972; **142**: 1–95.
*141. Weber H. Lumbar disc herniation: a controlled, prospective study with ten years of observation. *Spine*. 1983; **8**: 131–40.
*142. Weinstien JN, Lure JD, Tosteson TD *et al*. Surgical versus nonoperative treatment for lumbar disk herniation: the spine patient outcomes research trial (SPORT) observational cohort. *Journal of the American Medical Association*. 2006; **296**: 2451–9.
*143. Saal JA, Saal JS. Nonoperative treatment of herniated lumbar intervertebral disc with radiculopathy. *Spine*. 1989; **14**: 431–7.
144. Gibson JN, Waddell G. Surgery for degenerative lumbar spondylosis: updated Cochrane Review. *Spine*. 2005; **30**: 2312–20.
*145. Amundsen T, Weber H, Nordal HJ *et al*. Lumbar spinal stenosis: conservative or surgical management?: A prospective 10-year study. *Spine*. 2000; **25**: 1424–35; discussion 1435-6.
*146. Deyo RA, Nachemson A, Mirza SK. Spinal-fusion surgery – the case for restraint. *New England Journal of Medicine*. 2004; **350**: 722–6.
*147. Errico TJ, Gatchel RJ, Schofferman J *et al*. A fair and balanced view of spine fusion surgery. *Spine Journal*. 2004; **4** (Suppl.): S129–38.
*148. Fairbank J, Frost H, Wilson-MacDonald J *et al*. Randomised controlled trial to compare surgical stabilisation of the lumbar spine with an intensive rehabilitation programme for patients with chronic low back pain: the MRC spine stabilisation trial. *BMJ*. 2005; **330**: 1233.
149. Fritzell P, Hagg O, Wessberg P *et al*. Volvo Award winner in clinical studies: lumbar fusion versus nonsurgical treatment for chromic low back pain. A multicenter randomized controlled trial from the Swedish lumbar spine study group. *Spine*. 2001; **23**: 2521–34.
150. Weber H, Holme I, Amlie E. The natural course of acute sciatica with nerve root symptoms in a double-blind placebo-controlled trial evaluating the effect of piroxicam. *Spine*. 1993; **18**: 1433–8.
151. Dubourg G, Rozenberg S, Fautrel B *et al*. A pilot study on the recovery from paresis after lumbar disc herniation. *Spine*. 2002; **27**: 1426–31; discussion 1431.
152. Benoist M. The natural history of lumbar degenerative spinal stenosis. *Joint, Bone, Spine: Revue du Rhumatisme*. 2002; **69**: 450–7.

38

Chronic joint pain

TANYA BAQAI, ALI JAWAD, AND BRUCE KIDD

KEY LEARNING POINTS

- Biologic therapies have revolutionized the treatment of rheumatoid arthritis (RA).
- Approaches using multiple disease modifying drugs (including biologics) offer the possibility of disease remission in some patients with this disorder.
- RA is a major cardiovascular risk factor and therapy should be administered accordingly.
- Both pharmacologic and nonpharmacologic therapies play an equally important role in the management of osteoarthritis.
- Local or topical therapies may be as efficacious as systemic therapy in osteoarthritis with fewer adverse events.
- Soft tissue disorders are common and may become chronic if not treated at an early stage. Control of symptoms and maintenance of activity remains the mainstay of treatment for the majority of cases.

INTRODUCTION

Chronic joint pain is one of the leading causes of suffering and disability worldwide. Taken together, there are over 200 acute and chronic musculoskeletal disorders, some with multisystem involvement and some that affect specific regions only. The World Health Organization (WHO) classifies common rheumatic complaints under four headings, including inflammatory arthropathies, osteoarthritis and related disorders, regional periarticular or "soft-tissue" disorders, and back pain. A more detailed classification is given in **Table 38.1**.

Osteoarthritis is the most common musculoskeletal disorder, followed by neck and back pain, regional soft-tissue disorders, and finally rheumatoid arthritis (RA). Spinal disorders are covered elsewhere in this volume (see Chapter 37, Chronic back pain), and the three remaining groups of disorders will form the principal focus for this chapter.

ASSESSMENT

The history and examination of a patient presenting with arthritis or other musculoskeletal disease usually provide most of the key information required for diagnosis and treatment, without recourse to additional measures. Whereas the history provides information about the pathologic process and the impact upon the patient, the examination defines the anatomic structures involved.[1]

Although articular pain in adults is associated with many potential diagnoses, in practice the majority turn

Table 38.1 Classification of the rheumatic diseases.

	Type	Examples
1	Immune-based joint diseases	Rheumatoid arthritis; juvenile chronic arthritis; spondarthritis; (includes ankylosing spondylitis, plus reactive, psoriatic, and enteropathic arthritis)
2	Connective tissue diseases	Systemic lupus erythematosus; scleroderma; polymyositis, polyarteritis nodosa; Churg–Strauss syndrome; Wegener's granulomatosus; giant cell arteritis; Takayasu's disease
3	Infectious arthritis	Bacterial; viral; fungal diseases
4	Crystal deposition	Gout; chondrocalcinosis
5	Osteoarthritis	
6	Soft-tissue rheumatism	Tendinitis; capsulitis; enthesitis; bursitis; fasciitis
7	Miscellaneous	Bechet syndrome; Whipple's disease; fibromyalgia syndrome
8	Disorders of bone	Osteoporosis; osteomalacia; Paget's disease

out to have one of relatively few disorders. Around one-third of patients presenting with true inflammatory arthritis remain undiagnosed and have a relatively good prognosis, whereas the reminder mostly have either RA or spondyloarthropathy.[2] The most common causes of polyarticular pain include viral arthritis, osteoarthritis, inflammatory polyarthritis, fibromyalgia, and soft tissue problems whereas the differential diagnosis of pain in or around a single joint includes trauma, infection, and crystal disease.[3]

Important presenting symptoms in joint disease are pain, stiffness or locking, swelling, weakness or difficulty moving, fatigue, and emotional lability such as anxiety or depression.[4] When taking a history, particular attention should be given to the onset and subsequent temporal and spatial pattern of joint involvement as well as to the age and sex of the patient. Osteoarthritis is characterized by use-related pain, whereas inflammatory pain is most severe in the mornings and again towards the end of the day. Prolonged morning stiffness is usually present. However, it is not uncommon for symptoms to overlap and RA and osteoarthritis may be difficult to separate on symptoms alone.[5] The diagnosis of gout is more straightforward with symptoms beginning acutely with a pricking sensation and progressing to an intolerable burning pain. More constant severe pain throughout the day and night may indicate the presence of sinister bone pathology, but can also indicate important psychosocial influences.

RHEUMATOID ARTHRITIS

Definition

RA is a chronic systemic inflammatory disease of unknown etiology. It is characterized by a chronic polyarthritis affecting primarily the peripheral joints and related periarticular structures. It usually starts as an insidious symmetric polyarthritis, often with nonspecific systemic symptoms such as fatigue, low-grade temperatures, and loss of weight. It has an unpredictable and variable course and prognosis. Diagnostic and classification criteria have been proposed and are now widely used in both research and clinical practice (see **Box 38.1**).[6]

Epidemiology

The prevalence of RA varies from 0.5 to 1.5 percent of the population in Western countries and affects more women than men (ratio 2.5:1).[7] The annual incidence in women is estimated at 36/1,00,000 and in men 14/1,00,000, with the peak age of onset being between 30 and 55 years.[8]

Family studies demonstrate a modest genetic predisposition to the development of the disease. The concordance rate for monozygotic twins is about 25 percent, whereas fraternal twins and first-degree relatives of RA patients have a four-fold higher risk (2–5 percent) than the general population. HLA-DR4 and DR1 molecules are associated with an increased severity of the disease.[9]

Clinical features

The onset is usually insidious but can be episodic or acute. RA usually presents as a symmetrical polyarthritis affecting the small joints of the hands and feet. It rarely presents as a monoarthritis, in which case infection or crystal arthritis must be excluded.[10] In elderly patients, the onset of the disease may be indistinguishable from polymyalgia rheumatica, which is a relatively rare condition characterized by myalgia, morning stiffness, and a mostly transient arthritis lasting a few hours to days.[11]

Inflamed joints in RA become swollen, painful, and stiff. The cardinal symptoms and signs of inflammation are usually very obvious and include pain, heat, swelling,

Box 38.1 Criteria for the classification of RA

1. Morning stiffness in and around joints lasting one hour
2. Soft tissue swelling of three or more joint areas[a]
3. Swelling of the proximal interphalangeal, metacarpophalangeal or wrist joints[a]
4. Symmetrical arthritis[a]
5. Subcutaneous nodules
6. Positive test for rheumatoid factor
7. Radiographic erosions or periarticular osteopenia in hand or wrist joints

[a]Present for at least six weeks.
To be classified as having rheumatoid arthritis, a patient must meet at least four of the seven criteria. Adapted with permission of Wiley-Liss, Inc., a subsidiary of John Wiley & Sons, Inc., from *Arthritis and Rheumatism*, **31**, 1988, 315–24. © 1988 John Wiley & Sons, Inc.

Box 38.2 Laboratory features of rheumatoid arthritis

- Anemia
- Thrombocytosis
- Eosinophilia
- Large granular lymphocytes (especially in Felty syndrome)
- Elevated erythrocyte sedimentation rate
- Elevated C-reactive protein
- Decreased serum albumin
- Raised serum globulins
- Increased levels of alkaline phosphatase, aspartateaminotransferase, and γ-glutamyl transferase
- Rheumatoid factor (occurs in 75–80 percent)

loss of function, and, less commonly, erythema. Synovial fluid may accumulate, causing an effusion. Joint pain is usually more prominent and more persistent than in osteoarthritis, occurring at rest, at night, and on activity. Early morning stiffness is also a key feature suggestive of inflammatory joint disease and one of the diagnostic criteria of RA.

In addition to the symmetrical peripheral joint involvement, the cervical spine may also be involved. The synovium-lined atlantoaxial joint and/or the posterior apophyseal joints may become inflamed, causing pain in the neck and occipital headache. Pain may also occur as a result of temporomandibular joint disease.

Uncontrolled disease eventually results in inflammation spreading beyond the synovium of the joint to other nearby structures, including the tenosynovium of tendons, ligaments, other soft-tissue structures, and bone. Subcutaneous nodules can occur in more severe and advanced subsets of RA, which can cause pain, ulceration, and interference with functional activities. Extra-articular features are common and may involve multiple organ systems.[12]

Investigations

The laboratory features in RA reflect the acute-phase response and chronic inflammation of the joints and are listed in **Box 38.2**. Anemia, thrombocytopenia, leukopenia, or abnormal liver function tests may also be caused by drug toxicity.The earliest radiographic changes are seen in the hands in the form of soft-tissue swelling and periarticular osteopenia, but these are nonspecific signs. Erosions typical of RA develop in "bare" areas of bone (i.e. areas lacking articular cartilage) within three years of onset in 90 percent of those patients who ultimately develop erosive disease.[13] Late radiographic signs include narrowing of the joint space, severe erosions of subchondral bone, synovial cyst formation, and lack of bone repair. The distribution of radiologic disease in decreasing order of frequency is hands, feet, knees, hips, cervical spine, shoulders, and elbows.

Bone scintigraphy is helpful in confirming the presence of RA, the distribution of joint involvement, and in assessing disease activity.[14] The use of ultrasonography and extremity magnetic resonance imaging (MRI) is still being evaluated in RA but recent studies suggest that these techniques may be more sensitive for the detection of early disease than conventional assessments.[15]

Treatment

The aims of treatment for RA include:

- relief of symptoms, especially pain, joint stiffness, and general fatigue;
- prevention of or improvement in functional and vocational capabilities;
- prevention of deformity by joint protection and splintage;
- correction of existing deformity using surgery;
- halting the disease process.

Considerable progress has been made in developing validated instruments to assess disease activity and severity, which in turn allow for appropriate provision and monitoring of therapy. Two methods using numeric scoring systems are currently employed and assess a number of parameters including numbers of swollen and tender joints, inflammation markers, and global health and quality of life assessments. The Disease Assessment Score

(DAS28) score and the American College of Rheumatology (ACR) scores (20, 50, and 70) have both been validated for defining remission and disease activity.[16]

PHARMACOLOGIC THERAPY

Nonsteroidal anti-inflammatory drugs

The general pharmacology of nonsteroidal anti-inflammatory drugs (NSAIDs) is covered in Chapter 4, Clinical pharmacology: traditional NSAIDs and selective COX-2 inhibitors in the *Acute Pain* volume of this series and will not be discussed further. NSAIDs are used widely in the treatment of RA for their anti-inflammatory/analgesic properties. They reduce morning stiffness and the pain and swelling of inflamed joints but do not influence the acute-phase response or radiologic progression.[17] No individual NSAID has been shown to have a clear advantage over other NSAIDs with respect to efficacy, although selective cyclooxygenase (COX)-2 inhibitors have been reported to have less gastrointestinal toxicity than "classical" NSAIDs.[18][II], [19][II]

Other analgesic agents

The general principles for the use of analgesic agents in RA and other arthropathies are the same as for other disorders. Paracetamol (acetaminophen) with or without dextropropoxyphene, codeine, dihydrocodeine, or tramadol are all effective for symptom control. They may also be used singularly or in combination with NSAIDs, but tend not to be as effective in reducing morning stiffness.[20]

Antidepressants

The role of antidepressants in relieving pain and depression in RA is not clear. A randomized, double-blind, placebo-controlled study of 48 female outpatients with RA and depression/anxiety reported that dothiepin in doses up to 150 mg daily relieved pain and disability and reduced the duration of early morning stiffness.[21][II]

Disease-modifying antirheumatic drugs

All patients whose RA remains active despite adequate treatment with NSAIDs should be considered for disease-modifying antirheumatic drugs (DMARDs) (see **Table 38.2**). In broad terms, DMARDs are slow acting drugs with a delay of one to six months before a clinical response becomes evident. Efficacy cannot be predicted for an individual patient, but two-thirds of patients may respond. It should be noted that each drug has specific toxicity that requires monitoring.[59, 60]

The decision as to when to introduce DMARDs remains controversial. One randomized controlled trial (RCT) of 238 patients with recently diagnosed RA compared early (within one year of onset of symptoms) with delayed DMARD treatment.[61][II] Patients who received early treatment had significantly better outcome measures at 12 months although no differences were observed in radiologic progression between the early and delayed groups. In another prospective three-year follow-up study of 119 patients with early disease, a nine-month delay in starting hydroxychloroquine resulted in a detrimental effect on pain intensity and patient global well-being.[62][II] Combination therapy with up to three DMARDs is currently proposed as best practice for the initial management of RA compared with monotherapy or step-therapy, with studies suggesting that the response is superior in regimens that include methotrexate therapy.[63]

Biological DMARDs

The management of RA has been revolutionized by the development of biological DMARDs. These agents target a variety of small molecules and can be differentiated into four main categories:

1. tumor necrosis factor (TNF) α inhibitors;
2. interleukin 1 inhibitors;
3. T cell costimulation inhibitors;
4. B cell depleters.

The pro-inflammatory cytokine TNFα plays a key role in the pathophysiology of RA and TNF blocking agents have proved to be effective agents for the treatment of this disorder as well as other inflammatory arthritides including psoriatic arthritis, ankylosing spondylitis, and juvenile chronic RA.

Three main TNF-blocking agents exist at present; infliximab, etanercept, and adalimumab. Infliximab is a chimeric (human, murine) IgG1 monoclonal antibody against TNFα; etanercept is a soluble, recombinant fusion protein of the human TNF receptor and the Fc component of human IgG1 molecule, whilst adulimumab is a fully humanized IgG1 monoclonal antibody against TNFα. Several RCTs have now shown that the combination of anti-TNF agents with methotrexate is associated with significantly reduced radiographic progression, clinical disease activity scores, and improved functional status, compared to placebo and also compared to either the TNF-blocker or methotrexate alone (see **Table 38.2**). One recent study using combination therapy (including infliximab) demonstrated that in rheumatoid patients with less than two years of disease more than 50 percent were able to completely stop infliximab after one year of therapy, suggesting that medication-induced remission may be possible in some patients.[64][II]

Anakinra is a recombinant human interleukin-1 receptor antagonist (IL-1Ra) which has shown to improve clinical activity and radiographic scores compared to placebo, with various background therapy of DMARDs, steroids, and NSAIDs, at the discretion of clinicians. It is currently recommended for use in active RA after an adequate trial of another DMARD, usually methotrexate, and is also recommended in combination with methotrexate in Europe at present.[51][II]

Table 38.2 Summary of evidence from systematic reviews of disease-modifying drugs in RA.

Drug	Efficacy	Toxicity
Sulfasalazine	Improvements in the number of tender and swollen joints, pain score, and ESR. Evaluation of radiologic progression was inconclusive. Efficacy similar to other DMARDs, including parenteral gold and methotrexate (six RCTs[22][I])	Abdominal discomfort, skin rash, and abnormal liver function tests, but more serious hepatic dysfunction or marrow suppression uncommon. Discontinuation due to adverse side effects occurs less often than with other DMARDs, with the exception of hydroxychloroquine[23][I]
Penicillamine	Improvements in the number of swollen joints and ESR (six RCTs[24][I])	Adverse effects are common and potentially serious. They include skin rashes, mouth ulcers, altered taste, gastrointestinal reactions, proteinuria, bone marrow suppression, and autoimmune-mediated disorders such as myositis and myasthenia gravis[24][I]
Methotrexate	Improvement in the number of swollen and tender joints, pain score, physician and patient global assessment, and functional status (five RCTs[25][I]). Patients are more likely to continue taking methotrexate than other DMARDs[26][III], [27][III] and the magnitude of short-term improvement in disease activity is larger for methotrexate than for other DMARDs[28][I]	Adverse effects are common and include abnormal liver function tests, mouth ulcers, skin rashes, gastrointestinal, or hematological disorders. Infections may also occur even at low doses. More serious side-effects include pulmonary toxicity and hepatic fibrosis[29][I]
Parenteral gold	Improvement in the number of swollen joints in patient and physician global assessments and ESR (four RCTs[30][I]). Decreased rate of radiologic progression[31][I]	Dermatitis, stomatitis, proteinuria, and myelosuppression[30][I]
Azathioprine	Significant benefit from use of azathioprine (three RCTs[32][I]). It is useful as a corticosteroid-sparing agent	Increased risk of infection and tumor formation. Other side effects include nausea, vomiting, abnormal liver function tests, and bone marrow suppression[32][I]
Cyclophosphamide	Improvement in the number of tender and swollen joints, but no significant difference in ESR (three RCTs[33][I])	Nausea, vomiting, bone marrow suppression, alopecia, and increased risk of infection and cancer. Because of its toxicity, cyclophosphamide use is reserved for patients unresponsive to other DMARDs, and those with serious extra-articular complications such as systemic rheumatoid vasculitis[34][I]
Cyclosporine	Improvement in the number of tender and swollen joints and in functional status; reduced radiologic progression (three RCTs[35][I])	Patients develop nephropathy, which can be irreversible, and hypertension. Other adverse effects include nausea, dyspepsia, hypertrichosis, gingival hyperplasia, hepatic toxicity, and increased risk of infections and cancer. Because of its toxicity, cyclosporine is used for patients with severe disease or who are unresponsive to other DMARDs, or in combination with methotrexate[35][I]
Auranofin (oral gold)	Significantly less effective than other DMARDs[36][I]	Main adverse effects are diarrhea and abdominal discomfort. Serious adverse effects are rare[36][I]
Hydroxychloroquine	Improvements in swollen and tender joint counts, joint score, physician and patient global assessment, and ESR[37][I]	Ocular complications, with the risk being higher with chloroquine than hydroxychloroquine. Other adverse effects include gastrointestinal disturbances (the most common), skin rashes, renal abnormalities, vertigo, blurred vision, and

(Continued over)

Table 38.2 Summary of evidence from systematic reviews of disease-modifying drugs in RA (continued).

Drug	Efficacy	Toxicity
		very rarely cardiomyopathy and severe neurologic disorder[38][I]
Leflunomide	More effective than placebo in the treatment of rheumatoid arthritis and has similar efficacy to sulfasalazine. Radiographic progression was also significantly slower with leflunomide and sulfasalazine than with placebo (one RCT[39][I], [40, 41][II]). Improvements in the ACR responses after six months when used in combination with methotrexate therapy. There were more discontinuations due to adverse effects in the combination group versus placebo and more withdrawals due to lack of efficacy in the methotrexate plus placebo group.	Diarrhea, nausea, alopecia, rash, and transient abnormality in liver function tests[39][II]
TNF-α blockade	Infliximab produces improvements to both clinical and laboratory parameters of disease activity.[42][II], [43][II] Two RCTs have shown significant clinical benefit of etanercept with minimal toxicity in rheumatoid patients who had inadequate response to other DMARDs.[44][II], [45][II] In other trials, the combination of etanercept and low-dose weekly methotrexate was safe, well tolerated, and provided significantly greater clinical benefit than methotrexate alone.[46][II], [47][II] Adalumimab shows similar results with combination with methotrexate. Nonclinical trial study suggests restoration of good clinical response with adalimumab after secondary loss of efficacy from infliximab or etanercept[48][II], [49][II]	Long-term data not yet available. Preliminary data from the several TNF-α blockade registers show increased risk of respiratory infections, reactivation of latent tuberculosis. There is conflicting data about whether there is an increased risk of lymphoma and solid malignancies, such as skin cancers. Insufficient evidence for demyelinating-like syndromes, drug-induced lupus, viral hepatitis reactivation or exacerbation. Rarely, new onset interstitial lung disease with infliximab. Increased relative risk of worsening congestive cardiac failure with high dose infliximab (> 10 mg/kg). Rarely, pancytopenia and aplastic anemia
Anakinra	Five studies, including two clinical trials, to date show improvement in clinical response for treatment of rheumatoid arthritis (RA) alone or with MTX[50][II], [51][II]	Long-term data not yet available and no registries as yet. Serious infections are increased, higher incidence than in RA using other DMARDs, magnified by corticosteroid use. No data to date to suggest increased incidence of tuberculosis or malignancy
Abatacept	Reduced clinical activity, structural damage and radiographic progression with improved physical function in moderate-severe RA in those with inadequate response to one or more DMARDs such as MTX or TNF blocking agents, when used in combination with MTX[52][II], [53][II], [54][II]	Increased incidence of serious infection versus placebo (3 versus 1.9 percent) and 4.4 percent when in combination with other biological agents versus 1.5 percent in controls. No data when in combination with rituximab. Caution in use with chronic obstructive pulmonary disease patients due to increased incidence of adverse events than with placebo. Insufficent data as regards incidence of tuberculosis or malignancy[52][II], [53][II]
Rituximab	Improvement in patient global visual analog scale, fatigue, disability, quality of life and clinical signs, symptoms and/or laboratory measurements by 8–16 weeks in RA patients with an inadequate response to MTX who have failed conventional DMARDs or one or more TNF-inhibitors. RCTs show combination of rituximab and MTX have superior	Infusion reactions, although corticosteroids can reduce the incidence and severity of infusion reactions by 30 percent without changing efficacy. No cases of progressive multifocal leukoencephalopathy (PML) in RA, as regards at least two cases seen in systemic lupus erythematosus (SLE) (although PML also seen in

(Continued over)

Table 38.2 Summary of evidence from systematic reviews of disease-modifying drugs in RA (continued).

Drug	Efficacy	Toxicity
	clinical efficacy for RA when compared to monotherapy. Slows radiographic progression in patients who have had inadequate response to one or more TNF inhibitors[55][II], [56][II], [57][II], [58][II]	SLE without rituximab treatment). Small increased incidence of serious infections compared to placebo. No evidence as yet of increased frequency of tuberculosis in patients with lymphoma treated with rituximab or in RA patients. No evidence yet for increased risk of solid malignancy. Patients to be screened for hepatitis B and C prior to use as a case of hepatitis reactivation in oncological practice has been reported[55][II], [56][II]

DMARDs, disease-modifying antirheumatic drugs; ESR, erythrocyte sedimentation rate; TNF, tumor necrosis factor.

Abatacept is an example of a biological agent which modulates T cell activation. It is a soluble fusion protein of CTLA4 and human Ig, which competitively inhibits the CD28-B7 co-stimulation interaction. Phase III RCTs have demonstrated that its use in RA patients in association with methotrexate significantly reduces the rate of progression of erosions, joint space narrowing, and total radiographic scores. Its use is currently recommended in patients with active RA who have had an adequate trial of methotrexate, another DMARD or TNF inhibitor.[52][II], [53][II], [54][II]

Rituximab is a B cell depleting agent, used for years in the treatment of non-Hodgkin's lymphoma and more recently for systemic lupus erythematosus (SLE) and Wegener's granulomatosis, and now approved for use in the treatment of RA. It is a chimeric (human, murine) monoclonal antibody against CD20, present on B cell precursors before they differentiate into antibody-producing plasma cells. Two clinical trials to date have shown benefit of rituximab therapy in the treatment of rheumatoid patients whose disease is refractory to both methotrexate and TNF blockade, with significant improvement in clinical activity scores. Less strong data suggests that rituximab may also slow radiographic progression.[56][II], [65][II], [57][II]

Corticosteroids

Corticosteroids are often used for prompt relief of symptoms of inflammation. In practice, they are frequently given for acute exacerbations of the disease or as a "bridge therapy" until DMARDs become effective. They may be given directly into joints or as intramuscular/intravenous depot injections. The long-term use of oral steroids as a DMARD remains controversial because of the fear of side effects, particularly osteoporosis.

One systematic review comparing short-term (weeks) treatment using low-dose prednisolone (15 mg or less/day) with placebo or NSAIDs found that, in the short term, prednisolone had a greater effect than placebo or NSAIDs in controlling the activity and symptoms of the disease.[66][I] A second systematic review evaluating longer term (three months or more) steroid use drew the same conclusion.[67][I] Several RCTs have found a significant decrease in pain, disability, and the rate of progression of radiologic damage in patients treated with prednisolone 7.5 mg compared with placebo over two years, although joint destruction resumed after steroids were discontinued, often within one year of steroid withdrawl.[68][II]

Another study suggests that even prednisolone doses of as little as 5 mg per day for two years may improve clinical, functional and radiographic measures in DMARD naive, early RA patients, although it is unclear whether doses less than this have any beneficial effect.[69][II]

Medications addressing cardiovascular/atherosclerotic risk factors

Relatively recent studies have demonstrated an increased risk of coronary atherosclerosis and associated morbidity and mortality in patients with rheumatoid arthritis. Management of such patients should therefore include pharmacological and nonpharmacological measures to modify such risk factors as cigarette smoking, hyperlipidemia, hypertension, and a sedentary lifestyle.[70, 71] In addition to lipid lowering effects, HMG CoA reductase inhibitors (statins) may have clinically important anti-inflammatory properties, with beneficial effects on markers of inflammation in RA patients noted in one placebo-controlled trial of atorvastatin.[72][II]

NONPHARMACOLOGIC THERAPY

Physical therapy: rest versus exercise

Rest has long been recommended for patients with RA, especially during periods of active joint inflammation, although controlled studies of the effects of hospitalization and bed rest have not found this to be of benefit, unless the patient is seriously ill with active disease.[73][II], [74][II] The effects of joint immobilization in RA have been examined in several studies, which indicate that joint splintage may have short-term effects, such as reduced pain, that are not maintained in the longer term.[75][II] Overall, the evidence for effectiveness of massage and electrophysical modalities is absent or weak.

Available evidence suggests that range of motion, strengthening, and aerobic conditioning exercises are safe for patients with RA and improve muscle strength, cardiovascular fitness, and probably physical function. They do not seem to exacerbate joint symptoms. Preliminary evidence also suggests aerobic weight-bearing exercise may help prevent corticosteroid-associated osteoporosis.[76][III], [77][III], [78][III]

Diet

Patients should follow diets that help maintain a reasonable weight and that contain high amounts of polyunsaturated fatty acids, adequate calcium, vitamin D, and the recommended amounts of other vitamins and minerals. Food allergies may be a factor in RA in a very small number of patients.[79] Controlled studies have shown that omega-3 fatty acids (present in Pacific herring, king mackerel, salmon, and mullet) may reduce fatigue and joint tenderness in patients with RA.[80][II] Specifically, a diet enriched with eicosapentaenoic acid or docohexaenoic acid may result in decreased arachidonic acid metabolites and cytokines, with a concurrent decrease in symptoms.[81][II] Patients with RA may be deficient in zinc, copper, and magnesium, probably as a result of chronic inflammation, but there is no evidence that either wearing copper bracelets or taking zinc supplements improves symptoms.[82]

Patient education and other approaches

One meta-analysis of educational interventions for patients with RA or osteoarthritis has found a clinically small, but statistically significant, beneficial effect of patient education or counseling on both pain and disability in 17 trials.[83][I] Cognitive-behavioral therapies may also significantly reduce the patient's self-reported pain, functional disabilities, joint involvement, and disease activity, and feelings of low self-esteem.[84][II] Overall, further research into the use of nonpharmacological treatments and comprehensive arthritis service delivery models is required.[85]

Prognosis

It is difficult to predict the clinical course of RA.[86] Indicators of poor outcome are listed in **Box 38.3**. RA is mostly a persistent disease with slow progression. In a study of outcome of 50 patients seen within six months of the onset of symptoms, only 10 percent had no evidence of the disease after five years, another 10 percent had severe progression, whereas 80 percent had continuing disease.[87]

Box 38.3 Indicators of poor outcome in rheumatoid arthritis

- Gradual onset of disease
- Older women have a less favorable outcome
- Disease duration before consulting a physician
- Early development of rheumatoid nodules
- High titers of rheumatoid factor
- Persistently high ESR or CRP or plasma viscosity for more than a year
- Early development of erosions
- Extra-articular manifestations
- Severe functional impairment
- Early involvement of large joints

ESR, erythrocyte sedimentation rate; CRP, C-reactive protein.

In general terms, RA is characterized by progressive disability. One long-term follow-up study found that after 11 years 25 percent of patients with RA were severely disabled, and after 15 years 50 percent were similarly disabled.[88] Nearly half of all patients will be disabled or unable to work within ten years.[89] RA also shortens life expectancy by a few years in both men and women.[90]

More severe RA disease (more than 30 joints involved), is associated with higher mortality rates and has been compared to that of three-vessel coronary artery disease or stage IV Hodgkin's lymphoma.[91] Patients with RA that require hospital care have at least a two-fold increased mortality when compared to those without disease.[92] Patients who respond to therapy, particularly to DMARDs, may have a lower mortality, in particular with methotrexate which has a small, statistically significant survival advantage as regards cardiovascular risk factors.

OSTEOARTHRITIS

Definition

Osteoarthritis (OA) has been defined as a group of overlapping distinct diseases, which may have different etiologies but with similar biologic, morphologic, and clinical outcomes. The disease process not only affects articular cartilage but also involves the entire joint, including the subchondral bone, ligaments, capsule, synovial membrane, and periarticular muscles. There is gradual loss of articular cartilage, combined with thickening of the subchondral bone, bony overgrowths (osteophytes) at joint margins, and mild, chronic nonspecific synovial inflammation. Ultimately, the articular cartilage degenerates with fibrillation, fissure, ulceration, and full thickness loss of the joint surface.[93, 94]

Epidemiology

OA is an age-related condition and one of the most important causes of pain and disability in older people. However, the difference between physiologic aging of the cartilage and OA cartilage is not clear. Although radiographic evidence of OA is universal in at least some joints in people over the age of 60 years, significant symptomatic disease probably affects only about 10–20 percent of the population.[95] OA of the knee affects function in 10 percent of the population aged over 50, with the female–male ratio being 3:1.[96] OA of the hip is less common but is more likely to cause disability, with the prevalence increasing from less than 3 percent under the age of 65 through to 5 percent of people in their eighties.

OA is common worldwide, but the sites most commonly affected vary in different populations. Nodal OA of the hand is rare in black Africans and Malaysians, and OA of the hip is uncommon in black and Asian populations compared with white people.[97] These ethnic differences seem to reflect genetic rather than cultural factors.

Clinical features

It is important to stress that OA is symptomatic only in a minority of patients. Pain is generally activity related and is thought to arise from sites in and around the affected joint (see **Table 38.3**). Night pain usually occurs in advanced cases and may be caused by raised intraosseous pressure. Joint locking may indicate a loose body. In erosive OA, the pain is inflammatory in nature and is associated with erythema, tenderness, and stiffness, and is aggravated by rest. Sudden deterioration in a stable osteoarthritic joint may be caused by fracture, avascular necrosis, crystal synovitis, or even sepsis.[98]

Table 38.3 Possible causes of pain in osteoarthritis.

Tissue origin	Modifiers
Bone	
Periosteal elevation by osteophytes	Anxiety
Trabecular microfracture	Depression
Pressure on subchondral bone	Lack of social support
Hypertension in bone marrow	Secondary gain
Articular	
Synovitis	Physical demands
Pinching of synovial villi	Occupational
Joint capsule distension	Obesity
Periarticular	
Ligament damage	Neuromuscular integrity
Muscle spasm	Protective reflexes
Bursitis	Muscle weakness

Physical signs include crepitus on joint movement, bony enlargement, instability, deformity, restricted range of movement, and effusion. Periarticular tenderness is also common. Muscle weakness may contribute to joint instability and may aggravate the pain. Acute inflammatory signs may occur in crystal synovitis.

OA with deposition of calcium pyrophosphate dihydrate (pyrophosphate arthropathy) occurs predominantly in elderly women, but in younger patients it may be caused by an underlying metabolic disease, e.g. hemochromatosis, hyperparathyroidism, and Wilson's disease.[99] Apatite-associated destructive arthritis occurs usually in the hips and shoulders (Milwaukee shoulder) or knees of elderly women. It is usually associated with large amounts of apatite deposition. The outcome is poor.[100]

Investigations

Laboratory tests are not useful in the diagnosis of OA. The erythrocyte sedimentation rate (ESR) is usually normal; it may be slightly increased in the inflammatory stage but even then rarely exceeds 35 mm/hour.[101] The synovial fluid is generally relatively viscous and transparent and noninflammatory, with a cell count under $2000/mm^3$.[102]

The plain radiograph is the investigation most frequently used to confirm the clinical diagnosis. The radiologic features include narrowing of the joint space, osteophyte formation, sclerosis of the articular surfaces, and subchondral cyst formation. If plain radiographs do not show pathological alteration, a ^{99m}technetium phosphate radionuclide scan or MRI may be required to show earlier signs of disease.[103]

Treatment

Clinical guidelines for the management of hip and knee OA have been published.[104][V], [105][V], [106][V] Recommendations for pharmacologic therapy were broadly similar, although differences were apparent with respect to first-line choice of anti-inflammatory therapy. Both sets of guidelines stressed the importance of nonpharmacologic therapy including patient education and self-management programs.

PHARMACOLOGIC THERAPIES

Topical therapies

NSAID creams and gels

One systematic review of 86 clinical trials comparing topically applied NSAIDs with placebo found these agents had a relative benefit of 2.0 (95 percent confidence interval (CI) 1.5–2.7) for relief of chronic musculoskeletal pain caused by OA and tendonitis.[107][I] Topical NSAIDs have a good safety record. Large surveillance studies in general practice suggest good safety (adverse events <1.5 percent) with local skin reactions the principal side effect with no association between topical NSAIDs and upper gastrointestinal bleeding or perforation.[108][III]

Capsaicin cream

A nonsystematic meta-analysis of pooled data from three RCTs of topically applied capsaicin concluded that it was useful for pain relief.[109][IV] Active treatment with capsaicin results in significantly greater pain reduction than placebo.[110][II] Capsaicin may cause a mild, transient, burning sensation.

Intra-articular injections

Corticosteroid injections

These should be given as adjunctive therapy. Effusions, when present, should be aspirated before injections are administered. Periarticular injections of hydrocortisone are sometimes used to relieve painful bursitis associated with OA,[111] whereas injections of methylprednisolone or triamcinolone into the knee joint may relieve the pain of OA for a few months.[112]

Intra-articular hyaluronan injections

There is a reduction in the size and concentration of hyaluronan (hyaluronic acid) molecules present in synovial fluid in joints affected by OA. As a result, the capacity to absorb shock and to lubricate articulating surfaces is reduced.[113] A recent review concluded that injections of either preparation produce a small reduction in pain compared with placebo that may last several months.[113] There is evidence to support the efficacy of hyaluronan in the management of knee OA, both for pain reduction and functional improvement. However, although pain relief may be obtained for several months, rather than for several weeks as with steroid, this benefit may be offset by its slower onset of action and by the requirement of a course of three to five weekly injections with the logistical and cost issues. There is minimal evidence for a role in disease modification.

SYSTEMIC THERAPIES

If physical and/or local measures do not control pain in OA, oral analgesics or NSAIDs are considered next. Systematic reviews have found that simple analgesics such as paracetamol and NSAIDs produce short-term pain relief in OA.[94][I] However, there is no good evidence that NSAIDs are superior to simple analgesics such as paracetamol or that one NSAID is better than another.[94][I] There is some evidence that indometacin (and possibly other NSAIDs) may accelerate progression of OA.[114]

In practice, most physicians treat patients with paracetamol initially and an NSAID is added if symptoms remain uncontrolled. When used, NSAIDs are prescribed in the lowest effective dose and for a short time. There is some evidence to suggest a slight benefit if dextropropoxyphene is added to paracetamol but at a cost of increased toxicity.[115][V] An RCT of 90 patients showed that treatment of knee OA with tramadol allowed reduction of the naproxen dose among those patients with naproxen-responsive pain.[116][II]

CHONDROPROTECTIVE AGENTS

Glucosamine sulfate has received much attention in both the medical and popular press.[117] A number of controlled studies have been published, although many are small and of poor quality.[118] A larger three-year RCT has suggested that glucosamine retards the progression of symptomatic knee OA with no differences in safety or reasons for withdrawal between the treatment and placebo groups.[119] [II] Other studies have shown modest improvements in pain and function compared with placebo and current evidence supports a beneficial effect of glucosamine on OA although its exact role remains unclear.

Tetracyclines may offer some chondroprotection, but more data are awaited. Rumalon (a glucose aminoglycan peptide complex extracted from bovine cartilage), arteparon (glucosaminoglycan polysulfate with heparanoid actions), and chondroitin sulfate have not been shown to have chondroprotective actions.[120] The combination of glucosamine and chondroitin sulfate may be effective in patients with moderate to severe knee pain.[121][II]

NONPHARMACOLOGIC THERAPIES

Patient education and self-management

Education of the patient forms an integral part of the treatment plan for patients with OA. A meta-analysis of trials of patient education programs in comparison with standard NSAID use showed that education was 20 percent as effective as NSAIDs at providing pain relief.[122][I] Psychosocial support can improve general well-being by reducing the requirement for health care.[123][IV] Education of spouses or family members may improve social support to the patient.[124][IV] Regular telephone contact by a member of the multidisciplinary team can produce significant improvement in pain and functional status.[125][II]

Exercise therapy

A randomized controlled trial has been conducted that examined the effects of a structured exercise program on self-reported disability in 439 patients over 60 years old with knee OA.[126][II] The two exercise groups showed significant, but modest, reductions in disability and pain compared with the education group.

Physical therapy

Medical knee taping in patients with patellofemoral OA has been shown to be effective in reducing pain.[127][III] A walking stick or a cane of the correct height can improve function and reduce pain in patients with OA of the lower limbs.[128][IV] Weight loss has been shown to lead to a slower rate of development of symptomatic OA of the knees in women.[129][III]

Transcutaneous electrical nerve stimulation

Transcutaneous electrical nerve stimulation (TENS) has been shown to reduce pain and the use of analgesia compared with placebo in OA.[130][II] In another trial, no significant difference was found between TENS and oral naproxen in a placebo-controlled crossover study of 36 patients with OA of the knee.[131][II] Acupuncture has not been shown to be of benefit in OA, possibly because of relatively impressive responses in control groups.[132][II]

Splints and soles

A wedged insole changes the angle of the lower limb and may result in significant symptomatic improvement. Patients may also benefit from shoe orthoses to correct abnormal biomechanics due to leg length inequality, or vesicoplastic insoles that reduce the strain of impact loading.[133][IV] Trainers may also provide some relief for many people with lower limb and lumbar OA.[128]

Occupational therapy

In a trial of occupational therapy, patients with OA were assessed at baseline and then taught hand exercises both directly and with information sheets and were provided with appropriate adaptive devices.[134][IV] After 12 weeks, 49 percent of patients who previously perceived themselves as being disabled no longer felt so, with benefits that were additive to the use of NSAIDs.

Surgical treatment

Arthroscopic washout and cartilage debridement can relieve symptoms of OA of the knee for up to several months.[135] Closed tidal irrigation (nonarthroscopic washout) has also been shown to be effective in relieving pain.[136][II] Arthroscopic meniscal debridement may not improve outcome in OA of the knees.[137][II] Upper tibial osteotomy or supracondylar femoral osteotomy can provide effective pain relief in younger patients with OA of the medial compartment of the knees.[138]

Persistent, severe pain uncontrolled by medical and physical therapy is the best indication for joint replacement, especially when there is associated disability. Joint replacement is very effective for relief of pain and disability in patients with advanced OA of the hip and knee.[139] After such surgery, over 90 percent of patients can expect good function in a replaced joint for at least ten years.

REGIONAL SOFT-TISSUE DISORDERS

Definition

Many of the musculoskeletal conditions seen by clinicians are not primarily disorders of cartilage or synovium but arise as a result of problems within joint-related soft tissues such as tendons, ligaments, capsules, bursae, intervertebral disks, and meniscii. Guidelines for the diagnosis and treatment of these disorders are less well developed compared to RA and OA and whilst the outcome is mostly favorable, a significant proportion of cases progress to become chronic or resistant to therapy.

Shoulder

EPIDEMIOLOGY AND DIAGNOSIS

Shoulder pain is the second most common musculoskeletal complaint after back pain with a reported point prevalence of between 7 and 21 percent of adults.[140, 141, 142] Once present, shoulder pain may persist indefinitely, such that at least half of all patients presenting to a general practitioner with pain continue to have symptoms at one year.[143] Shoulder pain may be due to either intrinsic disorders or to referred pain syndromes although a standard history and examination should enable a diagnosis to be made in the majority of cases.[144] A longstanding comprehensive diagnostic system recognizing various independent entities such as frozen shoulder and tendonitis remains in widespread use today[145] and this approach is mirrored in more recent diagnostic criteria developed using a Delphi consensus approach[146] (see **Table 38.4**).

The site and distribution of pain usually provides important diagnostic information. Lateral or anterolateral shoulder pain is often associated with impingement syndromes involving the rotator cuff or with frozen shoulder. Posterior shoulder pain can arise from tendonitis of the external rotators but is more generally a reflection of referred cervical pain. Similarly, poorly localized pain, or pain that is referred below the elbow into the forearm of hand, should prompt a search for more central pathology.

Cluster analysis of examination findings has revealed three patterns based on range of movement.[147] The first includes patients with pain plus severely restricted passive range of glenohumeral movement who are most commonly suffering from frozen shoulder. Other patterns include mildly reduced passive range of movement and patients with pain but no restricted movement. The vast majority of patients exhibiting these features will have a rotator cuff disorder which is the largest single diagnostic category accounting for shoulder pain. In common with other tendinopathies, rotator cuff tendonitis is often characterized by pain on resisted movement with an

Table 38.4 Diagnostic criteria for upper limb disorders.

Disorder	Diagnostic criteria
Rotator cuff tendinitis	History of pain in the deltoid region and pain on resisted active movement (abduction, supraspinatus; external rotation, infraspinatus; internal rotation, subscapularis)
Bicipital tendinitis	History of anterior shoulder pain and pain on resisted active flexion or supination of forearm
Shoulder capsulitis	History of pain in the deltoid area and equal restriction of active and passive glenohumeral movement with capsular pattern (external rotation > abduction > internal rotation)
Lateral epicondylitis	Epicondylar pain and epicondylar tenderness and pain on resisted extension of the wrist
Medial epicondylitis	Epicondylar pain and epicondylar tenderness and pain on resisted flexion of the wrist
de Quervain's disease	Pain over the radial styloid and tender swelling of the first extensor of the wrist compartment and either pain reproduced by resisted thumb extension or a positive Finkelstein's test
Tenosynovitis of the wrist	Pain on movement localized to the tendon sheaths of the wrist and reproduction of pain by resisted active movement
Carpal tunnel syndrome	Pain or paresthesiae or sensory loss in the median nerve distribution and one of: positive Tinel's test; positive Phalen's test; nocturnal exacerbation of symptoms; motor loss with wasting of abductor pollicus brevis; abnormal nerve conduction time
Nonspecific diffuse	Pain in the forearm in the absence of a specific diagnosis or forearm pain pathology (sometimes includes loss of function, weakness, cramp, muscle tenderness, allodynia, or slowing of fine movements)

Adapted from *Annals of the Rheumatic Diseases*, 1998, **57**, 1–2, with permission of BMJ Publishing Group Ltd.

additional sign being that of a painful arc on active abduction of the affected side. The differential diagnosis includes true acromioclavicular joint disease arising from either OA or trauma, however, in these disorders glenohumeral movements are normal, there is no resisted pain, and symptoms are generally confined to the joint with the patient often pointing to the affected area (the "point sign").

TREATMENT

Frozen shoulder is considered to be a relatively benign self-limiting disorder, however, some patients may experience considerable pain and distress during the more acute stages which can prove difficult to control. Full recovery generally occurs between 12 and 42 months after onset of symptoms with less than 10 percent of patients requiring more aggressive surgical therapy. A wide variety of treatment options have been proposed although only a few approaches have been subjected to adequate clinical trials. There is evidence to support the use of intra-articular steroids in the more acute phases and the addition of physical therapy following injection may result in greater improvement than injection alone.[148][II] A role for intra-articular dilation has been shown in a number of studies although uncertainty remains as to whether capsular distention is superior to steroid injection alone.[149][II]

The goal of treatment of rotator cuff disorders is to control symptoms and maintain activity, relieve ongoing cuff impingement, and manage existing cuff tears. NSAIDs have been shown to be useful in the short term (within four weeks), but the long-term efficacy remains unclear.[150][I] Flexibility and strengthening exercises combined with joint mobilization are used widely and there is some evidence to support the use of these approaches.[151][I] Laser therapy and electromagnetic field therapy may also be useful but there is no evidence that other commonly used physical techniques are substantially better than placebo. Shoulder injections of local anesthetic may be helpful diagnostically and therapeutically, at least in the short term although this approach remains controversial, particularly given the risks of soft tissue atrophy associated with these agents.[152][I], [153][II] Cognitive-behavioral therapy may have a role to play in managing chronic symptoms, although this remains to be shown in clinical trials. Finally, surgical decompression and/or repair is warranted for patients who do not respond to conservative measures after three to six months with acromioplasty being the surgical procedure of choice for patients with refractory impingement.[154][III]

Forearm and hand

EPIDEMIOLOGY AND DIAGNOSIS

The prevalence of all types of elbow pain may be as high as 14 percent in older age groups.[155] A relationship to occupation is reported, with elbow pain being 1.6–1.8 times more common in those with strenuous jobs, such as packers and meat-cutters.[156] Lateral epicondylitis (tennis elbow) is the most common disorder of the elbow, being approximately six-fold more common than medial epicondylitis (golfer's elbow).[157]

Given problems with definitions, prevalence estimates for disorders of the forearm and hand vary widely, with the reported prevalence of nonspecific forearm pain ranging from 9 to 20 percent.[158] Reliable data for the prevalence of individual disorders such as tenosynovitis, trigger finger and thumb, and Dupuytren's contracture are not available. The relationship between occupation and many forearm/hand disorders (excluding tennis elbow) remains controversial although one meta-analysis has concluded that soft-tissue disorders of the neck and upper limb are associated with jobs involving prolonged abnormal postures, abnormally high forces, or frequent repetition.[159] As with other chronic disorders, psychosocial and cognitive factors probably play an important role in upper limb symptoms and disability, although evidence to support this remains indirect and the subject of continuing controversy.

The diagnosis of tennis elbow is based on a history of pain over the lateral epicondyle, together with local tenderness, pain on resisted wrist extension, or strong gripping in the presence of a normal range of elbow movement. Diagnosis of more distal tendinopathies is along similar lines with local symptoms and tenderness, together with provocation of pain on resisted movement of the relevant tendon. Local anesthetic blocks can play some role where the diagnosis is uncertain, however, laboratory and radiological investigations are generally used only to exclude other diagnoses.

TREATMENT

The most frequent treatments for soft-tissue disorders of the upper limb including tennis elbow include rest, oral analgesics, and NSAIDs. A review of physical therapies for forearm/hand pain is available,[160][I] although well-controlled RCTs demonstrating efficacy of most of the commonly used therapies are lacking. Somewhat surprisingly, a systematic review of topically applied NSAIDs found them to be effective in treating both acute and chronic soft-tissue disorders.[107][I] A pooled odds ratio for active drug against placebo in acute soft-tissue syndromes was 1.7, and that for chronic disorders was 2.0 in favor of the active drug.

Although evidence for inflammation is lacking in most soft-tissue disorders of the forearm and hand, locally injected steroids have been widely used and appear to provide better results than either placebo or local anesthetic alone.[158] The best evidence for the efficacy of corticosteroid injections has come from studies in patients with tennis elbow where treatment produces good short-term benefits, but no improvement in outcome at one year.[161][II] Other suggested therapies for which some evidence exists include the use of botulinum toxin,[162][II] autologous blood injection,[163][III] topical nitrates,[164][II] and acupuncture.[165][I] Unfortunately, relapse is common, with between 15 and 50 percent of patients with lateral epicondylitis having further symptoms and about 40 percent having prolonged discomfort over the next five years.[158][II] Surgery gives good results in the short term, but symptoms may recur.[166]

Lower limb

EPIDEMIOLOGY AND DIAGNOSIS

There are very few epidemiological data relating to soft-tissue disorders of the lower limb. Risk factors for the development of these disorders include trauma, unaccustomed exercise, obesity, poor footwear, and prolonged standing.[167]

In the hip, the most common soft-tissue disorders are due to problems associated with the numerous bursae that are found in this region. Trochanteric bursitis is the most prevalent condition and is often associated with other disorders, including osteoarthritis of the same hip, lumbar spondylosis, and RA.[168] Since no findings are pathognomonic of trochanteric bursitis, the diagnosis is generally based on the clinical picture, which includes pain along the lateral side of the upper thigh that is aggravated by activity or lying on the affected side. Physical examination reveals tenderness over the greater trochanter. Less frequent soft-tissue disorders in this area include iliopsoas bursitis, iliogluteal bursitis ("weaver's bottom"), and adductor tendinitis, which tends to occur as a sporting injury, particularly in gymnasts and horseback riders.[169]

Chronic knee pain is common at all ages: OA is the major determinant in the elderly, whereas anterior knee pain syndrome (chondromalacia patellae) is more important in adolescents and children. There are also a large number of soft-tissue structures within the knee giving rise to symptoms including ligamentous injuries, meniscal tears, bursitis, popliteal cysts, iliotibial band syndrome, and synovial plicae.[170] Prepatellar bursitis is among the most common of these and is usually related to repetitive trauma. Diagnosis is usually obvious, with a fluctuant swelling over the front of the patella. Anserine bursitis is also common, although in practice the term tends to be used loosely to describe any pain over the medial aspect of the upper tibia in the region of the bursa and so may include lesions of the medial ligament or pes anserus insertion.[171]

Soft-tissue disorders of the ankle include Achilles tendinitis, which is generally associated with repetitive trauma due to excessive use of the calf muscles during sporting activities. There may be an associated Achilles bursitis, which can also arise spontaneously or in association with a systemic arthropathy such as RA. One of the most common causes of pain around the heel is plantar fasciitis, which generally also results from repetitive microtrauma with risk factors being obesity, athletics, and poor footwear.[172] The disorder may coexist with subcalcaneal bursitis.

TREATMENT

Treatment options are similar to those discussed in the section on upper limb soft-tissue disorders, except that there are even fewer controlled trials demonstrating efficacy of particular therapeutic modalities. For the most part, primary care management consists of rest, simple analgesia, and NSAIDs. Physical therapy may be used in both acute and chronic disorders, but evidence for efficacy remains scant. Uncontrolled studies have shown infiltration of local anesthetics and steroids to be helpful in confirming the diagnosis and in bringing relief to a number of these disorders, but definitive studies are awaited.

REFERENCES

1. Doherty M, Dacre J, Dieppe P, Snaith M. The "GALS" locomotor screen. *Annals of the Rheumatic Diseases.* 1992; **51**: 1165–9.
2. El-Gabalawy HS, Duray P, Goldbach-Mansky R. Evaluating patients with arthritis of recent onset: studies in pathogenesis and prognosis. *Journal of the American Medical Association.* 2000; **284**: 2368–73.
3. Guidelines for the initial evaluation of the adult patient with acute musculoskeletal symptoms. American College of Rheumatology Ad Hoc Committee on Clinical Guidelines. *Arthritis and Rheumatism.* 1996; **39**: 1.
4. Dieppe P, Sergent J. History. In: Kippel JH, Dieppe PA (eds). *Rheumatology*, 2nd edn. Vol. 1. London: CV Mosby, 1998.
5. Helliwell PS. The semeiology of arthritis: discriminating between patients on the basis of their symptoms. *Annals of the Rheumatic Diseases.* 1995; **54**: 924–6.
6. Arnett FC, Edworthy SM, Bloch DA *et al.* The American Rheumatism Association 1987 revised criteria for the classification of rheumatoid arthritis. *Arthritis and Rheumatism.* 1988; **31**: 315–24.
7. Lawrence RC, Helmick CG, Arnett FC *et al.* Estimates of the prevalence of arthritis and selected musculoskeletal disorders in the United States. *Arthritis and Rheumatism.* 1998; **41**: 778–81.
8. Symmons DP, Barrett EM, Bankhead CR *et al.* The United Kingdom: results from the Norfolk Arthritis Register. *British Journal of Rheumatology.* 1994; **33**: 735–9.
9. Winchester R, Dwyer E, Rose S. The genetic basis of rheumatoid arthritis; the shared epitope hypothesis. *Rheumatic Diseases Clinics of North America.* 1992; **18**: 761–83.
10. Fleming A, Crown JM, Corbett M. Early rheumatoid disease. I. Onset. II. Patterns of joint involvement. *Annals of the Rheumatic Diseases.* 1976; **35**: 357–63.
11. Schumacher HR. Palindromic onset of rheumatoid arthritis: clinical, synovial fluid and biopsy studies. *Arthritis and Rheumatism.* 1982; **25**: 361–9.
12. Matteson EL, Cohen MD, Conn DL. Rheumatoid arthritis: clinical features and systemic involvement. In: Klippel JH, Dieppe PA (eds). *Rheumatology*, 2nd edn. London: Mosby, 1998: 5.4.1–8.
13. Resnick D. Rheumatoid arthritis. In: Resnick D (eds). *Bone and joint imaging*, 2nd edn. Philadelphia, PA: WB Saunders, 1996: 195–209.
14. Weissberg DL, Resnick D, Taylor A *et al.* Rheumatoid arthritis and its variants: analysis of scintiphotographic, radiographic and clinical examinations. *American Journal of Roentgenology.* 1978; **131**: 665–73.
15. * Freestan JE, Conaghnan PG, Dass S *et al.* Does extremity-MRI improve erosion detection in severely damaged joints? A study of long-standing rheumatoid arthritis using three imaging modalities. *Annals of the Rheumatic Diseases.* 2007; **66**: 1538–40.
16. Aletaha D, Ward MM, Machold KP *et al.* Remission and active disease in rheumatoid arthritis. Defining criteria for disease activity states. *Arthritis and Rheumatism.* 2005; **52**: 2625.
17. Donnelly S, Scott DL, Emery P. Management of early inflammatory arthritis. *Baillère's Clinical Rheumatology.* 1992; **6**: 251–60.
18. Silverstein FE, Faich G, Goldstein JL *et al.* Gastrointestinal toxicity with celecoxib vs nonsteroidal anti-inflammatory drugs for osteoarthritis and rheumatoid arthritis: the CLASS study. A randomized controlled trial. Celecoxib Long-term Arthritis Safety Study. *Journal of the American Medical Association.* 2000; **284**: 1247–55.
19. Bombardier C, Laine L, Reicin A *et al.* Comparison of upper gastrointestinal toxicity of rofecoxib and naproxen in patients with rheumatoid arthritis. VIGOR Study Group. *New England Journal of Medicine.* 2000; **343**: 1520–8.
20. Moreland LW, St Clair EW. The use of analgesics in the management of pain in rheumatic diseases. *Rheumatic Diseases Clinics of North America.* 1999; **25**: 153–91.
21. Ash G, Dickens CM, Creed FH *et al.* The effects of dothiopin on subjects with rheumatoid arthritis and depression. *Rheumatology.* 1999; **38**: 959–67.
22. Saurez-Almazor ME, Soskolne CL, Saunders LD, Russell AS. Use of second line drugs in the treatment of rheumatoid arthritis in Edmonton, Alberta: patterns of prescription and long-term effectiveness. *Journal of Rheumatology.* 1995; **22**: 836–43.
23. Felson DT, Anderson JJ, Meenan RF. The comparative efficacy and toxicity of second-line drugs in rheumatoid arthritis: results of two meta-analyses. *Arthritis and Rheumatism.* 1990; **33**: 1449–61.
24. Suarez-Almazor ME, Belseck E, Shea B *et al.* Rheumatoid arthritis (RA): penicillamine vs. placebo in RA. In: Tugwell P, Brooks P, Wells G *et al.* (eds). *Musculoskeletal Module of The Cochrane Database of Systematic Reviews*, issue 1. Oxford: Update Software, The Cochrane Library, 1999.
25. Suarez-Almazor ME, Belseck E, Shea B *et al.* Rheumatoid arthritis (RA): methotrexate vs. placebo. In: Tugwell P, Brooks P, Wells G *et al.* (eds). *Musculoskeletal Module of The Cochrane Database of Systematic Reviews*, issue 3. Oxford: Update Software, The Cochrane Library, 1998.
26. Pincus T, Marcum SB, Callahan LF. Long-term drug therapy for rheumatoid arthritis in seven rheumatology private practices. II. Second line drugs and prednisone. *Journal of Rheumatology.* 1992; **19**: 1885–94.
27. Wolfe F, Hawley DJ, Cathey MA. Termination of slow acting anti-rheumatoid therapy in rheumatoid arthritis: a

14 year prospective evaluation of 1017 starts. *Journal of Rheumatology.* 1990; **17**: 994–1002.
28. Gotzsche PC, Podenphant J, Olesen M, Halbert P. Meta-analysis of second-line anti-rheumatic drugs: sample size bias and uncertain benefit. *Journal of Clinical Epidemiology.* 1992; **45**: 587–94.
29. Alarcon GS, Lopez-Mendez A, Walter J *et al.* Radiographic evidence of disease progression in methotrexate treated and non-methotrexate disease modifying anti-rheumatic drug treated rheumatoid arthritis patients: a meta-analysis. *Journal of Rheumatology.* 1992; **19**: 1868–73.
30. Clark P, Tugwell P, Bennet K *et al.* Meta-analysis of injectable gold in rheumatoid arthritis. In: Tugwell P, Brooks P, Wells G *et al.* (eds). *Musculoskeletal Module of The Cochrane Database of Systematic Reviews*, issue 3. Oxford: Update Software, The Cochrane Library, 1998.
31. Rau R. Does parenteral gold retard radiological progression in rheumatoid arthritis? *Journal of Rheumatology.* 1996; **55**: 307–18.
32. Suarez-Almazor ME, Belseck E, Shea B *et al.* Rheumatoid arthritis (RA): azathioprine vs. placebo in RA. In: Tugwell P, Brooks P, Wells G *et al.* (eds). *Musculoskeletal Module of The Cochrane Database of Systematic Reviews*, issue 1. Oxford: Update Software, The Cochrane Library, 1999.
33. Suarez-Almazor ME, Belseck E, Shea B *et al.* Rheumatoid arthritis (RA): cyclophosphamide vs. placebo in RA. In: Tugwell P, Brooks P, Wells G *et al.* (eds). *Musculoskeletal Module of The Cochrane Database of Systematic Reviews*, issue 1. Oxford: Update Software, The Cochrane Library, 1999.
34. Jawad ASM, Scott DGI. Second-line agents in the treatment of systemic vasculitis. In: Dixon JS, Furst DE (eds). *Second-line agents in the treatment of rheumatic diseases.* New York: Marcel Dekker, 1992: 503–53.
35. Wells G, Haguenauer D, Shea B *et al.* Rheumatoid arthritis (RA): cyclosporine vs. placebo. In: Tugwell P, Brooks P, Wells G (eds). *Musculoskeletal Module of The Cochrane Database of Systematic Reviews*, issue 3. Oxford: Update Software, The Cochrane Library, 1998.
36. Felson DT, Anderson JJ, Meenan RF. Use of short-term efficacy/toxicity trade-offs to select second-line drugs in rheumatoid arthritis: a meta-analysis of published clinical trials. *Arthritis and Rheumatism.* 1992; **35**: 1117–25.
37. Saurez-Almazor ME, Belseck E, Shea B *et al.* Rheumatoid arthritis (RA): anti-malarials vs. placebo. In: Tugwell P, Brooks P, Wells G *et al.* (eds). *Musculoskeletal Module of The Cochrane Database of Systematic Reviews*, issue 3. Oxford: Update Software, The Cochrane Library, 1998.
38. Easterbrook M. The ocular safety of hydroxychloroquine. *Seminars in Arthritis and Rheumatism.* 1993; **23**: 62–7.
39. Smolen JS, Kalden JR, Scott DL *et al.* Efficacy and safety of leflunomide compared with placebo and sulphasalazine in active rheumatoid arthritis: a double-blind, randomised, multicentre trial. *Lancet.* 1999; **353**: 259–66.
40. Weinblatt ME, Kremer JM, Coblyn JS *et al.* Pharmacokinetics, safety, and efficacy of combination treatment with methotrexate and leflunomide in patients with active rheumatoid arthritis. *Arthritis and Rheumatism.* 1999; **42**: 1322.
41. Kremer JM, Genovese MC, Cannon GW *et al.* Concomitant leflunomide and methotrexate therapy for patients with active rheumatoid arthritis failing MTX monotherapy: open label extension of a randomised, double blind, placebo controlled trial. *Journal of Rheumatology.* 2004; **31**: 1521.
42. Maini R, St. Clair EW, Breedveld F *et al.* Infliximab (chimeric anti-tumour necrosis factor alpha monoclonal antibody) versus placebo in rheumatoid arthritis patients receiving concomitant methotrexate: A randomized phase III trial. *Lancet.* 1999; **354**: 1932.
43. St Clair EW, van der Heijde DM, Smolen JS *et al.* Combination of infliximab and methotrexate therapy for early rheumatoid arthritis: a randomized, controlled trial. *Arthritis and Rheumatism.* 2004; **50**: 3432.
44. Moreland LW, Baumgartner SW, Schiff MH *et al.* Treatment of rheumatoid arthritis with a recombinant human tumour necrosis factor receptor (p75)–Fc fusion protein. *New England Journal of Medicine.* 1997; **337**: 141–7.
45. Moreland LW, Schiff MH, Baumgartner SW *et al.* Phase III trial of DMARD failing rheumatoid arthritis patients with TNF receptor P75 Fc fusion protein (TNFR: Fc, ENBREL). *Journal of Investigative Medicine.* 1998; **46**: 228A.
46. Weinblatt ME, Kremer JM, Bankhurst AD *et al.* A trial of etanercept, a recombinant tumour necrosis factor receptor: Fc fusion protein, in patients with rheumatoid arthritis receiving methotrexate. *New England Journal of Medicine.* 1999; **340**: 253–9.
47. Bathon JM, Martin RW, Fleischmann RM *et al.* A comparison of etanercept and methotrexate in patients with early rheumatoid arthritis. *New England Journal of Medicine.* 2000; **343**: 1586–93.
48. Breedveld FC, Weisman MH, Kavanaugh AF *et al.* The PREMIER study: A multicenter, randomized, double-blind clinical trial of combination therapy with adalimumab plus methotrexate versus methotrexate alone or adalimumab alone in patients with early, aggressive rheumatoid arthritis who had not had previous methotrexate treatment. *Arthritis and Rheumatism.* 2006; **54**: 26.
49. Wick MC, Ernestam S, Lindblad S *et al.* Adalimumab (Humira®) restores clinical response in patients with secondary loss of efficacy from infliximab (Remicade®) or etanercept (Enbrel®): results from the STURE registry at Karolinska University Hospital. *Scandinavian Journal of Rheumatology.* 2005; **34**: 353–8.
50. Bresnihan B, Alvara-Gracia JM, Cobby M *et al.* Treatment of rheumatoid arthritis with recombinant human IL-1 receptor antagonist. *Arthritis and Rheumatism.* 1998; **41**: 2196.
51. Fleischmann RM, Schechtman J, Bennett R *et al.* Anakinra, a recombinant human interleukin-1 receptor antagonist (r-metHuIL-1ra), in patients with rheumatoid arthritis: A large, international, multicenter, placebo-controlled trial. *Arthritis and Rheumatism.* 2003; **48**: 927.

52. Kremer JM, Westhovens R, Leon M *et al.* Treatment of rheumatoid arthritis by selective inhibition of T-cell activation with fusion protein CTLA4Ig. *New England Journal of Medicine.* 2003; **349**: 1907.
53. Kremer JM, Genant HK, Moreland LW *et al.* Effects of abatacept in patients with methotrexate-resistant active rheumatoid arthritis: a randomized trial. *Annals of Internal Medicine.* 2006; **144**: 865.
54. Genovese MC, Becker JC, Schiff M *et al.* Abatacept for rheumatoid arthritis refractory to tumor necrosis factor alpha inhibition. *New England Journal of Medicine.* 2005; **353**: 1114.
55. Cohen SB, Emery P, Greenwald MW *et al.* Rituximab for rheumatoid arthritis refractory to anti-tumor necrosis factor therapy. *Arthritis and Rheumatism.* 2006; **54**: 2793.
56. Edwards JC, Szczepanski L, Szechinski J *et al.* Efficacy of B-cell-targeted therapy with rituximab in patients with rheumatoid arthritis. *New England Journal of Medicine.* 2004; **350**: 2572.
57. Fleischmann R, Racewicz A, Schechtman J *et al.* Rituximab efficacy in rheumatoid arthritis is independent of coadministration ofglucocorticoids: Results from the Dose-ranging Assessment International Clinical Evaluation of Rituximab in rheumatoid arthritis (DANCER) study. *Arthritis and Rheumatism.* 2005; **52**: 263.
58. Cohen SB, Emery P, Greenwald MW *et al.* Rituximab for rheumatoid arthritis refractory to anti-tumor necrosis factor therapy. *Arthritis and Rheumatism.* 2006; **54**: 2793–806.
59. The British Society for Rheumatology. *Guidelines for monitoring second line drugs in rheumatoid arthritis.* London: BSR Publications, 1993.
60. American College of Rheumatology ad hoc Committee on Clinical Guidelines. Guidelines for the management of rheumatoid arthritis. *Arthritis and Rheumatism.* 2002; **46**: 328–46.
61. Van Der Heide A, Jacobs JWG, Bijlsma JWJ *et al.* The effectiveness of early treatment with "second line" anti-rheumatic drugs: a randomised controlled trial. *Annals of Internal Medicine.* 1996; **124**: 600–07.
62. Egsmose C, Lund B, Borg G *et al.* Patients with rheumatoid arthritis benefit from early second line therapy: 5 year follow-up of a prospective double-blind placebo controlled study. *Journal of Rheumatology.* 1995; **22**: 2208–13.
* 63. Smolen JS, Aletaha D, Keystone E. Superior efficacy of combination therapy for rheumatoid arthritis. Fact or Fiction? *Arthritis and Rheumatism.* 2005; **52**: 2975.
* 64. Goekoop-Ruiterman YPM, de Vries-Bouwstra JK, Allaart CF *et al.* Clinical and radiographic outcomes of four different treatment strategies in patients with early rheumatoid arthritis (the BeSt study): a randomized, controlled trial. *Arthritis and Rheumatism.* 2005; **52**: 3381–90.
65. Emery P, Fleischmann R, Filipowicz-Sosnowska A *et al.* The efficacy and safety of rituximab in patients with active rheumatoid arthritis despite methotrexate treatment: results of a phase IIB randomized, double-blind, placebo-controlled, dose-ranging trial. *Arthritis and Rheumatism.* 2006; **54**: 1390.
66. Gotzsche PC, Johanson HK. Meta-analysis of short term low dose prednisolone vs. placebo and non-steroidal anti inflammatory drugs in rheumatoid arthritis. *British Medical Journal.* 1998; **316**: 811–18.
67. Criswell LA, Saag KG, Sems K *et al.* Rheumatoid arthritis (RA): moderate-term low dose corticosteroids. In: Tugwell P, Brooks P, Wells G *et al.* (eds). *Musculoskeletal Module of The Cochrane Database of Systematic Reviews*, issue 1. Oxford: Update Software, The Cochrane Library, 1999.
* 68. Kirwan JR. Arthritis and Rheumatism Council low dose glucocorticoid study group: the effect of glucocorticoids on joint destruction in rheumatoid arthritis. *New England Journal of Medicine.* 1995; **333**: 142–6.
69. Wassenberg S, Ram R, Steinfield P, Zeider H. Very low-dose prednisolone in early rheumatoid arthritis retards radiographic progression over two years: a multicenter, double-blind, placebo controlled trial. *Arthritis and Rheumatism.* 2005; **52**: 3371.
70. Kaplan MJ, McCune WJ. New evidence for vascular disease in patients with early rheumatoid arthritis. *Lancet.* 2003; **361**: 1068.
* 71. Hall FC, Dalbeth N. Disease modification and cardiovascular risk reduction: two sides of the same coin? *Rheumatology.* 2005; **44**: 1473.
72. McCarey DW, McInnes IB, Madhok R *et al.* Trial of Atorvastatin in Rheumatoid Arthritis (TARA): double-blind, randomised placebo-controlled trial. *Lancet.* 2004; **363**: 2015.
73. Alexander GJM, Hortas C, Bacon PA. Bed rest, activity and the inflammation of rheumatoid arthritis. *British Journal of Rheumatology.* 1983; **22**: 134–40.
74. Million R, Kellgren JH, Poole P, Jayson MIV. Long-term study of management of rheumatoid arthritis. *Lancet.* 1984; **1**: 812–16.
75. Gautt SJ, Spyker JM. Beneficial effect of immobilization of joints in rheumatoid and related arthritides: a splint study using sequential analysis. *Arthritis and Rheumatism.* 1969; **12**: 34–44.
76. Ytterberg SR, Mahowald KL, Krug HE. Exercise for arthritis. *Baillière's Clinical Rheumatology.* 1994; **8**: 161–89.
77. Machover S, Sapecky AJ. Effect of isometric exercise on the quadriceps muscle in patient with rheumatoid arthritis. *Archives of Physical Medicine and Rehabilitation.* 1996; **47**: 737–41.
78. Westby MD, Wade JP, Rangno KK, Berkowitz J. A randomized controlled trial to evaluate the effectiveness of an exercise program in women with rheumatoid arthritis taking low dose prednisolone. *Journal of Rheumatology.* 2000; **27**: 1674.
79. Panush RS, Webster EM. Food allergies and other adverse reactions to foods. *Medical Clinics of North America.* 1985; **69**: 533–46.
80. Conn DL, Arnold WJ, Hollister JR. Alternative treatments and rheumatic diseases. *Bulletin on the Rheumatic Diseases.* 1999; **48**: 1–4.

81. Geusens P, Wouters C, Nijs J *et al.* Long term effect of omega-3 fatty acid supplementation in active rheumatoid arthritis. A 12-month, double-blind, controlled study. *Arthritis and Rheumatism.* 1994; **37**: 824.
82. Simkin PA. Zinc, again (editorial). *Journal of Rheumatology.* 1997; **24**: 626–8.
83. Warsi A, LaValley MP, Wang PS *et al.* Arthritis self-management education programs: a meta-analysis of the effect on pain and disability. *Arthritis and Rheumatism.* 2003; **48**: 2207.
84. Bradley LA, Young LD, Anderson KO. Effects of psychological therapy on pain behaviour of rheumatoid arthritis patients. Treatment outcome and six-month followup. *Arthritis and Rheumatism.* 1987; **30**: 1105.
85. Theodora PM, Vliet Vlieland. Non-drug care for RA – is the era of evidence-based practice approaching? *Rheumatology.* 2007; **46**: 1397–404.
86. Scott DL, Long AF. An overview of studies of disease outcome. In: Long AF, Scott DL (eds). *Measuring outcomes in rheumatoid arthritis.* London: Royal College of Physicians, 1996: 35–44.
87. Masi AT. Articular patterns in the early course of rheumatoid arthritis. *American Journal of Medicine.* 1983; **75**: 16–26.
88. Rasker JJ, Cosh JA. The natural history of rheumatoid arthritis: a fifteen year follow-up study. *Clinical Rheumatology.* 1984; **3**: 11–20.
89. Yelin E, Henke C, Epstein W. The work dynamics of the person with rheumatoid arthritis. *Arthritis and Rheumatism.* 1987; **30**: 507–12.
90. Mutru O, Laakso M, Isomäki H, Koota K. Ten year mortality and causes of death in patients with rheumatoid arthritis. *British Medical Journal.* 1987; **30**: 507–12.
91. Scott DL, Symmons DPM, Coulton DL, Popert AJ. Long-term outcome of treating rheumatoid arthritis: Results after 20 years. *Lancet.* 1987; **1**: 1108.
92. Wolfe F, Mitchell DA, Sibley JT *et al.* The mortality of rheumatoid arthritis. *Arthritis and Rheumatism.* 1994; **37**: 481.
93. Pritzker KPH. Pathology of osteoarthritis. In: Brandt KD, Doherty M, Lohmander LS (eds). *Osteoarthritis*, 2nd edn. Oxford: Oxford University Press, 2003: 49–58.
94. Dieppe P, Chard J. Osteoarthritis. *Clinical Evidence.* 1999; **1**: 219–24.
95. Spector T, MacGregor AJ. Epidemiology of rheumatic diseases. In: Snaith ML (ed.). *ABC of rheumatology*, 2nd edn. London: BMJ Books, 1999: 82–6.
96. Silman AJ, Hochberg MC. *Epidemiology of the rheumatic diseases.* Oxford: Oxford University Press, 1993.
97. Pinals RS. Mechanism of joint destruction, pain and disability in osteoarthritis. *Drugs.* 1996; **52**: 14–20.
98. Doherty M, Dieppe P. Clinical aspects of calcium pyrophosphate crystal deposition. *Rheumatic Diseases Clinics of North America.* 1988; **14**: 395–414.
99. Dieppe PA, Doherty M, MacFarlane DG *et al.* Apatite-associated destructive arthritis. *British Journal of Rheumatology.* 1984; **3**: 84–91.
100. Campion J, Watt J. Imaging and laboratory investigations. In: Klippel JH, Dieppe PA (eds). *Rheumatology.* London: Mosby Year Book Europe, 1994: 7.5.1–14.
101. Freemont AJ, Denton J, Chuk A *et al.* Diagnostic value of synovial fluid microscopy: a reassessment and rationalisation. *Annals of the Rheumatic Diseases.* 1991; **50**: 101–07.
102. McCrae F, Should J, Dieppe P *et al.* Scintigraphic assessment of osteoarthritis of the knee joint. *Annals of the Rheumatic Diseases.* 1992; **51**: 938–42.
103. Pendleton A, Arden N, Dougados M *et al.* EULAR recommendations for the management of knee osteoarthritis: report of a task force of the Standing Committee for International Clinical Studies Including Therapeutic Trials (ESCISIT). *Annals of the Rheumatic Diseases.* 2000; **59**: 936–44.
104. Zhang W, Doherty M, Arden N *et al.* EULAR evidence based recommendations for the management of hip osteoarthritis: report of a task force of the EULAR Standing Committee for International Clinical Studies Including Therapeutics (ESCISIT). *Annals of the Rheumatic Diseases.* 2005; **64**: 669–81.
105. Jordan KM, Arden NK, Doherty M *et al.* EULAR Recommendations 2003: an evidence based approach to the management of knee osteoarthritis: Report of a Task Force of the Standing Committee for International Clinical Studies Including Therapeutic Trials (ESCISIT). *Annals of the Rheumatic Diseases.* 2003; **62**: 1145–55.
106. Zhang W, Doherty M, Leeb BF *et al.* EULAR evidence based recommendations for the management of hand osteoarthritis-report of a task force of the EULAR Standing Committee for International Clinical Studies Including Therapeutics (ESCISIT). *Annals of the Rheumatic Diseases.* 2007; **66**: 377–88.
*107. Moore RA, Tramer MR, Carroll D *et al.* Review: topical nonsteroidal anti-inflammatory drugs are effective and safe for pain. *British Medical Journal.* 1998; **316**: 333–8.
108. Evans JMM, McMahon AD, McGilchrist MM *et al.* Topical non-steroidal anti-inflammatory drugs and admission to hospital for upper gastrointestinal bleeding and perforation: a record linkage case control study. *British Medical Journal.* 1995; **311**: 22–6.
109. Zhang WY, Po ALW. The effectiveness of topically applied capsaicin: a meta-analysis. *European Journal of Clinical Pharmacology.* 1994; **46**: 517–22.
110. Deal CL, Schnitzer TJ, Lipstein JR *et al.* Treatment of arthritis with topically applied capsaicin; a double-blind trial. *Clinical Therapeutics.* 1991; **13**: 383–95.
111. Anonymous. What can be done about osteoarthritis? *Drug and Therapeutics Bulletin.* 1996; **34**: 33–5.
112. Anonymous. Articular and periarticular corticosteroid injections. *Drug and Therapeutics Bulletin.* 1995; **33**: 67–70.
113. Anonymous. Hyaluronan or hylans for knee osteoarthritis? *Drug and Therapeutics Bulletin.* 1999; **37**: 71–2.
114. Huskisson EC, Berry H, Gishen P *et al.* Effects of anti-inflammatory drugs on the progression of

osteoarthritis of the knee. *Journal of Rheumatology.* 1995; **22**: 1941–6.
115. Eccles M, Freemantle N, Mason J. North of England evidence based guideline development project: summary guideline for non-steroidal anti-inflammatory drugs versus basic analgesia in treating the pain of degenerative arthritis. The North of England Non-Steroidal Anti-Inflammatory Drug Guideline Development Group. *BMJ.* 1998; **317**: 526–30.
116. Schnitzer TJ, Kamin M, Olson WH. Tramadol allows reduction of naproxen dose among patients with naproxen-responsive osteoarthritis pain. *Arthritis and Rheumatism.* 1999; **42**: 1370–7.
117. Chard J, Dieppe P. Glucosamine for osteoarthritis: magic hype or confusion. *BMJ.* 2001; **322**: 1439–40.
118. Reginster JY, Deroisy R, Rovati LC *et al.* Long-term effects of glucosamine sulphate on osteoarthritis progression: a randomised, placebo-controlled clinical trial. *Lancet.* 2001; **357**: 251–6.
119. McAlindon TE, LaValley MP, Felson DT. Efficacy of glucosamine and chondroitin for treatment of osteoarthritis. *Journal of the American Medical Association.* 2000; **284**: 1241.
120. Wollheim FA. Current pharmacological treatment of osteoarthritis. *Drugs.* 1996; **52** (Suppl. 3): 27–38.
121. Clegg DO, Reda DJ, Harris CL *et al.* Glucosamine, chondroitin sulfate, and the two in combination for painful knee osteoarthritis. *New England Journal of Medicine.* 2006; **354**: 795–808.
122. Superio-Cabulslay E, Ward MM, Lorig KR. Patient education interventions in osteoarthritis and rheumatoid arthritis: a meta analytic comparison with nonsteroidal anti-inflammatory drug therapy. *Arthritis Care and Research.* 1996; **9**: 292–301.
123. Gallo F. The effects of social support networks on the health of the elderly. *Social Work in Health Care.* 1982; **8**: 65–74.
124. Keefe FJ, Caldwell DS, Baucom D *et al.* Spouse-assisted coping skills training in the management of osteoarthritic knee pain. *Arthritis Care and Research.* 1996; **9**: 279–91.
125. Rene J, Weinberger M, Mazzuca SA *et al.* Reduction of joint pain in patients with knee osteoarthritis who have received monthly telephone calls from lay personnel and whose medical treatment regimes have remained stable. *Arthritis and Rheumatism.* 1992; **35**: 511–15.
126. Ettinger Jr WH, Burns R, Messier SP *et al.* A randomized trial comparing aerobic exercise and resistance exercise with a health education program in older adults with knee osteoarthritis. *Journal of the American Medical Association.* 1997; **277**: 64–6.
127. Cushnaghan J, McCarthy C, Dieppe P. Taping the patella medially: a new treatment for osteoarthritis of the knee joint. *British Medical Journal.* 1994; **308**: 753–5.
128. Perrot S, Menkes CJ. Nonpharmacological approaches to pain in osteoarthritis: available options. *Drugs.* 1996; **52** (Suppl. 3): 21–6.
129. Felson DT, Zhang Y, Anthony JM *et al.* Weight loss reduces the risk for symptomatic osteoarthritis in women. The Framingham study. *Annals of Internal Medicine.* 1992; **116**: 535–9.
130. Taylor P, Hallett M, Flaherty L. Treatment of osteoarthritis of the knee with transcutaneous electrical nerve stimulation. *Pain.* 1981; **11**: 233–40.
131. Lewis B, Lewis D, Cumming G. The comparative analgesic efficacy of transcutaneous electrical nerve stimulation and a non-steroidal anti-inflammatory drug for painful osteoarthritis. *British Journal of Rheumatology.* 1994; **33**: 455–60.
132. Ernst E. Acupuncture as a symptomatic treatment of osteoarthritis. *Scandinavian Journal of Rheumatology.* 1997; **26**: 444–7.
133. Sasaki T, Yasuda K. Clinical evaluation of the treatment of osteoarthritic knees using a newly designed wedge insole. *Clinical Orthopaedics and Related Research.* 1987; **221**: 181–7.
134. Maratz V, Muncie Jr HL, Walsh MH. Occupational therapy in the multi-disciplinary assessment and management of osteoarthritis. *Clinical Therapeutics.* 1986; **9**: 24–9.
135. Anonymous. What can be done about osteoarthritis? *Drug and Therapeutics Bulletin.* 1996; **34**: 33–5.
136. Ike RW, Arnold WJ, Rothschild EW. Tidal irrigation versus conservative medical management in patients with osteoarthritis of the knee: a prospective randomised study. *Journal of Rheumatology.* 1992; **19**: 772–9.
137. Moseley JB, O'Malley K, Petersen NJ *et al.* A controlled trial of arthroscopic surgery for osteoarthritis of the knee. *New England Journal of Medicine.* 2002; **347**: 81–8.
138. Anonymous. Hip and knee joint replacements. *Drug and Therapeutics Bulletin.* 1992; **30**: 57–60.
139. Keuttner K, Goldberg VM (eds). *Osteoarthritic disorders.* Rosemont, IL: American Academy of Orthopedic Surgeons, 1995: 21–5.
140. Bradley EM, Tennant A. Changing profile of joint disorders with age; findings from a postal survey of the population of Calderdale, West Yorkshire, United Kingdom. *Annals of the Rheumatic Diseases.* 1992; **51**: 366–71.
141. Chard M, Hazleman R, Hazleman BL *et al.* Shoulder dislocations in the elderly: a community survey. *Arthritis and Rheumatism.* 1991; **34**: 766–9.
142. Allander E. Prevalence, incidence and remission rates of some common rheumatic diseases or syndromes. *Scandinavian Journal of Rheumatology.* 1974; **3**: 145–53.
143. Croft P, Pope D. Silman A The clinical course of shoulder pain: prospective cohort study in primary care. *British Medical Journal.* 1996; **313**: 601–02.
144. van der Heijden GJMG. Shoulder disorders: a state of the art review. *Baillière's Clinical Rheumatology.* 1999; **13**: 287–309.
145. Cyriax J. *Textbook of orthopaedic medicine.* London: Baillière Tindall, 1981.
*146. Palmer K, Coggon D, Cooper C, Doherty M. Work related upper limb disorders: getting down to specifics. *Annals of the Rheumatic Diseases.* 1998; **57**: 1–2.

147. Winters JC, Groenier HK, Sobel JS *et al.* Classification of shoulder complaints in general practice by means of cluster analysis. *Archives of Physical Medicine and Rehabilitation.* 1997; **78**: 1369–74.

*148. Carette S, Moffet H, Tardif J *et al.* Intraarticular corticosteroids, supervised physiotherapy, or a combination of the two in the treatment of adhesive capsulitis of the shoulder: a placebo-controlled trial. *Arthritis and Rheumatism.* 2003; **48**: 829–38.

149. Gam AN, Schydlowsky P, Rossel I *et al.* Treatment of "frozen shoulder" with distension and glucorticoid compared with glucorticoid alone. A randomised controlled trial. *Scandinavian Journal of Rheumatology.* 1998; **27**: 425–30.

150. van der Windt DAWM, van der Heijden GJMG, Scholten RJPM *et al.* The efficacy of non-steroidal anti-inflammatory drugs for shoulder complaints: a systemic review. *Journal of Clinical Epidemiology.* 1995; **48**: 691–704.

151. Green S, Buchbinder R, Hetrick S. Physiotherapy interventions for shoulder pain. *Cochrane Database of Systematic Reviews.* 2003; **CD004258**.

152. Buchbinder R, Green S, Youd JM. Corticosteroid injections for shoulder pain. *Cochrane Database of Systematic Reviews.* 2003; **CD004016**.

153. Plafki C, Steffen R, Willburger RE, Wittenberg RH. Local anaesthetic injection with and without corticosteroids for subacromial impingement syndrome. *International Orthopaedics.* 2000; **24**: 40.

154. Hyvonen P, Flinkkila T, Leppilahti J, Jalovaara P. Early recovery of isometric shoulder muscle strength after open acromioplasty in stage II impingement syndrome. *Archives of Orthopaedic and Trauma Surgery.* 2000; **120**: 290.

155. Takala J, Sievers K, Klaukka T. Rheumatic symptoms in the middle aged population in south-western Finland. *Scandinavian Journal of Rheumatology.* 1982; **47**: 15–29.

156. Linaker CH, Walker-Bone K, Palmer K, Cooper C. Frequency and impact of regional musculoskeletal disorders. *Baillière's Clinical Rheumatology.* 1999; **13**: 197–215.

157. Hamilton PG. The prevalence of humeral epicondylitis: a survey in general practice. *Journal of the Royal College of General Practitioners.* 1986; **36**: 464–5.

158. Helliwell PS. The elbow, forearm, wrist and hand. *Baillière's Clinical Rheumatology.* 1999; **13**: 311–28.

159. Stock SR. Workplace ergonomic factors and the development of musculoskeletal disorders of the neck and upper limbs: a meta-analysis. *American Journal of Industrial Medicine.* 1991; **19**: 87–107.

160. Green S, Buchbinder R, Barnsley L *et al.* Non-steroidal anti-inflammatory drugs (NSAIDs) for treating lateral elbow pain in adults (Cochrane Review). *Cochrane Database of Systematic Reviews.* 2002; **CD003686**.

*161. Smidt N, van der Windt DA, Assendelft WJ *et al.* Corticosteroid injections, physiotherapy, or a wait-and-see policy for lateral epicondylitis: a randomised controlled trial. *Lancet.* 2002; **359**: 657.

162. Hayton MJ, Santini AJ, Hughes PJ *et al.* Botulinum toxin injection in the treatment of tennis elbow. A double-blind, randomized, controlled, pilot study. *Journal of Bone and Joint Surgery. American volume.* 2005; **87**: 503–07.

163. Connell DA, Ali KE, Ahmad M *et al.* Ultrasound-guided autologous blood injection for tennis elbow. *Skeletal Radiology.* 2006; **35**: 371.

164. Paoloni JA, Appleyard RC, Nelson J, Murrell GA. Topical nitric oxide application in the treatment of chronic extensor tendinosis at the elbow: a randomized, double-blinded, placebo-controlled clinical trial. *American Journal of Sports Medicine.* 2003; **31**: 915.

165. Trinh KV, Phillips SD, Ho E, Damsma K. Acupuncture for the alleviation of lateral epicondyle pain: a systematic review. *Rheumatology (Oxford).* 2004; **43**: 1085.

166. Buchbinder R, Green S, Bell S *et al.* Surgery for lateral elbow pain (Cochrane Review). *Cochrane Database of Systematic Reviews.* 2002; **CD003525**.

167. Fedorczyk J. The role of physical agents in modulating pain. *Journal of Hand Therapy.* 1997; **10**: 110–21.

168. Chard MD, Hazelman BL. Tennis elbow: physical methods of treatment. In: Schlapback P, Gerber NJ (eds). *Physiotherapy: controlled trials and facts.* Basel: Karger, 1991: 99–107.

169. Shapira D, Nahir M, Scharf Y. Trochanteric bursitis: a common clinical problem. *Archives of Physical Medicine and Rehabilitation.* 1986; **67**: 470–8.

170. Mazieres B, Carette S. The hip. In: Kippel JH, Dieppe PA (eds). *Rheumatology,* 2nd edn. Vol. 1. London: CV Mosby, 1998: 4.10.1–4.10.8.

171. McAlindon TE. The knee. *Baillière's Clinical Rheumatology.* 1999; **13**: 329–44.

172. Graham GP, Fairclough JA. The knee. In: Kippel JH, Dieppe PA (eds). *Rheumatology,* 2nd edn. Vol. 1. London: CV Mosby, 1998: 4.11.1–4.11.14.

39

Therapies for chronic chest pain

IVAN N RAMOS-GALVEZ AND GLYN R TOWLERTON

KEY LEARNING POINTS

- Chest pain is common.
- A multidimensional approach to treatment helps to reduce its burden on health care and on the patient.
- Of all chest pains presenting to medical professionals, musculoskeletal etiologies are the most common.
- Cardiac rehabilitation programs have shown to reduce hospital admissions, improve mood, and increase activity in cardiac and noncardiac chest pain.
- Cardiac rehabilitation programs are associated with an equivalent or lower mortality than some conventional therapies.
- Spinal cord stimulation has shown to improve quality of life and reduce hospital admissions in patients with refractory angina, without masking symptoms of coronary events. It carries a similar mortality to medical treatments.

INTRODUCTION

In many ways, the approach to chest pain has mirrored that of axial pain. The reliance on the biomechanical model has now been coupled with a growing awareness of the cognitive aspects, their effect on disability, and quality of life in both the cardiac and noncardiac causes of chest pain.

When faced with this common clinical presentation, angina pectoris comes to mind and it is apposite to remember that etymologically this shares a common Greek origin with anxiety and anguish. Widening appreciation of this has been reflected in the initiation of a more multidisciplinary approach to the assessment of the cardiac patient in particular.

This chapter deals with pain originating in the anterior part of the chest cavity and with pain referred from somatic structures. Pain of a referred neuropathic nature is dealt with in Chapter 30, Chronic pain after surgery and Chapter 32, Herpes zoster pain including shingles and postherpetic neuralgia, as well as postcardiothoracic surgery pain, and will not be discussed here.

ETIOLOGY AND EPIDEMIOLOGY

There are multiple structures within the chest from where a pain may originate (**Table 39.1**). In a primary care setting:[1, 2]

- between 20 and 48 percent of consultations for chest pain were thought to be musculoskeletal in origin;
- 13–30 percent gastroesophageal reflux;
- 13 percent costochondritis;

- 10–17 percent cardiac cause/stable angina pectoris;
- 1.5 percent unstable angina pectoris/myocardial infarction;
- 9.5 percent undiagnosed.

It has been estimated that 12 percent of the population will experience chest pain lasting more than 24 hours in a six-month period.[3] The majority of resources are directed to the diagnosis, treatment, and exclusion of the cardiac causes.

The healthcare economics of chest pain have not been widely studied. In the United States, there are over 4.6 million visits a year to emergency departments for non-traumatic chest pain.[4] In 1998, Medicare beneficiaries were paid nearly US$11 billion for coronary artery disease.[5] A Swedish study of over 1000 patients attending a university hospital emergency department, with cardiac chest pain[6] for assessment and therapy, on average cost 26,800 SEK (€2900, US$3000, or £1900) per visit.

ASSESSMENT

Clinical history remains the main tool in the diagnosis of chest pain. Patients with clinical history suggestive of a cardiac origin undergo more extensive examination and diagnostic tests.[2]

The use of resources in health care is directed towards cardiac causes of chest pain despite its low frequency among chest pain diagnosis. Up to 30 percent of patients who present with chest pain lack coronary disease[7] in angiogram. However, work by Wright *et al.*[8] lends some justification towards this. They looked at the cost in health care generated by patients with chronic chest pain. They examined the impact of coronary artery angiography in subsequent requests for medical services and prescription drugs. They reported that over a period of 2.5 years postcoronary angiography there was a significant reduction in attendances to emergency services and prescription of oral and topical nitrates compared to the same length of time before angiography.

Psychological problems and coronary artery disease have been found to correlate. Anxiety, depression, and reduced quality of life are associated with angina and are independent outcome predictors of coronary angiographic findings. Patients with chest pain where no organic cause can be found have a higher proportion of panic disorders (15 percent), obsessive-compulsive disorder (21 percent), and major depressive episodes (28 percent).[9] Recurrent panic disorders may be linked to coronary artery disease,[10] and these patients have been found to be twice as likely to have coronary artery disease than the general population.[11] Patients with diagnosed depressive disorder and panic attacks have a tendency towards a three-fold increase in the risk of coronary artery disease, although that was not statistically significant.[11] Recently, a study carried out in the emergency room on patients diagnosed with nonspecific chest pain found that these patients scored highly for anxiety in the Hospital Anxiety and Depression Scale (HADS) and were more likely to report other symptoms accompanying the chest pain, such as dizziness, chills, hot flushes, or fear of dying.[12] Patients with chronic chest pain have been found to report passive pain-coping strategies, express an exaggerated degree of spouse reinforcement, and report a lower pain threshold when compared to other pain sufferers, including coronary arteriopaths.[13] There is a growing recognition that stable coronary pathology and chest pain of other origins deserves a more multidimensional approach to reduce its burden on patient and society alike.

ANATOMICAL NOTES

The human heart is estimated to contain more than 14,000 neurons[14] of autonomic origin. The sympathetic supply is via the cervical and upper thoracic sympathetic chains. The parasympathetic supply is via the vagus nerve. Both merge together to form the cardiac plexus which is an intricate network embedded in the tissues of the myocardium and the coronary and mediastinal vessels. This plexus is formed by afferent and efferent fibers that include chemoreceptors, pressoreceptors, mechanoreceptors, and pain receptors. These are connected by a number of pathways to the central nervous system (CNS). The stellate ganglion is the fusion of the inferior cervical and the superior thoracic. It can be identified consistently in normal persons.[15] There are four cardiac rami from the T2–T6 segment of the thoracic sympathetic trunk that

Table 39.1 Structures within the chest from where a chronic chest pain may originate.

Visceral	Somatic	Referred
Heart, pericardium, great vessels Upper gastrointestinal system: pharynx, esophagus, stomach, pancreas, liver, and gallbladder Respiratory system and pleura: trachea, bronchi, lungs, and pleura	Musculoskeletal system	Somatic from cervical or thoracic spine Neuropathic from thoracic nerves

also form part of the deep cardiac plexus.[16, 17] Recent work has elucidated more details of these pathways, but it is apposite to remember that silent ischemia often coexists with painful ischemia in the same patient. The evidence suggests that there is no correlation between the degree of pain and the severity of the lesion or ischemia.[18]

VISCERAL CHEST PAIN: CARDIAC

Refractory angina pectoris

The European Society of Cardiology defines refractory angina pectoris (RAP) as "a chronic condition characterized by the presence of angina caused by coronary insufficiency in the presence of coronary artery disease that cannot be controlled by a combination of medical therapy, angioplasty and coronary bypass surgery." The presence of reversible myocardial ischemia should be clinically established to be the cause of the symptoms. Chronic is defined as a duration of more than three months.[19, 20] Later definitions have included when revascularization is unfeasible or where the risks are unjustified.

INCIDENCE

As patients with angina pectoris live longer, the prevalence of this condition increases.[21] They often have good ventricular function and thus good prognosis. These patients are traditionally males in their sixties who have had multiple hospital admissions and high usage of healthcare resources. The incidence and admission rates of patients with myocardial infarction are both declining, but those of angina pectoris are on the increase.[20] The absolute prevalence of RAP is unknown, but may be in the region of 5:100,000 in the UK. It is estimated that 5–10 percent of patients with unstable angina will develop refractory angina.[20] In Europe, there are estimated to be 30–50,000 patients each year, and for the United States, 25–75,000.[19] In 1995, the Swedish Council of Technology Assessment in Healthcare showed that 9.6 percent of patients referred for revascularization were not suitable, despite severe symptoms.[22]

ASSESSMENT

This is essentially clinical. Assessment of these patients should be directed to determining the certainty of the diagnosis, the suitability of the medical therapy, revascularization procedures, and the assessment of other organic or psychological diagnosis. Patients with refractory angina pectoris often have a poor quality of life. Anxiety and depression[20] are prevalent in this population. Moore *et al.*[23] documented this to be up to 50 and 33 percent, respectively, for refractory angina, higher when compared to sufferers of other chronic painful conditions.[24]

The development of multidisciplinary teams and the growing realization of the palliative nature of several secondary cardiac interventions have helped increase awareness of refractory angina and the therapeutic options.[25] Specialist angina services provide a link between these disciplines and help provide a consistent message and approach to the patient.

THERAPEUTIC OPTIONS

Table 39.2 summarizes the evidence for the different therapeutic options for refractory angina pectoris.

Cardiac rehabilitation and angina plan

The aim of cardiac rehabilitation is to provide comprehensive care including secondary prevention through active risk factor management, physical reactivation, and psychosocial support.[51] This approach is recognized by the American College of Cardiologists (www.americanheart.org) and the European Society of Cardiology.[26] The UK Department of Health expects that chronic disease management programs will reduce emergency hospital bed day admissions by 5 percent by 2008.[52]

The benefit of mechanical enhancement of patients' own vasculature is often an embedded belief, as is the inevitability of further deterioration leading to increased

Table 39.2 Management of refractory angina pectoris.

Therapy	Supporting evidence
Angina plan	[26][I], [27][IV], [28][II], [29][II], [30][III]
Spinal cord stimulator	[19][III], [31][II], [32][I], [33][IV], [34][IV], [35][II], [36][III], [37][I], [38][IV]
Transmyocardial laser revascularization	[20][I], [39][II], [40][III]
Transcutaneous electrical nerve stimulation	[20, 41][II]
Transcutaneous laser revascularization	[42, 43, 44, 45][II]
Thoracic epidural	[20, 46][III]
Left stellate ganglion block	[20, 47, 48][III]
Thoracic sympathectomy	[20, 49][III]
Radiofrequency (RF) sympathectomy	[50][III]

morbidity and mortality. These often tightly held views should be addressed.[53] It would be interesting to speculate a more extensive cognitive approach earlier in the patients who go on to develop RAP, in parallel with traditional approaches of cardiac intervention which may effect a more enhanced quality of life and a reduction in use of healthcare resources. This would be supported by the work of Lewin[27] after the initial diagnosis of angina and the more recently proposed angioplasty plan.

The angina plan[27] is a cognitive-behavioral therapy (CBT) package developed to address the risk factor and belief misconceptions in angina sufferers. A facilitator interview is followed by telephone contacts. This has been demonstrated to reduce anxiety, glyceryl trinitrate (GTN) consumption, physical limitations, and enhance lifestyle modifications.[29] Brief disease management interventions have also shown reduced hospital admissions. A study of 271 chronic refractory angina patients showed that enrolment in a disease management course led to a reduction from 2.4 to 1.78 admissions per patient per year ($p<0.001$). The overall mortality during the study was lower than that of comparable groups treated with surgery. These disease-modification strategies resulted in a reduction of hospital costs per year of £1337 per patient per year.[53] Further cognitive-behavioral work in this patient group has shown that at six months follow up the differences in mood and activity were not as marked as before, but the attitude towards and understanding of their disease was more positive in the group that had undergone CBT,[28] which suggests that continued education might be necessary to maintain these benefits. Overall, there is level I evidence of the merits of this intervention.[29][II], [30][I]

Sympathetic blockade

Sympathectomies were first tried in 1964, when Apthorp *et al.*[54] reported that they relieved the angina pain in about 75 percent patients. Sympathetic blockade can be achieved by thoracic epidural, paravertebral block, sympathectomy, or stellate ganglion blockade.

Local anesthetic stellate ganglion blocks are reported to provide repeated benefit[47] for some patients, although the overall improvement only lasted a mean of 3.48 weeks.[48] In our own practice, the number of patients who experience a benefit longer than one month is low, but it can be used for acute exacerbations. It has a proven effect on symptoms, but not on ischemia.[36, 37][III] Thoracic paravertebral block are reported to provide satisfactory analgesia for a mean duration of 2.8 weeks with a follow up of up to two years, with a complication rate of 3 percent.[48]

There has been some interest in endoscopic thoracic sympathectomies,[49] despite the promising results shown by one study[20][III] as the number of patients included was small and the follow up was limited to six months. One case series looked at percutaneous radiofrequency thoracic sympathectomy as a less invasive technique with good results,[50] but further randomized evidence is lacking. High thoracic epidural anesthesia (HTEA) was initially described as a low-risk alternative to surgical thoracic sympathectomy.[46] Employing an indwelling catheter with intermittent boluses or continuous infusions that allowed the patients to be discharged from hospital, HTEA has an effect both on symptoms and on ischemia.[46][III] The evidence relates mainly to its use in acute unstable angina pectoris. Its use in a chronic setting is limited by the fact that it is usually administered via an infusion pump.

Transcutaneous electrical nerve stimulation

It is often thought that chest pain after provocation that disappears totally after 30–60 seconds of high-intensity stimulation is a strong indicator of ischemic origin. Manheimer *et al.*'s[41] randomized unblended study of 22 patients revealed a significant reduction in angina episodes (17 percent) and an increased exercise tolerance (15 percent).

The most frequent side effect of transcutaneous electrical nerve stimulation (TENS) is the development of skin reactions to the adhesive of the pads and skin sensitivity to the effect of the electrical current. Its efficacy may be limited if there is cutaneous change following left internal mammary artery (LIMA) harvest. These often limit the long-term use of this therapy, and spinal cord stimulation appears to be less problematic in this respect.[20] TENS has a documented effect on symptoms.[20][V]

Spinal cord stimulation

Spinal cord stimulation (SCS) has been used since the early 1970s and applied to refractory angina pain since 1985.[38] Studies have shown improved quality of life,[31, 32, 35, 38] reduction in hospital admission rates,[33, 38] comparable mortality for patients with similar degree of coronary artery disease, and symptoms controlled by medical or surgical means.[31, 55, 56] Studies have also demonstrated that these do not mask the symptoms of an acute coronary event.[33] A review by a Working Group of the European Society of Cardiology recommend spinal cord stimulation treatment for refractory angina pectoris.[34][V] Despite evidence in favor of the use of spinal cord stimulators, they are only effective in around 75 percent of patients with refractory angina pectoris.[19, 57] Factors predictive of good outcome have been suggested as left ventricular ejection fraction >40 percent, low cholesterol levels, fewer attempts at revascularization before the procedure, and a lower New York Heart Association (NYHA) grade.[55, 56, 58]

The mechanism of action is complex. An increase in myocardial perfusion during exercise is not thought to be the cause of the improvement as demonstrated by positron emission tomography (PET).[59] However, some authors still postulate that the mechanism of action is by increasing oxygen supply via vasodilatation of microvasculature.[57]

Bagger *et al.* conducted a study to evaluate the effect of long-term spinal cord stimulation at increasing the threshold for angina.[35, 60] They found that after performing atrial pacing, the pacing threshold for angina was increased by 50 percent in 70 percent of patients.[32, 35] However, this effect only lasted between three and nine months after which, despite paresthesia within the area of the pain, only 40 percent still had angina pain relief. These 40 percent still had benefit at 60-month follow up.

An Italian registry of SCS for RAP was established by Di Pedre and colleagues[36] who documented a reduction in weekly angina episodes in greater than 50 percent and an improvement in Canadian Cardiovascular Society angina class by at least one class in 80 percent.

The Electrical Stimulation versus Coronary Bypass Surgery (ESBY) study compared spinal cord stimulation with coronary artery bypass graft (CABG) in patients considered to derive only symptomatic benefit from CABG. There was no difference in long-term outcome between these therapies in terms of mortality or in improvement of quality of life, which significantly increased in both arms. The CABG group had significantly more cerebrovascular complications (16 versus 4 percent) and periprocedural morbidity (14 versus 2 percent). The CABG had less ischemic changes on stress testing, but the SCS group did not have active stimulation during the tests.[37] Larger studies have shown consistent findings with these results in regards of safety of the treatment,[38] reduction in nitroglycerin intake in follow up over 18 months, and reduction in the number of angina attacks.[19, 32, 35, 38]

Spinal cord stimulators are susceptible to failure. Studies quote that during these episodes the intake of nitrates escalated, as did the frequency of the angina attacks. Both variables returned to normal upon restitution of stimulation. No evidence of tolerance has been found, and the beneficial effects of spinal cord stimulation are suggested to be due to factors other than placebo.[35, 61]

Cost-effectiveness of spinal cord stimulation has been evaluated in several healthcare economies. Taking into consideration the reduction in hospital admissions, as well as the reduction in prescriptions, it is thought to be cost-effective.[38] The expense of the procedure and the device was recovered within 16 months of insertion. However, these conclusions were based on retrospective analysis.[38]

Enhanced external counter pulsation

Acting in the same way as aortic counter pulsation, this technique augments blood flow during diastole. The technique involves cuffs compressed in early diastole for up to 35 × 1-hour sessions. There have been several studies of enhanced external counter pulsation (EECP). A multicenter study (MUST-EECP) of 139 patients decreased anginal episodes by 25 percent ($p<0.035$) when compared to sham EECP.[62] The technique has a number of contraindications and is limited by availability, but has been licensed by the Food and Drug Administration (FDA) for RAP.

Pharmacological strategies

With emerging pharmaceutical strategies, optimization of the patient's medical regime should always be considered. Optimizing the medical treatment has shown to reduce the pain in 83 percent of patients with unstable angina and in 44 percent of patients referred for transmyocardial laser revascularization.[20] Fatty acid oxidation inhibitors, L-arginine, testosterone, and estrogens have all been used to impact on stable angina-like symptoms. Opioids have been advocated, but there is little formal evidence to support their use in RAP. In our center, antihyperalgesics have been employed with benefit, although it has been difficult to establish if these are addressing the pain or the associated anxiety and depression. Anecdotally, the tricyclics seem to be tolerated well in this patient cohort.

Other therapies

- **Intermittent urokinase**: 500,000 IU i.v. three times a week, for 12 weeks. There is limited evidence, but some studies have suggested that it could reduce angina episodes by 70 percent and the need for nitrates by 84 percent. Authors advocate that the benefit is from improvement in the rheological properties of blood and improved blood flow.[63] [IV]
- **Laser revascularization**: This consists of drilling channels into the myocardial wall with laser and has been performed transmyocardially (transmyocardial revascularization, TMR) via a minithoracotomy or percutaneously (percutaneous revascularization, PMR).
  - Randomized, but not sham, trials in TMR have shown significant improvements by two angina classes at 12 months by Allen *et al.*[39] (76 versus 32 percent; $p<0.001$) and Frazier *et al.*[40] (72 versus 13 percent; $p<0.001$). However, overall, no improvement in myocardial supply had been demonstrated and did not consistently improve exercise tolerance, dyspnea, or left ventricular function.[20] The placebo effect cannot be excluded as a mechanism.
  - In PMR, a laser fiberoptic lead is introduced through the peripheral artery into the left ventricle, and the channels are created with fluoroscopic and TOE guidance. A randomized unmasked trial looking at the effect of PMR, the PACIFIC trial, did reveal a reduction in angina class and an increase in exercise tolerance, but was associated with more morbidity in the PMR arm. However, sham randomized trials have not consistently reproduced this finding.[42, 43, 44, 45] On this basis, PMR has not gained FDA approval.
- **Gene therapy**: This is still experimental, although several studies have shown encouraging results in terms of decrease in angina class. The Angiogenic

Gene Therapy (AGENT-2) trial and the vascular endothelial growth factor in ischemia for vascular angiogenesis (VIVA) trial have included placebo arms and revealed significant changes in ischemic defect and angina class, respectively, but further work is needed with clinical efficacy and immunological security.[64, 65]

Syndrome X

Syndrome X is the combination of anginal chest pain, abnormal exercise testing, and normal coronaries on angiography. It appears to be more prevalent in women,[66] who tend to complain of symptoms after the menopause. Despite presenting angina on exertion and nearly 50 percent cases also at rest, only 40 percent benefit from sublingual nitrates during an episode of pain.[66] However, in a follow up of up to seven years, no acute coronary events or deterioration of cardiac function were found in a study that included 99 patients.[66]

The psychological impact of Syndrome X is widely acknowledged.[67] The use of a CBT approach has been shown to reduce symptom severity and frequency while improving mental state, quality of life, and increase social activities.[30, 68] Unlike RAP, a brief intervention CBT program did not show any benefit, although this was undertaken closely following angiographic assessment.[69]

An Italian group has tried spinal cord stimulation on the basis that it is an accepted therapy for refractory angina pain.[70] They found a reduced frequency of attacks and consumption of nitrates, and an increased exercise tolerance, threshold for angina pain, and overall improved quality of life. On this basis, they recommend that spinal cord stimulation be offered to patients with refractory angina pectoris and normal coronary arteries on angiography.

The management options for Syndrome X are summarized in **Table 39.3**.

VISCERAL CHEST PAIN: PERICARDIUM AND GREAT VESSELS

Pericarditis is an inflammation of the pericardium that is classically acute. A recurrent pericarditis with acute episodes lasting many years has been described. This term includes two clinical entities. Incessant pericarditis refers to pericarditis that relapses within six weeks of any attempt to reduce anti-inflammatory treatment. Intermittent pericarditis refers to those patients who have episodes where for more than six weeks while on no treatment they remain free from symptoms.[79] The incidence is 15–32 percent of the cases of acute pericarditis.[79, 80] Recurrent pericarditis is often associated with an autoimmune process.

Clinical features

Although they may have suffered an effusion, cardiac tamponade, cardiac failure, or cardiac arrhythmias during the first episode, they rarely suffer them during the relapses that often give only disabling chest pain with raised inflammatory markers in blood tests.[79] Constrictive pericarditis is not a feature of repeated episodes of recurrent pericarditis, and the prognosis is good with severe complications seen only rarely despite the severe impairment to quality of life.[79]

Diagnostic tests are not currently recommended unless there are multiple relapses and failure to improve with nonsteroidal anti-inflammatory drugs (NSAIDs). In those cases, aspiration of pericardial fluid may be indicated.[81]

Therapeutic options

The treatment hardly ever needs to be administered on an in-patient basis. Current evidence suggests treatment with NSAIDs and colchicine.[80, 82][II] Colchicine has reduced the incidence of recurrence at 18 months from 32.3 to 10.7 percent.[80, 82] High-dose steroids used to be advocated, but they have been abandoned as a routine treatment because of the side-effect profile. These are best reserved for cases resistant to conventional treatment and some authors suggest they are better administered intrapericardially.[83] A published case series of pericardiectomies failed to improve the symptoms,[84] suggesting surgical treatments are not routinely indicated.

Table 39.3 Management of Syndrome X.

Treatment	Supporting evidence	Treatment	Supporting evidence
β-blockers	[71, 72][III]	Estrogens	[III][73]
ACEI	[71, 72, 74][III]	Transcutaneous electrical nerve stimulation	[III][75]
Tricyclic antidepressants	[76][III]	PMP/cognitive-behavioral therapy	[III][77]
Spinal cord stimulation	[70, 75][III]	Nitrates	[V][66, 70]
Ca^{2+} channel blockers	[72, 78][III]	Adenosine antagonists	[V][78]

PMP, Pain Management Program.

VISCERAL CHEST PAIN: ESOPHAGEAL AND STOMACH

Pathophysiology

Both cardiac and esophageal causes of chest pain may coexist or have overlapping symptoms. Both can present with similar qualities, similar distribution, and dyspnea.[85] In order to establish that esophageal disease is the cause of angina-like chest pain, four criteria must be fulfilled.

1. The patient must have symptoms consistent with angina pectoris.
2. A cardiac basis for the symptoms must be excluded.
3. A cause–effect relationship between chest pain and esophageal abnormality must be established.
4. The correction of the esophageal problem should result in relief from the chest pain.[86]

Physiological stimuli in the healthy gastrointestinal tract are not painful. Some of the different etiologies that have been postulated for noncardiac chest pain related to the upper gastrointestinal tract include acid reflux, esophageal motor disorder, altered pain threshold/hypersensitivity, and psychiatric dysfunction.[87] Although 64 percent of the episodes of chest pain in different studies do not correlate with any esophageal abnormality that could be found on routine testing, 20 percent of the episodes could be correlated with pH abnormalities and 12 percent of the episodes could be correlated with motility abnormalities.[88]

Etiology and management

The most common etiology is thought to be occult gastroesophageal reflux disease that affects up to 40 percent of these patients.[7, 87, 89] Some of these patients have clinical features consistent with the disease, but pH studies have shown normal results,[87] although up to 53 percent of patients with undiagnosed noncardiac chronic chest pain have abnormal lower esophageal sphincter and up to 44 percent have abnormal pH proximal to the lower esophageal sphincter.[89] It is possible to have a negative pH study at rest that transforms into a positive study with an exercise-induced incompetent lower esophageal sphincter.[86]

Studies have suggested that in view of the high prevalence of gastroesophageal reflux disease in patients with noncardiac chest pain, it is recommended that a trial of proton-pump inhibitors (PPI) be conducted for four to eight weeks.[7, 87, 90] This has proven to be cost-effective beyond one year[7] when compared to investigations for gastrointestinal causes. Furthermore, when compared against placebo, the arms treated with PPI consistently showed a reduction in frequency and intensity of chest pain,[90] although some of the studies only included patients with known gastroesophageal reflux disease.

Very little relation has been found between chronic noncardiac chest pain and abnormal esophageal function.[91, 92] Based on the lack of correlation between chest pain and positive findings in esophageal motility tests, together with the demands imposed in patients for these tests and the poor cost–benefit ratio,[93] routine testing for esophageal motility in patients with undiagnosed chronic chest pain is not routinely recommended. Furthermore, although these tests can sometimes identify the esophagus as the cause of the pain, they do not direct therapy and they lack a gold standard to compare as normal reference point.[94]

Some studies have shown disappointing results when targeting chronic chest pain with therapies aimed at treating esophageal pain.[95, 96] These trials have not included PPI and the poor response rate may be related to the small proportion that has positive provocation studies in which a smooth muscle relaxant may prove beneficial. This benefit is seen in long-term follow up and the physiological benefit of a reduction in spasm of the esophageal wall does not always translate into a reduction in reported chest pain.[95] Another drug that has been used as part of diagnostic esophageal tests is the spasmomimetic agent edrophonium, but this appears to produce chest pain symptoms, as well as alterations in esophageal motility.[97]

Other patients have other esophageal motor disorders that do not fit into any diagnostic categories. One study reported that in 72 percent of these patients, botulinum toxin injections at the gastroesophageal junction can be beneficial for up to 18 months. The mean duration of a benefit >50 percent was just over seven months.[98] Stress can induce an increase in esophageal pressures and this increase seems to be greater when the stress is related to cognitive problems.[99]

Table 39.4 provides a comparison of angina and esophageal chest pain.

Table 39.4 Comparison of angina and esophageal chest pain.[100]

Pain description	Angina	Esophageal pain
Time-course	Short	Often prolonged
Site and radiation	Precordium, jaw, arm	Retrosternal, precordium, jaw, arm
Character	Pressure, tight, band-like, fear	Burning, pressure
Provoking factors	Exercise, stress, food, cold, rare at night	Food, posture, rare exercise, often at night
Relieving factors	Rest nitrates	Nitrates, antacids

SOMATIC CHEST PAIN: MUSCULOSKELETAL

After coronary artery disease and gastroesophageal reflux, the next most common cause is musculoskeletal chest wall syndromes. Around 70 percent of these patients have chest wall tenderness on palpation that in up to 16 percent can resemble classical angina.[101] The most common areas of musculoskeletal chest pain are sternum, xiphoid, left costosternal junctions, and left anterior chest wall.[101]

A musculoskeletal cause for a chest pain is suspected when the pain is specific of certain postures or movements or activities. Physical examination often finds tenderness to palpation over the structure that is the source of the pain.[102]

Etiology

The most common cause of musculoskeletal chest pain is costochondritis, with an incidence of up to 30 percent of all musculoskeletal chest pains,[103, 104] with inflammation of the costal cartilages and up to 42 percent of patients with recurrent costochondritis complaining of widespread pain.[103] In a number of patients the chest pain still prevails once the clinical signs of costochondritis have subsided. The incidence of costochondritis has risen steadily in the last few years because of an increase in the abuse of intravenous recreational drugs, mainly heroin.[105, 106, 107] Other conditions that predispose to costochondritis are diabetes, sepsis, following cardiothoracic surgery and medications. There have been an increasing number of case reports of patients with costochondritis secondary to *Pseudomonas aeruginosa*, *Candida albicans*,[106] *Salmonella pertusis*,[108] and *Escherichia coli*.[109]

The main symptom is pain or tenderness in the front of the chest that is normally sharp, exacerbated by pressure and movement of the chest wall. It can affect more than one costal cartilage. Tietze's syndrome is an entity similar to costochondritis. The main difference is the presence of swelling of the affected area with Tietze's syndrome that does not exist in costochondritis.

Treatments include conservative and interventional, and anti-inflammatory treatment both with steroids and nonsteroids has been described. Sulfasalazine (sulphazalazine) shows some evidence of being helpful in long-term treatment.[110][V] Interventional treatments that have been reported in four "illustrative" cases and include debridement, rib excision, chest wall en-bloc excision, and flap reconstructions[111] have been suggested in advanced cases. Most patients will achieve spontaneous resolution within a year,[112] so surgery must be regarded with considerable suspicion.

SOMATIC CHEST PAIN: REFERRED

With an estimated prevalence in the general population of 66 percent, spinal pain is another possible etiology of chronic thoracic pain.[113] It has been estimated that 15 percent of spinal pains originate in the thoracic spine.[114] Of those, it has been suggested that nearly half originated in the zygoapophyseal joints.[115, 116] Painful cervical facets were the cause of the pain in 55 percent of patients with neck pain and 42 percent patients with thoracic pain.[116] Manchikanti *et al.*[116] found this to be more prevalent in people with sedentary jobs. The diagnosis is made by exclusion of other pathologies and a high index of suspicion since there are no defined clinical or radiological features.[117] There have been descriptions of patterns of distribution of this pain in healthy volunteers, and these are mainly centered on the back.[118, 119]

Table 39.5 Other causes of chest pain.[120]

Common	Uncommon
Intercostal neuralgia	Bornholm's disease
Diabetic truncal neuropathy	Sternoclavicular syndrome
Fractures in osteoporosis/ malignancy	Sternalis syndrome
	Slipping rib syndrome
	Xyphodynia
	Winged scapula syndrome
	Vasculitis of pulmonary arteries (takayasu)

OTHER ETIOLOGIES OF CHEST PAIN

These are summarized in **Table 39.5**.

REFERENCES

1. Klinman MS, Stevens D, Gorenflo DW. Episodes of care for chest pain: a preliminary report from MIRNET. Michigan Research Network. *Journal of Family Practice*. 1994; **38**: 345–52.
2. Svavarsdottir AE, Jonasson MR, Gudmudsson GH *et al.* Chest pain in family practice. diagnosis and long-term outcome in a community setting. *Canadian Family Physician*. 1996; **42**: 1122–8.
3. Von Korff M, Dworkin SF, Le Resche L *et al.* An epidemiological comparison of pain complaints. *Pain*. 1988; **32**: 173–83.
4. Burt CW. Summary statistics for acute cardiac ischaemia and chest pain visits to United States' emergency departments in 1995–1996. *American Journal of Emergency Medicine*. 1999; **17**: 552–9.
5. McCord J, Nowack RM, McCullough PA *et al.* Ninety minute exclusion of acute myocardial infarction using quantitative point of care testing of myoglobin and troponin I. *Circulation*. 2001; **104**: 1454–6.

6. Forberg JL, Henriksen LS, Edenbrandt L *et al.* Direct hospital costs of chest pain patients attending the emergency department: a retrospective study. *BMC Emergency Medicine.* 2006; **6**: 6.
7. Borzecki AM, Pedrosa MC, Prashker MJ. Should noncardiac chest pain be treated empirically? A cost-effectiveness analysis. *Archives of Internal Medicine.* 2000; **160**: 844–52.
8. Wright RS, Monnahan RL, Kopeki SL *et al.* Cardiac catheterisation reduces resource utilisation in patients with chronic chest pain. *Catheterization and Cardiovascular Interventions.* 2000; **49**: 363–6.
9. Ho KY, Kang JY, Yeo B. Non-cardiac, non-oesophageal chest pain: the relevance of psychological factors. *Gut.* 1998; **43**: 105–10.
10. Katerndahl D. Panic and plaques: panic disorder and coronary artery disease in patiens with chest pain. *Journal of the American Board of Family Medicine.* 2004; **17**: 114–26.
11. Gomez-Caminero A, Blumenthals WA, Russo LJ *et al.* Does panic disorder increase the risk of coronary heart disease? A cohort study of a national managed care database. *Psychosomatic Medicine.* 2005; **67**: 688–91.
12. Demiryoguran NS, Karcioglu O, Topacoglu H *et al.* Anxiety disorder in patients with non-specific chest pain in the emergency setting. *Emergency Medicine Journal.* 2006; **23**: 99–102.
13. Bradley LA, Richter JE, Scarinci IC. Psychosocial and psychophysical assessments of patients with unexplained chest pain. *American Journal of Medicine.* 1992; **92**: 65–73.
14. Armour JA, Murphy DA, Yuan B-X *et al.* Gross and microscopic anatomy of the human intrinsic cardiac nervous system. *Anatomical Record.* 1997; **247**: 289–98.
15. Hogan QH, Erickson SJ. MR imaging of the stellate ganglion: normal appearance. *American Journal of Radiology.* 1992; **158**: 655–9.
16. Pather N, Partab P, Singh B *et al.* The sympathetic contributions to the cardiac plexus. *Surgical and Radiologic Anatomy.* 2003; **25**: 210–15.
17. Nonidez JF. Studies on the innervation of the heart. *American Journal of Anatomy.* 1939; **65**: 361–413.
18. Klein J, Chao S, Berman D, Rozanski A. Is 'silent' myocardial ischemia really as severe as symptomatic ischemia? The analytical effect of patient selection biases. *Circulation.* 1994; **89**: 1958–66.
19. Myran R, Jorgensen JV, Wiseth R. Epidural spinal cord stimulation in chronic refractory angina pectoris. *Tidsskr Nor Laegeforen.* 2004; **124**: 2754–6.
20. ∗ Mannheimer C, Camici P, Chester MR *et al.* The problem of chronic refractory angina. Report from the ESC on the treatment of refractory angina. *European Heart Journal.* 2002; **23**: 355–70.
21. ∗ Yusuf S. Design, baseline characteristics and preliminary clinical report of the organization to assess strategies for ischaemic syndromes-2 trial. *American Journal of Cardiology.* 1999; **85**: 20–5.
22. Brorsson B, Persson H, Landelius P *et al.* Smärtor i bröstet: Operation, ballongvidgning, medicinsk behandling. Report No. 140. Stockholm: Statens Beredning för Utvärdering av Medicinsk Metodik, 1998 (English translation).
23. Moore RK, Groves D, Bateson S *et al.* Health-related quality of life of patients with refractory angina before and one year after enrollment onto a refractory angina program. *European Journal of Pain.* 2005; **9**: 305–10.
24. Lyons RA, Lo SV Littlepage BN. Comparative health status of patients with 11 common illnesses in Wales. *Journal of Epidemiology and Community Health.* 1994; **48**: 388–90.
25. Wright C, Towlerton G, Fox K. Optimal treatment for complex artery disease and refractory angina. *British Journal of Cardiology.* 2006; **13**: 306–08.
26. ∗ Fox K, Garcia MA, Ardissino D *et al.* Guidelines on the management of stable angina pectoris; executive summary. *European Heart Journal.* 2006; **27**: 1341–81.
27. Lewin RJ. Improving quality of life in patients with angina. *Heart.* 1999; **82**: 654–5.
28. Mayou RA, Bryant BM, Sanders D. A controlled trial of CBT for non-cardiac chest pain. *Psychological Medicine.* 1997; **27**: 1021–31.
29. Lewin RJP, Furze G, Robinson J *et al.* A randomised controlled trial of a self-management plan for patients with newly diagnosed angina. *British Journal of General Practice.* 2002; **52**: 194–201.
30. ∗ Kisely S, Campbell LA, Skerritt P. Psychological interventions for symptomatic management of non-specific chest pain in patients with normal coronary anatomy. *Cochrane Database of Systematic Reviews.* 2005; **CD004101**.
31. Garcia-Moll M, Serra R, Garcia-Moll X. Refractory angina treated by spinal cord stimulation. The results of a long-term follow-up. *Revista Española de Cardiología.* 2000; **53**: 321–6.
32. De Jongste MJ, Hautvast RW, Hillege HL *et al.* Efficacy of spinal cord stimulation as adjuvant therapy for intractable angina pectoris: a prospective, randomized clinical study. Working Groups on Neurocardiology. *Journal of the American College of Cardiology.* 1994; **23**: 1592–7.
33. Murray S, Carson KG, Ewings PD *et al.* Spinal cord stimulation significantly decreases the need for acute hospital admission for chest pain in patients with refractory angina pectoris. *Heart.* 1999; **82**: 89–92.
34. ∗ Diedrichs H, Weber M, Voth E *et al.* Increased myocardial blood flow after spinal cord stimulation in patients with refractory angina pectoris. *Medizinische Klinik.* 2003; **98**: 146–50.
35. Hautvast RW, DeJongste MJ, Staal MJ *et al.* Spinal cord stimulation in chronic intractable angina pectoris: a randomized, controlled efficacy study. *American Heart Journal.* 1998; **136**: 1114–20.
36. Di Pedre F, Lanza GA, Zuin G *et al.* Immediate and long-term clinical outcome after spinal cord stimulation for refractory stable angina pectoris. *American Journal of Cardiology.* 2003; **91**: 951–5.

* 37. Mannheimer C, Eliasson T, Augustinsson LE *et al.* Electrical stimulation versus coronary artery bypass surgery in severe angina pectoris: the ESBY study. *Circulation.* 1998; **97**: 1157–63.
38. Yu W, Maru F, Edner M *et al.* Spinal cord stimulation for refractory angina pectoris: a retrospective analysis of efficacy and cost-benefit. *Coronary Artery Disease.* 2004; **15**: 31–7.
39. Allen KB, Dowling RD, Fudge TL *et al.* Comparison of transmyocardial revascularization with medical therapy in patients with refractory angina. *New England Journal of Medicine.* 1999; **341**: 1029–36.
40. Frazier OH, March RJ, Horvath KA. Transmyocardial revascularization with a carbon dioxide laser in patients with end-stage coronary artery disease. *New England Journal of Medicine.* 1999; **341**: 1021–8.
41. Mannheimer C, Carlsson CA, Emanuelsson H *et al.* The effects of transcutaneous electrical nerve stimulation in patients with severe angina pectoris. *Circulation.* 1985; **71**: 308–16.
42. Leon M. Direct myocardial revascularization in regeneration of endomyocardial channels trial (DIRECT). Paper presented at the Transcatheter Cardiovascular Therapeutics 2000 Meeting, Washington, DC, October 19, 2000.
43. Oesterle SN, Sanborn TA, Ali N *et al.* Percutaneous transmyocardial laser revascularisation for severe angina: the PACIFIC randomised trial. *Lancet.* 2000; **356**: 1705–10.
44. Stone GW, Teirstein PS, Rubenstein R *et al.* A prospective, multicenter randomized trial of percutaneous transmyocardial laser revascularization in patients with non-recanalizable chronic total occlusions. *Journal of the American College of Cardiology.* 2002; **39**: 1581–7.
45. Salem M, Rotevatn S, Stavnes S *et al.* Usefulness and safety of percutaneous myocardial laser revascularization for refractory angina pectoris. *American Journal of Cardiology.* 2004; **93**: 1086–91.
46. Gramling-Babb P, Miller MJ, Reeves ST *et al.* Treatment of medically and surgically refractory angina pectoris with high thoracic epidural analgesia: initial clinical experience. *American Heart Journal.* 1997; **133**: 648–55.
47. Hammond CM, Leach A. Long term benefits of stellate ganglion block in severe chronic refractory angina. *Pain.* 2000; **87**: 103–05.
48. Moore R, Groves D, Hammond C *et al.* Temporary sympathectomy in the treatment of chronic refractory angina. *Journal of Pain and Symptom Management.* 2005; **30**: 183–91.
49. Stritesky M, Dobias M, Demes R *et al.* Endoscopic thoracic sympathectomy – its effect in the treatment of refractory angina pectoris. *Interactive Cardiovascular and Thoracic Surgery.* 2006; **5**: 464–8.
50. Wilkinson H A. Percutaneous radiofrequency upper thoracic sympathectomy. Technique applications. *Neurosurgery.* 1996; **38**: 715–25.
51. World Health Organization. The rehabilitation of patients with cardiovascular diseases. Report on a seminar. EURO 0381. Copenhagen: World Health Organization, regional office for Europe, 1969.
52. Furze F, Lewin RJ, Murburg T *et al.* Does it matter what patients think? The relationship between changes in patients' beliefs about angina and their psychological and functional status. *Journal of Psychosomatic Research.* 2005; **59**: 323–9.
53. Moore RKG, David GG, Bridson JD *et al.* A brief cognitive-behavioural intervention reduces hospital admission in refractory angina pectoris. *Journal of Pain and Symptom Management.* 2007; **33**: 310–16.
54. Apthorp GH, Bhamberlain DA, Hayward GW. The effects of sympathectomy on the electrocardiogram and effort tolerance in angina pectoris. *British Heart Journal.* 1964; **26**: 218–26.
55. Jessurun GA, Ten Vaarwerk IA, De Jongste MJ *et al.* Sequelae of spinal cord stimulation for refractory angina pectoris. Reliability and safety profile of long-term clinical application. *Coronary Artery Disease.* 1997; **8**: 33–8.
56. Romano M, Auriti A, Cazzin R *et al.* Epidural spinal cord stimulation in the treatment of refractory angina pectoris. Its clinical efficacy, complications and long-term mortality. An Italian multicenter retrospective study. *Italian Heart Journal. Supplement.* 2000; **1**: 97–102.
57. Rapati D, Capucci R, Berti M *et al.* Spinal cord stimulation and quality of life in patients with refractory angina. *Minerva Anestesiologica.* 2001; **67**: 803–10.
* 58. Ten Vaarwerk IA, Jessurum GA, DeJongste MJ *et al.* Clinical outcome of patients treated with spinal cord stimulation for therapeutically refractory angina pectoris. The Working Group on Neurocardiology. *Heart.* 1999; **82**: 82–8.
59. De Landsheere C, Mannheimer C, Habets A. Effects of spinal cord stimulation on regional myocardial perfusion assessed by positron emission tomography. *American Journal of Cardiology.* 1992; **69**: 1143–9.
60. Bagger JP, Jensen BS, Johannses G. Long-term outcome of spinal cord electrical stimulation in patients with refractory chest pain. *Clinical Cardiology.* 1998; **21**: 286–8.
61. Ekre O, Norrsell H, Wahrborg P *et al.* Temporary cessation of spinal cord stimulation in angina pectoris – effects on symptoms and evaluation of long-term effect determinants. *Coronary Artery Disease.* 2003; **14**: 323–7.
62. Arora RR, Chou TM, Jain D *et al.* The multicenter study of enhanced externalcounterpulsation (MUST-EECP): effect of EECP on exercise-induced myocardialischemia and anginal episodes. *Journal of the American College of Cardiology.* 1999; **33**: 1833–40.
63. Schoebel F, Frazier H, Jessurum G *et al.* Refractory angina pectoris in end-stage coronary artery disease: Evolving therapeutic concepts. *American Heart Journal.* 1997; **134**: 587–602.
64. Grines CL, Watkins MW, Mahmarian JJ *et al.* Angiogene GENeTherapy (AGENT-2) Study Group. A randomized, double-blind, placebocontrolled trial of Ad5FGF-4 gene

therapy and its effect on myocardial perfusion in patients with stable angina. *Journal of the American College of Cardiology.* 2003; **42**: 1339–47.

65. Henry TD, Annex BH, McKendall GR *et al.* VIVA Investigators. The VIVA Trial: vascular endothelial growth factor in ischemia for vascular angiogenesis. *Circulation.* 2003; **107**: 1359–65.
66. Kaski JC, Rosano GM, Collins P. Cardiac syndrome X: clinical characteristics and left ventricular function. Long-term follow-up study. *Journal of the American College of Cardiology.* 1995; **25**: 807–14.
67. Asbury EA, Collins P. Psychosocial factors associated with noncardiac chest pain and cardiac syndrome X. *Herz.* 2005; **30**: 55–60.
68. * Peski-Oosterbaan AS, Spinhoven P, van Rood Y *et al.* Cognitive-behavioral therapy for noncardiac chest pain: a randomized trial. *American Journal of Medicine.* 1999; **106**: 424–9.
69. Sanders D, Bass CM, Mayou RA *et al.* Non-cardiac chest pain: why was a brief intervention apparently ineffective? *Psychological Medicine.* 1997; **27**: 1033–40.
70. Lanza GA, Sestito A, Sandric S *et al.* Spinal cord stimulation in patients with refractory angina pain and normal coronary arteries. *Italian Heart Journal. Supplement.* 2001; **2**: 25–30.
71. Ozcelik F, Altun A, Ozbay G. Antianginal and anti-ischaemic effects of nisoldipine and ramipril in patients with syndrome X. *Clinical Cardiology.* 1999; **22**: 361–5.
72. Lanza GA, Colonna G, Pasceri V *et al.* Atenolol versus Amlodipine versus ISMN on anginal symptoms in syndrome X. *American Journal of Cardiology.* 1999; **84**: 854–6.
73. Sitges M, Heras M, Roig E *et al.* Acute and mid-term combined hormone replacement therapy improves endothelial function in post-menopausal women with angina and angiographycally normal arteries. *European Heart Journal.* 2001; **22**: 2116–24.
74. Nalbantgil I, Onder R, Altintig A *et al.* Therapeutic benefits of cilazapril in patients with syndrome X. *Cardiology.* 1998; **89**: 130–3.
75. Jessurum GA, Hautvast RW, Tio RA *et al.* Electrical neuromodulation improves myocardial perfusion and ameliorates refractory angina pectoris in patients with syndrome X. *European Journal of Pain.* 2003; **7**: 507–12.
76. Cannon RO, Quyyumi AA, Mincemoyer R *et al.* Imipramine in patients with chest pain despite normal coronary angiograms. *New England Journal of Medicine.* 1994; **330**: 1411–17.
77. Mayou RA, Bryant BM, Sanders D *et al.* A controlled trial of cognitive behavioural therapy for non-cardiac chest pain. *Psychological Medicine.* 1997; **27**: 1021–31.
78. Kalsi JC, Valenzuela Garcia LF. Therapeutic options for the management of patients with cardiac syndrome X. *European Heart Journal.* 2001; **22**: 283–93.
79. Soler-Soler J, Sagrista-Sauleda J, Permanyer-Miralda G. Relapsing pericarditis. *Heart.* 2004; **90**: 1364–8.
80. Adler Y, Finkenstein Y, Guindo J. Colchicine treatment for recurrent pericarditis: A decade of experience. *Circulation.* 1998; **97**: 2138–85.
81. Zayas R, Anguita M, Torres F *et al.* Incidence of specific etiology and role of methods for specific etiologic diagnosis of primary acute pericarditis. *American Journal of Cardiology.* 1995; **75**: 378–82.
82. Imazio M, Bobbio M, Cocchi E *et al.* Colchicine in addition to conventional therapy for acute pericarditis: results of the COPE trial. *Circulation.* 2005; **112**: 2012–16.
83. Maisch B, Ristic AD, Seferovic PM *et al.* Intrapericardial treatment of autoreactive pericardial effusion with triamcinolone. The way to avoid side effects of systemic corticosteroid therapy. *European Heart Journal.* 2002; **23**: 1503–08.
84. Fowler NO, Harbin AD. Recurrent acute pericarditis: follow up study of 31 patients. *Journal of the American College of Cardiology.* 1986; **7**: 300–05.
85. Henderson RD, Wigle ED, Sample K *et al.* Atypical chest pain of cardiac or esophageal origin. *Chest.* 1978; **73**: 24–7.
86. DeMeester TR, O'Sullivan GC, Bermudez G *et al.* Esophageal function in patients with angina-type chest pain and normal coronary angiograms. Annual Meeting of the American Surgical Association, Boston, MA, 1982.
87. Botoman VA. Noncardiac chest pain. *Journal of Clinical Gastroenterology.* 2002; **34**: 6–14.
88. Peters L, Maas L, Petty D *et al.* Spontaneous noncardiac chest pain. Evaluation by 24-hour ambulatory esophageal motility and pH monitoring. *Gastroenterology.* 1988; **94**: 878–86.
89. Gastal OL, Castell JA, Castell DO. Frequency and site of gastroesophageal reflux in patients with chest symptoms. Studies using proximal and distal pH minitoring. *Chest.* 1994; **106**: 1793–6.
90. Achem SR, Kolts BE, Macmath T *et al.* Effects of omeprazole versus placebo in treatment of noncardiac chest pain and gastroesophageal reflux. *Digestive Diseases and Sciences.* 1997; **42**: 2138–45.
91. Frobert O, Funch-Jenses P, Bagger JP. Diagnostic value of esophageal studies in patients with angina-like chest pain and normal coronary angiograms. *Annals of Internal Medicine.* 1996; **124**: 959–69.
92. Limburg AJ, Beekhuis H, Van Dijk RB *et al.* Noncardiac chest pain: Is the esophagus really a frequent source? *Scandinavian Journal of Gastroenterology.* 1990; **25**: 793–8.
93. Meshkinpour H, Glick ME, Sanchez P *et al.* Esophageal manometry: a benefit and cost analysis. *Digestive Diseases and Sciences.* 1982; **27**: 772–5.
94. Richter JE. Overview of diagnostic testing for chest pain of unknown origin. *American Journal of Medicine.* 1992; **92**: 41–45.
95. Richter JE, Dalton CB, Bradley LA *et al.* Oral nifedipine in the treatment of noncardiac chest pain in patients with the nutcracker esophagus. *Gastroenterology.* 1987; **93**: 21–8.

96. Clouse RE, Lustman PJ, Eckert TC *et al.* Low-dose trazodone for symptomatic patients with esophageal contraction abnormalities. A double blind, placebo-controlled trial. *Gastroenterology.* 1987; **92**: 1027–36.
97. Richter JE, Hackshaw BT, Wu WC *et al.* Edrophonium: a useful provocative test for oesophageal chest pain. *Annals of Internal Medicine.* 1985; **103**: 14–21.
98. Miller LS, Pullela SV, Parkman HP *et al.* Treatment of chest pain in patients with noncardiac, nonreflux, nonachalasia spastic esophageal motor disorders using botulinum toxin injection into the gastroesophageal junction. *American Journal of Gastroenterology.* 2002; **97**: 1640–6.
99. Anderson KO, Dalton CB, Bradley LA *et al.* Stress induces alteration of esophageal pressures in healthy volunteers and non-cardiac chest pain patients. *Digestive Diseases and Sciences.* 1989; **34**: 83–91.
100. Collins A. Chronic chest pain. In: Rice A, Warfield C, Justins D, Eccleston C (eds). *Clinical pain management: chronic pain.* 1st edn. London: Hodder Arnold Publishers, 2002: 553–65.
101. Wise CM, Semble EL, Dalton CB. Musculoskeletal chest wall syndromes in patients with noncardiac chest pain: a study of 100 patients. *Archives of Physical Medicine and Rehabilitation.* 1992; **73**: 147–9.
102. Jensen S. Musculoskeletal causes of chest pain. *Australian Family Physician.* 2001; **30**: 834–9.
103. Disla E, Rhim HR, Reddy A *et al.* Costochondritis. A prospective analysis in an emergency department setting. *Archives of Internal Medicine.* 1994; **154**: 2466–9.
104. Fam AG, Smythe HA. Musculoskeletal chest wall pain. *Journal of the Canadian Medical Association.* 1985; **133**: 379–89.
105. Zapatero J, Lopez-Longo J, Monteagudo I *et al.* Costal chondritis in heroin addicts: a comparative study with post-surgical chondritis. *British Journal of Diseases of the Chest.* 1988; **82**: 341–6.
106. Gimferrer JM, Callejas MA, Sanchez-Lloret J. Candida albicans costochondritis in heroin addicts. *Annals of Thoracic Surgery.* 1986; **41**: 89–90.
107. Meyer CA, White CS. Cartilaginous disorders of the chest. *Radiographics.* 1998; **18**: 1109–23.
108. Caruana V, Swayne LC. Gallium detection of Salmonella costochondritis. *Journal of Nucleic Medicine.* 1988; **29**: 2004–07.
109. Alvarez F, Chocarro A, Garcia I *et al.* Primary costochondritis due to Escherichia coli. *Scandinavian Journal of Infectious Diseases.* 2000; **32**: 430–1.
110. Freestom J, Karim Z, Lindsay K *et al.* Can early diagnosis and management of costochondritis reduce acute chest pain admissions? *Journal of Rheumatology.* 2004; **31**: 2269–71.
111. Chicarilli ZN, Ariyan S, Stahl RS. Costochondritis: pathogenesis, diagnosis and management considerations. *Plastic and Reconstructive Surgery.* 1986; **77**: 50–9.
112. Disla E, Rhim HR, Reddy A *et al.* Costochondritis. A prospective analysis in an emergency department setting. *Archives of Internal Medicine.* 1994; **154**: 2466–9.
113. Linton SJ, Hellsing AL, Hallden K. A population-based study of spinal pain among 35–45-year-old individuals. *Spine.* 1998; **23**: 1457–63.
114. Manchikanti L, Pampati V. Research designs in interventional pain management: Is randomisation superior, desirable or essential? *Pain Physician.* 2002; **5**: 275–84.
115. Manchikanti L, Sing V, Pampati V. Evaluation of the prevalence of facet joint pain in chronic thoracic pain. *Pain Physician.* 2002; **5**: 243–9.
116. Manchikanti L, Boswell MV, Singh V *et al.* Prevalence of facet joint pain in chronic spinal pain of cervical, thoracic and lumbar regions. *BMC Musculoskeletal Disorders.* 2004; **5**: 15–21.
117. Dreyfuss P, Tibiletti C, Dreyer S *et al.* Thoracic zygoapophyseal joint pain: a review and description of an intraarticular block technique. *Pain Digest.* 1994; **4**: 46–54.
118. Dreyfuss P, Tibelitti C, Dreyer SJ. Thoracic zygoapophyseal joint pain patterns. A study in normal volunteers. *Spine.* 1994; **19**: 807–11.
119. Fukui S, Ohseto K, Shiotani M. Patterns of pain induced by distending the thoracic zygoapophyseal joints. *Regional Anaesthesia.* 1997; **22**: 322–36.
120. Swap CJ, Nagurney JT. Value and limitations of chest pain history in the evaluation of patients with suspected acute coronary syndromes. *Journal of the American Medical Association.* 2005; **295**: 2248–9.

40

Chronic abdominal, groin, and perineal pain of visceral origin

TIMOTHY J NESS

KEY LEARNING POINTS

- Abdominal, groin, and perineal pain can be of visceral, neuropathic, musculoskeletal, related to cancer or psychogenic origins.
- Visceral pain is poorly localized and evokes strong autonomic and emotional responses.
- There is poor correlation between visceral pathology and reports of visceral pain.
- The principles of the management of visceral pain are similar to those of other painful conditions.

INTRODUCTION

Scope

Chronic pain localized to the abdomen, groin, and/or perineum can have multiple etiologies ranging from focal sites of inflammation to idiopathic systemic diseases[1] (**Box 40.1**). These pains fall within the practice of virtually every medical specialty and are some of the most common presenting symptoms for the primary care physician. Pain experienced in the abdomen, groin, and/or perineum may arise from pathology of the nervous system innervating those structures or may originate in the viscera, vascular structures or musculoskeletal-articular stuctures in the region. Psychological disturbance frequently manifests as complaints of abdominal discomfort as evidenced by common usage of the term *hypochondria* as "imagined illness" when the term anatomically refers to the mid-upper abdomen. Stress clearly affects visceral sensation but acts more often as an exacerbator rather than generator of pain.[2] Other portions of this text address cancer-related pain, gynecological (pelvic) pain, chest (thoracic visceral) pain, neurological pain, psychogenic pain, spine-related pain, and pain syndromes occurring as complications of surgery (e.g. a neuroma following hernia repair); all of which can be causes of abdominal, groin, and perineal pain. As a consequence, this chapter will focus on pains arising from nongynecologic abdominal and pelvic viscera. The disease states of chronic pancreatitis, the irritable bowel syndrome and interstitial cystitis will then be discussed in depth as "archetype" chronic disease states, since these entities are illustrative of general phenomena present in patients presenting with chronic or recurrent abdominal, groin, and/or perineal symptomatology and therefore serve as examples of diagnostic workups and therapeutic modalities. Numerous other painful disorders with abdominal, groin, or perineal symptomatology will then

Box 40.1 Sources of chronic abdominal, groin, and perineal pain

Infectious-inflammatory pain states
- Esophagitis (XIX-4; XIX-5)
- Gastritis and duodenitis (XXI-14)
- Chronic gastric ulcer (XXI-4)
- Chronic duodenal ulcer (XXI-5)
- Radiation enterocolitis (XXI-16)
- Crohn's disease (XXI-9)
- Ulcerative colitis and other colitis/ulcer (XXI-17)
- Diverticular disease of the colon (XXI-12)
- Chronic pancreatitis (XXI-19)
- Ulceration of anus or rectum (XXV-5)
- Gallbladder disease (XXI-2)
- Pain from urinary tract – kidney stones (XXIV-10)
- Subphrenic abscess (XIX-1)
- Tuberculous peritonitis (NC)

Functional pain states
- Postgastric surgery syndrome, dumping (XXI-18)
- Postcholecystectomy syndrome (XXI-3)
- Dyspepsia and other dysfunctional disorders in stomach (XXI-15)
- Irritable bowel syndrome (XXI-11)
- Chronic constipation – fecal impaction (XXI-10)
- Proctalgia fugax (XXV-4)
- "Adhesions" (NC)

Musculoskeletal origin
- Thoracic, lumbar and sacral spinal disease (X, XXVI, XXVII)
- Slipping rib syndrome (XVII-10)
- Abdominal muscle wall (I-18, I-34)

Other pain states
- Herniated abdominal organs (XIX-2)
- Aneurysm of the aorta (XVII-7)
- Chronic mesenteric ischemia (XXI-8)
- Hepatic capsule distension secondary to cardiac failure (XXI-1)
- Injury of external genitalia (XXV-6)
- Pain due to hemorrhoids (XXV-3)
- Hydronephrosis – urinary bladder distension (XXIV-10)
- Interstitial cystitis (NC)

Abdominal pain of chest-related origin
- Cardiac (XVII-4,5)
- Pericarditis (XVII-6)
- Diaphram (XVII-8; XIX-2)
- Esophageal (XIX-3,4,5)

Generalized disease origin
- Familial Mediterranean fever (XXII-1)
- Intermittent acute porphyria (XXII-3)
- Variegate porphyria (XXII-5)
- Hereditary coproporphyria (XXII-4)
- Systemic rheumaticologic (I-8; I-27)
- Fibromyalgia (I-9)
- Lead poisoning (NC)
- Adrenal insufficiency (NC)

Due to cancer
- Esophagus (XVII-9)
- Stomach (XXI-6)
- Colon (XXI-13)
- Rectum (XXIX-5)
- Pancreas (XXI-7)
- Liver or biliary system (XXI-21)
- Kidney (XXI-22)
- Urinary bladder (XXIV-12)
- Prostate (XXV-7)
- Testicular (NC)
- Spinal involvement (X-3, XXVI-3, XXIX)
- Other metastatic including carcinomatosis (NC)

Gynecological pain
- Mittelschmerz (XXIV-1)
- Secondary dysmenorrhea (XXIV-2)
- Primary dysmenorrhea (XXIV-3)
- Endometriosis (XXIV-4)
- Posterior parametritis (XXIV-5)
- Tuberculous salpingitis (XXIV-6)
- Retroversion of the uterus (XXIV-7)
- Ovarian pain (XXIV-8)
- Injury of female external genitalia (XXV-6)
- Vaginismus or dyspareunia (XXIV-11)
- Chronic pelvic pain without obvious pathology (XXIV-9)

Neurologic origin
- Acute herpes zoster (XX-1)
- Postherpetic neuralgia (XX-2)
- Peripheral neuropathy (I-1)
- Central pain (I-6)
- Segmental or intercostal neuralgia (XX-3)
- 12th rib syndrome (XX-4)
- Abdominal cutaneous nerve entrapment syndrome (XX-5)
- Abdominal migraine (XXII-2)
- Postsurgical neuroma (NC)
- Painful scar (I-26)
- Neuralgias of iliohypogastric, ilioinguinal, genitofemoral nerves (XXV-1)
- Guillain–Barré syndrome (I-36)

Pain of psychological origin (XXIII-2; XXIII-3; XXIII-4; XXV-2)

Pain of uncertain origin (NC)

Roman numerals in parentheses indicate classification per Merskey and Bogduk.[1] NC indicates not classified.

briefly be discussed as "correlates" of the archetypal disorders. Various useful reviews are referenced in relation to the disorders discussed in this chapter and general statements will be referenced to those reviews. Prior to the discussion of "chronic" disorders, a brief discussion of pancreatic cancer will be presented as it serves as a contrast to most of the other conditions which are considered to be nonlife-threatening and associated with significant psychopathology such as anxiety, depression, and substance abuse.

General evaluation of abdominal pain

Abdominal pain is a common presenting symptom for the clinician. Primary evaluation includes an interview to assess the acute versus chronic nature of the complaints, exacerbating and ameliorating factors, and definition of coexisting disease. Chronic use of medications which alter bowel motility is meaningful. A detailed clinical history alone will result in a functionally accurate diagnosis in most patients.[3] Palpation of the abdomen can identify abdominal wall rigidity suggesting a peritoneal process, distended bowel, or underlying masses suggestive of neoplastic, infectious or obstructive processes and localizable tenderness which may suggest a particular organ system. Auscultation of bowel sounds may suggest the presence or absence of gastrointestinal motility and give evidence for obstruction. Rectal and pelvic exams may give additional information related to local pathology. Neurological examination may demonstrate evidence of neuropathy or localized radiculopathy. Basic laboratory examinations include testing for fecal blood, urinalysis, blood cell count with white cell differential, serum amylase/lipase levels, electrolytes, and liver function tests. Radiographic evaluations, other tests, endoscopic evaluations, ultrasonography, paracentesis, or advanced imaging studies would be dependent upon the persistence or progression of complaints.

ARCHETYPE DISORDERS

Pancreatic cancer

A full discussion of this subject is found in the *Cancer Pain* volume of this series.

Most tumors of the pancreas arise from exocrine tissue, primarily ductular epithelium with only rare cases of endocrine pancreatic tumors. In experimental animals, pancreatic cancer can be induced by several compounds (e.g. nitrosoureas) but no specific agent has been conclusively linked to its development. There is indirect evidence that tobacco use increases the incidence of pancreatic carcinoma and links have been made with hepatobiliary disease, diabetes mellitis, fatty foods, and alcohol ingestion, but conclusive evidence is still lacking. Nonsteroidal anti-inflammatories, increased intake of fruits and vegetables, and physical activity reduce risks of developing this cancer.[4] A premalignant condition for pancreatic cancer may be chronic pancreatitis but this has only been definitively demonstrated for patients with hereditary pancreatitis.[5] Pancreatic cancer occurs more frequently in males (2:1), in blacks, and in peoples of developed countries. The mean age at diagnosis is 55. It is the second most common cancer of the gastrointestinal tract and ranks fifth among cancers as a cause of death.

The classic presentation of pancreatic cancer[4] located at the head of the pancreas (70 percent of these tumors) is the triad of abdominal pain, weight loss, and jaundice due to obstruction of the biliary system. Epigastric tenderness and a palpable gallbladder or abdominal mass may be present, but in general there are no definitive findings on physical exam. Cancer in the body or tail of the pancreas may be associated with venous obstruction, portal hypertension, and/or bleeding. The abdominal pain is described as persistent and typically located in the middle of the upper abdomen and may have radiation through to the back. It can be dull and achy, gnawing, or have a cramping, colicky sensation. Pain is moderate to severe in 20–30 percent of patients at the time of presentation and is severe in >80 percent with advanced disease.[6] Weight loss may be profound and malabsorption is frequently noted. Due to its location and the typically asymptomatic nature of this cancer, tumors are often quite advanced and deemed unresectable at the time of presentation. Nonspecific and vague complaints such as nausea, aches, or weakness often attributed to anxiety or depression are often the earliest features.[4] Caraceni and Portenoy[6] have delineated several pancreatic cancer pain syndromes based on clinical characteristics and the pathology identified with approproptiate imaging modalities (**Box 40.2**). Abdominal computed tomography (CT) or ultrasonography followed by surgical or endoscopic biopsy are the most frequent diagnostic modalities. Findings from endoscopic retrograde cholangiopancreatography, arteriography, and/or pancreatic function tests may warrant progression to surgical treatment (curative resection versus palliative treatment) prior to definitive biopsy results. The prognosis of advanced disease is poor.

Once a patient has received a definitive diagnosis of pancreatic cancer, they may enter into palliative treatments in which the cancer may be treated surgically, with chemotherapy, or with radiation therapy.[4,7] The indications for their treatments are beyond the scope of this review, but are dependent upon precise localization and tumor differentiation. Ample use of opioids, anti-inflammatories, and adjuvant agents constitute medical therapies and are extensively employed, even to extremely high doses. Neuraxial opioids are considered appropriate. Psychological therapies and pastoral counseling become vitally important and the pharmacological treatment of anxiety and depression are considered to be standard care. Therapeutic options for pancreatic cancer pain are listed in **Box 40.3**.

Box 40.2 Pancreatic cancer pain syndromes

- Pain due to direct tumor involvement
  - Visceral pain
    - Infiltration of pancreas
    - Infiltration of duodenum/stomach
    - Liver metastases: capsule distension, diaphragmatic irritation
    - Biliary tree distension–obstruction
    - Bowel obstruction
    - Ischemic pain due to mesenteric vessel involvement
  - Somatic pain
    - Retroperitoneal involvement (direct, nodal)
    - Parietal peritoneum and abdominal wall involvement
    - Abdominal distension due to ascites
    - Bone metastases
  - Neuropathic pain
    - Radiculopathy from retroperitoneal spread
    - Radiculopathy from metastases
    - Lumbosacral plexopathy
    - Epidural spinal cord compression
- Pain due to cancer therapies
  - Postoperative pain syndromes
  - Biliary prosthesis complications
  - Postchemotherapy pain syndromes
  - Postradiation pain syndromes

Adapted from Caraceni and Portenoy.[6]

Box 40.3 Treatments for pancreatic cancer-related pain

- Analgesics and side-effect management[a]
  - Opioids[6][I]
  - Anti-inflammatories[6][I]
  - Antiemetics[6][V]
  - Adjuvants[b6][II]
    - Antidepressants
    - Stimulants (methyphenidate)
    - Anticonvulsants
    - Antiarrhythmics
- Curative surgery[c4][V]
- Palliative treatments (surgery, radiotherapy, chemotherapy)[4][IV], [7][IV]
- Neurolysis (neurolytic celiac plexus block)[8][I], [9][II]
- Biliary stenting procedures (for obstruction)[4][V]
- Psychological interventions[7][V]

[a]Assessed for cancer pain with pancreatic cancer patients as component.
[b]As indicated by side effects or nature of pain (e.g. neuropathic).
[c]Disease often unresectable at time of diagnosis – "curative" implies abolition of pain apart from that which is surgery-related.

A key modality of palliative treatment for patients with pancreatic cancer and other upper abdominal cancers is the neurolytic celiac plexus block (NCPB).[8] It has proven to be an effective neurolytic block in randomized controlled trials (RCTs),[10] which is safe and with few serious complications. The site of the tumor location appears to influence success rates of this treatment with a high probability of improvement with tumors involving the head of the pancreas, but poor responses in those involving the body and tail of the pancreas.[11] For this latter group it has been proposed that neurolysis of the splanchnic nerves may prove more efficacious.[12] Several percutaneous techniques of NCPB have been described,[13, 14, 15] including those which are guided by fluoroscopy or CT. The classic technique consists of the injection of a neurolytic agent (typically alcohol or phenol) into the retroperitoneal periaortic region of the upper abdomen/lower thorax. The nerve supply to the upper abdominal viscera traverse this region and so this technique results in deafferentation of sensory input from this region, but also affects bowel motility and systemic blood pressure due to efferent effects. Newer techniques such as videothoracoscopic splanchnicectomies have been described but have similar outcomes to the NCPB.[9] Commonly cited success rates range from 80 to 90 percent with success measured as a reduction of opioid requirement and improved quality of life but without profound effects on survival. When used alone, the NCPB abolishes the pain of pancreatic cancer in 10–24 percent of patients.[16] Quality of life measures show a progressive deterioration in patients with pancreatic cancer, but in a randomized, prospective study, Kawamata *et al.*[17] demonstrated that patients who received an NCPB as part of their pain management had less deterioration than those treated exclusively with systemic medications. Ischia *et al.*[16] evaluated three different techniques for percutaneous neurolysis (transaortic plexus block versus classic retrocrural versus bilateral splanchnicectomy) in a prospective randomized study of 61 patients and found no differences in the efficacy or morbidity of the various techniques. There is a case report of the effectiveness of bilateral vagotomy.[18]

The treatment of pain due to pancreatic cancer forms one end of the spectrum of pain management options. Aggressive surgical, medical, and other interventional treatments such as neuraxial opioids and neurolysis are considered not only acceptable, but ethically mandated in many cases. Presenting symptoms of pancreatic cancer may be protean in nature and similar to other abdominal pain disorders with a high incidence of anxiety and depression.

Chronic pancreatitis

Symptomatic pancreatitis can be associated with pancreatic cell death and/or with ductal fibrosis and calcification. Acute pancreatitis, such as that induced by passage of a gallstone, is thought to be pathogenetically and morphologically different from chronic pancreatitis[19] and generally resolves without permanent structural abnormalities. Chronic pancreatitis is associated with permanent abnormalities, but may present with an acute necrotic episode. Excessive alcohol consumption is the primary etiology in 70–80 percent of the cases of chronic pancreatitis in developed nations, although the precise mechanism of action of alcohol has not been determined. First described in 1788 by Cawley in his description of "a free living young man" who developed severe pancreatic disease, it has been described as a "drunkard's pancreas" since 1878. Only 5–10 percent of heavy drinkers develop symptomatic chronic pancreatitis and so there are likely genetic, infectious, and/or nutritional factors that also contribute to its development. The other 20–30 percent of cases of chronic pancreatitis are predominantly idiopathic in origin, although other etiologies include a pancreas divisum, genetic causes (hereditary-type), previous trauma, previous obstructive episodes, hyperparathyroidism, hyperlipidemia, statin use,[20] and α_1-antitrypsin deficiency. In certain Third World nations, a tropical variety of chronic pancreatitis is common and has been associated with specific dietary patterns.

Various theories have been put forward related to the precise pathophysiology of chronic pancreatitis. Experimentally, chronic pancreatitis may be induced in animals by the administration of toxins but similar links have not been conclusively identified in humans. Alterations in the protein components of pancreatic fluids have been noted which may result in the formation of "sludge" or intraductal "plugs" that become calcified into "stones" which produce inflammatory and fibrotic reactions.[21] It has been proposed that oxidative stress underlies chronic pancreatitis with periodic bursts of free radical formation leading to chronic injury. Genetic factors have been clearly identified in hereditary pancreatitis and in association with such diseases as cystic fibrosis, but no specific marker has been identified in association with other etiologies. Intraductal hypertension is a common sequel of stone formation/fibrosis and has been proposed as a source of the continuous pain that may develop in chronic pancreatitis. However, relief of ductal obstruction and hypertension does not invariably result in pain relief. Similarly, pancreatic intraparenchymal pressure, a correlate to myofascial compartment syndromes with associated ischemia and neural compression, has also been proposed as the source of pain. As stated before, for most cases of chronic pancreatitis a common finding is a high level of chronic alcohol ingestion. The average latent period is 18 years and a comorbidity is cirrhosis of the liver (to complement "cirrhosis" of the pancreas.) Cigarette smoking is associated with increased incidence of chronic pancreatitis[22] and diets with too much or too little fat and/or protein have been implicated.

Histopathologically, chronic pancreatitis is identified by the presence of intraductal calcification (stones), acinar cell loss, fibrosis, and inflammation. Proliferation of unmyelinated nerve fibers and mononuclear cell infiltrates around nerve sheathes has been noted and elevated levels of the neuropeptides have been identified[23] but, unfortunately, identifiable pathology does not firmly correlate with reports of pain.

The primary presenting complaint is pain. Classically, it is deep, boring, and epigastric with frequent radiation through to the back. It may be episodic in nature but may advance until it is continuous and may be precipitated by eating. Sitting upright or leaning forward may decrease the pain. It is often coupled with nausea and vomiting which may lead to dehydration, malnutrition, and an inability to take oral analgesics. Steatorrhea due to pancreatic insufficiency may result with advanced disease as may glucose intolerance and eventual diabetes mellitus with associated clinical history. Subjects with alcoholic chronic pancreatitis are generally thin individuals (often emaciated) and may have stigmata associated with extensive alcohol use and associated liver failure. An inflammatory mass may be palpable but typically abdominal guarding precludes adequate deep palpation. There are no definitive findings on physical exam.

Diffuse intraductal calcium deposition is pathognomonic of chronic pancreatitis and this may be demonstrated by plain abdominal radiographs in 30 percent of cases. Ultrasonagraphic evaluation is 60–70 percent sensitive for intraductal abnormalities and computed tomography is 90 percent sensitive. Endoscopic retrograde cholangiopancreatography (ERCP) is the "gold standard" for chronic pancreatitis based on ductal abnormalities which are graded by severity. Newer, noninvasive imaging studies include magnetic resonance cholangio-pancreatography. Elevated serum amylase and lipase levels indicate a pancreatic exocrine cell damaging process. Pancreatic function tests have found less utility with improved sensitivity of other diagnostic modalities.

A system of stratification or subgroupings of patients by morphological or functional criteria has never been agreed upon.[19] Differential diagnoses must include pancreatic cancer but also include peptic ulcer disease, irritable bowel syndrome, gallstones, and endometriosis. An initial first step in the management of pain in patients with chronic pancreatitis is the exclusion of complications that can be the cause of the pain such as pseudocysts or compression of adjacent visceral structures.[24]

The literature related to the treatment of pain in chronic pancreatitis consists of numerous retrospective collections of patients subjected to treatments determined by interest in applying a certain method.[19] Until recently, few studies of chronic pancreatitis pain have employed placebo-controlled methodologies. Those that have, generally demonstrated limited effects of the studied treatment. Interventional/procedural studies have generally not had controls performed. The symptomatology of chronic pancreatitis is episodic in nature with frequent exacerbations and spontaneous resolution. Hence, any "open" study which is initiated during an exacerbation (when the patient presents to the study physician for treatment) is likely to be deemed effective in some patients due to the natural course of the disease. Therapeutic options for chronic pancreatitis are listed in **Box 40.4** and a suggested treatment pathway given in **Figure 40.1**.

For alcoholic chronic pancreatitis, the initial treatment is abstinence from alcohol. If the patient continues to drink, their five-year mortality rate approaches 50 percent; if they do not drink, it takes 25 years to achieve a mortality rate of 50 percent. Psychological therapies directed toward developing alternative coping mechanisms and abstaining from alcohol are considered vitally necessary, but outcomes related to substance abuse treatment are mixed and not limited to this specific population. It has been commonly reported that total abstinence from alcohol achieves pain relief in up to 50 percent of patients, particularly those with mild to moderate disease,[24, 26] but even this tenet of care has been questioned.[33]

The endoscopic placement of stents, sphincterotomy, dilatation, and/or stone removal are well-established alternatives to surgery in the treatment of biliary tract diseases, and similar techniques for the relief of chronic pancreatic pain have developed.[28] However, recent randomized comparisons of endoscopic versus surgical management of ductal obstruction have suggested superiority of surgical intervention.[29, 32] Extracorporeal shock-wave lithotripsy with or without associated endoscopic procedures to remove stones from pancreatic ducts has been effective at reducing pain.[30, 34]

Box 40.4 Treatment options for chronic pancreatitis pain

- Abstinence from alcohol[25][IV], [26][III]
- Opioids[19][IV]
- Anti-inflammatories[26][IV]
- Antioxidants and micronutrients[27][V]
- Endoscopic management (stents, sphincterotomy, stone removal)[28][IV], [29][III], [30][III], [25][IV]
- Oral pancreatic enzyme treatment[25][IV]
- Neurolysis[21][V]
- Intraceliac steroid injections[31][V]
- Surgical diversion or resection[32][III]
- Pseudocystic drainage (percutaneous, endoscopic, surgical)[32][III]

Opioids are the primary analgesic therapy of advanced chronic pancreatitis,[25] although some have suggested use of "adjuvants" such as antidepressants. There is the unfortunate but common experience of clinicians that patients who have alcoholic pancreatitis may exchange their alcohol addiction for an opioid addiction. Patients with substance abuse histories develop painful diseases and ethically require treatment, but clinicians still experience significant angst in association with their patients' symptomatic treatment. Both corticosteroids and nonsteroidal anti-inflammatory drugs (NSAIDs) would seem logical choices in the treatment of a chronic inflammatory process. However, case reports[35, 36] of pancreatitis induced by these agents has temporized their use.

Based on the oxidative stress hypothesis, placebo-controlled medical trials of antioxidants and micronutrients such as vitamins C and E, β-carotene, S-adenosylmethionine, and selenium have produced favorable results.[25, 27] Oral pancreatic enzyme treatments have been utilized as inhibitors of pancreatic enzyme secretion with a resultant decrease in intraductal pressure. This negative feedback strategy has been effective at reducing pain and improving quality of life in some studies[37] but results overall have been mixed.[25] Negative feedback inhibition of pancreatic secretion can also be provided by somatostatin or its analogue octreotide and have similarly had mixed results related to pain, but they clearly affect some of the processes thought to be associated with complications of pancreatitis thought to be involved in the generation of pain (pseudocysts and fistulas).[25] Other pharmacological therapies that have undergone clinical trials with some measure of success related to pain include kappa opioid receptor agonists,[38] loxiglumide (a CCK-A receptor antagonist), and secretin which also improved pancreatic secretion viscosity[25] A notable failure in clinical trial was use of montelukast, a leukotriene receptor antagonist, which failed to have any effect on pain.[39]

Celiac plexus blocks with local anesthetics have been used for diagnostic purposes,[40] as part of protocols for the determination of eligibility for surgical treatment[41] and as primary therapies when coupled with steroids.[31, 40] It is notable that series reporting the efficacy of intraceliac plexus steroids did not compare their treatment with systemic steroids, although significant central nervous system effects of the steroids (i.e. acute mania) have been reported.[42] NCPBs have been performed using alcohol or phenol. NCPB for the treatment of nonmalignant pancreatic pain has both proponents[43] and opponents.[44] Fugere and Lewis[45] reviewed 20 series in which NCPBs were utilized for chronic pancreatitis and concluded that there were deficiencies in every report stating that most of the studies were not prospective, randomized, or controlled. They also noted that results of NCPB on chronic pancreatitis pain were not as good as those for cancer-related pain. Enthusiasm for NCPB for chronic pancreatitis has also been tempered by

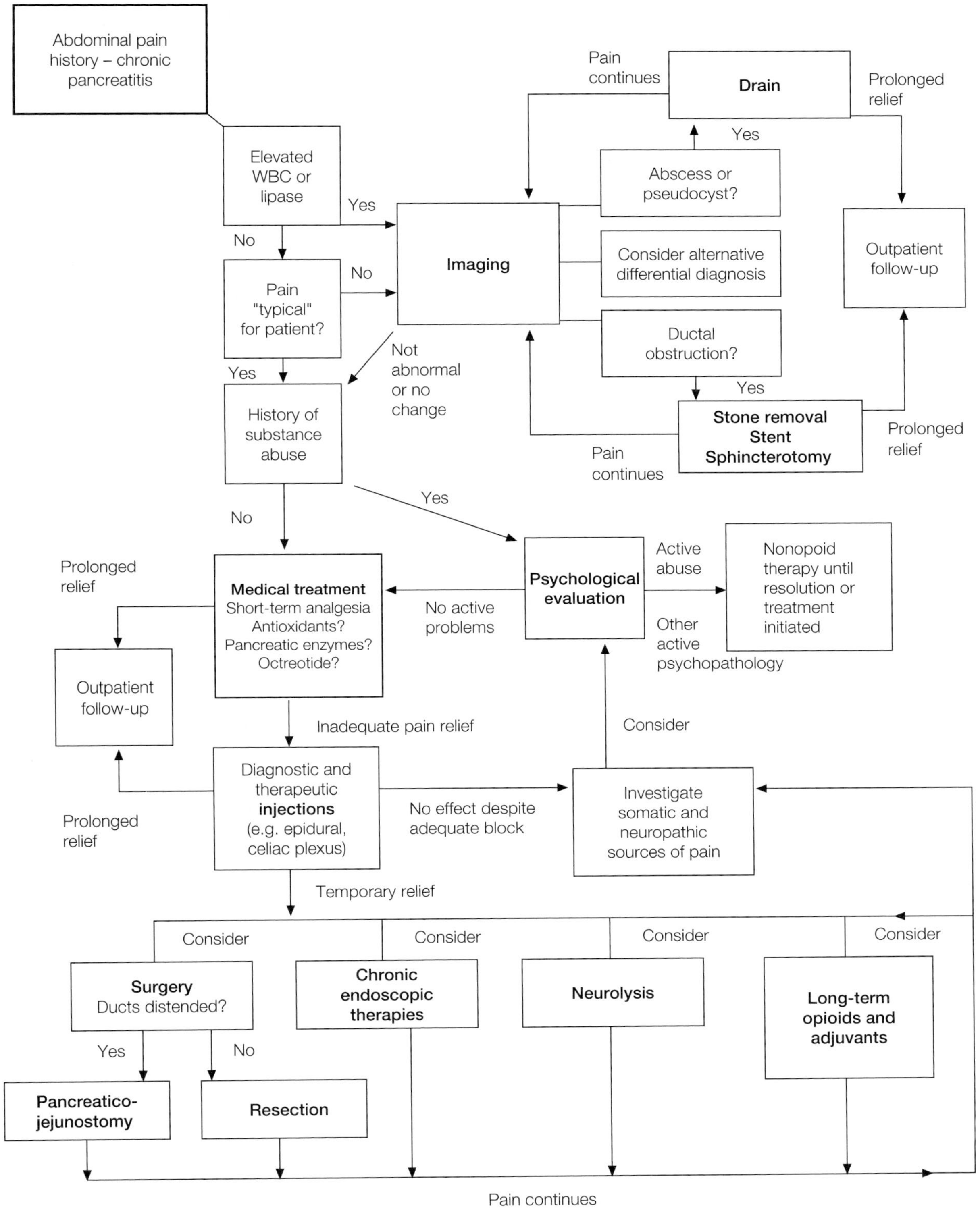

Figure 40.1 Proposed flow diagram for the evaluation and treatment of the patient presenting with chronic pancreatitis-related pain.

the apparent limited duration of effect requiring retreatment (e.g. two to six months),[44] secondary side effects such as chronic diarrhea,[46] and the occurrence of uncommon but catastrophic neurological sequelae.[47, 48, 49] Other forms of injection therapy have also been employed including bilateral splanchnic nerve blocks, intrapleural anesthetics, and epidural infusions in open trials and anecdotal reports.

Surgical treatment is often viewed as the definitive treatment of chronic pancreatitis despite the absence of prospective randomized studies. As noted before, when compared with endoscopic procedural therapies related to ductal decompression, surgical interventions proved superior at two- and/or five-year follow-ups.[29, 32] Relief of ductal hypertension/obstruction by surgical means is via pancreaticojejunostomy or by partial or total resection of the pancreas. Following total resection, the loss of the endocrine function of the pancreas leads to diabetes mellitus with its own associated morbidity and mortality.

Pancreatic pseudocysts are nonepithelialized sacs of pancreatic fluids and/or blood and necrotic debris with apparently inadequate drainage. They enlarge, are frequently painful, and risk rupture of their contents into the peritoneal cavity. Treatments have been predominantly procedural with open or percutaneous drainage, followed by marsupialization (connection of the cyst to nearby gastrointestinal structure) if recurrent. Following surgical drainage of pseudocysts, it has been reported that 96 percent of patients report short-term relief of pain and 53 percent remain pain free for many years.[50] No prospective, randomized studies related to pseudocyst drainage have been reported.

Visceral neurolysis via surgical splanchnicectomy or celiac ganglionectomy has been reported. The best results have been reported by Mallet-Guy[51] in a series of 215 patients treated with a combination of surgery and/or neurolysis. Ninety-eight patients had biliary diversions, biliary-enteric bypasses, or external drainage performed in addition to neurolysis; the other 117 patients had only exploratory surgery and neurolysis. Results were not stratified between groups. Five years after their surgery 5 percent of the patients had died, 8 percent had recurrence of their pain, 13 percent were lost to follow up and 74 percent were characterized as free from pain and relapsing effects (90 percent of living/available patients). Thoracoscopic splanchnic nerve resections have been reported.[52] Surgical neurolysis as a treatment for pain due to chronic pancreatitis has not been subjected to an RCT.

It has been proposed that the pain of chronic pancreatitis will eventually "burn out" and subside as the disease process progresses to total organ failure.[53] Whereas this may occur in some patients, it occurs at a variable rate and may not occur at all.[54] Hence, delay of treatment in the hopes of disease resolution is neither realistic nor ethical.

Interstitial cystitis

At present, there is no agreed upon etiology or pathophysiology for interstitial cystitis (IC). The only defining pathology is the presence of mucosal ulcers or "glomerulations" (small submucosal petechial hemorrhages) viewed cystoscopically after hydrodistension (sustained distension of the bladder). The presence of Hunner's (mucosal) ulcers, so named after the first clinician to describe them, separates IC patients into those with ulcerative versus nonulcerative types. Glomerulations are not unique to IC, but occur in other forms of cystitis (e.g. radiation cystitis). Theories related to the development of IC have centered around four primary hypotheses:

1. that a disruption of the normal urothelial barrier has occurred and bladder sensory nerves are being activated by urinary constituents;
2. that a systemic autoimmune disease is presenting as a local manifestation;
3. that abnormal mast cell activity occurs within the bladder; and
4. that alterations in peripheral and/or central nervous system structures have led to a neuropathic type of pain.

The frequent association of IC with other chronic diseases and pain syndromes such as inflammatory bowel disease, systemic lupus erythematosus, irritable bowel syndrome, "sensitive" skin, fibromyalgia, and allergies[55] speaks to the fact there may be multiple different pathophysiologies grouped together under one diagnosis. Recent studies have demonstrated some histopathological differences in bladder biopsies from patients with IC versus normal controls with increased expression of substance P-containing nerve fibers and substance P receptor-encoding mRNA,[56, 57] increased nerve growth factor content,[58] and altered mast cell activity.[59] The meaning of these findings is still to be determined.

Prevalence of IC is estimated to be 2 in 10,000.[60] It has a female to male ratio of 10:1 although some are proposing that in males it may have a higher prevalence but is given the diagnosis of prostatitis. Patients with IC are 10–12 times more likely to report childhood bladder problems than the general population. Although a history of urinary tract infection is twice as common in IC patients than non-IC patients, most report infrequent urinary tract infections (<1/year) prior to the onset of their IC symptoms. Urgency, frequency, nocturia, and associated pain are the primary symptoms of IC.[61] Pain may be localized to the lower abdomen, pelvis, groin, and/or perineum. The onset of the disease is normally abrupt with rapid progression of symptomatology, often following an "event" such as a prolonged episode of severe urgency while searching for a lavatory. Anxiety and depression are frequent comorbidities. Suprapubic tenderness to palpation may accompany a diagnosis of IC. As a diagnosis of exclusion, other physical findings and examinations should be negative for identifiable pathology with the exception of abnormal cystometry and cystoscopy.

A reasonable approach for evaluation and treatment has been proposed by Pontari *et al.*,[62] which includes urine cultures, pelvic and rectal exams, cystometry, and cystoscopy. Criteria for IC have been suggested by a consensus panel (**Table 40.1**). Parsons *et al.*[64] have proposed the use of intravesical potassium solutions as a provocative diagnostic test for IC with a sensitivity of 75 percent, but at present this serves only as a research tool.

The ultimate goal of therapy is to neutralize the factor(s) responsible for a disease process. In the absence of any known causative factors, the treatments for IC have been guided by prudence and a given patient's therapy typically progresses from the least invasive treatments and proceeds to the more invasive.[62] A listing of treatments for IC is given in **Box 40.5**. Some studies of treatments have employed placebo-controlled methodologies, but most have been open trials and generally without controls. Up to 50 percent of patients diagnosed with IC have spontaneous remissions with durations of 1–80 months.[60] Any treatment of IC must factor these patients into the "success" rate of that treatment.

Avoidance of foods that exacerbate symptoms (e.g. acidic foods such as cranberry juice) has proven to have great value in individuals, but has not been tested in a controlled fashion in large populations. As part of the diagnostic process, hydrodistension is performed and this procedure often proves to be therapeutic with short-term reductions in frequency and pain in more than half of the patients. Patients with symptomatic improvement for six months or more are considered candidates for repeat hydrodistension.[62] A controlled trial of amitriptyline reported a success rates of 64 percent.[69] Drugs such as oral antihistamines and the oral, renally excreted heparin-like agent, pentosanpolysulfate (Elmiron®) has been examined in placebo-controlled, double-blind studies with variable results.[66] Intravesical therapy with dimethyl sulfoxide (DMSO) and/or heparin and/or corticosteroids and/or bicarbonate has been proposed as effective therapies,[62] as has Clorpactin (a derivative of hypochlorous acid in a buffered base)[77] with success rates ranging from 50 to >90 percent. A controlled comparison of intravesical DMSO with intravesical saline by Perez-Marrero *et al.*[65] demonstrated improvements in symptomatology in 53 percent of the DMSO-treated group and only 18 percent of the saline-treated group. DMSO produces a distinct taste and smell in the patient's breath, so blinded comparisons were not performed. Based on the hypothesis that IC is a local manifestation of a systemic autoimmune disease, immunosuppressant therapies such as systemic cyclosporine[67] and intravesical Bacillus Calmette-Guerin immunotherapy[68] have been utilized in controlled trials with good success rates for the former and insignificant success rates reported for the latter.

Long-term treatment with opioids is an option in patients with IC, but this treatment remains controversial for all nonmalignant processes. Transcutaneous electrical nerve stimulation has been used in open trials and demonstrated to produce good results or remission in 26–54 percent of patients.[70] Behavioral therapies and self-care strategies such as timed voiding have proven to have value in some individuals.[76, 78] A report of a series of 13 patients by Irwin *et al.*[72] suggests that lumbar epidural local anesthetic blocks may have short-term efficacy in up to 75 percent of patients. Novel therapies that have demonstrated some success in controlled trials include the use of hyperbaric oxygen,[79] but the intravesical administration of the vanilloid, resiniferatoxin, proved disappointing.[71]

Neurolysis by percutaneous injection or surgical resection have been described. The most positive results are those of Gillespie[73] who reported on 175 women diagnosed with IC treated with laser obliteration of the

Table 40.1 Interstitial cystitis diagnostic criteria.[63]

Criteria	
I. Inclusion criteria (both required)	
1. Hunner's (mucosal) ulcer or glomerulations on cystoscopy	
2. Pain associated with the bladder or urinary urgency	
II. Exclusion criteria (any of the following)	
Age <18 years old	Symptomatic urethral diverticulum
Radiation cystitis	Uterine/cervical cancer
Cyclophoshamide cystitis	Vaginal or urethral cancer
Tuberculous cystitis	Benign or malignant bladder tumors
Bacterial cystitis or prostatitis in last three months	Bladder or lower ureteral calculi
Active genital herpes	Duration <9 months
Vaginitis	Absence of nocturia
Involuntary bladder contractions	Frequency <8 times per day
No urgency with bladder fill >350 cc	Symptoms relieved by antibiotics, urinary antiseptics, anticholinergics, or antispasmotics
Absence of urgency with 100 cc air or 150 cc water (fill rate 30–100 cc/min)	

Box 40.5 Interstitial cystitis treatment options

Hydrodistension[V]
Dietary modification[61][V]
Intravesical treatments
- Dimethyl sulfoxide[65][III]
- Heparin[66][V]
- Corticosteroids[66][V]
- Bicarbonate[66][V]
- Clorpactin[67][III]
- Bacillus Calmette–Guerin[68][III]

Antidepressants[69][III]
Antihistamines[66][V]
Cyclosporine[67][III]
Opioids[66][V]
Nonsteroidal anti-inflammatories[66][V]
Transcutaneous electrical nerve stimulation[70][V]
Pentosanpolysulfate[67][III]
Resinferatoxin[71][III]
Epidural local anesthetics[72][V]
Neurolysis[73][V]
Surgical resection/diversion[74][V], [75][V]
Behavioral[76][IV]
Physical therapies[61][V]

Criteria proposed by NIDDK Workshop on Interstitial Cystitis.[63]

vesicoureteric plexus bilaterally. One hundred and twelve patients reported complete relief and 58 partial relief following the procedure. Two-year follow-up in 45 patients in the "complete relief" group demonstrated no recurrence of symptoms. Considered a last resort, surgery in the form of supravesical diversions or cystectomy has also received mixed reports of efficacy. For example, Peeker *et al.*[74] reported excellent results in patients with classic (ulcerative) IC and poor results in nonulcerative IC. Webster *et al.*[75] reported that only two of their 14 patients treated surgically with urinary diversion and cystourethrectomy had symptom resolution, and Baskin and Tanagho[80] have reported on patients with continued bladder pain despite the absence of a bladder.

All clinical trials related to IC have been hampered by the inclusion of a likely heterogenous clinical population. This problem may become less problematic in the future with the advent of a diagnostic test that appears to have validity in the IC population. There is a presence of a specific peptide present within the urine of IC patients that impairs urothelial regrowth. Named the anti-proliferative factor (APF), this low molecular weight peptide is a member of the Frizzled 8 protein family and is present in bladder urine, but not renal pelvis urine of IC patients.[81] It has been identified in over 90 percent of rigorously diagnosed IC patients, is not present in other disorders, and is therefore viewed as the best laboratory diagnostic test for IC. The test itself will likely become available widespread pending further validation as a diagnostic test. Whether APF is present due to rheumatological, immunological, infectious, genetic, or neurological causes has not been determined, but it has been demonstrated to produce a downregulation of genes that stimulate epithelial proliferation and upregulates genes that inhibit cell growth. Future clinical trials may finally have a tool that allows for appropriate inclusion and exclusion of appropriate subjects for study.

Irritable bowel syndrome

Irritable bowel syndrome (IBS) is a diagnosis of exclusion that is based on symptomatology and has been demonstrated to have associated abnormalities of motility and/or sensation in different subpopulations. A frequent companion of other disorders without identifiable histopathology such as fibromyalgia, noncardiac chest pain, functional dyspepsia, and mixed headaches, it has similarly been associated with significant DSM-IV diagnoses such as anxiety and depression. There exist many diverse hypotheses related to the etiology of IBS. These propose that the pain may be psychosocial in origin, that the pain may be due to motility dysfunction at one or multiple sites in the gut (with dietary modifiers), or that the pain is a manifestation of visceral hyperalgesia. This visceral hyperalgesia may be due to peripheral sensitizers (e.g. mast cells) or altered central nervous system processing. Like many diagnoses of exclusion, it is likely that multiple pathophysiologies are present in different subgroups and that all of these hypotheses may be correct for different subgroups.

IBS is a common diagnosis given to 40–70 percent of referrals to gastroenterologists. In general populations, up to 20 percent of women and 10 percent of men experience symptomatology consistent with IBS, but most people with these symptoms do not seek medical care. Of those who do seek care, 50–60 percent have significant symptomatology consistent with depression and/or an anxiety disorder. IBS typically presents in the third or fourth decades of life and has a female to male ratio of 2:1. It is present in many cultures with similar prevalences noted in Britain, China, India, Japan, New Zealand, the United States, and South America.

At least three different clinical presentations are given the diagnosis of IBS, two of which have no pain or pain as a minor component (watery diarrhea group and alternating constipation–diarrhea group respectively). The third subgroup has abdominal pain as their primary symptom and altered bowel movements as a secondary or exacerbating complaint. In this group, pain is typically in the left lower quadrant or in the suprapubic region and may be precipitated by food ingestion and a need to defecate. Bloating, mucus in the stools, and flatulence are often prominent and anxiety may exacerbate symptoms. Although there is great variation between patients, the particular symptom complex for a given patient generally remains constant. Generalized abdominal tenderness to palpation is common. The classic physical finding is a tender, palpable mass (the sigmoid colon) in the left lower quadrant. As a diagnosis of exclusion, physical examination, imaging, and laboratory findings should be negative for neoplasm, inflammatory bowel disease, infection, diverticulosis, or other intra-abdominal process. Colonoscopy and/or barium enema radiography should not demonstrate focal lesions. Stool samples should not have occult blood or infectious agents present. It is generally agreed that the colons of patients with IBS are exceptionally reactive to physiological stimuli (e.g. eating) but the finding is not pathognomonic. There are no absolute criteria for the diagnosis of IBS except for a report of abdominal pain and altered bowel habit in the absence of identifiable pathology, but criteria have been proposed to facilitate a "positive" diagnosis (**Box 40.6**). Motility studies and sensation evocation with a distending balloon in the rectum or sigmoid colon may prove valuable in the stratification of patients to different groups, but at present still serve as research tools.

IBS has exacerbations and spontaneous resolution of pains and so "open" trials initiated when the patient presents with an exacerbation can easily demonstrate the effectiveness of virtually any therapy. Placebo rates of 40–70 percent have been quoted.[83] Unlike chronic pancreatitis or interstitial cystitis, procedural treatments have not been a major component of therapy because, by definition of the disease, there is no structural pathology to treat. Controlled studies have been performed, but are likely hampered by the multiple pathophysiologies that are all diagnosed as IBS. Without definitive, objective diagnostic criteria by which to stratify patients, it is likely that effective treatments will similarly be difficult to demonstrate. Due to the typically stable nature of a patient's symptom complex, once significant pathology has been ruled out, additional or repeat investigation is probably not necessary unless the symptom complex were to change.[84, 85]

As in any chronic pain disorder, an important (but not particularly testable) component to the management of IBS is a stable, trusting patient–physician relationship. Life-threatening pathology may be simply ruled out without an exhaustive investigation and the patient needs to be assured that their symptoms are believed. Therapeutic options for IBS are listed in **Box 40.7**. As part of a diagnostic/therapeutic trial, patients are generally advised to engage in dietary modifications such as avoiding milk products, avoiding excessive legume consumption (associated with gas production), increasing fiber and bran in those with constipation,[86, 93] avoiding caffeine- or sorbitol-containing foods, and establishing a stable dietary pattern in the hope of establishing a stable evacuation routine. Anticholinergics/antidiarrheals have been extensively employed clinically and extensively studied. Reviews of the efficacy of these agents have concluded that their benefit is unproven.[93] Traditional advice has been to keep analgesic therapy to a minimum with the use of opioids particularly discouraged. Recently, various antidepressants have been demonstrated to have efficacy in controlled studies.[90, 91, 92] Drugs acting via serotonin receptors as either 5HT-3 antagonists (alosetron) or 5HT-4 agonists (tegaserod) have been utilized in clinical practice[95] but ischemic colitis has proven to be a problematic side effect[96] resulting in some restriction of use. Peripherally restricted kappa opioid receptor agonists have found some utility in experimental trials.[94] Gastrokinetic agents, anti-diarrheals, serotonin receptor antagonists, osmotic laxatives, naloxone, cholecystokinin antagonists, and peppermint oil have all been proposed as effective. Injection therapies have not been generally employed in the treatment of IBS but a neurolytic

Box 40.6 Diagnostic criteria for irritable bowel syndrome

No identifiable neoplastic, infectious or inflammatory etiology for symptoms
Three months of continuous or recurrent symptoms of abdominal pain which is
- Relieved by defecation, *or*
- Associated with a change in stool consistency, *or*
- Associated with a change in stool frequency with two of the following:
  - Altered stool frequency (>3/day or <3/week)
  - Altered stool form
  - Altered stool passage (straining, urgency, incomplete evac.)
  - Passage of mucus
  - Abdominal bloating

From ROME II criteria.[82]

Box 40.7 Treatment options for irritable bowel syndrome

Dietary modification
- Food avoidance (caffeine, milk products, legumes)[84][V]
- Addition of fiber/bran/bulking agents[86][IV]

Behavioral therapies[87][III], [88][III], [89][II]
Antidepressants[90][III], [91][III], [92][III]
Anticholinergics/antispasmotics[93][II]
Kappa opioid receptor agonists[94][III]
Serotonin receptor agonists/antagonists[95][III]

celiac plexus block has been reported as useful in the treatment of idiopathic abdominal pain.[97] Behavioral treatments such as hypnosis, cognitive-behavioral therapy, and supportive psychotherapy have proven valuable, especially if pain is intermittent and there is identified psychiatric disease such as anxiety or depression.[87] Swedlund *et al.*,[88] in a prospective, randomized study of 99 patients with the diagnosis of IBS, demonstrated that those patients who received eight psychotherapy sessions (and antispasmotics and bulking agents) had less abdominal pain, better bowel movements, and less psychological distress at both three and 15 months following treatment than similar patients treated only with antispasmotics and bulking agents. Other studies have been less supportive of behavioral treatments.[89]

OTHER PAINFUL DISORDERS

General

The disorders of pancreatic cancer, chronic pancreatitis, IBS, and IC have been presented as archetypal examples illustrative of most of the problems facing the clinician in the diagnosis and management of this type of pain. In the case of pancreatic cancer, we have a disorder that has definable histopathology, is accepted as pain-producing by all caregivers, and elicits intensive and aggressive treatment. Palliative surgery, high dose narcotics, and therapeutic interventions such as neurolysis are considered standards of care. This contrasts with IC and IBS, disorders for which reassurance and "watchful waiting" are considered appropriate care, with aggressive treatments reserved for the patients who complain loudest and longest. For these disorders narcotics have been viewed as controversial at best and contraindicated in many patients. Chronic pancreatitis is somewhere intermediate to these other disorders in that definable pathology is present but this pathology does not correlate with pain symptomatology. Chronic pancreatitis has the additional factor of having a high incidence in substance abusers. It also has a frequent association with life-threatening complications such as pancreatic necrosis, malnutrition, and pseudocyst formation and so frequently may lead to hospitalization. Other sources of chronic abdominal visceral pain as well as urogenital and rectal pain syndromes producing groin and perineal symptomatology[98] all have correlates with these disorders and diagnostic work-ups and therapies are similar. A limited discussion of several of these painful disorders and their correlation to the above four archetype disorders will be given below.

Other visceral cancers

For a full discussion of this topic, see the *Cancer Pain* volume of this series.

Neoplasms can arise in all abdominal and pelvic structures. Symptomatology related to these neoplasms is similar for all sites with dull constant pain a common "early" symptom. Pain is generally localized to the chest or upper abdomen for upper gastrointestinal tract lesions and organs located in the upper abdomen. It is generally localized to lower abdomen/perineum for lower gastrointestinal tract lesions and pelvic organs. The key statement is "generally" since no symptomatology or location is pathognomonic for any specific disease site due to the frequent presence of metastatic extension prior to diagnosis. Visceral cancers are frequently asymptomatic until obstruction or invasion of other structures occurs. Anorexia, weight loss, fatigue, nausea, and virtually every other nonspecific symptom can be noted at presentation. Anemia, hematemesis, melena, hematuria, and palpable masses on physical exam may direct further investigation. Appropriate imaging and surgical exploration/biopsy are the definitive diagnostic modalities.

Sources of pain can be visceral due to the primary tumor or somatic/neuropathic due to local involvement and metastases. Cancer treatments themselves may be pain-producing. All of these sources of pain are similar to those described above under Pancreatic cancer (**Box 40.2**). Patterns of tumor spread differ between types of tumors and so general patterns of symptomatology related to metastases also differ. Gastrointestinal tumors tend to spread through the lymphatics towards the liver and may present with diffuse abdominal complaints. In contrast, prostatic tumors frequently spread relatively early to involve the lumbar spine and so may present as back pain. Pain treatment options for all cancers are similar to that described for pancreatic cancer (**Box 40.3**). Treatment of the cancer (surgery, chemotherapy, radiotherapy) may be curative or palliative. Neuroablation is an option with the particular site of treatment determined by the site of the symptomatic cancer (see **Figure 035.1** in Chapter 3, Applied physiology: persistent visceral pain). Celiac plexus blocks may be of benefit for tumors in the upper abdomen, superior hypogastric blocks for tumors in the pelvis and, recently, blockade of the ganglion of Impar[99] has been suggested as beneficial for perirectal/perineal symotomatology. Stenting of obstructed ureters or bowel segments may be necessary as well as potential surgical diversion (e.g. loop colostomy). Psychological interventions are always deemed appropriate in patients with an end-stage disease. Medical treatments are often empirically driven with the aggressive use of opioids, anti-inflammatories, antiemetics, and adjuvants appropriate for end-stage disease.

The "problems" that occur in cancer pain management are those that are present when the cancer has responded to treatment, but the treatment itself has proved to be pain-producing. Radiation enteritis/colitis, postsurgical phantoms, neuroma formation, neuropathies, altered biomechanics, adhesions/strictures, and other effects of "scarring" can all act as generators or modulators of pain that could also potentially represent tumor recurrence.

The associated roller coaster of emotions associated with the investigation, reinvestigation, or lack of investigation of symptoms can prove taxing to both the patient and clinician. Even definitive evidence of complications such as endoscopic confirmation of radiation changes or nerve conduction studies consistent with neuropathy do not absolve the clinician of the need for ongoing care. What constitutes appropriate care is somewhat fuzzy as the distinction between palliative care for pain due to metastatic cancer and that for chronic "benign" pain in a patient with a history of cancer is unclear and lapses into the realm of opinion.

Inflammatory bowel disease

Ulcerative colitis (UC) and Crohn's disease (CD) are two recurrent gastrointestinal inflammatory disorders with many similarities in symptomatology and histopathology, but significant differences in extent of the disease process, relapse incidence, and associated complications such as fistula formation. Common presenting symptoms include abdominal pain, fever, and altered bowel habits such as bloody diarrhea. Inflammatory bowel disease is more common in white than black people or Asians and three to six times more common in Jews than non-Jews. UC is three to five times more common than CD, but recurrent exacerbations are much less frequent. In UC, the gastrointestinal component of the disease process is restricted to the colon whereas in CD there is involvement in all portions of the gastrointestinal tract. Extracolonic features of inflammatory bowel disease include arthritis, skin changes, and evidence of liver disease. The diagnosis of inflammatory bowel disease is based on biopsy, colonoscopic/endoscopic appearances, and/or surgical evaluation. Other causes of inflammatory changes such as radiation enteritis or local infection (e.g. shigella, salmonella, amebiasis, *Clostridium difficile*) must be ruled out. Local complications of inflammatory bowel disease include the formation of fistulas, abscesses, strictures, perforation, and toxic dilation, all of which are more common in CD than UC. With a prolonged clinical course there is a potential for the development of carcinoma. There is a stated incidence of colon cancer of 1/2–1 percent per year for every year after the initial ten years of active inflammatory bowel disease. Surgical treatment of inflammatory bowel disease is normally reserved for the treatment of complications with 20–25 percent of UC patients requiring colectomy and 70 percent of patients with CD. Colectomy presumably resolves UC, but does not resolve all of the symptoms of CD since the disease process is panenteric.

Dietary alterations may have some acute effects during a "flare" but have not been demonstrated to alter overall disease progression. Neurolysis is typically avoided since symptoms may act as early indicators of life-threatening complications. Regional anesthetic techniques, although of possible short-term benefit during a flare, have the same risks as neurolysis in that they may mask disease complications. Surgery has remained an integral component in the management of inflammatory bowel disease. Pain treatment related to inflammatory bowel disease forms a limited-choice corollary to chronic pancreatitis (**Box 40.4**). Whereas UC is potentially "cured" by colectomy, CD continues for a lifetime. Overall, treatments are considered palliative for CD with varying degrees of evidence for implementation.[100] Surgical resection of portions of inflamed bowel, strictures, or abscesses/fistulas are not uncommon in CD but the strategies associated with surgical treatment continue to evolve. Surgical interventions may result in temporary relief until another site is affected but such resections may also result in a "short bowel" with associated nutritional compromise. Since reports of pain may be associated with life-threatening complications, these patients may have frequent hospitalizations. The use of opioids and other motility-altering drugs carries the perception of an increased risk of toxic dilation with an associated increase in morbidity and mortality. Similar to other diseases with unknown etiologies, genetic influences, immunologic abnormalities, and infectious agents have all been implicated and used as rationales for treatment. Primary treatment for exacerbations is typically bowel rest, anti-inflammatories (e.g. oral sulfasalazine, possible corticosteroids), nutritional/fluid/electrolyte management, and treatment of complications. No universal consensus appears to exist in relation to preventative treatment. Multiple therapies such as oral sulfasalazine, oral mesalazine, oral olsalazine, oral metronidazole, systemic corticosteroids, and mesalamine enemas/suppositories have been utilized not only as reactive treatments for exacerbations but as prophylactic measures. Although results related to use of these agents are encouraging for UC, a multicenter study failed to observe any decrease in the recurrence of CD exacerbations even with sulfasalazine. Immunosuppressants such as azothioprine, methotrexate, and cyclosporine have been used for a presumed immunologic etiology. Recent use of drugs known to affect inflammatory responses in rheumatological disorders has been encouraging[101] with successful clinical trials reported for infliximab[102] but not for etanercept.[103] Granulocyte-macrophage colony-stimulating factor has also had encouraging results related to improvements in quality of life and decreased disease severity.[104, 105] Novel anibiotics such as rifaximin[106] or probiotics[107] as treatments have been suggested, particularly for the prevention of extra-gastrointestinal symptoms such as arthralgias. Psychological treatments are justified by the presence of a life-long, recurrent disease process.[108]

Chronic mesenteric ischemia – ischemic colitis

Inadequate blood supply to meet the energy demands of viscera can lead to reports of pain, as occurs with cardiac angina. A similar phenomenon has been noted in the gastrointestinal system whereby severe abdominal pain may be precipitated by the ingestion of a meal.[109, 110] Fear of eating with subsequent weight loss and poor nutritional status may further compromise patients already in ill health due to atherosclerotic disease in multiple sites. Poor peripheral pulses, abdominal bruits, and arteriographic evidence of stenosis or occlusion in the three main mesenteric arteries are all consistent with the diagnosis of abdominal angina. Similar to cardiac disease, abdominal angina may precede infarction which has devastating life-threatening consequences. Arterial thrombosis, embolic events, venous occlusion, and low flow states due to poor cardiac output may all lead to the same disastrous results. Ischemic colitis represents approximately half of the cases of morbidity due to mesenteric vascular disease. Although usually diagnosed by colonoscopy, 20 percent of patients with ischemic colitis develop evidence of peritonitis requiring surgical diagnosis and treatment. Initial presentation may be with persistent diarrhea, rectal bleeding, or weight loss. Diagnostic work-up for mesenteric ischemia has angiography as the gold standard, but the less invasive magnetic resonance angiography and/or tonometry have diagnostic value.[111] Surgical revascularization, thrombectomy, thrombolytic therapy, or angioplasty are definitive treatments for mesenteric vasculopathy but, like all patients with widespread vascular disease, comorbidity may dictate outcome as much as the specific procedure performed. Pharmacologically, there can be short-term value of vasodilators such as papverine and, like most chronic processes with some low grade inflammatory component, there appears to be a role for the use of antioxidants and agents acting via cytokine mechanisms, but at present these treatments are experimental.[112]

Diverticular disease

Diverticuli can occur throughout the gastrointestinal tract but prove to be most common in the colon where they exist as small sac-like herniations of mucosa through the muscular wall, typically at the site of penetrating blood vessels. Duodenal, jejuna, and ileal diverticuli can occur with Meckel's diverticulum forming a special congenital abnormality present in 2 percent of the population. Meckel's diverticuli are particularly notable since they may contain acid-producing gastric mucosa and lead to enteral ulcer formation. Colonic diverticuli are generally pain free but with the development of inflammation and/or obstruction of their mouth, severe abdominal pain and infection may result. Peridiverticular abscesses, obstruction, colonic distension, bleeding, and altered bowel habit (diarrhea, constipation) are not uncommon. Painful diverticulosis classically presents as recurrent left lower quadrant colicky pain without evidence of inflammation. Like chronic pancreatitis, diverticular disease can produce pain which is episodic and which can have life-threatening consequences if ignored. Bleeding diverticuli are the most common sources of lower gastrointestinal tract bleeding[113] and segmental colonic resection has the highest success rate at stopping bleeding. However, effects on pain are unclear. Reports of pain do not always correlate with observable pathology and symptoms can be nonspecific. A European surgical consensus panel was not able to definitively state when surgery was indicated for symptomatic reasons and called for RCTs.[114] The poorly absorbed antibiotic rifaximin, normally used to treat traveller's diarrhea, has also been demonstrated to treat and prevent recurrences of symptomatic diverticular disease in controlled trials and large clinical series.[115, 116] Similar results have been noted with use of the anti-inflammatory mesalazine (mesalamine).[117]

Familial Mediterranean fever

An autosomal recessive genetic disease linked to chromosome 16, familial Mediterranean fever begins at age 5–15[118] (**Box 40.1**). Referred to as a trait of the sons of Shem (one of Noah's sons) due to its increased incidence in Sephardic Jews, Armenians, Turks, and Arabs, the known gene mutations have also been found in substantial numbers of people from other Mediterranean populations. Linked to alterations in the innate immune system involving the protein pyrin, the pathogenesis of this and other periodic fever syndromes is still being defined.[119] Features that are classic include periodic febrile episodes without identified triggering event, serous peritonitis, pleuritis, synovitis, and a rash that may resemble erysipelas. Abdominal pain of varying intensity occurs in 95 percent of the episodes with chest pain and arthralgias in 75 percent of episodes. The frequency of the episodes may vary from twice per week to once per year, but most commonly occur at two- to four-week intervals with acute episodes typically lasting between one and three days. Amyloidosis with associated kidney failure and athralgia are the most severe associated sequelae. Leukocytosis and elevated sedimentation rate may be present on laboratory exam. Typical treatment is episodic with the use of systemic analgesics although case reports support use of modalities such as intermittent spinal cord stimulation.[120] In controlled studies, daily colchicine has been demonstrated to decrease the frequency of attacks and risks of amyloidosis and is the treatment recommendation of a European consensus conference.[121] Prophylactic antibiotics, hormones, antipyretics, immunotherapy, psychotherapy, dietary alterations, chloroquine, and phenylbutazone have all been tried without success.

Porphyria

Several related genetic disorders, all characterized by the increased formation of porphyrins or their precursors, are termed porphyria[122, 123] (**Box 40.1**). Three subgroups have been identified which all have similar symptomatology: intermittent acute porphyria (IAP), hereditary coproporphyria, and variegate porphyria. Of these, IAP is the most frequently encountered with attacks of colicky abdominal pain that are intermittent, may be associated with environmental exposures, and which can last for days to months. Transmitted as an autosomal dominant disorder with incomplete penetrance, family history may or may not be helpful in the diagnosis. Certain drugs such as barbiturates, benzodiazepines, alcohol, phenytoin, ketamine, etomidate, meprobamate, and corticosteroids have been particularly implicated as "triggers" although use of many of these agents without the precipitation of a crisis has been reported. Constipation, abdominal distension, and profuse vomiting are common. Neurological dysfunction may occur principally due to demyelination effects with emotional disturbance a nonspecific symptom. Urine and blood tests related to porphyria may only be diagnostic during crises. Genetic testing of asymptomatic members in IAP families may allow for avoidance of triggers. Treatment is avoiding known triggers, treating crises with intravenous fluids, hemin, and/or increased carbohydrate intake, and treating pain and nausea with "safe" analgesics/antiemetics. Most opioids are alleged to be nontriggering, a notable exception is the mixed agonist–antagonist pentazocine. Chlorpromazine, promethazine, and droperidol have all been reported to be safe as antiemetics.

Orchialgia

Like abdominal pain, pain localized to the testes has a wide differential diagnosis.[124] Local processes such as tumor, infection (e.g. epididymitis), varicocele/hydrocele/spermatocele, and testicular torsion are all potentially acute and chronic sources of pain. Previous surgeries such as inguinal hernia repair and vasectomy, as well as non-iatrogenic trauma, can all lead to chronic inflammatory processes as well as altered sensation and associated chronic pain. Neuropathic etiologies ranging from diabetic neuropathy and entrapment neuropathies to spinal disk disease may all present with testicular pain. An uncommon side effect of statin drugs has been orchialgia.[125] Scrotal pain should be differentiated from testicular pain since the nerve supplies differ and may represent differing sites of pathology along sacral versus thoracolumbar pathways. Due to the "personal" nature of the site of pain, concerns related to psychological etiologies or sequelae of this chronic pain are maintained.

Treatment of chronic orchialgia forms a correlate to the disease entity of interstitial cystitis (**Box 40.5**) with numerous treatments proposed for a disease of unknown but presumably localized etiology. Traditional pain management has started with anti-inflammatories and/or antibiotics. Surgical procedures including epididymectomy, orchiectomy, or denervation procedures have been recommended,[126] but long-term outcomes are unknown and retrospective series have suggested limited benefit in "pain-prone" patients. Wesselmann *et al.*[98] have suggested that there may be benefit from low dose antidepressants, anticonvulsants, membrane-stabilizing agents, opiates and, in some patients, repeated lumbar sympathetic blocks, oral sympatholytics, and repeated infusions of phentolamine. Case reports support use of pulsed radiofrequency procedures.[127] Because of the wide differential diagnosis of testicular pain, no specific treatment will be universally effective, and no good interventional studies are available for guidance.

Chronic prostatitis/chronic pelvic pain syndrome

Chronic prostatitis/chronic pelvic pain syndrome (CP/CPPS) is defined as pain attributed to the prostate in the absence of identifiable pathology and has often been referred to as prostatodynia. Hallmark features consist of persistent complaints of urinary urgency, dysuria, poor urinary flow, and perineal discomfort without evidence of bacteria or white blood cells in prostatic fluids. It serves as a male-specific corollary to interstitial cystitis in that it has similar symptomatology, is a diagnosis of exclusion, and has a presumed site of pain generation. Infectious, inflammatory, neurological, and referred gastroenterological etiologies of the pain need to be ruled out. Cystoscopic findings of interstitial cystitis have been found in males with the diagnosis of prostatodynia.[61] Wesselmann *et al.*[98] have suggested that interstitial cystitis, CP/CPPS (male), and vulvodynia (female) may all be variations of a generalized disorder of the epithelium of the urogenital sinus. To further quote Wesselmann *et al.*,[98] no strikingly successful treatment options have been described. As with interstitial cystitis, treatments may be empiric trials of medications employed in the treatment of any other chronic pain. Antibiotics are commonly employed despite the absence of evidence for a microbiological etiology. Numerous clinical trials have been performed with improvement in symptoms associated with use of alpha adrenergic-blocking agents, transurethral microwave hyperthermia or dilation procedures, pelvic floor relaxation techniques, oral pentosan polysulfate, antioxidant therapies, and use of muscle-relaxing agents all with some efficacy in population subsets. Since monotherapies have proven to be of limited benefit in this disorder combination therapies are now being employed.[128]

Post cholecystectomy syndrome

Gallbladder inflammation, gallstones, and associated pathology of the biliary tract are known sources of acute pain that is typically coupled with dyspepsia and occasionally jaundice when obstructive. However, even after surgical resection of the gallbladder, pain may continue which is termed postcholecystectomy syndrome. In a follow-up study, Vetrhus *et al.*[129] found that 27 percent of patients who underwent cholecystectomy for uncomplicated gallstone disease or acute cholecystitis continued to have persistent abdominal pain five years after their surgery. Typically in the right upper quadrant of the abdomen, its symptomatology is similar to that of cholecystitis in that it may be exacerbated by eating, may be associated with nausea, and is described as continuous during the day, dull and frequently colicky. Appropriate workup will rule out definable pathology such as a retained bile duct stone or secondary pancreatitis. It is a correlate to chronic pancreatitis in that there may be abnormal pressures or motility within the biliary duct. Endoscopic demonstration of elevated sphincter of Oddi pressures suggest sphincter dysfunction as the cause of the syndrome which has also been termed a "functional" disorder.[130] During endoscopic retrograde cholangiopancreatography it may be possible to reproduce the pain by producing intraductal distension. Endoscopic or surgical sphinterotomy or sphinteroplasty have been beneficial in series reports and calcium channel blockers or long-acting nitrates have been proposed as therapeutic when sphincterotomy is not possible. Other treatment options are similar to chronic pancreatitis with dietary alterations, surgical re-explorations, focal injections/neurolysis, and traditional analgesics all suggested as therapeutic options. In many cases there is no objective identification of a site of pain generation so treatment is empiric. In many cases, the cholecystectomy was one aspect of this empiric treatment.

Proctalgia fugax

Episodic spasms (seconds to minutes) of pain localized to the rectum/anus, occurring at irregular intervals and without identifiable cause, are termed proctalgia fugax.[131] Highly prevalent, occurring in 14–19 percent of healthy subjects, the episodes are brief (seconds to minutes) and infrequent (normally <6/year). They may be precipitated by bowel movements, sexual activity, stress, and temperature changes and so may lead to avoidance behavior on the part of the patient. No etiology or method of treating/preventing proctalgia fugax has been universally accepted. Spasm of the sigmoid colon, levator ani, and/or pelvic floor musculature have been postulated as sources of the pain. If episodes are prolonged (>20 minutes) then the disorder is termed chronic proctalgia rather than proctalgia fugax and the likelihood of involvement of the levator ani musculature is increased, particularly if there is tenderness with posterior traction on the puborectalis during physical exam.[131] Local anorectal pathology such as fissures or abscesses need to be ruled out as alternate sources of pain and spasm. Due to the brief nature of most episodes, most reactive pharmacological treatments have usually proved inadequate although inhaled salbutamol, clonidine, nitroglycerin, antispasmotics, and calcium channel blockers have all been reported as effective. Heat or pressure applied to the perineum, food/drink consumption, dilation of the anal sphincter, assumption of a knee–chest position, and assumption of other postures have been anecdotally reported as beneficial.

Recurrent urolithiasis

Stones located within the urinary system (renal pelvis/calices, ureters, bladder, urethra) can produce severe pain (renal colic) and if sufficiently obstructive to urine flow can destroy kidney function. It occurs in 15 percent of white men and 6 percent of all women in industrialized countries.[132] Recurrent in "stone-formers," it may produce continuous pain when numerous or large renal pelvic (staghorn) calculi are present. Diagnosis is based on history of stone formation and/or imaging studies (intravenous pyelogram or computed tomography). The definitive treatment is the removal of the stone by spontaneous passage which may be assisted by fragmentation using lithotripsy or surgical removal. Drugs producing a relaxation effect in the ureters include NSAIDs, nifedipine, and tamsulosin. Pain treatments employed for renal colic are intended to be "temporizing" until stone removal occurs. As such, narcotics and NSAIDs are the mainstay of treatment. There may be particular benefit to the use of NSAIDs as they may produce ureteral relaxation in addition to analgesia. Therapies to reduce stone formation include alkalinization of urine, avoidance of certain drugs, use of thiazide diuretics, and dietary alterations.[133]

Polycystic kidney disease

This disorder is an autosomal-dominant genetic disease that eventually leads to kidney failure. Cyst formation, rupture, infection, and secondary compression/traction of neighboring structures may produce low back pain, abdominal pain, headache, chest pain, flank pain, and/or leg pain.[134] Renal stone formation and liver cyst formation are both common comorbidities and so reports of pain may require an assessment of those etiologies. Bajwa *et al.*[135] have proposed a general progression from non-pharmacological methods to non-narcotic analgesics and minimally invasive procedures to progressively more invasive procedures and use of opioids. Procedures unique to polycystic kidney disease include surgical or percutaneous drainage of the cysts with marsupialization to avoid fluid reaccumulation.[136]

Loin pain – hematuria syndrome

This is a descriptive diagnosis with the primary symptom of severe flank pain and the laboratory finding of hematuria. It is of obscure etiology and is associated with inconsistent pathology. It may be secondary to an immunoglobulin A nephritis but is predominantly a diagnosis of exclusion. Renal biopsies of subjects with this diagnosis by Spetie *et al.*[137] demonstrated a common finding of red blood cells in multiple tubules, suggesting a glomerular source of the hematuria. Glomerular basement membranes were observed to be commonly thick or thin but in general the glomeruli were without definable pathology. Accepted by some as a diagnosis that justifies aggressive interventions including nephrectomy or renal autotransplantation, its very existence as a discrete clinicopathological entity has been questioned. Recurrence of pain following surgical procedures including extensive surgical sympathectomy of the kidney has been common except in cases where there was meticulous screening of patients for other urological, nephrological, or psychiatric etiologies of the pain. Injection therapies have been normally viewed as short-lived. Transcutaneous electrical nerve stimulation has been reported to result in partial pain relief. Due to the limited success of other modalities of treatment, the use of narcotic analgesics may be considered.[138]

Other

Abdominal pain may also result from nonabdominal sites. Abdominal migraine is a variant of the more typical migraine. Rather than headache and nausea, symptomatology may consist of abdominal pain and nausea. Treatment is similar to that of other migraines.

Another source of abdominal pain may be cardiac failure, which produces congestion-related hepatomegaly and associated distension of the hepatic capsule. Similarly, low cardiac output may be associated with ischemia of the bowel.

Chronic ulceration of the stomach or duodenum may also produce recurrent epigastric pain. Potentially life-threatening due to their potential for hemorrhage and perforation they are generally viewed as acute events, diagnosed with endoscopy or contrast radiology and treated with antacids, mucosal coating agents, bowel rest, and drugs blocking gastric acid secretion/formation.

Nerve injury or entrapments can occur after any abdominal or pelvic surgery resulting in neuralgias, neuroma formation, or referred pains (e.g. testicular pain following an inguinal hernia repair). Evaluation and treatment are similar to those of other neuropathic pains. The surgical demonstration of adhesions in post-abdominal surgery patients may be attributed as a source of abdominal or pelvic pain but the role of these adhesions in producing pain is a matter of debate. It would appear that unless adhesions are producing bowel obstruction, adhesiolysis appears unlikely to produce reliable benefit. Treatment is episodic and symptomatic, but the use of narcotic analgesics may lead to further bowel dysfunction and so may be viewed as a late option.

SUMMARY

Chronic pain with abdominal, groin, or perineal localization is a common clinical entity with multiple etiologies both known and unknown. Four archetypal disorders have been presented in depth, as well as multiple other disorders as correlates. Each of the sources of pain listed in **Box 40.1** have their own unique aspects but similarities in evaluation and treatment are apparent. All forms of cancer have their correlate in pancreatic cancer with defined pathology and a desire for aggressive palliative treatment. Infectious and inflammatory pain states are correlates to chronic pancreatitis in that they have definable pathology but variable symptomatology. They also have associated potentially life-threatening complications such as abscess formation, fistula formation, and hemorrhage. Functional and undefined pain conditions have their correlates in IBS and IC with presumably defined sites of pain generation but minimal or absent definable pathology at those sites. All therapies are both disorder dependent and patient dependent. Outcome studies for many therapies are nonexistent and so the challenge for the clinician treating pain is to define the most appropriate therapy for an individual patient. It is beyond the scope of the present article to delineate every option ever tried, but the general maxim of starting "simple" and advancing as needed is prudent for all of the disorders.

REFERENCES

1. Merskey H, Bogduk N (eds). *Classification of chronic pain*, 2nd edn. Seattle: IASP Press, 1994.
2. Bhatia V, Tandon RK. Stress and the gastrointestinal tract. *Journal of Gastroenterology and Hepatology.* 2005; **20**: 332–9.
3. Silen W. Abdominal pain. In: Kaspar DL, Fauci AS, Longo DL *et al.* (eds). *Harrison's principles of internal medicine*, 16th edn. New York: McGraw-Hill, 2005: 82–4.
4. Freelove R, Walling AD. Pancreatic cancer: diagnosis and managment. *American Family Physician.* 2006; **73**: 485–92.
5. Andren-Sandberg A, Dervenis C, Lowenfels B. Etiologic links between chronic pancreatitis and pancreatic cancer. *Scandinavian Journal of Gastroenterology.* 1997; **32**: 97–103.
6. Caraceni A, Portenoy RK. Pain management in patients with pancreatic carcinoma. *Cancer.* 1996; **78**: 639–53.
7. * Fazal S, Saif MW. Supportive and palliative care of pancreatic cancer. *Journal of the Pancreas.* 2007; **8**: 240–53.
8. * Yan BM, Myers RP. Neurolytic celiac plexus block for pain control in unresectable pancreatic cancer. *American Journal of Gastroenterology.* 2007; **102**: 430–8.
9. Stefaniak T, Basinski A, Vingerhoets A *et al.* A comparison of two invasive techniques in the management of

intractable pain due to inoperable pancreatic cancer: neurolytic celiac plexus block and videothorascopic splanchnicectomy. *European Journal of Surgical Oncology.* 2005; **31**: 768–73.

10. Wong GY, Schroeder DR, Carns PE *et al.* Effect of neurolytic celiac plexus block on pain relief, quality of life, and survival in patients with unresectable pancreatic cancer: a randomized controlled trial. *Journal of the American Medical Association.* 2004; **291**: 1092–9.
11. Rykowski JJ, Hilgier M. Efficacy of neurolytic celiac plexus block in varying locations of pancreatic cancer: influence on pain relief. *Anesthesiology.* 2000; **92**: 347–54.
12. Ozyalcin NS, Talu GK, Camlica H, Erdine S. Efficacy of coelic plexus and splanchnic nerve blockades in body and tail located pancreatic cancer pain. *European Journal of Pain.* 8: 539–45.
13. Kappis M. Sensibilitat und lokale anaesthesic im chirugischen gobect der bauchhohle mit besonder berucksichrtigung der splanchnicusanethesia. *Beiträge zur Klinischen Chirurgie.* 1919; **115**: 161–75.
14. Moore DC. *Regional block: a handbook for use in the clinical practice of medicine and surgery,* 3rd edn. Springfield: Charles C. Thomas, 1961.
15. Sharfman WH, Walsh TD. Review article: Has the analgesic efficacy of neurolytic celiac plexus block been demonstrated in pancreatic cancer pain? *Pain.* 1990; **41**: 267–71.
16. Ischia S, Ishia A, Polati E, Finco G. Three posterior percutaneous celiac plexus block techniques. A prospective, randomized study in 61 patients with pancreatic cancer pain. *Anesthesiology.* 1992; **76**: 534–40.
17. Kawamata M, Ishitani K, Ishikawa K *et al.* Comparison between celiac plexus block and morphine treatment on quality of life in patients with pancreatic cancer pain. *Pain.* 1996; **64**: 597–602.
18. Merandino KA. Vagotomy for the relief of pain secondary to pancreatic carcinoma. *American Journal of Surgery.* 1964; **108**: 1–2.
19. * Warshaw AL, Banks PA, Fernandez-Del Castillo C. AGA Technical review: treatment of pain in chronic pancreatitis. *Gastroenterology.* 1998; **115**: 765–76.
20. Johnson JL, Loomis IB. A case of simvastatin-associated pancreatitis and review of statin-associated pancreatitis. *Pharmacotherapy.* 2006; **26**: 414–22.
21. Gupta V, Toskes PP. Diagnosis and management of chronic pancreatitis. *Postgraduate Medical Journal.* 2005; **81**: 491–7.
22. Maisonneuve P, Lowenfels AB, Mullhaupt B *et al.* Cigarette smoking accelerates progression of alcoholic chronic pancreatitis. *Gut.* 2005; **54**: 510–14.
23. Vera-Portocarrero L, Westlund KN. Role of neurogenic inflammation in pancreatitis and pancreatic pain. *Neurosignals.* 2005; **14**: 158–65.
24. Malfertheiner P, Dominguez-Munoz JE, Buchler MW. Chronic pancreatitis: management of pain. *Digestion.* 1994; **55**: 29–34.
25. van Esch AAJ, Wilder-Smith OHG, Jansen JBMJ *et al.* Pharmacological management of pain in chronic pancreatitis. *Digestive and Liver Disease.* 2006; **38**: 518–26.
26. Gullo L, Barbara L, Labo G. Effect of cessation of alcohol use on the course of pancreatic dysfunction in alcoholic pancreatitis. *Gastroenterology.* 1988; **95**: 1063–8.
27. Kirk GR, White JS, McKie L *et al.* Combined antioxidant therapy reduces pain and improves quality of life in chronic pancreatitis. *Journal of Gastrointestinal Surgery.* 2006; **10**: 499–503.
28. Monkemuller K, Kahl S, Malfertheiner P. Endoscopic therapy of chronic pancreatitis. *Digestive Diseases.* 2004; **22**: 280–91.
29. Dite P, Ruzicka M, Zboril V, Novoty I. A prospective, randomized trial comparing endoscopic and surgical therapy for chronic pancreatitis. *Endoscopy.* 2003; **35**: 553–8.
30. Dumonceau J-M, Costamagna G, Tringali A *et al.* Treatment for painful calcified chronic pancreatitis: extracorporeal shock wave lithotripsy versus endoscopic treatment: a randomized controlled trial. *Gut.* 2007; **56**: 545–52.
31. Busch EH, Atchison SR. Steroid celiac plexus block for chronic pancreatitis: results in 16 cases. *Journal of Clinical Anesthesia.* 1989; **1**: 431–3.
32. Cahen DL, Gouma DJ, Nio Y *et al.* Endoscopic versus surgical drainage of the pancreatic duct in chronic pancreatitis. *New England Journal of Medicine.* 2007; **356**: 727–9.
33. Lankisch PG. Natural course of chronic pancreatitis. *Pancreatology.* 2001; **1**: 3–14.
34. Guda NM, Partington S, Freeman ML. Extracorporeal shock wave lithotripsy in the management of chronic calcific pancreatitis: a meta-analysis. *Journal of the Pancreas.* 2005; **6**: 6–12.
35. Castiella A, Lopez P, Bujanda L, Arenas JI. Possible association of acute pancreatitis with naproxen. *Journal of Clinical Gastroenterology.* 1995; **21**: 258.
36. Felig DM, Topazian M. Corticosteroid-induced pancreatitis (letter). *Annals of Internal Medicine.* 1996; **124**: 1016.
37. Czako L, Takacs T, Hegyi P *et al.* Quality of life assessment after pancreatic enzyme replacement therapy in chronic pancreatitis. *Canadian Journal of Gastroenterology.* 2003; **17**: 597–603.
38. Eisenach JC, Carpenter R, Curry R. Analgesia from a peripherally active k-opioid receptor agonist in patients with chronic pancreatitis. *Pain.* 2003; **101**: 89–95.
39. Cartmell MT, O'Reilly DA, Porter C, Kingsnorth AN. A double-blind placebo-controlled trial of a leukotriene receptor antagonists in chronic pancreatitis in humans. *Journal of Hepato-biliary-pancreatic Surgery.* 2004; **11**: 255–9.
40. Hanowell ST, Kennedy SF, MacMamara TF, Lees DE. Celiac plexus block: diagnostic and therapeutic application in abdominal pain. *Southern Medical Journal.* 1980; **73**: 1330–2.

41. Little JM. Chronic pancreatitis: results of a protocol of management. *Australian and New Zealand Journal of Surgery.* 1983; **53**: 403–09.
42. Fishman SM, Catarau EM, Sachs G *et al.* Corticosteroid-induced mania after single regional application at the celiac plexus. *Anesthesiology.* 1996; **85**: 1194–6.
43. Bell SN, Cole R, Roberts-Thomson IC. Coeliac plexus block for control of pain in chronic pancreatitis. *British Medical Journal.* 1980; **281**: 1604.
44. Leung JWC, Bowen-Wright M, Aveling W *et al.* Coeliac plexus block for pain in pancreatic cancer and chronic pancreatitis. *British Journal of Surgery.* 1983; **70**: 730–2.
45. Fugere F, Lewis G. Coeliac plexus block for chronic pain syndromes. *Canadian Journal of Anaesthesia.* 1993; **40**: 954–63.
46. Chan VWS. Chronic diarrhea: an uncommon side effect of celiac plexus block. *Anesthesia and Analgesia.* 1996; **82**: 205–07.
47. Takeda J, Namai H, Fukushima K. Anterior spinal artery syndrome after left celiac plexus block. *Anesthesia and Analgesia.* 1996; **83**: 178–9.
48. Cherry DA, Lamberty J. Paraplegia following coeliac plexus nerve block. *Anaesthesia and Intensive Care.* 1984; **12**: 59–61.
49. Galiazia EJ, Lahiri SK. Paraplegia following celiac plexus block with phenol. *British Journal of Anaesthesia.* 1974; **46**: 539–40.
50. Lohr-Happe A, Peiper M, Lankisch PG. Natural course of operated pseudocysts in chronic pancreatitis. *Gut.* 1994; **35**: 1479–82.
51. Mallet-Guy PA. Late and very late results of resections of the nervous system in the treatment of chronic relapsing pancreatitis. *American Journal of Surgery.* 1983; **145**: 234–8.
52. Maher JW, Johlin FC, Pearson D. Thoracoscopic splanchnicectomy for chronic pancreatitis pain. *Surgery.* 1996; **120**: 603–10.
53. Ammann RW, Akovbiantz A, Largiader F, Schueler G. Course and outcome of chronic pancreatitis. *Gastroenterology.* 1984; **86**: 820–88.
54. Lankisch PG, Lohr-Happe A, Otto J, Creutzfeld W. Natural course in chronic pancreatitis: pain, exocrine and endocrine pancreatic insufficiency and prognosis of the disease. *Digestion.* 1993; **54**: 148–55.
* 55. Alagiri M, Chottiner S, Ratner V *et al.* Interstitial cystitis: unexplained associations with other chronic disease and pain syndromes. *Urology.* 1997; **49**: 52–7.
56. Pang X, Marchand J, Sant GR *et al.* Increased number of substance P positive nerve fibres in intersitial cystitis. *British Journal of Urology.* 1995; **75**: 744–50.
57. Marchand JE, Sant GR, Kream RM. Increased expression of substance P receptor-encoding mRNA in bladder biopsies from patient with interstitial cystitis. *British Journal of Urology.* 1998; **81**: 224–8.
58. Lowe EM, Anand P, Terenghi G *et al.* Increased nerve growth factor levels in the urinary bladder of women with idiopathic sensory urgence and interstitial cystitis. *British Journal of Urology.* 1997; **79**: 572–7.
59. Theoharides TC, Sant GR, el-Mansoury M *et al.* Activation of bladder mast cells in interstitial cystitis: a light and electron microscopic study. *Journal of Urology.* 1995; **153**: 629–36.
60. Held PJ, Hanno PM, Wein AJ. Epidemiology of interstitial cystitis. In: Hanno PM (ed.). *Interstitial cystitis.* London: Springer-Verlag, 1990: 29–48.
* 61. Bogart LM, Berry SH, Clemens JQ. Symptoms of interstitial cystitis, painful bladder syndrome and similar diseases in women: a systematic review. *Journal of Urology.* 2007; **177**: 450–6.
62. Pontari MA, Hanno PM, Wein AJ. Logical and systematic approach to the evaluation and management of patients suspected of having interstitial cystitis. *Urology.* 1997; **49**: 114–20.
63. Wein AJ, Hanno PM, Gillenwater JY. Interstitial cystitis: an introduction to the problem. In: Hanno PM, Staskin DR, Krane RJ, Wein AJ (eds). *Interstitial cystitis.* New York: Springer-Verlag, 1990: 3–16.
64. Parsons CL, Greenberger M, Gaball L *et al.* The role of urinary potassium in the pathogenesis and diagnosis of interstitial cystitis. *Journal of Urology.* 1998; **159**: 1862–7.
65. Perez-Marrero R, Emerson LE, Feltis JT. A controlled study of dimethyl sulfoxide in interstitial cystitis. *Journal of Urology.* 1988; **140**: 36–9.
66. Theoharides TC. Treatment approaches for painful bladder syndrome/interstitial cystitis. *Drugs.* 2007; **67**: 215–35.
67. Sairanen J, Tammella TL, Leppilahti M *et al.* Cyclosporine A and pentosan polysulfate sodium for the treatment of interstial cystitis: a randomized comparative study. *Journal of Urology.* 2005; **174**: 2235–8.
68. Mayer R, Propert KJ, Peters KM *et al.* A randomized controlled trial of intravesical bacillus calmette-guerin for treatment refractory interstial cystitis. *Journal of Urology.* 2005; **173**: 1186–91.
69. van Ophoven A, Pokupic S, Heinecke A, Hertle L. A prospective, randomized, placebo controlled, double-blind study of amitriptyline for the treatment of interstitial cystitis. *Journal of Urology.* 2004; **172**: 533–6.
70. Fall M, Lindstrom S. Transcutaneous electrical nerve stimulation in interstitial cystitis. *Urologic Clinics of North America.* 1994; **21**: 131–9.
71. Payne CK, Mosbaugh PG, Forrest JB *et al.* Intravesical resiniferatoxin for the treatment of interstitial cystitis: a randomized, double-blind, placebo controlled trial. *Journal of Urology.* 2005; **173**: 1590–04.
72. Irwin PP, Hammonds WD, Galloway NTM. Lumbar epidural blockade for management of pain in interstitial cystitis. *British Journal of Urology.* 1993; **71**: 413–6.
73. Gillespie L. Destruction of the vesicoureteric plexus for the treatment of hypersensitive bladder disorders. *British Journal of Urology.* 1994; **74**: 40–3.
74. Peeker R, Aldenborg F, Fall M. The treatment of interstitial cystitis with supratrigonal cystectomy and

ileocystoplasty: difference in outcome between classic and nonulcer disease. *Journal of Urology.* 1998; **159**: 1479–82.
75. Webster GD, MacDiarmid SA, Timmons SL. Impact of urinary diversion procedures in the treatment of interstitial cystitis and chronic bladder pain. *Neurourology and Urodynamics.* 1992; **11**: 417.
76. Chaiken DC, Blaivas JG, Blaivis ST. Behavioral therapy for the treatment of refractory interstitial cystitis. *Journal of Urology.* 1993; **149**: 1445–8.
77. Messing EM, Stamey TA. Interstitial cystitis, early diagnosis, pathology and treatment. *Urology.* 1978; **12**: 381–92.
78. Whitmore KE. Self-care regimens for patients with interstitial cystitis. *Urologic Clinics of North America.* 1994; **21**: 121–30.
79. van Ophoven A, Rossbach G, Pajonk F, Hertle L. Safety and efficacy of hyperbaric oxygen therapy for the treatment of initerstitial cystitis: a randomized, sham controlled, double-blind trial. *Journal of Urology.* 2006; **176**: 1442–6.
80. Baskin LS, Tanagho EA. Pelvic pain without pelvic organs. *Journal of Urology.* 1992; **147**: 683–6.
81. Keay SK, Szekely Z, Conrads TP *et al.* An antiproliferative factor from interstitial cystitis patients is a frizzled 8 protein-related sialoglycopeptide. *Proceedings of the National Academy of Sciences of the United States of America.* 2004; **101**: 11803–08.
82. Drossman DA, Corazziari E, Talley J *et al.* ROME II: A Multinational Consensus Document on Functional Gastrointestinal Disorders. *Gut.* 1999; **45**: 1–81.
83. Maxwell P, Mendall MA, Kumar D. Irritable bowel syndrome. *Lancet.* 1997; **350**: 1691–5.
84. Cremoni F, Talley NJ. Irritable bowel syndrome: epidemiology, natural history, health care seeking and emerging risks. *Gastroenterology Clinics of North America.* 2005; **34**: 189–204.
85. Farthing MJG. Treatment options in irritable bowel syndrome. *Best Practice and Research. Clinical Gastroenterology.* 2004; **18**: 773–86.
86. Bijkerk CJ, Muris JW, Knottnerus JA *et al.* Systematic review: the role of different types of fibre in the treatment of irritable bowel syndrome. *Alimentary Pharmacology and Therapeutics.* 2004; **19**: 245–51.
87. Guthrie E, Creed F, Dawson D, Tomenson B. A controlled trial of psychological treatment for the irritable bowel syndrome. *Gastroenterology.* 1991; **100**: 450–7.
88. Swedlund J, Sjoden L, Ottosson JO, Doteval G. Controlled study of psychotherapy in irritable bowel syndrome. *Lancet.* 1983; **2**: 589–91.
89. Talley NJ, Owen BK, Boyce P, Paterson K. Psychological treatments for irritable bowel syndrome: a critique of controlled treatment trials. *American Journal of Gastroenterology.* 1996; **91**: 277–83.
90. Vahedi H, Merat S, Rashidioon A *et al.* The effect of fluoxetinein patients with pain and constipation-predominant irritable bowel syndrome: a double-blind randomized-controlled study. *Alimentary Pharmacology and Therapeutics.* 2005; **22**: 381–5.
91. Tabas G, Beaves M, Wang J *et al.* Paroxetine to treat irritable bowel syndrome not respondinig to high-fibre diet: a double-blind, placebo-controlled trial. *American Journal of Gastroenterology.* 2004; **99**: 914–20.
92. Tack J, Broekaert D, Fischler B *et al.* A controlled crossover study of the selective serotonin reuptake inhibitor citalopram in irritable bowel syndrome. *Gut.* 2006; **55**: 1095–103.
* 93. Quartero AO, Meineche-Schmidt V, Muris J *et al.* Bulking agents, antispasmodic and antidepressant medication for the treatment of irritable bowel syndrome. *Cochrane Database of Systematic Reviews.* 2005; **CD003460**.
94. Delvaux M, Beck A, Jacob J *et al.* Effect of asimadoline, a kappa opioid agonist, on pain induced by colonic distension in patients with irritable bowel syndrome. *Alimentary Pharmacology and Therapeutics.* 2004; **20**: 237–46.
95. Tonini M, Pace F. Drugs acting on serotonin receptors for the treatment of functional GI disorders. *Digestive Diseases.* 2006; **24**: 59–69.
96. Camilleri M. Is there an experimental basis for the development of ischaemic colitis as a result of 5-HT3 antagonist treatment? *Neurogastroenterology and Motility.* 2007; **19**: 77–84.
97. Hastings RH, McKay WR. Treatment of benign chronic abdominal pain with neurolytic celiac plexus block. *Anesthesiology.* 1991; **75**: 156–8.
* 98. Wesselmann U, Burnett AL, Heinberg LJ. The urogenital and rectal pain syndromes. *Pain.* 1997; **73**: 269–94.
99. Plancarte RB, Velaquez R, Patt RB. Neurolytic blocks of the sympathetic asis. In: Patt RB (ed.). *Cancer pain.* Philadelphia: Lippincott-Raven, 1993: 377–425.
100. Gerson LB, Triadafilopoulos G. Palliative care in inflammatory bowel disease: an evidence-based approach. *Inflammatory Bowel Diseases.* 2000; **6**: 228–43.
101. Chang JT, Lichtenstein GR. Drug insight: antagonists of tumor-necrosis factor-alpha in the treatment of inflammatory bowel disease. *Nature Clinical Practice. Gastroenterology and Hepatology.* 2006; **3**: 220–8.
102. Panaccione R. Infliximab for the treatment of Crohn's disease: review and indications for clinical use in Canada. *Canadian Journal of Gastroenterology.* 2001; **15**: 371–5.
103. Sanborn WJ, Hanauer SB, Katz S *et al.* Etanercept for active Crohn's disease: a randomized, double-blind, placebo-controlled trial. *Gastroenterology.* 2001; **121**: 1088–94.
104. Korzenik JR, Dieckgraefe BK, Valentine JF *et al.* Sargramostim for active Crohn's disease. *New England Journal of Medicine.* 2005; **352**: 2193–201.
105. Dieckgraefe BK, Korzenik JR. Treatment of active Crohn's disease with recombinant human granulocyte-macrophage colony-stimulating factor. *Lancet.* 2002; **360**: 1478–80.
106. Shafran I, Johnson LK. An open-label evaluation of rifaximin in the treatment of active Crohn's disease. *Current Medical Research and Opinion.* 2005; **21**: 1165–9.

107. Karimi O, Peña AS. Probiotics in arthralgia and spondyloarthropathies in patients with inflammatory bowel disease. *Revista Española Enfermedades Digestivas.* 2005; **97**: 570–4.
108. Garcia-Vega E, Fernandez-Rodriguez C. A stress management programme for Crohn's disease. *Behaviour Research and Therapy.* 2004; **42**: 367–83.
109. Kolkman JJ, Mensink PB, van Petersen AS *et al.* Clinical approach to chronic gastrointestinal ischaemia: from "intestinal angina" to the spectrum of chronic splanchnic disease. *Scandinavian Journal of Gastroenterology.* 2004; **241** (Suppl.): 9–16.
110. Sreenarasimhaiah J. Chronic mesenteric ischemia. *Best Practice and Research. Clinical Gastroenterology.* 2005; **19**: 283–95.
111. van Boekel JH, Geelkerken RH, Wasser MN. Chronic splanchnic ischaemia. *Best Practice and Research. Clinical Gastroenterology.* 2001; **15**: 99–119.
*112. Kozuch PL, Brandt LJ. Review article: diagnosis and management of mesenteric ischaemia with an emphasis on pharmacotherapy. *Alimentary Pharmacology and Therapeutics.* 2005; **21**: 201–15.
113. Place RJ, Simmang CL. Diverticular disease. *Best Practice and Research. Clinical Gastroenterology.* 2002; **16**: 135–48.
114. Kohler L, Sauerland S, Neugebauer E. Diagnosis and treatement of diverticular disease: results of a consensus development conference. The Scientific Committee of the European Association for Endoscopic Surgery. *Surgical Endoscopy.* 1999; **13**: 430–6.
115. Papi C, Ciaco A, Koch M, Capurso L. Efficacy of rifaximin in the treatment of symptomatic diverticular disease of the colon. A multicentre double-blind, placebo-controlled trial. *Alimentary Pharmacology and Therapeutics.* 1995; **9**: 33–39.
116. Latella G, Pimpo MT, Sottili S *et al.* Rifaximin improves symptoms of acquired uncomplicated diverticular disease of the colon. *International Journal of Colorectal Disease.* 2003; **18**: 55–62.
117. Comparato G, Fanigliulo L, Cavallaro LG *et al.* Prevention of complications and symptomatic recurrences in diverticular disease with mesalazine: a 12-month follow-up. *Digestive Diseases and Sciences.* 2007; **52**: 2934–41. epub.
118. Onen F. Familial Mediterranean fever. *Rheumatology International.* 2006; **26**: 489–96.
119. Simon A, van der Meer JWM. Pathogenesis of familial periodic fever syndromes or hereditary autoinflammatory syndromes. *American Journal of Physiology. Regulatory, Integrative and Comparative Physiology.* 2007; **292**: R86–98.
120. Kapur S, Mutagi H, Raphael J. Spinal cord stimulation for relief of abdominal pain in two patients with familial Mediterranean fever. *British Journal of Anaesthesia.* 2006; **97**: 866–8.
121. Kallinich T, Haffner D, Niehues T *et al.* Colchicine use in children and aldolescents with familial Mediterranean fever: literature review and consensus statement. *Pediatrics.* 2007; **119**: 474–83.
122. Dombeck TA, Satonik RC. The porphyrias. *Emergency Medicine Clinics of North America.* 2005; **23**: 885–99.
123. Herrick AL, McColl KE. Acute intermittent porphyria. *Best Practice and Research. Clinical Gastroenterology.* 2005; **19**: 235–49.
124. Granitsiotis P, Kirk D. Chronic testicular pain; an overview. *European Urology.* 2004; **45**: 430–6.
125. Linnebur SA, Hiatt WH. Probable statin-induced testicular pain. *Annals of Pharmacotherapy.* 2007; **41**: 138–42.
126. Nariculum J, Minhas S, Adeniyi A *et al.* A review of the efficacy of surgical treatment for and pathological changes in patients with chronic scrotal pain. *BJU International.* 2007; **99**: 1091–3.
127. Cohen SP, Foster A. Pulsed radiofrequency as a treatment for groin pain and orchialgia. *Urology.* 2003; **61**: 645.
128. Ness TJ. Pelvic pain in women and men: recent findings. *Current Opinion in Anaesthesiology.* 2005; **18**: 555–62.
129. Vetrhus M, Berhane T, Soreide O, Sondenaa K. Pain persists in many patients five years after removal of the gallbladder: observations from two randomized controlled trials of symptomatic, noncomplicated gallstone disease and acute cholecystitis. *Journal of Gastrointestinal Surgery.* 2005; **9**: 826–31.
*130. Behar J, Corazziari E, Guelrud M *et al.* Functional gallbladder and sphincter of Oddi disorders. *Gastroenterology.* 2006; **130**: 1498–509.
*131. Bharucha AE, Wald A, Enck P, Rao S. Functional anorectal disorders. *Gastroenterology.* 2006; **130**: 1510–18.
132. Bihl G, Meyers A. Recurrent renal stone disease – advances in pathogenesis and clinical management. *Lancet.* 2001; **358**: 651–6.
133. Micali S, Grande M, Sighinolfi MC *et al.* Medical therapy of urolithiasis. *Journal of Endourology.* 2006; **20**: 841–7.
134. Bajwa ZH, Sial KA, Malik AB, Steinman TI. Pain patterns in patients with polycystic kidney disease. *Kidney International.* 2004; **66**: 1561–9.
*135. Bajwa ZH, Gupta S, Warfield CA, Steinman TI. Pain management in polycystic kidney disease. *Kidney International.* 2001; **60**: 1631–44.
136. Badani KK, Hemal AK, Menon M. Autosomal dominant polycystic kidney disease and pain – A review of the disease from aetiology, evaluation, past surgical treatment options to current practice. *Journal of Postgraduate Medicine.* 2004; **50**: 222–6.
137. Spetie DN, Nadasdy T, Nadasdy G *et al.* Proposed pathogenesis of idiopathic loin-pain-hematuria syndrome. *American Journal of Kidney Diseases.* 2006; **47**: 419–27.
138. Weisberg LS, Bloom PB, Simmons RL *et al.* Loin pain hematuria syndrome. *American Journal of Nephrology.* 1993; **13**: 229–37.

41

Chronic pelvic pain

ANDREA J RAPKIN AND MONICA LEE

KEY LEARNING POINTS

- Chronic pelvic pain (CPP) is pelvic pain that has persisted for six months or more. The amount of pain is often greater than the degree of pathology.
- Gynecologic causes of CPP can be divided into noncyclic and cyclic.
- Primary and secondary dysmenorrhea are cyclic. Primary dysmenorrhea is best treated with nonsteroidal anti-inflammatory drugs (NSAID) and hormonal contraceptives; treatment of secondary dysmenorrhea depends on the etiology, but both may respond to menstrual supression.
- The most prevalent cyclic gynecologic cause of CPP is endometriosis.
- The pain with endometriosis is most likely associated with deeply infiltrating lesions. Numerous medical and surgical techniques are available for treatment.
- Pelvic pain, urinary urgency, urinary frequency, and frequent nocturia without evidence of urinary tract infection are suggestive of painful bladder syndrome or interstitial cystitis.
- Eliciting a trigger point or localizing tenderness to a specific branch of a somatic nerve is indicative of neuropathic pain. Injection of local anesthetic can be diagnostic as well as therapeutic.
- Psychological factors impact the perception and maintenance of pain. Depression and a history of physical and/or sexual abuse are common and should be addressed. Cognitive behavioral therapy is an important component of multidisciplinary management.
- Physical examination should encompass not only the pelvic viscera system, but also the musculoskeletal and neurologic systems.
- Management of CPP should involve a multidisciplinary approach for maximal benefit. Individual components of therapy may include:
  - pharmacologic therapy: NSAIDs, antidepressants, anticonvulsants, and possibly narcotics, depending on the presumed etiology of the pain, trigger point injections, and local anesthetic nerve blocks.
  - physical therapy including consideration of transcutaneous electric nerve stimulation (TENS) unit device in cases where there is a myofascial contribution to the pain.
- Vulvar vestibulitis, vestibulodynia vulvar dermatoses, cyclic vulvovaginitis, and dysesthetic vulvodynia are subtypes of vulvodynia.
- The etiology of vulvodynia may be infectious, trauma, allergens, underlying dermatologic, neurologic, urologic, or systemic conditions.
- Vulvar vestibulitis is vulvar pain characterized by entry dyspareunia, vestibular erythema, and vestibular tenderness.

- Therapies for vulvodynia depend on results of evaluation, and may include antifungal agents, antihistamines, topical corticosteroids, topical or injected local anesthetics, and estrogen.
- Tricyclic antidepressants, anticonvulsants, biofeedback and physical therapy of pelvic floor muscles, and cognitive-behavioral therapy may enhance the above therapies.
- Surgical intervention (perineoplasty – total or subtotal) should be offered in cases of vulvar vestibulitis resistant to medical therapy.

INTRODUCTION

Chronic pelvic pain (CPP) is defined as pelvic pain that persists for more than six months in the same location. It may occur in individuals with no apparent visceral or somatic abnormalities or, if disease is present, the pain is frequently more pronounced than the degree of pathology might suggest. Chronic pelvic pain is often associated with depression, anxiety (hopelessness and helplessness) and other mood disturbances, catastrophizing, somatizing, and dependent personality styles, marital and social discord, including sexual dsysfunction. The purpose of this chapter is to review the pelvic anatomy, differential diagnosis, and management, including the role of multidisciplinary assessment and treatment of CPP.

EPIDEMIOLOGY

In the USA, an estimated 12–15 percent of women report signs and symptoms suggestive of CPP, or have been diagnosed with CPP,[1, 2] and up to 15 percent have vulvodynia.[3] Approximately 10 percent of referrals to gynecologists and 44 percent of laparoscopies are performed to evaluate CPP.[4, 5] The impact of CPP on society is not measured only by the amount spent on the diagnosis and treatment, but also by the opportunity cost it exacts. For example, Mathias and colleagues[1] reported a 45 percent reduction in work productivity and a 15 percent increase in time lost from work in women with CPP.

ETIOLOGY AND PATHOPHYSIOLOGY

Neuroanatomy

VISCERAL INNERVATION

The reproductive organs have a dual innervation via the sympathetic (thoracolumbar) and parasympathetic (sacral) autonomic, with contributions from the somatic sensory nervous system.[6, 7] The visceral afferent fibers travel the same route as their corresponding efferent autonomic fibers (**Table 41.1**). The afferent innervation of the upper vagina, cervix, uterus, proximal fallopian tubes, upper bladder, terminal ileum, and distal large bowel travels with the thoracolumbar sympathetics through the inferior hypogastric plexus to the hypogastric nerve to the superior hypogastric plexus and on to the lower thoracic and lumber splanchnic nerves which enter the spinal cord at T10–L1. Other pathways of afferent innervation from the pelvis travel via the pelvic (parasympathetic) splanchnic nerves (nervi erigentes) to

Table 41.1 Pelvic structures and their innervations.

Organ	Spinal segment	Nerves
Outer two-thirds of fallopian tubes, upper ureter	T9–10	Thoracolumbar splanchnic nerves through mesenteric plexus
Ovaries	T9–10	Thoracolumbar splanchnic nerves traveling with ovarian vessels via renal and aortic plexus and celiac and mesenteric ganglia
Uterine fundus, proximal fallopian tubes, broad ligament, upper bladder, cecum, appendix, terminal large bowel	T11–12, L1	Thoracolumbar splanchnic nerves through uterine and hypogastric plexus
Lower abdominal wall	L1–2	Iliohypogastric, ilioninguinal
Perineum, vulva, lower vagina, anus, rectum	L1–L2, S2–S4	Pudental, ilioninguinal, genitofemoral, posterior femoral cutaneous, anococcygeal
Upper vagina, cervix, lower uterine segment, posterior urethra, bladder trigone, uterosacral and cardinal ligaments, rectosigmoid, lower ureters	S2–S4	Sacral afferents traveling through the pelvic plexus

S2–4. The perineum, anus, and pelvic floor muscles are supplied by somatic branches of the pudendal nerve (S2–4). Urogenital sinus structures, including the lower vagina, lower bladder, and rectosigmoid, are innervated by both the thoracolumbar and sacral afferents.[6]

The outer fallopian tube, ovary, and upper ureter are innervated by sympathetic nerves traveling with the ovarian artery, and enter the sympathetic nerve chain at L4, ascend with the chain, and enter the spinal cord at T9 and T10. The afferents from the ovary and outer fallopian tube therefore bypass the inferior hypogastric nerve and superior hypogastric plexus. Visceral conditions are characterized by referred pain to the dermatomes associated with pelvic organ innervation, i.e. T10–L2 (anterior abdominal wall and anterior thighs) and dorsal rami of L1–L2 (lower back).[8, 9, 10] Referred pain is well localized, superficial in location, and appears to arise in the same spinal cord segment receiving the pain input.

MECHANISMS OF SOMATIC AND VISCERAL PAIN

A complete description may be found in Chapter 3, Applied physiology: persistent visceral pain.

PERIPHERAL CAUSES OF CHRONIC PELVIC PAIN

Table 41.2 lists the differential diagnosis of the peripheral (outside of the central nervous system (CNS)) etiology of chronic pelvic pain. It is helpful to consider pain as either "cyclic" or "noncyclic," based on whether the pain is exacerbated premenstrually or with menses. Although not all cyclic pain derives from the reproductive system, suppression of gonadal steroids or menses is often useful for the management of cyclic pelvic pain.

Gynecologic: cyclic pelvic pain

Dysmenorrhea or painful menses is the most common category of cyclic pelvic pain. It is a common disorder of the female reproductive tract and affects approximately 50 percent of menstruating women.[11] Dysmenorrhea may be described as primary or secondary, depending on its etiology. Primary dysmenorrhea refers to pain with menses in the absence of an underlying pathology. Secondary dysmenorrhea refers to pain in the presence of an underlying disorder such as adenomyosis or endometriosis.

PATHOPHYSIOLOGY

Several mechanisms are likely to activate the thoracolumbar and pelvic afferents invoking dysmenorrhea. These include: (1) myometrial contractions leading to intense intrauterine pressure and uterine hypoxia; (2) hyperproduction of prostaglandins and leukotrienes and other hormonal factors which increase afferent terminal excitability; (3) altered CNS processing of the afferent barrage possibly mediated by opioid or gamma aminobutyric acid (GABA)-ergic mediations; and (4) environmental and behavioral factors.[12] In primary dysmenorrhea, an increase in endometrial prostaglandin production is seen in the secretory phase of the cycle.[12]

SYMPTOMS AND SIGNS

As retrospective history may be inaccurate, the diagnosis of cyclic exacerbation of pain often depends on the review of a daily pain ratings and menstrual calendar to confirm the cyclic nature of the pain.

Primary dysmenorrhea

In primary dysmenorrhea, onset of pain generally occurs approximately one year following menarche when ovulatory cycles are established. The pain starts near or at the onset of menses, lasting for 48–72 hours, is suprapubic and cramping, radiating to the lumbosacral region and anterior thighs. Associated gastrointestinal symptoms including nausea, vomiting, and diarrhea are common.

Secondary dysmenorrhea usually occurs years after menarche, and pain may occur up to two weeks prior to the onset of menses and last until the cessation of menses. In primary dysmenorrhea, the physical examination is unremarkable, although at the time of dysmenorrhea some suprapubic and uterine tenderness is common, whereas with secondary dysmenorrhea, careful pelvic examination may reveal abnormalities in adnexal structures, uterine size, contour, mobility and/or tenderness, and nodularity of the uterosacral ligaments and rectovaginal septum.

DIAGNOSIS

Evaluation includes cervical studies to rule out gonorrhea or chlamydial infection, a complete blood count (CBC), and erythrocyte sedimentation rate (ESR). Transvaginal ultrasound should be performed as it may suggest an anatomic disorder underlying the cyclic pain. Secondary dysmenorrhea is discussed in detail under Secondary dysmenorrhea below.

TREATMENT

The standard treatment for primary dysmenorrhea is prostaglandin synthetase inhibitors. Dosing requires around-the-clock administration at the onset of menses or, preferably, one to two days prior to onset of pain for the first few days of menses. Treatment is effective in up to

Table 41.2 Peripheral causes of chronic pelvic pain.

Gynecologic		Gastrointestinal	Genitourinary	Neurologic	Musculoskeletal	Systemic
Noncyclic	**Cyclic**					
Adhesions	Primary dysmenorrhea	Irritable bowel syndrome	Recurrent or relapsing systourethritis	Nerve entrapment syndrome	Low back pain syndrome	Acute intermittent porphyria
Endometriosis Salpingo-oophoritis	Secondary dysmenorrhea Imperforate hymen or transverse vaginal septum	Ulcerative colitis Granulomatous colitis (Crohn's disease)	Urethral syndrome Interstitial cystitis	Neuroma Trigger points	Myofascial syndrome Fibromyalgia	Abdominal migraine Systemic lupus erythematosus
Ovarian remnant syndrome	Cervical stenosis	Carcinoma	Ureteral diverticula or polyps		Pelvic floor muscle tension/spasm or trigger points	Lymphoma
Pelvic congestion syndrome (varicosities)	Uterine anomalies (congenital malformation, bicornuate uterus, blind uterine horn)	Infectious diarrhea	Carcinoma of the bladder		Hernia	Neurofibromatosis
Ovarian neoplasms	Intrauterine synechiae (Asherman syndrome)	Recurrent partial small bowel obstruction	Ureteral obstruction			
Pelvic relaxation	Endometrial polyps Uterine leiomyoma Adenomyosis	Diverticulitis Hernia Abdominal angina Recurrent appendiceal colic	Pelvic kidney			
	Pelvic congestion syndrome (varicosities) Endometriosis Atypical cyclic Endometriosis Adenomyosis Ovarian remnant syndrome Chronic functional ovarian cyst formation					

80 percent of cases.[13] A recent Cochrane review[14] found that nonsteroidal anti-inflammatory drugs (NSAID) were significantly more effective than placebo for pain relief (OR 7.91), but were not found to be significantly more effective than paracetamol.

Further benefit may be obtained by adding an oral contraceptive pill (OCP) with relief noted in more than 90 percent.[15] A meta-analysis of four randomized controlled trials (RCTs) found that combined OCPs provide effective pain relief.[16] Contraceptive rings, patches, and progestin containing intrauterine devices and implants may also be effective. High-dose oral or depot progestins and gonadotropin-releasing hormone (GnRH) agonists (with low-dose add-back therapy) are other forms of hormonal suppression.[17] If more aggressive medical therapy including narcotic analgesia is necessary, laparoscopy should be considered to rule out endometriosis.

Other alternative forms of treatment include acupuncture or transcutaneous electric nerve stimulation (TENS).[18, 19, 20] A meta-analysis of nine RCTs found that high frequency TENS was effective for treatment of dysmenorrhea, but that there was insufficient evidence to assess the efficacy of low frequency TENS.[21] Surgical management can be considered once conservative medical management has failed or if an underlying disorder is present. Surgical approaches to dysmenorrhea may include laparoscopic uterosacral nerve ablation or presacral neurectomy. In selected cases of dysmenorrhea, after childbearing has been completed, hysterectomy may be appropriate. These interventions are further discussed later in this chapter. There is currently no evidence that spinal manipulation is effective for the treatment of primary or secondary dysmenorrhea.[22]

Secondary dysmenorrhea

Secondary dysmenorrhea most commonly arises when a woman is in her twenties or thirties, after years of less painful cycles. Elevated prostaglandins may also play a role in secondary dysmenorrhea but, by definition, concomitant pelvic pathology must also be present. Common causes include endometriosis (see below under Endometriosis), adenomyosis, endometrial polyps, endometritis, pelvic inflammatory disease, copper intrauterine devices (IUDs), ovarian cysts, congenital pelvic malformations, and cervical stenosis.

Adenomyosis

Adenomyosis refers to the presence of endometrial glands and stroma within the uterine musculature. It can be a diffuse disease or it can form nodules that resemble myomas. The ectopic endometrial tissue stimulates the surrounding myometrium to hypertrophy, causing an enlarged globular uterus.

INCIDENCE

Incidence is generally estimated to be 20 percent of women, but has been found in up to 65 percent of women in one study and cannot be accurately estimated.[23] Patients are typically between 40 and 50 years of age. Adenomyosis may be more common in parous women and those who have had prior uterine surgery. Fibroids and endometriosis often coexist with adenomyosis.[24]

SIGNS AND SYMPTOMS

Abnormal uterine bleeding, primarily menorrhagia, and premenstrual and menstrual pain are the most common symptoms.

DIAGNOSIS

Definitive diagnosis is by histological examination of hysterectomy specimen. The preoperative diagnosis can be suggested when there is menorrhagia and dysmenorrhea, particularly if the uterus is enlarged but has a heterogenous echo texture on ultrasound, but no myomata. The sensitivity and specificity of transvaginal ultrasound were 81 and 71 percent, respectively.[25] Magnetic resonance imaging (MRI) may show areas of decreased signal intensity in areas of adenomyosis, and is the best way to distinguish adenomyosis from normal myometrium or fibroids, but is an expensive modality for diagnosis.[26]

TREATMENT

Hormonal treatment for adenomyosis is similar to that of endometriosis and includes OCPs, progestins or GnRH analog (also see below under Treatment under Endometriosis). However, six months after cessation of therapy, the enlargement of the uterus and symptoms usually recur. Uterine artery embolization may be effective and hysterectomy is curative.

Endometriosis

INCIDENCE

In the general female population, prevalence is estimated at approximately 10 percent and with infertile women it is 15–25 percent, and 28–74 percent of women undergoing diagnostic laparoscopy for CPP.[27, 28, 29] In the past decade, the incidence has increased, perhaps reflecting delayed childbearing but also the increasing use of laparoscopy and greater awareness of subtle endometriotic lesions.[30] Endometriosis may present in any age group (from adolescents to postmenopausal women on hormonal therapy), however most diagnoses are made in women in their thirties or forties.[31] Endometriosis has been suggested by one study to be the etiology in up to 70 percent of adolescents with CPP unresponsive to medical treatment.[32]

ETIOLOGY

In women with endometriosis, endometrial glands and stroma are located outside the uterine cavity, most commonly at the cul-de-sac, ovaries, and the pelvic visceral and parietal peritoneum. The favored theory, proposed by Sampson in the 1920s, is that endometriosis results from retrograde menses with implantation of endometrium on the peritoneum and nearby organs. Retrograde menses occur in 70–90 percent of women. However, endometriosis does not necessarily result. It may be that altered peritoneal immune function contributes to the progression of endometriosis, and the eutopic endometrium may also differ in women prone to endometriosis.[33] Proliferation occurs with each menstrual cycle, with resultant inflammation, scarring, fibrosis, and adhesion formation. Thus, the risk of endometriosis is thought to increase with abnormal menstrual activity, such as shorter menstrual cycle, menorrhagia, obstruction to outflow, and reduced parity.[31] The estrogenic hormonal environment further permits proliferation. Further theories include celomic metaplasia of the peritoneum and hematogenous/lymphatic spread to extrapelvic sites.[33]

SYMPTOMS AND SIGNS

The most common symptoms of endometriosis are:

- Dysmenorrhea: pelvic pain may be present all month but is is invariably associated with menstruation, and may start seven days prior. Pain is sharp/pressure-like and located in the lower abdomen, back, and rectum.
- Deep (pelvic as opposed to introital) dyspareunia.
- Infertility.
- Abnormal uterine bleeding: usually from a secretory endometrium.
- Nongynecologic symptoms: dyschezia (pain during bowel movements) or cyclic hematochezia with involvement of intestine/rectum. Urinary urgency, frequency, bladder pain, and hematuria with urinary tract involvement. Patients rarely can develop bowel or ureteral obstruction.

Classic physical findings include uterosacral nodularity and focal tenderness on bimanual and rectovaginal examination. With severe disease, fibrosis can result in a fixed, retroverted uterus. Adnexal masses may be palpated, consistent with endometriomata.[33]

DIAGNOSIS

A definitive diagnosis is made by laparoscopy or laparotomy.[34] Typical endometriotic lesions range from the early, active petechial lesions to the older and less active powder-burn, fibrotic lesions.[35] Clinical diagnosis of endometriosis is accurate approximately 50 percent of the time.[30] Deep infiltrating lesions are most prevalent in the pouch of Douglas and the uterosacral ligaments and may cause pain by infiltrating nerve endings.[36] Sensory innervation of endometriotic implants may also contribute to pain sensations.[37] Other diagnostic options include ultrasound (however this is limited to diagnosis of ovarian endometriomas), and an elevated CA-125 and ESR (however the specificity is low).

TREATMENT

The chronic, recurring nature of endometriosis makes effective treatment difficult. There are several medical and surgical options. Untreated, minimal to moderate endometriosis may progress in 30 percent of patients, regress in 30 percent, or remain static in 40 percent.[38] With medical treatment, the goal is to induce a pseudomenopause or pseudopregnancy state to reduce the hormonal/cyclic stimulation of endometriotic lesions, and to decidualize or atrophy the lesions.

No studies have compared medical versus surgical treatment of endometriosis, but costs and side effects often dictate the choice of medical treatment. Initial therapy according to an expert consensus panel recommendations include a trial of NSAIDs with or without combined estrogen–progestin formulations.[39,40,41] A recent Cochrane review[42] found only one applicable RCT comparing NSAIDs to placebo in women with endometriosis; it had only 24 patients and found that there was no evidence of a positive effect on pain relief. However, NSAIDs have a low risk side-effect profile and are available over the counter. Hormonal combined OCPs have been used in both a cyclic and continuous fashion.[43] Traditionally, low estrogen dose OCPs containing more androgenic progestogens have been used but OCPs with new generation progestogen, desogestrol, has also been proven effective.[44]

If unsuccessful, high-dose progestins, androgenic hormones (danazol), or gonadotropin-releasing hormone (GnRH) agonists and GnRH plus aromatase inhibitors are used to induce atrophy of implants.[33] The most commonly used progestogens are medroxy-progesterone acetate and norethindrone acetate.[43,45] The levonorgestrol-releasing intrauterine system (Lng-IUS) is a novel approach to endometriosis. Its mechanism is unknown but it has been found to be more effective than expectant management in an RCT.[46] Danazol acts primarily by inhibiting the LH surge and steroidogenesis and by increasing free testosterone levels.[43]

GnRH agonists bind to GnRH receptors and down-regulates, eventually causing hypoestrogenism and amenorrhea.[45] Methods of delivery include nasal spray twice daily or a depot formulation. Side effects include those of a hypoestrogenic state: mood swings, vaginal dryness, decreased libido, myalgias, and headache. In an RCT of six-month GnRH-agonist therapy in laparoscopically confirmed endometriosis, decreased pain was associated with GnRH-agonist treatment as well as a decrease in the size of the endometriotic lesions.[47] GnRH-agonist therapy may be initiated without laparoscopically confirmed endometriosis if it is clinically suspected. Hormonal add-back therapy (i.e. norethindrone acetate 2–5 mg daily with or without estrogen) has also been utilized to prevent the long-term hypoestrogenic side effects (bone loss) of long-term (12 months) therapy, with continued relief of pelvic pain.[48] After discontinuation of GnRH-agonist treatment, recurrence of symptoms may return in up to 36–75 percent of patients over a five-year period, most commonly in patients with severe disease.[49] An RCT comparing Lng-IUS with depot GnRH analog for the treatment of CPP-associated endometriosis found that both were effective treatments and one was not significantly better than the other.[50] The Lng-IUS does not provoke hypoestrogenism and it requires only one medical intervention for its introduction every five years.

Surgical intervention involves laparotomy or laparoscopy. At the time of the laparoscopy, endometriosis lesions should be ablated or preferably removed. There have been no randomized trials to compare the efficacy of these methods with each other. Endometriomas should be removed with their capsule to prevent recurrence.[51] In an RCT of minimal to moderate endometriosis, laparoscopic laser treatment was noted to benefit 90 percent of women at one-year follow-up.[38] A prospective cohort study on patients with stage III–IV endometriosis found that 87.7 percent of the patients were satisfied with the results of ablative surgery at 12 months postoperatively.[52] An RCT with endometriosis to either diagnostic laparoscopy only or immediate excisional procedure found that laparoscopic excision of endometriosis (80 percent) is more effective than placebo (32 percent) at reducing pain and improving quality of life.[53] A review of the literature shows that in comparison to expectant management there is a significant amount of pain relief at six months after surgery with laser laparoscopic surgery for minimal, mild, and moderate endometriosis.[54] Recurence rate of pain after 24 months is around 50 percent.

In women who have finished childbearing, a hysterectomy with bilateral salpingo-oophorectomy, appendectomy, and removal of any residual gastrointestinal, genitourinary, or peritoneal disease can be performed. Hysterectomy without bilateral salpingo-ophorectomy is found to be less effective, with more disease recurrence and higher re-operation rates of approximately 30 percent.[55] Additional benefit in pain reduction may be derived from adjunctive acupuncture or multidisciplinary pain management (**Box 41.1**).[56]

Box 41.1 Treatment approach when endometriosis is suspected

- Trial of low-dose monophasic combination oral contraceptive pills (one pill/day for three to six months)
- If no improvement, three-month therapy with a GnRH agonist; if pain improves continue for three additional months, may consider hormonal add-back therapy
- Surgery to evaluate for pathology if no improvement with GnRH agonist:
  - excision/thermal ablation/laser of endometriotic lesions;
  - excision of endometriomas;
  - ± presacral neurectomy (for central pain);
  - ± hysterectomy and bilateral salpingo-oophorectomy;
- Endometriosis confirmed; hormonal management with one of following if pain persists/recurs following surgery:
  - continuous monophasic oral contraceptive pills to induce amenorrhea;
  - progestins:
    - medroxyprogesterone acetate (MPA) 30 mg p.o. q.d.;
    - depot MPA 150 mg i.m. q.3mo.
    - megestrol 40 mg p.o. q.d.;
    - norethindrone acetate 2–5 mg p.o. q.d.
- Levonorgestrol-releasing intrauterine device:
  - danazol 400–800 mg p.o. q.d.;
  - GnRH agonist:
    - nafarelin 200–400 g intranasal b.i.d.;
    - leuprolide 3.75 mg i.m. q.mo. or 11.25 mg i.m. q.3mo.
- ± Add-back therapy with norethindrone 2–5 mg p.o. q.d. or conjugated/esterified estrogen 0.625 mg p.o. q.d. and MPA 2.5 mg p.o. q.d.
- Multidisciplinary pain management – may be considered early in the management.

OUTCOME WITH RESPECT TO CPP

The relationship of endometriosis to chronic pelvic pain is unclear as endometriosis is a common finding in reproductive-age women without pain, and other pathology (i.e. adhesions, interstitial cyctitis, pelvic floor muscle spasm, abdominal wall pain) may be simultaneously present.[34] Classically, the severity of disease does not significantly correlate with the degree of pain.[57, 58] However, vaginal and uterosacral endometriosis was highly associated with complaints of deep dyspareunia[58] and deeply infiltrating lesions, particularly of the uterosacral ligaments were strongly associated with pain.[36] In contrast, Stovall *et al.*[59] found at a mean follow-up of 15 years that stage of disease was associated with persistence and intensity of chronic pelvic pain. In summary, pain that is not cyclical and/or does not respond to adequate surgical and medical management of endometriosis should be reevaluated for another source of pain and/or other contributing factors.

Pelvic congestion

PATHOPHYSIOLOGY

The syndrome of pelvic congestion was first proposed in the 1950s by Taylor,[60] who stated that autonomic nervous system dysfunction from emotional stress could cause smooth muscle spasm and congestion of the ovarian and uterine–pelvic venous plexes. Beard *et al.*[61, 62] investigated the prevalence of pelvic venous congestion in a blinded study on patients with CPP with no other obvious cause found at the time of laparoscopy. On transuterine pelvic venography, women with CPP had a larger mean ovarian vein diameter, delayed disappearance of contrast medium, and greater ovarian plexus congestion than controls.

SYMPTOMS AND SIGNS

Dull/aching pelvic pain accentuated with postural changes, ambulation, menstruation, and coitus; gastrointestinal symptoms characteristic of irritable bowel syndrome; genitourinary symptoms without evidence of infection; significant emotional disturbance; and on examination, tenderness over the adnexa, uterus, parametria, and especially the uterosacral ligaments.[60, 61]

DIAGNOSIS

Prior to carrying out invasive measures, symptomatic treatment to differentiate gastrointestinal, genitourinary, or myofascial etiology of CPP should be performed. Different techniques are now available to diagnose pelvic congestion, but none are as accurate as the transuterine venogram which is not widely available. On transvaginal ultrasound or MRI there may be uterine enlargement, thickened endometrium, cystic ovaries, and dilated pelvic veins. Laparoscopy can reveal varicosities[62] but false negative findings may occur.

TREATMENT

Hormonal suppression with progestin, medroxyprogesterone acetate (MPA) 30 mg may improve the symptoms of pelvic congestion, especially if combined with cognitive-behavioral therapy.[63, 64] OCPs have not been proven to be effective in treatment of pelvic congestion.[65] An RCT of GnRH analog, goserelin versus MPA found that one year following six months of treatment, goserelin was superior to MPA.[66] Several small, noncontrolled studies have looked at transcatheter embolization of pelvic veins with good short-term success.[67, 68] Further studies are indicated to evaluate the risks and long-term benefits.[69] Hysterectomy with bilateral salpingo-oophorectomy may be considered in women who have failed medical management. In a prospective study, 12 of 36 women on hormone replacement therapy following a hysterectomy with bilateral salpingo-oophrectomy (for pelvic congestion) were noted to have residual pain at one-year follow-up.[70]

Ovarian remnant syndrome

PATHOPHYSIOLOGY

The ovarian remnant syndrome is a rare complication resulting from ovarian cortical tissue left *in situ* during a difficult salpingo-oophorectomy, generally in the setting of extensive inflammation from tubo-ovarian abscess or endometriosis.[71, 72] In this situation, the remnants of the ovarian tissue may become functional and cystic.[73]

SYMPTOMS AND SIGNS

Pelvic pain usually arising one to five years after surgery is often cyclic, accompanied by flank pain. Associated genitourinary and gastrointestinal symptoms are common.[74] Pelvic examination may reveal a tender mass in the lateral region of the pelvis.

DIAGNOSIS

The diagnosis is suspected on the basis of history, physical examination, ultrasound, and hormonal evaluation.[71, 75] In a patient who has had a bilateral salpingo-oophorectomy and is not on hormone replacement, premenopausal levels of estradiol and follicle-stimulating hormone (FSH) levels should be present, although on occasion the remaining ovarian tissue may not be active enough to suppress FSH levels. Clomiphene citrate may be used to stimulate ovarian tissue to enhance diagnosis by ultrasound.

TREATMENT

Hormonal therapy may be utilized to suppress the ovarian remnant. GnRH agonists have shown superior results over oral contraceptives, progestins, and danazol in providing relief. The patients who achieved relief with the GnRH agonist were also noted to have subsequent relief with surgery.[76] Exploratory laparotomy is the method of choice for removal of residual ovarian tissue.[77] Surgical management via laparoscopy is controversial given the presence of extensive adhesions and potential complications, including hemorrhage, ureteral, bladder, and bowel damage.[74] Recurrent remnants occur in 15 percent of cases.

Residual ovary syndrome

Residual ovary syndrome consists of recurrent functional ovarian cysts in an individual who has undergone hysterectomy. The ovaries may be adherent to the pelvic side wall or vaginal cuff. Pain is usually limited to episodes of cyst formation. The treatment is ovarian suppression with combined estrogen/progestin contraceptives, high-dose progestins, or salpingo-oophorectomy.

GYNECOLOGIC NONCYCLIC PAIN

Adhesions

INCIDENCE

The precise role of adhesions in the genesis of CPP is unclear. The incidence of adhesions in patients undergoing laparoscopy for CPP ranges from 16–51 percent.[27, 78] The marked variation in incidence of adhesions noted in these studies may relate to the use of dissimilar control groups and/or a failure to recognize other causes of "occult" pelvic pain (abdominal wall or pelvic floor muscle pain, pelvic congestion, irritable bowel syndrome, and interstitial cystitis) prior to laparoscopy. Rapkin reported adhesions in 26 percent of CPP patients and 39 percent of asymptomatic infertility patients, with no significant differences in the location or density of adhesions between the two groups.[27] One cannot conclude that adhesions are causal, or even highly associated with CPP, as other populations (i.e. infertility patients) have been demonstrated to have substantial adhesions.

SYMPTOMS AND SIGNS

Abdominal/pelvic pain in women with adhesions is generally noncyclical, and commonly associated with dyspareunia. A clinical presentation synonymous with partial or complete obstruction of the bowel may be seen. Uterine immobility and adnexal mass/tenderness may be noted during physical examination.[79]

DIAGNOSIS

Diagnosis is by exploratory laparoscopy or laparotomy. The technique, known as "pain mapping" (office microlaparoscopy with local anesthesia/conscious sedation), was thought to allow physicians to better locate the adhesions associated with pelvic pain.[80] In an observational pain mapping study of 50 women under local anesthesia, manipulation of appendiceal and pelvic adhesions was observed to contribute significantly to pelvic pain.[28] However, correlation between lysis of adhesions or removal of these adhesions and long-term pain outcome could not be established.

TREATMENT

The mechanism by which adhesions contribute to chronic pain is thought to be secondary to the restriction of bowel mobility and distention.[81] Therefore, adhesiolysis should improve subjective pain symptoms; indeed, in several retrospective, noncontrolled studies, pain was improved in 50–90 percent of these patients.[81, 82, 83] An RCT of adhesiolysis for pelvic pain found that surgery did not benefit women with mild or moderate degrees of pelvic adhesions.[84] Adhesiolysis was of no more benefit than expectant management, except in those patients with severe, vascularized, and dense adhesions involving the small bowel. These patients tended to have symptoms and physical findings consistent with intermittent partial small bowel obstruction.[84] The lack of benefit of adhesiolysis was confirmed in another RCT of 100 patients who had laparoscopically documented adhesions and CPP and were randomly assigned to either adhesiolysis or no adhesiolysis at the time of diagnostic laparoscopy.[85] Patients were evaluated for 12 months postoperatively. The authors concluded that laparoscopic adhesiolysis was not more beneficial than diagnostic laparoscopy alone, demonstrating the substantial placebo effect of surgical intervention.

The patient's degree of psychosocial functioning and other signs which may be a proxy for an abnormal pain amplification state may also influence the effectiveness of adhesiolysis. For example, a small prospective, but uncontrolled study found that after eight months, chronic pelvic pain patients with "CPP syndrome" had not benefited from surgery.[86] They defined women with "CPP syndrome" as those presenting with four or more of the following: (1) pain duration greater than six months; (2) incomplete relief by previous treatments; (3) impaired physical functioning secondary to pain; (4) vegetative signs of depression; and (5) altered family roles.

Tumors and cysts of the reproductive organs and salpingo-oophoritis

Other gynecologic pathology that may present with symptoms of chronic discomfort include adnexal masses and uterine leiomyomata (fibroids). Vague lower abdominal discomfort and fullness and bladder or gastrointestinal symptoms may be related to leiomyomata or ovarian neoplasm. On examination, a pelvic mass is generally palpated, which is confirmed by ultrasound. A myomectomy or hysterectomy may be therapeutic for uterine myomata, especially if associated with abnormal bleeding or if uterine size is greater than 14 cm. An adnexal mass larger than 6 cm is concerning for malignancy and should be referred to a gynecologist. Solid or complex components and bilaterality are also more suspicious for malignancy, and a persistent mass should also be concerning for inflammatory mass, endometrioma or malignancy as functional cysts (follicles and corpus luteum cysts) usually resolve over four to eight weeks. One way of preventing functional cysts from recurring is ovulation suppression with hormonal contraception.

Salpingo-oophoritis/pelvic inflammatory disease (PID) generally presents as an acute process. Chronic pelvic pain can develop secondary to subacute infections with chlamydia for example, or possibly related to past salpingo-oophoritis with large hydrosalpinges and adhesion formation, causing restriction of pelvic organs and stretching of the pelvic peritoneum or an inflammatory insult leading to chronic up-regulation of neural processing.[87] Diagnosis of acute PID is made by clinical criteria proposed by Sweet and Gibbs.[88] Two of the three must be present: lower abdominal pain as well as lower abdominal tenderness (with or without rebound), cervical motion tenderness, and adnexal tenderness. In addition, one of the following minor criteria must be present: (1) temperature greater than 38°C, leukocytosis (>10,500 white blood cells/mm^3); (2) culdocentesis fluid containing white cells and bacteria on Gram stain; (3) presence of an inflammatory mass; (4) elevated ESR; (5) a Gram stain from the endocervix revealing Gram-negative intracellular diplococci; or (6) studies of endocervical secretions revealing chlamydia or gonorrhea. However, clinical diagnosis leads to error in 50 percent of cases[88] and, in repeated episodes of pain suggestive of salpingo-oophoritis, laparoscopy may be performed to verify the diagnosis.

GASTROENTEROLOGIC CAUSES OF CHRONIC PELVIC PAIN

Gastrointestinal disease may mimic the features of chronic gynecologic pelvic pain, due to the common innervation tract (T10–L1) between the cervix, uterus, adnexa, and lower ileum, sigmoid colon, and rectum. The complete differential diagnosis and management of pain of enterocolic origin is presented in Chapter 10, The psychological assessment of pain in patients with chronic pain.[89, 90, 91, 92, 93]

Endometriosis affecting the bowel

Implantation of endometriotic lesions on the intestine can cause cyclic abdominal pain. In severe cases, partial or complete bowel obstruction may develop. The incidence of a significant bowel involvement with endometriosis is approximately 5 percent.

Hernia

Although infrequent in the female population, the presence of an abdominal wall hernia in a patient with chronic pelvic pain should be included in the differential diagnoses.[94] These include inguinal (indirect or direct), femoral, spigelian, incisional, and umbilical. Symptoms and signs include history of an abdominal or groin mass and pain or discomfort with an increase in intra-abdominal pressure. Spigelian hernias result from a defect through the transversalis fascia, just lateral to rectus muscle at the level of the semicircular line of Douglas.[95] Incisional hernias generally occur at fascial defects with vertical incisions. Other types of hernias include sciatic hernias secondary to atrophy of the piriformis muscle, which may include the ipsilateral ovary in its hernia sac, and vaginal hernias (cystocele, rectocele, and enterocele).[96] Treatment of abdominal hernias includes surgical repair through the laparoscope or through a skin incision. Vaginal hernias are repaired surgically or a pessary may be used.

Irritable bowel syndrome

Irritable bowel syndrome (IBS) accounts for 7–60 percent of referrals to gynecologists[97] and 48 to 79 percent of patients with chronic pelvic pain, dyspareunia, dysmenorrhea, or a history of numerous abdominal surgeries also have IBS.[98] Women who have undergone hysterectomy for CPP are twice as likely to have IBS.[99]

A full discussion of IBS appears in Chapter 40, Chronic abdominal, groin, and perineal pain of visceral origin.

UROLOGIC CAUSES OF CHRONIC PELVIC PAIN

Many chronic pelvic pain cases are primary urinary tract disorders.[100, 101] The overlap in clinical presentation in part relates to the close development and anatomic relationship of the urinary and genital tracts. Urologic symptoms can stem from a primary gynecologic cause, including bladder and ureteral involvement of endometriosis or external bladder compression with a uterine leiomyomata. The differential diagnosis in urologic causes of chronic pelvic pain should include the following.

Recurrent infectious cystitis

Suprapubic pain, dysuria, frequency, and urgency comprise the classic presentation of cystitis. Microscopic analysis with pyuria and a positive urine culture are diagnostic. Women frequently produce "clean catch" urine specimens that are still contaminated with vaginal secretions, as evidenced by squamous epithelial cells. Catheterized specimens are therefore recommended if repeated bouts of infectious symptoms occur. In cases of recurrent infection, repeat culture and test of cure cultures will aid in diagnosis and management. Further history should be elicited to determine the etiology; if associated with intercourse, voiding following intercourse and prophylactic antibiotics may be used after coitus. Recurrent infections in peri- and postmenopausal women may benefit from vaginal estrogen cream by altering the vaginal pH and modifying the vaginal flora.[102] Chlamydial infection is responsible for approximately 25 percent of cases of pyuria and urethritis in women with a sterile urine culture.[101]

Urethral syndrome

ETIOLOGY

The diagnosis of urethral syndrome is one of exclusion. Its unknown etiology makes the diagnosis and treatment difficult. Subclinical infection, chronic inflammation of the periurethral glands, or urethral spasticity with periurethral muscle fatigue have been suggested as possible etiologies.

SYMPTOMS AND SIGNS

Classically, urethral syndrome presents with irritative lower urinary tract symptoms – dysuria, suprapubic discomfort, urinary frequency, and dyspareunia.[101, 103] Voiding dysfunction such as stranguria, the slow and painful discharge of urine, may occur. A careful physical examination should be performed to evaluate for possible structural causes of pain. The urethra should be evaluated for discharge, tenderness, or a mass suggestive of a urethral diverticulum or Skene's cyst.

DIAGNOSIS

Diagnostic studies include urinalysis with urine culture and sensitivity, urethral evaluation for chlamydia, mycoplasma, or ureaplasma infection, and a wet mount for infectious or atrophic vaginitis.

TREATMENT

Treatment consists of reeducation of voiding habits through pelvic floor muscle biofeedback,[101] antibiotic therapy with doxycycline or erythromycin for 10–14 days if chlamydia is suspected, or chronic suppression with a three- to six-month low-dose course of broad-spectrum antibiotics. Urethral dilation has been performed in recalcitrant cases. In a prospective study, Bergman and colleagues[103] assigned 60 women to serial urethral dilation, antibiotic treatment, or placebo. Seventy-five percent of women in the urethral dilation group had absence of symptoms, which was significantly higher than in the placebo (20 percent) or tetracycline group (50 percent). Improvement in the uroflowmetry dynamics was also noted only in the dilation group. Vaginal estrogen for peri- and postmenopausal women should also supplement treatment. Other treatments have included muscle relaxants, alpha-antagonists (terazosin and doxazosin), and psychotherapy.

Interstitial cystitis

SYMPTOMS

This is a symptom complex characterized by pelvic pain, urinary urgency, urinary frequency, and nocturia.[104] Symptoms of dyspareunia and perimenstrual exacerbation with negative laboratory studies are consistent with both interstitial cystitis (IC) and urgency/frequency syndrome.[105] The National Institutes of Health (NIH) Consensus Criteria from 1988 for the diagnosis of IC includes at least two of the following: pain on bladder filling relieved by emptying; pain in the suprapubic, pelvic, urethral, vaginal, or perineal region; glomerulations on endoscopy or decreased compliance on cystometrogram.[106] Symptoms that do not meet IC criteria can be termed "painful bladder syndrome" and are probably a variant of interstitial cystitis.

A full discussion of this condition appears in Chapter 40, Chronic abdominal, groin, and perineal pain of visceral origin.

MUSCULOSKELETAL CAUSES OF CHRONIC PELVIC PAIN

In women with CPP, isolated back pain without pelvic pain is rarely a presentation of primary gynecologic pathology. Generally, the etiology of low back pain results from an imbalance of muscle groups related to repetitive movements, fatigue, or faulty posture (lordosis and kyphosis). Back pain may be caused by gynecologic, vascular, neurologic, psychogenic, or spondylogenic (related to the axial skeleton and its structures) pathology.[107, 108]

Myofascial pain

Reports of the prevalence of myofascial pain as a cause of pelvic pain vary from 15 to 89 percent.[10, 100, 109] This discrepancy in part reflects the overlap in innervation and referred pain sites in the musculoskeletal structures and the visceral pelvic structures. Whether pain is primarily myofascial or is a manifestation of referred pain is not known. Myofascial pain syndrome and fibromyalgia should be ruled out with history and physical examination.[110]

SYMPTOMS AND SIGNS

Musculoskeletal pain typically presents as a dull aching pain that is difficult to localize. Structures including the rectus muscle, iliopsoas, quadratrus lumborum, piriformis, and obturators, innervated via T12–L4, and levator ani, innervated via S2–4, can refer pain to the lower abdomen pelvis and vulva or vagina. This pain is further enhanced if there is a primary pelvic pathology or irritation, including bladder and colon activity, menses, and intercourse, as these organs also have a similar innervation of T10–S4,[10, 108, 109, 111] therefore, myofascial pain is often worse during menses. On digital examination of the abdominal, back, or vaginal dermatomes, pressure on a trigger point evokes local and referred pain. Performing a straight leg raising maneuver tensing the abdominal wall muscles exacerbates abdominal wall pain.

TREATMENT

Physical therapy to evaluate posture, muscle length, strength, and flexibility as well as trigger point injections are critical in the treatment of myofascial pain.[112] Psychological factors should also be assessed and treated. The comorbid factors of depression, anxiety, and maladaptive behavior may potentiate the pain.[10, 111] Medications such as low-dose tricyclic antidepressants and anticonvulsants may also be useful.

Neuropathic pain/nerve entrapment or injury

PATHOPHYSIOLOGY

Injury to or cutaneous nerve entrapment of the ilioinguinal (T12, L1), iliohypogastric (T12, L1), genitofemoral (L1, L2), and pudendal (S2–4) nerves may result in chronic lower abdominal and perineal pain. Generally, the iliohypogastric/ilioinguinal nerve pain develops following a Pfannensteil skin incision or other lower abdominal skin incision which results in nerve entrapment or stretch.[113, 114] This syndrome may also occur spontaneously by muscular impingement of the nerve between the transverse and internal oblique muscles from repetitive activity, physical trauma, or poor posture.

Neurologic injury may also occur at the time of gynecological surgery due to: (1) improper placement or positioning of retractors, especially retractors with deep lateral retractor blades; (2) improper positioning of patients in lithotomy position preoperatively; and (3) radical surgical dissection and subsequent autonomic nerve disruption.

SYMPTOMS AND SIGNS

Stabbing, sharp pain, typically elicited by exercise and chronic dull aching pain that is relieved by bed-rest, may reflect nerve entrapment.[113, 115] In a series of 46 women with a clinical diagnosis of ilioinguinal nerve entrapment, 88 percent had hyperesthesiae and 53 percent dysesthesia.[116] The site of maximal pain with ilioinguinal or iliohypogastric nerve entrapment is along the lateral edge of the rectus margin and may radiate to the hip or sacroiliac region.

DIAGNOSIS

Nerve entrapment is diagnosed by eliciting focal tenderness over the site of the nerve entrapment.[117] This is carried out by having the patient tense her abdominal muscles in the supine position by raising either her shoulders or legs while pressing with a single finger medial and below the anteriosuperior iliac spine or along the course of the involved nerve. If the abdominal pain is secondary to abdominal nerve entrapment, the pain will worsen with this maneuver and is located in the characteristic dermatome distribution for that nerve.[118]

TREATMENT

Relief of pain with a peripheral nerve block is both diagnostic and often therapeutic. Approximately 5 mL of bupivacaine 0.25 percent or other local anesthetic is injected into the tender point using a 22–26 gauge 1.5-inch-long needle. The needle is placed such that the fat pad is slowly penetrated until the needle tip reproduces the pain.[108, 109, 111, 116] Initially, severe pain may occur; however, relief (five to ten minutes for onset of the local anesthetic) will follow and is continued by repeating biweekly injections, up to five, as needed.[119] Other forms of more long-standing treatment include cryoneurolysis and nerve transection. Hahn[116] reported a 76 percent improvement in pain with surgical transection at one year of follow-up in 51 cases of treated trapped nerves. Two other studies have reported complete relief after surgical management in over 70 percent of patients.[120, 121] As with all neurolytic techniques, however, there is a high probability of failure over time, painful neuroma formation, and anesthesia dolorosa. Other therapeutic options include topical local anesthetic creams or patches, low-dose tricyclic antidepressants, anticonvulsants, physical therapy (to strengthen muscles, mobilize nerves, and avoid traction on nerves), and acupuncture. Narcotic medications are relatively ineffective.

CHRONIC PELVIC PAIN WITHOUT OBVIOUS PATHOLOGY

The International Association for the Study of Pain (IASP) classification includes a category entitled chronic pelvic pain without obvious pathology. This category is useful because it allows the assignment of a diagnosis in situations where the etiology of the pain, even after an exhaustive evolution, remains elusive. This diagnosis should not imply, however, that the pain is psychogenic in nature, yet unrecognized neurophysiologic or biochemical perturbations may in the future be identified in women with pelvic pain without obvious pathology. Dysmenorrhea, for example, was thought to be a neurotic affectation until the discovery of prostaglandins. Furthermore, the multifactorial etiology of most unexplained chronic pain conditions is just beginning to be recognized.[122] The management of pelvic pain without obvious pathology is similar to that of any enigmatic pain process: multidisciplinary management including pharmacological and psychological interventions, although specific studies are lacking.

Psychological factors in chronic pelvic pain

Factors can promote the chronicity of pain. Women with CPP have higher levels of depression, anxiety, and somatization, as well as emotional, physical, and sexual abuse.[123, 124, 125, 126, 127, 128] Catastrophizing, pain-related anxiety and fear, depression (hopelessness), and loss of control (helplessness) can lead to persistent pain; whereas self-efficacy, pain-coping strategies, readiness to change, and acceptance can help prevent or break the cycle of chronic pain.[129]

A woman's response to an acute pain experience may therefore be more likely to progress to a chronic process based on a current or previous emotional experience, catastrophizing personality style, expectations, mechanism or thinking, and/or habits. This process likely involves alterations in central processing. The stimulus for these alterations and mechanisms underlying the maintenance of changes in central processing without an inflammatory stimulus or nerve damage are unknown. Other factors may include alterations in the hypothalamic–pituitary–adrenal axis and cortisol levels.[122, 130]

DEPRESSION

Major depression and other dysthymic, panic, and somatization disorders have been associated with CPP of unknown etiology.[131, 132] Higher depression scores and family histories of affective disorder were described in women with CPP without pathology than in women with chronic pelvic pain and pathology as established by laparoscopy.[131] Often, the depression preceded the onset of the pain; however, no prospective or outcome studies have been performed.[89, 131, 132] A recent systematic review found depression to be correlated with pelvic pain with an OR of 2.59.[133]

Sexual and physical abuse

Women with CPP have a higher incidence of sexual and/or physical abuse in childhood and adulthood with prevalence rates of approximately 50 percent.[132, 134, 135, 136, 137] A history of sexual and physical abuse is an independent risk factor for CPP.[138] A recent systematic review found a strong association of sexual abuse with CPP with an OR of 2.67.[133] A higher incidence of substance abuse has been reported in the CPP population.[135]

CLINICAL EVALUATION

History

Critical to the evaluation and management of CPP is a detailed history. A pain questionnaire may assist in helping the patient express issues that she may otherwise be unable to verbally express.

The history should include:

- The chronology of the pain. In what context did the pain arise? Was there an eliciting event? Has the pain changed? What does the patient think is causing the pain?
- The nature of the pain: character, intensity, location and radiation, aggravating and alleviating factors, and the effect of menses, exercise, work, stress, intercourse, and orgasm.
- The severity of pain, rated from 0 to 10 on a verbal or visual analog scale.
- Associated somatic symptoms. Specifically related to the:
  - genital tract (abnormal vaginal bleeding, discharge, mittelschmerz, dysmenorrhea, dyspareunia, infertility);
  - gastrointestinal tract (constipation, diarrhea, flatulence, tenesmus, alterations to pain before and after a bowel movement, blood, changes in color or caliber of stool);
  - musculoskeletal system (pain distribution, radiation, association with injury, fatigue, postural changes, exercise, lifting);
  - urologic tract (dysuria, urgency, frequency, nocturia, hematuria, suprapubic pain).
- Neurologic system (burning, lancinating pain, allodynia, and or numbness in the distribution of a particular peripheral nerve).
- Prior evaluations for the pain including treatment history, operative and pathology reports, as well as side effects/success or failure of prior treatments.
- Impact on family, work, daily activities. Is the degree of pain such that the pain prevents the patient from performing a family role or occupation? Is litigation or worker's compensation an issue? What is the attitude of the patient and family toward the pain and resultant behavior?

- Past medical, surgical, gynecologic, obstetric history, and medication intake including pain medication.
- Current and past psychological history. History of past or current physical, sexual, and/or emotional abuse, history of hospitalization, suicide attempts, and chemical (drug or alcohol) dependence.
- Patient's expectations. What is the goal of treatment?

Prospective daily pain ratings or calendars to note the occurrence and intensity of pain, menstrual bleeding, and mood rating (0–10) are very helpful in the evaluation of CPP. Aggravating factors should be noted in the daily rating, utilizing an analog scale from 0 (no pain) to 10 (most severe pain ever) for at least two months or two menstrual cycles, and is best continued until pain has resolved. Daily rating increases self-efficacy, demonstrates compliance, allows for diagnosis of atypical (luteal phase as opposed to just with menses) cyclic pain, demonstrates improvement with treatment, and allows the patient to recognize the connection between pain and stress or physical activities.

Examination

Perform a complete physical examination, with particular attention to the abdomen, back, vagina, vulva, and pelvic floor muscles, and pelvic viscera. Prior to the examination, the patient should carefully localize the area(s) of pain, as this can help differentiate the tissues involved in the genesis of pain. The examination should include evaluation of:

- General: The patient's general body habitus, posture while sitting, standing, and walking, and anxiety level.
- Abdomen: Evaluate for scars and sites of hypersensitivity in specific dermatome regions and for trigger points or nerve entrapment. A bilateral straight leg raising or abdominal crunch maneuver performed to discern abdominal wall sources of pain, as abdominal wall pain (myofascial and neuropathic) is augmented and visceral pain is diminished with the above maneuver.[109, 111, 118] The quality of bowel sounds should be noted as well as distension, sites of tenderness to palpation, and guarding. While the patient is standing, evaluate visually and by palpation for hernias (inguinal, femoral, and Spigelian).
- Musculoskeletal: The patient should be evaluated for concurrent fibromyalgia or scoliosis. Discrepancy in leg length, muscle strength, and range of motion should be assessed and pelvic floor muscle tenderness, trigger points, and hernias should be elicited by palpation of tender sites.
- Neurological: It should be determined if there are signs of hyperalgesia and allodynia in the distribution of a particular nerve. Neurological examination including sensation of pinprick, cold and light touch is useful as is assessment of perineal and lower extremity strength, sensation, and reflexes.
- Gynecologic: Assess the vulva for lesions, rashes, evidence of trauma and old scars (episiotomy). A cotton-tipped swab should then be used to evaluate for sites of hypersensitivity within the vulva and vestibule. A unidigital examination is then performed to palpate the urethra, bladder base, vaginal sidewalls, levator ani, pubococcygeus, coccygeus, piriformis, obturator internus, cervix, and uterosacral ligament to elicit any tenderness. Evaluate for pelvic floor relaxation (cystocele, rectocele, enterocele) and vaginal atrophy. Bimanual examination may elicit uterine or adnexal tenderness, and/or abnormalities in size, shape, or mobility. A rectovaginal examination is then performed to further assess uterosacral tenderness, nodularity, and rectal disease/occult blood. Speculum examination should be performed to inspect visually for vaginal or cervical lesions, hypoestrogenization, and to rule out vaginitis.

DIAGNOSTIC STUDIES

Diagnostic work-up includes a CBC, ESR, clean catch or catheterized urine for urinalysis and culture, cervical and urethral studies for gonorrhea and chlamydia, pregnancy test (if indicated), wet mount of vaginal secretions, Pap smear if indicated, stool guaiac, and, if diarrhea is present, stool culture. Pelvic ultrasound is warranted but abdominal/pelvic computed tomography (CT) scan or pelvic or lower back MRI should only be performed if other pathology is suspected. Other studies (i.e. cystoscopy, colonoscopy) should be based on patient symptomatology or on consultation with other specialists (urologist, gastroenterologist, neurologist, orthopedist, and physical therapist). Surgical evaluation with diagnostic laparoscopy or hysteroscopy may be considered if initial therapy fails or if pelvic examination is abnormal.

EVIDENCE-BASED EVALUATION OF MANAGEMENT

Pharmacological

NSAIDs, narcotics, antidepressants, and anticonvulsants have been utilized in the treatment of CPP as in other types of chronic pain. NSAIDs are also widely used in patients with cyclic pelvic pain. They act as inhibitors of prostaglandin production and may also act on local cytokines. A Cochrane review[14][I] found that NSAIDs in patients with dysmenorrhea were significantly more effective than placebo for pain relief (OR 7.91). Another Cochrane review[42][II] found only one applicable RCT comparing NSAIDs to placebo in women with endometriosis and found that there was no evidence of a positive effect.

Only one RCT has looked at the effect of a selective serotonin reuptake inhibitor (SSRI) on pelvic pain[139][II] and found no significant difference between sertraline and placebo in the measures of pain and functional disability. CPP patients treated with gabapentin alone or in combination with amitriptyline was better than with amitriptyline alone.[140] Treatment of CPP with narcotics should include a narcotic contract between provider and patient as well as regularly scheduled appointments for follow-up. Tricyclic antidepressants and serotonin/norepinephine reuptake inhibitor would be theoretically more effective than SSRIs but studies for CPP are lacking.

Cyclic pelvic pain should respond to menstrual suppression with continuous oral contraceptive pills, high-dose progestins, or gonadotropin-releasing hormone agonists with hormone add-back therapy to minimize bone loss. These hormones act by suppressing ovulation and lessening the endometrial lining of the uterus. Menstrual volume is thus decreased as well as the amount of prostaglandins produced, in effect reducing dysmenorrhea by decreasing uterine motility, and thus cramping. A Cochrane review of five RCTs of OCPs for primary dysmenorrhea found OCPs more effective than placebo.[16] [I] There have been two RCTs looking at medroxyprogesterone acetate in patients with pelvic congestion syndrome or adhesions, but not endometriosis or dysmenorrheal, and pain scores were improved at the end of treatment.[141][I]

Physical therapy

There are few randomized studies in the area of physical therapy and pelvic pain. One open randomized study found that distention of painful pelvic structures in women with CPP resulted in significant relief of pain and improvement in quality of life measures.[142][II] However, in the multidisciplinary approach of treatment for CPP, physical therapy is often incorporated in the management,[143] especially in cases of myofascial syndrome. TENS and biofeedback are often used in conjunction by the physical therapist.[144] A meta-analysis of seven randomized controlled trials found that high frequency TENS is more effective for pain relief than placebo.[21][I] Intravaginal TENS provides electrical stimulation to the pelvic floor muscles and is also available.[145][III]

Injection therapies

TRIGGER POINT INJECTIONS

Trigger point injections may provide prolonged relief by interfering with transmission of the pain impulse and thus eliminating the positive feedback arc.[10] No RCTs specifically looked at chronic pelvic pain and trigger point injections. One small RCT compared trigger point injections in patients with myofascial syndrome with bupivacaine 0.5 percent, etidocaine 1 percent, or saline. Subjective improvement was noted with the local anesthetic treatment over saline.[146][II] Slocumb[10][III] studied the response of 122 women with abdominal pelvic pain characterized by dermatome hypersensitivity and trigger points: 89.3 percent reported relief or improvement in pain, such that no further therapy was required over the duration of the study (3–36 months). Further management of myofascial pain is described in Chapter 12, Diagnostic procedures in chronic pain. Botulinum toxin injections were effective in reducing pain in patients with myofascial pain syndrome but the difference in pain between the two modes was not significantly different.[147][II]

LOCAL ANESTHETIC NERVE BLOCKS

In some cases, with multiple trigger points in the vaginal wall, back, and abdominal wall, a series of abdominal nerve, caudal, pudendal or epidural blocks may prove to be more fruitful in treating the pain than multiple trigger point injections.[10][III] Nerve blocks with local anesthetics may provide relief of neuralgia due to nerve injury. Prolonged partial pain relief may occur for weeks or months following one or more nerve blocks beyond the anticipated duration of the local anesthetic. The explanation for prolonged pain relief may be secondary to reduced capacity of the nerve to maintain repetitive impulses, decreased excitability of the nerve fiber, and systemic uptake of the anesthetic. Nerve blocks have also been used as a prerequisite for evaluating potential effectiveness prior to neurectomy.[148][III] Superior hypogastric plexus block by CT guidance and at the time of microlaparoscopy may provide further evaluation and management in chronic pelvic pain.[149, 150][III] CT guidance has also been found to be useful for needle guidance in pudendal nerve blocks.[151][III]

Surgery

Very few RCTs evaluate the surgical management of chronic pelvic pain. However, a large prospective observational cohort study with 370 participants found that patients improved modestly with either medical or surgical therapy.[152][III]

LAPAROSCOPY

Laparoscopy has an important role in the diagnosis and management of acute pelvic pain. Its exact role in the evaluation of patients with chronic pelvic pain is more controversial and limited.[153] Of patients with CPP 14–77 percent have no obvious pathology and two-thirds of patients have findings of adhesions, which may or may not play a role in their pain.[29, 154] In a review on the use of laparoscopy in chronic pelvic pain, Howard[4, 155] found that CPP patients had approximately twice the incidence of pelvic pathology compared with the 28 percent incidence of pathology in the non-CPP population.

Indications

Prior to proceeding with laparoscopy, a thorough evaluation of the patient's pelvic pain should be carried out to exclude other nongynecologic etiologies of CPP, as outlined above under Gastroenterologic causes of chronic pelvic pain; Urologic causes of chronic pelvic pain; Musculoskeletal causes of chronic pelvic pain; Neuropathic pain/nerve entrapment or injury; and Chronic pelvic pain without obvious pathology. An abnormal pelvic examination prior to laparoscopy is associated with pathology 70–90 percent of the time, and abnormal pathology is present in one-half of patients with normal preoperative pelvic examinations.[4] During the operative procedure, specific attention should be directed at sites of increased tenderness on physical examination. Laparoscopy should be performed when one believes it will help in the management:

- failure of medication (hormonal and analgesic) to relieve pain over a minimum of three months;
- surgical management of adhesions, endometriosis, or hernias;[29, 156][III]
- for pain mapping. Under conscious sedation and local anesthesia, direct visualization by minilaparoscopy can be performed to evaluate intra-abdominal sites associated with pelvic pain to help isolate sources of somatic and visceral pain. However, no outcome studies exist as to whether pain management guided by pain mapping is more efficacious.[80, 157][III]

Adverse effects

One may erroneously attribute the source of pain to "pathology" visualized at the time of laparoscopy when a nongynecologic source, such as irritable bowel syndrome, myofascial pain, or nerve entrapment, may be the true etiology. The patient must also be clear that she may still have some degree of pain following the procedure. Surgical injury to bowel, bladder, ureter, vessels, and nerves are potential complications.

Evidence for efficacy

The use of laparoscopy is controversial, as nonsurgical management of chronic pelvic pain is successful in 65–90 percent of patients regardless of the presence of "pathology".[10, 47, 143, 158] The only RCT of the use of laparoscopy randomized women with CPP to one of two treatment modalities.[143][II] The standard approach in 49 patients involved routine laparoscopy. The other 57 patients underwent an integrated approach, including assessment of somatic, psychological, dietary, environmental, and physiotherapeutic factors. Laparoscopy was not routinely performed in this group.[143] Of the 49 patients in the standard group, 65 percent had no abnormality, 5 percent had endometriosis, 18 percent had adhesions, and the remainder had myomata, ovarian cysts, or pelvic varices. The integrated approach was significantly more effective in the reduction of pelvic pain (75 versus 41 percent).[143] The authors concluded that laparoscopy provided too little a benefit to warrant its routine use in the management of CPP. Although there was a 35 percent incidence of pelvic pathology, these abnormalities overall were considered negligible and minimally additive to the preoperative diagnosis.[143]

Hysterectomy

Thirty percent of patients presenting to pelvic pain clinics have already undergone hysterectomy without experiencing relief of pain.[5] A decline in the incidence of hysterectomy for the indication of CPP from 16.3 to 5.8 percent was rated after the initiation of a multidisciplinary approach to the diagnosis and treatment of chronic pelvic pain.[158] Additionally, preoperative pelvic pain is a major risk factor for postsurgical pain one year after hysterectomy.[159]

INDICATIONS

Patients with cyclic pain or dysfunctional uterine bleeding are excellent candidates for hysterectomy, especially if they have relief of pain with hormonal suppression. The American College of Obstetricians and Gynecologists (ACOG) criteria set on hysterectomy for pelvic pain states the following as indications for hysterectomy:[160] no remediable pathology found on laparoscopic examination and presence of pain for more than six months with a negative effect on the patient's quality of life. However, unless there is uterine pathology, endometriosis, secondary dysmenorrhea, or significant prolapse, hysterectomy is unlikely to be helpful for CPP. Prior to hysterectomy, medical management and multidisciplinary therapy should be tried, and other nongynecologic etiologies should be evaluated, including the patient's psychological and psychosexual status.[160]

CONTRAINDICATIONS

Desire for future fertility and known medical or psychological risks that exceed benefit are contraindications.[160]

ADVERSE EFFECTS

Preoperatively, one needs to discuss with the patient the potential outcomes of the surgery – including the possibility of posthysterectomy pelvic pain – secondary to nerve entrapment, new trigger points, irritable bladder or bowel, postoperative adhesions, residual ovary, ovarian remnant, recurrent endometriosis, and vaginal cuff pain.[73]

EVIDENCE OF EFFICACY

No RCTs have compared hysterectomy with no surgery in CPP patients. From the limited nonrandomized studies, one may estimate that one in four women will continue to have persistent pain following hysterectomy for CPP.[160, 161, 162, 163][III] The success rate of hysterectomy for the treatment of CPP is better with cyclic pelvic pain. Stovall *et al.*,[162] in a retrospective study of 99 women, and Hillis *et al.*[163] in a prospective cohort of 308 women, noted a 77 and 74 percent response rate, respectively, in woman who underwent hysterectomy for CPP felt to be of uterine origin. At one-year follow-up, however, 25 percent of women in Stovall's group noted a persistence of worsening of pain. Hillis observed that persistent pain was associated with multiparity, prior history of PID, lack of pathology, and Medicare payer status.[163] A retrospective study of 98 women with a history of CPP who underwent abdominal hysterectomy found that 96% of women reported improvement in pain and 87% were satisfied with their surgery.[164] A large prospective cohort study of women with pain and depression or pain only who underwent hysterectomy for benign conditions found that both groups had significant and substantial pain reduction 24 months after surgery.[165] There was a smaller reduction in the pain in the depression group.

Presacral neurectomy/uterosacral transection

Presacral neurectomy involves transection of the superior hypogastric plexus at the level of the sacrum. This differs from uterosacral transection (laparoscopic uterine nerve ablation (LUNA)) in which the nerves are cut at the level of the uterus. LUNA involves the destruction of the uterine nerve fibers as they exit the uterus through the uterosacral ligament.

INDICATIONS

Cotte[166] documented the use of presacral neurectomy (PSN) or sympathectomy as a treatment for intractable dysmenorrhea in 1937. PSN has since been recommended as a surgical treatment for women with deep central pain secondary to refractory primary dysmenorrhea or endometriosis. Afferent innervation from the cervix, uterus, and proximal fallopian tubes (T11–L12) travels through the superior hypogastric plexus. PSN interrupts pain from these organs by transection of these nerves.

Preoperative evaluation/requirements should include:

- failure in the past to respond to medical management;
- interference with daily activities secondary to the pain;
- assessment for structural abnormalities likely contributing to the pain;
- evaluation for somatic (nonvisceral) causes of pain;
- possible trial of paracervical or fluoroscopic guided hypogastric plexus blockade to assess whether surgery may benefit;
- a discussion of the expectations/long-term relief of pain with the procedure.

CONTRAINDICATIONS

Afferents from the adnexal structures travel with the sympathetic fibers along the infundibulopelvic ligament to enter the spinal cord at T9–T10. Therefore, lateralizing pain of visceral origin will not be relieved by PSN or LUNA.

ADVERSE EFFECTS

Risks of the procedure include: ureteral injury secondary to the close proximity of these structures necessitating laparotomy[167][V] and dysfunction of the bladder and rectum with PSN due to the common pathway of their sympathetic afferent nerves along the superior hypogastric plexus.[168] With uterosacral nerve ablation, a theoretical risk of uterine prolapse exists.[169, 170][V]

EVIDENCE FOR EFFICACY

Generally quoted statistics on the efficacy of PSN or LUNA report a 70–80 percent improvement in primary and less for secondary dysmenorrhea.[168, 171, 172, 173, 174][III]

The addition of uterosacral ligament resection to conservative laparoscopic surgery for endometriosis did not reduce the medium- or long-term frequency and severity of recurrence of dysmenorrhea.[175] An RCT of LUNA decreased dysmenorrhea in women with no evidence of endometriosis at the one year mark. However, the addition of LUNA in patients with endometriosis did not add to pain relief.[176] Zullo *et al.*[177][II] randomized patients suffering from severe dysmenorrhea associated with endometriosis to either receive PSN or no PSN at the time of laparoscopic surgery. They found significantly more pain relief with PSN at both six (87.3 versus 60.3 percent) and 12 months (85.7 versus 57.1 percent).

A Cochrane database meta-analysis[178][I] concluded that there was evidence that uterine nerve ablation was more effective for primary dysmenorrhea as compared to no treatment. When comparing LUNA with PSN, there was no pain relief difference in the short term, however,

PSN was better in the long term. LUNA combined with surgical treatment of endometrial implants as compared to surgical treatment without LUNA did not result in further relief. The same results were true for PSN but there was a significant difference in relief of midline abdominal pain.

Psychological therapies

Psychological evaluation should be performed early in the evaluation of CPP. Stress reduction, relaxation, and behavioral therapies should also be addressed.[143][II] Assessment should evaluate the pain complaint, impact on life circumstances, controlling factors, and coping mechanisms. Issues often involve relationship dysfunction requiring family and marital therapy, presence of past or current physical or sexual abuse, and the negative effects on self-esteem and independence. Prolonged psychotherapy for these issues is generally not part of pain management but can be used in conjunction. No RCTs have assessed the effect of psychological approaches on chronic pelvic pain, however, a randomized trial of multidisciplinary management of CPP (which involves a component of psychological assessment and therapy) has demonstrated significant improvement in pain and well-being with the multidisciplinary approach compared with standard gynecologic treatment. Standardized psychological testing is helpful to determine whether affective disturbance is present, as well as to establish a baseline against which to measure treatment response and guide treatment approaches.

There have been studies looking at cognitive-behavioral therapy and chronic pain, although not specifically with respect to CPP.[179]

Alternative medicine

Nontraditional approaches to CPP include chiropractic treatment, hypnosis, and acupuncture.[18, 180] A prospective study on chiropractic treatment in 18 CPP patients demonstrated significant improvement in pain and functioning over a six-week treatment period of flexion/distraction and trigger point techniques.[180][III] A randomized controlled study found a 90 percent improvement in dysmenorrhea with acupuncture compared with only 36 percent in the placebo group.[181][II] A Cochrane review[21][I] of acupuncture for pain relief with dysmenorrhea concluded that there was insufficient evidence to determine the effectiveness of acupuncture in reducing dysmenorrhea.

Multidisciplinary pain management

Numerous studies have demonstrated the utility of an interdisciplinary pain management program in treating CPP.[180, 182, 183][III] This approach involves simultaneous evaluation of somatic and psychological components of chronic pelvic pain by different health care specialists. One program utilizing cognitive-behavioral therapy, acupuncture, and tricyclic antidepressants was successful in reducing pain by at least 50 percent in 85 percent of the subjects.[180] Other studies have suggested that similar results may be obtained with a multidisciplinary team.[143, 158, 182, 183, 184] In a prospective randomized, controlled study, the multidisciplinary approach combining the traditional gynecologic treatment with psychological, dietary, and physical therapy input was found to be more effective than traditional gynecologic (medical and surgical) management of cure.[143][II]

VULVODYNIA

Definition

The most recent classification of vulvar pain, agreed upon at the 2003 Congress of the International Society for the Study of Vulvovaginal Disease (ISSVD), consists of two major categories:[185] (1) vulvar pain related to a specific disorder: a) infection, b) inflammation, c) neoplasm, d) neurologic disease or (2) vulvodynia: vulvar discomfort usually described as burning pain occurring in the absence of a specific disorder. Vulvodynia is called "generalized", involving the entire vulva, or "localized," involving a portion or component of the vulva (e.g. vestibule, clitoris, hemivulva). It may be termed "provoked," i.e. by sexual and/or nonsexual contact or "unprovoked," i.e. spontaneous or "mixed" (provoked and unprovoked). Common causes of vulvodynia include those described below.

VULVAR VESTIBULITIS/VESTIBULODYNIA

Entry dyspareunia with vestibule erythema and tenderness to light touch. The term vestibulitis signifies the presence of inflammation, which was thought to be misleading since much evidence suggests no such presence. Therefore, the ISSVD voted to discontinue use of this term in favor of localized vulvar pain or, more specifically, vestibulodynia.

CHRONIC VULVOVAGINITIS

Symptoms include vulvar burning and itching. On examination, vulvar erythema is diffuse and associated with vulvar swelling. The etiology is unclear, but candidiasis or estrogen deficiency is often a contributing factor.

ALLERGIC DERMATITIS

Contact dermatitis is an inflammatory reaction of the skin to a primary irritant or to an allergenic substance.

Vulvar dermatitis (vulvar eczema) is the most common vulvar inflammatory skin disease in women.

VULVAR DERMATOSES

The dermatoses include lichen sclerosus, lichen planus, and lichen simplex chronicus. Vulvar pain is noncyclic and associated with significant pruritus. On examination, hypopigmentation or hyperpigmentation is present with atrophic or hyperplastic tissue. A stenotic introitus, flattening of the labial folds, vulvar fissures, with white plaques and erythema may be present. Biopsy is required to make the diagnosis and eliminate a malignant process. Treatment depends on the specific dermatosis (high-potency topical corticosteroids, testosterone ointment).[186]

DYSESTHETIC VULVODYNIA

Generally considered a diagnosis of exclusion, it presents commonly in perimenopausal and postmenopausal women as nonspecific superficial vulvar burning or perineal discomfort with intermittent, deep, aching pain. Patients deny entry dyspareunia. Physical examination is normal, with no tenderness on palpation. Pudendal nerve tenderness, hyperesthesiae, or hypoesthesiae in a saddle distribution extending from the mons pubis to the upper inner thighs and posteriorly across ischial tuberosities may be noted on examination.[187] The etiology may be secondary to an aberration in cutaneous nerve perception (pudendal nerve distribution S2–S4) at either the central or peripheral level. Tricyclic antidepressants starting at 10 mg q.d. to 40–60 mg q.d. may be of benefit in this condition.[188] Topical 5 percent lidocaine may provide additional benefit. Other reported treatments, although of unproven effectiveness, include acupuncture, pelvic floor muscle, physical therapy, TENS, regional nerve blocks, and anticonvulsants.[188]

Epidemiology

The typical patient with vulvodynia used to be described as a nulliparous woman in her twenties or early thirties who often develops symptoms suddenly.[189] In a survey of over 4900 women aged 18–64, it was reported that 16 percent of the 3000 respondents had experienced vulvar pain lasting at least three months and 7 percent had vulvar pain at the time of the survey and, many had seen up to five different doctors for this problem.[190] Unexplained vulvar pain was found to be of similar incidence among white and African-American women. Hispanic women were 80 percent more likely than white women to have experienced chronic vulvar pain.

Etiology

Vulvar pain is multifactorial in many cases (**Table 41.3**) A detailed history and examination is important to help direct diagnosis and treatment.[191]

Clinical evaluation

HISTORY

Assess the onset, the type of pain, timing (constant or cyclic), associated activities (i.e. intercourse), inciting agents (perfumes, lotions, detergents, clothing), and relieving factors (i.e. antifungal medications). A pain diary may better define these characteristics.

In addition, past or current infections (human papillomavirus, herpes, candida), medications, local and systemic dermatologic disorders, neurologic disorders (i.e. herniated disks, herpes zoster, pudendal or genitofemoral neuralgia), urologic disorders (interstitial cystitis, urethral syndrome), and physical trauma (vaginal deliveries,

Table 41.3 Etiologies of vulvodynia.

Etiologies of vulvodynia	
Infections	Bartholin's gland abscess, vulvovaginal candidiasis, herpes, herpes zoster, human papillomavirus, molluscum contagiosum, Trichomonas
Trauma	Sexual assault, prior vaginal deliveries, hymenectomy, vaginal surgery
Systemic illness	Bechet's disease, Crohn's disease, Sjögren syndrome, systemic lupus erythematosus
Neoplasia	Vulvar intraepithelial neoplasia and invasive squamous cell carcinoma
Allergens/toxic medications	Soaps, fabric softeners, bubble bath, sprays, douches, antiseptics, sanitary pads, suppositories, creams, laser treatment, podophyllin, trichloroacetic acid (TCA), 5-fluorouracil (5-FU)
Dermatological conditions	Allergic and contact dermatitis, eczema, hidradenitis suppurativa, lichen planus, lichen sclerosus, pemphigoid, pemphigus, psoriasis, squamous cell hyperplasia
Urinary tract syndromes	Interstitial cystitis and urethral syndrome
Neurological	Referred pain from urethra, vagina, and bladder, dysesthesiae secondary to herpes zoster, spinal disk problems, specific neuralgias (pudendal, genitofemoral)
Psychological	Sexual/physical abuse sexual history

episiotomy, vaginal surgery) should be ascertained. Sexual history evaluating lubrication, ability to achieve orgasm, whether the pain is primary or secondary, and a history of sexual abuse should be assessed.

EXAMINATION

In many cases, the vulva appears normal. Evaluate for discoloration, ulcers, fissures, and atrophy. Tenderness should be outlined using a cotton-tipped swab. Tone and tenderness of the pelvic floor muscles should be assessed.

Vaginal pH, "whiff" test, and microscopic examination of vaginal secretions with potassium hydroxide (KOH) and normal saline can help evaluate for vaginitis and estrogen deficiency. Vaginal fluid may be cultured for Candida (as microscopic evaluation may reveal candidias is in only 50 percent of cases).[192] Acetowhite changes or lesions should be biopsied to evaluate for an underlying dermatosis or infectious or neoplastic process.

VESTIBULODYNIA (FORMERLY VULVAR VESTIBULITIS SYNDROME)

The vestibule is the nonpigmented, nonkeratinized, squamous epithelium of the vulva between the labia minora and the hymen. The ductal orifices from Bartholin's, Skene's, and the minor vestibular glands open onto the vestibule.

The etiology is unknown. On biopsy, the subepithelial tissue often demonstrates a nonspecific, chronic inflammatory infiltrate, consisting predominately of lymphocytes without direct glandular inflammation.[193] A recent model of vulvar vestibulitis places the disorder within the concept of chronic pain disorder, similar to fibromyalgia and irritable bowel disorder and temporomandibular disorder.[194] This theory describes vestibulitis as a group of conditions characterized by varying degrees of pain and dysfunction in the mucosa, underlying musculature, and associated dysfunction in pain-regulatory systems.[195, 196, 197, 198, 199, 200, 200, 201, 202] The belief is that a convergence of a variety of pathophysiological mechanisms, including a predisposition of the mucosa toward heightened inflammatory response, pelvic muscle dysfunction, previous trauma, intrinsic CNS dysregulation, and modulation of psychologic traits result in the clinical manifestations of vulvar vestibulitis. The underlying pathophysiologic disorder resulting in vulvar pain likely involves autonomic nerve dysfunction, resulting in altered immune function, increased tissue vascularity, nerve endings, vascular injury, and histamine release in the surrounding tissue (**Figure 41.1**).[203, 204, 205] Treatment should therefore be based at all levels of the neuraxis.

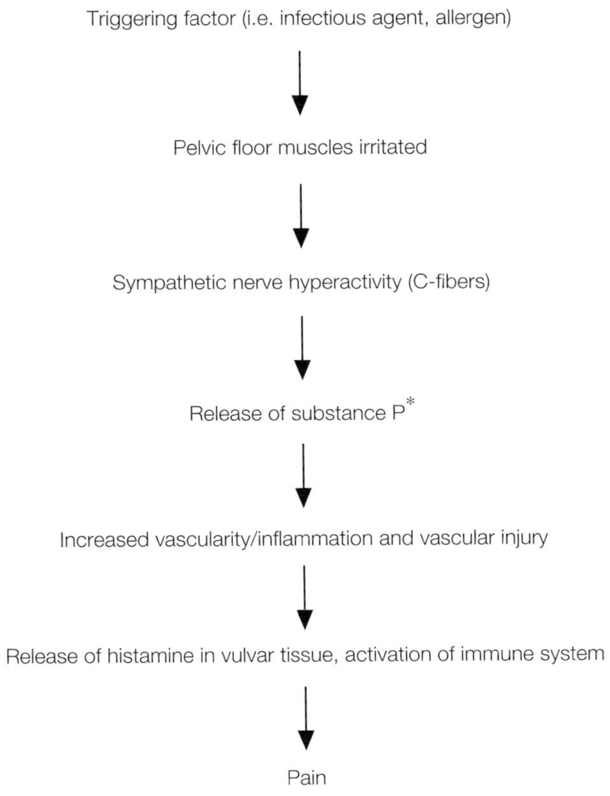

Figure 41.1 Potential mechanisms of vulvodynia. *Important in the transmission and modulation of the pain response.

Symptoms

Pain with vestibular touch especially intercourse and sometimes chronic burning/irritation are common presenting symptoms. Vestibulodynia typically presents as persistent introital or contact-related burning. Urinary symptoms with a negative urine culture may be present in 11–44 percent of women.[192, 205] The coexistence of interstitial cystitis and vestibulitis has been defined as the "urogenital sinus syndrome."[205]

Diagnosis

Vulvar vestibulitis is characterized by three criteria:[206] (1) introital pain on vestibular or vaginal entry (entry dyspareunia), (2) vestibular erythema, commonly involving the posterior fourchette, and (3) vestibular tenderness – gentle pressure from a cotton-tipped applicator at the vestibule reproduces the pain (allodynia).

EVIDENCE-BASED EVALUATION OF MANAGEMENT OF VULVODYNIA

Few RCTs have evaluated the different treatment modalities for vulvodynia or vulvar vestibulitis. Given the potential for multiple etiologies, successful treatment is often difficult (**Table 41.4**). Numerous medical options are available for treatment. Supportive measures include sitz baths or ice and proper vulvar hygiene (cotton underwear, keeping area dry, avoidance of constrictive garments, prolonged sanitary pad usage, and irritating agents).

Pharmacological

ANTIFUNGALS

Vulvovaginal candidiasis has often been implicated in vulvodynia. Antifungals, including fluconazole 150 mg orally once a week for six weeks then once a month for six months, may provide relief in cases of cyclic monilial culture-positive vulvodynia. However, even in culture-positive cases of vulvar vestibulitis, improvement may not occur, as Ledger *et al.*[192][V] reported only a 16 percent success.

ANTIHISTAMINES/CORTICOSTEROIDS

Allergens may also be an inciting agent for vulvodynia. In addition to avoiding the noxious substance, antihistamines (i.e. hydroxyzine) as well as topical corticosteroids (hydrocortisone 1 percent cream b.i.d.) may help alleviate the discomfort. Ledger *et al.*[192][V] observed a 48 percent response to hydroxyzine, however, no significant difference was noted between IgE-negative and -positive groups, although the histology revealing inflammatory changes suggests that an anti-inflammatory applied topically for up to four weeks would be helpful. There are no data to support this approach. Steroid creams also thin tissue.

ESTROGENS

In cases of pain secondary to atrophied tissue which may occur postpartum, on low-dose oral contraceptives, or peri- or postmenopausally, estrogen vaginal cream or oral hormone replacement therapy as indicated should be utilized.[207][I]

TRICYCLIC ANTIDEPRESSANTS

Tricyclic antidepressants in doses of 25–75 mg at night or at divided amounts throughout the day have been utilized successfully in cases of vulvodynia.[188][V]

ANTICONVULSANTS

Gabapentin (GBP) is an anticonvulsant that has been used successfully in many different types of chronic pain conditions, especially those with neuropathic pain.[208, 209][V]

LOCAL ANESTHETICS

Lidocaine 5 percent to the vestibule nightly, significantly improves pain and dysparenia.[210][III] Local anesthetic nerve blocks (caudal, pudendal, and perineal) have been used successfully in one pilot study for vestibulodynia.[211][III]

Table 41.4 Treatment of vulvodynia.

Treatment of vulvodynia	
Supportive measures	Warm sitz baths, Burrow's solution, topical anesthetic agents (2 percent topical xylocaine gel or 5 percent ointment) and other lubricants with intercourse
Vulvar hygiene	Cotton underwear, avoid constrictive garments
Treat underlying cause	Human papillomavirus (HPV)[a] – TCA 30 percent, topical 5-FU, interferon 1 million IU per injection to painful site with total of 12 injection sites over four weeks[a]
	Candida – fluconazole 150 mg once a week for six weeks then once a month for six months
	Allergens – avoid agent (these patients should also avoid local creams and suppositories containing propylene glycol), hydroxyzine or other antihistamine, hydrocortisone 1 percent cream b.i.d., 5 percent aspirin cream q.i.d.
	Atrophy – topical estrogen vaginal cream, oral hormone replacement therapy
Diet modification	Low-oxalate diet with calcium citrate 400 mg p.o. t.i.d.
Tricyclic antidepressants	Amitriptyline, desipramine, nortriptyline, 10–50 mg h.s.
Psychological and behavioral pain management	
Biofeedback	
Surgery	Vestibuloplasty, partial or total vestibuloectomy with vaginal advancement

[a]Current studies do not substantiate human papillomavirus as a causative factor in vulvodynia, however its treatment, in particular interferon, is still supported in the literature.
5-FU, 5-fluorouracil.

BOTULINUM TOXIN

Botulinum toxin A has been used in refractory pain conditions associated with skeletal muscle hypertonicity.[212, 213][III] One case report found that botulinum toxin A was useful when the patient was refractory to many other therapies including gabapentin, carbamazepine, physical therapy, and local anesthetic injections.[211] After injection of botulinim toxin, the area of diffuse allodynia became more refined to the vestibule so that she was able to receive a vestibulectomy.

Surgical

PERINEOPLASTY/VESTIBULECTOMY

Surgery is often performed in cases of severe vulvar vestibulitis recalcitrant to medical management.[214] Excision of a localized painful area, such as the anterior and posterior vestibule, or the lateral vestibule with vaginal advancement can be performed. The Woodruff procedure is a U-shaped excision that includes the hymeneal ring and the adjacent 0.5 cm of tissue. The incision extends from 5 mm beneath the urethra to the fourchette and is 2–5 mm in depth. The adjacent vaginal tissue is then mobilized to cover the excised area. In the literature, success rates based on nonrandomized, retrospective studies range from 47 to 100 percent. Success, however, diminishes to 40–60 percent as the length of follow-up increases.[191, 192][III] One study that randomized patients to either vestibuloplasty or perineoplasty found no improvements in all ten patients who had vestibuloplasty and complete resolution of symptoms in patients who received a perineoplasty.[215] [III] Progressive introital dilation using vaginal dilators is also recommended by some and should be used for six weeks prior to intercourse.[192] Patients with vestibulitis associated with dyspareunia since their first sexual episode tend to have an incomplete response.[214] Complications include bleeding, infection, hematoma, complete or partial wound separation, Bartholin duct cyst formation, anal sphincter weakness, uneven healing requiring further surgery, vaginismus, and vaginal stenosis.[214]

Psychological and behavioral pain management

Meana *et al.*[216] observed that women with physical findings of vestibulitis did not have significant psychological findings. However, women with no apparent findings on examination were more likely to have psychological issues or relationship and sexual dysfunction. One randomized trial observed a beneficial effect when cognitive-behavioral therapy was incorporated either with or without surgical treatment.[217][II]

Diet modification

Hyperoxaluria has been implicated in aggravating vulvar pain through the formation of sharp oxalate crystals.[218] A prospective study noted a 10 percent objective (pain-free sexual intercourse) decrease in women following a low-oxalate diet (avoiding such foods as tea, coffee, cocoa, wine, chocolate, peanuts, peanut butter, all berries, prunes, all beans, eggplant, sweet potatoes, spinach, spicy food, vinegar, wheat germ, tofu) with calcium citrate (400 mg t.i.d.) to inhibit formation of calcium oxalate crystals.[219][III] Further investigation is needed as other studies report up to a 75 percent significant improvement on a low-oxalate diet and calcium citrate.[220]

Biofeedback

Pelvic floor muscle irritability may aggravate the underlying cause of vulvar vestibulitis. A decrease in subjective vulvar pain in 83 percent of women followed 16 weeks of electromyographic biofeedback in a prospective, nonrandomized uncontrolled trial. Pelvic floor muscle physical therapy may also be useful.

Prognosis

Up to two-thirds of patients may be cured following a variety of treatments.[192] Recalcitrant pain subsequent to surgery warrants further medical management prior to surgery.[221]

REFERENCES

1. Mathias SD, Kuppermann M, Liberman RF *et al.* Chronic pelvic pain: prevalence, health-related quality of life, and economic correlates. *Obstetrics and Gynecology.* 1996; **87**: 321–7.
2. Walker EA, Katon WJ, Katon WS, Alfrey H. The prevalence of chronic pain and irritable bowel syndrome in two university clinics. *Journal of Psychosomatic Obstetrics and Gynaecology.* 1991; **12** (Suppl.); 66–9.
3. Bachmann GA, Rosen R, Arnold LD *et al.* Chronic vulvar and other gynecologic pain: prevalence and characteristics in a self-reported survey. *Journal of Reproductive Medicine.* 2006; **51**: 3–9.
4. Howard FM. The role of laparoscopy in chronic pelvic pain: Promise and pitfalls. *Obstetrics and Gynecological Survey.* 1993; **48**: 357–87.
5. Reiter RC. A profile of women with chronic pelvic pain. *Clinical Obstetrics and Gynecology.* 1990; **33**: 130–6.
6. Kumazawa T. Sensory innervation of reproductive organs. In: Cervero F, Morrison J (eds). *Visceral sensation.* New York: Elsevier Science Publications, 1986: 115–31.

7. Cervero F, Tattersall JEH. Somatic and visceral sensory integration in the thoracic spinal cord. In: Cervero F, Morrison J (eds). *Visceral sensation*. New York: Elsevier Science Publications, 1986: 189–205.
8. Wesselmann U, Lai J. Mechanisms of referred visceral pain: uterine inflammation in the adult virgin rat results in neurogenic plasma extravasation in the skin. *Pain*. 1997; **73**: 209–317.
9. Giamberardino MA, Berkley KJ, Lezzi S *et al*. Changes in skin and muscle sensitivity in dysmenorrheic vs normal women as a function of body site and monthly cycle. *Social Neuroscience*. 1995; **21**: 1638.
* 10. Slocumb JC. Neurological factors in chronic pelvic pain: Trigger points and the abdominal pelvic pain syndrome. *American Journal of Obstetrics and Gynecology*. 1984; **149**: 536–43.
11. The American College of Obstetricians and Gynecologists. Dysmenorrhea. *ACOG Technical Bulletin*. 1983; Number **68**.
12. Rapkin AJ, Rasgon NL, Berkley KJ. Dysmenorrhea. In: Yaksh TL, Lynch C, Zapol WM *et al*. (eds). *Anesthesia: biologic foundations*. Philadelphia, PA: Lippincott-Raven, 1997: 785–93.
13. The Medical Letter: Drugs for dysmenorrhea. *Medical Letter on Drugs and Therapeutics*. 1979; **21**: 81–4.
14. Marjoribanks J, Proctor ML, Farquhar C. Nonsteroidal anti-inflammatory drugs for primary dysmenorrhea. *Cochrane Database of Systematic Reviews*. 2003; **CD001751**.
15. Chan WY, Dawood MY. Prostaglandin levels in menstrual fluid of non-dysmenorrheic and of dysmenorrheic subjects with and without oral contraceptive or ibuprofen therapy. *Advances in Prostaglandin and Thromboxane Research*. 1980; **8**: 1443–7.
16. Proctor ML, Roberts H, Farquhar CM. Combined oral contraceptive pill (OCP) as treatment for primary dysmenorrhea. *Cochrane Database of Systematic Reviews*. 2001; **CD002120**.
17. Smith RP. Cyclic pelvic pain and dysmenorrhea. In: Ling FW (ed.). *Obstetrics and gynecology clinics of North America*, Vol. 4. Philadelphia, PA: W.B. Saunders Company, 1993: 753–64.
18. Helms JM. Acupuncture for the management of primary dysmenorrhea. *Obstetrics and Gynecology*. 1987; **69**: 51–6.
19. Mannheimer JS, Whaler EC. The efficacy of transcutaneous electrical nerve stimulation in dysmenorrhea. *Clinical Journal of Pain*. 1985; **1**: 75–83.
20. Witt CM, Reinhold T, Brinkhaus B *et al*. Acupuncture in patients with dysmenorrhea: a randomized study on clinical effectiveness and cost-effectiveness in usual care. *American Journal of Obstetrics and Gynecology*. 2008; **198**: 166. e1–8.
21. Proctor ML, Smith CA, Farquhar CM, Stones RW. Transcutaneous electrical nerve stimulation and acupuncture for primary dysmenorrhea. *Cochrane Database of Systematic Reviews*. 2002; **CD002123**.
22. Proctor ML, Hing W, Johnson TC, Murphy PA. Spinal manipulation for primary and secondary dysmenorrhea. *Cochrane Database of Systematic Reviews*. 2006; **CD002119**.
23. McElin TW, Bird CC. Adenomyosis of the uterus. *Obstetrics and Gynecology Annual*. 1974; **3**: 425–41.
24. Molitor JJ. Adenomyosis: A clinical and pathological appraisal. *American Journal of Obstetrics and Gynecology*. 1971; **110**: 275–84.
25. Atri M, Reinhold C, Mehio AR *et al*. Adenomyosis: US features with histologic correlation in an in vitro study. *Radiology*. 2000; **215**: 783–90.
26. Reinhold C, Tafazoli F, Mehio A *et al*. Uterine adenomyosis: endovaginal US and MR imaging features with histopathologic correlation. *Radiographics*. 1999; **19**: S147–60.
* 27. Rapkin AJ. Adhesions and pelvic pain: a retrospective study. *Obstetrics and Gynecology*. 1986; **68**: 13–15.
28. Almeida OD, Val-Gallas JM. Conscious pain mapping. *Journal of the American Association of Gynecologic Laparoscopists*. 1997; **4**: 587–90.
29. Reese KA, Reddy S, Rock JA. Endometriosis in an adolescent population: the Emory experience. *Journal of Pediatric and Adolescent Gynecology*. 1996; **9**: 125–8.
30. Martin DC, Hubert GD, VanderZwaag R. Laparoscopic appearances of peritoneal endometriosis. *Fertility and Sterility*. 1989; **51**: 63–7.
31. Eskenazi B, Warner ML. Epidemiology of endometriosis. *Obstetrics and Gynecology Clinics of North America*. 1997; **24**: 235–58.
32. Probst AM, Laufer MR. Endometriosis in adolescents. Incidence, diagnosis and treatment. *Journal of Reproductive Medicine*. 1999; **44**: 751.
33. D'Hooghe TM, Hill JA. Endometriosis. In: Berek JS, Adashi EY, Hillard PA (eds). *Novak's gynecology*, 12th edn. Baltimore, MD: Williams & Wilkins, 1996: 887–914.
34. Hurd WJ. Criteria that indicate endometriosis in the cause of chronic pelvic pain. *Obstetrics and Gynecology*. 1998; **92**: 1029–32.
35. Redwine DB. Age-related evolution on colour appearance of endometriosis. *Fertility and Sterility*. 1987; **48**: 1062–3.
36. Cornillie FJ, Oosterlynck D, Lauweryns JM *et al*. Deeply infiltrating pelvic endometriosis: histology and clinical significance. *Fertility and Sterility*. 1990; **53**: 978–83.
37. Berkley KJ, Rapkin AJ, Papka RE. The pains of endometriosis. *Science*. 2005; **308**: 1587–9.
* 38. Sutton CJ, Pooley AS, Ewen SP, Haines P. Follow-up report on a randomized controlled trial of laser laparoscopy in the treatment of pelvic pain associated with minimal to moderate endometriosis. *Fertility and Sterility*. 1997; **68**: 1070–4.
* 39. Rice VM. Conventional medical therapies for endometriosis. *Annals of the New York Academy of Sciences*. 2002; **955**: 343–52.
* 40. Gambone JC, Mittman BS, Munro MG *et al*. Consensus statement for the management of chronic pelvic pain and endometriosis: proceedings of an expert panel consensus process. *Fertility and Sterility*. 2002; **78**: 961–72.

41. Rouff G, Lema M. Strategies in pain management: New and potential indications for COX-2 specific inhibitors. *Journal of Pain and Symptom Management.* 2003; **S2**: S21–31.
42. Allen C, Hopewell S, Prentice A. Non-steroidal anti-inflammatory drugs for pain in women with endometriosis. *Cochrane Database of Systematic Reviews.* 2005; **CD004753**.
43. The Practice Committee of the American Society for Reproductive Medicine. Treatment of pelvic pain associated with endometriosis. *Fertility and Sterility.* 2006; **86**: S18–27.
44. Vercellini P, De Giorgi O, Mosconi P *et al.* Cyproterone acetate versus a continuous monophasic oral contraceptive in the treatment of recurrent pelvic pain after conservative surgery for symptomatic endometriosis. *Fertility and Sterility.* 2002; **77**: 52–61.
45. Olive DL. Medical therapy of endometriosis. *Seminars in Reproductive Medicine.* 2003; **21**: 209–22.
46. Vercellini P, Frontino G, De Giorgi O *et al.* Comparison of a levonorgestrel-releasing intrauterine device versus expectant management after conservative surgery for symptomatic endometriosis: a pilot study. *Fertility and Sterility.* 2003; **80**: 305–09.
47. Bergqvist A, Bergh T, Hogstrom L *et al.* Effects of triptorelin versus placebo on the symptoms of endometriosis. *Fertility and Sterility.* 1998; **69**: 702–08.
48. Hornstein MD, Surrey ES, Weisberg GW, Casino LA. Leuprolide acetate depot and hormonal add-back in endometriosis: a 12-month study. *Obstetrics and Gynecology.* 1998; **91**: 16–24.
49. Waller KG, Shaw RW. Gonadotropin-releasing hormone analogues for the treatment of endometriosis: long-term follow-up. *Fertility and Sterility.* 1993; **59**: 511–15.
50. Petta CA, Ferriani RA, Abrao MS *et al.* Randomized clinical trial of a levonorgestrel-releasing intrauterine system and a depot GnRH analogue for the treatment of chronic pelvic pain in women with endometriosis. *Human reproduction.* 2005; **20**: 1993–8.
51. Saleh A, Tulandi T. Reoperation after laparoscopic treatment of ovarian endometriomas by excision and by fenestration. *Fertility and Sterility.* 1999; **72**: 322–4.
52. Jones KD, Sutton C. Patient satisfaction and changes in pain scores after ablative laparoscopic surgery for stage III-IV endometriosis and endometriotic cysts. *Fertility and Sterility.* 2003; **79**: 1086–90.
53. Abbott J, Hawe J, Hunter D *et al.* Laparoscopic excision of endometriosis: a randomized, placebo-controlled trial. *Fertility and Sterility.* 2004; **82**: 878–84.
54. Jacobson TZ, Barlow DH, Garry R, Koninckx P. Laparoscopic surgery for pelvic pain associated with endometriosis. *Cochrane Database of Systematic Reviews.* 2001; **CD001300**.
55. Namnoun AB, Hickman TN, Goodman SB *et al.* Incidence of symptom recurrence after hysterectomy for endometriosis. *Fertility and Sterility.* 1995; **64**: 898–902.
56. Rapkin AJ, Kames LD. The pain management approach to chronic pelvic pain. *Journal of Reproductive Medicine.* 1987; **32**: 323–7.
57. Fukaya T, Hoshiai H, Yajima A. Is pelvic endometriosis always associated with chronic pain? A retrospective study of 618 cases diagnosed by laparoscopy. *American Journal of Obstetrics and Gynecology.* 1993; **169**: 719–22.
58. ∗ Vercellini P, Trespidi L, De Giorgi O *et al.* Endometriosis and pelvic pain: relation to disease stage and localization. *Fertility and Sterility.* 1996; **65**: 299–304.
59. Stovall DW, Bowser LM, Archer DF, Guzick DS. Endometriosis-associated pelvic pain: evidence for an association between the stage of the disease and a history of chronic pelvic pain. *Fertility and Sterility.* 1997; **68**: 13–18.
60. Taylor Jr JC. Pelvic pain based on a vascular and autonomic nervous system disorder. *American Journal of Obstetrics and Gynecology.* 1954; **67**: 1177–96.
61. Beard RW, Reginald PW, Wadworth J. Clinical features of women with chronic lower abdominal pain and pelvic congestion. *British Journal of Obstetrics and Gynaecology.* 1988; **95**: 153–61.
62. Beard RW, Highman JH, Pearce S, Reginald PW. Diagnosis of pelvic varicosities in women with chronic pelvic pain. *Lancet.* 1984; **2**: 946–9.
63. Farquhar CM, Rogers V, Frank S *et al.* A randomized controlled trial of medroxyprogesterone acetate and psychotherapy for the treatment of pelvic congestion. *British Journal of Obstetrics and Gynaecology.* 1989; **96**: 1153–62.
64. Regional PW, Adams J, Franks S *et al.* Medroxyprogesterone acetate in the treatment of pelvic pain due to venous congestion. *British Journal of Obstetrics and Gynaecology.* 1989; **96**: 1148–52.
65. Allen WM. Chronic pelvic congestion and pelvic pain. *American Journal of Obstetrics and Gynecology.* 1971; **109**: 198–202.
66. Soysal ME, Soysal S, Vicdan K *et al.* A randomized controlled trial of goserelin and medroxyprogesterone acetate in the treatment of pelvic congestion. *British Journal of Obstetrics and Gynecology.* 2001; **16**: 931–9.
67. Sichlau MJ, Yao JST, Vogelzang RL. Transcatheter embolotherapy for the treatment of pelvic congestion syndrome. *Obstetrics and Gynecology.* 1994; **83**: 892–6.
68. Tarazov PG, Prozorovskij KV, Ryzhkov VK. Pelvic pain syndrome caused by ovarian varices. Treatment by transcatheter embolization. *Acta Radiologica.* 1997; **38**: 1023–5.
69. Venbrux AC, Lambert DL. Embolization of the ovarian veins as a treatment for patients with chronic pelvic pain caused by pelvic venous incompetence (pelvic congestion syndrome). *Current Opinion in Obstetrics and Gynecology.* 1999; **11**: 395.
70. Beard RW, Kennedy RG, Gangar KF *et al.* Bilateral oophorectomy and hysterectomy in the treatment of intractable pelvic pain associated with pelvic congestion.

British Journal of Obstetrics and Gynaecology. 1991; **98**: 988–92.
71. Steege JF. Ovarian remnant syndrome. *Obstetrics and Gynecology.* 1987; **70**: 64–7.
* 72. Siddall-Allum J, Rae T, Rogers V *et al.* Chronic pain caused by residual ovaries and ovarian remnants. *British Journal of Obstetrics and Gynaecology.* 1994; **101**: 979–85.
73. Steege JF. Pain after hysterectomy. In: Steege JF, Metzger DA, Levy BS (eds). *Chronic pelvic pain – an integrated approach.* Philadelphia, PA: W.B. Saunders Company, 1998: 135–44.
74. Lafferty HW, Angioli R, Rudolph J, Penalver MA. Ovarian remnant syndrome: experience at Jackson Memorial Hospital, University of Miami, 1985 through 1993. *American Journal of Obstetrics and Gynecology.* 1996; **174**: 641–5.
75. Price FV, Edwards R, Buchsbaum HJ. Ovarian remnant syndrome: difficulties in diagnosis and management. *Obstetrics and Gynecological Survey.* 1990; **45**: 151–6.
76. Carey MP, Slack MC. GnRH analogue in assessing chronic pelvic pain in women with residual ovaries. *British Journal of Obstetrics and Gynaecology.* 1996; **103**: 150–3.
77. Pettit PD, Lee RA. Ovarian remnant syndrome. *Diagnostic dilemma and surgical challenge. Obstetrics and Gynecology.* 1988; **71**: 580–3.
78. Hughes JM. Psychological aspects of pelvic pain. In: Rocker I (ed.). *Pelvic pain in women. Diagnosis and management.* London: Springer-Verlag, 1990: 13–20.
79. Stovall TG, Elder RF, Ling FW. Predictors of pelvic adhesions. *Journal of Reproductive Medicine.* 1989; **34**: 345–8.
* 80. Howard FM, El-Minawi AM, Sanchez RA. Conscious pain mapping by laparoscopy in women with chronic pelvic pain. *Obstetrics and Gynecology.* 2000; **96**: 934–9.
81. Duffy DM, diZerega GS. Adhesion controversies; pelvic pain as a cause of adhesions, crystalloids on preventing them. *Journal of Reproductive Medicine.* 1996; **41**: 19–26.
82. Saravelos HG, Li T-C, Cooke ID. An analysis of the outcome of microsurgical and laparoscopic adhesiolysis for chronic pelvic pain. *Human Reproduction.* 1995; **10**: 2895–901.
83. Fayez JA, Clark RR. Operative laparoscopy for the treatment of localized chronic pelvic-abdominal pain caused by postoperative adhesions. *Journal of Gynecologic Surgery.* 1994; **10**: 79–83.
* 84. Peters AAW, Trimbos-Kemper GCM, Admiral C, Trimbos JB. A randomized clinical trial on the benefit of adhesiolysis in patients with intraperitoneal adhesions and chronic pelvic pain. *British Journal of Obstetrics and Gynaecology.* 1992; **99**: 59–62.
* 85. Swank DJ, Swank-Bordewijk SC, Hop WC *et al.* Laparoscopic adhesiolysis in patients with chronic abdominal pain: A blinded randomised controlled multi-centre trial. *Lancet.* 2003; **361**: 1247–51.
86. Steege JF, Scott AL. Resolution of chronic pelvic pain after laparoscopic lysis of adhesions. *American Journal of Obstetrics and Gynecology.* 1991; **165**: 278–83.
87. Lipscomb GH, Ling FW. Relationship of infection and chronic pelvic pain. *Obstetrics and Gynecology Clinics of North America.* 1993; **20**: 699–708.
88. Sweet RL, Gibbs RS. Pelvic inflammatory disease. In: Sweet RL, Gibbs RS (eds). *Infectious diseases of the female genital tract.* Baltimore, MD: Williams & Wilkins, 1990: 241–66.
89. Thompson WG. Irritable bowel syndrome: Pathogenesis and management. *Lancet.* 1993; **341**: 1569–72.
90. Whitehead WE, Cheskin LJ, Heller BR *et al.* Evidence for exacerbation of irritable bowel syndrome during menses. *Gastroenterology.* 1990; **98**: 1485–9.
91. Longstreth GF, Preskill DB, Youkeles L. Irritable bowel syndrome in women having diagnostic laparoscopy or hysterectomy. Relation to gynecologic features and outcome. *Digestive Diseases and Sciences.* 1990; **35**: 1285–90.
* 92. Drossman DA, Thompson WG. The irritable bowel syndrome. Review and a graduated multicomponent treatment approach. *Annals of Internal Medicine.* 1992; **116**: 1009–16.
93. Lee AW, Bell RM, Griffen Jr WO, Hagihara P. Recurrent appendiceal colic. *Surgery, Gynecology and Obstetrics.* 1985; **161**: 21–4.
94. Hightower NC, Roberts JW. Acute and chronic lower abdominal pain of enterologic origin in chronic pelvic pain. In: Renaer MR (ed.). *Chronic pelvic pain in women.* New York: Springer-Verlag, 1981: 110–37.
95. Spangen L. Spigelian hernia. *Surgical Clinics of North America.* 1984; **64**: 351–66.
96. Miklos JR, O'Reilly MJ, Saye WB. Sciatic hernia as a cause of chronic pelvic pain in women. *Obstetrics and Gynecology.* 1998; **91**: 998–1001.
97. Reiter RC. Occult somatic pathology in women with chronic pelvic pain. *Clinical Obstetrics and Gynecology.* 1990; **33**: 154–60.
98. Smith RP. Lower gastrointestinal disease in women. *Obstetrics and Gynecology Clinics of North America.* 2001; **28**: 351–61.
99. Longstreth GF. Irritable bowel syndrome: diagnosis in the managed care era. *Digestive Diseases and Sciences.* 1997; **42**: 1105–11.
100. Reiter RC. Occult somatic pathology in women with chronic pelvic pain. *Clinical Obstetrics and Gynecology.* 1990; **33**: 154–60.
101. Summit RL. Urogynecologic causes of chronic pelvic pain. In: Ling FW (ed.). *Obstetrics and gynecology clinics of North America: contemporary management of chronic pain.* Philadelphia, PA: W.B. Saunders Company, 1993: 685–98.
102. Raz R, Stamm WE. A controlled trial on intravaginal estriol in postmenopausal women with recurrent urinary tract infections. *New England Journal of Medicine.* 1993; **329**: 753–6.
103. Bergman A, Karram M, Bhatia NN. Urethral syndrome: a comparison of different treatment modalities. *Journal of Reproductive Medicine.* 1989; **34**: 157–60.

104. Nigro DA, Wein AJ, Foy M *et al.* Associations among cystoscopic and urodynamic findings in women enrolled in the Interstitial Cystitis Data Base (ICDB) Study. *Urology.* 1997; **49** (Suppl. 5AS): 86-92.
105. Karram MM. Frequency, urgency, and painful bladder syndrome. In: Walters MD, Karram MM (eds). *Clinical urogynecology.* St Louis, MO: Mosby, 1993: 285–98.
*106. Gillenwater JY, Wein AJ. Summary of the National Institute of Arthritis, Diabetes, Digestive and Kidney Diseases Workshop on Interstitial Cystitis. National Institutes of Health, Bethesda, MD, August 28–29. *Journal of Urology.* 1988; **140**: 203–06.
107. Morscher E. Low back pain in women. In: Renaer MR (ed.). *Chronic pelvic pain in women.* New York: Springer-Verlag, 1981: 137–54.
108. Baker PK. Musculoskeletal origins of chronic pelvic pain. In: Ling FW (ed.). *Obstetrics and gynecology clinics of North America: contemporary management of chronic pain.* Philadelphia, PA: W.B. Saunders Company, 1993: 719–42.
109. Slocomb JC. Chronic somatic myofascial and neurogenic abdominal pelvic pain. In: Porreco RP, Reiter RC (eds). *Clinical obstetrics and gynecology.* Philadelphia, PA: J.B. Lippincott and Co, 1990: 145–53.
110. Staud R. Biology and therapy of fibromyalgia: Pain in fibromyalgia syndrome. *Arthritis Research and Therapy.* 2006; **8**: 208. Epub 2006 April 24.
111. Travell J. Myofascial trigger points. Clinical view. *Advances in Pain Research and Therapy.* 1976; **1**: 919–26.
112. Weiss JM. Pelvic floor myofascial trigger points: Manual therapy for interstitial cystitis and the urgency-frequency syndrome. *Journal of Urology.* 2001; **166**: 2226–31.
113. Sippo WC, Burghardt A, Gomez AC. Nerve entrapment after pfannenstiel incision. *American Journal of Obstetrics and Gynecology.* 1987; **157**: 420–1.
114. Irwin W, Anderson W, Taylor P, Rice L. Minimizing the risk of neurologic injury in gynecologic surgery. *Obstetrics and Gynecology.* 2004; **103**: 374–82.
115. Hameroff SR, Carlson GL, Brown BR. Ilioinguinal pain syndrome. *Pain.* 1981; **10**: 253–7.
116. Hahn L. Clinical findings and results of operative treatment in ilioinguinal nerve entrapment syndrome. *British Journal of Obstetrics and Gynaecology.* 1989; **96**: 1080–3.
*117. McDonald JS. Management of chronic pain. In: Ling FW (ed.). *Obstetrics and gynecology clinics of North America: contemporary management of chronic pain.* Philadelphia, PA: W.B. Saunders Company, 1993: 817–39.
118. Thomson H, Francis DMA. Abdominal-wall tenderness: a useful sign in the acute abdomen. *Lancet.* 1977; **2**: 1053–4.
119. Srinivasan R, Greenbaun DS. Chronic abdominal wall pain: a frequently overlooked problem. Practical approach to diagnosis and management. *American Journal of Gastroenterology.* 2002; **97**: 824–30.
120. Hahn L. Clinical Findings and results of operative treatment in ilioinguinal nerve entrapment syndrome. *British Journal of Obstetrics and Gynecology.* 1989; **96**: 1080–3.
121. Ivica Ducic, Michael Moxley, Ali Al-Attar. Algorithm for Treatment of postoperative incisional groin pain after cesarean delivery or hysterectomy. *Obstetrics and Gynecology.* 2006; **108**: 27–31.
*122. Diatchenko L, Nackley AG, Slade GD *et al.* Idiopathic pain disorders – Pathways of vulnerability. *Pain.* 2006; **123**: 226–30.
123. Renaer M, Vertommen H, Nijs P *et al.* Psychosocial aspects of chronic pelvic pain in women. *American Journal of Obstetrics and Gynecology.* 1979; **134**: 75–80.
124. Duleba AJ, Jubanyik KJ, Greenfeld DA, Olive DL. Changes in personality profile associated with laparoscopic surgery for chronic pelvic pain. *Journal of American Association of Gynecologic Laparoscopists.* 1998; **5**: 389–95.
125. Harrop-Griffiths J, Katon W, Walker E *et al.* The association between chronic pelvic pain, psychiatric diagnoses, and childhood sexual abuse. *Obstetrics and Gynecology.* 1988; **71**: 589–94.
126. Rapkin AJ, Kames LD, Darke LL. History of physical and sexual abuse in women with chronic pelvic pain. *Obstetrics and Gynecology.* 1990; **76**: 92–6.
127. Walling MK, Reiter RC, O'Hara MW *et al.* Abuse history and chronic pain in women: I. Prevalence of sexual abuse and physical abuse. *Obstetrics and Gynecology.* 1994; **84**: 193–9.
128. McGowan LPA, Pitts MK, Clarke-Carter DD. Chronic pelvic pain: A meta-analytic review. *Psychology and Health.* 1999; **13**: 937–51.
129. Keefe FJ, Rumble ME, Scipio CD *et al.* Psychological aspects of persistent pain: Current state of the science. *J Pain.* 2004; **5**: 195–211.
130. Heim C, Ehlert U, Hanker JP, Hellhammer DH. Abuse-related posttraumatic stress disorder and alterations of the hypothalamic–pituitary–adrenal axis in women with chronic pelvic pain. *Psychosomatic Medicine.* 1998; **60**: 309–18.
131. Magni G, Salmi A, deLeo D, Ceola A. Chronic pelvic pain and depression. *Psychopathology.* 1984; **17**: 132–6.
132. Walker E, Katon W, Harrop-Griffiths J. Relationship of chronic pelvic pain of psychiatric diagnoses and childhood sexual abuse. *American Journal of Psychiatry.* 1988; **145**: 75–80.
133. Latthe P, Mignini L, Gray R *et al.* Factors predisposing women to chronic pelvic pain: systematic review. *British Medical Journal.* 2006; **332**: 749–55.
134. Gross RJ, Doerr H, Caldirola D *et al.* Borderline syndrome and incest in chronic pelvic pain patients. *International Journal of Psychiatry in Medicine.* 1980; **10**: 79–96.
135. Harrop-Griffiths J, Katon W, Walker E *et al.* The association between chronic pelvic pain, psychiatric diagnoses and childhood sexual abuse. *Obstetrics and Gynecology.* 1988; **71**: 589–94.
136. Rapkin AJ, Kames LD, Darke LL. History of physical and sexual abuse in women with chronic pelvic pain. *Obstetrics and Gynecology.* 1990; **76**: 90–6.

137. Walling MK, Reiter RC, O'Hara MW *et al.* Abuse history and chronic pain in women. 1. Prevalence of sexual abuse and physical abuse. *Obstetrics and Gynecology.* 1994; **84**: 193–9.
138. Abramson LY, Seligman MEP, Teasdale JD. Learned helplessness in human: critique and reformation. *Journal of Abnormal Psychology.* 1978; **87**: 49–74.
139. Engel Jr CC, Walker EA, Engel AL *et al.* A randomized, double-blind crossover trial of sertraline in women with chronic pelvic pain. *Journal of Psychosomatic Research.* 1998; **44**: 203–07.
140. Sator-Katzenschlager SM, Scharbert G, Kress HG *et al.* Chronic pelvic pain treated with gabapentin and amitriptyline: a randomized controlled pilot study. *Wiener klinische Wochenschrift.* 2005; **117**: 761–8.
141. Stone W, Mountfield J. Interventions for treating chronic pelvic pain in women. *Cochrane Database of Systematic Reviews.* 2000; **CD000387**.
142. Heyman J, Ohrvik J, Leppert J. Distension of painful structures in the treatment for chronic pelvic pain in women. *Acta Obstetricia et Gynecologica Scandinavica.* 2006; **85**: 599–603.
*143. Peters AA, van Dorst E, Jellis B *et al.* A randomized clinical trial to compare two different approaches in women with chronic pelvic pain. *Obstetrics and Gynecology.* 1991; **77**: 740–4.
144. Morris L, Newton RA. Use of high voltage pulsed galvanic stimulation for patients with levator ani syndrome. *Physical Therapy.* 1987; **67**: 1522–5.
145. de Oliveira Bernardes N, Bahamondes L. Intravaginal electrical stimulation for the treatment of chronic pelvic pain. *Journal of Reproductive Medicine.* 2005; **50**: 267–72.
146. Hameroff SR, Crago BR, Blitt CD *et al.* Comparison of bupivacaine, etidocaine, and saline for trigger point therapy. *Anesthesia and Analgesia.* 1981; **60**: 752–5.
147. Graboski CL, Gray DS, Burnham RS. Botulinum toxin A versus bupivacaine trigger point injections for the treatment of myofascial pain syndrome: A randomised double blind crossover study. *Pain.* 2005; **118**: 170–5.
148. Starling JR, Harms BA. Diagnosis and treatment of genitofemoral and ilioinguinal neuralgia. *World Journal of Surgery.* 1989; **13**: 586–91.
149. Wechsler RJ, Maurer PM, Halpern EJ, Frank ED. Superior hypogastric plexus block for chronic pelvic pain in the presence of endometriosis: CT techniques and results. *Radiology.* 1995; **196**: 103–06.
150. Steege JF. Superior hypogastric block during microlaparoscopic pain mapping. *Journal of the American Association of Gynecologic Laparoscopists.* 1998; **5**: 265–7.
151. McDonald JS, Spigos DG. Computed tomography-guided pudendal block for treatment of pelvic pain due to pudendal neuropathy. *Obstetrics and Gynecology.* 2000; **95**: 306–09.
152. Lamvu G, Williams R, Zolnoun D *et al.* Long-term outcomes after surgical and nonsurgical management of chronic pelvic pain: One year after evaluation in a pelvic pain specialty clinic. *American Journal of Obstetrics and Gynecology.* 2006; **195**: 591–8; discussion 598-600.
153. Lamvu G, Tu F, As-Sanie S *et al.* The role of laparoscopy in the diagnosis and treatment of conditions associated with chronic pelvic pain. *Obstetrics and Gynecology Clinics of North America.* 2004; **31**: 619–30.
154. Stout AL, Steege JF, Dodson WC, Hughes CL. Relationship of laparoscopic findings to self-report of pelvic pain. *American Journal of Obstetrics and Gynecology.* 1991; **164**: 73–9.
155. Howard FM. Chronic pain as a diagnosis. In: Howard FM, Perry PC, Carter JE *et al.* (eds). *Pelvic pain diagnosis and management.* Philadelphia, PA: Lippincott Williams & Wilkins, 2000: 493–508.
156. Baker PN, Symonds MD. The resolution of chronic pelvic pain after normal laparoscopy findings. *American Journal of Obstetrics and Gynecology.* 1992; **166**: 835–6.
157. Swanton A, Iyer L, Reginald PW. Diagnosis, treatment and follow up of women undergoing conscious pain mapping for chronic pelvic pain: a prospective cohort study. *BJOG.* 2006; **113**: 792–6.
158. Reiter RC, Gambone JC, Johnson SR. Availability of a multidisciplinary pelvic pain clinic and frequency of hysterectomy for pelvic pain. *Journal of Psychosomatic Obstetrics and Gynaecology.* 1991; **12** (Suppl.): 109.
159. Brandsborg B, Nikolajsen L, Hansen CT *et al.* Risk factors for chronic pain after hysterectomy: a nationwide questionnaire and database study. *Anesthesiology.* 2007; **106**: 1003–12.
160. ACOG criteria set. Hysterectomy, abdominal or vaginal for chronic pelvic pain. Number 29, November 1997. Committee on Quality Assessment. American College of Obstetricians and Gynecologists. *International Journal of Gynaecology and Obstetrics.* 1998; **60**: 316–17.
161. Carlston KJ, Miller BA, Fowler Jr FJ. The Maine women's health study. II. Outcomes of nonsurgical management of leiomyomas, abnormal bleeding, and chronic pelvic pain. *Obstetrics and Gynecology.* 1994; **83**: 566–72.
162. Stovall TG, Ling FW, Crawford DA. Hysterectomy for chronic pelvic pain of presumed uterine etiology. *Obstetrics and Gynecology.* 1990; **75**: 676–9.
*163. Hillis SD, Marchbanks PA, Peterson HB. The effectiveness of hysterectomy for chronic pelvic pain. *Obstetrics and Gynecology.* 1995; **86**: 941–5.
164. Tay SK, Bromwich N. Outcome of hysterectomy for pelvic pain in premenopausal women. *Australian and New Zealand Journal of Obstetrics and Gynaecology.* 1998; **38**: 72–6.
165. Hartmann KE, Ma C, Lamvu GM *et al.* Quality of life and sexual function after hysterectomy in women with preoperative pain and depression. *Obstetrics and Gynecology.* 2004; **104**: 701–9.
166. Cotte G. Resection of the presacral nerves in the treatment of obstinate dysmenorrhea. *American Journal of Obstetrics and Gynecology.* 1937; **33**: 1034–40.

167. Chen F-P, Soong Y-K. The efficacy and complications of laparoscopic presacral neurectomy in pelvic pain. *Obstetrics and Gynecology.* 1997; **90**: 974–7.
168. Candiani GB, Fedele L, Vercellini P *et al.* Presacral neurectomy for the treatment of pelvic pain associated with endometriosis: a controlled study. *American Journal of Obstetrics and Gynecology.* 1992; **167**: 100–03.
169. Davis GD. Uterine prolapse after laparoscopic uterosacral transection in nulliparous airborne trainees. A report of three cases. *Journal of Reproductive Medicine.* 1996; **41**: 279–80.
170. Good MC, Copas Jr PR, Doody MC. Uterine prolapse after laparoscopic uterosacral transection. A case report. *Journal of Reproductive Medicine.* 1992; **37**: 995–6.
171. Ingersoll FM, Meigs JV. Presacral neurectomy for dysmenorrhea. *New England Journal of Medicine.* 1948; **238**: 357–60.
172. Polan ML, DeCherney A. Presacral neurectomy for pelvic pain in infertility. *Fertility and Sterility.* 1980; **34**: 557–60.
173. Vercellini P, Fedele L, Bianchi S, Candiani GB. Pelvic denervation for chronic pain associated with endometriosis. Fact or fancy? *American Journal of Obstetrics and Gynecology.* 1991; **165**: 745–9.
174. Nezhat CH, Seidman DS, Nezhat FR, Nezhat CR. Long-term outcome of laparoscopic presacral neurectomy for the treatment of central pelvic pain attributed to endometriosis. *Obstetrics and Gynecology.* 1998; **91**: 701–04.
175. Vercellini P, Aimi G, Busacca M *et al.* Laparoscopic uterosacral ligament resection for dysmenorrhea associated with endometriosis: results of a randomized, controlled trial. *Fertility and Sterility.* 2003; **80**: 310–19.
176. Johnson NP, Farquhar CM, Crossley S *et al.* A double-blind randomised controlled trial of laparoscopic uterine nerve ablation for women with chronic pelvic pain. *BJOG.* 2004; **111**: 950–9.
177. Zullo F, Palomba S, Zupi E *et al.* Effectiveness of presacral neurectomy in women with severe dysmenorrhea caused by endometriosis who were treated with laparoscopic conservative surgery: a 1-year prospective randomized double-blind controlled trial. *American Journal of Obstetrics and Gynecology.* 2003; **189**: 5–10.
*178. Proctor ML, Latthe PM, Farquhar CM *et al.* Surgical interruption of pelvic nerve pathways for primary and secondary dysmenorrhea. *Cochrane Database of Systematic Reviews.* 2005; **CD001896**.
179. Vlaeyen JW, Morley S. Cognitive-behavioral treatments for chronic pain: what works for whom? *Clinical Journal of Pain.* 2005; **21**: 1–8. Review.
180. Kames LD, Rapkin AJ, Naliboff BD *et al.* Effectiveness of an interdisciplinary pain management program for the treatment of chronic pelvic pain. *Pain.* 1990; **41**: 41–6.
181. Helms JM. Acupuncture for the management of primary dysmenorrhea. *Obstetrics and Gynecology.* 1987; **69**: 51–6.
182. Hawk C, Long C, Azad A. Chiropractic care for women with chronic pelvic pain: A prospective single-group intervention study. *Journal of Manipulative and Physiological Therapeutics.* 1997; **20**: 73–9.
183. Milburn A, Reiter RC, Rhomberg AT. Multidisciplinary approach to chronic pelvic pain. In: Ling FW (ed.). *Obstetrics and gynecology clinics of North America: contemporary management of chronic pelvic pain.* Philadelphia, PA: W.B. Saunders Company, 1993: 643–61.
184. Gambone JC, Reiter RC. Nonsurgical management of chronic pelvic pain: A multidisciplinary approach. *Clinical Obstetrics and Gynecology.* 1990; **33**: 205–11.
*185. Moyal-Baracco M, Lynch PJ. 2003 ISSVD terminology and classification of vulvodynia: a historical perspective. *Journal of Reproductive Medicine.* 2004; **49**: 772.
186. Foster DC. Vulvar disease. *Obstetrics and Gynecology.* 2002; **100**: 145–63.
187. Turner MLC, Marinoff SC. Pudendal neuralgia. *American Journal of Obstetrics and Gynecology.* 1991; **165**: 1233–6.
188. McKay M. Dysesthetic ("essential") vulvodynia – treatment with amitriptyline. *Journal of Reproductive Medicine.* 1993; **38**: 9–13.
189. Welsh BM, Berzins K N, Cook KA, Fairley CK. Management of common vulval conditions. *Medical Journal of Australia.* 2003; **178**: 391–5.
190. Harlow BL, Stewart EG. A population-based assessment of chronic unexplained vulvar pain: have we underestimated the prevalence of vulvodynia? *Journal of the American Medical Women's Association.* 2003; **58**: 82–8.
191. Baggish MS, Miklos JR. Vulvar pain syndrome: a review. *Obstetrics and Gynecological Survey.* 1995; **50**: 618–27.
192. Ledger WJ, Kessler A, Leonard GH, Witkin SS. Vulvar vestibulitis – A complex clinical entity. *Infectious Diseases in Obstetrics and Gynecology.* 1996; **4**: 269–75.
193. Pyka RE, Wilkinson EJ, Friedrich Jr EG *et al.* The histopathology of vulvar vestibulitis syndrome. *International Journal of Gynecological Pathology.* 1998; **7**: 249–57.
*194. Zolnoun D, Hartmann K, Lamvu G *et al.* A conceptual model for the pathophysiology of vulvar vestibulitis syndrome. *Obstetrics and Gynecological Survey.* 2006; **61**: 395–401.
195. Bornstein J, Goldschmid N, Sabo E. Hyperinnervation and mast cell activation may be used as histopathologic diagnostic criteria for vulvar vestibulitis. *Gynecologic and Obstetric Investigation.* 2004; **58**: 171–8.
196. Eva LJ, MacLean AB, Reid WMN *et al.* Estrogen receptor expression in vulvar vestibulitis syndrome. *American Journal of Obstetrics and Gynecology.* 2003; **189**: 458–61.
197. Foster DC, Hasday JD. Elevated tissue levels of interleukin-1 beta and tumor necrosis factor-alpha in vulvar vestibulitis. *Obstetrics and Gynecology.* 1997; **89**: 291–6.
198. Foster DC, Stodgell CJ. Impact of genetic variation in interleukin-1 receptor antagonist and melanocortin-1 receptor genes on vulvar vestibulitis syndrome. *Journal of Reproductive Medicine.* 2004; **49**: 503–09.
199. Gerber S, Bongiovanni AM, Ledger WJ *et al.* A deficiency in interferon-alpha production in women with vulvar

vestibulitis. *American Journal of Obstetrics and Gynecology.* 2002; **186**: 361–4.

200. Gerber S, Bongiovanni AM, Ledger WJ *et al.* Defective regulation of the proinflammatory immune response in women with vulvar vestibulitis syndrome. *American Journal of Obstetrics and Gynecology.* 2002; **186**: 696–700.
201. Gerber S, Bongiovanni AM, Ledger WJ *et al.* Interleukin-1beta gene polymorphism in women with vulvar vestibulitis syndrome. *European Journal of Obstetrics, Gynecology, and Reproductive Biology.* 2003; **107**: 74–7.
202. Jeremias J, Ledger WJ, Witkin SS. Interleukin 1 receptor antagonist gene polymorphism in women with vulvar vestibulitis. *American Journal of Obstetrics and Gynecology.* 2000; **182**: 283–5.
203. Glazer HI, Rodke G, Swencionis c *et al.* Treatment of vulvar vestibulitis syndrome with electromyographic biofeedback of pelvic floor musculature. *Journal of Reproductive Medicine.* 1995; **40**: 283–90.
204. Stewart EG, Berger BM. Parallel pathologies? Vulvar vestibulitis and interstitial cystitis. *Journal of Reproductive Medicine.* 1997; **42**: 131–4.
205. Zolnoun D, Hartmann K, Lamvu G *et al.* A conceptual model for the pathophysiology of vulvar vestibulitis syndrome. *Obstetrical and Gynecological Survey.* 2006; **61**: 395–401; quiz 423.
206. Friedrich EG. Vulvar vestibulitis syndrome. *Journal of Reproductive Medicine.* 1987; **32**: 110–15.
207. Suckling J, Lethaby A, Kennedy R. Local oestrogen for vaginal atrophy in postmenopausal women. *Cochrane Database of Systematic Reviews.* 2003; **CD001500**.
208. Ben-David B, Friedman M. Gabapentin therapy for vulvodynia. *Anesthesia and Analgesia.* 1999; **89**: 1459–60.
209. Scheinfeld N. The role of gabapentin in treating diseases with cutaneous manifestations and pain. *International Journal of Dermatology.* 2003; **42**: 491–5.
210. Zolnoun D, Hartmann KE, Steege JF. Overnight 5% lidocaine ointment for treatment of vulvar vestibulitis. *Obstetrics and Gynecology.* 2003; **102**: 84–7.
211. Rapkin AJ, McDonald JS, Morgan M. Multilevel local anesthetic nerve blockade for the treatment of vulvar vestibulitis syndrome. *American Journal of Obstetrics and Gynecology.* 2008; **198**: 41–5.
212. Gunter J, Brewer A, Tawfik O. Botulinum toxin a for vulvodynia: a case report. *Journal of Pain.* 2004; **5**: 238–40.
213. Yoon H, Chung WS, Shim BS. Botulinum toxin A for the management of vulvodynia. *International Journal of Impotence Research.* 2007; **19**: 84–7.

*214. Haefner HK. Critique of new gynecologic surgical procedures: Surgery for vulvar vestibulitis. *Clinical Obstetrics and Gynecology.* 2000; **43**: 689–700.

215. Bornstein J, Zarfati D, Goldik Z, Abramovici H. Perineoplasty compared with vestibuloplasty for severe vestibulitis. *British Journal of Obstetrics and Gynaecology.* 1995; **102**: 652–5.
216. Meana M, Yitzchak MB, Samir K, Cohen D. Biopsychosocial profile of women with dyspareunia. *Obstetrics and Gynecology.* 1997; **90**: 583–9.
217. Schultz WC, Gianotten WL, van der Meijden WI *et al.* Behaviour approach with or without surgical intervention to the vulvar vestibulitis syndrome: A prospective randomized and intervention to the vulvar vestibulitis syndrome: a prospective randomized and non-randomized study. *Journal of Psychosomatic Obstetrics and Gynaecology.* 1996; **17**: 143–8.
218. Solomon CC, Melmed MH, Heitler SM. Calcium citrate for vulvar vestibulitis. *Journal of Reproductive Medicine.* 1991; **36**: 879–2.
219. Baggish MS, Sze EHM, Johnson R. Urinary oxalate excretion and its role in vulvar pain syndrome. *American Journal of Obstetrics and Gynecology.* 1997; **177**: 507–11.
220. Melmed HM. A low calcium oxalate diet and calcium citrate administration are effective treatments for vulvar pain syndrome. *Journal of Gynecologic Surgery.* 1996; **12**: 217–18.
221. Bornstein J, Goldik Z, Alter Z *et al.* Persistent vulvar vestibulitis: the continuing challenge. *Obstetrics and Gynecological Survey.* 1998; **53**: 39–44.

42

Fibromyalgia and myofascial pain: mechanisms to management

SERENA F CARVILLE AND ERNEST H CHOY

KEY LEARNING POINTS

- Fibromyalgia is characterized by chronic widespread pain, whereas pain in myofascial pain is localized.
- Fibromyalgia is a syndrome associated with a wide range of symptoms and other conditions, one of which is myofascial pain
- Fibromyalgia arises at least in part due to an alteration in central pain processing.
- Elevated levels of substance P, central sensitization, wind-up and extrinsic factors are all involved in the pathophysiology.
- There are (at least) three different subgroups of fibromyalgia patients who respond differently to management strategies.
- Treatment must be tailored to the individual needs of the patient depending on their range of symptoms.
- The ideal management is generally a multidisciplinary approach.

INTRODUCTION

Fibromyalgia syndrome (FMS) and myofascial pain (MFP) are two common chronic pain disorders, which frequently coexist. MFP is the most common cause of regional pain in clinical populations[1, 2] and FMS is one of the most common causes of widespread pain. Both conditions are characterized by reduced pain threshold, presence of tender points, and evidence of central sensitization. This has led to the hypothesis that both conditions share similar pathogenic mechanisms.

In FMS, chronic widespread pain that persists in all four quadrants of the body is often accompanied by a range of symptoms including fatigue, sleep disturbance, functional impairment, cognitive dysfunction, variable bowel habits, depression, stiffness, and more. One-third of FMS patients experience significant minor depression or anxiety, which may contribute to the severity of the symptoms or may be a result of suffering from chronic pain. FMS patients have reduced pain thresholds (hyperalgesia) and feel pain with normally innocuous stimuli (allodynia). FMS shares many common features with, and often coexists with, other syndromes such as irritable bowel syndrome (IBS), chronic fatigue syndrome (CFS), and dysmenorrhagia, leading to the suggestion that it is part of a spectrum of disorders characterized by somatization. FMS also occurs concomitantly with other conditions such as rheumatoid arthritis and systemic lupus erythematosus. In the past, this form has been called secondary FMS, suggesting that these conditions predispose patients to develop FMS. However, this has not been used recently as the precise relationship between FMS and these chronic painful conditions remains unclear.

MFP is characterized by regional areas of chronic pain, arising from "taut bands" of muscle. It can include neck and shoulder pain, tension headaches, and lower back pain. Trigger points are found at discrete regions across the body, which are hypersensitive. Palpation of these causes local and referred pain. It has been proposed that MFP is a "precursor" to FMS, or that it is one of the many factors contributing to the "syndrome" of FMS. In the past there has been confusion over the distinction between FMS and MFP, however, they can both exist as distinct entities and research has led to differential diagnosis becoming clearer.

DIAGNOSIS

Fibromyalgia syndrome

Since first being described in the 1800s, FMS has been labeled by various different titles, including muscular rheumatism, myalgia, interstitial fibrositis, myofascitis, and myofascial pain. In 1977, Smythe and Moldofsky[3] applied the term fibrositis to patients with localized or generalized musculoskeletal pain associated with tender points. This is a misnomer since the term implies an inflammatory process in fibrous tissue which has never been demonstrated by biopsy. The diagnosis of FMS has been problematic in the absence of an objective test. In 1990, Wolfe *et al.*[4] defined the American College of Rheumatology (ACR) classification criteria, which are currently the standard used to diagnose this syndrome in clinical and therapeutic research. They state that patients must have a history of widespread pain lasting more than three months, defined as: pain in both sides of the body, pain above and below the waist. In addition, axial skeletal pain (cervical spine, anterior chest, thoracic spine, or low back) must be present. Low back pain is considered lower segment pain. They must also have pain in at least 11 of 18 tender point sites on digital palpation with an approximate force of 4 kg (until the color under the nail blanches). These must be reported as "painful" not just "tender" (see **Figure 42.1**).

Although the ACR criteria are useful for providing uniform populations for research and clinical trials, there is significant controversy about the diagnosis. Some clinicians have argued that FMS is not a distinct disease entity. Labeling patients with FMS encourages chronic illness behavior and would increase healthcare consumption. However, recent research in the UK showed the contrary to be true. Using the General Practice Research

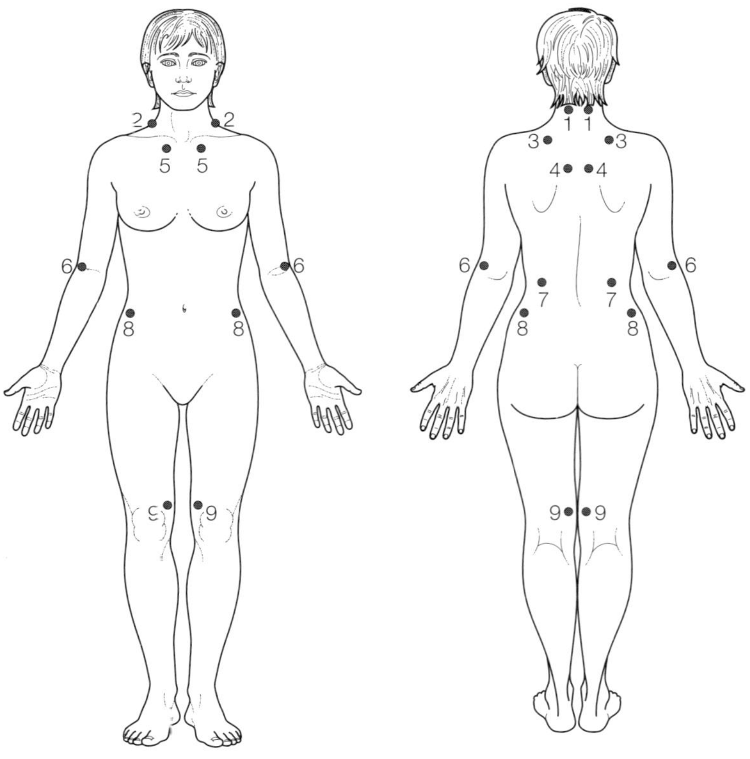

Figure 42.1 Bilateral tender point locations for fibromyalgia: 1, occiput; 2, low cervical; 3, trapezius; 4, supraspinatus; 5, second rib; 6, lateral epicondyle; 7, gluteal; 8, greater trochanter; 9, knee. At least 11 of these must be present.

Database, Gallagher *et al.*[5] showed that healthcare utilization amongst FMS patients was already very high in the eight years preceding the diagnosis. Interestingly, healthcare utilization decreased after the diagnosis indicting that the diagnosis of FMS could be used constructively to reassure and educate patients.

While research has shown that the diagnosis of FMS has positive benefits, the validity of the ACR classification criteria in routine clinical practice is less certain. The key area of contention is the validity and sensitivity of the tender point count. Although intuitively tender point count is a measure of pressure pain threshold, recent research has shown that the number of tender points is largely influenced by psychological distress and is therefore not necessarily the best measure of overall tenderness or means of categorizing patients.[6, 7] A recent study in the UK demonstrated that ≥ 11 tender points can be demonstrated in 40 percent of people with chronic widespread pain, 20 percent of people with regional pain, and 5 percent with no pain. Conversely, 29 percent of people with chronic widespread pain only had ≤ 4 tender points. The presence of tender points without pain was confirmed by Schochat and Raspe.[8] Furthermore, although the tender points are frequently present in FMS patients, pain is not restricted to these areas.[9, 10] MFP trigger points are also not restricted to these 18 locations. In addition, men inherently have a higher pain threshold than women. It is consequently possible that the guide of 4 kg pressure may not be great enough to detect positive tender points in men, which may account for the lower prevalence of FMS diagnosis in males.[11, 12] Cumulatively, these factors are likely to reduce the sensitivity of the ACR classification criteria and lead to underdiagnosis of the condition.

Indeed, a recent study by Katz *et al.*[13] has demonstrated this problem. In this study, the ACR classification criteria were compared with clinical diagnosis by experienced clinicians and survey criteria for FMS. Only a moderate degree of agreement was found. Importantly, it showed that the cut-off point of 11 out of 18 tender points was insensitive. A better balance of sensitivity versus specificity would have been achieved by using a threshold of six tender points.

Aside from tender point count, others have criticized that the ACR criteria ignore other important features of FMS such as pain threshold, mood, sleep disturbance, and fatigue. Many of the collaborators involved in defining these criteria have expressed concern about their use in clinical practice.

Subtypes of FMS

Due to the wide range of symptoms associated with FMS, it has been hypothesized that FMS patients can be divided into three different subgroups, reflecting the "syndrome" aspect of this condition.[14, 15]

These three groups were identified by cluster analysis and could be identified as those exhibiting:

1. moderate anxiety, depression, catastrophizing, and poor control over pain, the highest pain thresholds and low tenderness;
2. high levels of anxiety, depression and catastrophizing, low pain control, and considerable tenderness; and
3. low levels of anxiety, depression, and catastrophizing, good control over pain but very low pain threshold and the most tenderness.[15]

In the analysis by Giesecke *et al.*,[15] the first subgroup was considered to represent "typical FMS," as more than half of the patients fell within this category. It is important to note that the patients in this study were recruited from the community. The proportion of patients in each subtype may change if patients in secondary care were studied since the latter tends to include a higher incidence of mood disturbance and psychosocial stress.

Myofascial pain

Similar to FMS, MFP has many different labels. It has been cited under different headings over the years including fibrositis and myofibrositis when distinction between FMS was not so clear. MFP was first defined in the 1950s as was the "trigger point" which characterizes the condition.[16] More research into its pathophysiology has led to clearer definition between MFP and FMS. However, research into this condition has been hampered by the lack of classification/diagnostic criteria. Heterogeneity in patient populations across studies is always a potential confounder which may explain different observations. This problem has been addressed by the publication of Long and Kephort's modified criteria (**Box 42.1**) in 1998 which are now commonly used.[17]

The trigger point feels harder than the surrounding muscle, as within the trigger point the muscle has formed a tense "knot." Palpation of a trigger point causes local and referred pain, the latter of which is not a feature of FMS tender points. This trigger point can also be associated with a twitch response which is termed the "jump sign." It can be active or latent, a latent trigger point will not be associated with referred or spontaneous pain, but is still sensitive to palpation.

MFP can be labeled under different terms depending on the area of the body that it affects such as temporomandibular disorder (TMD), low back pain, and tension headache. It is also associated with limited movement, weakness, and autonomic dysfunction.

Box 42.1 Long and Kephort's modified criteria for the MFP.[17]

All of the following must be present:

1. regional pain;
2. presence of a taut palpable band;
3. distinct pattern of referred pain;
4. exquisite local tenderness at one or more points in the taut band;
5. limited range of motion in the affected area.

Plus one of the following:

1. local twitch response to snapping palpation or needling;
2. pressure on myofascial trigger points reproduces pain;
3. pain alleviated by deactivating the myofascial trigger point.

EPIDEMIOLOGY

Epidemiology of chronic widespread pain

The prevalence of chronic widespread pain in population studies is approximately 3–16 percent.[18] It is more common in women compared with men. Prevalence increases with age with the highest prevalence found between the age group of 59–74 years. However, children also suffer from chronic widespread pain with a prevalence of 7.5 percent.

FMS

Estimates of the prevalence of fibromyalgia varies significantly depending on the classification/diagnostic criteria. Whilst many secondary care studies utilized the ACR classification criteria, many community studies investigated patients with chronic widespread pain. In population-based studies, prevalence varies from 0.1 to 3 percent and 2 to 16 percent in clinical situations.[19] The mean age was 50. Women are affected more frequently than men with a ratio of 3:1[20] but it has been reported to be as high as 9:1 in a US study. As discussed above, the prevalence of FMS may be an underestimate while the gender ratio is biased toward a higher female predisposition due to the drawbacks of the ACR classification criteria.

Furthermore, prevalence can be influenced by social, economic, cultural, and ethnic factors, therefore epidemiology may show significant geographical variation. In 1987, the General Practice Research Database (GPRD) in the UK began recording all visits to general practice surgeries. Between 1990 and 2001 the incidence of FMS increased, most probably due to the instigation of the ACR diagnostic criteria and increased awareness in general practices. Although it is predominantly a disease of middle age, all ages can be affected. The mean age of onset recorded by the GPRD was 49.[21]

MFP

MFP is the most common cause of chronic regional pain.[22] It can include low back pain, shoulder pain, tension headaches, and facial pain, amongst others. It is again more common in women. Studies have suggested that many people attending general practitioner (GP) or pain clinics with other complaints may actually suffer from MFP. For example, 85 percent with low back pain and >90 percent with chronic neck pain and tension headaches may in some cases arise from referred MFP.[1, 23, 24] As mentioned above, varying diagnoses make epidemiological studies hard to interpret for the prevalence of this condition.

ASSOCIATED CONDITIONS

There are a group of disorders that have been termed "affective spectrum disorders" which frequently coexist with one another. These include fibromyalgia, but also irritable bowel syndrome, chronic fatigue syndrome, depression and anxiety disorders, and migraine. These are all associated with psychological distress. It had been thought that depression may lead to the development of widespread pain, and although it is commonly reported in fibromyalgia (in 20–30 percent of patients) it is more likely that it in fact occurs the other way round (the pain results in depression) as the majority of patients do not suffer from any psychiatric illness and, when present, the depression can be treated without improving the pain state.

RISK FACTORS

Fibromyalgia

Many studies have shown that psychological features are risk factors for chronic generalized musculoskeletal pain and/or fibromyalgia. These include somatization, having a mental disorder, presence of psychological distress, major depression, panic disorder, and familial major mood disorder. Sociocultural factors such as a low level of income, being divorced, being disabled, being an immigrant, smoking, and/or lower social class have been implicated but definitive evidence linking these to the development of fibromyalgia is lacking.

MFP

Similar to FMS, some studies[25, 26] of MFP in patients with temporomandibular disorder, high baseline somatization score, anxiety, and depression were significant risk factors for development of chronic MFP.

PATHOPHYSIOLOGY

Fibromyalgia

The exact pathophysiological mechanisms behind FMS remain unknown although a number of hypotheses and contributing factors have been identified and proposed.[27, 28]

MUSCLE ANOMALIES

The generalized muscle pain frequently appears to be exhibited following suffering of localized muscle pain,[29] often due to injury, such as whiplash[30] or low back pain.[31] Although no obvious muscle or tissue damage is present in FMS patients, some changes within the muscle have been reported. The microcirculation of muscles appears to be altered resulting in reduced muscle tissue oxygenation.[32, 33] This is not specific to FMS, but may be important for onset of pain and hypersensitivity in chronic pain conditions. This can cause other muscle changes which have also been observed in fibromyalgia patients, including "red ragged and moth-eaten" fibers, possibly due to distribution and proliferation of mitochondria and various metabolic effects. Hypoxia of muscle tissue may lead to the release of pain substances including serotonin, bradykinin, substance P, and histamine, which sensitize nociceptive fibers, and is exacerbated during contraction of the muscle.

GENETICS

Buskila *et al.*[34] suggested a possible genetic factor in the development of FMS by demonstrating that 28 percent of offspring of mothers with FMS suffered from chronic widespread pain. Offspring with and without FMS did not differ on anxiety, depression, global well-being, quality of life, and physical functioning.[34] In a case controlled study in which the frequency of FMS in 533 relatives of 78 probands with FMS was compared with 272 relatives of 40 probands with rheumatoid arthritis (RA), Arnold *et al.*[35] found that FMS aggregated strongly in families. The risk of suffering from FMS in a relative of a proband with FMS was increased eight-fold when compared with probands of RA. They also tended to have significantly higher number of tender points and major mood disorders.[35] More recently, a study compared the prevalence of chronic widespread pain in monozygotic and dizygotic twins. They found that genetic factors accounted for 50 percent of the total variance.[36] This provides persuasive evidence supporting the importance of genetic factor in the pathogenesis of FMS.

A number of candidate genes have been examined in more details which include HLA, polymorphism of catechol-O-methyltransferase (COMT),[34, 37, 38] and more recently polymorphism in the 5HT2A receptor,[39] serotonin transporter gene.[40] Overall, it is likely that FMS is a polygenetic disorder, due to the many different factors that may be involved. It is possible that genetic factors may act in collaboration with environmental factors (or mechanical/psychological traumas) to contribute to the development of FMS.

NEUROENDOCRINE ALTERATIONS

In patients with FMS, a reduced hypothalamic-pituitary-adrenal (HPA) axis response to stress has been demonstrated.[41, 42, 43] The neuroendocrine response acts normally under baseline conditions, but not when subjected to stress or even normal activities of daily living. However, this deficit might have more impact on depression, a common associated feature of FMS as well as chronic pain. Patients with FMS often report experiencing previous stressful or traumatic events. A reduced HPA axis response to stress can contribute to FMS development or worsening of FMS. The HPA axis is also linked to the autonomic nervous system, which is involved in modulating sleep, mood, pain, and cardiovascular activities (including microcirculation of muscles). This could explain many clinical features and the association of FMS with sympathetic nerve system over activity, although more detailed mechanistic studies will be needed to confirm a causative relationship. Abnormal HPA axis activity has also been observed to a lesser extent in chronic low back pain sufferers, therefore it does appear to be linked to chronic pain.

Hormones such as cortisol, growth hormone (GH), and thyroid hormone can be affected particularly in patients with an altered HPA axis. Studies have reported increased levels of adrenocortical trophic hormone (ACTH) and decreased levels of insulin-like growth factor (IGF-1), triiodothyronine (T3), GH, estrogen, and urinary cortisol.[44]

A reduction in IGF-1 levels has also been proposed as a contributing factor for FMS development/symptomatology. Bennett *et al.*[45] observed that FMS patients had declining levels over the following one to two years. These patients with a low level of IGF-1 also failed to secrete GH after stimulation with clonidine and L-dopa suggesting that low IGF-I levels in patients with FMS are a secondary phenomenon due to hypothalamic-pituitary-GH axis dysfunction.

Some have suggested that the HPA deficit may be a secondary phenomenon rather than having a causative role as it has been observed in people with sleep disturbances. FMS patients have been reported to have a reduction of stage 4 non-REM, or deep sleep, which also leads to reduced pressure pain thresholds, increased aching and fatigue.[46] FMS patients are frequently more painful and tender in the morning and experience significant morning stiffness, this is lessened after nights where they have had more restful sleep. Although a cause and effect relationship has not been established, this does appear to be an important factor in FMS.

Another hypothesis involves the role of proinflammatory cytokines which could induce hyperalgesia in the central nervous system (CNS). Release of these cytokines can be triggered by chronic stress. They are known to directly contribute to peripheral and central neuropathic pain as well as depression and can lead to exaggerated pain states similar to those seen in FMS.[47] A recent study in 40 patients with chronic widespread pain, including 26 with FMS and 40 age- and sex-matched healthy controls, found lower relative gene expression for the anti-inflammatory cytokines interleukin-4 and interleukin-10.[48]

NEURONAL PLASTICITY

A characteristic feature of FMS is hyperalgesia (increased sensitivity to mechanical, thermal, and electrical stimuli) and allodynia (painful response to normally non-noxious stimuli). These are likely to be due to altered mechanisms within the CNS such as "wind-up" and central sensitization which have been demonstrated in FMS patients.[49, 50] Altered pain processing has been illustrated by studies using functional magnetic resonance imaging (fMRI) where painful pressure stimuli result in increased cerebral blood flow in areas associated with activation by noxious stimuli. This is exaggerated in FMS patients at stimulus intensities that may otherwise be seen as non-noxious.[51] High levels of catastrophizing were also associated with increased activity in similar areas,[52] as was depression.[15] (See **Table 42.1**.) Neither catastrophizing nor depression affects hyperalgesia, therefore other mechanisms must also be involved in fibromyalgia.[52, 53]

One of the models proposed is a "bottom to top" approach in which regional musculoskeletal pain (for example MFP) leads to widespread and persistent pain, generalized hypersensitivity, and consequently FMS. This is based on neural plasticity of the CNS, in which persistent input or activation of peripheral nociceptors causes a change in CNS function and eventually structural changes. Although FMS appears to be due to a central dysfunction, it is the peripheral factors that are the most debilitating for the individuals affected, and the activation of the peripheral pain receptors undoubtedly plays some role in the central sensitization observed, possibly as an instigating factor.

Repetitive activation of muscle nociceptors leads to peripheral sensitization, therefore decreasing the excitation threshold and increasing the response to low level noxious stimuli (hyperalgesia). Wind-up occurs in the spinal dorsal horn, when repetitive input from the C-fiber nociceptors increases the response of the neurones. This causes increased release of substance P and glutamate activating the *N*-methyl-D-aspartic acid (NMDA) receptors by removing the magnesium block. Temporal summation studies have been carried out in FMS patients with intramuscular electrical stimulation. The results showed that temporal summation was more pronounced in FMS patients compared to controls, indicating central sensitization.[54] Similar results were reported for FMS and whiplash patients,[55] again supporting the hypothesis that localized pain (or trauma) can develop into FMS.

An epidural injection of lignocaine relieves pain and tender points in FMS,[56] which supports the involvement of peripheral nociception causing the pain. In a study population of FMS patients, 87 percent reported that they suffered from localized pain before FMS. A further study demonstrated that 25 percent of chronic back pain sufferers and 21.6 percent with neck trauma went on to develop FMS.

Research also supports central sensitization in FMS as injections of ketamine in responders with FMS reduced the pain and allodynia experienced. However, not all FMS patients responded to ketamine suggesting that FMS is heterogenous and one mechanism is not universally responsible for FMS.

An alternative theory is that the model works from "top to bottom." In this case chronic stress and pain catastrophizing lead to FMS in the periphery. It has been

Table 42.1 Regional cerebral blood flow following various stimuli.

Brain region	Stimuli that increase blood flow	Painful or nonpainful?
Contralateral primary somatosensory cortex (S1)	Mechanical	Painful and nonpainful
Contralateral secondary somatosensory cortex (S2)	Mechanical	Painful and nonpainful
Anterior cingular cortex	Mechanical Catastrophizing	Painful
Insula	Mechanical Aversive stimuli Depression	Painful
Thalamus	Mechanical	Painful

observed that pain catastrophizing is higher in FMS patients than in controls and other chronic pain conditions, but this may not be the preceding factor.[57] Recent research has shown that fibromyalgia patients have elevated levels of substance P in the cerebrospinal fluid (CSF),[58, 59] which could be due to an increased release from neurones in the periphery and/or CNS.

Descending inhibition is also altered or impaired in FMS.[60] Research into the diffuse noxious inhibitory control system (DNIC) has revealed that FMS and MFP patients appear to lack this function, in which normally a noxious stimuli applied to one body site would suppress pain at another site. (See **Figure 42.2**.)

Myofascial pain

In MFP, the muscle which causes the pain is said to be a "taut band" which has contracted abnormally. Electrophysiological evidence suggests that the responsible factor is a dysfunctional motor end-plate.[61, 62] For an unknown reason, excess amounts of acetylcholine (ACh) are released into the synaptic cleft even when the muscle is at rest. This leads to depolarization of the membrane of the motor fiber, causing cross-bridge activation and muscle contraction. Because of the excess ACh present, the depolarization is sustained and the muscle can become maximally contracted with the sarcomeres at their shortest, causing the muscle to become "taut" and resulting in a trigger point (see **Figure 42.3**). This contraction increases the energy consumption of the muscle, putting increased demand on the microcirculation and leading to local ischemia and hypoxia. As previously discussed this can initiate a pain state. MFP is also associated with enhanced pain sensitivity and wind-up, due to the persistent stimulation of the nociceptors. Similar to FMS, TMD patients have reduced pressure pain thresholds and decreased descending inhibition of nociceptive reflexes.

MANAGEMENT

Fibromyalgia

In order to improve the outcome of FMS, first one must acknowledge the problem. Regardless of whether FMS is a single condition/disease or not, it is a major healthcare

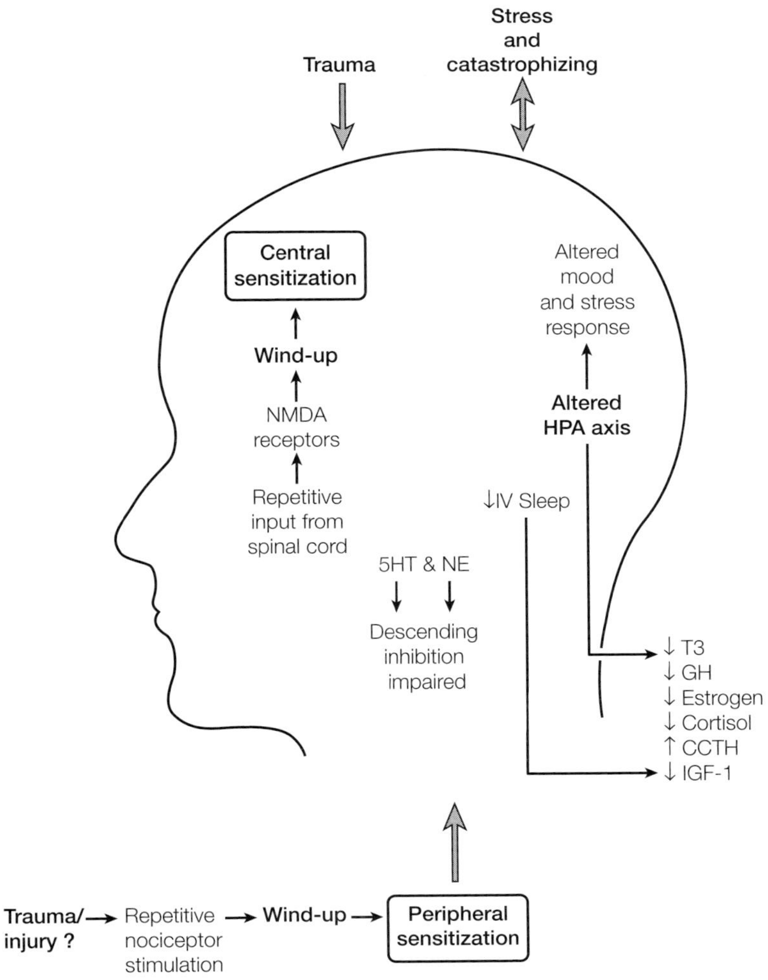

Figure 42.2 Contributing factors to the pathophysiology of fibromyalgia.

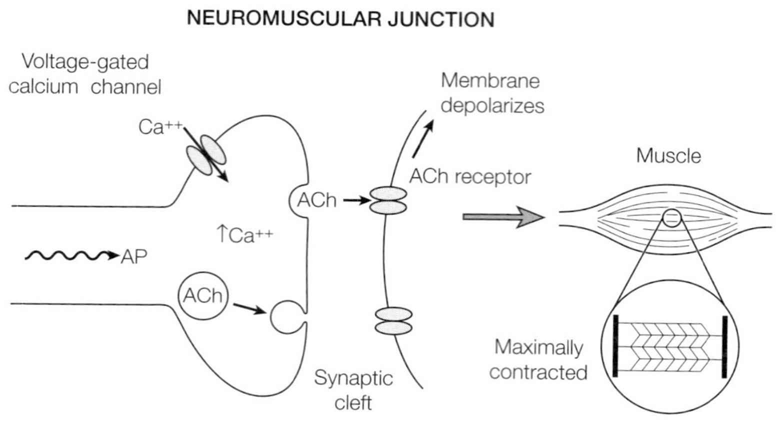

Figure 42.3 Mechanisms of development of myofascial pain by increased release of ACh.

burden and must be addressed. As previously mentioned, diagnosis of FMS can help reduce the healthcare burden through reduced investigations and referral to specialists.[21] Therefore, ignoring the problem is not the solution. Clearly, the diagnosis of FMS can be used constructively to reassure patients, thereby reducing healthcare utilization.

As FMS is a complex syndrome associated with a wide range of symptoms, treatment should be tailored to the individual, addressing their particular needs and targeting their most distressing symptoms. The best strategy is to use a multidisciplinary approach to treatment, using both pharmacological and nonpharmacological interventions as required. It is unlikely that a single treatment will target all of the different symptoms involved. The different subgroups of patients with FMS respond differently to treatment strategies,[63] highlighting the fact that patients should be managed according to their individual needs, rather than following a generalized approach.

In the following section we aim to discuss the current evidence for treatment of FMS, which can be selected to suit the individual concerned. This is based on evidence gained from studies using the 1990 ACR criteria for FMS diagnosis in order to study a more homogenous population. The European League Against Rheumatism have also produced guidelines for management of FMS.[64]

Nonpharmacological

Due to the lack of a "gold standard" treatment for FMS, a wide range of nonpharmacological approaches have been tested with varying success and more research is required. These include; exercise, cognitive-behavioral therapy, homeopathy, physiotherapy, acupuncture, magnetism, dietary alterations, and laser therapy, amongst others.

By the nature of the interventions, the study quality is inevitably rated as poorer in quality than the pharmacological trials, since double-blind trials are not possible. However these interventions are safe as they are not associated with potential adverse events and therefore long-term use is not detrimental.

EXERCISE

The literature on exercise is extensive: over 20 studies since the 1990 ACR criteria, but the majority of these are of relatively poor quality as they are often open studies, although a limited number are investigator blinded. These studies reported mixed results.[65, 66, 67] However, most experts concurred that aerobic exercise and strength training are beneficial for some FMS patients and this is supported by systematic reviews.[68, 69, 70, 71][III] It should be noted that exercise rarely improves pain, and this symptom can in fact be worsened at first.[72] Other factors including function, tender point count, aerobic performance, and global well-being have all been reported to improve. FMS patients are equally able to carry out exercise as healthy people, at levels tailored to each individual. When performing strength training they can experience the same strength gains,[73] which may in turn lead to functional improvements and/or quality of life. Adherence to a program may be a limiting factor, but otherwise long-term use is without risks.

Heated pool-based exercise is particularly beneficial and is supported by one randomized controlled trial and one open randomized trial.[72, 74, 75] Heated pools or hydrotherapy are effective for pain relief even without exercise.[76, 77][III] Buoyancy reduces pressure load from the muscles, and the heated water provides relaxation. Pain relief may only be temporary, but treatment can be maintained long term without any safety concerns. Treatment improves pain and function and reduces tender point count, although availability of a hydrotherapy pool and cost are limiting factors.

COGNITIVE-BEHAVIORAL THERAPY

Cognitive-behavioral therapy (CBT) and/or patient education may help improve pain and function in some individuals, either as sole therapy or in combination with exercise.[49, 78, 79, 80, 81][III] It may be particularly beneficial to provide CBT early after diagnosis to help patients understand FMS and learn how they themselves can be actively involved in its management. As FMS is a chronic condition without a permanent remedy, patient education is an important aspect of management as patients have to learn to manage their pain better even if they also receive other therapy. This therefore may help to improve their long-term prognosis by providing more realistic health beliefs. The quality of published trials in this area is relatively poor, but its use has been supported by previous reviews[71, 72, 82] and expert opinion supports its use.

With regard to the subgroups of FMS patients that have been proposed, the second group who experience the highest levels of distress may respond best to this approach,[15] whereas the other two groups with moderate and low mood disturbances and distress are less likely to require CBT. Variation in trial reports and/or success may be compounded by this factor.

OTHER THERAPIES

A range of dietary interventions has been studied in fibromyalgia, however, no one treatment has more than one study. A randomized controlled trial using *Chlorella pyrenoidosa* supplements showed improvements in the treated group for pain and function, however, the patients also continued their usual treatment.[83] Vegan and vegetarian diets have also been reported to show some nonsignificant improvements, as have ascorbigen (with broccoli power) supplements.[84, 85, 86] Complementary therapies including homeopathic remedies[87, 88, 89] and acupuncture[90, 91] have also been reported to have benefits for pain, tenderness, quality of life, and well-being for FMS patients. However, there have also been negative studies for acupuncture, but it may be of benefit to some patients. A number of miscellaneous treatments have also been used in FMS including therapy with lasers, magnets, ultrasound, and music vibration. Clearly, the paucity of evidence does not allow a firm conclusion and recommendations to be made regarding these therapies.

Pharmacological

A number of pharmacological interventions have been shown to be efficacious in randomized controlled trials for FMS, despite the fact that at this point in time only one treatment is specifically licensed for its management (in the US). These can be used with or without combination with a nonpharmacological intervention in the management of FMS.

ANALGESICS

Tramadol is a useful moderately potent opioid analgesic that can help to improve pain and function.[92, 93][II] It is a centrally acting analgesic which inhibits norepinephrine and serotonin reuptake whilst also being an agonist for the mu opioid receptor. The most commonly reported adverse events include nausea, somnolence, constipation, and dizziness. However, it should be prescribed with caution as typical opiate withdrawal can be experienced at termination so careful down-titration must be observed. Dependence and abuse are also potential issues to bear in mind when prescribing.[94] Other systemic analgesics have been used in short-term studies including lidocaine, ketamine, and morphine. While ketamine and lidocaine have received some support for short-term pain relief (postinjection), there is doubt over their efficacy for treating a chronic condition such as FMS.[95, 96] Topical analgesics (including xylocaine and capsaicin) are not of benefit in this condition.

ANTIDEPRESSANTS

Antidepressants should be considered for FMS patients.[71, 82, 97][I] Tricyclic antidepressants (TCAs), selective serotonin reuptake inhibitors (SSRIs), dual reuptake inhibitors, mono-amine oxidase inhibitors, and serotonin antagonists have all been reported to have benefits. The evidence is strongest for amitriptyline and fluoxetine, but recently trials of a newer class of dual reuptake inhibitors have reported good positive results.

TCAs such as amitriptyline (the most widely used and studied in FMS) inhibit serotonin (5HT3) and norepinephrine (NE) reuptake, but also affect glutaminergic neurotransmission by acting on histamine, ACh and NMDA channels. Positive results are reported for sleep, fatigue, and pain in FMS.[98, 99, 100] The effect is independent to the drugs antidepressant action as the doses prescribed are much lower than those for depression. Despite the positive results, tolerance is variable due to the anticholinergic effects of this class of treatment. Adverse events can include dry mouth, digestive disturbances, and neuropsychiatric disturbances. SSRIs lack these actions, so are better tolerated, but results are mixed. Fluoxetine has had two positive studies for a variety of symptoms including pain, function, fatigue, and depression.[100, 101] Dual reuptake inhibitors, however, have a similar efficacy as TCAs for NE and 5HT but lack the anticholinergic effects. Their tolerance is good (headaches and nausea are the most commonly reported adverse events) and studies for milnacipran, duloxetine, and venlafaxine have all reported positive effects on pain, function, pain threshold, fatigue, and quality of life (although the study on venlafaxine was open and nonrandomized).[102, 103, 104]

Tropisetron and ondansetron are 5HT3 receptor antagonists which have shown pain and tender point count improvements in FMS patients but only in short-term studies (five to ten days).[105, 106, 107] Further investigation is required into long-term use of these medications.

OTHER PHARMACOLOGICAL INTERVENTIONS

Anti-epileptics such as pregabalin increase inhibitory neurotransmission and block calcium and/or sodium channels.

A large recent controlled study in FMS patients reported good effects for sleep, pain, and fatigue and good tolerability with most adverse events being dizziness or somnolence, mild to moderate in severity.[108][II] This is the first treatment to be licensed by the FDA for FMS in the US.

Pramipexole is a dopamine agonist that was developed for the treatment of Parkinson's disease, however, its action within the mesolimbic system (particularly on sleep control) provided the potential for treatment in FMS. Results from a placebo controlled trial have supported its use with improvements in pain, fatigue, function, and global wellbeing with good tolerance, however, patients were allowed to continue with current medications if at a stable dose.[109] [II] Further research is warranted.

Hypnotics including zolpidem act on benzodiazepine receptors. In FMS they are effective for sleep and fatigue, but not pain, so should only be used in combination with another approach. Sodium oxybate (a commercial form of gammahydroxybutyrate) is known to increase slow-wave sleep and GH levels (both impaired in FMS patients). It has been shown to improve pain as well as fatigue and sleep in FMS.[110][II] There is the potential for abuse with this medication, however, and it has been associated with date rape, so its use in FMS should be considered with caution.

Tizanidine, an alpha 2 adrenergic central agonist, probably acts by reducing levels of substance P in the CNS and has been reported to reduce pain and improve sleep and quality of life in FMS. However, the study was not controlled or blinded.[111][III]. Adverse events can include tiredness, somnolence, dizziness, and dry mouth. It should be used with caution in women receiving oral contraceptives, which can reduce its clearance.

GH has been studied in FMS due to research showing reduced levels in FMS patients. Although results were positive for quality of life and tender points, its usefulness is limited by potential side effects and high cost.[112][II]

There has been a suggestion that FMS patients benefit from thyroid hormone therapy and that perhaps patients (or a subgroup of them) suffer from a subclinical deficiency in this hormone. Three small studies by Lowe *et al.*[113, 114, 115][III] suggest that tri-iodothyronine is beneficial for pain and function following up to eight months treatment in euthyroid female FMS patients. Long-term toxicity remains a significant safety concern.

Nonsteroidal anti-inflammatory drugs (NSAID) may be useful for short-term pain relief when used in addition to other therapies (e.g. stretching exercises), however, they should not be considered as an option for long-term management due to their gastrointestinal effects. Most studies of NSAIDs have produced negative results in FMS.

Myofascial pain

There are few placebo-controlled trials into managements for MFP, therefore most evidence is based on clinical experience. As with FMS, treatment should be tailored to the individual, bearing in mind the muscles involved, contributing factors, and any concomitant diseases.

The first-line approach should be nonpharmacological treatment. Physiotherapy involving stretching the muscle to release the tension is the most commonly used method. The "spray and stretch" approach is sometimes used where a vapocoolant spray is applied to the muscle whilst it is stretched gently which can produce relief from the pain. This aims to deactivate the trigger point by restoring the muscle to its full length.[116][III] For long-term relief, the patient should also be taught home management, including stretching exercises, to prevent the trigger point recurring. Education should be given to help avoid triggering activities, such as posture, sitting positions, etc., and to learn to recognize situations which might increase muscle tension and try to avoid them. These interventions have not been studied directly in MFP. Exercise has not received support in clinical trials for MFP, however, clinicians often support the idea that stretching and strengthening should be included in exercise programs.[117][V] Postural training has been seen to produce benefits, as have range-of-motion exercises and relaxation.[118]

Acupuncture has been researched in MFP, partly due to the proximity of acupuncture points and common MFP trigger points. Results have been promising, but further research is needed.[119]

Trigger point injections have been used to directly deactivate trigger points for patients who are not responsive to stretching and/or exercise techniques alone. It has been suggested that these should be combined with exercise so that the patients do not become dependent on the injections. Dry needling, anesthetics, steroid, and botulinum toxin have all been used. One study showed that dry needling was equally effective as lidocaine, but caused more postinjection soreness.[120] It is thought that perhaps dry needling acts by mechanically disrupting the trigger point until it relaxes.

Local tender point injection of drugs such as procaine, lidocaine, and corticosteroids may reduce the pain or prolong the relief although a systematic review suggested that the choice of drug did not affect outcome.[121] There is no evidence to support the use of corticosteroids as local inflammation is absent, and they have been reported to be no more effective than saline injections.[122]

Recent research has suggested the use of botulinum toxin. This acts by blocking ACh release at the neuromuscular junction. This would therefore theoretically reduce the muscle activity at the trigger point and help to restore the local microcirculation to normal levels. Reports in the literature have been mixed with efficacy over steroids and saline being reported, but not compared to lidocaine.[123] Further research is warranted.

Benzodiazepines have been studied in MFP with support for their use in the short term,[124] but long-term use has not been researched.

PROGNOSIS

Long-term cohort studies in the Americas and Europe found no significant change in FMS prognosis over a six- to eight-year period.[6, 125] Severity of pain, fatigue, disability, and quality of life remains unchanged. In America, the annual healthcare cost of FMS in 1996 was $2274 per patient. Confronted by such worrying statistics, the Chief Medical Officer in the UK wrote to all the doctors in the UK emphasizing the healthcare burden of chronic widespread pain, urging that more research is essential to address the problem and improve outcome.

For FMS, although it is rare for symptoms to subside completely, if patients are able to learn to manage their chronic pain and adopt effective coping behavior, it is unlikely that the pain will progress and may in fact reduce, although the patients remain symptomatic. Unfortunately, the lack of an effective treatment for all symptoms, or all sufferers, means that a multidimensional approach will most likely be required and a number of interventions may have to be used before the most appropriate for each individual is determined. The prognosis is linked to the severity or range of symptoms experienced by the individual concerned. Those with fewer symptoms may be better able to manage their syndrome with education and coping behaviors, whereas patients with a more wide range of FMS-related symptoms, or more severe spectrum, are more likely to require a more complex approach which may have a less positive long-term prognosis. It is important that the patients realize that complete remission is rare for them to be able to manage the pain better.

In MFP the prognosis is generally good.[22] With effective treatment and education in postural and/or mechanical behaviors to reduce recurrence of the trigger point, it is likely that once treated the pain may not return.

SUMMARY

Fibromyalgia is a chronic syndrome of widespread pain that is associated with a variable spectrum of symptoms and concomitant disorders. It is characterized by allodynia and hyperalgesia with the presence of $\geq$11 out of 18 positive tender points and widespread pain in all four quadrants of the body that has persisted for over three months. In contrast, myofascial pain is a regional pain syndrome that can affect one muscle in isolation. It is caused by a "taut band" of muscle in which the muscle becomes maximally contracted and fails to relax of its own accord. In the past, the two have been seen to overlap and research has led to differential diagnosis, although MFP can occur within the spectrum of FMS-related syndromes. Management of both is likely to require a multidisciplinary approach with a combination of pharmacological and nonpharmacological approaches. With MFP this can be effective in relieving the symptoms and education of preventative behaviors can stop recurrence of the pain. However, in FMS the goal of treatment is currently to reduce symptoms to a more tolerable level as remission is rare. More research into FMS pathogenesis and treatment will hopefully lead to more promising medical development in this area.

REFERENCES

1. Skootsky SA, Jaeger B, Oye RK. Prevalence of myofascial pain in general internal medicine practice. *Western Journal of Medicine*. 1989; **151**: 157–60.
2. Aronoff GM, Evans WO, Enders PL. A review of follow-up studies of multidisciplinary pain units. *Pain*. 1983; **16**: 1–11.
3. Smythe HA, Moldofsky H. Two contributions to understanding of the "fibrositis" syndrome. *Bulletins of Rheumatic Diseases*. 1977; **28**: 928–31.
* 4. Wolfe F, Smythe HA, Yunus MB *et al.* The American college of rheumatology 1990 criteria for the classification of fibromyalgia. *Arthritis and Rheumatism*. 1990; **33**: 160–72.
* 5. Gallagher AM, Thomas JM, Hamilton WT, White PD. Incidence of fatigue symptoms and diagnoses presenting in UK primary care from 1990 to 2001. *Journal of the Royal Society of Medicine*. 2004; **97**: 571–5.
6. Wolfe F, Anderson J, Harkness D *et al.* A prospective, longitudinal, multicentre study of service utilization and costs in fibromyalgia. *Arthritis and Rheumatism*. 1997; **40**: 1560–70.
7. Petzke F, Gracely RH, Park KM *et al.* What do tender points measure? Influence of distress on 4 measures of tenderness. *Journal of Rheumatology*. 2003; **30**: 567–74.
8. Schochat T, Raspe H. Elements of fibromyalgia in an open population. *Rheumatology*. 2003; **42**: 829–35.
9. Kosek E, Ekholm J. Modulation of pressure pain thresholds during and following isometric contraction. *Pain*. 1995; **61**: 481–6.
10. Kosek E, Ekholm J, Hansson P. Sensory dysfunction in fibromyalgia patients with implications for pathogenic mechanisms. *Pain*. 1996; **68**: 375–83.
11. Yunus MB, Inanici F, Aldag JC, Mangold RF. Fibromyalgia in men: comparison of clinical features with women. *Journal of Rheumatology*. 2000; **27**: 485–90.
12. Buskila D, Neumann L, Alhoashle A, Abu-Shakra M. Fibromyalgia syndrome in men. *Seminars in Arthritis and Rheumatism*. 2000; **30**: 47–51.
* 13. Katz RS, Wolfe F, Michaud K. Fibromyalgia diagnosis: A comparison of clinical, survey, and American College of Rheumatology criteria. *Arthritis and Rheumatism*. 2006; **54**: 169–76.
14. Turk DC, Okifuji A, Sinclair JD, Starz TW. Pain, disability, and physical functioning in subgroups of patients with fibromyalgia. *Journal of Rheumatology*. 1996; **23**: 1255–62.

* 15. Giesecke T, Williams DA, Harris RE *et al.* Subgrouping of fibromyalgia patients on the basis of pressure-pain thresholds and psychological factors. *Arthritis and Rheumatism.* 2003; **48**: 2916–22.
16. Travell JG, Simons DG, Simons LS. *Myofascial pain and dysfunction: The trigger point manual*, 2 edn. Vol. 1. Baltimore: Williams & Wilkins, 1999.
* 17. Long SP, Kephort W. Myofascial pain syndrome. In: Ashburn MA, Rice CJ (eds). *The management of pain.* Philadelphia: Churchill Livingstone, 1998: 299–321.
18. Gran TJ. The epidemiology of chronic generalized musculoskeletal pain. *Best Practice and Research Clinical Rheumatology.* 2003; **17**: 547–61.
19. Neumann L, Buskila D. Epidemiology of fibromyalgia. *Current Pain and Headache Reports.* 2003; **7**: 362–8.
20. White KP, Speechley M, Harth M, Ostbye T. The London fibromyalgia epidemiology study: The prevalence of fibromyalgia syndrome in London, Ontario. *Journal of Rheumatology.* 1999; **26**: 1570–6.
21. Hughes G, Martinez C, Myon E *et al.* The impact of a diagnosis of fibromyalgia on health care resource use by primary care patients in the UK: An observational study based on clinical practice. *Arthritis and Rheumatism.* 2006; **54**: 177–83.
22. Fricton JR. Myofascial pain. *Baillière's Clinical Rheumatology.* 1994; **8**: 857–80.
23. Rosomoff HL, Fishbain DA, Goldberg M *et al.* Physical findings in patients with chronic intractable benign pain of the neck and/or back. *Pain.* 1989; **37**: 279–87.
24. Davidoff RA. Trigger points and myofascial pain: toward understanding how they affect headaches. *Cephalagia.* 1998; **18**: 436–48.
25. Velly AM, Gornitsky M, Philippe P. Contributing factors to chronic myofascial pain: A case-control study. *Pain.* 2003; **104**: 491–9.
26. Rammelsberg P, LeResche L, Dworkin S, Mancl L. Longitudinal outcome of temporomandibular disorders: a 5-year epidemiologic study of muscle disorders defined by research diagnostic criteria for temporomandibular disorders. *Journal of Orofacial Pain.* 2003; **17**: 9–20.
27. Staud R. Fibromyalgia pain: do we know the source? *Current Opinion in Rheumatology.* 2004; **16**: 157–63.
28. Price DD, Staud R. Neurobiology of fibromyalgia syndrome. *Journal of Rheumatology.* 2005; **75**: 22–8.
29. Bengtsson A, Henriksson K-G, Jorfeldt L. Primary fibromyalgia. A clinical and laboratory study of 55 patients. *Scandinavian Journal of Rheumatology.* 1986; **15**: 340–7.
30. Buskila D, Neumann L, Vaisberg G *et al.* Increased rates of fibromyalgia following cervical spine injury. A controlled study of 161 cases of fibromyalgia following cervical spine injury. *Arthritis and Rheumatism.* 1997; **40**: 446–52.
31. Lapossy E, Maleitzke R, Hrycaj P *et al.* The frequency of transition of chronic low back pain to fibromyalgia. *Scandinavian Journal of Rheumatology.* 1995; **24**: 29–33.
32. Lindman R, Hagberg M, Bengtsson A *et al.* Capillary structure and mitochondrial volume density in the trapezius muscle of chronic trapezius myalgia, fibromyalgia and healthy subjects. *Journal of Musculoskeletal Pain.* 1995; **3**: 5–22.
33. Sandberg M, Larsson B, Lindberg L-G, Gerdle B. Different patterns of blood flow response in the trapezius muscle following needle stimulation (acupuncture) between healthy subjects and patients with fibromyalgia and work-related trapezius myalgia. *European Journal of Pain.* 2005; **9**: 497–510.
34. Buskila D, Neumann L, Hazanov I, Carmi R. Familial aggregation in the fibromyalgia syndrome. *Seminars in Arthritis and Rheumatism.* 1996; **26**: 605–11.
* 35. Arnold LM, Hudson JI, Hess EV *et al.* Family study of fibromyalgia. *Arthritis and Rheumatism.* 2004; **50**: 944–52.
36. Kato K, Sullivan PF, Evengard B, Pedersen NL. Importance of genetic influences on chronic widespread pain. *Arthritis and Rheumatism.* 2006; **54**: 1682–6.
37. Buskila D, Neumann L. Fibromyalgia syndrome (FM) and nonarticular tenderness in relatives of patients with FM. *Journal of Rheumatology.* 1997; **24**: 941–4.
38. Gursoy S, Erdal E, Herken H *et al.* Significance of catechol-O-methyltransferase gene polymorphism in fibromyalgia syndrome. *Rheumatology International.* 2003; **23**: 104–7.
39. Bondy B, Spaeth M, Offenbaecher M *et al.* The T102C polymorphism of the 5-HT2A-receptor gene in fibromyalgia. *Neurobiology of Disease.* 1999; **6**: 433–9.
40. Offenbaecher M, Bondy B, De Jonge S *et al.* Possible association of fibromyalgia with a polymorphism in the serotonin transporter gene regulatory region. *Arthritis and Rheumatism.* 1999; **42**: 2482–8.
41. Maes M, Lin A, Bonaccorso S *et al.* Increased 24-hour urinary cortisol excretion in patients with post-traumatic stress disorder and patients with major depression, but not in patients with fibromyalgia. *Acta Psychiatrica Scandinavica.* 1998; **98**: 328–35.
42. Crofford LJ. The hypothalamic pituitary adrenal stress axis in fibromyalgia and chronic fatigue syndrome. *Zeitschrift fur Rheumatologie.* 1998; **57**: 67–71.
* 43. Adler GK, Kinsley BT, Hurwitz S *et al.* Reduced hypothalamic-pituitary and sympathoadrenal responses to hypoglycaemia in women with fibromyalgia syndrome. *American Journal of Medicine.* 1999; **106**: 534–43.
* 44. Mease P. Fibromyalgia syndrome: review of clinical presentation, pathogenesis, outcome measures, and treatment. *Journal of Rheumatology.* 2005; **75**: 6–21.
45. Bennett RM. Disordered growth hormone secretion in fibromyalgia: a review of recent findings and a hypothesized etiology. *Zeitschrift fur Rheumatologie.* 1998; **57**: 72–6.
46. Moldofsky H, Scarisbrick P, England R, Smythe H. Musculoskeletal symptoms and non-REM sleep disturbance in patients with "fibrositis syndrome" and healthy subjects. *Psychosomatic Medicine.* 1975; **37**: 341–51.
47. Kelley KW, Bluthe R-M, Dantzer R *et al.* Cytokine-induced sickness behavior. *Brain, Behavior, and Immunity.* 2003; **17**: S112–8.

48. Ueceyler N, Valenza R, Stock M *et al.* Reduced levels of antiinflammatory cytokines in patients with chronic widespread pain. *Arthritis and Rheumatism.* 2006; **54**: 2656–64.
* 49. Desmeules JA, Cedraschi C, Rapiti E *et al.* Neurophysiologic evidence for a central sensitization in patients with fibromyalgia. *Arthritis and Rheumatism.* 2003; **48**: 1420–9.
50. Staud R, Vierck CJ, Cannon RL *et al.* Abnormal sensitization and temporal summation of second pain (wind-up) in patients with fibromyalgia syndrome. *Pain.* 2001; **91**: 165–75.
* 51. Gracely RH, Petzke F, Wolf JM, Clauw DJ. Functional magnetic resonance imaging evidence of augmented pain processing in fibromyalgia. *Arthritis and Rheumatism.* 2002; **46**: 1333–43.
52. Gracely RH, Geisser ME, Giesecke T *et al.* Pain catastrophizing and neural responses to pain among persons with fibromyalgia. *Brain.* 2004; **127**: 835–43.
53. Giesecke T, Gracely RH, Williams DA *et al.* The relationship between depression, clinical pain, and experimental pain in a chronic pain cohort. *Arthritis and Rheumatism.* 2005; **52**: 1577–84.
54. Sorensen J, Graven-Nielsen T, Henriksson KG *et al.* Hyperexcitability in fibromyalgia. *Journal of Rheumatology.* 1998; **25**: 152–5.
55. Banic B, Petersen-Felix S, Andersen OK *et al.* Evidence for spinal cord hypersensitivity in chronic pain after whiplash injury and in fibromyalgia. *Pain.* 2004; **107**: 7–15.
56. Bengtsson M, Bengtsson A, Jorfeldt L. Diagnostic epidural opioid blockade in primary fibromyalgia at rest and during exercise. *Pain.* 1989; **39**: 171–80.
57. Geisser ME, Casey KL, Brucksch CB *et al.* Perception of noxious and innocuous heat stimulation among healthy women and women with fibromyalgia: Association with mood, somatic focus, and catastrophizing. *Pain.* 2003; **102**: 243–50.
58. Vaeroy H, Sakurada T, Forre O *et al.* Modulation of pain in fibromyalgia (fibrositis syndrome): cerebrospinal fluid (CSF) investigation of pain related neuropeptides with special reference to calcitonin gene related peptide (CGRP). *Journal of Rheumatology – Supplement.* 1989; **19**: 94–7.
59. Russell IJ, Orr MD, Littman B *et al.* Elevated cerebrospinal fluid levels of substance P in patients with the fibromyalgia syndrome. *Arthritis and Rheumatism.* 1994; **37**: 1593–601.
60. Julien N, Goffaux P, Arsenault P, Marchand S. Widespread pain in fibromyalgia is related to a deficit of endogenous pain inhibition. *Pain.* 2005; **114**: 295–302.
61. Mense S. Pathophysiologic basis of muscle pain syndromes. *Physical Medicine Rehabilitation Clinics of North America.* 1997; **8**: 179–96.
62. Simons DG, Hong CZ, Simons LS. Endplate potentials are common to midfiber myofascial trigger points. *American Journal of Physical Medicine and Rehabilitation.* 2002; **81**: 212–22.
63. Turk DC, Okifuji A, Sinclair JD, Starz TW. Differential responses by psychosocial subgroups of fibromyalgia syndrome patients to an interdisciplinary treatment. *Arthritis Care and Research.* 1998; **11**: 397–404.
64. Carville SF, Arendt-Nielsen S, Bliddal H *et al.* EULAR evidence based recommendations for the management of fibromyalgia syndrome. *Annals of the Rheumatic Diseases.* 2008; **67**: 536–41.
65. Valim V, Oliveria L, Suda A *et al.* Aerobic fitness effects in fibromyalgia. *Journal of Rheumatology.* 2003; **30**: 1060–9.
66. Richards SC, Scott DL. Prescribed exercise in people with fibromyalgia: parallel group randomised controlled trial. *British Medical Journal.* 2002; **325**: 185.
67. Jones KD, Burckhardt CS, Clark SR *et al.* A randomized controlled trial of muscle strengthening versus flexibility training in fibromyalgia. *Journal of Rheumatology.* 2002; **29**: 1041–8.
68. Busch A, Schachter CL, Peloso PM, Bombardier C. Exercise for treating fibromyalgia syndrome. *Cochrane Database of Systematic Reviews.* 2002; **CD003786**.
69. Crofford LJ, Appleton BE. The treatment of fibromyalgia: a review of clinical trials. *Current Rheumatology Reports.* 2000; **2**: 101–3.
70. Sim J, Adams N. Systematic review of randomized controlled trials of nonpharmacological interventions for fibromyalgia. *Clinical Journal of Pain.* 2002; **18**: 324–36.
* 71. Goldenberg DL, Burckhardt C, Crofford L. Management of fibromyalgia syndrome. *Journal of the American Medical Association.* 2004; **292**: 2388–95.
* 72. Adams N, Sim J. Rehabilitation approaches in fibromyalgia. *Disability and Rehabilitation.* 2005; **27**: 711–23.
73. Hakkinen A, Hakkinen K, Hannonen P, Alen M. Strength training induced adaptations in neuromuscular function of premenopausal women with fibromyalgia: Comparison with healthy women. *Annals of the Rheumatic Diseases.* 2001; **60**: 21–6.
74. Altan L, Bingol U, Aykac M *et al.* Investigation of the effects of pool-based exercise on fibromyalgia syndrome. *Rheumatology International.* 2004; **24**: 272–7.
75. Jentoft ES, Kvalvik AG, Mengshoel M. Effects of pool-based and land-based aerobic exercise on women with fibromyalgia/chronic widespread muscle pain. *Arthritis and Rheumatism-Arthritis Care and Research.* 2001; **45**: 42–7.
76. Evcik D, Kizilay B, Gokcen E. The effects of balneotherapy on fibromyalgia patients. *Rheumatology International.* 2002; **22**: 56–9.
77. Yurkuran M, Celiktas M. A randomized, controlled trial of balneotherapy in the treatment of patients with primary fibromyalgia syndrome. *Physikalische Medizin Rehabilitationsmedizin Kurortmedizin.* 1996; **6**: 109–12.
78. Rivera RJ, Moratalla JC, as MF *et al.* Long-term efficacy of therapy in patients with fibromyalgia: a physical exercise-based program and a cognitive-behavioral approach. *Arthritis Care and Research.* 2004; **51**: 184–92.

79. Singh BB, Berman BM, Hadhazy VA, Creamer P. A pilot study of cognitive behavioral therapy in fibromyalgia. *Alternative Therapies in Health and Medicine*. 1998; **4**: 67–70.
80. Nielson RW, Walker C, McCain GA. Cognitive behavioral treatment of fibromyalgia syndrome: Preliminary findings. *Journal of Rheumatology*. 1992; **19**: 98–103.
81. Fors EA, Gotestam KG. Patient education, guided imagery and pain related talk in fibromyalgia coping. *European Journal of Psychiatry*. 2000; **14**: 233–40.
82. Rossy LA, Buckelew SP, Dorr N *et al.* A meta-analysis of fibromyalgia treatment interventions. *Annals of Behavioral Medicine*. 1999; **21**: 180–91.
83. Merchant RE, Andre CA, Wise CM. Nutritional supplementation with Chlorella pyrenoidosa for fibromyalgia syndrome: A double-blind, placebo-controlled, crossover study. *Journal of Musculoskeletal Pain*. 2001; **9**: 37–54.
84. Azad KA, Alam MN, Haq SA *et al.* Vegetarian diet in the treatment of fibromyalgia. *Bangladesh Medical Research Council Bulletin*. 2000; **26**: 41–7.
85. Bramwell B, Ferguson S, Scarlett N, Macintosh A. The use of ascorbigen in the treatment of fibromyalgia patients: a preliminary trial. *Alternative Medicine Reviews*. 2000; **5**: 455–62.
86. Kaartinen K, Lammi K, Hypen M *et al.* Vegan diet alleviates fibromyalgia symptoms. *Scandinavian Journal of Rheumatology*. 2000; **29**: 308–13.
87. Bell IR, Lewis DA, Lewis SE *et al.* EEG alpha sensitization in individualized homeopathic treatment of fibromyalgia. *International Journal of Neuroscience*. 2004; **114**: 1195–220.
88. Bell IR, Lewis DA, Brooks AJ *et al.* Individual differences in response to randomly assigned active individualized homeopathic and placebo treatment in fibromyalgia: implications of a double-blinded optional crossover design. *Journal of Alternative and Complementary Medicine*. 2004; **10**: 269–83.
89. Bell IR, Lewis DA, Brooks AJ *et al.* Improved clinical status in fibromyalgia patients treated with individualized homeopathic remedies versus placebo. *Rheumatology (Oxford)*. 2004; **43**: 577–82.
90. Deluze C, Bosia L, Zirbs A *et al.* Electroacupuncture in fibromyalgia: results of a controlled trial. *British Medical Journal*. 1992; **305**: 1249–52.
91. Sprott H. Efficiency of acupuncture in patients with fibromyalgia. *Clinical Bulletin of Myofascial Therapy*. 1998; **3**: 37–43.
92. Bennett RM, Kamin M, Karim R, Rosenthal N. Tramadol and acetaminophen combination tablets in the treatment of fibromyalgia pain: a double-blind, randomized, placebo-controlled study. *American Journal of Medicine*. 2003; **114**: 537–45.
93. Russell J, Kamin M, Bennett RM *et al.* Efficacy of tramadol in treatment of pain in fibromyalgia. *JCR: Journal of Clinical Rheumatology*. 2000; **6**: 250–7.
94. Senay EC, Adams EH, Geller A *et al.* Physical dependence of Ultram (tramadol hydrochloride): Both opioid-like and atypical withdrawal symptoms occurr. *Drug and Alcohol Dependence*. 2003; **69**: 233–41.
95. Graven-Nielsen T, Aspegren KS, Henriksson KG *et al.* Ketamine reduces muscle pain, temporal summation, and referred pain in fibromyalgia patients. *Pain*. 2000; **85**: 483–91.
96. McCleane G. Does intravenous lidocaine reduce fibromyalgia pain?: A randomized, double-blind, placebo controlled cross-over study. *Pain Clinic*. 2000; **12**: 181–5.
* 97. Arnold LM, Keck Jr PE, Welge JA. Antidepressant treatment of fibromyalgia. A meta-analysis and review. *Psychosomatics*. 2000; **4**: 104–13.
98. Carette S, Oakson G, Guimont C, Steriade M. Sleep electroencephalography and the clinical response to amitriptyline in patients with fibromyalgia. *Arthritis and Rheumatism*. 1995; **38**: 1211–7.
99. Ginsberg F, Mancaux A, Joos E *et al.* A randomized placebo-controlled trial of sustained-release amitriptyline in primary fibromyalgia. *Journal of Musculoskeletal Pain*. 1996; **4**: 37–47.
100. Goldenberg D, Mayskiy M, Mossey C *et al.* A randomized, double-blind crossover trial of fluoxetine and amitriptyline in the treatment of fibromyalgia. *Arthritis and Rheumatism*. 1996; **39**: 1852–9.
101. Arnold LM, Hess EV, Hudson JI *et al.* A randomized, placebo-controlled, double-blind, flexible-dose study of fluoxetine in the treatment of women with fibromyalgia. *American Journal of Medicine*. 2002; **112**: 191–7.
102. Gendreau RM, Thorn MD, Gendreau JF *et al.* Efficacy of milnacipran in patients with fibromyalgia. *Journal of Rheumatology*. 2005; **32**: 1975–85.
103. Arnold LM, Lu Y, Crofford LJ *et al.* A double-blind, multicenter trial comparing duloxetine with placebo in the treatment of fibromyalgia patients with or without major depressive disorder. *Arthritis and Rheumatism*. 2004; **50**: 2974–84.
104. Sayar K, Aksu G, Ak I, Tosun M. Venlafaxine treatment of fibromyalgia. *Annals of Pharmacotherapy*. 2003; **37**: 1561–5.
105. Farber L, Stratz T, Bruckle W *et al.* Efficacy and tolerability of tropisetron in primary fibromyalgia – A highly selective and competitive 5-HT3 receptor antagonist. *Scandinavian Journal of Rheumatology – Supplement*. 2000; **29**: 49–54.
106. Hrycaj P, Stratz T, Mennet P, Muller W. Pathogenetic aspects of responsiveness to ondansetron (5-hydroxytryptamine type 3 receptor antagonist) in patients with primary fibromyalgia syndrome – A preliminary study. *Journal of Rheumatology*. 1996; **23**: 1418–23.
107. Spath M, Stratz T, Neeck G *et al.* Efficacy and tolerability of intravenous tropisetron in the treatment of fibromyalgia. *Scandinavian Journal of Rheumatology*. 2004; **33**: 267–70.
108. Crofford LJ, Rowbotham MC, Mease PJ *et al.* Pregabalin for the treatment of fibromyalgia syndrome: Results of a

randomized, double-blind, placebo-controlled trial. *Arthritis and Rheumatism*. 2005; **52**: 1264–73.

109. Holman AJ, Myers RR. A randomized, double-blind, placebo-controlled trial of pramipexole, a dopamine agonist, in patients with fibromyalgia receiving concomitant medications. *Arthritis and Rheumatism*. 2005; **52**: 2495–505.
110. Scharf MB, Baumann M, Berkowitz DV. The effects of sodium oxybate on clinical symptoms and sleep patterns in patients with fibromyalgia. *Journal of Rheumatology*. 2003; **30**: 1070–4.
111. McLain D. An open label dose finding trial of tizanidine [Zanaflex] for treatment of fibromyalgia. *Journal of Musculoskeletal Pain*. 2002; **10**: 7–18.
112. Bennett RM, Clark SC, Walczyk J. A randomized, double-blind, placebo-controlled study of growth hormone in the treatment of fibromyalgia. *American Journal of Medicine*. 1998; **104**: 227–31.
113. Lowe JC, Garrison RL, Reichman AJ *et al*. Effectiveness and safety of T3 (Triiodothyronine) therapy for euthyroid fibromyalgia: A double-blind placebo-controlled response-driven crossover study. *Clinical Bulletin of Myofascial Therapy*. 1997; **2**: 31–57.
114. Lowe JC, Reichman AJ, Yellin J. The process of change during T3 treatment for euthyroid fibromyalgia: A double-blind placebo-controlled crossover study. *Clinical Bulletin of Myofascial Therapy*. 1997; **2**: 91–124.
115. Lowe JC, Garrison RL, Reichman AJ, Yellin J. Triiodothyronine (T3) treatment of euthyroid fibromyalgia: A small-N replication of a double-blind placebo-controlled crossover study. *Clinical Bulletin of Myofascial Therapy*. 1997; **2**: 71–88.

*116. Simons DG. Myofascial pain syndrome due to trigger points. In: Goodgold J (ed.). *Rehabilitation medicine*. St Louis: C.V. Mosby, 1988: 686–723.

117. Rosen NB. Physical medicine and rehabilitation approaches to the management of myofascial pain and fibromyalgia syndromes. *Baillières Clinical Rheumatology*. 1994; **8**: 881–916.
118. Wright EF, Domenech MA, Fischer Jr JR. Usefulness of posture training for patients with temporomandibular disorders. *Journal of the American Dental Association*. 2000; **131**: 202–10.
119. Myers CD, White BA, Heft MW. A review of complementary and alternative medicine use for treating chronic facial pain. *Journal of the American Dental Association*. 2002; **133**: 1189–96.
120. Hong C-Z. Lidocaine injection versus dry needling to myofascial trigger point: The importance of the local twitch response. *American Journal of Physical Medicine and Rehabilitation*. 1994; **73**: 256–63.

*121. Simons DG, Travell JG, Simons PT. *Travell and Simons' myofascial pain and dysfunction: the trigger point manual*. Vol. 1. Baltimore: Williams & Wilkins, 1999.

122. Frost FA, Toft B, Aaboe T. Isotonic saline and methyl prednisolone acetate in blockade treatment of myofascial pain. [Danish]. *Ugeskrift for Laeger*. 1984; **149**: 652–4.
123. Pereda CA, Uson JJ, Carmona L. Systematic review: Can botulinum toxin be recommended as treatment for pain in myofascial syndrome? [Spanish]. *Reumatologia Clinica*. 2006; **2**: 173–82.
124. Singer E, Dionne R. A controlled evaluation of ibuprofen and diazepam for chronic orofacial muscle pain. *Journal of Orofacial Pain*. 1997; **11**: 139–46.
125. Baumgartner E, Finckh A, Cedraschi C, Vischer TL. A six year prospective study of a cohort of patients with fibromyalgia. *Annals of the Rheumatic Diseases*. 2002; **61**: 644–5.

43

Psychiatric diagnosis and chronic pain

STEPHEN P TYRER

KEY LEARNING POINTS

- Most patients with a psychiatric disorder seen in a pain clinic will have had a preexisting psychiatric illness or will have developed mental illness because of their chronic painful illness.
- Depression and anxiety are the most common psychiatric illnesses affecting people with chronic pain.
- In many cases, it is appropriate to treat depression with antidepressant drugs, particularly if there is pervasive loss of pleasure. The selective serotonin reuptake inhibitor (SSRI) drugs are usually employed first, but tricyclic antidepressants and serotonin-norepinephrine reuptake inhibitors (SNRI) drugs are more appropriate if there is evidence of a neuropathic pain state.
- Posttraumatic stress disorder is a poor prognostic sign in people with chronic pain who have developed pain following an injury.
- People with borderline or dependent personality disorders require specialized attention in a pain clinic service. In these individuals, a contract needs to be established early in therapy, applying particular care to the administration of drugs. Psychodynamic treatment has been shown to be of assistance in selected patients with borderline states.
- Both cognitive behavior therapy (CBT) and tricyclic antidepressants have been shown to be effective in the treatment of persistent somatoform pain disorder.
- Substance misuse, which includes both alcohol and drugs, occurs in between one in eight and one in four people attending pain clinics, respectively. Those with a history of previous misuse or likelihood of misuse should have their drugs monitored closely.

INTRODUCTION

Although not usually considered by the uninitiated, it is now accepted clearly that psychological and psychiatric factors are of prime importance in the evaluation of pain. Thirty years ago, the International Association for the Study of Pain (IASP) stated categorically that "activity induced in the nociceptor and nociceptive pathways by a noxious stimulus is not pain, which is always a psychological state ..."[1] Psychological issues are discussed in Chapter 10, The psychological assessment of pain in patients with chronic pain and Chapter 13, Psychological effects of chronic pain: an overview and this chapter will be primarily concerned with psychiatric issues in chronic pain.

Psychiatric disorders are frequently manifest in patients suffering from chronic pain. This is the situation in patients attending general medical clinics, family practices, and pain clinics.[2] In some cases, psychiatric disorders may present with pain as the prime symptom.

This is certainly known for chest pain in adolescents,[3] abdominal pain in childhood,[4] panic disorder,[5] post-traumatic stress disorder,[6] and the rare presentation of psychotic disorders with delusional pain.[7] However, it is unlikely that most physicians involved with patients with chronic pain will be presented with such patients at the time that they see the patient concerned. It is much more common for patients with chronic pain to develop psychiatric disorders and increased functional impairment because of their widespread pain.[8] Pain affects enjoyment, reduces the opportunity to take part in pleasurable activities, and fundamentally changes the whole direction of a person's life. Furthermore, if patients believe that there is no cure for this symptom, they are understandably downcast and affected adversely in their emotional state. The chronic pain physician needs to know which psychiatric diagnoses are likely to be found in patients with chronic pain, how these may be identified, and what actions should be taken when these are encountered.

SCHEDULES FOR CLASSIFYING PSYCHIATRIC DISORDERS IN PAIN

There are two widely used schedules for the classification of psychiatric disorders:

1. the International Classification of Diseases, 10th edition (ICD-10);[9]
2. the Diagnostic and Statistical Manual for Mental Disorder, 4th edition (DSM-IV).[10]

In addition, the IASP has developed its own classification for painful conditions.[11] A comparison of the diagnoses used in all three systems is shown in **Table 43.1**.

PSYCHIATRIC DIAGNOSES

Depression

Depressive illness is the most common associated psychiatric disorder that is found in patients with chronic pain. Between 20 and 50 percent of patients attending chronic pain clinics fulfil the criteria for this diagnosis.[2, 12, 13] The three most typical symptoms of a depressive illness are:

1. depressed mood;
2. loss of interest and pleasure;
3. loss of energy and increased fatigue.[9]

Loss of appetite and/or weight, change in sleep pattern, and poor concentration are also usually present. These latter symptoms are commonly found in patients with chronic pain who are not necessarily depressed. It has therefore been recommended in physically unwell patients that these somatic symptoms be replaced with nonsomatic alternatives.[14] If changes in appetite or weight are replaced by a depressed appearance, sleep disturbances by social withdrawal, fatigue by brooding, and diminished concentration by a lack of reactivity to pleasant events, the diagnostic confidence of depression in patients with chronic pain is increased.[15]

Table 43.1 Comparison of three schedules used in diagnosing emotional aspects of pain.

Symptoms and signs	ICD-10	DSM-IV	IASP
Emotional conflict or psychosocial problems associated with pain disorder	Persistent somatoform pain disorder	Pain disorder associated with psychological factors	Monosymptomatic (if pain in single site)
Belief of disease. Unable to accept medical reassurance	Hypochondriacal disorder	Hypochondriasis	Hypochondriacal subtype
Multiple and variable symptoms for at least two years	Somatization disorder	Somatization disorder	Multiple complaints, usually from at least five systems of the body
Symptoms of depression	Depressive episode	Major depressive episode or dysthymia	Pain associated with depression
Severe depression with delusions of disease, torture, or deserved punishment	Severe depressive episode with psychotic symptoms	Major depressive episode with psychotic features	Pain associated with depression
Delusions of physical defect, disorder, or disease	Delusional disorder	Delusional disorder (somatic type)	Delusional or hallucinatory pain
Pain due to persistent muscle contraction	Psychological factors associated with diseases	Psychological factors affecting medical condition	Muscle tension pain

DSM-IV, Diagnostic and Statistical Manual for Mental Disorder, 4th edition; IASP, International Association for the Study of Pain; ICD-10, International Classification of Diseases, 10th edition.

It is rare for pain (except for headaches and facial pain) to be a presenting symptom of a patient with depressive illness in the absence of any existing or past organic findings. If such a symptom is found in association with any suggestion of psychotic ideation, enquiry should be made of possible delusional beliefs.[7]

The risk of death by suicide is increased in patients with chronic pain. In a recent systematic review, it was found that relative to controls, risk of death by suicide was doubled in chronic pain patients.[16] A number of risk factors for suicidal intent in chronic pain were identified in this review, including:

- the type, intensity, and duration of pain;
- sleep-onset insomnia co-occurring with pain;
- hopelessness about pain;
- the desire for escape from pain; and
- specifically, pain catastrophizing (negative thoughts in which pain is seen in terms of extremes, e.g. "I worry it will never end"), which is highly related to hopelessness about pain.

In patients with these symptoms, who have not responded well to treatment and who are depressed, it is appropriate to ask about suicidal intent. Positive responses to questions such as "Do you wish you would not wake up in the morning?" should be followed by "Have you had thoughts of suicide?" and "Have you planned how you would do this?" If the patient replies yes to this last question and other risk factors are present, active suicidal risk is a definite possibility. In such cases, and if there is any doubt, it is vital to contact the local mental health team, which may include an assertive outreach team or the local psychiatric clinic, to discuss the person concerned as soon as possible. It may be appropriate and advisable in rare instances to do this without informing the patient if there is concern about the safety of the patient and the individual's ability or motivation to follow through on the recommended plan of treatment. In cases where safety cannot be established, it may be necessary to arrange supervised transportation to a psychiatric treatment facility or emergency service.

There is debate about how far to treat depression in people with chronic pain. Cognitive behavior therapy (CBT) is sometimes utilized, but usually in the context of treatment aimed at altering attributions arising from the chronic painful state. Although there is a belief by some that standard antidepressant drugs are not effective in such patients,[17] based in part on limited evidence that these agents are no more effective in depressed compared to nondepressed patients,[18] studies have shown that depression is ameliorated in such patients[19][I] and the effects of these drugs on the degree of pain is clearly evident.[20, 21, 22][I] One reason for the belief of poor efficacy of antidepressants is because the standard drugs of this type used in psychiatric practice, the selective serotonin reuptake inhibitor (SSRI) group of drugs have virtually no analgesic effect *per se*,[22][I] whereas the older tricyclic drugs have been shown to be effective in neuropathic pain,[21, 22][I] despite the fact that their value in nociceptive pain states is not so firmly based.[20][II] The newer monamine inhibitors that inhibit the reuptake of both serotonin and norepinephrine, the serotonin-norepinephrine reuptake inhibitors (SNRIs), are more effective than the SSRIs in reducing neuropathic pain[23] [II], [24] and there is evidence that these drugs are more effective in treating depressive symptoms in severe depressive disorders.[25]

ANXIETY AND STRESS-RELATED DISORDERS

Anxiety disorders have recently been found to be correlated more closely than depression with chronic painful conditions in a large US sample of chronic pain patients.[26] In particular, people who are fearful of anxiety-related sensations, who interpret somatic symptoms as harmful and who avoid situations where these feelings are likely to arise, have greater disability.[27] The term "anxiety sensitivity" has been used to describe this condition in these individuals.[28]

The diagnoses included under this rubric comprise generalized anxiety disorder (GAD), panic disorder, phobias, posttraumatic stress disorder, adjustment disorders, and obsessive compulsive disorder.

Generalized anxiety disorder

The symptoms of this disorder include excessive anxiety and worry, occurring frequently for a period of at least six months with difficulty in controlling this. Additionally, the person concerned has at least three additional symptoms including restlessness, becoming tired easily, difficulty in concentrating, irritability, muscle tension, or disturbed sleep.[29] Early work suggested that female patients with chronic pain and who were not seeking compensation had a higher frequency of GAD than expected,[30] although women with anxiety were not found to have a poorer prognosis compared with men in a recent investigation.[31] Higher degrees of anxiety were related to greater intensity of pain in this study.[31] This same study showed that patients with this symptom have a poorer prognosis and this has been shown by others.[32] It has been suggested that patients with chronic pain may use worry to reduce the physical sensations associated with pain, and thus fulfil the diagnostic criteria for GAD.[33] This hypothesis does not have experimental proof.

CBT has been shown to be effective in chronic painful conditions.[34][I] This treatment is also used in GAD associated with pain.[35] It has been shown that in patients with low back pain who have pain-related anxiety receiving CBT combined with physical therapy, that improvement in anxiety was more important than changes in physical capacity in predicting outcome.[36] Similar benefits when reducing anxiety in patients with back pain were shown in a Finnish study.[37] In a recent World Health Organization (WHO) survey, people with back and neck pain were over 2.5 times more likely to have GAD than controls without this condition.[38] This survey was not able to show the temporal relationship between pain and anxiety, but other studies have strongly suggested that anxiety sensitivity is a feature in this population.[27, 36]

Panic disorder

Panic disorder comprises severe unpredictable anxiety episodes that can occur "out of the blue," although they are usually more common in one situation than another. The symptoms include intense fear and apprehension, often with a fear of dying. There is usually a desire to escape to an alternative place where the person believes the symptom will be less intense. Patients with panic disorder always have intense somatic symptoms of anxiety. If these symptoms are associated with a very frightening experience, the condition should be classified separately as a stress disorder.

Although the pain sensitivity of patients with panic disorder has been reported to be no different from that of controls,[39] patients with chronic painful conditions are more likely to have panic than average.[26] People with migraine attacks may be particularly prone.[40] These findings suggest that panic and migraine may be directly related through a single mechanism.

Treatment of panic disorder is best achieved with either CBT or with medication. In normal practice, the SSRI group of antidepressants should be the first line of pharmacological treatment for patients with panic disorder.[41][I]

Phobias

When anxiety symptoms occur in response to a specific environmental situation, the term "phobia" is used. Most people encountered in a pain clinic who have phobic disorders will have had such disorders beforehand. However, a phobia may develop because of the experience of the event leading to the pain, e.g. travel phobia following a road traffic accident.[42] The condition known as "social phobia," in which sufferers feel anxious in social situations and avoid such engagements, has been found to be over-represented in disabled workers with chronic musculoskeletal pain.[43]

Stress disorders

The psychiatric disorders classified in ICD-10 and DSM-IV as resulting from stress include acute stress reactions, posttraumatic stress disorder (PTSD), and adjustment disorder. Acute stress reactions and PTSD develop in response to exceptionally threatening experiences, but acute stress subsides within days (and is not considered further), whereas PTSD is more prolonged. This disorder consists of persistent, intrusive recall or reenactment of the traumatic event in memories, dreams, and flashbacks. Restriction of the emotions, avoidance of situations that might provoke memories of the trauma, and increased arousal to particular perceptual stimuli, e.g. sudden loud sounds, are associated symptoms.

There is clear evidence that the experience and management of pain can be aggravated by PTSD. One of the main reasons for this is because PTSD is associated with high anxiety and we have seen that anxiety is associated comorbidly with chronic pain.[26] Furthermore, the presence of PTSD is a poor prognostic sign.[44, 45] Hyperarousal, excessive attention to changes in the environment, and an inclination to focus on bodily symptoms are frequent accompaniments of both PTSD and chronic pain, which may explain these findings.[46]

If PTSD is identified, treatment should be carried out by a specialized team who are familiar with treatment procedures in this condition. Debriefing and superficial treatments of this type are not valuable and have been found to worsen the prognosis in those who have more intense symptoms.[47][II] Trauma-focused CBT and eye movement desensitization and reprocessing (EMDR), a technique that involves movement of the patient's eyes in a systematic way whilst recalling disturbing memories, have been found to be effective in treating PTSD in a recent meta-analysis.[48] Either of these treatments is recommended as first-line in the treatment of PTSD according to a recent national guideline.[49] If facilities for such treatment are not available or if these therapies are not successful, treatment with the antidepressant drugs, amitriptyline, mirtazapine, or phenelzine has been shown to be effective.[49]

Adjustment disorders consist of states of emotional distress that arise following a major life change or stressful life event. The symptoms accompanying this disorder include excessive worrying, mild depressed mood, poor sleep, inability to cope, and some difficulties in carrying out daily routines. However, the symptoms are not usually persistent and do not reach the threshold to enable an alternative psychiatric illness to be diagnosed. These disorders are considered to develop in response to a variety of stressful events, the symptoms representing an adaptation to these stressors or to their continuing effects. The difficulty is in deciding what is abnormal or delayed adaptation. By definition, these disorders would not have developed but for the stressful event. Symptoms last for less than six months, except in the case of prolonged depressive reaction, otherwise an alternative diagnosis should be sought. In an early study of patients with chronic pain, male patients had adjustment disorder significantly more frequently than females, but this may have been more related to change in work status.[50] In most cases, it is not thought that specific intervention is necessary.

Personality disorders

Personality disorders refer to a long-standing manner of handling life circumstances that adversely affects the person's social, occupational, or domestic life. Although it has been said that personality disorders are more common in chronic pain patients,[51] there has been a dearth of good research in this area. People without any previous history of personality disorders may appear to suffer from such a condition because of the exacerbation of premorbid personality characteristics resulting from pain and subsequent stresses.[52] Originally, it was thought that some patients who developed chronic pain had a "pain-prone personality," but there is very little evidence for such a label.[53]

Table 43.2 illustrates the main types of personality disorders described together with associated behaviors. An early study suggested patients with chronic pain had compulsive personality features.[54] More recently, a study of outpatients attending a chronic pain clinic in Germany showed that more than one in ten subjects had a paranoid or a borderline personality disorder, with passive-aggressive, avoidant, and obsessive-compulsive personality disorders being significantly over-represented compared to a control group.[55]

Individuals with borderline personality disorder and other cluster B personality disorders (see **Table 43.2**) are at greater risk of misusing medication, and benzodiazepines and opioid drugs should be prescribed very carefully in this group. In these patients it is essential to explain clearly the aims and likely outcomes of treatment strategies proposed, concentrating on one treatment intervention at a time. A big problem is treatment compliance and consistent clinic attendance and a contract should be established at the start. There have been recent trials that show benefit of psychotherapeutic interventions in the treatment of personality disorder.[56] However, there is inadequate evidence to confidently recommend any particular therapy. There is limited evidence that antidepressants, particularly the selective serotonin reuptake inhibitors and the monoamine oxidase inhibitors, have some benefits in the management of this condition, and lesser evidence for the advantages of antipsychotic drugs and mood stabilizers.[57] There is no basis to recommend different treatments for the different personality disorders. All these treatments should be carried out by psychiatrists and it may be necessary to refer these patients to a specialized psychiatric unit.

A recent structured evidence-based review warns all pain clinicians to be skeptical about the assessment of personality in patients who are in pain.[58] Personality profiles of patients who have chronic pain usually alter considerably if pain is reduced. This was shown more than 30 years ago, but is not generally realized.[59] This change has been shown convincingly for the widely quoted Minnesota Multiphasic Personality Inventory (MMPI) schedule.[60] These findings illustrate that many personality questionnaires are influenced by the current state of the individual, including physical and mental health.

Table 43.2 Personality types, associated symptoms and behaviors.

Personality cluster	Personality disorders included in the cluster	Symptoms and behaviors
Cluster A	Paranoid	Long-standing mistrust and suspiciousness
	Schizoid	No desire for social relationships
	Schizotypal	Discomfort in social contact together with perceptual distortions
Cluster B	Antisocial	Irresponsible behavior. Lack of regard for others
	Borderline	Unstable interpersonal relationships; impulsive
	Histrionic	Attention-seeking, shallow emotions
	Narcissistic	Grandiose ideation, needs admiration; lacks empathy
Cluster C	Avoidant	Avoids social contact; inhibited; feelings of inadequacy
	Dependent	Submissive behavior, fearful of separation
	Obsessive-compulsive	Preoccupation with orderliness and control

Somatoform disorders

For a diagnosis of a somatoform disorder to be made, there should be continued presentation of physical symptoms together with persistent requests for medical investigations, despite negative findings of organic illness and reassurance by doctors that the symptoms have no physical basis. In some patients, physical disorders may have been present, but these do not explain the nature and extent of the present symptoms, or the distress and preoccupation of the patient.

Guidelines have been published on the management of patients with somatoform disorders who present in general hospitals,[61, 62] which include addressing psychological and psychiatric issues.

These disorders are frequent. In a recent survey of patients attending a general practice clinic in Holland, the prevalence of somatoform disorders was as high as 21.9 percent.[63] Many of these patients are severely disabled, but it is only the minority that are likely to be assessed by clinical psychologists or psychiatrists, despite a recent recommendation advocating joint working between liaison psychiatrists and pain physicians.[64]

The value of the present classifications of these syndromes has been brought into question because of the imprecise categorization of such disorders and the fact that many patients fall into the category of undifferentiated somatoform disorder, a watered-down version of somatization disorder. Pain is only one of the symptoms that can occur in a somatoform disorder. Other symptoms include palpitations, breathlessness, cough, swallowing air, and frequency of micturition. Those somatoform disorders that are concerned with painful conditions are indicated below, together with their ICD-10 codes.

PERSISTENT SOMATOFORM PAIN DISORDER (F45.4)

The main complaint in this disorder is of persistent, severe, and distressing pain, which cannot be explained fully by any bodily process or physical disorder. Furthermore, this occurs in association with emotional conflict or psychosocial problems that are considered to be the main cause.[9] In a different diagnostic classificatory schedule, DSM-IV,[10] the diagnosis of pain disorder can be made as long as "psychological factors are judged to have an important role in the onset, severity, exacerbation or maintenance of the pain." It can be seen that the threshold for a diagnosis of pain disorder in DSM-IV is lower than in ICD-10.

Particular skills are required to manage these patients. An agenda should be set early on, with a limit on investigations. It is essential to allocate one single treating doctor, who communicates directly with all other therapists and advises on all proposed treatment.

There are two established treatments for this condition, antidepressants and CBT. Antidepressants that inhibit both serotonin and norepinephrine uptake, such as amitriptyline and venlafaxine, are more effective than the SSRI group of antidepressants.[19, 25][II] CBT has been shown to be of definite value in those who have reached the stage to accept that medical or surgical interventions are not indicated.[34][I] The value of biofeedback is yet to be established, despite suggestions that this treatment may be valuable in chronic headache.[65][II]

HYPOCHONDRIACAL DISORDER (F45.2)

In this condition, the patient believes that he or she has a serious or progressive physical disorder that persists despite negative investigations and reassurance. Between 1 and 2 percent of the patients in the general population have been found to have hypochondriacal features and these are more evident in older people.[66] Fear of disease (disease phobia) is associated with anxiety, whereas a false belief of having a disease (disease conviction) is associated more with somatic symptoms. Although this condition may seem to be more frequent in patients with chronic pain, there has been no recent survey of this condition in a pain clinic. It has been found that a hypochondriacal attitude is considered the least desirable quality if one has chronic pain.[67]

SOMATIZATION DISORDER (F45.0)

Somatization disorder, formerly known as Briquet's syndrome, is by far the most crippling somatoform disorder. Its main features are multiple, recurrent, and frequently changing physical symptoms, which have been present for many years. Most patients have a long and complicated history of contact with both primary and specialist medical care services, during which time many negative investigations have been carried out. These patients have major impairment in social or occupational functioning. Personality disorders, particularly of the passive-dependent and histrionic types, are considerably over-represented compared to control subjects with anxiety and depression.[68] The gender ratio of patients with this condition is 5:1, female:male. The prevalence rate has been estimated to be 0.5 percent, but this is probably an underestimate, the true rate is probably higher.[69]

In practice, the diagnosis of undifferentiated somatoform disorder (F45.1), which has a lower criteria for diagnosis, is found to be much the most frequent diagnosis in standard populations.[70, 71] This category comprises a raft of heterogeneous conditions in which physical and psychiatric disorders intermingle.

Psychoactive substance use

There is a higher rate of alcohol and analgesic misuse in patients with chronic pain. Between 12 and 28 percent of patients attending specialized pain clinic facilities reach the criterion for diagnosis under this category.[12] High average alcohol consumption before developing a chronic painful state was found to be a poor prognostic sign in a large follow-up study of patients with lower limb pain.[72]

Despite these findings of an increased prevalence of substance misuse generally, there has been a change in attitude about the use of opioid medication for patients with chronic nonmalignant pain. Although it has been argued that long-term opioid use leads to increased drug dependency and further functional impairment in patients who have disproportionate pain and disability,[73] recent work has not found clear evidence that this is the case. In a large study of patients with chronic pain comparing opioid users with nonusers, there was no increase in illness behavior exhibited by the opioid users after controlling for other variables.[74] Benzodiazepine use, on the other hand, was associated with reduced activity and disability.

It seems that prior alcohol and substance abuse are likely risk factors in leading to what is described as a "downhill spiral" in patients with chronic pain involving escalating doses and abuse of opioid therapy. Notwithstanding this, opioid use is not contraindicated in this population, except for those who have evidence of previous drug dependency or who are found to regularly ask for additional medication ahead of schedule. If there is definite evidence of opioid misuse, it is normally advisable to refer the patient to a specialized substance misuse center. Brief psychosocial interventions and contingency management (which consists of payment of money or tokens to patients if they succeed in reducing opiate use) have been found to improve compliance with therapy.[75] Drug detoxification may be needed before these strategies are employed; the decision rests with the substance misuse team, to whom the patient should be referred if such treatments are being considered.

A specialized tool, the current opioid misuse measure (COMM),[76] has very recently been developed to identify people who are prone to abuse opioids. The use of this instrument needs further assessment in more pain clinic settings.

Factitious disorder

In factitious disorder, patients consciously fabricate symptoms and may even physically injure themselves in order to produce symptoms and signs that are typical of an organic illness. The motivation for exhibiting such symptoms in factitious disorder is to obtain medical care. Abdominal pain, often suspected to be due to renal or biliary colic, is the most frequent presentation of a painful factitious disorder. Most people encountered in clinical practice with this disorder are healthcare professionals with a considerable female preponderance.[77] They are often found to have a number of different diagnoses at different times. Their families are closely involved and are convinced of an organic etiology. Frequent attendance at emergency departments, coupled with negative investigations, raises suspicions that this disorder may be present.

Malingering

In malingering, there is also a conscious wish to fabricate symptoms. However, the reason why malingerers behave in this way is to obtain financial gain or avoid situations for responsibilities that they wish to avoid.

CONCLUSIONS

The difficulty for the nonpsychiatric physician in examining a patient with long-standing pain is in differentiating distress from illness. The majority of patients seen are in understandable emotional discomfort, but most do not have a psychiatric illness that requires alternative treatment other than for the pain itself. Warning symptoms and signs of psychiatric illness include a recent major change in emotional functioning, in particular withdrawal and change in interest, persistent memories of traumatic events, and sudden behavioral changes. It is valuable to have mental health professionals attached to pain clinics so that accurate evaluation can be made of these patients. These individuals also improve the diagnostic confidence of physicians attending such clinics.[78]

REFERENCES

1. Merskey H. Pain terms; a list with definitions and notes on the usage. *Pain.* 1979; **6**: 249–52.
2. Tyrer SP, Capon N, Peterson DN *et al.* The detection of psychiatric illness and psychological handicaps in a British pain clinic population. *Pain.* 1989; **36**: 63–74.
3. Hotopf M, Mayou R, Wadsworth M, Wessely S. Psychosocial and developmental antecedents of chest pain in young adults. *Psychosomatic Medicine.* 1999; **61**: 861–7.
4. Garber J, Zeman J, Walker LS. Recurrent abdominal pain in children: psychiatric diagnoses and parental psychopathology. *Journal of the American Academy of Child and Adolescent Psychiatry.* 1990; **29**: 648–56.
5. Meuret A, White KS, Ritz T *et al.* Panic attack symptom dimensions and their relationship to illness characteristics in panic disorder. *Journal of Psychiatric Research.* 2006; **40**: 520–7.
6. Palyo S, Beck JG. Post-traumatic stress disorder symptoms, pain, and perceived life control: associations with psychosocial and physical functioning. *Pain.* 2005; **117**: 121–7.
7. Fisher C. The reach of neurology. *Archives of Neurology.* 2003; **60**: 173–7.
8. Tyrer S. Psychosomatic pain. *British Journal of Psychiatry.* 2006; **188**: 91–3.
9. WHO. *The ICD-10 classification of mental and behavioural disorders: clinical descriptions and diagnostic guidelines.* Geneva: World Health Organization, 1992.
10. American Psychiatric Association. *Diagnostic and statistical manual of mental disorders DSM-IV-TR*, 4th edn (text revision). Washington DC: American Psychiatric Association, 2000.
11. Merskey H, Bogduk N. *Classification of chronic pain: descriptions of chronic pain syndromes and definitions of pain terms*, 2nd edn. Seattle: IASP Press, 1994.

12. Polatin P, Kinney RK, Gatchel RJ *et al.* Psychiatric illness and chronic low back pain. The mind and the spine – which goes first? *Spine.* 1993; **18**: 66–71.
13. Fishbain D, Cutler R, Rosomoff HL, Rosomoff RS. Chronic pain-associated depression: Antecedent or consequence of chronic pain? A review. *Clinical Journal of Pain.* 1997; **13**: 116–37.
14. Endicott J. Measurement of depression in patients with cancer. *Cancer.* 1984; **53**: 2243–8.
15. Wilson K, Mikail SF, D'Eon JL, Minns JE. Alternative diagnostic criteria for major depressive disorder in patients with chronic pain. *Pain.* 2001; **91**: 227–34.
16. Tang N, Crane C. Suicidality in chronic pain: a review of the prevalence, risk factors and psychological links. *Psychological Medicine.* 2006; **36**: 575–86.
17. Stimmel G, Escobar JI. Antidepressants in chronic pain: a review of efficacy. *Pharmacotherapy.* 1986; **6**: 262–7.
18. Richeimer S, Bajwa ZH, Kahraman SS *et al.* Utilization patterns of tricyclic antidepressants in a multidisciplinary pain clinic: a survey. *Clinical Journal of Pain.* 1997; **13**: 324–9.
* 19. Fishbain D. Evidence-based data on pain relief with antidepressants. *Annals of Medicine.* 2000; **32**: 305–16.
20. Sullivan M, Robinson JP. Antidepressant and anticonvulsant medication for chronic pain. *Physical Medicine and Rehabilitation Clinics of North America.* 2006; **17**: 381–400.
21. Onghena P, Van Houdenhove B. Antidepressant-induced analgesia in chronic non-malignant pain: a meta-analysis of 39 placebo-controlled studies. *Pain.* 1992; **49**: 205–19.
* 22. McQuay H, Moore RA. Antidepressants and chronic pain. *British Medical Journal.* 1997; **314**: 763–4.
23. Barkin R, Barkin S. The role of venlafaxine and duloxetine in the treatment of depression with decremental changes in somatic symptoms of pain, chronic pain, and the pharmacokinetics and clinical considerations of duloxetine pharmacotherapy. *American Journal of Therapeutics.* 2005; **12**: 431–8.
24. Stahl S, Grady MM, Moret C, Briley M. SNRIs: their pharmacology, clinical efficacy, and tolerability in comparison with other classes of antidepressants. *CNS Spectrums.* 2005; **10**: 732–47.
25. McAllister-Williams RH, Tyrer SP. Antidepressants for the treatment of depression and anxiety disorders: the same mechanism of action?. In: Kasper S, den Boer JA, Sitsen JMA (eds). *Handbook of depression and anxiety*, 2nd edn. New York: Marcel Dekker, 2003: 443–56.
* 26. McWilliams L, Goodwin RD, Cox BJ. Depression and anxiety associated with three pain conditions: results from a nationally representative sample. *Pain.* 2004; **111**: 77–83.
27. Asmundson GJG, Vlaeyen JWS, Crombez G. *Understanding and treating fear of pain.* Oxford: Oxford University Press, 2004.
28. Reiss S, Peterson RA, Gursky DM, McNally RJ. Anxiety sensitivity, anxiety frequency and the prediction of fearfulness. *Behaviour Research and Therapy.* 1986; **24**: 1–8.
* 29. Tyrer P, Baldwin D. Generalised anxiety disorder. *Lancet.* 2006; **368**: 2156–66.
30. Fishbain DA, Goldberg M, Labbe E *et al.* Compensation and non-compensation chronic pain patients compared for DSM-III operational diagnoses. *Pain.* 1988; **32**: 197–206.
31. Keogh E, McCracken LM, Eccleston C. Gender moderates the association between depression and disability in chronic pain patients. *European Journal of Pain.* 2006; **10**: 413–22.
32. Hadjistavropoulos HD, Hadjistavropoulos T. The relevance of health anxiety to chronic pain: Research findings and recommendations for assessment and treatment. *Current Pain and Headache Reports.* 2003; **7**: 98–104.
33. Borkovec TD, Alcaine O, Behar E. Avoidance theory of worry and generalized anxiety disorder. In: Heimberg RG, Turk CL, Mennin DS (eds). *Generalized anxiety disorder in research and practice.* New York: Guilford Press, 2004: 77–108.
* 34. Morley S, Eccleston C, Williams A. Systematic review and meta-analysis of randomized controlled trials of cognitive behaviour therapy and behaviour therapy for chronic pain in adults, excluding headache. *Pain.* 1999; **80**: 1–13.
35. Raudenska J, Javurkova A. Cognitive-behavioral therapy of depression, generalized anxiety disorder and panic disorder in chronic pain. *Bolest.* 2003; **6**: 8–16.
36. McCracken LM, Gross RT, Eccleston C. Multimethod assessment of treatment process in chronic low back pain: Comparison of reported pain-related anxiety with directly measured physical capacity. *Behaviour Research and Therapy.* 2002; **40**: 585–94.
37. Riipinen M, Niemistö L, Lindgren KA, Hurri H. Psychosocial differences as predictors for recovery from chronic low back pain following manipulation, stabilizing exercises and physician consultation or physician consultation alone. *Journal of Rehabilitation Medicine.* 2005; **37**: 152–8.
* 38. Demyttenaere K, Bruffaerts R, Lee S *et al.* Mental disorders among persons with chronic back or neck pain: Results from the world mental health surveys. *Pain.* 2007; **129**: 332–42.
39. Roy-Byrne P, Uhde TW, Post RM *et al.* Normal pain sensitivity in patients with panic disorder. *Psychiatry Research.* 1985; **14**: 77–84.
40. Breslau N, Davis GC. Migraine, physical health and psychiatric disorder: A prospective epidemiologic study in young adults. *Journal of Psychiatric Research.* 1993; **27**: 211–21.
41. Katon W. Panic disorder. *New England Journal of Medicine.* 2006; **354**: 2360–7.
42. Mayou R, Bryant BM. Effects of road traffic accidents on travel. *Injury.* 1994; **25**: 457–60.
43. Asmundson G, Jacobson SJ, Allerdings MD, Norton GR. Social phobia in disabled workers with chronic musculoskeletal pain. *Behaviour Research and Therapy.* 1996; **34**: 939–43.
* 44. Mason S, Turpin G, Woods D *et al.* Risk factors for psychological distress following injury. *British Journal of Clinical Psychology.* 2006; **45**: 217–30.

45. Geisser ME, Roth RS, Bachman JE, Eckert TA. The relationship between symptoms of post-traumatic stress disorder and pain, effective disturbance and disability among patients with accident and non-accident related pain. *Pain.* 1996; **66**: 207–14.
46. Asmundson G, Coons MJ, Taylor S, Katz J. PTSD and the experience of pain: research and clinical implications of shared vulnerability and mutual maintenance models. *Canadian Journal of Psychiatry.* 2002; **47**: 930–7.
* 47. Mayou R, Ehlers A, Hobbs M. Psychological debriefing for road traffic accident victims. Three-year follow-up of a randomised controlled trial. *British Journal of Psychiatry.* 2000; **176**: 589–93.
48. Bradley R, Greene J, Russ E *et al.* A multidimensional meta-analysis of psychotherapy for PTSD. *American Journal of Psychiatry.* 2005; **162**: 214–27.
* 49. National Institute for Clinical Excellence. Management of post-traumatic stress disorder in adults in primary, secondary and community care. Clinical guideline 26. Cited March 2005. Available from: www.nice.org.uk.
50. Fishbain DA, Goldberg M, Meagher BR *et al.* Male and female chronic pain patients catagorised by DSM-III psychiatric diagnostic criteria. *Pain.* 1986; **26**: 181–97.
51. Weisberg JN. Personality and personality disorders in chronic pain. *Current Review of Pain.* 2000; **4**: 60–70.
52. Polatin P, Gatchel RJ, Fishbain DA *et al.* Personality disorders in the chronic pain population: Basic concepts, empirical findings, and clinical implications. *Pain Forum.* 1997; **6**: 1–21.
53. Turk D, Salovey P. Chronic pain as a variant of depressive disease. A critical reappraisal. *Journal of Nervous and Mental Disease.* 1984; **172**: 398–404.
54. Fishbain DA, Goldberg M, Labbe E *et al.* Compensation and non-compensation chronic pain patients compared for DSM-III operational diagnoses. *Pain.* 1988; **32**: 197–206.
* 55. Conrad R, Schilling R, Bausch C *et al.* Temperament and character personality profiles and personality disorders in chronic pain patients. *Pain.* 2007; **130**: 144–56.
56. Bateman A, Fonagy P. Treatment of borderline personality disorder with psychoanalytically oriented partial hospitalisation: an 18-month follow-up. *American Journal of Psychiatry.* 2001; **158**: 36–42.
57. Tyrer P, Bateman AW. Drug treatment for personality disorders. *Advances in Psychiatric Treatment.* 2004; **10**: 389–98.
58. Fishbain DA, Cole B, Cutler RB *et al.* Chronic pain and the measurement of personality: Do states influence traits?. *Pain Medicine.* 2006; **7**: 509–29.
59. Sternbach R, Timmermans G. Personality changes associated with reduction of pain. *Pain.* 1975; **1**: 177–81.
* 60. Love PW, Peck CL. The MMPI and psychological factors in chronic low back pain: a review. *Pain.* 1987; **28**: 1–12.
61. Royal College of Physicians and Psychiatrists. *The psychological care of medical patients.* Council Report CR35. London: Royal College of Psychiatrists, 1995.
62. Royal College of Surgeons and Psychiatrists. *Report of the Working Party on the Psychological Care of Surgical Patients.* Council Report CR55. London: Royal College of Psychiatrists 1997.
63. De Waal M, Arnold IA, Eekhof JAH. Somatoform disorders in general practice: prevalence, functional impairment and comorbidity with anxiety and depressive disorders. *British Journal of Psychiatry.* 2004; **184**: 470–6.
64. Dolin S, Stephens J. Pain clinics and liaison psychiatry. *Anaesthesia.* 1998; **53**: 317–9.
65. Silver N. Headache (chronic tension-type). *Clinical Evidence.* 2005; **14**: 1610–9.
66. Kellner R, Hernandez J, Pathak D. Hypochondriacal fears and beliefs, anxiety, and somatisation. *British Journal of Psychiatry.* 1992; **160**: 525–32.
67. Large R, Strong J. The personal constructs of coping with chronic low back pain: is coping a necessary evil? *Pain.* 1997; **73**: 245–52.
68. Stern J, Murphy M, Bass C. Personality disorders in patients with somatisation disorder. A controlled study. *British Journal of Psychiatry.* 1993; **163**: 785–9.
69. Bhui K, Hotopf M. Somatization disorder. *British Journal of Hospital Medicine.* 1997; **58**: 145–9.
70. Bass C, Peveler R, House A. Somatoform disorders: severe psychiatric illnesses neglected by psychiatrists. *British Journal of Psychiatry.* 2001; **179**: 11–14.
* 71. Sharpe M, Mayou R. Somatoform disorders: a help or hindrance to good patient care? *British Journal of Psychiatry.* 2004; **184**: 465–7.
72. Castillo R, MacKenzie EJ, Wegener ST, Bosse MJ. Prevalence of chronic pain seven years following limb threatening lower extremity trauma. *Pain.* 2006; **124**: 321–9.
73. Schofferman J. Long-term use of opioid analgesics for the treatment of chronic pain of nonmalignant origin. *Journal of Pain and Symptom Management.* 1993; **8**: 279–88.
* 74. Ciccone D, Just N, Bandilla EB *et al.* Psychological correlates of opioid use in patients with chronic nonmalignant pain: a preliminary test of the downhill spiral hypothesis. *Journal of Pain and Symptom Management.* 2000; **20**: 180–92.
* 75. National Institute for Health and Clinical Excellence. Interventions to reduce substance misuse among vulnerable young people. (Public health intervention guidance), 2007. Available from: www.nice.org.uk/PHI004.
76. Butler SF, Budman SH, Fernandez KC *et al.* Development and validation of the Current Opioid Misuse Measure. *Pain.* 2007; **130**: 144–56.
77. Allanson J, Bass C, Wade DT. Characteristics of patients with persistent severe disability and medically unexplained neurological symptoms: a pilot study. *Journal of Neurology, Neurosurgery and Psychiatry.* 2002; **73**: 307–09.
78. Michie MH, Tyrer SP, Charlton JE, Thompson JW. The assessment of psychiatric illness by physicians in patients with chronic pain. In: Bond MR, Charlton JE, Woolf J (eds). *Proceedings of the VIth World Congress on Pain.* Amsterdam: Elsevier, 1991: 235–40.

44

Chronic pain in children

NAVIL F SETHNA, ALYSSA LEBEL, AND LISA SCHARFF

KEY LEARNING POINTS

- The chronic pain experience in childhood presents a multifaceted challenge to clinicians, as it not only causes suffering and interruption to daily living, but also has distinctive issues that are individual to each child and family.
- Evaluation of the many factors (physiological, individual, family, school and peers, healthcare system) within the child's immediate environment and in the community at large that have an impact on the pain experience, is an important aspect of pain management.
- Biological, psychological, and functional aspects of pain should be considered in the management of diverse childhood persistent and recurrent pain experiences.
- Management plans should, where possible, be based on the current best evidence for efficacy of specific interventions for chronic pain conditions in childhood.

BASIC CONSIDERATIONS

Chronic and recurrent pain in children is a major health concern that significantly affects most aspects of children's daily lives. Those affected become physically inactive, dependent on others for basic daily tasks, reduce socialization with their peers, suffer strained family relationship, and lag behind in school attendance.[1][III], [2][III] Whether the pain is persistent, episodic, or both, it fluctuates in severity, quality, frequency, and predictability and involves a single or multiple body regions. The various different types of pediatric chronic pain conditions have not been systematically examined and infrequently followed in longitudinal studies. However, it is known that tissue injury may sensitize the nervous system and invoke variable biological and behavior responses that are uniquely determined by the complex interplay between each child's genetic composition, developmental stage, and environmental influence.[3][IV], [4]

PATHOPHYSIOLOGY

Acute injury or disease may cause the pain and nervous system sensitization and this often resolves after healing of the tissue. Such pain and hypersensitivity may persist past resolution of the underlying cause, becomes a self-sustained condition independent of the original pathology that initiated it and becomes in itself a disease entity; a chronic pain.[5] Irrespective of the cause of the pain it is associated with negative affect and psychological distress that has been recognized in many pain syndromes of organic origin and of uncertain causes.[4] Although the underlying pathophysiology of unexplained pain in which the nociceptive substrate is difficult to find, and enhanced sensitivity to pain are incompletely understood, mechanism-based research suggests a biological plausibility of a common denominator of neural plasticity at different levels of integration that may be important to understand the interplay of body and mind in chronic pain conditions.[6]

EPIDEMIOLOGY

Despite the growing knowledge in the field of childhood pain, limited data are available about the prevalence of chronic pain, the probability of its presentation in association with specific somatic or psychological disorders, natural history of pain syndromes, and how developmental challenges and risk factors affect diagnosis, treatment, and outcomes.[7] Epidemiological studies indicate disease-related, recurrent, and chronic pain are common in childhood, and the frequency estimates range from 15 to 25 percent and approximately 30 percent of randomly selected school-age children.[8][III], [9][III], [10][III], [11][III] A similar prevalence of medically unexplained physical symptoms accounts for 25–35 percent of adult outpatient clinic studies.[12][III], [13][III]

PRINCIPLES AND GOALS OF MANAGEMENT

In the absence of a cure or treatable cause, the major goal of care for children with chronic and recurrent pain conditions is to restore health and function through interdisciplinary rehabilitative (biopsychosocial) programs. Although most patients' priority is relief from pain, healthcare providers are presented with challenges of biological, psychological, and social difficulties in children with chronic pain. The biopsychosocial model addresses the multidimensional dynamic interplay of psychophysiological antecedents and consequences of pain, and facilitates functional restoration to activities of daily living through modulation of cognitive, emotional, and physical status, which often occurs before the patient perceives pain reduction.

As with adult interdisciplinary pain treatment programs, pediatric research supports the effectiveness of interdisciplinary cognitive-behavioral[14][III] and physical therapy interventions in improving self-reported functioning through positive changes in the child's cognitions and coping responses.

ARCHETYPE DISORDERS

In this review, we will address the overall assessment and management of three most common pain conditions arising from musculoskeletal (fibromyalgia, complex regional pain syndromes), nervous system (headaches) disorders, and viscera (recurrent abdominal pain), as archetypes of the complex nature of chronic and recurrent pain syndromes in children.

MUSCULOSKELETAL PAIN

Musculoskeletal pain (MSP) constitutes a large group of joint, muscle, tendon, and bone disorders. It is a common presenting complaint in pediatric practice, affects 6–15 percent of school children, and is frequently associated with benign causes.[15][V], [16][III] Chronic and recurrent pain may present a diagnostic challenge to the practitioner and a source of great anxiety to the child and parents.[17][III] While most MSP complaints are not of serious origin, early diagnosis of the primary cause of the pain should be the goal of the clinician to avoid delaying the detection of treatable underlying conditions. The differential diagnosis of MSP includes an exhaustive list of many possible causes and is beyond the scope of this chapter, but they should be considered when screening for disease causes in children with MSP. In general, the source of MSP in childhood can be attributed to broad categories of noninflammatory (mostly benign), inflammatory due to abnormal immune responses (e.g. rheumatologic diseases), infection, malignancies, and trauma. This section focuses specifically on isolated common MSP conditions that present with persistent pain as the most prominent symptom and reason to seek consultation.

Diagnostic evaluation

The clinician's primary objective is to obtain general and relevant comprehensive medical history, including psychological status, to distinguish noninflammatory pain from other possible causes of MSP. Performance of a thorough physical examination with special attention to, but not limited to, the painful musculoskeletal site(s) along with appropriate diagnostic studies can facilitate and support the final diagnosis.[18] Careful characterization of the pain will greatly aid in narrowing the differential diagnosis. Given the mutual relationship between chronic pain and mood, the initial assessment of a child with chronic pain also warrants special consideration of a comprehensive psychosocial assessment.[19] Children should be permitted to self-report pain using a developmentally appropriate rating scale, the family members should report their observations regarding child's pain and special approaches of surrogate measures should be used for the assessment of pain of children with special needs (neurologically impaired and noncommunicating).[20][V]

Juvenile fibromyalgia syndrome

The prevalence of juvenile fibromyalgia syndrome (JFS) is approximately 1.3 percent in children aged 9–17 years.[21]

[V] A population-based prospective study of schoolchildren reported a widespread pain prevalence of 14.6 percent among the ages of 11 and 14 years. At one-year follow up, the new onset of such a pain was 7.7 percent. The widespread pain was associated with behavioral and emotional difficulties, and somatic symptoms of frequent headaches and high level of sports activity; these factors predicted increased short-term risk of developing widespread pain at follow up.[22][III]

CLINICAL PRESENTATION

The primary presenting symptoms are diffuse persistent or intermittent MSP involving the extremities, back, and neck that may not manifest concurrently and are present for at least three months duration. Earlier criteria proposed for the diagnosis of JFS emphasized the combined importance of symptoms and tender points.[23][III] Subsequent revised criteria from multicenter adult study, the American College of Rheumatology (ACR) criteria, showed that concurrent presence of widespread pain and tenderness on palpation in at least 11 of 18 tender point sites have better sensitivity (88 percent) and specificity (81 percent).[24][IV] However, the proper diagnostic criteria of tender points are subject to assessors' training and performance of a thorough physical examination.[23][III] The pain is often associated with many subjective symptoms; some investigators have noted overlapping complaints of fatigue ranging from 20 to 100 percent.[25][V], [26][V] A recent study suggested that a combination of a high level of fatigue and many regional painful areas are equally useful symptoms in the diagnosis of fibromyalgia.[27] The diagnosis of primary fibromyalgia is established in the absence of evidence for other conditions that may be associated with fibromyalgia-like symptoms, such as connective tissue disease, hypermobility, and somatoform pain conditions.[24][IV]

ETIOLOGY

The cause of fibromyalgia is unknown. Hypermobility may contribute to musculoskeletal pain in JFS, a high incidence (81 percent) of schoolchildren with JFS were found to have hypermobility by blinded assessors compared with 1 percent of children without JFS.[28][III] Recent adult psychophysical studies suggest that the widespread MSP could be due to central sensitization and enhanced perceptual wind-up phenomenon as a possible etiology or predisposing factor.[29]

Sleep disturbance is common among children with JFS ranging from 67 to 96 percent in those under the age of 17 years[23][III], [26][V], [30][III] and is confirmed by a polysomnographic study and a subset of 38 percent of JFS children had a primary sleep disorder of periodic limb movements in sleep.[31][III] In one study, a high prevalence (28 percent) of JFS was observed among offspring of mothers with fibromyalgia. Because psychological and familial factors were not different in children with and without fibromyalgia, the high familial occurrence of JFS may be attributable to genetic factors.[32][V] Some studies have reported more behavioral and emotional (e.g. anxiety, depression) problems in children with JFS than controls and so it has been speculated that psychological factors may contribute to increased sensitivity to pain and associated disability.[21][V], [33][III] On the other hand, a number of studies failed to demonstrate significant differences in psychological issues between children with fibromyalgia and their families, compared to children with other illnesses and their families. Occurrence of depressive symptoms is relatively comparable in children with JFS and juvenile rheumatoid arthritis.[34][V], [35][III]

PROGNOSIS

Little is known about the natural history of JFS. A large epidemiological study of 338 schoolchildren prospectively followed 28 children (21 with fibromyalgia fulfilling ACR adult criteria and 7 with tender point count criteria of 11 of 18 points) over a 30-month period. At the end of the study, 11 of the 15 (73 percent) children with fibromyalgia no longer fulfilled the fibromyalgia criteria and showed significant reduction in the mean tenderness threshold at the painful and control sites. None of the seven children who experienced only tender points criteria, without diffuse pain, developed fibromyalgia over the follow-up period.[36][III]

MANAGEMENT

There are no randomized placebo-controlled trials of the use of analgesics and other medications in JFS. An earlier study of JFS involving 15 children, with a mean age of 13 years, demonstrated ineffectiveness of salicylate and other anti-inflammatory medications; most (73 percent) children responded to cyclobenzaprine (a muscle relaxant), at a mean dose 12.75 mg (range 5–25 mg at bedtime). An additional two patients who did not respond to cyclobenzaprine improved with amitriptyline (10–30 mg at bedtime) and trazodone 50 mg at bedtime.[37][V] Tricyclic antidepressants are used primarily to improve sleep, other medications such as selective serotonin reuptake inhibitor (SSRI) antidepressants, tramadol, gabapentin, and pregabalin are also used empirically and based on adult empirical experiences. There are very few data on the usefulness of trigger-point or tender-point injections, or the use of transcutaneous electrical nerve stimulator.

A general and individualized rehabilitative approach for management of chronic pain disorders is applicable to children with JFS.

- Patient and family education, cardiovascular fitness (low impact aerobic exercise), weight control, and physical therapy for flexibility training.

- Psychological interventions are used to reduce pain perception, and improve functional ability and quality of life. Children taught cognitive-behavioral therapies can effectively manage chronic and disabling musculoskeletal pain.[38][III]

Complex regional pain syndromes

Complex regional pain syndromes (CRPS) type 1 and 2 are recent terminologies that refer to what was previously known as reflex sympathetic dystrophy (RSD) and causalgia, respectively. CRPS type 1 occurs without a definable nerve lesion, whereas type 2 follows a definable nerve lesion. These diagnostic criteria were standardized by an International Association for the Study of Pain (IASP) consensus development conference in 1995 to encompass the minimal criteria.[39] In adults, studies have attempted validation of the original[40][IV] and modified[41] [IV] IASP criteria of CRPS as compared to established painful neuropathic disorders and have found relatively weak interobserver agreement or sensitivity and specificity based on clinical examination and quantitative sensory evaluation.[42][IV], [43][III] These criteria are yet to be validated in children with CRPS.

CLINICAL PRESENTATION

The typical presentation of CRPS usually follows an injury, albeit trivial, and affects distal extremities characterized by pain, altered skin sensitivity, swelling, cutaneous autonomic changes, pronounced guarding of the affected limb, and functional disability. Although involvement of lower limbs is consistently reported in children and has occurred as frequently as 87 percent,[44][V] it may involve an upper extremity or contralateral corresponding limbs.[44][V], [45][V] These findings fluctuate over time and the objective findings may not be present at the time of examination and may spread to other extremities and body regions.[44][V], [46][V]

Most of the criteria of CRPS 1 were developed on the basis of clinical experience alone for which there is no distinctive biomarker characteristic of the disorder. Diagnostic tests are performed to primarily exclude other pathologies. None of these tests provide consistent positive findings of altered specific function(s), therefore, questions have been raised about their validity. A preliminary study confirms altered central processing using quantitative thermal and mechanical tests in children with CRPS, the diagnostic specificity of these tests is yet to be determined.[47][III]

ETIOLOGY

There is no single theory that explains the intricate presentation of CRPS, usually initiated by a noxious event that is disproportionate to the ensuing pain, and several mechanisms have been proposed including neurological disorder,[48][V] inflammation,[49][V] sympathetic nervous system dysregulation,[50][V], [51][III] anticipatory pain and immobilization (fear avoidance),[52][V] genetic predisposition, higher incidence associated with histocompatability antigens HLA-DQ1 and HLA-A3, B7, and DR2,[53] [III], [54][III] and sensitization of the neurons at various levels of integration from the periphery to central nervous system.[55][III], [56][III], [57][III]

Psychological factors are implicated in the causation and/or maintenance of CRPS 1 because the proposed mechanisms outlined above fail to account fully for the patient's pain and are considered by some as a somatoform pain disorder; somatoform pain disorders may account for some of the cases, but certainly do not account for all CRPS sufferers.[58][V], [59][V], [60]

AGE AT ONSET

Complex regional pain syndrome 1 has been reported in children as young as 30 months, but predominantly occurs in preadolescence and adolescence.[44][V], [58][V], [61][V], [62][V]

GENDER DIFFERENCES

The findings from most pediatric studies of CRPS/RSD suggest that it is more frequent in girls than boys and the prevalence ratios ranges from 5 to 13:1.[44][V], [58][V], [62][V], [63][II]

TREATMENT

For the purpose of this discussion, hereafter the term CRPS also refers to pediatric studies that used the previous definition of RSD. There are numerous diverse therapies reported in the literature for management of CRPS in children, but none has been examined in well-controlled randomized controlled trials to be reliably effective. There is only one prospective randomized controlled trial that has examined the effectiveness of physical therapy and cognitive-behavioral treatment to improve pain and overall (89 percent) excellent improvement in functional status for short-term symptoms with a duration of 1–18 weeks.[63] Most practitioners recommend early intervention to prevent refractoriness, disability, and to enhance favorable outcome. The initial therapeutic strategies include patient and family education, physical therapy, and cognitive-behavioral therapy.[45][V], [58][V], [62][V], [63][II]

The primary goal of management is to restore normal function through activity irrespective of severity of the pain as follows:

- Aggressive step-wise mobilization of the affected limb by eliminating guarding postures and assistive

devices, posture correction, encouraging range of motion, flexibility exercise and gradual weight bearing, normalizing motor, gait control and increase ambulation, and strengthening hand grip and dexterity to avoid undesirable immobilization contractures.
- Improve overall physical deconditioning through age-specific aerobic training programs to reduce fatigue, increase endurance, and avoid reinjury.
- Desensitize allodynia by warm/cold contrast bath, hydrotherapy, compression sleeves to reduce edema and touch intolerance, and gentle massage by self-touch of sensitive skin with application of inert creams/gels.

PHARMACOLOGICAL THERAPIES

Various analgesics have been proposed, but no specific treatment has been consistently effective in children with CRPS.[64] The appropriate role for medication is to alleviate pain, improve sleep, and facilitate physical therapy.

- Tricyclic antidepressants are offered primarily to ameliorate para-insomnia and reactive depression that are often associated with persistent pain.[65, 66]
- Anticonvulsants have a promising benefit, but the data on their use in CRPS are experience-based and anecdotal.[67][V], [68][V], [69][II]
- Nonsteroidal anti-inflammatory drugs (NSAIDs) may alleviate pain from inflammation and even partial pain relief is desirable to mobilize the painful limb.
- Opioid use is controversial and efficacy is yet to be demonstrated. Opioids are prescribed for short-term treatment of acute pain or on time-contingent schedule prior to physical therapy in order to maximize compliance with mobilization of the painful limb.
- Other therapies including antagonist of calcium channel, sodium channel, beta-adrenergic, and alpha-adrenergic receptors, calcitonin, steroids, and Lidoderm (5 percent) patches have shown to produce short-term relief of pain in uncontrolled trials.[68][V], [70][IV], [71][IV], [72][V], [73][III], [74][III], [75][V]
- Baclofen and clonazepam have been prescribed for symptomatic treatment of dystonia and muscle spasms with variable success.[76]

SYMPATHETIC BLOCKADE

Sympathetic blockade is considered when the pain is not sufficiently controlled to restore regular function after use of the conservative therapy described above under Pharmacological therapies. The site of action of selective sympathetic blockade and long-term efficacy are yet to be validated in placebo-controlled trials.[77, 78][V], [79][V]

The experience with nerve blockade for management of pediatric CRPS is limited in the form of case reports and is based on uncontrolled studies.[80][V], [81][V] A trial of selective sympathetic and/or somatic nerve blockade is worth considering when overwhelming pain and allodynia hinder progress of an active exercise program despite pharmacological and psychological therapy or poor circulation particularly associated with impending infection. In a controlled trial, 35 percent of children with CRPS required lumbar epidural infusion of a local anesthetic to control intense pain and allow effective mobilization of the affected limb in a hospitalized setting.[63][II]

A preliminary prospective trial in a small number of hospitalized children with CRPS 1 reported favorable two-month benefit from combination of continuous peripheral blockade, physical therapy, and psychological support.[82][III] Further controlled and longitudinal studies are needed to confirm the effectiveness of such an approach.

Invasive therapies of dorsal column and peripheral nerve stimulators with implanted programmable generators, intrathecal baclofen, and chemical and surgical sympathectomies have been examined with variable success in adults in prospective trials but have not been studied in children.[83][III], [84][III], [85][III] These procedures potentially can worsen or produce a new pain syndrome, e.g. postsympathectomy neuralgia.[86][I], [87][I]

Psychological counseling should include individual cognitive-behavioral and family intervention to eliminate reinforcement of maladaptive behaviors and promote positive coping skills.[44][V], [63][II]

PROGNOSIS

Childhood CRPS presents with a wide clinical spectrum that ranges from a mild self-limited course to severe pain and disability. In contrast to adult CRPS, the time course of illness in childhood CRPS is shorter and the prognosis is favorable in most children.[44][V], [45][V], [58][V], [62][V], [63][II], [88][V] Early treatment may shorten the course of the illness and disability, and may prevent osseous growth deformities.[89][V], [90][V] In three retrospective pediatric trials, aggressive therapy of active mobilization, analgesics and/or psychological therapy yielded functional improvement ranging from 60, 69, and 92 percent, respectively.[45][V], [62][V], [91][V] A long-term follow-up study of 70 children with CRPS reported the presence of some degree of residual pain and dysfunction in 54 percent of children at a median follow-up interval of three years and 50 percent of those children who were engaged in competitive sport before treatment were unable to return to sports because of residual pain.[44][V] A recent controlled trial of pediatric CRPS showed a response rate of 89 percent to conservative therapy, including resolution of musculoskeletal signs, improvement in function, and return to school. Although recurrent episodes were frequent, most patients continued to respond to conservative therapy more readily than with the initial therapy after onset of the CRPS.[63][II]

PRIMARY HEADACHE DISORDERS

Headaches are common during childhood. In one Swedish interview study of 9000 schoolchildren,[92][II] 40 percent of children before age seven years reported having at least one memorable headache. In a later review by the same author, 10 percent of children reported having recurrent headaches. In another Canadian study,[93][IV] 85 percent of children aged five to seven years reported headaches, as did 100 percent of adolescents aged 14–16 years. Most of these pain experiences were reported as mild to moderate in intensity, of short duration, and not disruptive to daily activities. However, an increasingly recognized minority of children is reported to have daily headaches associated with significant disability. These patients present with decreased academic performance and school absenteeism, reactive anxiety, depression, disrupted family interactions, and increased healthcare costs.[94][III] Fortunately, most childhood headaches are benign, not associated with underlying organic pathology, and amenable to pharmacological and cognitive-behavioral interventions, and lifestyle changes that enhance functional behavior, such as dietary support, regular sleep hours, and adequate hydration. Secondary headaches, such as related to central nervous infection, mass, vascular anomalies or venous sinus thrombosis, hydrocephalus, obstructive Arnold–Chiari malformation, or pseudotumor cerebri, are generally eliminated by a thorough history and examination. Warning signals on history include:

- onset at age less than five years, without a family history of migraines;
- sudden and severe onset of a new headache;
- mental status change during headache course;
- recent infection or fever;
- pain beginning during vigorous exercise or head/neck trauma;
- pain radiation to posterior thorax (meningeal);
- history of toxic exposure/substance use.

On examination, careful consideration should be given to (1) change in consciousness, attention, language, and memory, (2) papilledema, (3) cranial nerve asymmetry, (4) motor strength asymmetry, (5) abnormal tone, (6) involuntary movements (dysmetria), (7) gait ataxia, (8) nuchal rigidity, (9) toxic appearance, or (10) new neurologic abnormality.

Management of primary headaches in a patient free of the above considerations, especially with a positive family history, is unlikely to change following neuroimaging, electroencephalogram (EEG), or lumbar puncture.[95]

Primary headache disorders in childhood predominantly include migraine headaches and tension-type headaches. The reported prevalence for migraine headache is estimated at 3 percent for children aged 3–7 years, 4–11 percent for ages 7–11 years, and 8–23 percent for ages 11–15 years. The mean age of onset for boys is 7.2 years and for girls 10.9 years.[96][IV] Of note, some researchers[97][V] suggest that children less than three years may have an early common migraine headache which presents as periodic irritability, head-banging or holding, change in sleep and behavioral patterns, abdominal pain, recurrent vomiting, and pallor. These migraine variants now referred to as childhood periodic syndromes and include cyclic vomiting, abdominal migraine, benign paroxysmal vertigo, benign paroxysmal torticollis, acute confusional migraine, and acephalgic migraine.

Diagnosis

The diagnosis of primary headache in children, including migraine with and without aura, is based on clinical criteria modified in 2004 by the International Headache Society (**Tables 44.1** and **44.2**).[98] Tension-type headache criteria for children are still evolving, but are based on the adult description (**Table 44.2**).

Headache assessment

The clinical interview is essential and includes both open-ended and structured questions about headache duration, location, frequency, intensity, quality, triggers (puberty, diet, worries), associated affect ("How did you feel when you had your last headache?"), and accompanying symptoms. Such a symptom checklist[93][IV] may include feeling:

- aches or pins and needles in arms and legs;
- dizziness: spinning; near-fainting;
- soreness in neck and shoulders;
- light bothering the eyes;
- seeing of bright white or colored spots, flashes, wavy lines, or dark/blank;
- spots described as a puzzle where a piece has been removed;
- sounds are bothersome;
- tired, wanting to sleep;
- sick to the stomach and/or vomiting;
- hot and sweaty;
- the heart beating very fast.

These symptoms may accompany the pain or may occasionally present independent of the headache.

For chronic pain problems, data related to childhood disability, such as pain interfering with school work and attendance, socializing with peers, sports activity,

Table 44.1 Criteria for migraine without aura.

Criterion	
A. Five attacks or greater, fulfilling B–D	
B. Headache attack lasting 1–72 hours	
C. Headache has at least two of the following four features:	1. Either the bilateral or unilateral (front/temporal) location 2. Pulsating quality 3. Moderate to severe intensity 4. Aggravated by physical activities
D. At least one of the following accompanies headache:	1. Nausea and/or vomiting 2. Photophobia and phonophobia (may be inferred by behavior)
E. Both of the following:	1. History and physical and neurological examinations do not suggest an organic disorder, including head trauma, vascular disorders, nonvascular intracranial disorder, substances or their withdrawal, noncephalic infection, metabolic disorder, disorder of the cranium, neck, eyes, ears, nose, sinuses, teeth, mouth, or other facial or cranial structures; 2. History and/or physical and/or neurological examinations suggest an organic disorder, but migraine attacks do not occur for the first time in close temporal relation to the disorder.

Table 44.2 Tension-type headache criteria.

Criterion	
A. At least ten previous headache episodes fulfilling criteria B–D. Number of days with such headache <180 per year (<15 per month)	
B. Headache lasting from 30 minutes to 7 days	
C. Headache with at least two of the following pain characteristics:	1. Pressing/tightening (nonpulsating) quality 2. Mild or moderate intensity (may inhibit, but not prohibit, activities) 3. Bilateral location 4. No aggravation by walking, stair-climbing, or similar routine physical activity
D. Both of the following:	1. No nausea or vomiting (may have anorexia) 2. Photophobia and phonophobia are absent, or one but not the other occurs
E. Same as for migraine without aura (as above)	

performing domestic chores and leisure activities, watching television, playing video games, should be elicited.

Differential diagnosis

Migraines in children generally present without aura (prevalence of 70 versus 15 percent for migraine with aura). It is important to recognize some migraine syndromes which present more commonly in pediatrics, including ophthalmoplegic migraine (third nerve paresis or palsy); complex migraine (transient neurological abnormalities); basilar artery migraine (Bickerstaff's migraine); confusional migraine (most common in adolescence, with aphasia); and Alice-in-Wonderland syndrome (headache with visual illusion and spatial distortions). Both epilepsy and migraine headaches, two paroxysmal disorders, may coexist in an individual. However, nonepileptiform EEG abnormalities are also common in migraineurs and do not constitute a seizure diagnosis. As in adults, particularly female, adolescents may have visual symptoms not associated with headache – "migraine sine hemicrania." Acute confusional migraine, which may present with unexpected stroke-like symptoms (dysphasia and aphasia), is a benign migraine variant but always prompts a neurological evaluation in children. Migraine variants are much more prevalent in pediatrics, may precede the development of common migraine, and may occur in a patient with a family history of migraines. In these cases, headache may not be initially a prominent symptom. Such disorders are benign; paroxysmal vertigo (brief episodes presenting before age six years with transient instability with or without nystagmus), paroxysmal torticollis (recurrent head tilt with occasional nausea and vomiting), and cyclic vomiting (recurrent cycles of abdominal pain, nausea, and vomiting with negative gastrointestinal and metabolic evaluations). In one recent report of 5848 children over eight years, 1106 migraineurs were identified, of whom 108 (9.8 percent) had "migraine equivalents," i.e. transient neurological symptoms between headaches.[99]

Genetics

Familial hemiplegic migraine (FHM), the first clearly-defined genetic pediatric headache disorder, is a possible window into the still enigmatic molecular and cellular origins of migraine headache. Migraine susceptibility is believed to be inherited, with its presentation modified by both internal and environmental factors, although specific generic loci are not readily identified in most families with migraine headaches. However, in FHM, at least three loci have been documented by linkage analysis. FHA4 is a rare autosomal dominant form of migraine with aura, with a variable presentation of hemiparesis, ataxia, and nystagmus. Some headache episodes may resemble confusional migraine. Cerebellar atrophy may be seen on magnetic resonance imaging. The first gene identified with FHM was CACNAlA on chromosome 19p13 (FHM1). It encodes for the alpha-1A subunit of the PIQ-type, voltage-gated calcium channel. Another specific FHM polymorphism involves ATP 1A2 (FHM2) on chromosome lq23, which encodes the alpha-2 subunit of the NA^+/K^+ pump. Further FHM linkage studies have excluded these two loci, suggesting additional heterogeneity of this disorder.[100][III]

Therapeutic options

Treatment includes pharmacologic and non-pharmacologic therapies and is initiated with patient and family education, removal of possible triggers, and if appropriate, changes in a disrupted lifestyle (school attendance, physical activity, sleep, dietary habits). Overuse of particularly symptomatic and centrally acting analgesics is prevalent in children with chronic daily headache. Attempts to discontinue the overused medications may cause rebound. If prophylactic medication is prescribed, it should be given every day, whether or not a headache is present. Attention to the following good health habits remains the primary therapy.

Hydration: Children need at least four to eight glasses of fluid without caffeine per day. During a headache or increased activity, sports drinks (with sugar and salt) are recommended.

Sleep: Fatigue and overexertion may trigger headaches. Most children require eight to ten hours of uninterrupted sleep each night and a regular sleep schedule.

Diet: Children do best with regular and balanced meals. Foods that trigger headache are unique to individuals, and general exclusionary diets are not indicated.

Activity: Sensible child activity schedules, without overcrowding or exposure to stressful and upsetting situations, are reasonable.

PRACTICE PARAMETER

Systematic review of 166 articles by the American Academy of Neurology[101][I] from 1980 to 2003 with an age qualifier of 3–18 years, and a four-tiered scheme of evidence classification (class I–IV) and recommendation (levels A–C, U). Acute treatment recommendations were:

- ibuprofen effective (level A);
- paracetamol (acetaminophen) probably effective (level B);
- sumatriptan nasal spray effective for adolescents (level A);
- no data for oral triptans (level U);
- inadequate data for subcutaneous sumatriptan (level U).

For preventive treatment:

- flunarizine probably effective (level B); not available in USA;
- insufficient evidence to recommend cyproheptadine, amitriptyline, valproate semisodium (divalproex sodium), topiramate, or levetiracetum (level U);
- pizotifen, nimodipine, and clonidine showed no efficacy (level B); not recommended;
- there is conflicting evidence for the use of propranolol and trazodone (level U).

The review also concluded that there is a need for "multicenter, placebo-controlled clinical trials to assess the safety, tolerability, and efficacy of medications used for the acute and preventive treatment of pediatric migraine."

The present practice of pediatric headache therapy is based on adult guidelines. According to the US Headache Consortium in 2000,[102][I] the adult agents that show the best balance of efficacy, evidence, and adverse effects are amitriptyline, valproate semisodium, propranolol, and timolol. There is lower efficacy and less evidence for aspirin, NSAID, gabapentin, verapamil, other beta-blockers, riboflavin, magnesium, and feverfew. Consensus efficacy is available for cyproheptadine, diltiazem, nortriptyline, and doxepin. No efficacy greater than placebo is present for carbamazepine, indometacin, nifedipine, and lamotrigine.

Acute treatment

The goal of acute therapy is to abort an attack of severe pain and suppress pain, nausea, and vomiting. For mild–moderate pain and minimal nausea, preferred agents are NSAIDs and paracetamol. For severe pain, opioids may be judiciously used, as well as nasal sumatriptan.[103][II] As previously noted, we have little pediatric data regarding the safety and efficacy of subcutaneous sumatriptan and oral triptans.[104][II] Adverse effects of the 5-HT 1B/1D receptor agonists include initial selective constriction of intracranial extracerebral vessels and inhibition of release of vasoactive neuropeptides from trigeminal nerve terminals in the intracranial vessels and meninges. Secondary effects include inhibition of nociceptive neurotransmission in the brain stem and cervical spinal descending trigeminal sensory nucleus.[105] For nausea and vomiting, diphenhydramine and hydroxyzine are least associated with adverse effects, such as the mood changes and dystonia potentially seen with chlorpromazine and metoclopramide. The dosing regimens shown in **Table 44.3** are suggested for pediatric dosing.

PARACETAMOL AND NSAIDS

Paracetamol is the most commonly and widely used analgesic and antipyretic in children. It has no peripheral anti-inflammatory effects and it putatively acts on cyclooxygenase (COX-1 more than COX-2) through central nervous system mechanisms. Although a weak analgesic, it is a generally safe agent, if proper pediatric doses are administered. The recommended single doses are 15–20 mg/kg and 10–15 mg/kg for repeated dosing. Maximum recommended doses are 90 mg/kg in children and adolescents, 60 mg/kg in infants, and 45 mg/kg in preterm infants. Paracetamol is available in multiple formulations and administration routes.

NSAIDs act primarily at peripheral sites and have a prominent anti-inflammatory effect, as well as analgesia and antipyresis. Their selection is guided by their adverse effects, including gastritis, bleeding, and platelet and renal dysfunction.

The major mechanisms of action of NSAIDs are through inhibition of prostaglandin synthesis by blockade of constitutive and expressed COX. The pharmacology of most NSAIDs has been studied in children aged two years and older and in general, the elimination half-lives are similar to adults for most of the agents. In children 3–30 months, the volume of distribution and clearance of ibuprofen and ketorolac are increased, suggesting a possible need for a higher initial dose.[106][II], [107][III]

Aspirin, although used for acute pain, is contraindicated in the presence of fever in children due to an association with Reye's syndrome. For severe pain, parenteral ketorolac is effective. The oral formulation of paracetamol and ibuprofen is similar in efficacy to other NSAIDs with markedly fewer adverse effects. Intravenous ketorolac at a dose of 0.5 mg/kg every six hours has been shown to be safe and effective for short-term post-operative pain management (48 hours) in children as young as two years.[108][III]

For acute intravenous treatment of severe headache, one to two doses of ketorolac (0.5–1 mg/kg) in the emergency department or intramuscularly in the primary physician's office may break a headache attack. Intravenous valproate semisodium (10–15 mg/kg intravenously over 30 minutes) has also shown promise in adult studies and for controlling seizure activity in children. Intravenous magnesium is currently under investigation.[109][II]

OPIOIDS

Oral opioids, administered for mild to moderate pain, include oral opioid preparations (codeine, oxycodone, morphine elixir, and rapid-release tablets) and opioid–NSAID combinations (paracetamol with codeine or oxycodone). Tramadol is an unusual opioid, with weak mu-l-receptor agonism and modulates the GABAergic, noradrenergic, and serotonergic systems which may account for the headache-alleviating effect. It has a safe and effective profile in children.[110][II]

Rectal suppositories of morphine and hydromorphone are available for management of severe pain in patients in whom the oral route is unavailable or where there is presence of nausea and vomiting.

The recommend oral opioid doses are shown in **Table 44.4**.

For prophylactic treatment of pediatric headaches, pharmacologic choices are still currently based on adult studies including anticonvulsants, with the caveats of slow titration and anticipation of greater side effects. Current adult literature supports beta-blockers, amitriptyline, and valproic acid as the most effective agents for headache

Table 44.3 Dosing recommendations for specific migraine and adjuvant medications.

Drug	Dosing regimen
Sumatriptan	Initial doses: intranasal 5–20 mg; oral 25 mg in adolescents; subcutaneous 3–6 mg
Zolmitripan	Oral 2.5 mg, peaks in 2 hours, nasal 5 mg
Eletriptan	Oral 20–40 mg, peaks in 1.3 hours
Diphenhydramine and hydroxyzine	Oral 1–1.5 mg/kg/dose; 6.25–25 mg every 6 hours
Chlopromazine	Oral 1 mg/kg every 8 hours
Metaclopromide	1–2 mg/kg/dose every 6 hours

Table 44.4 Recommend oral opioid doses.

Oral opioid	Dose
Morphine	0.3 mg/kg every 3–4 hours
Hydromorphone	0.02–0.08 mg/kg every 3–4 hours
Methadone	0.2 mg/kg every 4–8 hours
Codeine	0.5–1 mg/kg every 3–4 hours
Oxycodone	0.1–0.2 mg/kg every 3–4 hours

Table 44.5 Calcium channel blockers dosing.

Calcium channel blocker	Recommended dose
Propranolol	1–3 mg/kg/24 hours, in two or three divided doses
Verapamil	4–8 mg/kg/24 hours, in three divided doses

prophylaxis. Second tier agents include other anticonvulsants, such as gabapentin, topiramate, and levetiracetam, which are considered to block nerve discharge by binding to inappropriately active sodium and neuronal calcium channels. Beta-blockers, such as propranolol, may decrease reactive vasodilation of intracranial arterioles but may also effect an earlier step in the neuroinflammatory cascade associated with migraines. Pediatric anecdotal experience suggests that these agents are most effective for patients with severe but infrequent migraines. Calcium channel blockers, such as verapamil, bind directly to inappropriately active ion channels. The recommended dosing is shown in **Table 44.5**.

Tricyclic antidepressants, such as amitriptyline and nortriptyline, potentiate the analgesic actions of serotonin and norepinephrine at nerve terminals in the central nervous system, especially in the trigeminal nucleus caudalis. They are recommended for migraines that are frequent but less severe and often associated with sleep disturbance. Their side effects are due to additional cholinergic, histaminergic, and adrenergic actions, resulting in possible dry mouth, constipation, urinary retention, sedation, weight gain, orthostatic hypotension, increased intraocular pressure, tachycardia, and heart block. Although the cardiac risks for children are low, it is recommended that an electrocardiogram be taken before initiation of the therapy to exclude rhythm abnormalities and during dose escalation to monitor QT-interval prolongation. Amitriptyline is the most effective agent, but also has the highest anticholinergic side effects of sedation and orthostatic dizziness. Therefore, nortriptyline with milder anticholinergic untoward effects is often the first choice.

Recommended dosing

The recommended dosing for amitriptyline and nortriptyline is 0.2–0.4 mg/kg orally at bedtime with titrations upwards by 0.25 mg/kg every five to seven days. The dose may be administered twice a day at 0.2–0.3 mg/kg.

Other antidepressants, such as fluoxetine, sertraline, citalopram, escitalopram, venlafaxine, and trazodone, are best used for associated symptoms, such as anxiety, mood disorder, and sleep disturbance. The data regarding their analgesic efficacy remain anecdotal; however, trazodone has shown some efficacy in pediatric trials.[111][I]

Anticonvulsants are used for management of headaches because they depress abnormal neuronal discharges and raise the inappropriately lowered threshold of sensitized neurons. They are variably active at voltage-gated ion channels, and at glutamate, *N*-methyl-D-aspartic acid (NMDA), gamma-aminobutyric acid, and glycine receptors. Much of pediatric experience with these agents is for seizure management. Their use as analgesics is extrapolated from adult experience. The first-generation agents, such as phenytoin and carbamazepine, are associated with serious adverse effects and require regular blood level monitoring. The second-generation medications, such as gabapentin, lamotrigine, topiramate, zonisamide, levetiracetam, and pregabalin, may not require laboratory monitoring, have fewer sedation or cognitive effects, and fewer overall adverse effects. Recommended oral dosing is given in **Table 44.6**. Caution is advised with their use as the pediatric experience with these agents is limited and the true incidence of serious side-effect profile is not fully known.

NMDA receptor antagonists show promise as regulators of the central nervous sensitization that occurs during pathologic or excessive NMDA-receptor activation, as postulated to occur during chronic headaches. Activation of NMDA receptor and release of glutamate, a primary excitatory amino acid of central nervous system (CNS), prevents magnesium from reentering and blocking the channel pore resulting in a chronically open state and excessive calcium influx. NMDA-receptor antagonists bind to the magnesium site as an effective receptor blocker. However, the safety and efficacy of NMDA-receptor antagonists for clinical use are yet to be demonstrated. Anticonvulsants with NMDA-receptor antagonist effects are used for chronic headache prophylaxis. Pediatric use may be particularly limited due to developmental regulation of these receptor subtypes.

Dosing of NMDA antagonists

The dose of dextromethorphan in children over the age 12 years is 30 mg every six to eight hours up to a maximum dose of 120 µg/24 hours. The adult recommended dose of memantine is 5 mg/24 hours, up to a maximum dose of 20 mg/24 hours. Future studies are needed to demonstrate the efficacy and safety of botulinum toxins for pediatric tension headache and other complementary therapies of magnesium, riboflavin, feverfew, and butterbur.[112][V]

Table 44.6 Anticonvulsants: recommended oral dosing.

Anticonvulsant	Recommended dose
Carbamazepine	5–10 mg/kg/24 hours divided into two doses; incremental increase of 10 mg/kg/24 hours per week; maximum dose for children over the age of 12 years is 1.6–2.4 g/24 hours
Oxcarbazepine	For children over the age of 12 years, dose is 300–600 mg/24 hours; maximum dose 900–2400 mg/24 hours
Phenytoin	2–3 mg/kg divided into two to three doses per day, incremental increase of 0.5 mg/kg every 3–4 weeks; maximum dose 5 mg/kg per day (1000 mg per day)
Valproic acid	5–15 mg/kg administered in a single night-time dose or three divided doses per day; incremental increase of 5–10 mg/kg every 5–7 days; maximum dose 60 mg/kg/day
Gabapentin	5–10 mg/kg administered either once, twice, or three times a day; maximum dose 2400–3600 mg/24 hours
Lamotrigine	0.15–0.6 mg/kg/24 hours administered in a single night-time dose or twice-a-day divided dose; slow incremental increase every 2 weeks
Levetiracetam	10 mg/kg/24 hours, prescribed in twice-a-day divided doses
Topiramate	1–3 mg/kg/24 hours; maximum dose 600 mg/24 hours
Zonisamide	2–4 mg/kg/24 hours; maximum dose 400 mg/24 hours

Nonpharmacologic therapies

Unencumbered by significant side effects and efficacious, nonpharmacologic therapies are highly recommended in the treatment of both acute and chronic pediatric headaches. Such modalities include biofeedback with relaxation and cognitive-behavioral therapies and may modify the multiple factors that trigger and/or exacerbate the migraine headaches and disability cycle.[113][I] Less information is currently available for acupuncture and alternative medicine therapies.[114][II], [115][III]

FUNCTIONAL ABDOMINAL PAIN

Another frequent complaint in children is functional abdominal pain (FAP). FAP is a broad category of functional diagnostic entities, taking the place of recurrent abdominal pain (RAP).[116][V] The newest criteria for pediatric functional gastrointestinal disorders define a broad FAP category and include diagnoses, such as functional dyspepsia, irritable bowel syndrome (IBS), and abdominal migraine.[117][V] Because these definitions are relatively new, the majority of research has used the traditional RAP label and definition. Thus, the research described below applies to FAP as a general category.

Prevalence

Between 4 and 25 percent of school-age children complain of abdominal pain severe enough to interfere with daily activities.[118][IV], [119][V], [120][IV] There appears to be an increase in prevalence in children aged four to six years and again in early adolescence,[121][IV], [122][IV] with a higher prevalence in females, particularly after the age of 12 years.[123][V] There is also a higher prevalence of FAP in locations with more social stressors,[119][V], [124][IV] indicating a strong psychosocial component. The majority of children with FAP probably have IBS and many children with abdominal pain without the hallmark symptom of altered bowel habit may develop this over time (for review, see Ref. 125).

Between 30 and 60 percent of these children will likely experience symptom remission.[123][V], [126][V] Long-term follow-up studies have noted, however, that children with FAP are more likely to report abdominal pain several years after evaluation than healthy controls[127][V]and may be at greater risk of developing psychiatric disorders.[128][V] The continuation of pain in children with FAP is associated with psychological distress,[129][IV] family members with irritable bowel syndrome,[130][IV] and high levels of healthcare utilization.[131][II]

Diagnosis

Organic causes are rarely found in FAP, only about 10 percent of these children are diagnosed with pain that is not functional. Warning signs that need to be investigated include:[132][V], [133][V]

- involuntary weight loss;
- deceleration of linear growth;
- gastrointestinal blood loss;
- significant vomiting;
- chronic severe diarrhea;
- persistent right upper or right lower quadrant pain;
- unexplained fever;
- family history of inflammatory bowel disease;
- pain far from umbilicus;
- pain awakening the child at night;
- nocturnal diarrhea;
- dysuria.

These warning signs are generally absent in FAP, and the subcategories of FAP have specific positive symptom criteria that should be applied for diagnostic purposes. FAP is not the "wastebasket diagnosis" it is often thought to be, but rather a broad diagnostic category with specific syndrome subsets.[132][V]

Psychological symptoms

FAP has been associated with elevated anxiety and depression;[134][IV], [135][IV] however, the presence of abdominal pain, regardless of identification of a functional or organic problem, is associated with increased levels of distress.[136][IV] Stressful life events and/or a lack of coping skills are triggers of symptom flares in both irritable bowel syndrome and inflammatory bowel disease.[137][IV]

Psychological issues need to be assessed in FAP; however, the simplistic view that these issues are responsible for the pain is no longer an acceptable conclusion. An interactive biopsychosocial model is currently employed to understand FAP. An underlying abnormal bowel reactivity to physiological changes, such as gut distension, inflammatory processes, as well as the physiological changes associated with psychological stressors is likely taking place in these patients.[132][V]

Psychological symptoms are associated with the presence of pain, regardless of diagnosis; however, functional status and parental psychological symptoms appear to be strongly related to treatment-seeking behavior. Levy *et al.* identified maternal psychopathology as a significant factor in treatment seeking for FAP[138][II] and treatment seekers are significantly more likely to be missing school than nontreatment seekers.[139][II] Disability may depend on the ability of the child's parents to facilitate school attendance rather than any specific characteristic of the pain or the child.

Treatment

The traditional treatment of choice for FAP has been support and reassurance that no organic pathology exists and that the child will likely improve with time. This approach tends to fare no better than no treatment at all for children with FAP because of the relatively high remission rate (see Ref. 140 for review).

Many different categories of medication are used clinically in the treatment of FAP and antidepressants, in particular, are frequently used.[141][V] A recent Cochrane review concluded that there is little evidence to support the use of pharmacology in FAP outside clinical trials.[142][II]

There are currently only two published controlled medication trials in children with FAP. See *et al.*[143][II] conducted a double-blind placebo-controlled crossover trial of famotidine in 25 children with dyspepsia and found that the medication trial was associated with significant improvement in the dyspeptic symptoms; however, pain ratings were no different between the trials. Symon *et al.*[144][II] conducted a double-blind crossover placebo-controlled trial of pizotifen syrup in 14 children diagnosed with abdominal migraine. The medication trial was associated with less pain frequency and severity than the placebo trial. Thus, specific medications do show some promise in the treatment of FAP subtypes; however, there is a dearth of information regarding popularly utilized medications, such as antidepressants.

Clinically, children and parents often associate their FAP symptoms with specific foods, and eating is frequently cited as a pain trigger. Lactose intolerance is a potential cause of RAP and is worth investigation in children with a potential predisposition; however, a positive test result and elimination of lactose from the diet is not necessarily associated with pain relief.[145][II] Sorbital malabsorption has similarly been cited as a potential cause of chronic abdominal pain.[146][V]

It is relatively easy and economical to maintain food diaries that may assist in determining the relationship between specific foods, mealtimes, and pain. Many families will initiate dietary restrictions or food challenges on their own. It is not uncommon to find at least a clinical relationship between greasy foods and/or large meals and altered bowel habits. If the child has constipation, the inclusion of fiber supplements or increasing dietary fiber has been demonstrated to be effective.[147][II]

Unfortunately, very little evidence exists to support the role of most dietary treatments in FAP.[148][I] Despite the common associations made between specific foods and FAP, there are few investigations regarding dietary restrictions in these syndromes, and there is often a strong placebo response in controlled studies of dietary change. In one promising study, peppermint oil supplementation was investigated for use in children with irritable bowel syndrome.[149][II] Seventy-six percent of patients who received peppermint oil reported decreases in the severity of symptoms, compared with only 19 percent who received placebo.

The majority of research in the treatment of FAP has been focused on psychological treatment, specifically cognitive-behavioral therapy, that is designed to teach coping skills and relaxation, as well as to teach the parents to reinforce healthy functional behavior. Such treatments generally report good results.

Sanders and colleagues[150][I] conducted a controlled study of CBT in 16 children with recurrent abdominal pain consisting of stress management and parent training. Both groups reported symptom improvement; however, 75 percent of the treated group became pain-free compared to 25 percent of the controls. In a second study, Sanders *et al.*[151][I] randomized 44 children with RAP into CBT or standard assurance treatment. Again both groups showed a significant pain decrease; however, over half the patients receiving CBT were reportedly pain free at posttreatment compared to 23.8 percent of controls. Improvement was maintained at 12 months.

In a more recent study, Robins *et al.*[152][I] randomized 69 children into standard medical follow up or CBT and standard medical groups. The CBT treatment consisted of relaxation training, problem-solving training related to pain symptoms, and parent training. Significantly less pain and school absences were found in the CBT group compared to controls, and improvement was maintained one year later.

Continued research is clearly necessary; however, in general, the use of psychological therapies can be considered probably useful in the treatment of FAP. The above studies utilized the following elements in their active treatments:

- relaxation training;
- cognitive-behavioral stress management;
- parent training to address reinforcement of symptoms and sick role.

Other psychology-based treatment elements described in the research literature show promise, but have not been investigated as thoroughly. These include:

- self-hypnosis training;[153][IV]
- biofeedback.[154][II]

Other treatment options

Several other treatment options are available for the child with FAP; however, little is known about the efficacy of most. Acupuncture has been increasingly utilized; however, the one controlled study assessing acupuncture in adults with irritable bowel syndrome[155][II] reported no significant differences between groups treated with true versus sham acupuncture. Reflexology massage, similarly investigated in adult IBS patients, has demonstrated no clear benefit.[156][IV] Mechanical treatment through the use of transcutaneous electrical nerve stimulation is also often clinically used,[157][V] but has not been researched in a controlled manner.

Conclusions

Despite an increase in interest in FAP by researchers in recent years, there are few well-researched options for treatment. The most progress has been made in refining and developing diagnostic criteria to establish subtypes of FAP that are defined by specific symptoms. Pharmacological research has been disappointing in this area and diet treatments, while having a certain amount of face validity, also remain questionable. Treatments that have the most promise are the psychologically based ones with cognitive-behavioral approaches that incorporate parent training.

REFERENCES

1. Hunfeld JA, Perquin CW, Duivenvoorden HJ *et al.* Chronic pain and its impact on quality of life in adolescents and their families. *Journal of Pediatric Psychology.* 2001; **26**: 145–53.
2. Perquin CW, Hazebroek-Kampschreur AA, Hunfeld JA *et al.* Chronic pain among children and adolescents: physician consultation and medication use. *Clinical Journal of Pain.* 2000; **16**: 229–35.
3. Mulder EJ, Van Baal C, Gaist D *et al.* Genetic and environmental influences on migraine: a twin study across six countries. *Twin Research.* 2003; **6**: 422–31.
4. * Bursch B, Walco GA, Zeltzer L. Clinical assessment and management of chronic pain and pain-associated disability syndrome. *Journal of Developmental and Behavioral Pediatrics.* 1998; **19**: 45–53.
5. * Coderre TJ, Melzack R. The contribution of excitatory amino acids to central sensitization and persistent nociception after formalin-induced tissue injury. *Journal of Neuroscience.* 1992; **12**: 3665–70.
6. * Pockett S. Spinal cord synaptic plasticity and chronic pain. *Anesthesia and Analgesia.* 1995; **80**: 173–9.
7. * McGrath PA. Chronic pain in children. In: Crombie IK (ed.). *Epidemiology of pain.* Seattle: IASP Press, 1999: 81–101.
8. Mikkelsson M, Salminen JJ, Kautiainen H. Non-specific musculoskeletal pain in preadolescents. Prevalence and 1-year persistence. *Pain.* 1997; **73**: 29–35.
9. McGrath PA, Speechley KN, Seifert CE *et al.* A survey of children's acute, recurrent, and chronic pain: validation of the pain experience interview. *Pain.* 2000; **87**: 59–73.
10. Perquin CW, Hunfeld JA, Hazebroek-Kampschreur AA *et al.* The natural course of chronic benign pain in childhood and adolescence: a two-year population-based follow-up study. *European Journal of Pain.* 2003; **7**: 551–9.
11. Groholt EK, Stigum H, Nordhagen R, Kohler L. Recurrent pain in children, socio-economic factors and accumulation in families. *European Journal of Epidemiology.* 2003; **18**: 965–75.
12. Peveler R, Kilkenny L, Kinmonth AL. Medically unexplained physical symptoms in primary care: a comparison of self-report screening questionnaires and clinical opinion. *Journal of Psychosomatic Research.* 1997; **42**: 245–52.
13. Hamilton J, Campos R, Creed F. Anxiety, depression and management of medically unexplained symptoms in medical clinics. *Journal of the Royal College of Physicians of London.* 1996; **30**: 18–20.
14. Eccleston C, Malleson PN, Clinch J *et al.* Chronic pain in adolescents: evaluation of a programme of interdisciplinary cognitive behaviour therapy. *Archives of Disease in Childhood.* 2003; **88**: 881–5.
15. Schappert SM, Nelson C. National ambulatory medical care survey: 1995–96 summary. *Vital and Health Statistics*, Series 13. 1999; **10**: i–vi, 1–122.
16. McGhee JL, Burks FN, Sheckels JL, Jarvis JN. Identifying children with chronic arthritis based on chief complaints: absence of predictive value for musculoskeletal pain as an

indicator of rheumatic disease in children. *Pediatrics.* 2002; **110**: 354–9.

17. Konijnenberg AY, De Graeff-Meeder ER, Kimpen JL *et al.* Children with unexplained chronic pain: do pediatricians agree regarding the diagnostic approach and presumed primary cause? *Pediatrics.* 2004; **114**: 1220–6.
* 18. Malleson PN, Beauchamp RD. Rheumatology: 16. Diagnosing musculoskeletal pain in children. *Canadian Medical Association Journal.* 2001; **165**: 183–8.
* 19. Scharff L, Langan N, Rotter N *et al.* Psychological, behavioral, and family characteristics of pediatric patients with chronic pain: a 1-year retrospective study and cluster analysis. *Clinical Journal of Pain.* 2005; **21**: 432–8.
20. Fanurik D, Koh JL, Schmitz ML *et al.* Children with cognitive impairment: parent report of pain and coping. *Journal of Developmental and Behavioral Pediatrics.* 1999; **20**: 228–34.
21. Mikkelsson M, Sourander A, Piha J, Salminen JJ. Psychiatric symptoms in preadolescents with musculoskeletal pain and fibromyalgia. *Pediatrics.* 1997; **100**: 220–7.
22. Jones GT, Silman AJ, Macfarlane GJ. Predicting the onset of widespread body pain among children. *Arthritis and Rheumatism.* 2003; **48**: 2615–21.
23. Yunus MB, Masi AT. Juvenile primary fibromyalgia syndrome. A clinical study of thirty-three patients and matched normal controls. *Arthritis and Rheumatism.* 1985; **28**: 138–45.
24. Wolfe F, Smythe HA, Yunus MB *et al.* The American College of Rheumatology 1990 criteria for the classification of fibromyalgia. Report of the Multicenter Criteria Committee. *Arthritis and Rheumatism.* 1990; **33**: 160–72.
25. Gedalia A, Garcia CO, Molina JF *et al.* Fibromyalgia syndrome: experience in a pediatric rheumatology clinic. *Clinical and Experimental Rheumatology.* 2000; **18**: 415–9.
26. Siegel DM, Janeway D, Baum J. Fibromyalgia syndrome in children and adolescents: clinical features at presentation and status at follow-up. *Pediatrics.* 1998; **101**: 377–82.
* 27. Katz RS, Wolfe F, Michaud K. Fibromyalgia diagnosis: a comparison of clinical, survey, and American College of Rheumatology criteria. *Arthritis and Rheumatism.* 2006; **54**: 169–76.
28. Gedalia A, Press J, Klein M, Buskila D. Joint hypermobility and fibromyalgia in schoolchildren. *Annals of the Rheumatic Diseases.* 1993; **52**: 494–6.
* 29. Price DD, Staud R. Neurobiology of fibromyalgia syndrome. *Journal of Rheumatology. Supplement.* 2005; **75**: 22–8.
30. Roizenblatt S, Tufik S, Goldenberg J *et al.* Juvenile fibromyalgia: clinical and polysomnographic aspects. *Journal of Rheumatology.* 1997; **24**: 579–85.
31. Tayag-Kier CE, Keenan GF, Scalzi LV *et al.* Sleep and periodic limb movement in sleep in juvenile fibromyalgia. *Pediatrics.* 2000; **106**: E70.
32. Buskila D, Neumann L, Hazanov I, Carmi R. Familial aggregation in the fibromyalgia syndrome. *Seminars in Arthritis and Rheumatism.* 1996; **26**: 605–11.
33. Walco GA, Ilowite NT. Cognitive-behavioral intervention for juvenile primary fibromyalgia syndrome. *Journal of Rheumatology.* 1992; **19**: 1617–9.
34. Vandvik IH, Forseth KO. A bio-psychosocial evaluation of ten adolescents with fibromyalgia. *Acta Paediatrica.* 1994; **83**: 766–71.
35. Reid GJ, Lang BA, McGrath PJ. Primary juvenile fibromyalgia: psychological adjustment, family functioning, coping, and functional disability. *Arthritis and Rheumatism.* 1997; **40**: 752–60.
36. Buskila D, Neumann L, Hershman E *et al.* Fibromyalgia syndrome in children – an outcome study. *Journal of Rheumatology.* 1995; **22**: 525–8.
37. Romano TJ. Fibromyalgia in children; diagnosis and treatment. *West Virginia Medical Journal.* 1991; **87**: 112–4.
38. Degotardi PJ, Klass ES, Rosenberg BS *et al.* Development and evaluation of a cognitive-behavioral intervention for juvenile fibromyalgia. *Journal of Pediatric Psychology.* 2006; **31**: 714–23.
* 39. Stanton-Hicks M, Janig W, Hassenbusch S *et al.* Reflex sympathetic dystrophy: changing concepts and taxonomy. *Pain.* 1995; **63**: 127–33.
40. Bruehl S, Harden RN, Galer BS *et al.* External validation of IASP diagnostic criteria for complex regional pain syndrome and proposed research diagnostic criteria. International Association for the Study of Pain. *Pain.* 1999; **81**: 147–54.
41. Harden RN, Bruehl S, Galer BS *et al.* Complex regional pain syndrome: are the IASP diagnostic criteria valid and sufficiently comprehensive? *Pain.* 1999; **83**: 211–9.
42. Galer BS, Bruehl S, Harden RN. IASP diagnostic criteria for complex regional pain syndrome: a preliminary empirical validation study. International Association for the Study of Pain. *Clinical Journal of Pain.* 1998; **14**: 48–54.
43. van de Vusse AC, Stomp-van den Berg SG, de Vet HC, Weber WE. Interobserver reliability of diagnosis in patients with complex regional pain syndrome. *European Journal of Pain.* 2003; **7**: 259–65.
44. Wilder RT, Berde CB, Wolohan M *et al.* Reflex sympathetic dystrophy in children. Clinical characteristics and follow-up of seventy patients. *Journal of Bone and Joint Surgery. American Volume.* 1992; **74**: 910–9.
45. Bernstein BH, Singsen BH, Kent JT *et al.* Reflex neurovascular dystrophy in childhood. *Journal of Pediatrics.* 1978; **93**: 211–5.
46. Maleki J, LeBel AA, Bennett GJ, Schwartzman RJ. Patterns of spread in complex regional pain syndrome, type I (reflex sympathetic dystrophy). *Pain.* 2000; **88**: 259–66.
47. Sethna NF, Meier PM, Zurakowski D, Berde CB. Cutaneous sensory abnormalities in children and adolescents with complex regional pain syndromes. *Pain.* 2007; **131**: 153–61.
48. van der Laan L, ter Laak HJ, Gabreels-Festen A *et al.* Complex regional pain syndrome type I (RSD): pathology of skeletal muscle and peripheral nerve. *Neurology.* 1998; **51**: 20–5.

49. Oyen WJ, Arntz IE, Claessens RM *et al.* Reflex sympathetic dystrophy of the hand: an excessive inflammatory response? *Pain.* 1993; **55**: 151–7.
50. Wasner G, Schattschneider J, Heckmann K *et al.* Vascular abnormalities in reflex sympathetic dystrophy (CRPS I): mechanisms and diagnostic value. *Brain.* 2001; **124**: 587–99.
51. Wasner G, Heckmann K, Maier C, Baron R. Vascular abnormalities in acute reflex sympathetic dystrophy (CRPS I): complete inhibition of sympathetic nerve activity with recovery. *Archives of Neurology.* 1999; **56**: 613–20.
52. Galer BS, Butler S, Jensen MP. Case reports and hypothesis: a neglect-like syndrome may be responsible for the motor disturbance in reflex sympathetic dystrophy (complex regional pain syndrome-1). *Journal of Pain and Symptom Management.* 1995; **10**: 385–91.
53. Kemler MA, van de Vusse AC, van den Berg-Loonen EM *et al.* HLA-DQ1 associated with reflex sympathetic dystrophy. *Neurology.* 1999; **53**: 1350–1.
54. Mailis A, Wade J. Profile of Caucasian women with possible genetic predisposition to reflex sympathetic dystrophy: a pilot study. *Clinical Journal of Pain.* 1994; **10**: 210–7.
55. Rommel O, Malin JP, Zenz M, Janig W. Quantitative sensory testing, neurophysiological and psychological examination in patients with complex regional pain syndrome and hemisensory deficits. *Pain.* 2001; **93**: 279–93.
56. Thimineur M, Sood P, Kravitz E *et al.* Central nervous system abnormalities in complex regional pain syndrome (CRPS): clinical and quantitative evidence of medullary dysfunction. *Clinical Journal of Pain.* 1998; **14**: 256–67.
57. Eisenberg E, Chistyakov AV, Yudashkin M *et al.* Evidence for cortical hyperexcitability of the affected limb representation area in CRPS: a psychophysical and transcranial magnetic stimulation study. *Pain.* 2005; **113**: 99–105.
58. Sherry DD, Weisman R. Psychologic aspects of childhood reflex neurovascular dystrophy. *Pediatrics.* 1988; **81**: 572–8.
59. Ochoa JL, Verdugo RJ. Reflex sympathetic dystrophy. A common clinical avenue for somatoform expression. *Neurologic Clinics.* 1995; **13**: 351–63.
* 60. Lynch ME. Psychological aspects of reflex sympathetic dystrophy: a review of the adult and paediatric literature. *Pain.* 1992; **49**: 337–47.
61. Guler-Uysal F, Basaran S, Geertzen JH, Goncu K. A 2 1/2-year-old girl with reflex sympathetic dystrophy syndrome (CRPS type I): case report. *Clinical Rehabilitation.* 2003; **17**: 224–7.
62. Stanton RP, Malcolm JR, Wesdock KA, Singsen BH. Reflex sympathetic dystrophy in children: an orthopedic perspective. *Orthopedics.* 1993; **16**: 773–9; discussion 9–80.
63. Lee BH, Scharff L, Sethna NF *et al.* Physical therapy and cognitive-behavioral treatment for complex regional pain syndromes. *Journal of Pediatrics.* 2002; **141**: 135–40.
* 64. Sethna NF. Complex regional pain syndromes I and II (reflex sympathetic dystrophy, causalgia). In: Jones HR, De Vivo DC, Darras BT (eds). *Neuromuscular disorders of infancy, childhood, and adolescence. A clinician's approach.* New York: Butterworth Heinemann, 2003: 1185–96.
* 65. Sethna NF. Pharmacotherapy in long-term pain: Current experience and future direction. In: McGrath P, Finley A (eds). *Chronic and recurrent pain in children and adolescents, progress in pain research and management.* Seattle: IASP, 1999: 243–66.
* 66. Wilens TE, Biederman J, Baldessarini RJ *et al.* Cardiovascular effects of therapeutic doses of tricyclic antidepressants in children and adolescents. *Journal of the American Academy of Child and Adolescent Psychiatry.* 1996; **35**: 1491–501.
67. Mellick GA, Mellick LB. Reflex sympathetic dystrophy treated with gabapentin. *Archives of Physical Medicine and Rehabilitation.* 1997; **78**: 98–105.
68. Rusy LM, Troshynski TJ, Weisman SJ. Gabapentin in phantom limb pain management in children and young adults: report of seven cases. *Journal of Pain and Symptom Management.* 2001; **21**: 78–82.
69. van de Vusse AC, Stomp-van den Berg SG, Kessels AH, Weber WE. Randomised controlled trial of gabapentin in complex regional pain syndrome type 1 [ISRCTN84121379]. *BMC Neurology.* 2004; **4**: 13.
70. Christensen K, Jensen EM, Noer I. The reflex dystrophy syndrome response to treatment with systemic corticosteroids. *Acta Chirurgica Scandinavica.* 1982; **148**: 653–5.
71. Ghostine SY, Comair YG, Turner DM *et al.* Phenoxybenzamine in the treatment of causalgia. Report of 40 cases. *Journal of Neurosurgery.* 1984; **60**: 1263–8.
72. Davis KD, Treede RD, Raja SN *et al.* Topical application of clonidine relieves hyperalgesia in patients with sympathetically maintained pain. *Pain.* 1991; **47**: 309–17.
73. Devers A, Galer BS. Topical lidocaine patch relieves a variety of neuropathic pain conditions: an open-label study. *Clinical Journal of Pain.* 2000; **16**: 205–8.
74. Scadding JW, Wall PD, Parry CB, Brooks DM. Clinical trial of propranolol in post-traumatic neuralgia. *Pain.* 1982; **14**: 283–92.
75. Bickerstaff DR, Kanis JA. The use of nasal calcitonin in the treatment of post-traumatic algodystrophy. *British Journal of Rheumatology.* 1991; **30**: 291–4.
* 76. Schwartzman RJ, Kerrigan J. The movement disorder of reflex sympathetic dystrophy. *Neurology.* 1990; **40**: 57–61.
* 77. Nelson DV, Stacey BR. Interventional therapies in the management of complex regional pain syndrome. *Clinical Journal of Pain.* 2006; **22**: 438–42.
78. Hogan QH, Erickson SJ, Haddox JD, Abram SE. The spread of solutions during stellate ganglion block. *Regional Anesthesia.* 1992; **17**: 78–83.
79. Cooper DE, DeLee JC, Ramamurthy S. Reflex sympathetic dystrophy of the knee. Treatment using continuous

epidural anesthesia. *Journal of Bone and Joint Surgery. American Volume.* 1989; **71**: 365–9.
80. Doolan LA, Brown TC. Reflex sympathetic dystrophy in a child. *Anaesthesia and Intensive Care.* 1984; **12**: 70–2.
81. Okada T, Maeda M, Takechi T *et al.* Reflex sympathetic dystrophy in childhood: a case report. *Acta Paediatrica Japan.* 1997; **39**: 690–3.
82. Dadure C, Motais F, Ricard C *et al.* Continuous peripheral nerve blocks at home for treatment of recurrent complex regional pain syndrome I in children. *Anesthesiology.* 2005; **102**: 387–91.
83. Hassenbusch SJ, Stanton-Hicks M, Schoppa D *et al.* Long-term results of peripheral nerve stimulation for reflex sympathetic dystrophy. *Journal of Neurosurgery.* 1996; **84**: 415–23.
84. van Hilten BJ, van de Beek WJ, Hoff JI *et al.* Intrathecal baclofen for the treatment of dystonia in patients with reflex sympathetic dystrophy. *New England Journal of Medicine.* 2000; **343**: 625–30.
85. Kemler MA, Barendse GA, van Kleef M *et al.* Spinal cord stimulation in patients with chronic reflex sympathetic dystrophy. *New England Journal of Medicine.* 2000; **343**: 618–24.
86. Mailis A, Furlan A. Sympathectomy for neuropathic pain. *Cochrane Database of Systematic Reviews.* 2003; **CD002918**.
87. Turner JA, Loeser JD, Deyo RA, Sanders SB. Spinal cord stimulation for patients with failed back surgery syndrome or complex regional pain syndrome: a systematic review of effectiveness and complications. *Pain.* 2004; **108**: 137–47.
88. Rush PJ, Wilmot D, Saunders N *et al.* Severe reflex neurovascular dystrophy in childhood. *Arthritis and Rheumatism.* 1985; **28**: 952–6.
89. Dangel T. Chronic pain management in children. Part II: Reflex sympathetic dystrophy. *Paediatric Anaesthesia.* 1998; **8**: 105–12.
90. Lloyd-Thomas AR, Lauder G. Lesson of the week. Reflex sympathetic dystrophy in children. *BMJ.* 1995; **310**: 1648–9.
91. Sherry DD, Wallace CA, Kelley C *et al.* Short- and long-term outcomes of children with complex regional pain syndrome type I treated with exercise therapy. *Clinical Journal of Pain.* 1999; **15**: 218–23.
92. Billie BS. Migraine in school children. A study of the incidence and short-term prognosis, and a clinical, psychological and electroencephalographic comparison between children with migraine and matched controls. *Acta Paediatrica Supplement.* 1962; **136**: 1–151.
93. McGrath PA, Speechley KN, Seifert CE *et al.* A survey of children's acute, recurrent, and chronic pain: validation of the pain experience interview. *Pain.* 2000; **87**: 59–73.
94. Konijnenberg AY, Uiterwaal CS, Kimpen JL *et al.* Children with unexplained chronic pain: substantial impairment in everyday life. *Archives of Disease in Childhood.* 2005; **90**: 680–6.
* 95. Lewis DW, Ashwal S, Dahl G *et al.* Practice parameter: evaluation of children and adolescents with recurrent headaches: report of the Quality Standards Subcommittee of the American Academy of Neurology and the Practice Committee of the Child Neurology Society. *Neurology.* 2002; **59**: 490–8.
96. Stewart WF, Linet MS, Celentano DD *et al.* Age- and sex-specific incidence rates of migraine with and without visual aura. *American Journal of Epidemiology.* 1991; **134**: 1111–20.
97. Barlow CF. Migraine in the infant and toddler. *Journal of Child Neurology.* 1994; **9**: 92–4.
* 98. Anonymous. The international classification of headache disorders. 2nd edn. *Cephalalgia.* 2004; **24**: 9–160.
* 99. Al-Twaijri WA, Shevell MI. Pediatric migraine equivalents: occurrence and clinical features in practice. *Pediatric Neurology.* 2002; **26**: 365–8.
100. Montagna P. Molecular genetics of migraine headaches: a review. *Cephalalgia.* 2000; **20**: 3–14.
101. Lewis D, Ashwal S, Hershey A *et al.* Practice parameter: pharmacological treatment of migraine headache in children and adolescents: report of the American Academy of Neurology Quality Standards Subcommittee and the Practice Committee of the Child Neurology Society. *Neurology.* 2004; **63**: 2215–24.
102. Silberstein SD. Practice parameter: evidence-based guidelines for migraine headache (an evidence-based review): report of the Quality Standards Subcommittee of the American Academy of Neurology. *Neurology.* 2000; **55**: 754–62.
103. Ahonen K, Hamalainen ML, Rantala H, Hoppu K. Nasal sumatriptan is effective in treatment of migraine attacks in children: A randomized trial. *Neurology.* 2004; **62**: 883–7.
104. Ahonen K, Hamalainen ML, Eerola M, Hoppu K. A randomized trial of rizatriptan in migraine attacks in children. *Neurology.* 2006; **67**: 1135–40.
*105. Tepper SJ, Rapoport AM, Sheftell FD. Mechanisms of action of the 5-HT1B/1D receptor agonists. *Archives of Neurology.* 2002; **59**: 1084–8.
106. Hamalainen ML, Hoppu K, Valkeila E, Santavuori P. Ibuprofen or acetaminophen for the acute treatment of migraine in children: a double-blind, randomized, placebo-controlled, crossover study. *Neurology.* 1997; **48**: 103–7.
107. Kelley MT, Walson PD, Edge JH *et al.* Pharmacokinetics and pharmacodynamics of ibuprofen isomers and acetaminophen in febrile children. *Clinical Pharmacology and Therapeutics.* 1992; **52**: 181–9.
108. Dsida RM, Wheeler M, Birmingham PK *et al.* Age-stratified pharmacokinetics of ketorolac tromethamine in pediatric surgical patients. *Anesthesia and Analgesia.* 2002; **94**: 266–70.
109. Cete Y, Dora B, Ertan C *et al.* A randomized prospective placebo-controlled study of intravenous magnesium sulphate vs. metoclopramide in the management of acute migraine attacks in the Emergency Department. *Cephalalgia.* 2005; **25**: 199–204.
110. Silberstein SD, Freitag FG, Rozen TD *et al.* Tramadol/acetaminophen for the treatment of acute migraine pain:

findings of a randomized, placebo-controlled trial. *Headache.* 2005; **45**: 1317–27.
111. Victor S. Drugs for preventing migraine headache in children. *Cochrane Database of Systematic Reviews.* 2003; **CD002761**.
112. Tepper SJ, Bigal ME, Sheftell FD, Rapoport AM. Botulinum neurotoxin type A in the preventive treatment of refractory headache: a review of 100 consecutive cases. *Headache.* 2004; **44**: 794–800.
113. Eccleston C, Yorke L, Morley S *et al.* Psychological therapies for the management of chronic and recurrent pain in children and adolescents. *Cochrane Database of Systematic Reviews.* 2003; **CD003968**.
114. Diener HC, Kronfeld K, Boewing G *et al.* Efficacy of acupuncture for the prophylaxis of migraine: a multicentre randomised controlled clinical trial. *Lancet Neurology.* 2006; **5**: 310–6.
115. Scharff LMD, Masek BJ. A controlled study of minimal-contact thermal biofeedback treatment in children with migraine. *Journal of Pediatric Psychology.* 2002; **27**: 109–19.
116. Apley J. The child with recurrent abdominal pain. *Pediatric Clinics of North America.* 1967; **14**: 63–72.
117. Rasquin A, Di Lorenzo C, Forbes D *et al.* Childhood functional gastrointestinal disorders: child/adolescent. *Gastroenterology.* 2006; **130**: 1527–37.
118. Apley J, Naish N. Recurrent abdominal pains: A field study of 1,000 schoolchildren. *Archives of Disease in Childhood.* 1958; **33**: 165–70.
119. Faull C, Nicol AR. Abdominal pain in six-year-olds: An epidemiological study in a new town. *Journal of Child Psychology and Psychiatry and Allied Disciplines.* 1986; **27**: 251–60.
120. Malaty HM, Abudayyeh S, O'Malley KJ *et al.* Development of a multidimensional measure for recurrent abdominal pain in children: population-based studies in three settings. *Pediatrics.* 2005; **115**: e210–5.
121. Chitkara DK, Rawat DJ, Talley NJ. The epidemiology of childhood recurrent abdominal pain in Western countries: a systematic review. *American Journal of Gastroenterology.* 2005; **100**: 1868–75.
122. Ramchandani PG, Hotopf M, Sandhu B, Stein A. The epidemiology of recurrent abdominal pain from 2 to 6 years of age: results of a large, population-based study. *Pediatrics.* 2005; **116**: 46–50.
123. Stickler GB, Murphy DB. Recurrent abdominal pain. *American Journal of Diseases of Childhood.* 1979; **133**: 486–9.
124. Alfven G. The covariation of common psychosomatic symptoms among children from socio-economically differing residential areas. An epidemiological study. *Acta Paediatrica.* 1993; **82**: 484–7.
125. Burke P, Elliott M, Fleissner R. Irritable bowel syndrome and recurrent abdominal pain. A comparative review. *Psychosomatics.* 1999; **40**: 277–85.
126. Bury RG. A study of 111 children with recurrent abdominal pain. *Australian Paediatric Journal.* 1987; **24**: 117–9.
127. Walker LS, Garber J, Van Slyke DA, Greene JW. Long-term health outcomes in patients with recurrent abdominal pain. (Special Issue: Pediatric chronic conditions). *Journal of Pediatric Psychology.* 1995; **20**: 233–45.
128. Campo JV, Di Lorenzo C, Chiappetta L *et al.* Adult outcomes of pediatric recurrent abdominal pain: do they just grow out of it? *Pediatrics.* 2001; **108**: E1.
129. Mulvaney S, Lambert EW, Garber J, Walker LS. Trajectories of symptoms and impairment for pediatric patients with functional abdominal pain: a 5-year longitudinal study. *Journal of the American Academy of Child and Adolescent Psychiatry.* 2006; **45**: 737–44.
130. Pace F, Zuin G, Di Giacomo S *et al.* Family history of irritable bowel syndrome is the major determinant of persistent abdominal complaints in young adults with a history of pediatric recurrent abdominal pain. *World Journal of Gastroenterology.* 2006; **12**: 3874–7.
131. Lindley KJ, Glaser D, Milla PJ. Consumerism in healthcare can be detrimental to child health: lessons from children with functional abdominal pain. *Archives of Disease in Childhood.* 2005; **90**: 335–7.
132. Subcommittee on Chronic Abdominal Pain. Chronic abdominal pain in children. *Pediatrics.* 2005; **115**: 212–815.
133. Scharff L, Leichtner AM, Rappaport LA. Recurrent abdominal pain. In: Schechter NL, Berde CB, Yaster M (eds). *Pain in infants, children, and adolescents,* 2nd edn. New York: Lippincott Williams & Wilkins, 2002: 719–31.
134. Hodges K, Kline JJ, Barbero G, Woodruff C. Anxiety in children with recurrent abdominal pain and their parents. *Psychosomatics.* 1985; **26**: 859–66.
135. Campo JV, Bridge J, Ehmann M *et al.* Recurrent abdominal pain, anxiety, and depression in primary care. *Pediatrics.* 2004; **113**: 817–24.
136. Walker LS, Greene JW. Children with recurrent abdominal pain and their parents: More somatic complaints, anxiety, and depression than other patient families? *Journal of Pediatric Psychology.* 1989; **14**: 231–43.
137. Jones MP, Wessinger S, Crowell MD. Coping strategies and interpersonal support in patients with irritable bowel syndrome and inflammatory bowel disease. *Clinical Gastroenterology and Hepatology.* 2006; **4**: 474–81.
138. Levy RL, Langer SL, Walker LS *et al.* Relationship between the decision to take a child to the clinic for abdominal pain and maternal psychological distress. *Archives of Pediatrics and Adolescent Medicine.* 2006; **160**: 961–5.
139. Venepalli NK, Van Tilburg MA, Whitehead WE. Recurrent abdominal pain: what determines medical consulting behavior? *Digestive Diseases and Sciences.* 2006; **51**: 192–201.
*140. Scharff L. Recurrent abdominal pain in children: a review of psychological factors and treatment. *Clinical Psychology Review.* 1997; **17**: 145–66.
141. Olden KW. The use of antidepressants in functional gastrointestinal disorders: new uses for old drugs. *CNS Spectrums.* 2005; **10**: 891–6.

142. Huertas-Ceballos A, Macarthur C, Logan S. Pharmacological interventions for recurrent abdominal pain (RAP) in childhood. *Cochrane Database of Systematic Reviews.* 2002; **CD003017**.
143. See MC, Birnbaum AH, Schechter CB *et al.* Double-blind, placebo-controlled trial of famotidine in children with abdominal pain and dyspepsia: global and quantitative assessment. *Digestive Diseases and Sciences.* 2001; **46**: 985–92.
144. Symon DN, Russell G. Double blind placebo controlled trial of pizotifen syrup in the treatment of abdominal migraine. *Archives of Disease in Childhood.* 1995; **72**: 48–50.
145. Barr RG, Levine MD, Watkins JB. Recurrent abdominal pain of childhood due to lactose intolerance. *New England Journal of Medicine.* 1979; **300**: 1449–52.
146. Hyams JS. Sorbitol intolerance: an unappreciated cause of functional gastrointestinal complaints. *Gastroenterology.* 1983; **84**: 30–3.
147. Feldman W, McGrath P, Hodgson C *et al.* The use of dietary fiber in the management of simple, childhood, idiopathic, recurrent, abdominal pain. Results in a prospective, double-blind, randomized, controlled trial. *American Journal of Diseases of Children.* 1985; **139**: 1216–8.
148. Huertas-Ceballos A, Macarthur C, Logan S. Dietary interventions for recurrent abdominal pain (RAP) in childhood. *Cochrane Database of Systematic Reviews.* 2002; **CD003019**.
149. Kline RM, Kline JJ, Di Palma J, Barbero GJ. Enteric-coated, pH-dependent peppermint oil capsules for the treatment of irritable bowel syndrome in children. *Journal of Pediatrics.* 2001; **138**: 125–8.
150. Sanders MR, Rebgetz M, Morrison M *et al.* Cognitive-behavioral treatment of recurrent nonspecific abdominal pain in children: An analysis of generalization, maintenance, and side effects. *Journal of Consulting and Clinical Psychology.* 1989; **57**: 294–300.
151. Sanders MR, Shepherd RW, Cleghorn G, Woolford H. The treatment of recurrent abdominal pain in children: A controlled comparison of cognitive-behavioral family intervention and standard pediatric care. *Journal of Consulting and Clinical Psychology.* 1994; **62**: 306–14.
152. Robins PM, Smith SM, Glutting JJ, Bishop CT. A randomized controlled trial of a cognitive-behavioral family intervention for pediatric recurrent abdominal pain. *Journal of Pediatric Psychology.* 2005; **30**: 397–408.
153. Anbar RD. Self-hypnosis for the treatment of functional abdominal pain in childhood. *Clinical Pediatrics.* 2001; **40**: 447–51. 2001-18302-002.
154. Humphreys PA, Gevirtz RN. Treatment of recurrent abdominal pain: components analysis of four treatment protocols. *Journal of Pediatric Gastroenterology and Nutrition.* 2000; **31**: 47–51.
155. Fireman Z, Segal A, Kopelman Y *et al.* Acupuncture treatment for irritable bowel syndrome. A double-blind controlled study. *Digestion.* 2001; **64**: 100–03.
156. Tovey P. A single-blind trial of reflexology for irritable bowel syndrome. *British Journal of General Practice.* 2002; **52**: 19–23.
157. Sylvester K, Kendall GP, Lennard-Jones JE. Treatment of functional abdominal pain by transcutaneous electrical nerve stimulation. *BMJ.* 1986; **293**: 481–2.

45

Principles of chronic pain therapy in elderly patients

JOHN HUGHES AND CHRIS DODDS

KEY LEARNING POINTS

- The elderly population is growing with up to 50 percent suffering chronic pain.
- The physiological reserve of an individual reduces with time and at the extreme of age, this limitation may become apparent as part of normal activity.
- Assessment is essential and requires adequate time as mental processing changes.
- Psychological, social, and environmental factors must be considered as part of pain management.
- Cognitive deficit is common at the extremes of age, but most patients can self-report their pain.
- Drugs can be used with good benefit at adequate dosing. Starting with a low dose and slowly titrating to effect minimizes side effects.
- Nondrug interventions are frequently beneficial.
- Pain management in the elderly provides both challenges and rewards. The process cannot be rushed and requires patience and perseverance.

INTRODUCTION

Pain in the elderly is common and poses both challenges and rewards for its management. The International Association for the Study of Pain (IASP) Global Year Against Pain in Older Persons was in 2006. There is also a summary publication by the IASP[1] as part of the Progress in Pain Research and Management series. This provides an up-to-date and comprehensive review of the issues relating to pain in the older population.

The aim of this chapter is to examine some of the key areas related to elderly pain and its management. All of us are at risk of suffering from painful conditions, with the older person having the potential to suffer from several painful conditions at once. Specific conditions are covered in Chapter 5, Epidemiology of chronic pain: classical to molecular approaches to understanding the epidemiology of pain. Here we discuss the issues specific to the older population, including epidemiology, before reviewing the physiological and psychological consequences of aging and discuss their relevance to pain management. Assessment poses particular difficulties and is a vital component of pain management. This is further complicated when the effects of cognitive deficit and dementia are considered. Our discussion of the interventions used in pain management focus on those that are of particular importance to the elderly.

EPIDEMIOLOGY

The world population continues to grow and with increasing life expectancy the older population is expected to continue increasing. The percentage of people over

65 years in 2007 varies from 3.3 percent in the least-developed countries to over 15 percent in the developed countries. The overall percentage of over 60 year olds is currently 11 percent and expected to rise to 22 percent by 2050. The fastest growing group of elderly people are those over 80 years, growing at a rate of almost 4 percent per annum.[2]

Estimates suggest that up to 50 percent of elderly adults living in the community suffer from chronic pain.[3] Thomas *et al.*,[4] looking at pain in the previous four weeks, found a prevalence of 66 percent in the older population. They show that the prevalence of some pains decrease across age groups, but those in the lower limb increase in the oldest age group, thus the overall prevalence remains similar across older age groups. They also demonstrate that pain which interferes with daily life rises with increasing age from 32 percent in 50–59-year-old women to 50 percent in the over 80 year olds. For men, the rise was from 33 to 41 percent. This work recognizes that pain has a greater impact on daily living with increasing age for those living in the community, but does not explain what factors contribute to these increases. A study from Catalonia, looking at pain in the general population (592 respondents) over 65 years, found a prevalence of any pain at 73.5 percent and for pain lasting more than three months at 71.4 percent, with both rates consistent across age groups. This study also identified low back pain, joints, and lower limb pain as causing most problems.[5] A European study involving 1520 subjects with a mean age of 82.1 years assessed nonmalignant pain present every day for the previous seven days and disability in performing activities of daily living. Approximately 46 percent of subjects reported daily pain and these subjects had a higher risk of developing disability, an association which was stronger with increased severity of pain and number of painful sites.[6]

Chronic back pain is common in the community in general and in the elderly specifically. An Italian study looking at frequent low back pain in the over 65 year age group demonstrated a prevalence of 31.5 percent, which is consistent with other studies. Interestingly, only 7.5 percent had functional limitations due to back pain and 76 percent had no back pain-related impairment.[7] A recent review of the back pain literature suggests that benign back pain prevalence reduces with increasing age, but severe back pain increases with increasing age. However, these conclusions require further research in older age groups, which is currently limited, and standardization of definitions to allow more appropriate comparisons to be made between studies.[8][IV]

Visceral pain in the elderly is reported to decline with increasing age, with one recent study reporting a prevalence in the 50–59-year age group of 11.7 percent that fell to 9.7 percent in the oldest age groups (70–79 years and >80 years).[4] This may account for delays in diagnoses and appropriate intervention in older patients with pathology, but little or no associated pain.

A large number of elderly people live in the community, but require sheltered or nursing home care. These individuals frequently have complex medical problems, as well as social issues. A significant number of nursing home residents also have varying degrees of cognitive impairment. Pain assessment and management in these settings is complex and poses challenges for the care providers. It is estimated that 45–80 percent of nursing home residents have pain that interferes with their functional ability and quality of life.[9]

Many chronic pain studies do not examine age explicitly or specifically study older age groups, so the true impact of pain for older individuals is not understood. Typically, the older population is defined as being over 60 years of age and all participants are grouped together. Few papers look specifically at the very elderly or stratify across the older age groups. This is often due to limited numbers of individuals in each older age group and the frequent presence of confounders, such as comorbidity, that make it difficult to interpret the results.

PHYSIOLOGICAL INFLUENCES

The well-documented physiological changes that occur as a result of the ageing process develop at different rates and do not strictly follow chronological age. They are further influenced by concomitant medical conditions and the polypharmacy that accompanies their management. This often means that older individuals respond less predictably than their younger counterparts as the degree of physiological change is more varied in the older population. The correlation between comorbidity and pain in the older patient[10] is associated with increased pain severity, reduced activity, and increased depressive symptoms. The physiological reserve of an individual reduces with time and at the extreme of age, this limitation may become apparent as part of normal activity. Even a minor illness, acute or chronic, may be sufficient to reduce function. Many elderly patients adapt their behavior and expectations to this failing reserve and avoid challenging their fragile physiological reserve. This may make identifying such high-risk patients very difficult from the history alone.

The elderly show altered pharmacokinetics and pharmacodynamics with regard to drug handling. For example, decreases in lean body mass influence the volume of distribution of drugs, such that maintenance doses of many pharmacological agents may need reducing. Renal function deteriorates with age and by the age of 80 years may approximate to renal insufficiency. Reductions in blood flow and glomerular filtration rate will influence drug clearance. Liver metabolism is rarely an issue in the elderly, but enzyme systems may not be as easily induced as in younger patients.

As in the larger pain literature, genetic factors contributing to pain in the elderly have begun to be investigated, but the findings to date in the elderly suggest genetic factors are not important. A study looking at the development of neck pain in the elderly failed to demonstrate a significant influence of genetic factors.[11] [IV] Similar work on back pain in the over 70 age group suggests a small genetic effect in men but not women. Significant predictors for back pain found in this latter study included previous or current diagnosis of osteoporosis, arthritic or lumbar disk disease, as well as environmental effects.[12][IV]

Pain mechanisms

There is a growing understanding of altered neural processing with increasing age,[13, 14] which has been well reviewed by Gagliese and Farrell.[15] It is clear that there are neurobiological changes with ageing at the neuronal level, including reductions in myelination, axonal atrophy, and altered electrophysiological responses. These are not linear with age, but the degree of neuronal regeneration following injury is slowed with increasing age[16] and the deterioration in the endogenous inhibitory systems that occurs with age[17] starts in middle age.[18]

Not all nociceptive modalities reduce in sensitivity with age. A study by Lautenbacher *et al.*[19] found an enhancement of pain pressure thresholds. They postulate that superficial pain (heat) is not significantly different in the elderly and is processed differently from deeper pain (pressure), which is influenced to a greater degree by descending inhibition in the dorsal horn. Reduced descending inhibition[17] may account for the enhanced pressure pain in the older subject, which may help explain why older patients are more likely to develop musculoskeletal (deeper) pain than younger patients, as seen in the epidemiology studies reviewed (see above under Epidemiology).

Visceral pain perception does appear to reduce with increasing age.[4] The atypical presentation of abdominal, cardiac, or thoracic pain is well known, but poorly understood. The consequences of this atypical presentation can include delayed diagnosis with concomitant complications and a higher mortality risk. Atypical pain may lead to misdiagnosis and thus inappropriate management. The understanding of visceral mechanisms is increasing, but age-related effects are poorly understood.[20] Most of the research is on somatic mechanisms that may not be directly transferable to visceral nociception.

Dementia and cognitive deficits are common in the older population, including Alzheimer's disease which is commonly seen in residential care home settings. A study looking at heat pain perception and cerebral event-related potentials in cognitively impaired older adults demonstrated a significant difference in threshold for just noticeable sensations, but no difference for painful heat thresholds. Patients with Alzheimer's disease may be slightly less reliable witnesses with longer cortical latencies, but with similar levels of activation. This suggests slower cortical processing in the cognitively impaired subjects.[21] This supports the thought that patients with Alzheimer's disease do experience pain, but the processing is altered. Cardiovascular disease and diabetes mellitus are incriminated in the development of vascular dementia and Alzheimer's disease. A pilot study looking at cognitively impaired nursing home patients demonstrated higher pain prevalence in patients with cardiovascular disease (hypertension) or diabetes mellitus (65 percent) compared to those without (36.4 percent). The difference is significant despite the limitations in the study. Although further work is needed, these authors postulate that cortical and subcortical changes resulting from these conditions may be responsible for the difference in pain.[22]

Postoperative pain

There is debate as to the severity of postoperative pain in the older patient, since there is some suggestion that postoperative pain intensity reduces after the age of 60 years.[23] A study using cannulation as a standardized clinical painful stimulus found both statistical and clinical reductions in pain in patients over 65 years.[24] A study looking at morphine requirements postoperatively did not show a significant difference in reported pain score in the elderly compared to younger patients.[25][III] The sex differences in morphine dose, with women requiring higher morphine doses to provide adequate analgesia, were not apparent in the elderly patients suggesting a hormonal influence on pain modulation in the postoperative setting.

Postoperative cognitive deficit is well recognized as a complication of surgery and may be more pronounced in the elderly population. Postoperative pain is considered to be one of the factors influencing this, and there may be particular concerns about the influence of analgesic techniques on postoperative cognition. A recent review of the postoperative pain literature showed pethidine (meperidine) to have a direct influence on cognitive deficit, but other commonly used postoperative opioids did not show significant effects on delirium or cognitive deficits and no differences were found between intravenous or epidural techniques. Further studies are required with sufficient power to detect a difference, as well as more standardized techniques.[26][II]

PSYCHOLOGICAL INFLUENCES

The role of psychology and the psychological make up of individuals has become increasingly recognized as important at both a research and clinical level. Cognitive factors, such as attitudes, beliefs, and coping, are known to influence pain perception and behaviors, as well as response to treatment.[27] Stoicism and cautiousness also play a role in pain reporting and response to illness. Stoicism may account for some of the underreporting of pain and may be a barrier to adequate pain management.[28] This work has examined age effects, finding that pain reporting reduced with age, but that this could be accounted for by alterations in stoic and cautious attitude. This suggests that psychological factors may play an important role in determining age-related changes in pain rather than age itself.

The social circumstances of patients will influence the effect pain has on their ability to perform daily activities. This is a complex area, as the same circumstances influence factors such as anxiety and depression. Pain and depression are associated with pain being more persistent.[29] It is then difficult to evaluate if the depression is modifying the ability to perform daily activities or the pain. There are, however, trends suggesting that individuals in pain who have few or no social ties experience greater degrees of interference in daily living. This is true for the older postretirement population, as well as the preretirement age group (50–64 years). The same group found that the exception to this were patients with children who are in frequent contact, which increased the degree of interference caused by pain and was particularly true in men. Despite limitations, these findings have implications beyond primary and secondary health care and extend into the role of public health.[30]

ASSESSMENT

Assessing pain in the elderly requires an understanding that pain also influences a person's ability to perform tasks of daily living, their emotional wellbeing, and ability to interact with friends, family, etc. Assessment, therefore, has to take these factors into account. There is a need to examine the past medical history, as well as social and psychological components of pain. Past interventions and their outcomes, as well as the patient's willingness to engage in any proposed new interventions, has to be understood. Self-report is typically more reliable as compared to proxy reports, and allowing time for patients to express themselves is important along with simple and clear questions.

Any pain scales should be explained clearly and if one is not understood then consideration should be given to using a different one. Most elderly patients are able to use one of the common self-assessment tools, such as the Faces Scale or verbal rating scale, even if they have more difficulty with the numerical rating scale or the visual analog scale. These simple tools will give an insight to the severity of the pain and can be managed by individuals with moderate cognitive impairment.[31] There is evidence to suggest that using assessment scales increases the frequency of diagnosing pain in the elderly. One study compared asking patients "do you have pain" with three assessment scales. The scales group diagnosed a greater incidence of pain. This was particularly noticeable in the over 85-year age group and to a lesser extent in those with cognitive deficit.[32] Older patients commonly have more than one painful complaint and each requires assessment on its own merits. Examination can then be focused according to the history and discussion of the current complaint.

Patient's attitudes to pain influence their responses to assessment. Research by Yong *et al.*,[33] validating a pain attitude questionnaire, has demonstrated both similarities and differences in stoicism and cautiousness across the ages in chronic pain patients.[33] It is postulated that older patients may be more accepting of their pain (as part of the ageing process) compared to the younger generation. Other dimensions will also influence the pain experience, including mood and self-esteem, as well as actual or perceived biological changes.

A consensus document has been produced with the aim of helping researchers and clinicians assess pain in older people.[34][V] This report includes self-reporting and observational methods that can be used in elderly patients, including those with dementia. Which assessment methods are best suited in a specific situation will depend on the context of the assessment. These authors recommend a short ten-minute battery of assessment tools that can be used in the clinic setting.

In support of this multidimensional approach, the evaluation of eight measures that distinguish between elderly patients with chronic low back pain and pain-free individuals yielded a brief functional and medical assessment battery for research into this area and feel it could easily be adapted for clinical practice.[35][II] Dimensions included in the self-report and observation of function include mood as measured by the Geriatric Depression Scale, as well as the presence of comorbidities.

A full discussion of assessment tools currently available, along with the benefits and limitations, is beyond the scope of this text. A complete discussion is available in a recent IASP publication devoted to pain in the elderly.[1] Many assessment tools are currently available and have been validated in specific patient groups, but many are cumbersome and better suited to the research environment.

Barriers to assessment

Making complete pain assessments can be complicated in any population, but there are particular difficulties with the older patient, including barriers and misconceptions on the part of the public and healthcare profession. Clinicians, nurses, and psychologists with an interest in pain surveyed the ethical issues relating to pain management, finding that the undertreatment of pain in the elderly and pain management at the end of life were both major dilemmas.[36] Underlying these were a range of themes, including concern about barriers inhibiting care, conflicts with others, inappropriate pain management, and regulatory issues.

Specific barriers in the postoperative assessment of pain in the elderly include issues related to patients and/or healthcare workers.[37] Recent work identifies similar issues (see **Table 45.1**). Language can also be a barrier, as an older patient may not describe a sensation as painful, but may describe it as an ache or unpleasant sensation. Other research suggests that older patients are reluctant to label some sensations as painful[38] and there are limited investigations of language in the postoperative setting.[39] Multiple barriers remain despite developments over recent years, including outdated attitudes, poor assessment, and inadequate use of medications.[40]

Surveys of nursing homes suggest a lack of written policies and absence of standardized assessments, low rates of staff education, and low rates of access to pain specialists.[41] Surveys assessing nursing responses to two scenarios of pain in elderly patients highlights that a patient's self-report alone was not enough for staff to report pain, with the more experienced nurses being least likely to believe self-reports of pain. Under half the nurses involved indicated they would alter the analgesic dose in response to the scenarios.[42] When staff and patient reports of pain have been compared, a UK study found reasonable concordance between staff and patients when interviews of patients and staff were compared to reviews of medical records. Differences in reporting were greater in the severely cognitively impaired patients, and patients reported more back and wound pain, while staff reported cardiac and stroke pain. Staff reported they could tell if a patient was in pain, but less than one-third asked patients about pain. In this study there was little difference between qualified and unqualified staff assessments.[43] As has been shown in other groups, the assessment of pain in the elderly by different health professionals may yield different results. The degree of agreement of assessment between nurses and physicians was 32 percent in medicine and 44 percent on the geriatric wards.[44] The prevalence of pain in a group assessed by proxy was 65 percent on the medical wards and 20 percent on the geriatric wards. Clearly, barriers remain with regard to providing consistent pain assessment across settings and across modalities of assessment.

There are several areas of poor understanding with regard to pain management in this population that persist at all levels (professional and public alike). Education is the link if these barriers are to be addressed before there is the opportunity to improve the delivery of interventions aimed at managing the patient's pain. Recent guidelines on pain assessment in the elderly provide practical skills for use in hospital and domestic settings.[45][V]

Postoperative pain

Postoperative pain is experienced by the elderly and can be severe, and underreporting of pain is common. Satisfaction with postoperative pain management has been shown to be high (87 percent) even in the context of severe postoperative pain (62 percent).[46] Predictors associated with satisfaction included preoperative education, younger age, oral medication, and type of surgery. These authors concluded that there is still significant undermanagement that may be addressed by better preoperative education.

The assessment principles regarding postoperative pain are the same as discussed above under Assessment. Comparisons of pain scales in older patients often reveal problems with visual analog scales. For example, in one study comparing three pain scales in younger and older patients following radical prostatectomy, the visual analog scale was not sufficiently sensitive to detect alterations in pain quality in the older patient and the verbal rating scale was more appropriate.[39] Although the older age group reported lower pain on two pain descriptor scales,

Table 45.1 Barriers to pain management in the elderly.

Category	Barrier
Patient related	Fear of bothering or angering caregivers
	Belief that caregiver is doing all they can to relieve the pain
	Anxiety in using unfamiliar equipment
	Access to health care
	Cost of health care
Healthcare team related	Lack of understanding and training of pain assessment tools
	No expression of pain means no pain is experienced
	Pain perception decreases with increasing age
	Opioids are poorly tolerated in the elderly
Barriers relating to patient, family, and healthcare team	Lack of training in pain management for elderly patients
	Lack of awareness regarding use of language
	Belief that pain is inevitable with ageing
	Fear of side effects from medications
	Fear of addiction to opioids

Modified from Pasero C, McCaffery M. Postoperative pain management in the elderly. In BR Ferrell, BA Ferrell (Eds). IASP Press, Seattle, WA, 1996.[37]

the visual analog scale did not detect this. Given that up to 35 percent of the elderly are visually impaired, the visual analog scale should generally be avoided in the elderly.

IMPAIRED COGNITION

Cognitively impaired elderly patients are harder to assess but continue to have significant pain. In a cross-sectional study of nursing home residents, patients with cognitive impairment had more frequent pain in fewer sites with greater severity.[47] Although nursing home residents demonstrate similar levels of pain across the spectrum of cognitive impairment, analgesic use reduces as cognitive impairment increases.[48] Similarly, an Italian study of the over 85-year age group in care also demonstrated a correlation between low cognitive performance and inadequate analgesia.[9]

Behavioral disturbances were more common in patients with cognitive deficit. The relationship between behavior and pain in cognitively impaired individuals suggest that pain has a greater influence on dysfunctional behavior in patients with severe dementia compared to those with less severe forms.[49] Careful assessment of dementia, behavioral dysfunction, and pain, and treatment of the physical suffering may address the behavioral disturbance.[49]

Assessment of patients with dementia can be difficult. Assessment tools including self-assessment tools are available for cognitively impaired patients.[50][I], [51] Pautex *et al.*[52] assessed four self-assessment scales with one observational scale in patients with mild, moderate, and severe dementia. They found that the majority (over 90 percent) of mild and moderately impaired patients and 40 percent of the severely impaired patients were able to use at least one scale. There was only moderate correlation between the observational and self-assessment scales, demonstrating that self-assessment should be used where possible. Other studies have also demonstrated that patients with dementia are often able to use self-assessment tools for rating their pain.[53] In 2004, Closs *et al.*[54] looked at five assessment scales in nursing home residents with varying degrees of cognitive impairment. There was good consistency generally between the scales, although there was poor consistency with the severely impaired residents. The verbal rating scale was the most consistent across the spectrum of cognitive impairment. The assessment of pain by proxy is complicated and generally should be avoided. Manfredi *et al.*[55] examined the validity of facial expression as an indicator of pain during dressing changes for decubitus ulcers in patients with and without severe dementia. Nurses and medical students watching videotapes of facial expression and vocalization during the dressing changes showed reasonable agreement for the presence of pain, but not for its intensity.

PAIN MANAGEMENT CONSIDERATIONS

The frequent comorbidities seen in the elderly often results in polypharmacy. The effect of drug interactions and the altered handling of drugs in the elderly increases the risk of complications. Caution has to be exercised in developing a management plan with appropriate consideration to side effects and potential interactions.[56] Other chapters detail the management of specific conditions and discuss the pharmacology of individual drug groups. In a general sense, the World Health Organization (WHO) analgesic ladder can guide initial pain management. There is a principle in prescribing, particularly in the elderly, to start with a low dose and slowly titrate to benefit or side effects. The aim of pain management is to improve pain and optimize function, particularly with regard to daily activities. The eradication of pain is usually unrealistic and the lowest drug dose will often not provide optimal analgesia. Optimal treatment typically combines pharmacological and nonpharmacological interventions, including the home remedies that patients utilize for themselves. Most elderly patients use a variety of pain management methods, including prescribed medication, rest, and distraction and identify cold, exercise, hot bath/shower, and alcohol as effective.[57] Longitudinal studies of nursing home residents suggest that the use of long-acting opioids in a nursing home setting is relatively safe.[58]

A qualitative study looking at elderly patients preference for pain management strategies and barriers to management found that patients wanted to be actively involved in their management and make informed decisions. They were happy to try new methods and interventions. Conventional medication, exercise, and physiotherapy were the least liked options.[59] These studies suggest a need to involve patients more closely and discuss management options with regard to the patient's perspective and preferred strategies.

The use of nondrug interventions is of great importance in optimizing management. Many patients are aware of the interventions they can use at home to ease their pain and optimize function. These may include the use of heat and cold, position, and mobility, as well as aids for moving, dressing, or performing activities of daily living. There is also a role for physical therapy.

Paracetamol

Paracetamol (acetaminophen) is a well-tolerated drug with few side effects in all age groups. It has a role as an opioid and anti-inflammatory sparing agent. Evidence suggests that it may be as efficacious as other agents, while also being cost effective.[60][V] It is therefore prudent to consider its use as part of a pain management plan. There are, however, no studies looking specifically at the very elderly or frail with regard to altered drug handling. This is a group where physiological reserve is limited and altered dosing may be required.

Nonsteroidal anti-inflammatory drugs

Nonsteroidal anti-inflammatory drugs (NSAIDs) are commonly used for arthritic and musculoskeletal conditions with good analgesic efficacy. The Cox-2-specific agents have a reduced incidence of gastrointestinal side effects, but increased cardiovascular side effects resulted in the voluntary withdrawal of rofecoxib from the market in 2004.[61][I] There had been previous work suggesting NSAIDs had an increased risk in susceptible patients to develop congestive cardiac failure.[62][III] A more detailed discussion can be found in Chapter 15, The use of NSAIDs and paracetamol (acetaminophen) in chronic pain.

There is evidence that the elderly are at increased risk of gastrointestinal complications with NSAID use. This risk returns to baseline on withdrawal of the agent.[63][I] The elderly are also at risk of the renal and cardiovascular complications of these drugs, which appear to be dose related. There is therefore an argument to minimize the duration of treatment and use the lowest effective dose.[64] It has been suggested that other analgesics with fewer side effects should also be considered as alternatives to the NSAIDs.[65] Consideration should also be given to using the NSAIDs for exacerbations of pain and for short duration only. The use of an NSAID with a proton pump inhibitor may be as effective as a Cox-2 antagonist alone.

Opioids

The use of opioids for nonmalignant pain has increased over recent years. There have been several publications regarding opioid use[66][V], [67][V], [68] and other organizations have published consensus documents. There are theoretical reasons why older patients may have an altered response to opioids and the adage of "start low and go slow" with regard to titration is important. This does not negate the requirement for adequate analgesia. An earlier paper by Aubrun *et al.*[69] demonstrated lower subcutaneous dosing with morphine on the wards in older patients, but not intravenous dosing titrated to effect in the recovery ward. There have been studies demonstrating reduced opioid requirements in elderly patients, but the variability of dose is wide and individual titration is suggested.[70][V]

When opioids are used chronically, there is a potential for dose escalation, possibly as a result of tolerance. A small retrospective review of 206 patients demonstrated that initial opioid doses were the same, but that escalation over approximately 15 months was almost 50 percent lower in the older population (60 years and above). The older patients also had a sustained reduction in visual analog pain score compared to the younger patients. The postulate is that older patients may have a reduced rate of tolerance.[71] The use of slow-release opioids over a six-month period demonstrated improved functional ability and social engagement and failed to demonstrate a higher rate of side effects in a nursing home population compared to short-acting opioids. The authors suggest that slow-release opioids may have a role in the long-term management of nonmalignant pain in the nursing home population.[58]

Coanalgesics

The incidence of neuropathic pain is common in the elderly. Conditions including painful diabetic neuropathy, postherpetic neuralgia, central poststroke pain, and trigeminal neuralgia are all seen in this age group. Despite multidisciplinary pain management, there remains a role for drug therapy. The commonly used agents have been studied, but not specifically in the older population.

The antidepressants have long been used in managing neuropathic pain. A systematic review suggests that the best evidence is for amitriptyline with a number needed to treat (NNT) of 2.0 for moderate pain relief and number needed to harm (NNH) for minor harm of 4.6.[72][I] The elderly are poorly tolerant of these agents due to the side effects, notably, sedation, postural hypotension, falls, and urinary retention. Nortriptyline may be better tolerated than amitriptyline. The analgesic effects are independent of the antidepressant effects with benefit often in the 50–100-mg dose range for amitriptyline.

Systematic reviews have also been performed for anticonvulsants demonstrating that there is no role for these agents in acute pain, with the exception of trigeminal neuralgia. They should be withheld until other interventions have been tried.[73][I] Gabapentin has been shown to have an effect on neuropathic pain with an NNT of 2.9 for diabetic neuropathy and 3.9 for postherpetic neuralgia and an NNH for minor harm of 3.7.[74][I] There is no clear research date demonstrating improved efficacy of gabapentin over the older agents. Other anticonvulsants continue to be studied, but as yet clear evidence is awaited.

Psychological strategies

As part of pain management, the role of psychological strategies must not be forgotten. As described above, there are several psychological variables that influence pain. If these can be understood then they may be used to improve a patient's quality of life and provide appropriate pain management.

Self-help focused on improving physical functioning, mood, and pain over seven weeks compared to an educational booklet group demonstrated improvements in function and pain intensity with a three-month follow up.[75] Self-management strategies to control emotions were shown to alter pain intensity in the older population.[76] There were differences in the patients' ability to regulate their emotions, with the oldest group (over 80 years), men, and those living alone being less able to control their emotions.[76] Those who did benefit have a potential tool to manage their pain without the risks and costs associated with pharmacological interventions. Depression has an influence on pain. A study looking at musculoskeletal pain in elderly women and the effect on activities of daily living found that an outpatient integrative psychotherapeutic programme for depression provided improvements in daily activities and quality of life compared to the untreated group.[77][II]

Physiotherapy and exercise

Many of the common pains related to the elderly involve the musculoskeletal system. There is, therefore, a role for physiotherapy both from the perspective of recovery from injury or following surgery, but also in optimizing and maintaining function or improving fitness in the frail elderly.

In a small study looking at osteoarthritis of the knee, a common condition in the elderly, a 12-week exercise and walking protocol improved physical function, symptom severity, and the limitation of function by pain for up to six months.[78] A more recent study compared community physiotherapy to a pharmacy review and demonstrated benefits compared to controls who received an information leaflet. At three-month follow up, 40 percent of the physiotherapy group, 33 percent of the pharmacy group, and 19 percent of controls responded to treatment with reduction in pain scores and improvement in function.[76] Although these benefits were not sustained at 6- and 12-month follow up, there was a reduction in general practitioner consultation rates in the physiotherapy group at six months, and an overall reduction in the use of NSAIDs and high patient satisfaction in the treatment groups.[79] Exercise is often considered beneficial for many reasons. A study looking at pain as a barrier to exercise over a 12-month period has shown that walking for exercise can increase with time. They found no significant alteration in pain and that the initial pain level was not a barrier to walking. The patients did however self-report their level of exercise.[80] A larger physiotherapy-based study looking at exercise in elderly patients with low back pain followed them up at two years (70 percent response rate). The numbers performing some exercise at two years was 72 percent compared to 49 percent before the rehabilitation program, which had an exercise orientation to it. Those who failed to maintain the exercise gave the reason of no benefit or aggravated pain. Of those who continued to exercise, the majority did so for its health benefits.[81]

GUIDELINES FOR PAIN MANAGEMENT IN THE ELDERLY

There have been several publications that provide guidelines for managing pain in the elderly. Some are aimed specifically at the elderly and others are more general, but incorporate recommendations relating to the older population. The Australian and New Zealand College of Anaesthetists and Faculty of Pain Medicine have produced an evidence-based text on acute pain management with specific reference to the elderly.[70] Other guidelines have been published with regard to chronic pain.[82, 83][V]

CONCLUSIONS

Pain in the older person is a real and increasing problem as the proportion of the population over the age of 70 years increases. Many live independently, but increasing numbers will be in sheltered or residential care. There are aging effects on the physiological systems that influence functional reserve and pain processing. Psychological adaptations with increasing age also affect both pain perception and strategies used in managing pain.

Assessment of pain and its impact on the individual is vital if an appropriate management plan is to be developed with the aim of providing improved quality of life and function. This is made more complex in patients with cognitive deficit who may have great difficulty in clearly communicating their pain. There are many assessment methods available, some of which are validated. At a practical level such tools need to be easy to administer and provide reproducible and reliable results when administered by different members of staff. This requires further research to find assessment tools that are appropriate for the clinic or in the care home.

Education is a key to providing appropriate management for these patients and involves carers, as well as healthcare professionals and the patients themselves. This is where guidelines have a role in providing a basic level of understanding and intervention in the first instance. There remain a variety of barriers to providing care relating to all members of the team, some have been overcome with time, but others remain.

Interventions need to be focused on what is achievable. A biopsychosocial approach is important with support for the patient to reach their potential. Traditional drug interventions have a place in management with appropriate consideration being taken with regard to side effects and interactions between medications. An approach of starting with a low dose and titrating slowly to benefit or side effects is often suggested. Nondrug interventions are also of great benefit and are often already used with effect by patients, including heat, cold, physical activity, etc. The psychological treatments, including self-help, may be used with clear benefits seen in function and quality of life.

Pain management in the elderly provides both challenges and rewards. The process cannot be rushed and requires patience and perseverance. A significant amount of education is required to increase awareness of the size of the problem, as well as to its management and assessment.

REFERENCES

* 1. Gibson SJ, Weiner DK. *Pain in older persons.* Progress in pain research and management 35. Seattle: IASP Press, 2005: 432.
2. United Nations. *World population aging 2007.* New York: United Nations, 2007.
3. Helme RD, Gibson SJ. Pain in older people. In: Crombie IK (ed.). *Epidemiology of pain.* Seattle: IASP Press, 1999: 103–12.
4. Thomas E, Peat G, Harris L *et al.* The prevalence of pain and pain interference in a general population of older adults: cross-sectional findings from the North Staffordshire Osteoarthritis Project (NorStOP). *Pain.* 2004; **110**: 361–8.
5. Miro J, Paredes S, Rull M *et al.* Pain in older adults: a prevalence study in the Mediterranean region of Catalonia. *European Journal of Pain.* 2007; **11**: 83–92.
6. Soldato M, Liperoti R, Landi F *et al.* Non malignant daily pain and risk of disability among older adults in home care in Europe. *Pain.* 2007; **129**: 304–10.
7. Cecchi F, Debolini P, Lova RM *et al.* Epidemiology of back pain in a representative cohort of Italian persons 65 years of age and older: the InCHIANTI study. *Spine.* 2006; **31**: 1149–55.
8. Dionne CE, Dunn KM, Croft PR. Does back pain prevalence really decrease with increasing age? A systematic review. *Age and Ageing.* 2006; **35**: 229–34.
9. Frondini C, Lanfranchi G, Minardi M, Cucinotta D. Affective, behavior and cognitive disorders in the elderly with chronic musculoskelatal pain: the impact on an aging population. *Archives of Gerontology and Geriatrics.* 2007; **44** (Suppl. 1): 167–71.
10. Leong IY, Farrell MJ, Helme RD, Gibson SJ. The relationship between medical comorbidity and self-rated pain, mood disturbance, and function in older people with chronic pain. *Journals of Gerontology. Series A, Biological Sciences and Medical Sciences.* 2007; **62**: 550–5.
11. Hartvigsen J, Petersen HC, Frederiksen H, Christensen K. Small effect of genetic factors on neck pain in old age: a study of 2,108 Danish twins 70 years of age and older. *Spine.* 2005; **30**: 206–08.
12. Hartvigsen J, Christensen K, Frederiksen H, Petersen HC. Genetic and environmental contributions to back pain in old age: a study of 2,108 Danish twins aged 70 and older. *Spine.* 2004; **29**: 897–901; discussion 902.
13. Gibson SJ, Farrell M. A review of age differences in the neurophysiology of nociception and the perceptual experience of pain. *Clinical Journal of Pain.* 2004; **20**: 227–39.
14. Edwards RR, Fillingim RB. Effects of age on temporal summation and habituation of thermal pain: clinical relevance in healthy older and younger adults. *Journal of Pain.* 2001; **2**: 307–17.
15. Gagliese L, Farrell MJ. The neurobiology of aging, nociception, and pain: an integration of animal and human evidence. In: Gibson SJ, Weiner DK (eds). *Pain in older persons.* Progress in Pain Research and Management. Seattle: IASP Press, 2005: 25–44.
16. Verdu E, Ceballos D, Vilches JJ, Navarro X. Influence of aging on peripheral nerve function and regeneration. *Journal of the Peripheral Nervous System.* 2000; **5**: 191–208.
17. Edwards RR, Fillingim RB, Ness TJ. Age-related differences in endogenous pain modulation: a comparison of diffuse noxious inhibitory controls in healthy older and younger adults. *Pain.* 2003; **101**: 155–65.
18. Lariviere M, Goffaux P, Marchand S, Julien N. Changes in pain perception and descending inhibitory controls start at middle age in healthy adults. *Clinical Journal of Pain.* 2007; **23**: 506–10.
19. Lautenbacher S, Kunz M, Strate P *et al.* Age effects on pain thresholds, temporal summation and spatial summation of heat and pressure pain. *Pain.* 2005; **115**: 410–18.
20. Moore AR, Clinch D. Underlying mechanisms of impaired visceral pain perception in older people. *Journal of the American Geriatrics Society.* 2004; **52**: 132–6.
21. Gibson SJ, Voukelatos X, Ames D *et al.* An examination of pain perception and cerebral event-related potentials following carbon dioxide laser stimulation in patients with Alzheimer's disease and age-matched control volunteers. *Pain Research and Management.* 2001; **6**: 126–32.
22. Achterberg WP, Scherder E, Pot AM, Ribbe MW. Cardiovascular risk factors in cognitively impaired nursing home patients: a relationship with pain? *European Journal of Pain.* 2007; **11**: 707–10.
23. Thomas T, Robinson C, Champion D *et al.* Prediction and assessment of the severity of post-operative pain and of satisfaction with management. *Pain.* 1998; **75**: 177–85.
24. Li SF, Greenwald PW, Gennis P *et al.* Effect of age on acute pain perception of a standardized stimulus in the emergency department. *Annals of Emergency Medicine.* 2001; **38**: 644–7.
25. Aubrun F, Salvi N, Coriat P, Riou B. Sex- and age-related differences in morphine requirements for postoperative pain relief. *Anesthesiology.* 2005; **103**: 156–60.
26. Fong HK, Sands LP, Leung JM. The role of postoperative analgesia in delirium and cognitive decline in elderly patients: a systematic review. *Anesthesia and Analgesia.* 2006; **102**: 1255–66.
27. Jensen MP, Ehde DM, Hoffman AJ *et al.* Cognitions, coping and social environment predict adjustment to phantom limb pain. *Pain.* 2002; **95**: 133–42.
28. Yong HH. Can attitudes of stoicism and cautiousness explain observed age-related variation in levels of self-rated pain, mood disturbance and functional interference

in chronic pain patients? *European Journal of Pain.* 2006; **10**: 399–407.

29. Geerlings SW, Twisk JW, Beekman AT *et al.* Longitudinal relationship between pain and depression in older adults: sex, age and physical disability. *Social Psychiatry and Psychiatric Epidemiology.* 2002; **37**: 23–30.
30. Peat G, Thomas E, Handy J, Croft P. Social networks and pain interference with daily activities in middle and old age. *Pain.* 2004; **112**: 397–405.
31. Kaasalainen S, Crook J. A comparison of pain-assessment tools for use with elderly long-term-care residents. *Canadian Journal of Nursing Research.* 2003; **35**: 58–71.
32. Kamel HK, Phlavan M, Malekgoudarzi B *et al.* Utilizing pain assessment scales increases the frequency of diagnosing pain among elderly nursing home residents. *Journal of Pain and Symptom Management.* 2001; **21**: 450–5.
33. Yong H-H, Bell R, Workman B, Gibson SJ. Psychometric properties of the Pain Attitudes Questionnaire (revised) in adult patients with chronic pain. *Pain.* 2003; **104**: 673–81.
34. Hadjistavropoulos T, Herr K, Turk DC *et al.* An interdisciplinary expert consensus statement on assessment of pain in older persons. *Clinical Journal of Pain.* 2007; **23**: S1–43.
35. Rudy TE, Weiner DK, Lieber SJ *et al.* The impact of chronic low back pain on older adults: a comparative study of patients and controls. *Pain.* 2007; **131**: 293–301.
36. Ferrell BR, Novy D, Sullivan MD *et al.* Ethical dilemmas in pain management. *Journal of Pain.* 2001; **2**: 171–80.
37. Pasero C, McCaffery M. Postoperative pain management in the elderly. In: Ferrell BR, Ferrell BA (eds). *Pain in the elderly.* Seattle: IASP Press, 1996: 45–68.
38. Yong HH, Gibson SJ, Horne DJ, Helme RD. Development of a pain attitudes questionnaire to assess stoicism and cautiousness for possible age differences. *Journals of Gerontology. Series B, Psychological Sciences and Social Sciences.* 2001; **56**: P279–84.
39. Gagliese L, Katz J. Age differences in postoperative pain are scale dependent: a comparison of measures of pain intensity and quality in younger and older surgical patients. *Pain.* 2003; **103**: 11–20.
40. Closs SJ. What can be done to meet the needs of older people experiencing pain? *Professional Nurse.* 2004; **20**: 29–31.
41. Allcock N, McGarry J, Elkan R. Management of pain in older people within the nursing home: a preliminary study. *Health and Social Care in the Community.* 2002; **10**: 464–71.
42. Katsma DL, Souza CH. Elderly pain assessment and pain management knowledge of long-term care nurses. *Pain Management Nursing.* 2000; **1**: 88–95.
43. Closs SJ, Barr B, Briggs M. Reporting of painful conditions in nursing homes. *Journal of Clinical Nursing.* 2006; **15**: 1203–05.
44. Rainfray M, Brochet B, de Sarasqueta AM, Michel P. [Assessment of pain in elderly hospitalised patients. A transversal descriptive survey]. *La Presse Médicale.* 2003; **32**: 924–9.
45. Collett B, O'Mahoney S, Schofield P *et al.* The assessment of pain in older people. *Clinical Medicine.* 2007; **7**: 496–500.
46. Sauaia A, Min SJ, Leber C *et al.* Postoperative pain management in elderly patients: correlation between adherence to treatment guidelines and patient satisfaction. *Journal of the American Geriatrics Society.* 2005; **53**: 274–82.
47. Leong IY, Nuo TH. Prevalence of pain in nursing home residents with different cognitive and communicative abilities. *Clinical Journal of Pain.* 2007; **23**: 119–27.
48. Closs SJ, Barr B, Briggs M. Cognitive status and analgesic provision in nursing home residents. *British Journal of General Practice.* 2004; **54**: 919–21.
49. Cipher DJ, Clifford PA, Roper KD. Behavioral manifestations of pain in the demented elderly. *Journal of the American Medical Directors Association.* 2006; **7**: 355–65.
50. Zwakhalen SM, Hamers JP, Abu-Saad HH, Berger MP. Pain in elderly people with severe dementia: a systematic review of behavioural pain assessment tools. *BMC Geriatrics.* 2006; **6**: 3.
51. Cohen-Mansfield J. Pain Assessment in Noncommunicative Elderly persons – PAINE. *Clinical Journal of Pain.* 2006; **22**: 569–75.
52. Pautex S, Herrmann F, Le Lous P *et al.* Feasibility and reliability of four pain self-assessment scales and correlation with an observational rating scale in hospitalized elderly demented patients. *Journals of Gerontology. Series A, Biological Sciences and Medical Sciences.* 2005; **60**: 524–9.
53. Manz BD, Mosier R, Nusser-Gerlach MA *et al.* Pain assessment in the cognitively impaired and unimpaired elderly. *Pain Management Nursing.* 2000; **1**: 106–15.
54. Closs SJ, Barr B, Briggs M *et al.* A comparison of five pain assessment scales for nursing home residents with varying degrees of cognitive impairment. *Journal of Pain and Symptom Management.* 2004; **27**: 196–205.
55. Manfredi PL, Breuer B, Meier DE, Libow L. Pain assessment in elderly patients with severe dementia. *Journal of Pain and Symptom Management.* 2003; **25**: 48–52.
56. Shimp LA. Safety issues in the pharmacologic management of chronic pain in the elderly. *Pharmacotherapy.* 1998; **18**: 1313–22.
57. Jakobsson U, Rahm Hallberg I, Westergren A. Pain management in elderly persons who require assistance with activities of daily living: a comparison of those living at home with those in special accommodations. *European Journal of Pain.* 2004; **8**: 335–44.
58. Won A, Lapane KL, Vallow S *et al.* Long-term effects of analgesics in a population of elderly nursing home residents with persistent nonmalignant pain. *Journals of Gerontology. Series A, Biological Sciences and Medical Sciences.* 2006; **61**: 165–9.

59. Lansbury G. Chronic pain management: a qualitative study of elderly people's preferred coping strategies and barriers to management. *Disability and Rehabilitation.* 2000; **22**: 2–14.
60. Nikles CJ, Yelland M, Del Mar C, Wilkinson D. The role of paracetamol in chronic pain: an evidence-based approach. *American Journal of Therapy.* 2005; **12**: 80–91.
61. Garner SE, Fidan DD, Frankish RR, Maxwell LJ. Rofecoxib for osteoarthritis. *Cochrane Database of Systematic Reviews.* 2005; **CD005115**.
62. Page J, Henry D. Consumption of NSAIDs and the development of congestive heart failure in elderly patients. An underrecognized public health problem. *Archives of Internal Medicine.* 2000; **160**: 777–84.
63. Hernandez-Diaz S, Rodriguez LA. Association between nonsteroidal anti-inflammatory drugs and upper gastrointestinal tract bleeding/perforation: an overview of epidemiologic studies published in the 1990s. *Archives of Internal Medicine.* 2000; **160**: 2093–9.
64. Savage R. Cyclo-oxygenase-2 inhibitors: when should they be used in the elderly? *Drugs and Aging.* 2005; **22**: 185–200.
65. Langford RM. Pain management today – what have we learned? *Clinical Rheumatology.* 2006; **25** (Suppl. 1): S2–8.
66. The Pain Society. *Recommendations for the appropriate use of opioids for persistent non-cancer pain. A consensus statement prepared on behalf of the Pain Society, the Royal College of Anaesthetists, the Royal College of General Practitioners and the Royal College of Psychiatrists.* London: The Pain Society, 2004.
67. Kalso E, Allan L, Dellemijn PL *et al.* Recommendations for using opioids in chronic non-cancer pain. *European Journal of Pain.* 2003; **7**: 381–6.
68. Auret K, Schug SA. Underutilisation of opioids in elderly patients with chronic pain: approaches to correcting the problem. *Drugs and Aging.* 2005; **22**: 641–54.
69. Aubrun F, Bunge D, Langeron O *et al.* Postoperative morphine consumption in the elderly patient. *Anesthesiology.* 2003; **99**: 160–5.
70. Australian and New Zealand College of Anaesthetists and Faculty of Pian Medicine. *Acute pain management: scientific evidence.* Canberra: National Health and Medical Research Council, 2005.
71. Buntin-Mushock C, Phillip L, Moriyama K, Palmer PP. Age-dependent opioid escalation in chronic pain patients. *Anesthesia and Analgesia.* 2005; **100**: 1740–5.
72. Saarto T, Wiffen PJ. Antidepressants for neuropathic pain. *Cochrane Database of Systematic Reviews.* 2005; **CD005454**.
73. Wiffen P, Collins S, McQuay H *et al.* Anticonvulsant drugs for acute and chronic pain. *Cochrane Database of Systematic Reviews.* 2005; **CD001133**.
74. Wiffen PJ, McQuay HJ, Edwards JE, Moore RA. Gabapentin for acute and chronic pain. *Cochrane Database of Systematic Reviews.* 2005; **CD005452**.
75. Ersek M, Turner JA, McCurry SM *et al.* Efficacy of a self-management group intervention for elderly persons with chronic pain. *Clinical Journal of Pain.* 2003; **19**: 156–67.
76. Paquet C, Kergoat MJ, Dube L. The role of everyday emotion regulation on pain in hospitalized elderly: insights from a prospective within-day assessment. *Pain.* 2005; **115**: 355–63.
77. Nickel MK, Lahmann C, Muehlbacher M *et al.* Change in instrumental activities of daily living disability in female senior patients with musculosceletal pain: a prospective, randomized, controlled trial. *Archives of Gerontology and Geriatrics.* 2006; **42**: 247–55.
78. Dias RC, Dias JM, Ramos LR. Impact of an exercise and walking protocol on quality of life for elderly people with OA of the knee. *Physiotherapy Research International.* 2003; **8**: 121–30.
79. Hay EM, Foster NE, Thomas E *et al.* Effectiveness of community physiotherapy and enhanced pharmacy review for knee pain in people aged over 55 presenting to primary care: pragmatic randomised trial. *British Medical Journal.* 2006; **333**: 995.
80. Rhudy JL, Dubbert PM, Kirchner KA, Williams AE. Efficacy of a program to encourage walking in VA elderly primary care patients: the role of pain. *Psychology, Health and Medicine.* 2007; **12**: 289–98.
81. Mailloux J, Finno M, Rainville J. Long-term exercise adherence in the elderly with chronic low back pain. *American Journal of Physical Medicine and Rehabilitation.* 2006; **85**: 120–6.
82. Anonymous. The management of persistent pain in older persons. *Journal of the American Geriatrics Society.* 2002; **50**: S205–24.
83. Australian Pain Society. *Pain in residential aged care facilities: management strategies.* North Sydney: Australian Pain Society, 2005.

46

Pain management and substance misuse

CATHY STANNARD

KEY LEARNING POINTS

- Opioids have been shown in clinical trials to be effective for a number of chronic pain conditions.
- The degree to which prescribed opioids predispose to substance misuse problems is not known.
- Risk factors associated with propensity to develop substance misuse problems should be evaluated and therapy monitored appropriately.
- Patients with a past or current history of substance misuse should be offered opioid therapy, if appropriate, for their pain condition. Close evaluation of therapy needs to be supported by collaboration between appropriate healthcare professionals.

INTRODUCTION

The use of opioid drugs for the management of acute pain states and for the management of pain associated with cancer is well established. There is now a considerable and wide-ranging literature on the use of these drugs in persistent pain conditions not associated with malignant disease.[1] The concerns of clinicians regarding the propensity of these drugs to cause problems of tolerance, dependence, and addiction remain largely unanswered. These concerns become sharply focused when prescribing opioid analgesic drugs for patients in pain who have a past or current history of substance misuse.[2]

This chapter outlines the burdens of substance misuse to individuals and society and discusses the relevant neurobiology in order to explain why use of opioid drugs may lead to medical and legal problems. Definitions of addiction, dependence, and tolerance to opioid drugs in the context of pain management are discussed and data regarding risks of iatrogenic problem drug use are presented. The discussion supports the safe use of opioids for long-term pain control by giving guidance on identification and management of problem drug use and outlines principles of management of persistent pain in patients with addictive disease.

BACKGROUND

Psychoactive substances and the law

A psychoactive substance changes the way a person thinks and may modify mood and level of consciousness. The medicinal use of such substances, particularly the opioids, is well established, but their nonmedical (illicit) use is widespread with individuals using the drugs for the perceived benefit of the psychoactive experience.

A legal framework exists for the control and regulation of drugs that are considered to be dangerous or harmful to individuals or to society. Some of the medical and legal issues in the United States have been considered by Bloodworth.[3] There are three international conventions under which most countries (within their own legislative framework) agree to restrict nonmedical use of and trade in certain classes of drugs, including opioids, cannabis, cocaine, hallucinogens, and various hypnotics and sedatives.[4] Individual countries may prohibit other substances, such as alcohol.

Epidemiology of substance misuse

Dependence on psychoactive substances is a common global problem. The British Crime Survey 2005/6 showed that a third of 15–59-year-olds have used illegal drugs at some stage with the figure rising to 45.1 percent in the 16–24 age group with cannabis being the most frequently used drug, cocaine powder or crack cocaine being used by 2.4 percent of individuals, and heroin or methadone being used by 0.1 percent of this age group.[5] Other surveys of developed countries paint a similar picture. Data from Canada, the USA, and European countries suggest that more than 2 percent of young people report heroin use and almost 5 percent reported smoking cocaine at some stage. More than 20 percent of those surveyed in the USA report using at least one illicit drug other than cannabis.[6] More recent data give a substance dependence or abuse prevalence in the US population over the age of 12 years of 9.4 percent, with the vast majority of these not receiving treatment for addiction.[7] The United Nations World Drug Report 2006 estimated that 200 million people, or 5 percent of the global population age 15–64 years, have used illicit drugs at least once in the previous year.[8]

The problem of substance misuse imposes significant burdens on the individual and on society. The effects on an individual have been classified into four groups:[9]

1. chronic health effects (cirrhosis, HIV, hepatitis);
2. acute health effects (overdose, injury whilst intoxicated);
3. acute social problems (arrest, disruption of relationship);
4. chronic social problems (disruption of family role, effect on employment, low income).

Substance misuse places a significant burden on society in terms of healthcare costs of both acute and chronic illness, criminal behavior and the burden of poor productivity and absenteeism from work, as well as unemployment.[7]

Definitions in relation to substance misuse

Existing diagnostic criteria, whilst of considerable applicability in the field of substance misuse, serve to cause confusion when prescribing opioids for pain relief and have acted both as a barrier to appropriate prescribing and a source of concern to patients and their carers. A more pragmatic set of criteria, applicable to individuals being prescribed opioids for pain were developed by Portenoy[10] (**Table 46.1**).

The confusion regarding nomenclature has prompted production of a clarifying consensus statement from the American Pain Society, the American Society for

Table 46.1 Criteria for diagnosing addiction in the context of patients taking opioids for chronic pain.

Criteria		
1.	An intense desire for the drug and overwhelming concern about its continued availability (psychological dependence)	
2.	Evidence of compulsive drug use, characterized, for example by	a. Unsanctioned dose escalation b. Continued dosing despite significant side effects c. Use of drugs to treat symptoms not targeted by therapy, or d. Unapproved use during periods of no symptoms
	and/or	
3.	Evidence of one or more of a group of associated behaviors, including:	a. Manipulation of the treating physician or medical system for the purpose of obtaining additional drug (altering prescriptions, for example) b. Acquisition of drugs from other medical sources or from nonmedical sources c. Drug hoarding or sales d. Unapproved use of other drugs (particular alcohol or other sedatives/hypnotics) during opioid therapy

Reprinted from Journal of Pain and Symptom Management, 5, Portenoy RK, Chronic opioid therapy in non-malignant pain, S46–62, Copyright Elsevier (1990), with permission.

Addiction Medicine and the American Academy of Pain Medicine.[11, 12] Addiction is defined by the observation of impaired control over drug use, craving, or compulsion, regarding drug use and continued use despite harm. The consensus statement highlights problems of evaluating addiction in the presence of unrelieved pain, which may itself be accompanied by apparently aberrant patterns of drug use. The term "pseudoaddiction" is clarified and describes a pattern of behaviors, such as drug hoarding and attempts to procure extra supplies, as well as more worrisome behaviors including illicit drug use and deception, that might usually be indicative of an addiction problem but which resolve on adequate treatment of pain.

Neurobiology of substance misuse

Addiction is a chronic relapsing brain disorder in which repeated exposure to certain substances induces plastic change in motivational and reward systems of the brain. Not all individuals exposed to these substances will develop an addiction disorder: the propensity to addiction and the manifestations of the disorder are shaped by genetic, psychologic, environmental, and social factors. Further discussion is available on the website of the National Institute on Drug Abuse.[13]

Modification of motivation and reward signaling systems is so powerful that the addicted patient will continue to use drugs when the cost of doing so in terms of physical, psychological, social, and emotional harm is high. Over time, secondary stimuli associated with drug taking (specific venues, drug-taking paraphernalia, etc.) become powerfully conditioned and can trigger relapse, even after a prolonged period of abstinence.[14] There is evidence that this persistence of drug-seeking behavior over time may be related to mechanisms of learning and memory.[15]

CLINICAL ISSUES

Risk of addiction to prescribed opioids

Not all patients exposed to reward-inducing psychoactive drugs will develop an addiction syndrome. Many patients using these drugs appropriately for pain relief will develop tolerance to one or more of the effects of the drug (including analgesia). They are also likely to develop physical dependence as manifest by withdrawal on dose tapering or cessation. However, the potential for pain-relieving medicines, particularly opioids to be used for purposes other than pain relief (by the patient or by others), and for the development of true addiction, remains a concern for prescribing physicians.

A number of questions need to be answered to inform the decision to prescribe or be prescribed opioids.

WHAT IS THE PREVALENCE OF ADDICTION TO OPIOIDS IN A PATIENT WITH NO HISTORY OF SUBSTANCE MISUSE?

The risk of becoming addicted in patients without a known history of addiction during opioid treatment for pain is not known. Clinical trials of opioid efficacy are often of insufficient duration to detect development of a substance misuse problem. The historical study of Porter and Jick is often quoted as reassurance that addiction to prescribed opioids is unlikely.[16][V] More recent publications describe methods of identifying substance misuse, including validated and unvalidated behavioral observations, Diagnostic and Statistical Manual of Mental Disorders (DSM)-III and -IV criteria,[17] Portenoy criteria, and urine toxicology. From these data, overall prevalence rates vary considerably. Several prospective studies of cancer and of noncancer patients identify no substance misuse on behavioral criteria,[18, 19][V], [20][V], [21][V] although some studies in whom no substance misuse problems were detected had previous substance misuse as an exclusion criterion.[22][II], [23][V] In contrast, prevalence rates of up to 50 percent are also reported in one retrospective[24] and one cross-sectional study[25] of noncancer pain patients. Overall, the published literature would suggest that prevalence rates from problem drug use are lower in patients with cancer-related pain, with a notable exception being one study which described a prevalence of 44.2 percent, although this was from a study of inpatients who had undergone urine toxicology during their hospital stay.[26]

WHAT ARE THE RISK FACTORS THAT INCREASE THE LIKELIHOOD OF OPIOID ADDICTION?

The degree to which an individual is at risk of becoming addicted to opioids is shaped by genetic, environmental, social, and cultural factors. It is generally agreed that a family history of substance misuse is an important risk factor for addiction to prescribed drugs.[9] The relative contributions from environmental and genetic influences within a family have been characterized by family, twin, and adoption studies.[27, 28] Such studies suggest that heritability for opioid dependence is high.[29] The specific contribution of environmental and cultural factors that render an individual likely to be at risk of substance misuse are difficult to quantify, but are likely to include social class, occupation, and educational factors, as well as cultural perceptions (and legislation) relating to substance misuse.[30]

Misuse of opioids is frequently associated with a current or previous history of other substance misuse, including alcohol and nicotine.[31, 32] Nonsubstance misuse psychiatric disorders are also common in the substance-misusing population with lifetime rates of psychiatric disorders being reported as greater than 40 percent in most studies and up to over 80 percent in a smaller number of studies.[33] Depressive, anxiety, and substance misuse disorders are also associated with increased use of prescribed opioids in the general population.[34, 35] Although repeated use of psychoactive substances can give rise to symptoms of other psychiatric disorders, such as sleep, perceptual, and mood disturbance, and similarly people with mental illness may use psychoactive substance to alleviate unpleasant experiences, an independent relationship between substance misuse and other mental illness has been demonstrated.[36]

HOW CAN PRESCRIBERS IDENTIFY WHO MIGHT RUN INTO PROBLEMS?

A patient who is being considered for opioid therapy must be assessed by means of the usual triad of medical history, clinical examination, and, where necessary, relevant special investigations.

Medical history

It is essential to take a detailed medical, family, social, and occupational history from the patient, including an assessment of their beliefs regarding their presenting complaint and their expectations regarding the outcome of the consultation. It is helpful to explain that a full picture of all substances, prescribed or otherwise (including alcohol and tobacco), used by the patient, is important to support the safe prescribing of medications for pain relief.

Substance misusing patients may have come into contact with a number of other healthcare providers who may have documented concerns in the medical case record or in correspondence. It is important to take note of this information, but the clinician considering a trial of opioid therapy must place most weight on the results of his or her own evaluation of the patient as the context of previous discussions is rarely known. If the relationship between a patient and a previous healthcare provider has broken down, it may be helpful to explore this from the patient's perspective. No long-term pain management plan will succeed without the support of the patient's family members and others currently involved in their care, particularly the primary care practitioner. It is useful to solicit opinion from these individuals.

Clinical examination

There are no characteristics of the patient with a past or current substance misuse problem that are pathognomonic.[37] Signs of current intoxication with or withdrawal from alcohol or opioids may be obvious in the clinic and, if present, should be discussed with the patient. A more detailed examination may reveal signs of chronic alcohol use (hepatomegaly, spider naevi) or signs suggestive of previous or current intravenous drug use. Features in the clinical presentation which may suggest a history of substance misuse are summarized in **Box 46.1**.

Box 46.1 Features in the clinical presentation that may suggest a history of substance misuse

- Current intoxication/withdrawal.
- Patient has assertive personality, often demanding immediate action.
- Patient may show unusual knowledge of controlled substances.
- Patient gives medical history with textbook symptoms or gives evasive or vague answers to questions regarding medical history.
- Patient reluctant or unwilling to provide reference information. May have no General Practitioner.
- Patient will often request a specific controlled drug and is reluctant to try a different drug.
- Patient generally has no interest in diagnosis, fails to keep appointments for further diagnostic tests, or refuses to see another practitioner for consultation.
- Cutaneous signs of drug abuse-skin tracks and related scars on the neck, axilla, groin, neck, forearm, wrist, foot and ankle. Such marks are usually multiple, hyper-pigmented and linear. New lesions may be inflamed. Shows signs of "pop" scars from subcutaneous injections.

The British Pain Society. Pain and substance misuse: improving the patient experience. A consensus document for consultation, 2006, The British Pain Society.

Screening instruments for addiction

If the patient has a current diagnosis of addiction, this may need to be managed separately (by appropriately trained professionals) in parallel with ongoing pain management. Additionally, a past or current history of an addiction problem is a significant predictor of likelihood of running into problems when prescribing controlled substances for pain. A number of tools are available to screen for the presence of an addictive disorder. The CAGE questionnaire was developed to screen for alcohol misuse and has been adapted to screen for other drug use.[38] The questionnaire is simple to administer and has been demonstrated to be both sensitive and specific as a screening tool. The Screening Tool for Addiction Risk (STAR) questionnaire is a validated tool that has been developed to evaluate addiction problems in chronic pain patients and includes questions regarding prior treatment in a drug or alcohol rehabilitation facility, as well as questions regarding nicotine use and treatment in another pain clinic.[39]

Urine toxicology and other laboratory tests

Because the validity of self-reported drug use may be limited,[40] it is helpful to document objective information regarding drug use. Such information is more likely to identify the occurrence of problems when combined with behavioral observations.[41]

HOW CAN PRESCRIBERS RECOGNIZE WHEN A PROBLEM IS DEVELOPING?

At the time of initiation of opioid therapy, a plan for monitoring progress towards agreed outcome goals, adverse effects of medication, and appropriateness of use of medication should be agreed with the patient. Patients should be reminded that tolerance to the analgesic effect of drugs may be expected.

Savage[42] has described behaviors relating to addiction domains which may be observed during opioid therapy and distinguishes between behaviors suggestive of addiction and behaviors concordant with therapeutic use of medications. A single observation of an apparently aberrant behavior should not prompt an immediate diagnosis of an addiction problem: a pattern of aberrant behaviors over time would give rise to more concern. Clinicians do not always agree regarding which behaviors are most worrisome.[43] Portenoy[44] has grouped behaviors into those more or less likely to be indicative of aberrancy (**Table 46.2**).

A number of screening tools for aberrant drug-related behavior have been developed. These include the Prescription Opiate Abuse Checklist,[45] The Prescription Drug Use Questionnaire,[46] and a more recent multidimensional tool, the Screener and Opioid Assessment for Patients with Pain.[47,48] The Pain Medication Questionnaire asks questions relating to behaviors and attitudes regarding the use of pain medication.[49] This latter is nonopioid-specific so can be used to evaluate patients taking a range of pain medications.

An instrument for predicting compliance and efficacy of opioids and risk/benefit of continuing an opioid trial was recently developed by Belgrade and colleagues.[50] Although this has only been validated retrospectively to date, it is the only instrument that addresses the three important clinical dimensions of chronic opioid prescribing. For their own as well as their patients' safety, clinicians have to make judgments about:

- likely compliance with the therapeutic regimen and likelihood of aberrant behaviors;
- likely efficacy of opioid analgesia; and
- the decision to continue or discontinue opioids at each review.

The DIRE score[50] had good sensitivity, specificity, and inter-rater reliability.

IS THE OPIOID PRESCRIPTION BEING USED BY THE INTENDED RECIPIENT?

Diversion of prescribed medications may occur by patients receiving drugs for pain relief and also by individuals who do not have genuine symptoms, but purport to do so as a means of obtaining a supply of saleable drugs.

Table 46.2 Aberrant drug-related behaviors that raise concern about the potential for addiction in medical patients prescribed opioids for chronic pain.

Probably more predictive of addiction	Probably less predictive of addiction
Selling prescription drugs	Aggressive complaining about the need for more drug
Prescription forgery	Drug hoarding during periods of reduced symptoms
Stealing or "borrowing" drugs from others	Requesting specific drugs
Injecting oral formulations	Openly acquiring similar drugs from other medical sources
Obtaining prescription drugs from nonmedical sources	Unsanctioned dose escalation
Concurrent abuse of alcohol or illicit drugs	Unapproved use of the drug to treat another symptom
Multiple dose escalation or other noncompliance with therapy despite warnings	
Multiple episodes of prescription "loss"	
Repeatedly seeking prescription from other clinicians or from emergency rooms without informing prescriber or after warning to desist	
Evidence of deterioration in the ability to function at work, in the family, or socially that appear to be related to the drug use	
Repeated resistance to changes in therapy, despite clear evidence of adverse physical or psychological effects from the drug	

Diversion can include:[37]

- transfer of prescription drugs from intended recipient to others in pain;
- unlawful transfer of prescription drugs from legitimate to illegal channels of distribution;
- theft from manufacturers or wholesalers;
- theft from pharmacies, hospitals, surgeries, veterinary practices, care homes, hospices;
- prescription fraud;
- use of over-the-counter or prescription medicines to synthesize more potent drugs with a higher street value;
- use of over-the-counter medicines to augment the effect of prescribed or street drugs, i.e. the sedating antihistamines such as cyclizine, promethazine, or dyphenhydramine to produce a "buzz" with methadone.

Diversion may be difficult to detect, particularly in those without symptoms who are attempting to acquire drugs for subsequent monetary or other gain.[42, 51]

Management of the patient with a history of substance misuse

Both persistent pain and problem drug use are common and are therefore likely to co-occur in patients referred for chronic pain management. There are, however, reasons why individuals who use illicit substances may have greater than expected needs for pain relief:[37]

- Compared to those who are not dependent, the presence of a drug misuse syndrome seems to worsen the experience of pain and individuals may have previous experiences of self-medication to remove pain and psychological distress.
- Drug misusers have a low tolerance of nonpharmacological interventions to achieve pain control.
- By nature of their chronically relapsing condition, drug misusers have frequent episodes of intoxication and withdrawal, which may alter the intensity of the pain experience.
- Virtually all forms of addiction are associated with sleep disturbance and this is a well-established exacerbating factor in chronic pain.
- Depression and anxiety are common features in addiction and these have an important influence on the pain experience.
- Drug users are more likely to suffer from accidental and nonaccidental injury, and medical complications related to their drug use. This places them at high risk from physical problems that may require analgesia.
- For patients receiving opioid substitution therapy for addiction, there is evidence that supports increased sensitivity to experimental pain.[52, 53] This hyperalgesia may recognize a state of central sensitization to pain involving neurobiological phenomena similar to those associated with tolerance.[54]

A full assessment of both pain and addiction (see above under Medical history) is mandatory.

The patient should be given a clear explanation of the nature of their pain complaint and the rationale for the available therapeutic interventions should be discussed.

PRESCRIBING OPIOIDS FOR THE ADDICTED PATIENT

The mainstay of drug therapy for opioid addiction is substitution with either methadone or buprenorphine. Opioid substitution therapy is effective in decreasing misuse of opioids and other substances, improving adherence to treatment, reducing criminal activity, and improving individual function.[55]

Patients using a long-term illicit opioid or those receiving a maintenance prescription for addiction management will not derive analgesic benefit from their regular dose. For those using unprescribed medications, prescribed doses must include replacement of the patient's usual opioid and other chemical consumption.

There must be a frank discussion between the patient and team members regarding acceptable and unacceptable behavior in relation to prescribed drugs and the therapeutic goals. The patient must agree that adherence to the prescribed regimen will be monitored appropriately, including by means of random urine toxicology screening. Consequences of noncompliance with any part of the program must be explicit at the outset. All such discussions with the patient should be carefully documented and a copy given to the patient if necessary. This may take the form of a formal treatment contract, although the legal status of these documents is variable.[56]

PATIENTS RECOVERING FROM ADDICTION

A key feature of addiction is the relapsing nature of the condition. There is, therefore, the potential for reactivation of a substance misuse problem if scheduled drugs need to be prescribed for pain and symptom control. Patients and clinicians need to understand that drug exposure is only one component of relapse and that a careful plan for pain management with involvement of appropriate support should allow safe management of pain and other symptoms.

SPECIALIST SUPPORT FOR THE PAIN MANAGEMENT TEAM

Direct collaboration between addiction specialists, pain physicians, and primary care teams is mandatory when managing patients with a past or current history of substance misuse. In this way, the ongoing management of both pain and addiction can proceed optimally. It is also helpful for teams involved in the management of pain in the addicted patient to communicate regarding family and social issues which may have a bearing on the pain complaint and its management.

CONCLUSIONS

Opioid drugs have an established role in the management of persistent pain. Concerns regarding the possibility that these drugs may cause harm to those for whom they are prescribed or to others are substantiated by the published literature. However, the risk of an individual patient running into problems cannot be quantified. Prescribing practice can be guided by an understanding of the relevant laws and regulations, role of opioids in a pain management plan, and an awareness of predisposing factors for problem drug use. Screening tools are now available to supplement the clinical impression and similarly, instruments now exist to identify when problems are occurring.

If a patient with pain has a past or current history of substance misuse, he or she should be managed with the same tools, supported by clinical evidence, as those without a history of addiction. Management of pain in the substance-misusing patient poses particular challenges for the healthcare team, but an open and collaborative relationship between the patient, his or her carers, and all relevant healthcare professionals should allow pain to be managed safely and effectively.

REFERENCES

1. Eisenberg E, McNicol E, Carr DB. Opioids for neuropathic pain. *Cochrane Database of Systematic Reviews.* 2006; **CD006146**.
2. Ballantyne JC. Opioids for chronic pain: Taking stock. *Pain.* 2006; **125**: 3–4.
* 3. Bloodworth D. Opioids in the treatment of chronic pain: legal framework and therapeutic indications and limitations. *Physical Medicine and Rehabilitation Clinics of North America.* 2006; **17**: 355–79.
4. United Nations Office on Drugs and Crime (UNODC). Drug control treaties and related resolutions. New York: United Nations Office on Drugs and Crime. Available from: http://www.unodc.org/unodc/en/drug_and_crime_conventions.html
5. Roe S, Man L. *Drug misuse declared: findings from the 2005/6 British Crime Survey.* London: Home Office, 2006.
6. United Nations Office for Drug Control and Crime Prevention. *Global illicit drug trends 2002.* New York: UNODCCP, 2002.
7. Chou I, Narasimhan K. Neurobiology of addiction. *Nature Neuroscience.* 2005; **8**: 1427.
8. United Nations Office on Drugs and Crime. *World drug report.* New York: UNODC, 2006.
* 9. World Health Organization. *Neuroscience of psychoactive substance use and dependence.* Geneva: WHO, 2004.
* 10. Portenoy RK. Chronic opioid therapy in non-malignant pain. *Journal of Pain and Symptom Management.* 1990; **5**: S46–62.
* 11. American Academy of Pain Medicine, the American Pain Society and the American Academy of Pain Medicine. *Consensus statement: Definitions related to the use of opioids for the treatment of pain.* Glenview, IL: American Pain Society. Last updated February 2001, cited February 2008. Available from: www.ampainsoc.org/advocacy/opioids2.htm
* 12. Savage SR, Joranson DE, Covington EC *et al.* Definitions related to the medical use of opioids: evolution towards universal agreement. *Journal of Pain and Symptom Management.* 2003; **26**: 655–67.
* 13. National Institute on Drug Abuse. Drugs, brains, and behavior – the science of addiction. Last updated April 2007, cited December 2007. Available from: www.nida.nih.gov/scienceofaddiction/.
14. O'Brien CP, Childress AR, Ehrman R, Robbins SJ. Conditioning factors in drug abuse: can they explain compulsion? *Journal of Psychopharmacology.* 1998; **12**: 15–22.
15. Hyman SE. Addiction: a disease of learning and memory. *American Journal of Psychiatry.* 2005; **162**: 1414–22.
16. Porter J, Jick H. Addiction is rare in patients treated with narcotics. *New England Journal of Medicine.* 1980; **302**: 123.
17. American Psychiatric Association. *Diagnostic and statistical manual of mental disorders (DSM-IV)*, 4th edn. Washington, DC: American Psychiatric Association, 1994.
* 18. Zenz M, Strumpf M, Tryba M. Long-term oral opioid therapy in patients with chronic malignant pain. *Journal of Pain and Symptom Management.* 1992; **7**: 77.
19. Evans PJD. Narcotic addiction in patients with chronic pain. *Anaesthesia.* 1981; **36**: 597–602.
20. Cowan DT, Allan L, Griffiths P. A pilot study into the problematic use of opioid analgesics in chronic non-cancer pain patients. *International Journal of Nursing Studies.* 2002; **39**: 59–69.
21. Dellemijn PLI. Opioids in non-cancer pain: a life-time sentence? *European Journal of Pain.* 2001; **5**: 333–9.
22. Moulin DE, Lezzi A, Amireh R *et al.* Randomized trial of oral morphine for chronic non-cancer pain. *Lancet.* 1996; **347**: 143–7.
23. Schofferman J. Long-term opioid analgesic therapy for refractory lumbar spine pain. *Clinical Journal of Pain.* 1999; **15**: 136–40.
24. Saper JR, Lake AE, Hamel RL *et al.* Daily scheduled opioids for intractable head pain: long-term observations of a treatment program. *Neurology.* 2004; **62**: 1687–94.

25. Michna E, Ross EL, Hynes WL *et al.* Predicting aberrant drug behavior in patients treated for chronic pain: importance of abuse history. *Journal of Pain and Symptom Management.* 2004; **28**: 250–8.
26. Passik SD, Schreiber J, Kirsh KL. A chart review of the ordering of urine toxicology screen in a cancer center: do they influence on pain management? *Journal of Pain and Symptom Management.* 2000; **19**: 44.
27. Heath AC, Martin NG, Lynskey MT *et al.* Estimating two-stage models for genetic influences on alcohol, tobacco or drug use initiation and dependence vulnerability in twin and family data. *Twin Research.* 2002; 5: 113–24.
28. Vanyukov MM, Tarter RE. Genetic studies of substance abuse. *Drug and Alcohol Dependence.* 2000; **59**: 101–23.
29. Tsuang MT, Bar JL, Harley RM, Lyons MJ. The Harvard Twin Study of Substance Abuse: what we have learned. *Harvard Review of Psychiatry.* 2001; **9**: 267–79.
30. Compton WM, Thomas YF, Conway KP, Colliver JD. Developments in the epidemiology of drug use and drug use disorders. *American Journal of Psychiatry.* 2005; **162**: 1494–502.
31. Strain EC, Brooner RK, Bigelow GE. Clustering of multiple substance use and psychiatric diagnoses in opiate addicts. *Drug and Alcohol Dependence.* 1991; **27**: 127–34.
32. Edlund MJ, Steffict D, Hudson T *et al.* Risk factors for clinically recognized opioid abuse and dependence among veterans using opioids for chronic non-cancer pain. *Pain.* 2007; **129**: 355–62.
33. Strain EC. Assessment and treatment of comorbid psychiatric disorders in opioid-dependent patients. *Clinical Journal of Pain.* 2002; **18** (4 Suppl): S14–27.
34. Sullivan MD, Edlund MJ, Steffick D, Unutzer J. Regular use of prescribed opioids: association with common psychiatric disorders. *Pain.* 2005; **119**: 95–103.
35. Sullivan MD, Edlund MJ, Zhang L *et al.* Association between mental health disorders, problem drug use, and regular prescription opioid use. *Archives of Internal Medicine.* 2006; **166**: 2087–93.
36. Khantzian EJ. The self-medication hypothesis of substance use disorders: a reconsideration and recent applications. *Harvard Review of Psychiatry.* 1997; **4**: 231–44.
* 37. The British Pain Society. *Pain and substance misuse: improving the patient experience.* London: The British Pain Society, last updated April 2007, cited February 2008. Available from: www.britishpainsociety.org/pub_professional.htm#misuse
38. Brown R, Rounds L. Conjoint screening questionnaire for alcohol and drug abuse. *Wisconsin Medical Journal.* 1995; **94**: 135–40.
39. Friedman R, Li V, Mehrotra D. Treating pain patients at risk: evaluation of a screening tool in opioid-treated pain patients with and without addiction. *Pain Medicine.* 2003; **4**: 186–9.
* 40. Katz N, Fanciullo GJ. Role of urine toxicology testing in the management of chronic opioid therapy. *Clinical Journal of Pain.* 2002; **18** (4 Suppl): S76–82.
41. Katz NP, Sherburne S, Beach M *et al.* Behavioral monitoring and urine toxicology testing in patients receiving long-term opioid therapy. *Anesthesia and Analgesia.* 2003; **97**: 1097–102.
* 42. Savage SR. Assessment for addiction in pain-treatment settings. *Clinical Journal of Pain.* 2002; **18** (4 Suppl): S28–38.
43. Passik SD, Kirsh KL, Whitcomb L *et al.* Pain clinician's rankings of aberrant drug taking behaviours. *Journal of Pain and Palliative Care Pharmacotherapy.* 2002; **16**: 39–49.
* 44. Portenoy RK. Opioid therapy for chronic non-malignant pain: a review of the critical issues. *Journal of Pain and Symptom Management.* 1996; **11**: 203–17.
45. Chabal CMD. Prescription opiate abuse in chronic pain patients: Clinical criteria, incidence, and predictors. *Clinical Journal of Pain.* 1997; **13**: 150–5.
46. Compton P, Darakjian J, Miotto K. Screening for addiction in patients with chronic pain and "problematic" substance use: Evaluation of a pilot assessment tool. *Journal of Pain and Symptom Management.* 1998; **16**: 355–63.
47. Butler SF, Budman SH, Fernandez K, Jamison RN. Validation of a screener and opioid assessment measure for patients with chronic pain. *Pain.* 2004; **112**: 65–75.
48. Akbik H, Butler SF, Budman SH *et al.* Validation and clinical application of the Screener and Opioid Assessment for Patients with Pain (SOAPP). *Journal of Pain and Symptom Management.* 2006; **32**: 287–93.
49. Adams LL, Gatchel RJ, Robinson RC *et al.* Development of a self-report screening instrument for assessing potential opioid medication misuse in chronic pain patients. *Journal of Pain and Symptom Management.* 2004; **27**: 440–59.
50. Belgrade MJ, Schamber CD, Lindgren BR. The DIRE score: Predicting outcomes of opioid prescribing for chronic pain. *Journal of Pain.* 2006; **7**: 671–81.
51. Inciardi JA, Surratt HL, Kurtz SP *et al.* Mechanisms of prescription drug diversion among drug-involved club- and street-based populations. *Pain Medicine.* 2007; **8**: 171–83.
52. Compton P, Charuvastra VC, Kintaudi K, Ling W. Pain responses in methadone-maintained opioid abusers. *Journal of Pain and Symptom Management.* 2000; **20**: 237–45.
53. Compton P, Charuvastra VC, Ling W. Pain intolerance in opioid-maintained former opiate addicts: effect of long-acting maintenance agent. *Drug and Alcohol Dependence.* 2001; **63**: 139–46.
* 54. Mao J. Opioid-induced abnormal pain sensitivity: implications in clinical opioid therapy. *Pain.* 2002; **100**: 213–17.
* 55. Alford DP, Compton P, Samet JH. Acute pain management for patients receiving maintenance methadone or buprenorphine therapy. *Annals of Internal Medicine.* 2006; **144**: 127–34.
* 56. Fishman SM, Kreis PG. The opioid contract. *Clinical Journal of Pain.* 2002; **18** (4 Suppl): S70–5.

Index

This index covers the chapters in this volume only. A combined index covering all four volumes in the *Clinical Pain Management* series is available as a pdf on the accompanying website: www.clinicalpainmanagement.co.uk

An *F* following a page reference indicates that the reference is to a figure; a *T* indicates that the reference is to a table.

Notes

To save space in the index, the following abbreviations have been used:

CAM – complementary and alternative medicine
CBT – cognitive-behavior(al) therapy
CPSP – chronic postsurgical pain
CRPS – complex regional pain syndrome
MRI – magnetic resonance imaging
NSAIDs – nonsteroidal anti-inflammatory drugs
TENS – transcutaneous electrical nerve stimulation